Immunohistochemistry and Ancillary Studies in Diagnostic Dermatopathology

Second Edition

Immunohistochemistry and Ancillary Studies in Diagnostic Dermatopathology

Second Edition

Edited by
Mai P. Hoang
Harvard Medical School

CAMBRIDGE
UNIVERSITY PRESS

CAMBRIDGE
UNIVERSITY PRESS

Shaftesbury Road, Cambridge CB2 8EA, United Kingdom

One Liberty Plaza, 20th Floor, New York, NY 10006, USA

477 Williamstown Road, Port Melbourne, VIC 3207, Australia

314–321, 3rd Floor, Plot 3, Splendor Forum, Jasola District Centre, New Delhi – 110025, India

103 Penang Road, #05-06/07, Visioncrest Commercial, Singapore 238467

Cambridge University Press is part of Cambridge University Press & Assessment, a department of the University of Cambridge.

We share the University's mission to contribute to society through the pursuit of education, learning and research at the highest international levels of excellence.

www.cambridge.org
Information on this title: www.cambridge.org/9781009549226

DOI: 10.1017/9781009549240

When citing this work, please include a reference to the DOI 10.1017/9781009549240

First published 2017
Reprinted 2019
Second edition 2025

Printed in Great Britain by Ashford Colour Press Ltd

A catalogue record for this publication is available from the British Library

A Cataloging-in-Publication data record for this book is available from the Library of Congress

ISBN 978-1-009-54922-6 Hardback

To Hòa and Talya

Contents

Contributors

Kristine M. Cornejo
Associate Professor of Pathology
Harvard Medical School
Massachusetts General Hospital
Boston, MA, USA

María Teresa Fernández Figueras
Professor of Anatomic Pathology
International University of Catalonia
Chair, Department of Anatomic Pathology
General University Hospital of Catalonia, Quirónsalud Group
Barcelona, Spain

Emily M. Hartsough
Clinical Fellow in Pathology
Massachusetts General Hospital
Boston, MA, USA

Mai P. Hoang
Professor of Pathology
Harvard Medical School
Director of Dermatopathology
Massachusetts General Hospital
Boston, MA, USA

Gregory Hosler
Clinical Professor, Departments of Dermatology and Pathology
University of Texas Southwestern Medical Center
Dallas, TX, USA

Soma Jobbagy
Clinical Fellow in Pathology
Massachusetts General Hospital
Boston, MA, USA

Jakob M. T. Moran
Clinical Fellow in Pathology
Massachusetts General Hospital
Boston, MA, USA

Joana Pardal
Consultant Pathologist
Braga Hospital
Braga, Portugal

M. Angelica Selim
Professor of Pathology and Dermatology
Director of Dermatopathology
Department of Pathology
Duke University Medical Center
Durham, NC, USA

Wun Ju Shieh
Visiting Professor
Department of Microbiology and Immunology, School of Medicine
College of Medicine, Taipei Medical University
Taipei, Taiwan

Preface and Acknowledgments

Building on the foundation of antigen-antibody interaction and epitope retrieval technique, immunohistochemistry has become an indispensable diagnostic tool. Molecular diagnostic techniques have identified numerous novel gene alterations, complementing immunohistochemistry in recognition and classification of distinct tumor entities. Yet few textbooks are dedicated to diagnostic immunohistochemistry and ancillary studies in the subspecialty of dermatopathology. In this second edition, we aim to bridge this gap by updating readers with these helpful diagnostic tests. The text is divided into twelve chapters that cover entities based on lineage, including epithelial, melanocytic, lymphoid, adnexal, and soft tissue. Synopses of applicable antibodies, tables outlining the staining patterns of the entities in the differential diagnosis, applicable panels of immunostains, as well as molecular findings that are deemed helpful are included. The role of immunohistochemistry as a screening test for underlying molecular alteration and genetic syndromes, diagnosing immunobullous diseases, and detection of infectious agents is discussed. A synopsis of applicable antibodies is outlined when applicable. Each chapter ends with a case study in which clinical presentation and work-up are outlined.

We hope this book will serve the readers as a helpful diagnostic guide in rendering diagnoses for cutaneous neoplasms and disorders.

Special thanks to all contributing authors and the Cambridge University Press team, including Rebecca Illidge, Lucy Edwards, Helen Kitto, and Reshma Venkatachalapathy of Integra, for their invaluable help.

We sincerely hope that this book will serve as a useful resource for the readers.

Chapter 1

Introduction to Immunohistochemistry

Mai P. Hoang

Introduction

Immunohistochemistry is an interdisciplinary set of scientific techniques used for the visualization of tissue-level and cellular architecture. It exists at the intersection of the fields of immunology, histology, and chemistry. Immunohistochemical staining plays a critical role in clinical diagnostic pathology. Seeing the dispersion of various proteins and other cellular components in a tissue sample allows pathologists to render or corroborate a clinical diagnosis. In order to visualize the localization of cellular components, the field exploits the natural ability of antibody proteins from the immune system to bind to a specific antigen. A parallel field, immunocytochemistry, involves the same set of techniques applied to cells, not full tissue sections. However, the two terms are sometimes used interchangeably by researchers.

In the early 1940s, scientists at Harvard Medical School, led by Dr. Albert Coons, demonstrated that antibodies that were labeled with a fluorescent tag maintained specificity for their antigen.[1] Building on this discovery, scientists then incubated tissues with these fluorescently labeled antibodies and examined the tissues for the label under fluorescence microscopy. The localization of antibodies, and thus their tags, to the antigens allowed them to directly determine the presence and location of antigens within the tissue samples.

Over the last few decades, the techniques used in immunohistochemical staining have become exponentially more complex. Several milestones have accelerated the growth of the field of immunohistochemistry with the first one being the introduction of enzyme-labeled antibodies that allow visualization of targeted antigens by bright-field microscopy.[2] The production of monoclonal antibodies with greater specificity results in countless types of antibodies, tags, and reagents available for use.[3] Signal strength can be improved with antigen retrieval methods that enhance the ability of antibodies to bind to epitopes in formalin-fixed paraffin-embedded tissues.[4] Archival tissue samples can be stained, allowing for potential retrospective research. Other recent developments include sensitive secondary detection systems,[5] automated staining systems,[6] and digital imaging analysis.[7] The strength of the signal can be further amplified using indirect epitope detection, in which tagged secondary antibodies that are specific against the untagged primary antibody are applied to the tissue. Improvements in consistency, reproducibility, and stain quality, made possible with automated systems and image analysis technologies, allow for accurate quantification of staining in tissue samples. All of these developments in turn advance clinical diagnoses and propel research.

As the complexity of immunohistochemical techniques has progressed, so has their utility. The exploitation of the specificity of these interactions enables us to detect molecules of interest in tissue samples through immunohistochemical methods. In addition to being adjunct diagnostic tools, which are discussed in subsequent chapters, immunohistochemical markers can now be used as screening tests for hereditary syndromes (**see Chapter 10**). In the era of personalized medicine, biomarker expression can guide risk stratification and therapeutic decision. The association of these molecules with certain disease presentations allows us to use information gathered through staining as biomarkers for diseases. Thus, an entire line of study within the field of immunohistochemistry involves the discovery of these biomarkers and their clinical relevance.[8] Currently, several biomarkers are approved by the Food and Drug Administration (FDA) for diagnostic use in cancer, including Her2, estrogen receptor, epidermal growth factor receptor, and PDL1.[9] An ever-growing body of literature catalogues the relationships between expressions of various proteins and diseases. The presence of these biomarkers within a tumor can be used by the medical team to guide and personalize treatment.[8]

Immunohistochemical techniques are growing progressively more sensitive and specific. Our understanding and manipulation of antibody-epitope interactions have allowed immunohistochemistry and other related technologies to grow into fields of their own, including immunofluorescence (IF) (**see Chapter 11**) and *in situ* hybridization (ISH) using both deoxyribonucleic acid (DNA) and ribonucleic acid (RNA) probes. Antibodies have grown into powerful clinical and research tools. This chapter will describe the conceptual framework of immunohistochemistry, outline technical mechanisms, and explain its clinical relevance.

1.1 Antibody Structure and Function

Antibodies, or immunoglobulins, are polypeptide structures that are involved in humoral immune response. They are clonally produced in the body by B-lymphocytes. Antibodies recognize and bind with high specificity to another molecule, called an antigen. Often, this antigen is a region of a protein comprised of five to six amino acid residues, called an epitope. Antigens can be homopolymeric or multivalent with multiple identical epitopes or heteropolymeric with multiple distinct epitopes.[10] In the body, antibodies might bind to a virus to prevent it from infecting a cell. They also might form an agglutination reaction, causing a clump of antigens to form, which can then be eliminated by the immune system.

Antibodies are Y-shaped polypeptide heterotetramers composed of two "heavy" chains and two "light" chains. The quaternary structure is maintained by disulfide linkages in cysteine-rich moieties of the polypeptide chains. The structure can be further divided into the constant, or fixed, region (Fc) and the antigen-binding domain (Fab). The antigen-binding domain contains a variable region and a hypervariable region, which is on the end of the protein. It is the hypervariable region of the antigen-binding domain that determines the epitope specificity of the antibody (**Figure 1.1**).[11]

In the body, recombination of genomic DNA accounts for the high variability of antibody structure and, thus, the vast range of antigens against which specificity is conferred. Antibodies can be engineered to have an affinity for a countless array of antigens. Antibodies recognize epitopes based on a unique shape-size-charge profile. Antibody-antigen recognition occurs via

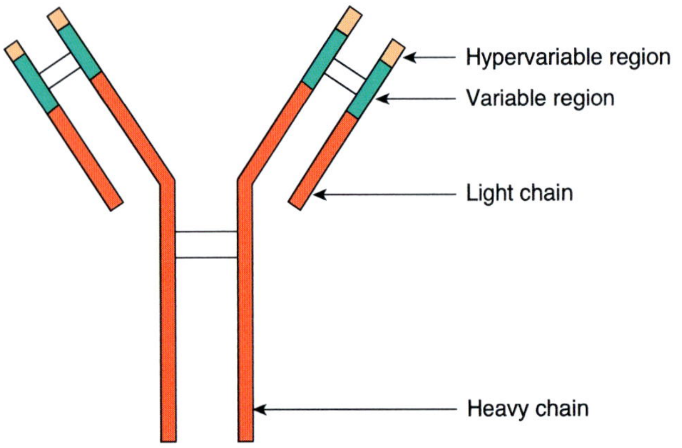

Figure 1.1 Structure of an antibody. An antibody protein is a heterotetramer, containing two heavy chains and two light chains. Disulfide bonds link the four polypeptides. The variable and hypervariable regions confer specificity against a certain antigen.

ionic/electrostatic (non-covalent) intermolecular forces, and follows an induced-fit model.[11] For this reason, it is critical that the structural integrity of the epitope is maintained even after the tissue has been excised. Epitopes can be linear or conformational.[12] Linear epitopes are five to seven contiguous amino acids while conformational or discontinuous epitopes are made of small groups of amino acids brought into close proximity through conformational folding or binding.[11] While epitopes in immune responses are conformational, those in formalin-fixed paraffin-embedded tissues are invariably linear.[13] Therefore, if the antigen of interest is denatured or undergoes a conformational change, the structure of the epitope may be disrupted, and the antibody may no longer be able to bind to it.

Common sources of antibodies for clinical and research use include mouse, rat, rabbit, goat, sheep, chicken, and horse. The source of the antibody is important for indirect antigen detection. Antibodies can be produced that are specific against another species' antibodies. This can enhance signal strength and improve technical efficiency. There are a wide variety of commercially available antibodies. Advances in molecular biology and genetic techniques have provided us with the technology necessary to engineer antibodies specific to nearly any biological macromolecule.[14] Western blotting and/or immunoprecipitation are often used to determine whether or not an antibody is specific for an antigen. By engineering antibodies, specificity can be enhanced, and they can be tailored to work well in preserved tissue samples.[14]

Further complicating the process of antibody selection is the availability of mono- and polyclonal antibodies. *Polyclonal antibodies* are groups of antibodies raised against multiple epitopes of a single antigen. *Monoclonal antibodies*, in contrast, are raised against a single epitope of a single antigen. They are usually produced from a mouse using the technique of Kohler and Milstein.[3] Rabbit monoclonal antibodies have higher affinity than mouse monoclonal antibodies, likely as a result of high glycosylation. Immunohistochemistry using polyclonal antibodies is far more sensitive. However, the use of a monoclonal antibody is a more specific process. Fittingly, different research questions can influence antibody selection. For example, if a researcher is looking simply for the presence of a protein in a cell that might exist in low concentration, it is likely advisable to use a polyclonal antibody. However, if you are looking for a specific domain of a specific protein, use of a monoclonal antibody would likely be superior. The balance between sensitivity and specificity is something that all laboratories struggle with in developing immunohistochemical assays. In addition, test volume, reagent cost, and which antibody clone to use when more than one monoclonal antibody is available are additional factors that a clinical immunohistochemical laboratory must consider.

1.2 Tissue Preservation and Antigen Retrieval

The antigenicity of a molecule, or its ability to be recognized by its antigen, is an important factor to consider in any immunohistochemical protocol. Because antigens are recognized by antibodies based on their unique properties, it is crucial that they remain structurally intact. If an antigen is present in a cell, but any of its properties (including size, shape, charge, and amino acid sequence) are compromised, the staining could fail, leading to a false negative result.[15]

Frequently, immunohistochemical staining is performed on archival tissue samples. Fixation stabilizes and protects the tissue from the rigorous processing and immunohistochemical staining. The most commonly used technique for tissue preservation is formalin fixation.[16] For over one hundred years, formalin-fixed paraffin-embedded tissues (FFPE) have been the standard tissue preparation. While the exact mechanism by which this preservation works is yet unknown, it is thought that formalin preserves tissue by inducing methylene cross-links between different protein moieties. It is very important that the preservation process is performed correctly to prevent degradation of the tissue over time. After the tissue has been fixed in formalin, it must be embedded in a wax block for storage and sectioning. The fixed tissue is first submerged in a concentrated ethanol solution. This process dehydrates the tissue. Water molecules are reactive, and their presence within a tissue could reduce the quality of preservation.[17] If dehydration is incomplete, there can be a detrimental effect on the integrity of the macromolecules within the cells. Oxidation caused by any residual water in the sample can be devastating to tissue quality. Therefore, it is crucial that dehydration is completed. The ethanol is then exchanged with xylenes, then finally paraffin. The fixed tissue is then embedded in a paraffin wax and mounted onto a block. However, the addition of methylene cross-links, in conjunction with the highly hydrophobic environment created by the paraffin coating, facilitate a conformational shift in various macromolecules in the preserved tissue sample. Thus, this process maintains the integrity of the tissue structure at the cellular level over time, but it does so at the cost of molecular structural integrity. Proteins within preserved tissues can be returned to their native state, as the reactions presumed to be underlying fixation are reversible processes. Another important consideration for maintaining tissue integrity is the ischemic time, or the time elapsed between excision from the body and fixation. The longer that unpreserved tissue is cut off from the blood stream, the less likely it is that cellular architecture will be conserved, as the tissue may begin to degrade from within the paraffin block.

One of the major limitations of using IHC on preserved tissue samples is the decreased antigenicity of epitopes in fixed tissue. At some point in the fixation process, the structure of proteins within the tissue is altered. If this affects the structure of the intracellular molecular target, then the antibody will not be able to recognize and bind to it. Antibodies recognize their targets based on the unique size, shape, and charge profile of the epitope.[11] Alteration of any of these properties diminishes the strength of the antibody-antigen interaction. In formalin-fixed, paraffin-embedded tissue, methylene cross-links induced by the fixation process and the hydrophobic environment of the wax alter protein conformation. This might mask the epitope. Alternatively, if the epitope consists of amino acids from different parts of the polypeptide that are brought together only when the protein is folded properly into its three-dimensional structure, the epitope could be completely compromised. Therefore, mitigating antigenicity loss with antigen retrieval methods is a crucial step in any immunohistochemical staining protocol.

It was demonstrated by Shi that by incubating tissue samples at high temperature prior to incubation with primary and secondary antibodies, the strength of the signal was dramatically enhanced.[4] While the exact mechanism by which this works has yet to be determined, it is thought that antigen retrieval methods disrupt the cross-linkage between formalin and protein and restore the epitopes to their native conformations, thus enabling the antibody to bind to them with enhanced specificity. Because a macromolecule's tertiary (three-dimensional) structure of polypeptides is environmentally sensitive, the temperature and pH at which antigen retrieval is performed will influence the efficacy of the procedure. Originally, antigen retrieval was performed by boiling formalin-fixed tissue slides in a pressure cooker prior to staining. It is believed that the high temperature of the boiling water returned epitopes to their natural state, allowing antibodies to bind in the intended manner. Later, it was demonstrated that this same enhancement of antigenicity occurred in tissues warmed in a microwave oven prior to incubation with antibodies.[4] It is possible that the high temperature hydrolyzes the cross-links that were induced during the initial preservation process, thereby allowing the renaturation of proteins into their native states.[18]

Currently, there are two commonly used antigen retrieval techniques: Heat Induced Epitope Retrieval (HIER) and Protease Induced Epitope Retrieval (PIER). The latter uses an enzymatic reaction catalyzed by Proteinase K, Trypsin, Pepsin, Pronase, and others to restore antigens to their original conformations, again through an unknown mechanism. Other techniques, including incubation with peroxide, detergents, or other solvents, are less frequently used. High pH retrieval solutions are often used for antibodies with cytoplasmic or membranous staining, while low pH retrieval solutions are used for antibodies with nuclear staining. It is crucial that the conditions of antigen retrieval process be tailored to the specific antigen of interest. The variability of ideal conditions by target antigen limits the number of potential targets that can be detected on a single slide. Multiple staining is possible but must be carefully optimized.

1.3 Methods of Antigen Detection

As Coons et al. demonstrated in 1941,[1] antibodies retain their properties even after the addition of a detectable tag. This allows us to directly detect the presence of antigens in tissue. However, detection of tags attached directly to antibodies binding their epitopes leads to relatively low levels of detectable staining. The staining intensity can be amplified by adding a step to the procedure. Instead of hybridizing a labeled antibody to the antigen, an unlabeled primary antibody is used. Then, after rinsing and another round of antigen retrieval, a labeled secondary antibody, specific against the primary antibody is added to the slide. Typically, these antibodies are raised in separate species. The primary antibody might be raised in a rabbit, while the secondary antibody is a mouse, anti-rabbit antibody. By adding this second layer of staining, the signal is amplified. Multiple secondary antibodies can bind to each single primary antibody.

The enhanced stain quality is startlingly apparent under bright-field microscopy. Additionally, because the secondary antibody can bind to any antibody raised in the species to which it is specific, the use of this second layer can increase efficiency. When a secondary antibody is utilized, the primary antibody can be applied to the tissue in low concentrations, thereby reducing reagent consumption.[19]

Though Coons originally labeled his antibodies with fluorescent labels, many immunohistochemical staining protocols utilize another method. The introduction of enzymes as antibody tags greatly expanded the utility of immunohistochemistry for pathology.[19] This method allows for the simultaneous detection of multiple cellular elements within the same tissue. In this process, the antibody is conjugated to an enzyme. The enzyme retains the ability to catalyze its reaction, while the antibody retains its specificity. Typically, the enzymes catalyze a reaction that forms a colored precipitate. The common enzymes used for this method are horseradish peroxidase and alkaline phosphatase. When staining a tissue with an enzyme-conjugated antibody, the tissue must be incubated with a chromogen reagent that reacts with the enzyme to form a colored product.

To prevent nonspecific staining and false positive results, further steps must be taken. Depending on the cell or tissue type, the enzyme that is bound to the antibody might exist in the cells. Background staining can be attributed to either non-specific antibody staining in the setting of polyclonal antibodies or endogenous enzymes. Therefore, it is necessary to block the action of endogenous enzymes with homologous functions. Some form of peroxidase block containing hydrogen peroxide is generally used to neutralize endogenous peroxidase activity.[20] Depending on the tissue type of interest, there may also be endogenous immunoglobulins within the tissue. Brown et al.[21] demonstrated that conjugating the antibodies that were applied experimentally to Fab fragments from antibodies of interest prevents the interaction of experimental secondary antibodies with endogenous antibodies, thereby avoiding false positive results.

Detection systems attach reporter molecules or labels to primary or secondary antibodies to visualize the antibody-antigen reaction in the tissue sections by bright-field microscopy. There have been several detection methods developed over the years with the polymer-based labeling method being currently the most widely used by the automated systems. The most common labels are enzymes such as horseradish peroxidase and alkaline phosphatase. In the presence of substrate and chromogen, enzymes produce a colored precipitate at the site of antigen-antibody reaction. 3,3'-diaminobenzidine tetrahydrochloride (DAB) is the brown chromogen for horseradish peroxidase. For alkaline phosphatase, 5-bromo-4-chloro-3-indolyl phosphate/nitro blue tetrazolium chloride (blue), fast red (red), and new fuchsin (fuchsia) are the common chromogens.

In *direct method* (**Figure 1.2A**), the label is attached directly to the antibody that targets the epitope of interest. Although rapid, this method requires a high concentration of primary antibody. The *indirect or sandwich method* (**Figure 1.2B**) allows the use of the same secondary antibody with several different primary antibodies. Since the number of labels is higher than primary antibody, this method requires less amount of primary antibody and improves the specificity of the secondary antibody. The *enzyme bridge method* is used mainly in research.[22] The *peroxidase-antiperoxidase method* (**Figure 1.2C**) is similar to the enzyme bridge method yet with hundred-fold to thousand-fold sensitivity; however, this indirect method is a

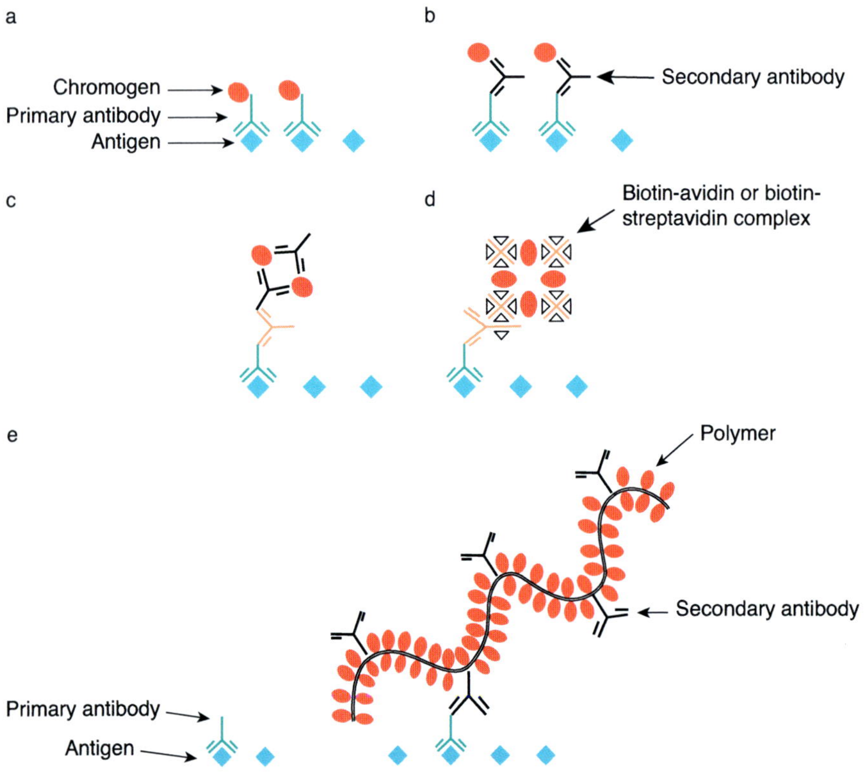

Figure 1.2 Models of different detection methods in immunohistochemical staining: (A) direct method, (B) indirect method, (C) peroxidase-antiperoxidase method or alkaline phosphatase-antialkaline phosphatase method, (D) biotin-avidin method or biotin-streptavidin method, and (E) polymer labeling two-step method.

laborious method.[23] In the *biotin-avidin method* (**Figure 1.2D**), biotin is linked to the primary antibody. Avidin is linked to peroxidase and has high affinity for biotin. The increased sensitivity is seen due to the large number of biotin molecules attached to the primary antibody.[24] One disadvantage is that nonspecific or false positive staining can be seen due to endogenous biotin. Streptovidin is substituted for avidin in the *biotin-streptavidin method* (**Figure 1.2D**). The multistep includes incubation with primary antibody, reaction with biotinylated secondary antibody, binding with an enzyme (peroxidase or alkaline phosphatase) conjugated streptavidin, and detection with chromogen substrate. It has higher sensitivity than the biotin-avidin method.[25] *Alkaline phosphatase-antialkaline phosphatase method* (**Figure 1.2C**) employs a similar principle to the peroxidase-antiperoxidase method.[26] This method is essential for double stain in order to avoid the cross-reactivity when two immunoperoxidase methods are used together.[27]

The above methods are multistep, complex, and time consuming. It is difficult to standardize and to achieve desirable sensitivity. Furthermore, recent methods including tyramine signal amplification,[28] immunopolymerase chain reaction,[29] and end-product amplification[30] are complex and have nonspecific staining. With the availability of automated staining systems, two-step indirect polymer kits from several manufacturers including Roche/Ventana, Novovastra/Leica, Agilent/Dako, Thermo Scientific/Lab Vision, and others are widely used currently. In the *polymer labeling 2-step method* (**Figure 1.2E**) antibodies and marker systems are linked to synthetic polymer or polymerized proteins such as micropolymers, dextran, polypeptides, and DNA branches. Approximately 4–70 molecules of enzymes (peroxidase or alkaline phosphatase) and 10–20 molecules of secondary antibody are attached to a polymer.[31] This method increases the number of enzymes that can be coupled to the linking antibodies. The main advantages include the elimination of biotinylated secondary antibody and higher specificity.

1.4 Standardization and Quality Control

While immunostains are still done by hand in many research laboratories, automated systems are routinely used in clinical immunohistochemical laboratories. The currently available autostainers include Ventana Benchmark Ultra (Ventana Medical Systems, Tucson, Arizona), Leica Bond Max (Leica Biosystems, Buffalo Grove, Illinois), Dako Omnis (Dako North America, Carpinteria, California), and Biocare IntelliPath FLX (Biocare Medical, Concord, Massachusetts). *Open systems* are used in research environments since they offer flexibility in used reagents, whereas *closed systems* are ideal in clinical laboratories since only certain ready-to-use reagents are allowed, resulting in standardization and consistency. In an automated system with *sequential processing* the slides remain within the instrument throughout the staining process. On the other hand, in *parallel processing*, one or more steps of the staining process are performed on a separate instrument. Greater flexibility is achieved with *continuous slide loading* while high capacity is possible with *batch slide loading*. These automated systems perform antigen retrieval, antibody incubation, and chromogen application with consistency.[6] They allow accurate, consistent, and reproducible staining by reducing human dependent errors; therefore, they have dramatically increased the efficiency in clinical and research settings and have greatly enhanced standardization.

Outlined in **Table 1.1** are the preanalytic, analytic, and postanalytic phases of a "total" clinical immunohistochemical test.[16,32] The fixation process is a key determinant of the outcome of immunohistochemistry with variables including types of fixative, delayed fixation, inadequate length of fixation, and over-fixation. During tissue processing, wax with a lower melting temperature (45°C) is preferred over one with a high melting temperature (65°C). Tissue sections with thickness greater than 5 micrometers often increased background staining. Clinical immunohistochemical laboratories must perform analytical validation of immunohistochemical tests prior to implementation for clinical use in accordance with the Clinical Laboratory Improvement Act of 1988.[33] They must demonstrate performance characteristics of these tests including accuracy, precision/reproducibility, sensitivity, and specificity.[34] **Table 1.2** outlines the recent guidelines for validating clinical immunohistochemical assays.[34]

Once an immunohistochemical test has been successfully validated, positive as well as negative control tissues must be included in every staining process, ideally on the same glass slide with the patient's tissue sample. Nuclear staining has always been regarded as more reliable than cytoplasmic staining.

Table 1.1 Preanalytic, analytic, and postanalytic phases of a "total" immunohistochemical test (adapted from Engel and Moore and Goldstein et al.)[16, 32]

Phase	Factors	Variables
Preanalytic	Tissue obtainment	Delayed fixation, prolonged ischemia
	Fixation	Types of fixative, degree of cross-linking, duration of fixation
	Tissue processing	Paraffin-embedded or frozen
	Tissue sectioning	Section thickness, drying temperature and duration
Analytic	Deparaffination	Dewaxing reagent
	Antigen retrieval	Heat, enzyme, detergent, low versus high pH retrieval solutions
	Blocking	Endogenous enzymes and nonspecific protein interaction
	Wash buffers	Tris- or phosphate-buffered saline
	Primary antibody	Polyclonal or monoclonal
	Detection system	Avidin-biotin or polymer-based methods
	Enzyme-substrate-chromogen	peroxidase or alkaline phosphatase
	Control tissues	
Postanalytic	Interpretation	Control tissues, manual interpretation, image analyses
	Quality control	Internal and external agency
	Results report	Qualitative or quantitative results

Table 1.2 Guidelines for analytic validation of clinical immunohistochemical assays (adapted from the College of American Pathologists, www.cap.org)

Recommendation: Laboratories must validate all laboratory developed immunohistochemical tests
Strong recommendation: At least 90% overall concordance between the new test and expected results
Good practice statement: A minimum of 10 positive and 10 negative tissues for non-predictive markers
Good practice statement: A minimum of 20 positive and 20 negative for predictive markers
Good practice statement: Using validation tissues that have been fixed and processed similar to the tested clinical cases
Good practice statement: A minimum of 1 known positive and 1 known negative for validation of new reagent lot
Good practice statement: A minimum of 2 known positive and 2 known negative for validation when changing antibody dilution, antibody vendor yet same antibody clone, incubation or retrieval time yet same method
Good practice statement: Confirm assay performance when changing fixative type, tissue processing, antigen retrieval method, antigen detection system, and laboratory water supply

Internal positive control and negative control are the ideal ways to assess for false negative staining and false positive staining, respectively.

Once the tissue samples have been stained, they can be used for diagnostic or research purposes. Depending on the stain, antigen, tissue sample, and type of information needed, the qualitative data of the stain can be interpreted differently. For certain stains and questions, knowing simply whether the sample is positive or negative for the antigen in question is sufficient. For other diagnostic purposes, a certain threshold of positive cells is necessary for definitive diagnosis. In some cases, pathologists will approximate visually the percentage of positive-staining cells. In other situations, an accurate count of positive cells is necessary. Whole slide scanning together with digital imaging analysis assist in providing consistent, reproducible, and quantitative immunohistochemical results and counting nuclear staining signals (such as Ki67, p53, estrogen receptor, and progesterone receptor).

The regulatory efforts of both the FDA and College of American Pathologists (CAP) have been focused on ensuring consistency and reliability of diagnostic tests. Participation in External Quality Assessment (EQA) and Proficiency Testing Programs is essential to maintain quality assurance. The College of American Pathologists offers a number of proficiency testing programs in the evaluation of immunohistochemical assay methodology and performance. International EQA programs designed for immunohistochemistry include Nordic Immunohistochemical Quality Control (independent scientific organization, Denmark, www.nordiqc.org) and United Kingdom National External Quality Assessment Service (UK NEQAS, Sheffield, England, www.ukneqas.org.uk).

To find the best practice in immunohistochemistry, one must know the diagnostic sensitivity and specificity of each immunostain, track the immunostain utilization data in one's own laboratory, and replace new and better stains with the existing ones.

1.5 Immunohistochemistry in the Detection of Molecular Abnormality

With our currently growing knowledge of tumor molecular genetics as well as the effectiveness of targeted therapy, IHC is playing an increasingly important role as diagnostic, therapeutic, and prognostic marker since it is cost-effective, rapid, and more accessible in the routine practice especially when limited tissue is available for genetic studies. IHC can currently detect the following types of molecular alterations in tumors which will be discussed in detail in the respective chapters: (1) chromosomal translocations/fusion, (2) gene overexpression, (3) gene amplification, (4) specific mutations, (5) gene deletion or loss of function, and (6) epigenetics changes (**Table 1.3**).

Detection of gene rearrangement can be done by different methods including IHC, fluorescence *in situ* hybridization (FISH), and reverse transcription-polymerase chain reaction (RT-PCR). In some cases, rearrangements involve a growing number of fusion partners, thus multiple primer sets are required for RT-PCR screening and novel rearrangements will be missed. Fluorescence *in situ* hybridization would require special microscope and technical expertise thus is not available in many laboratories. IHC is less laborious, cost-saving, and more

Table 1.3 Immunostains for the detection of molecular alterations

Immunostain	Antibody clone	Tumor type	Detected fusion(s)
Fusion			
ALK	5A4, 1A4, D5F3	Anaplastic large cell lymphoma	*NPM::ALK*
		Inflammatory myofibroblastic tumor	*TPM3::ALK, RANBP2::ALK, CLTC::ALK*
BCOR	c-10	*BCOR::CCNB3* round cell sarcoma	*BCOR::CCNB3*
		Primitive myxoid mesenchymal tumor of infancy	*BCOR* internal tandem duplication
CAMTA1	polyclonal	Epithelioid hemangioendothelioma	*WWTR1::CAMTA1*
CCNB3	polyclonal	*BCOR::CCNB3* round cell sarcoma	*BCOR::CCNB3*
CSF1	21113	Tenosynovial giant cell tumor	*CSF1* rearrangement
DDIT3	JM10-31	Myxoid liposarcoma	*DDIT3* rearrangement
DUX4	P4H2	*CIC::DUX4* round cell sarcoma	*CIC::DUX4*

Table 1.3 (cont.)

Immunostain	Antibody clone	Tumor type	Detected fusion(s)
FLI1	MRQ-1	Ewing sarcoma	*EWSR1/FLI1*
FOSB	5g4	Pseudomyogenic hemangioendothelioma	*SERPINE1::FOSB* *ACTB::FOSB*
		Epithelioid hemangioma	*ZFP36::FOSB*
NUT	C52B1	NUT carcinoma porocarcinoma	*YAP1::NUTM1* *WWTR1::NUTM1*
MYB	Epy69y	Adenoid cystic carcinoma	*MYB::NFIB*
Pan-TRK	EPR17341	Infantile fibrosarcoma Spitz neoplasms Lipofibromatosis-like neural tumor	*ETV6::NTRK3*
PAX3	GT1210	Biphenotypic sinonasal sarcoma	*PAX3::MAML3, PAX3::NCOA2, PAX3::FOXO1*
PLAG1	3b7	Pleomorphic adenoma	*CTNNB1::PLAG1, LIFR::PLAG1, CHCHD7::PLAG1*
ROS1	D4d6	Inflammatory myofibroblastic tumor	*YWHAE::ROS1, TFG::ROS1*
SS18-SSX	E9X9V	Synovial sarcoma	*SS18::SSX1, SS18::SSX2, SS18::SSX4*
SSX (c-terminus)	E5A2C	Synovial sarcoma	*SS18::SSX1, SS18::SSX2, SS18::SSX4*
STAT6	polyclonal	Solitary fibrous tumor	*NAB2::STAT6*
TFE3	polyclonal	Alveolar soft part sarcoma	*TFE3::ASPSCR1*
		Epithelioid hemangioendothelioma	*YAP1::TFE3*
WT1 (c-terminus)	Wt49	Desmoplastic small round cell tumor	*EWSR1::WT1*
YAP1 (c terminus)	D8H1X	Poroma, porocarcinoma	*YAP1::MAML2* *MAML2::YAP1* *YAP1::NUTM1*
Overexpression			
ETV4	16	CIC::DUX4 round cell sarcoma	*CIC::DUX4*
MUC4	8G7	Low-grade fibromyxoid sarcoma	*FUS::CREB3L2*
NKX2.2	d-4	Ewing sarcoma	*EWSR1::FLI1, EWSR1::ERG*
TLE1	1F5	Synovial sarcoma	t(X;18), *SSX1* or *SSX2::SYT*
WT1	Wt49	CIC::DUX4 round cell sarcoma	*CIC::DUX4*
Amplification			
CDK4	DCS-35	Well-differentiated liposarcoma	12q13-15 amplification
MDM2	If2	Well-differentiated liposarcoma	12q13-15 amplification
c-MYC	Ep121	Radiation-induced angiosarcoma	*c-MYC* amplification
HER2	4B5		*HER2* amplification
Mutation			
BAP1	Bsb-109	BAP1-inactivated melanocytic tumor	*BAP1* mutation
Beta-catenin	14, EP35	Desmoid fibromatosis	*CTNNB1* or *APC* mutation
BRAFV600E	VE1	Various tumors with *BRAF*V600E mutation	*BRAF*V600E mutation
NRASQ61 R	SP174	Various tumors with *NRAS*Q61 R mutation	*NRAS*Q61 R mutation
PRKAR1A	OTI6C7	Pigmented epithelioid melanocytoma	*PRKAR1A* mutation
PTEN	6H2.1	Cowden syndrome	*PTEN* mutation
SDHB	211a11ae7	Pheochromocytoma-paraganglioma	*SDHB* mutation
Deletion			
SMARCB1/INI1	25/baf47	Malignant rhabdoid tumor	*SMARCB1* inactivation
		Epithelioid sarcoma	*SMARCB1* inactivation
PRKAR1A	OTI6C7	Melanotic schwannoma	*PRKAR1A* inactivation
Epigenetic			
H3K27me3	(lys27)(c36b11)	Malignant peripheral nerve sheath tumor	*NF1* inactivation

widely available than FISH and RT-PCR assays. It would be a cost-effective means to screen for gene translocation which is uncommon. IHC can detect gene fusions in vascular neoplasms (CAMPTA1, FOSB, and TFE3), fibroblastic and myofibroblastic neoplasms (ALK, pan-TRK, ROS1, and STAT6), melanocytic neoplasms (ALK, pan-TRK, ROS1), and round cell tumor (BCOR, CCNB3, DUX4, and WT1). There is strong correlation between protein expression by IHC and *ROS1* rearrangement detected either by FISH or next-generation sequencing (NGS).[35] Several antibody clones including ALK1 (Dako), 5A4 (Leica Microsystem), and D5F3 (Cell Signaling Technology) have been shown to exhibit high sensitivity and specificity in comparison to NGS in detecting ALK fusions.[36]

BRAFV600E and NRASQ61R immunostains can detect specific *BRAF* and *NRAS* mutations. A number of studies have demonstrated monoclonal antibody VE1 to exhibit 85–100% sensitivity and 86–100% specificity in detecting BRAFV600E mutation in melanomas.[37] Cytoplasmic expression is the typical staining pattern and background nuclear staining can be observed in some *BRAF* variant mutations (**Figures 1.3 and 1.4**).[37] In series of 171 tumors from 64 patients by Menzies et al.[38] and 230 tumors from 99 patients by Boursault et al.,[39] homogeneity of BRAFV600E expression in the primary and metastatic tumors was observed. Therefore, testing any patient's samples with adequate viable tumor would be sufficient for determining *BRAF* mutation status.

NRAS mutation usually occurs in codon 61 where glutamine is replaced by arginine (NRASQ61R) or leucine (NRASQ61L). Molecular detection of *NRAS* mutations involving codon 61, codon 12, and codon 13 can be time consuming. NRAS IHC is faster and more cost effective and has been shown to have high sensitivity and specificity.[40,41] The NRASQ61R immunostain (clone SP174) has 100% sensitivity and specificity, while NRASQ61L (clone 26193 from New East Bioscience) immunostain exhibits lower sensitivity (80%) and good specificity (100%).[41] NRASQ61R or NRASQ61L antibody binds to a cytoplasmic protein. Positivity is considered when a strong, diffuse and homogeneous cytoplasmic staining is present (**Figures 1.5 and 1.6**). The positive percentage is around 80% which is easily visualized at low magnification.[40]

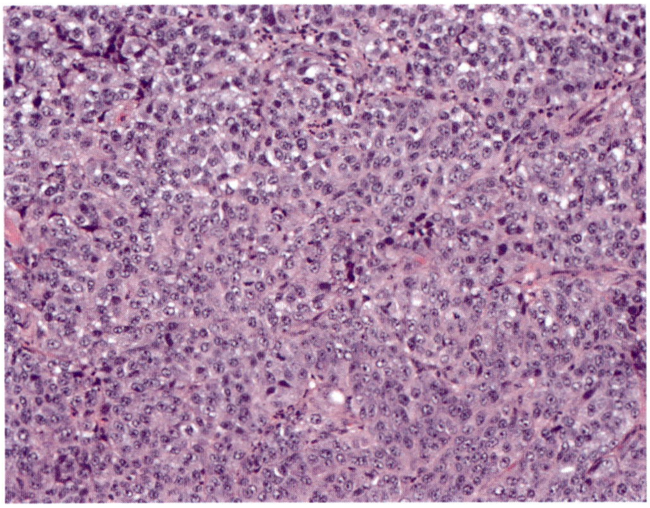

Figure 1.3 A proliferation of atypical epithelioid tumor cells characteristic of melanoma (X200).

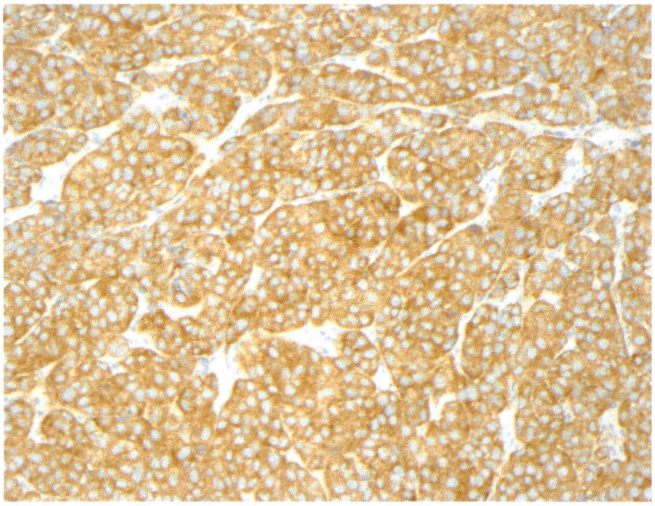

Figure 1.4 Diffuse cytoplasmic BRAFV600E expression (X200).

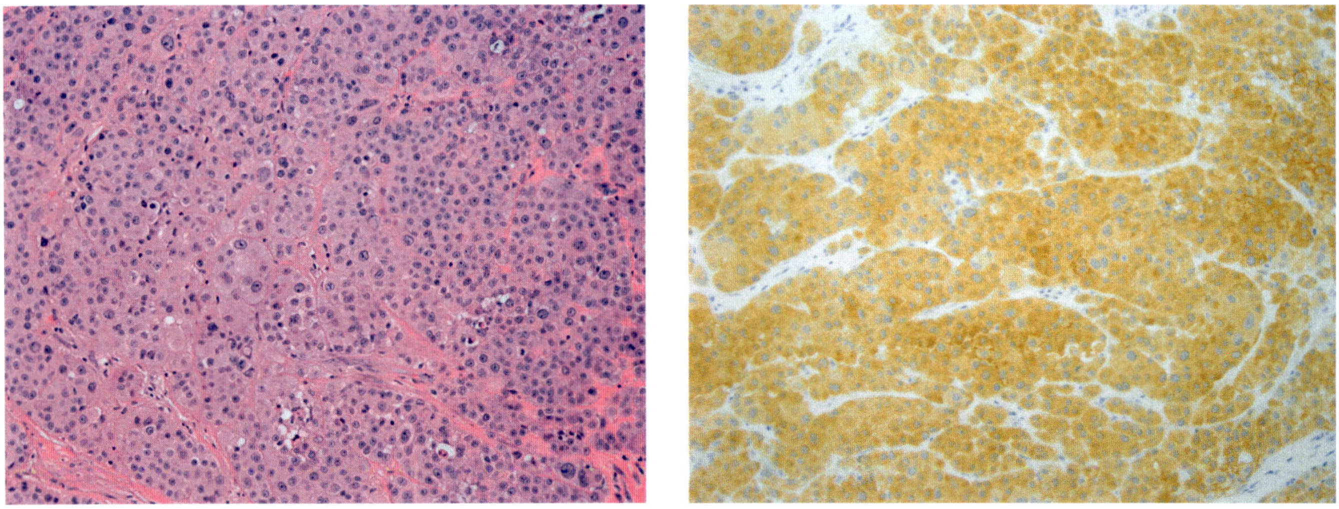

Figures 1.5 and 1.6 A melanoma with strong cytoplasmic NRASQ61R expression (X200, X200)

CDK4 and MDM2 immunostains can detect gene amplifications in well-differentiated and dedifferentiated liposarcomas. Other immunostains can detect gene deletion (SMARCB1/INI1), epigenetic alterations (H3K27me3), and increased expression discovered via gene expression profiling (ETV4, MUC4, NKX2.2, TLE1, and WT1) (**Table 1.3**).

1.6 Chromogenic *In Situ* Hybridization

RNA ISH assay (RNAscope) targeting high-risk HPV E6/E7 mRNA transcript has been reported to be a sensitive assay. HPV mRNA ish probes targeting E6 and E7 mRNA transcript of HPV6, HPV11, HPV16, HPV18 and HPV33 have shown to be helpful tests in detecting papillomavirus in formalin-fixed paraffin-embedded tissue.[42]

1.7 Dual Chromogenic Immunohistochemistry

Dual chromogenic immunostain is comprised of DAB (brown) chromogen labeling one target and red chromogen for the other. Examples of clinical diagnostic stains include combined Melan-A and Ki67, combined S100 and D2-40, and combined CD4 and CD8 immunostains. In clinical practice a combined PDL1 and CD8 combined immunostain can guide treatment decision (**Figure 1.7**).[43] Programmed death (PD)-1 is an immunoglobulin superfamily member expressed on the surface of activated T cells and B cells, while PD-L1 is present on the surface of tumor cells. Although PD1 has two ligands, it exhibits greater affinity with PD-L1 than PD-L2. When PD-L1 expressed on tumor cells binds to PD-1 expressed on activated T-cells, an inhibition of tumor immune destruction by activated T-cells occurs.[44] Blocking the interaction between PD1 and its ligand PD-L1 has resulted in improvements in antitumor responses.[45] Pembrolizumab (Keytruda®) and nivolumab (Opdivo®) are two anti-PD1/PD-L1 inhibitors that targeted the PD-1 pathway and have recently been approved by the FDA (Foods and Drugs Administration) for the treatment of advanced metastatic melanoma. A landmark publication showed that patients with metastatic melanoma treated with tumor infiltrating lymphocytes (TIL) followed by high-dose IL-2 demonstrated a 34% overall response rate.[46] Studies on the role of tumor infiltrating lymphocytes/immune response as prognostic markers and predictor of response to immunomodulators have shown that in melanoma CD8+ T-cell density is the best predictive marker of response to PD1 blockade therapy.

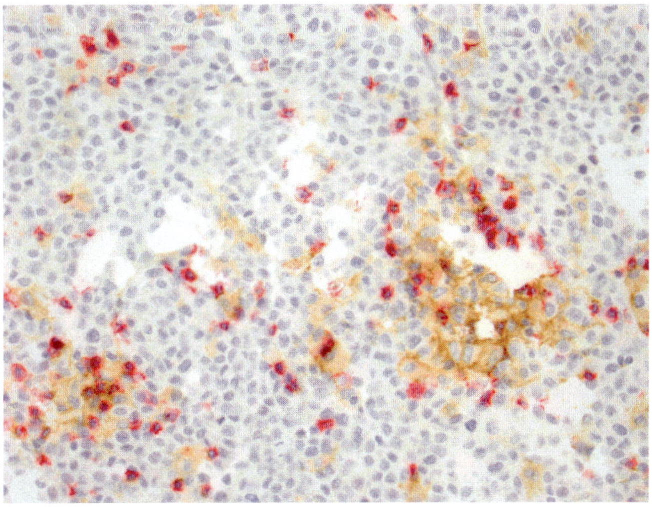

Figure 1.7 Membranous PDL1 staining (brown) by melanoma cells and intratumoral CD8-positive (red) T-lymphocytes (X400).

1.8 Multiplex Immunohistochemistry and Immunofluorescence

Recent novel techniques including multiplexed immunohistochemistry and immunofluorescence, automated multispectral analysis, and advanced quantitation software can allow one to quantitate and assess co-expression and spatial relationship through simultaneous detection of multiple markers; whereas traditional IHC can only evaluate 1–2 proteins or 2–3 DNA/RNA molecules.[47] Multiplex techniques can be cyclic immunofluorescence,[48] tyramide-base,[47] epitope-targeted mass spectrometry,[49] or RNA detection.[50] These techniques are currently utilized mainly in the research settings.

1.9 Future Direction

Bright-field RNA *in situ* hybridization using techniques similar to those of immunohistochemistry have allowed the detection of messenger RNA as well as long non-coding RNA with sensitivity to single RNA molecules in formalin-fixed paraffin-embedded tissues.[51,52] Recent studies have reported the potential of formalin-free, non-crosslinking fixatives to replace formalin in diagnostic pathology and research.[53] Quantum dots are semiconductor nanoparticles that emit different wavelengths depending on their size, shape, and composition.[54] Due to their narrow emission spectra and higher fluorescent signal per unit of light absorbed, quantum dots has been reported to be more accurate and precise at low concentration than traditional IHC.[55] In addition to detecting proteins, new immunostains will continue to play an important role in diagnostic pathology with an increased availability of novel techniques, sensitive and specific biomarkers, predictive markers, and mutation-specific antibodies.

References

1. Coons AH, Creech HJ, Jones RN. Immuno-logical properties of an antibody containing fluorescent group. *Pro Soc Exp Biol Med* 1941; **47**: 200–2.
2. Nakane PK. Simultaneous localization of multiple tissue antigens using the peroxidase-labeled antibody method: a study on pituitary glands of the rat. *J Histochem Cytochem* 1968; **16**: 557–60.
3. Kohler G, Milstein C. Continuous cultures of fused cells secreting antibody of predefined specificity. *Nature* 1975; **256**: 495–7.
4. Shi SR, Key ME, Kalra KL. Antigen retrieval in formalin-fixed,

paraffin-embedded tissues: an enhancement method for immunohistochemical staining based on microwave oven heating of tissue sections. *J Histochem Cytochem* 1991; **39**: 741–8.

5. Hsu SM, Raine L, Fanger H. A comparative study of the peroxidase-antiperoxidase method and an avidin-biotin complex method for studying polypeptide hormones with radioimmunoassay antibodies. *Am J Clin Pathol* 1981; **75**: 734–8.
6. Moreau A, Le Neel T, Joubert M, Truchaud A, Laboisse C. Approach to automation in immunohistochemistry. *Clin Chim Acta* 1998; **278**: 177–84.
7. Feldman MD. Beyond morphology: whole slide imaging, computer-aided detection, and other techniques. *Arch Pathol Lab Med* 2008; **132**: 758–63.
8. Howat WJ, Wilson BA. Tissue fixation and the effect of molecular fixatives on downstream staining procedures. *Methods* 2014; **70**: 12–19.
9. O'Hurley G, Sjostedt E, Rahman A, et al. Garbage in, garbage out: a critical evaluation of strategies used for validation of immunohistochemical biomarkers. *Mol Oncol* 2014; **8**: 783–98.
10. Lipman NS, Jackson LR, Trudel LJ, et al. Monoclonal versus polyclonal antibodies: distinguishing characteristics, applications, and information resources. *Inst Lab Anim Res J* 2005; **46**: 258–68.
11. Janeway CA, Travers P, Walport M, Shlomchik MJ. Chapter 3: antigen recognition by B-cell and T-cell receptors. *Immunobiology*, 5th ed. Garland Science, New York, 2001.
12. Bogen SA, Vani K, Sompuram SR. Molecular mechanisms of antigen retrieval: antigen retrieval reverses steric interference caused by formalin-induced cross-links. *Biotech Histochem* 2009; **84**: 207–15.
13. Sompuram SR, Vani K, Hafer LJ, et al. Antibodies immunoreactive with formalin-fixed tissue antigens recognize linear protein epitopes. *Am J Clin Pathol* 2006; **125**: 82–90.
14. Schofield DJ, Lewis AR, Austin MJ. Genetic methods of antibody generation and their use in immunohistochemistry. *Methods* 2014; **70**: 20–7.
15. Khoury T, Sait S, Hwang H, et al. Delay to formalin fixation effect on breast biomarkers. *Mod Pathol* 2009; **22**: 1457–67.
16. Goldstein NS, Hewitt SM, Taylor CR, et al. Recommendations for improved standardization of immunohistochemistry. *Appl Immunohistochem Mol Morphol* 2007; **15**: 124–33.
17. Xie R, Chung J-Y, Ylaya K, et al. Factors influencing the degradation of archival formalin-fixed paraffin-embedded tissue sections. *J Histochem Cytochem* 2011; **59**: 356–65.
18. Warford A, Akbar H, Riberio D. Antigen retrieval, blocking, detection and visualisation systems in immunohistochemistry: a review and practical evaluation of tyramid and rolling circle amplification systems. *Methods* 2014; **70**: 28–33.
19. Brandtzaeg P. The increasing power of immunohistochemistry and immunocytochemistry. *J Immunol Methods* 1998; **216**: 49–67.
20. Pitts A, Williams EE. Destruction of endogenous peroxidase activity in order to locate cellular antigens by peroxidase-labeled antibodies. *J Histochem Cytochem* 1974; **22**: 51–4.
21. Brown KJ, Pemberton AD, Wright SH, Miller HRP. Primary antibody-Fab fragment complexes: a flexible alternative to traditional direct and indirect immunolabeling techniques. *J Histochem Cytochem* 2004; **52**: 1219–30.
22. Mason TE, Phifer RF, Spicer SS, Swallow RA, Dreskin RB. An immunoglobulin enzyme bridge method for localizing tissue antigens. *J Histochem Cytochem* 1969; **17**: 563–9.
23. Sternberger LA, Hardy PH, Cuculis JJ, et al. The unlabeled antibody enzyme method of immunohistochemistry: preparation and properties of soluble antigen-antibody complex (horseradish peroxidase-antihorseradish peroxidase) and its use in identification of spirochetes. *J Histochem Cytochem* 1970; **18**: 315–33.
24. Hsu S-M, Raine L, Fanger H. Use of avidin-biotin peroxidase complex (ABC) in immunoperoxidase techniques: a comparison between ABC and unlabeled antibody (PAP) procedures. *J Histochem Cytochem* 1981; **29**: 577–80.
25. Elias JM, Margiotta M, Gaborc D. Sensitivity and detection efficiency of the peroxidase antiperoxidase (PAP), avidin-biotin peroxidase complex (ABC), and peroxidase-labeled avidin-biotin (LAB) methods. *Am J Clin Pathol* 1989; **92**: 62–7.
26. Cordell JL, Falini B, Erber WN, et al. Immunoenzymatic label of monoclonal antibodies using immune complexes of alkaline phosphatase and monoclonal anti-alkaline phosphatase (APAAP complexes). *J Histochem Cytochem* 1984; **32**: 219–29.
27. Wagner L, Worman CP. Color-contrast staining of two different lymphocyte subpopulations: a two-color modification of alkaline phosphatase monoclonal anti-alkaline phosphatase complex technique. *Stain Technol* 1988; **63**: 129–36.
28. Stack EC, Wang C, Roman KA, Hoyt CC. Multiplexed immunohistochemistry, imaging, and quantitation: a review, with an assessment of tyramide signal amplification, multispectral imaging and multiplex analysis. *Methods* 2014; **70**: 46–58.
29. Sano T, Smith CL, Cantor CR. Immuno-PCR: very sensitive antigen detection by means of specific antibody-DNA conjugates. *Science* 1992; **258**: 120–2.
30. Chen B-X, Szabolcs MJ, Matsushima AY, Erlanger BF. A strategy for immunohistochemical signal enhancement by end-product amplification. *J Histochem Cytochem* 1996; **44**: 819–24.
31. Wiedorn KH, Goldmann T, Henne C, Kuhl H, Vollmer E. EnVision+, a new dextran polymer-based signal enhancement technique for in situ hybridization (ISH). *J Histochem Cytochem* 2001; **49**: 1067–71.
32. Engel KB, Moore HM. Effects of preanalytical variable on the detection of proteins by immunohistochemistry in formalin-fixed, paraffin-embedded tissue. *Arch Pathol Lab Med* 2011; **135**: 537–43.
33. Fetsch PA, Abati A. The clinical immunohistochemistry laboratory: regulations and troubleshooting guidelines. *Methods Mol Biol* 2010; **588**: 399–412.
34. Fitzgibbons PL, Bradley LA, Fatheree LA, et al. Principles of analytic validation of immunohistochemical assays. Guideline from the College of American Pathologists Pathology and Laboratory Quality Center. *Arch Pathol Lab Med* 2014; **138**: 1432–43.
35. Su Y, Goncalves T, Dias-Santagata D, Hoang MP. Immunohistochemical detection of ROS1 fusion. *Am J Clin Pathol* 2017; **147**: 77–82.
36. Wakuda K, Morita M, Sekikawa M, Morikawa N, Miura K, Doshita K, Iida Y, Kodama H, Mamesaya N, Kobayashi H, Ko R, Ono A, Kenmotsu H, Naito T, Murakami H, Muramatsu K, Kawata T, Mori K, Shimizu T, Gon Y, Takahashi T. Concordance of ALK fusion gene-rearrangement between

immunohistochemistry and next-generation sequencing. *Int J Clin Oncol.* 2024; **29**: 96–102.

37. Routhier CA, Mochel MC, Lynch K, et al. Comparison of 2 monoclonal antibodies for immunohistochemical detection of BRAFV600E mutation in malignant melanoma, pulmonary carcinoma, gastrointestinal carcinoma, thyroid carcinoma, and gliomas. *Hum Pathol* 2013; **44**: 2563–70.
38. Menzies AM, Lum T, Wilmott JS, et al. Intrapatient homogeneity of BRAFV600E expression in melanoma. *Am J Surg Pathol* 2014; **38**: 377–82.
39. Boursault L, Haddad V, Vergier B, et al. Tumor homogeneity between primary and metastatic sites for BRAF status in metastatic melanoma determined by immunohistochemical and molecular testing. *PLoS One* 2013; **8**: e70826.
40. Dias-Santagata D, Su Y, Hoang MP. Immunohistochemical detection of NRASQ61 R mutation in diverse tumor types. *Am J Clin Pathol* 2016; **145**: 29–34.
41. Kakavand H, Walker E, Lum T, et al. BRAF (V600E) and NRAS (Q61L/Q61 R) mutational analysis in metastatic melanoma using immunohistochemistry: a study of 754 cases highlighting potential pitfalls and guidelines for interpretation and reporting. *Histopathology* 2016; **69**: 680–6.
42. Luk PP, Selinger CI, Cooper WA, Mahar A, Palme CE, et al. Clinical utility of in situ hybridization assays in head and neck neoplasms. *Head Neck Pathol* 2019; **13**: 397–414.
43. Tumeh PC, Harview CL, Yearley JH, et al. PD-1 blockade induces responses by inhibiting adaptive immune resistance. *Nature* 2014; **515**: 568–71.
44. Zou W, Chen L. Inhibitory B7-family molecules in the tumour microenvironment. *Nat Rev Immunol* 2008; **8**: 467–77.
45. Topalian SL, Hodi FS, Brahmer JR, et al. Safety, activity, and immune correlates of anti-PD1 antibody in cancer. *N Engl J Med* 2012; **366**: 2443–54.
46. Rosenberg SA Yannelli JR, Yang JC, et al. Treatment of patients with metastatic melanoma with autologous tumor-infiltrating lymphocytes and interleukin 2. *J Natl Cancer Inst* 1994; **86**: 1159–66.
47. Stack EC, Wang C, Roman KA, Hoyt CC. Multiplexed immunohistochemistry, imaging, and quantitation: a review, with an assessment of Tyramide signal amplification, multispectral imaging and multiplex analysis. *Methods* 2014; **70**: 46–58.
48. Zrzazhevskiy P, Gao X. Quantum dot imaging platform for single-cell molecular profiling. *Nat Commun* 2013; **4**: 1619. https://doi.org/10.1038/ncomms2635.
49. Giesen C, Wang HA, Schapiro D, et al. Highly multiplex imaging of tumor tissues with subcellular resolution by mass cytometry. *Nat Methods* 2014; **11**: 417–22.
50. Ke J, Chen RZ, Ban T, et al. Structural basis for RNA recognition by a dimeric PPR-protein complex. *Nat Struct Mol Biol* 2013; **20**: 1377–82.
51. Tubbs RR, Wang H, Wang Z, et al. Ultrasensitive RNA in situ hybridization for detection of restricted clonal expression of low-abundance immunoglobulin light chain mRNA in B-cell lymphoproliferative disorders. *Am J Clin Pathol* 2013; **140**: 736–46.
52. Ricciuti B, Mencaroni C, Paglialunga L, Paciullo F, Crino L, Chiari R, Metro G. Long noncoding RNAs: new insights into non-small cell lung cancer biology, diagnosis and therapy. *Med Oncol* 2016; **33**: 10. doi: 10.1007/s12032-016-0731-2.
53. Kothmaier H, Rohrer D, Stacher E, Quehenberger F, Becker KF, Popper HH. Comparison of formalin-free tissue fixative: a proteomic study testing their application for routine pathology and research. *Arch Pathol Lab Med* 2011; **135**: 744–52.
54. Jin Z, Hildebrandt N. Semiconductor quantum dots for in vitro diagnostics and cellular imaging. *Trends Biotech* 2012; **30**: 394–403.
55. Chen C, Sun SR, Gong YP, et al. Quantum dots-based molecular classification of breast cancer by quantitative spectroanalysis of hormone receptors and HER2. *Biomaterials* 2011; **32**: 7592–9.

Chapter 2

Molecular Studies

Gregory A. Hosler and Mai P. Hoang

Introduction

Deoxyribonucleic acid (DNA) → ribonucleic acid (RNA) → protein is the central dogma of molecular biology. In pathology, and dermatopathology, each step along this progression can be used to engineer ancillary tests for the purposes of diagnosis, prognosis and therapy.[1] The previous chapter focused on "protein" through the use of immunohistochemistry (IHC). This chapter moves forward by taking steps backward in the progression discussing dermatopathology-applicable assays that use nucleic acids at their core.

Molecular testing is useful in dermatopathology and is not cost-effective but has become increasingly necessary for the diagnosis of soft tissue tumors. For diagnosis, testing should be considered a progression, beginning with readily available and inexpensive tools (the naked eye, for example, with clinical inspection) and then progressing to more esoteric or complex testing (such as IHC then molecular, for example), only as indicated. [1,2] Appropriate use criteria are needed and available for specific scenarios but continue to rapidly evolve.[3,4]

2.1 Chromogenic *In Situ* Hybridization

There are variations of *in situ* hybridization (ISH) based on detection methods. Chromogenic *in situ* hybridization, or CISH, is used synonymously with ISH and is discussed here. Fluorescence *in situ* hybridization, or FISH, is the other main type of ISH and is discussed separately.

DNA and RNA ISH assays are a good segue from IHC as they are often performed in the same laboratories and are in wide use. They are also similar in that the assays produce a signal on cells or tissue while maintaining tissue architecture and integrity (i.e., *in situ*). This allows for the evaluation of cells of interest in the context of the entire assayed tissue. Moreover, the workflows of IHC and ISH are similar, and, in some cases, the same laboratory machinery can be used. Commercial kits are available for commonly used targets. Cross-training (IHC and ISH) among laboratory personnel is commonplace.

Principles

The basic principle of all ISH assays is to use labeled oligonucleotide probes to detect complementary sequences in frozen or formalin-fixed paraffin-embedded (FFPE) tissue. ISH assays may be designed to be DNA → DNA, DNA → RNA, RNA → DNA or RNA → RNA. In today's laboratories, RNA ISH assays are the most commonly employed due to their superior sensitivity. For example, DNA ISH assays for the detection of human papillomavirus (HPV) have a reported sensitivity/specificity of 83%/89%, but this increases to 96%/97% using RNA ISH.[5]

DNA and RNA ISH are similar but with some notable differences. In DNA ISH, small oligonucleotide probes are designed to DNA target sequences, which, typically, are specific to infectious organisms or tumors. RNA ISH also uses small oligonucleotide probes but targets mRNA. By targeting mRNA, RNA ISH can detect active transcripts as opposed to targets embedded in the genome. Moreover, some tumors have characteristic genetic rearrangements resulting in gene fusions, which, in some cases, can be detected by mRNA probes but not DNA probes.

In the more common diagnostic RNA ISH assays used today, the tissue is first made permeable to give access to the RNA. Oligonucleotide probes are hybridized to the target RNA. Hybridization requires optimized conditions (buffers, temperature, etc.). A signal can be produced by labeling the oligonucleotide probe with biotin and adding avidin or streptavidin conjugated to horseradish peroxidase or alkaline phosphatase, similar to IHC. Other signal-producing techniques are available including ones using amplification processes. The signals can be visualized in the context of the cellular morphology and tissue architecture by a light microscope or by digital means.

Advantages and Disadvantages

One advantage of ISH over IHC is that, in general, the sensitivity is higher. The main disadvantage is the limited repertoire of probes for diagnostic dermatopathology. Other challenges with ISH (when compared with IHC) include the higher cost of materials, the slight increased complexity of the assay, and potential for failed tests. The latter is due to the unstable nature of RNA which becomes more important when using older archived material.

Applications

The most common use for ISH in today's dermatopathology practice is for the detection of HPV (**see Case Study 1**). Because HPV cannot be cultured, serologic testing cannot distinguish between active disease and previous exposure, and p16 immunostain lacks desired sensitivity, direct detection of the virus using HPV-ISH is preferred in certain diagnostic settings.[5,6] Specifically, HPV-ISH is used for the diagnosis of condylomata and more high-grade lesions like high-grade vulvar intraepithelial neoplasia and Bowen disease. In theory, ISH can be used to detect other HPV-driven lesions like verruca vulgaris, verruca palmoplantaris and epidermodysplasia verruciformis, for example, and are used in research settings, but those HPV serotypes are not covered in the cocktails designed for most commercially available products. Available cocktails include low-risk HPV, high-risk HPV, and pan-HPV, which may contain some combination of low-risk and high-risk but not all HPV serotypes. For reporting, it is important to disclose the specific serotypes included in each assay so not to mislead clinicians. For example, "pan-HPV" can lead one to think all HPV serotypes are tested but this is not the case.

The use of RNA ISH is becoming more commonplace as conditions are optimized and performance parameters improve. In hematopathology-dermatopathology, kappa and lambda ISH is replacing IHC. Evaluating kappa and lambda mRNA or protein can be a surrogate for clonality as most reactive/inflammatory processes contain a mixture of light chains. A kappa:lambda ratio determination can be useful because skewed, or restricted, light chain mRNA or expression is suggestive of clonal expansion and neoplasia. This principle has been employed for decades by using IHC but IHC is limited to detecting protein expression, which only occurs on certain mature B cells and plasma cells. Many neoplastic B cells produce light chain mRNA that does not lead to surface protein, and therefore RNA ISH is more sensitive than IHC. RNA ISH has the added advantage over IHC in that it can detect both primitive B cells (with a light, dusty mRNA signal) and more mature B cells and plasma cells (heavy signal), allowing for scrutiny of different populations (Figure 2.1). Therefore, kappa/lambda ISH can be useful for evaluating not only plasma cell-rich processes (marginal zone B-cell

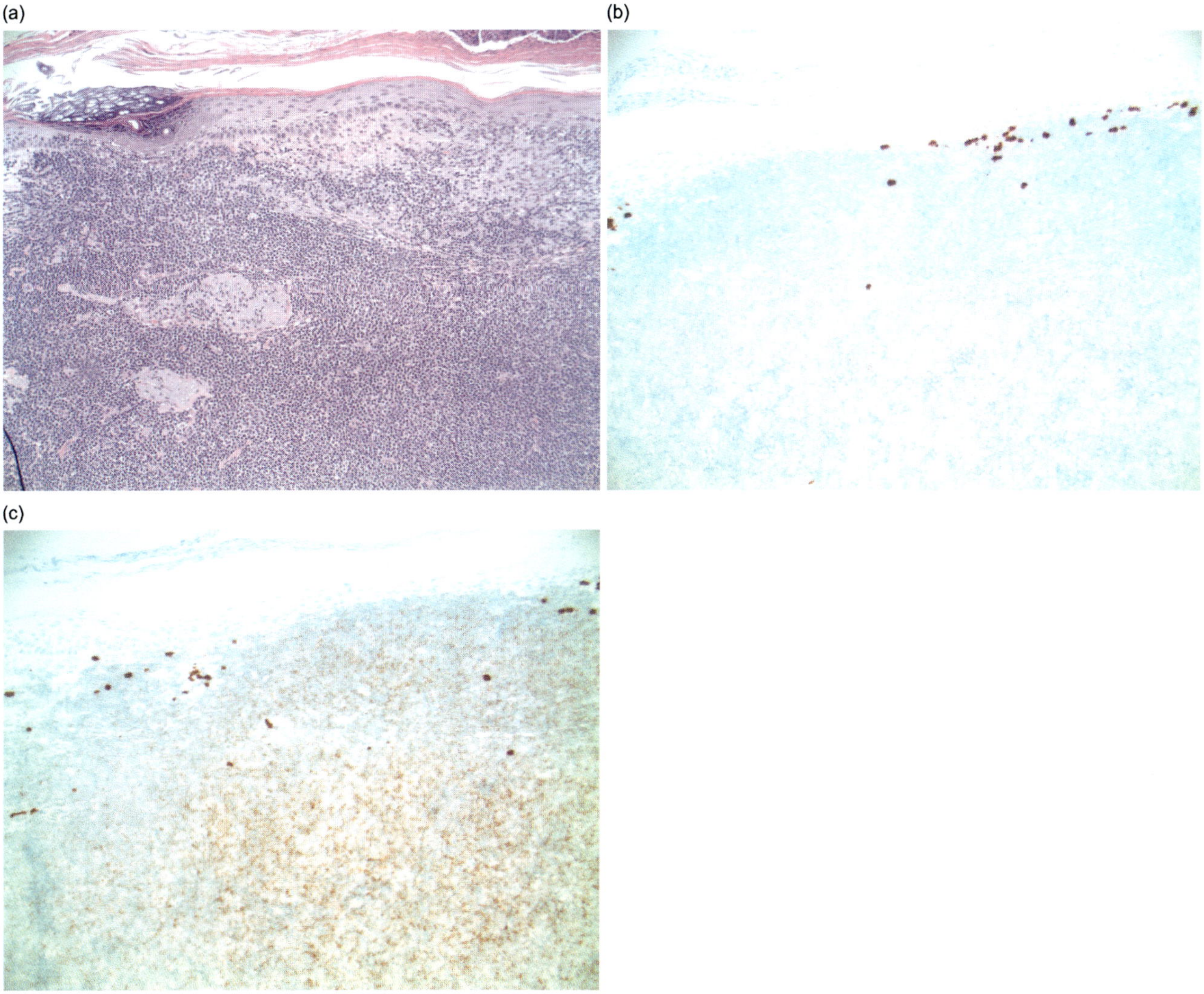

Figure 2.1 Kappa and lambda *in situ* hybridization (ISH). ISH can be a surrogate for clonality for hematolymphoid infiltrates. This 55-year-old man presented with a nodule on his torso. The infiltrate extends from the undersurface of the epidermis into the dermis in a nodular pattern. The infiltrate contains mildly enlarged mononuclear cells (A, H&E, X100). Kappa (B, X100) and lambda (C, X100) *in situ* hybridization show lambda restriction, consistent with clonality. Lambda exhibits light, dusty-appearing signal corresponding to the more primitive B cells. Both kappa and lambda show superficial cells with darker signal corresponding to reactive plasma cells.

Table 2.1 EBV-positive lymphoproliferative disorders possibly encountered in skin

B-cell disorders	EBV-positive diffuse large B-cell lymphoma
	EBV-positive mucocutaneous ulcer
	Lymphomatoid granulomatosis
	Plasmablastic lymphoma
	Endemic Burkitt lymphoma
	Post-transplant lymphoproliferative disorder*
T/NK-cell disorders	EBV-positive hemophagocytic lymphohistiocytosis
	Systemic chronic active EBV infection
	Hydroa vacciniforme-like lymphoproliferative disorder
	Systemic (and peripheral) EBV-positive T-cell lymphoma
	Aggressive NK-cell leukemia
	Extranodal NK/T-cell lymphoma, nasal type
	Angioimmunoblastic T-cell lymphoma

* Can be B-cell or T-cell proliferations

EBV: Epstein-Barr virus, NK: natural killer

lymphoma, plasmacytoma) but a wide spectrum of B-cell neoplasia (to include follicle center lymphoma, diffuse large B-cell lymphoma and other systemic/nodal B-cell malignancies).

Various other uses for ISH have been surfacing in dermatopathology. For example, Epstein-Barr virus (EBV) detection is useful in the diagnosis of various EBV-related hematopoietic lymphoproliferative disorders and malignancies (**Table 2.1**). IHC for EBV proteins, such as EBV nuclear antigens (EBNAs) and latent membrane proteins (LMPs), can be useful but lack the sensitivity of EBV-ISH directed to lymphocyte mRNA from *EBER1/EBER2* genes.[7] Probes for other infectious agents (CMV, SARS-CoV-2) are also available. MYB is a transcription factor that is overexpressed in certain adnexal tumors, such as adenoid cystic carcinoma, which often carries a rearrangement driving expression. MYB ISH is replacing MYB IHC due to its improved performance parameters.[8] Probes to other targets continue to be released but the scope of RNA ISH remains fairly narrow.

2.2 Fluorescence *In Situ* Hybridization

Fluorescence *in situ* hybridization (FISH) uses many of the same principles as CISH but is discussed separately given its unique requirements and applications. While IHC and ISH are widely implemented and used in diagnostic laboratories, FISH is often limited to large reference laboratories since the costs of specialized equipment and labor require sufficient volumes to justify an otherwise uncommonly employed assay. Moreover, reliance on FISH has waned in recent years as high-throughput sequencing achieves many of the same goals, and the cost of sequencing is trending downwards. Nonetheless, FISH remains resilient as these targeted assays can be turned around more quickly than extensive sequencing panels and the cost/reimbursement for FISH currently may be more favorable than sequencing in some settings.

Principles

Similar to CISH, FISH is based on using labeled oligonucleotide probes to detect targeted sequences within cells or intact tissue allowing for the direct visualization of signals within the cells of interest. FISH can be used on aspirates, peripheral blood and bone marrow, frozen tissue, and FFPE tissue, the latter of which is the most common source for dermatopathology applications. FISH uses single-stranded DNA probes which complement cellular DNA targets. The hybridization of the target probe and denatured target DNA occurs under optimized conditions (buffer, temperature, etc.). In contrast to CISH, the FISH probes are labeled for the purpose of fluorescence and can simultaneously use multiple fluorochromes to evaluate multiple targets in the same assay. The labeled probes will bind to complementary sequences and unbound probes are washed. The bound and labeled probes can be visualized within nuclei (highlighted by DAPI) under a fluorescence microscope or via specialized digital scanners.

Depending on the application and design of the probes, this technique can be used to detect target copy number gains and losses (as normal cells are diploid and should provide two signals per probe per nucleus) as well as amplifications, deletions, inversions, and unique rearrangements, or translocations. In the case of rearrangements, two different probe strategies can be employed. In one strategy, two probes are designed to flank a potential breakpoint, moving two juxtaposed differentially colored probes apart if the DNA is rearranged (i.e., "break-apart" FISH). Or, a single probe can be engineered to be complementary to, or spanning, the rearranged DNA, a so-called "dual fusion FISH" assay.

Advantages and Disadvantages

FISH has an advantage over cytogenetics, which is also used to evaluate for chromosomal aberrations, because it does not require dividing cells for analysis. It is also easier to technically perform. FISH assays can be performed within days and have designated codes for reimbursement. FISH allows for direct visualization and testing of cells of interest, which can be very important with inflamed lesions (background normal inflammatory cells) and heterogeneous lesions (melanoma arising in a nevus, for example), which is an advantage over other molecular techniques, such as cytogenetics, comparative genomic hybridization, gene expression profiling and sequencing. It can also be performed on small samples, requiring only a few cells to score.

The main disadvantage of FISH is that it is limited by the specific probes used for a given assay. For example, testing for copy number variations (CNVs), rearrangements, deletions, or insertions will only yield a positive result if the targets tested are altered. This means that false negative results will occur if there are CNVs involving nontargeted parts of the genome or if there are pathogenic minor breakpoints undetectable using probes directed to major breakpoints, for example. Therefore, FISH is most efficient and effective when there is a specific molecular question being asked. Another disadvantage of FISH is that it remains a fairly expensive, labor-intensive assay requiring a high level of training to perform and is only available in larger reference-type laboratories.

Applications

There are three main categories of uses of FISH in dermatopathology: (1) evaluating for CNVs in histopathologically ambiguous melanocytic lesions; (2) evaluating for amplifications, deletions, and/or rearrangements in (cutaneous) soft tissue neoplasms; and (3) evaluating for rearrangements in hematopoietic tumors, specifically diffuse large B-cell lymphomas. Other rarer uses include evaluating for amplifications, deletions and/or rearrangements in adnexal tumors (*MAML2* rearrangement in low-grade mucoepidermoid carcinoma and *EWRS1* or *FUS* rearrangements in myoepithelioma, for example), melanocytic tumors (Spitz kinase fusions and the *CRTC1::TRIM11* in rare melanocytomas, for example), and tumors metastatic to the skin.

FISH assays designed to distinguish melanoma from benign histopathologic mimickers have been available for several decades (**see Case Study 5**).[9] This assay took discovery data from comparative genomic hybridization studies to select a limited panel of target areas, or genes, to probe. Most assays use a combination of *RREB1*, *MYC*, *CCND1*, *CDKN2A*, and/or *MYB* (+/- centromere) probes. CNVs at any locus (specifically gains of *RREB1*, *MYC*, *CCND1*, losses of *MYB*, or homozygous loss of *CDKN2A*) would suggest malignancy since normal human DNA and the DNA of benign tumors maintain diploid status. An exception is Spitz nevi, which can, on occasion, have reduplicated genomes resulting in tetraploidy and therefore CNV. Outside of Spitz tumors and desmoplastic melanoma, FISH has high sensitivity and specificity when distinguishing melanoma from nevi. Because it allows for direct visualization of the cells (*in situ*), it can be effective for evaluating heterogeneous lesions (melanoma arising in association with a nevus, for example) because the cells of interest can be selectively scored.

There are numerous soft tissue neoplasms which harbor characteristic genetic aberrations which can be detectable by FISH (**Table 2.2**). While high-throughput sequencing is replacing FISH in the evaluation of soft tissue neoplasms, FISH remains an efficient assay in terms of cost and turn-around time when the pre-test probability is high for a specific diagnosis and a confirmation molecular test is needed.

FISH remains commonly used by hematopathologists to evaluate hematopoietic neoplasia. In dermatopathology, FISH may be useful when evaluating intermediate- or high-grade tumors for the presence of characteristic rearrangements, specifically those involving *BCL2*, *BCL6*, or *MYC*. Detection of rearrangements can be helpful diagnostically as they are often observed in diffuse large B-cell lymphoma (leg type) and systemic diffuse large B-cell lymphomas. These rearrangements can have negative prognostic implications, and this information can be useful to oncologists when designing treatment plans.

There are some other uncommon uses for FISH in dermatopathology. While the melanoma FISH assay is primarily diagnostic, it can provide prognostic information. For example, Spitz tumors with homozygous loss of *CDKN2A* often portends a poor prognosis. Similarly, melanomas with *CCND1* and *MYC* copy number gains may behave more aggressively. FISH can also be used to confirm kinase fusions (involving *ALK*, for example) associated with tumors along the Spitz nevus → Spitz melanocytoma → Spitz melanoma spectrum. FISH for *CRTC1::TRIM11* may be used to differentiate the *CRTC1::TRIM11* rearranged melanocytoma from melanoma and clear cell sarcoma of soft tissue.

Table 2.2 Rearrangements in cutaneous soft tissue neoplasms

Diagnosis	Rearrangement
Alveolar rhabdomyosarcoma	*FOXO1* rearrangement
Alveolar soft part sarcoma	*ASPSCR1::TFE3**
Angiofibroma of soft tissue	*AHRR::NCOA2*
Angiomatoid fibrous histiocytoma	*EWSR1::CREB1**
Angiosarcoma (post-radiation)	*MYC* amplification
Atypical lipomatous tumor/well-differentiated liposarcoma	*MDM2* amplification
Atypical spindle cell/pleomorphic lipomatous tumor	*RB1* deletion
Calcifying aponeurotic fibroma	*FN1::EGF*
Clear cell sarcoma of soft tissue	*EWSR1::ATF1**
Composite hemangioendothelioma	*YAP1::MAML2, PTB1::MAML2, EPC1::PCH2*
Dermatofibrosarcoma protuberans	*COL1A1::PDGFB**
Desmoplastic small round cell tumor	*EWSR1::WT1*
Epithelioid hemangioma	*FOSB* rearrangement
Epithelioid hemangioendothelioma	*WWTR1::CAMTA1**
Epithelioid hemangioendothelioma, subset	*YAP1::TFE3*
Ewing sarcoma	*EWSR1::FLI1**
Extraskeletal myxoid chondrosarcoma	*EWSR1::NR4A3**
Giant cell fibroblastoma	*COL1A1::PDGFB**
Hemosiderotic fibrolipomatous tumor	*TGFRB3::OGA**
Hybrid nerve sheath tumors	*VGLL3* rearrangement
Infantile fibrosarcoma	*ETV6::NTRK3**
Inflammatory myofibroblastic tumor	*ALK* or *ROS* rearrangements*
Lipofibromatosis-like neural tumor	*NTRK* rearrangement
Low grade fibromyxoid sarcoma	*FUS::CREB3L2**
Mesenchymal chondrosarcoma	*HEY1::NCOA2*
Myxoid liposarcoma	*FUS::DDIT3**
Nodular fasciitis	*MYH9::USP6**
Ossifying fibromyxoid tumor of soft parts	*PHF1* rearrangements*
Pseudomyogenic hemangioendothelioma	*SERPINE1::FOSB**
Retiform hemangioendothelioma	*YAP1::MAML2* or *YAP* rearrangement
Sclerosing epithelioid fibrosarcoma	*EWSR1::CREB3L1**
Superficial CD34-positive fibroblastic tumor	*PRDM10* rearrangement
Synovial sarcoma	*SS18* rearrangements*
Undifferentiated small round cell sarcoma	*CIC* and *BCOR* rearrangements*

* Most common rearrangement but minor rearrangements also occur

2.3 Comparative Genomic Hybridization

In the near future, discussions on comparative genomic hybridization (CGH) may be reserved for discovery and historical purposes only as high-throughput sequencing is largely replacing its utility in the diagnostic setting.

Principles

Similar to FISH, CGH evaluates for CNVs in the tumor genome. Different from FISH, which evaluates only specific targeted loci, CGH can be designed to evaluate the entire tumor genome. Historically, CGH was performed by using metaphase spreads but current methods use segments of the genome tiled to chips called oligonucleotide arrays, or array CGH (aCGH). When the arrays use stretches of DNA with single nucleotide polymorphisms (SNPs), they are designated SNP arrays, and can detect CNVs and copy-neutral loss of heterozygosity.

In dermatopathology applications, aCGH is performed by extracting DNA from FFPE tissue. The lesional DNA and normal, or control, DNA are differentially labeled and hybridized to the DNA on the chip array. Unbound DNA is washed and CNVs are determined by the relative signals of test and control DNA at each position on the array. Based on the library tiled to the chip, aCGH assays can be designed to evaluate the entire tumor genome, specific chromosomes or parts of chromosomes, or other specific targets with variable resolution.

Advantages and Disadvantages

The main advantage of aCGH over FISH, for example, is that it can generate abundant CNV data. Depending on chip design, aCGH is capable of analyzing the entire genome. Breadth of coverage often comes at the expense of resolution, however. For example, a whole-genome chip may identify areas of the genome with CNVs, but not the specific gene, which may be important in some settings. Therefore, the strategy behind chip design is highly dependent on the question being asked.

aCGH is a fairly complex assay, requiring specialized equipment and interpretations, and, therefore, it is only available in a few large reference laboratories or academic centers. It is an expensive assay with variable reimbursement and can take several weeks to perform. Although it is effective for identifying CNVs, it will not detect balanced translocations and inversions. Another limitation of aCGH is that it requires relatively good quantity and quality of DNA from the test sample. Because the DNA is extracted from scrolls off the paraffin block or slides, short of macrodissection, the test DNA is often diluted by normal DNA which may impact results.

Applications

Outside of the research setting, the only current significant use for aCGH in dermatopathology is in the evaluation of histopathologically ambiguous melanocytic lesions. CNVs are common in melanoma and, with the exception of Spitz nevi, are uncommon in nevi.[10] Spitz nevi can have gains in 11p and a phenomenon termed tetraploidy (reduplication of entire genome). These known changes in melanocytic lesions can be exploited for diagnostic purposes and can be particularly useful in characterizing Spitz tumors. Compared with FISH, which only analyzes a few targeted loci, aCGH can evaluate the entire genome, and because of this, many prefer aCGH over FISH in the evaluation of Spitz tumors. However, as mentioned above, because aCGH requires a fairly significant amount of tumor DNA (most assays require at least 0.5 mm of tumor depth), and, in most cases, the entire tissue is assayed, aCGH may not be reliable for small samples, thin lesions, and heterogeneous lesions (melanoma at a nevus, for example).

2.4 Gene Expression Profiling

Gene expression profiling (GEP) can be a powerful technique with the ability to provide diagnostic and prognostic information and other data on cellular function. Therefore, there is potential for a broad range of applications, but in dermatopathology, its scope remains fairly narrow.

Principles

GEP essentially assesses a snapshot of the function of tested cells by identifying and quantifying mRNA transcripts. This is in stark contrast to CGH and FISH, which assess relative quantities of DNA. GEP analysis can be performed on normal cells, tumors, or inflammatory conditions. Given the numerous potential transcripts in a sample and the transcripts' various biological functions, the development of GEP assays can be very labor intensive.

In the example of analyzing a tumor from FFPE tissue, RNA is extracted from either scrolls from the paraffin block or from scraped off tissue from newly generated slides from the block. The RNA is (often) labeled and bound to a tiled chip containing a library of complementary sequences, and the relative signals from the label (fluorescence, for example) and location of the signals on the chip are recorded and analyzed. Some assays may use quantitative reverse-transcription polymerase chain reaction as a stand-alone assay or in combination with chip-based technology.

Advantages and Disadvantages

Because GEP evaluates the transcriptome, it offers information which is different and potentially complementary (or even superior in some cases) to DNA-based assays. While the technologies around RNA extraction have vastly improved in recent decades, failed tests remain more common in RNA-based assays compared with DNA-based assays due to the inherent instability of RNA. This is magnified when using archived material. The other disadvantage of GEP is the complexity of analysis. Interpretation of types and quantities of mRNA requires extensive development of complex algorithms. Commercial tests are available and optimized but making updates or other changes to the proprietary assays as more data become available has major constraints.

Applications

The most common application of GEP in dermatopathology is in the evaluation of melanocytic lesions. Commercial assays are available for both prognosis and diagnosis.[11,12] Prognostic assays are developed by analyzing RNA from melanomas which have known clinical outcomes. The specific types and relative quantities of transcripts can be compared between tumors with indolent behavior and more aggressive tumors, and this principle is used to create prognostic GEP algorithms. Prognostic assays are requested by clinicians to provide patients with more data for planning and potentially management purposes. For example, in North America a clinically validated and commercially available GEP method (DecisionDx-UM) is used to classify primary uveal melanomas into prognostic class 1 (with low metastatic risk) and class 2 (with high metastatic risk).[13] The histopathologic features of melanoma provide data on its likely behavior and contribute to the pathologic stage. Specifically, the tumor (Breslow) depth and presence/absence of ulceration impact the stage. GEP assays, because they evaluate transcripts, and are a snapshot of the biological function of the tumor, may provide additional independent data for prognosis including the likelihood for sentinel lymph node involvement, distant metastases, and/or survival.

Diagnostic GEP assays are also commercially available.[12] These assays are designed to help with histopathologically ambiguous melanocytic lesions, and, therefore, are often utilized by dermatopathologists. Diagnostic assays are developed by analyzing the types and quantities of transcripts from known benign nevi, known melanoma, and ambiguous lesions with known clinical outcomes. The transcripts may be specific to melanocytes or to the microenvironment. These data are used to create algorithms for assessing the transcripts from histopathologically ambiguous lesions and help predict a benign or malignant clinical course. Commercially available assays have fairly high sensitivity and specificity over a broad range of melanocytic lesions. Similar to aCGH, testing is usually performed on scrolls or whole slides from formalin-fixed, paraffin-embedded tissue, and, therefore, outside of macrodissection, the test transcripts may get diluted by normal mRNA, which could impact interpretation of heterogeneous lesions. Another limitation for the commercially available GEP assay is that it is not validated on recurrent lesions and metastatic lesions.

While these diagnostic and prognostic assays for melanocytic lesions are the most common applications for GEP in dermatopathology, there are other emerging examples. GEP has been used to evaluate cutaneous carcinoma of unknown primary.[14] GEP using limited gene panels can be used to assess RNA directly taken off the cutaneous surface. This has been termed "tape-stripping" as RNA is extracted from material stuck to tape which was adhered to the skin surface. This method has been used to evaluate pigmented lesions in order to help guide the decision to biopsy.[15] For example, if the clinician or patient is reluctant to biopsy (perhaps because the site is cosmetically sensitive, the patient has poor wound healing, etc.), the GEP assay could be performed, and if it yields a benign profile, the clinician and patient may opt to monitor. By design, as screening assays, these assays have relatively high sensitivity and low specificity.[16] A current commercially available assay uses a limited gene panel (*PRAME*, *LINC*, control) and reports of its utility are variable. This tape-stripping approach can also be used to help with ambiguous inflammatory conditions, such as psoriasis vs eczema, when biopsy is not possible, or biopsy results fail to yield a definitive diagnosis.[17]

2.5 Polymerase Chain Reaction (Non-Sequencing Assays, Including RT-PCR Fusion Detection)

The polymerase chain reaction (PCR) and its variants are simple and powerful techniques which have been widely used in the research and diagnostic setting for decades. Amplification of small amounts of nucleic acids allows for broad applications, including but not limited to disease-specific mutation detection (tumors, genodermatoses, etc.) and identifying infectious agents. PCR components are incorporated into other assays such as gene expression profiling, clonality testing, microsatellite instability testing, and sequencing assays, which are all discussed separately.

Principles

PCR utilizes small oligonucleotide DNA primers which are complementary to nucleotide sequences flanking areas of interest for the purposes of amplification and detection. When amplifying DNA, the target could be human, tumor, or microorganism genomic material, for example. The primers are hybridized to the target, and with the addition of a DNA polymerase and nucleotides, the internal sequence is replicated. The strands of DNA are denatured by increasing the temperature, and annealed by decreasing the temperature, in a process termed thermocycling. Therefore, by cycling between optimized denaturing and annealing (and DNA polymerase activity) conditions, the target DNA is replicated in a logarithmic fashion. The amplified PCR product is then detected by its sequence and/or size. Capillary electrophoresis can be used to determine its size. Labeled probes directed to the amplified PCR product can be used to determine the target's presence and/or its sequence.

PCR can also be used to amplify and detect RNA using a variant of the assay called reverse-transcription PCR, or RT-PCR. With RT-PCR, the RNA is converted to cDNA before thermocycling, and the rest of the process is the same as standard PCR. RT-PCR can be used to detect types and quantities of transcripts, including gene-fusion transcripts. Quantitative assays using fluorescence binders, or qRT-PCR, also exist and quantitation can occur in "real time". Nested PCR and allele-specific PCR are other variations.

Advantages and Disadvantages

The main advantage of PCR testing and its variants is its relative simplicity and low cost. If designed appropriately (primer selection, for example), these assays are remarkably sensitive and specific with broad applications. To perform standard PCR, the sequence must be known in order to design primers, and the size of the PCR product (interval sequence) must be limited to a few hundred base pairs. RT-PCR is more sensitive than FISH and useful when testing samples with low levels of tumor. It is still used in the detection of gene fusions, particularly when a tumor type has variability in its DNA breakpoints. RT-PCR may suffer from an increased failure rate (when compared to DNA assays) due to degraded RNA, similar to other RNA-based assays.

Applications

As mentioned, the applications for PCR are broad. The most common uses are for the detection of a specific mutation (genodermatosis or tumor-specific mutation), a specific pathogen (histopathologically undetectable mycobacteria or speciation, for example), or identity testing (possible switched samples). Because of the amplification component, PCR and its variants are very useful for analyzing samples with low levels of targets (minimal residual disease and pathogens, for example). RT-PCR is still used to detect gene fusions, such as rearrangements associated with synovial sarcoma and other tumors with variability in breakpoints (**see Case Study 3**). PCR is often incorporated into other assays, such as gene expression profiling, clonality testing, microsatellite instability testing, and sequencing assays.

2.6 Sequencing

Sequence analysis has evolved over the past decades, with many technologies incorporating PCR. Examples include Sanger sequencing, pyrosequencing, and high-throughput (or next-generation) sequencing.

Principles

Sanger sequencing has largely been replaced by newer technologies but is still used in research and diagnostic settings. With Sanger sequencing, the target area is small and amplified by PCR. Once a template is created, DNA polymerase replicates DNA using a combination of normal nucleotides and chain-terminating nucleotides. The chain-terminating nucleotides are fluorescently labeled, with each nucleotide (A, C, G, or T) labeled with a different fluorochrome. This results in many DNA products with different lengths, each ending with a differentially labeled chain-terminating nucleotide. If these products are separated in a gel based on size, the sequence of the PCR template can be decoded.

Pyrosequencing also utilizes PCR. During the polymerase activity, nucleotides are added to the mix one at a time (A, C, G, or T). If a nucleotide is incorporated into the growing strand, light ("pyro") is detected and the nucleotide recorded. This process is repeated until the sequence of interest is generated.

Next-generation sequencing (NGS) refers to a sequencing platform that performs numerous simultaneous PCR reactions and then aligns all the overlapping sequences for a single interpretation. Based on these simultaneous reactions and reads, other terms used to describe NGS are "massively parallel," "deep," and "ultra-deep" sequencing. All forms of NGS begin with the design of a sequencing library. The library is based on the NGS strategy. For example, the library may be designed to assay the entire human genome, the entire exome, the entire transcriptome, or targeted arrays designed to detect disease-specific hot-spot mutations (melanoma driving mutations, soft tissue tumor fusions, mechanobullous disease mutations, etc.), for example. The library is created by fragmenting the desired components of genomic DNA (or other template) and preparing it for sequencing. Usually this is accomplished by ligating adaptors to the fragmented library and amplifying the fragments. Sequencing can be performed using different technologies. Examples include fluorescently labeled dNTPs (Illumina), pyrosequencing (454), and the detection of hydrogen, or pH, with the addition of dNTPs (Ion Torrent). Once all the fragments are sequenced, the sequences from all the products are aligned and software algorithms are used to make calls for each base. The "depth" refers to the number of aligned overlapping sequences for a given stretch of DNA. Increased depth is needed to analyze the transcriptome and to detect low-level mutations (i.e., low levels of tumor among many normal cells), emphasizing the importance of the overall NGS design strategy.

Advantages and Disadvantages

For Sanger sequencing, because it has been around for so many years, there is familiarity with the assay and comfort with interpreting results, and therefore many laboratories still use Sanger sequencing to confirm results from newer technologies. It is a relatively expensive assay with fairly high limits of detection (approximately 20% of mutant alleles). Pyrosequencing does not use fluorescence and is therefore less expensive to perform. The limits of detection are better (approximately 5% mutant alleles) than Sanger sequencing. Pyrosequencing is an effective assay when analyzing a mutation that is fairly consistent and in a localized area but not if the mutation potentially spans multiple exons or genes.

NGS has many advantages over other sequencing platforms and other molecular assays. The cost per sequenced base pair is significantly lower for NGS than other sequencing methods. This technology has a large scope of applications as it has the capability to not only detect point mutations, but also insertions, deletions, fusions, tumor mutational burden, and CNVs. And, with the ability to evaluate the transcriptome, NGS will likely supplant other sequencing methods along with FISH, aCGH, GEP, and traditional clonality and microsatellite instability platforms. Before this happens, however, there needs to be heavy investment in bioinformatics. Distinguishing biologically relevant alterations from innocuous variations, or polymorphisms, is one of the largest remaining challenges with NGS. Additionally, while the cost per base pair has plummeted, sequencing assays remain relatively expensive, including the cost of data storage, and the technology has outpaced payors' understanding and willingness to reimburse in many scenarios. Moreover, due to the complexity of the NGS assays, including interpretation, results may take several weeks, which can impact patient management in some cases.

Applications

In dermatopathology, sequencing remains uncommon. Sequencing is the test of choice for genodermatoses, but testing is often performed off buccal swabs or peripheral blood and not from biopsy specimens. Sequencing is also the test of choice for tumor mutational analysis to determine candidate targeted therapies for patients with advanced disease, but this is often ordered by dermatologists or oncologists. In these scenarios, Sanger sequencing or pyrosequencing may be used to identify specific mutations, but NGS is becoming more commonly used, particularly for sequencing entire genes or panels of genes (germline or tumor).

NGS is beginning to play a larger role in the assessment of soft tissue tumors. While FISH remains useful for relatively quickly identifying specific rearrangements or other genetic alterations, NGS is the test of choice when the scope of possible mutations is large. This is particularly true for diagnostically ambiguous low-grade lesions with distinctive histopathologic patterns as they often harbor detectable rearrangements. Identifying mutations may help with diagnosis but also may drive management if the detected mutation has an available targeted therapy (**see Case Study 2**).

Sequencing has had a very limited role in the diagnosis of melanocytic lesions until recently. This is largely because common mutations are shared between benign and malignant lesions (*BRAF* V600E, for example) or because the mutations are not specific or consistently observed in a given melanocytic lesion. The emergence of NGS has offered new potential in the diagnostic arena. As mentioned, NGS can detect a wide range of genetic alterations including but not limited to point mutations, deletions, rearrangements, and CNVs. With this NGS scope, distinguishing melanoma from nevus through the identification of nevus-specific mutations, oncogenic driver mutations, quantity of mutations, patterns of mutations, or CNVs is now possible. NGS has been used to distinguish Spitz nevi from Spitz (or Spitzoid) melanoma, to distinguish desmoplastic nevus from desmoplastic melanoma, and for many other applications.[18–20]

2.7 Microsatellite Instability

Microsatellite instability (MSI) is not commonly used in dermatopathology but is arguably underutilized. IHC is by far more commonly employed but largely due to access. These assays can be complementary if used appropriately. Conventional MSI testing is by PCR and capillary electrophoresis but tumor mutational burden (TMB) can now be assessed by high-throughput sequencing.

Principles

A subset of tumors have mutations which cause defects in the machinery required to repair errors created during the normal DNA replication process of cell division. The most common genes affected are *MLH1*, *MSH2*, *MSH6*, and *PMS2*. In normal cells, the protein products from these genes form heterodimers, specifically MLH1/PMS2 and MSH2/MSH6. These heterodimers are integral to the DNA repair process, and when not present or functioning normally, cells accumulate genetic mutations which may or may not be biologically relevant but can be detected.

When there is a functional defect in the mismatch repair process, mutations accumulate. Microsatellites are small stretches of DNA which contain tandem repeats of 1–6 base pair segments.[1] Because of the repetitive sequences, these loci are susceptible to "slippage" during replication, leading to changes of their size, and PCR primers designed to these regions can detect the size alterations. In normal DNA replication with repaired errors, the sizes of microsatellites remain constant, but, with slippage (and no repair), the size of these regions vary leading to a wider distribution of sizes, which can be detected by capillary electrophoresis (Figure 2.2). Errors can also be detected and quantified by sequencing analysis.

Advantages and Disadvantages

The advantage of MSI testing (over IHC) is that it is a functional assay. Because IHC detects the presence of mismatch repair proteins, false-negative results may occur when the proteins are not functional or if the mutated gene/protein is not part of the panel. MSI testing will identify all functional defects. The main disadvantage of MSI testing compared with IHC is that MSI testing is agnostic to the defect. Therefore, if there is an abnormality, the specific mutation is not known. This is less of an issue as the cost of sequencing has dropped and NGS panels covering multiple candidate genes are available. Other disadvantages of MSI testing include its limited availability, its relative unfamiliarity among dermatopathologists, and its requirement for comparison normal tissue/DNA, which is not always present in the biopsy specimen.

Applications

MSI testing has narrow use in dermatopathology. Muir-Torre syndrome is characterized by defects in mismatch repair and is allelic to Lynch syndrome. Muir-Torre syndrome patients develop sebaceous tumors along with visceral tumors and are often diagnosed following a cutaneous biopsy. Sebaceous neoplasms are often sporadic but patients who have sebaceous neoplasms at a young age, sebaceous neoplasms outside the head and neck region, sebaceous adenomas (anywhere), sebaceous carcinomas outside of the eyelid region, and any cystic or otherwise unusual sebaceous neoplasm are at high risk for having Muir-Torre syndrome. The risk increases with personal or family history of certain visceral tumors, such as colon and endometrial cancers.

Sebaceous neoplasms in these settings will often lead to an evaluation for Muir-Torre syndrome, preferably following dialogue with the clinician and consent from the patient. When embarking on a workup for mismatch repair defects, most dermatopathologists begin with IHC. Most laboratories test MLH-1 and MSH-2 but some test MLH-1, MSH-2, MSH-6, and PMS-2. When using the full panel, a positive test often has loss of both MSH-2 and MSH-6 (because these are heterodimers and when one is lost or not functional, the other degrades quickly). Less commonly, there is loss of both MLH-1 and PMS-2. When loss of expression is observed, this can be suggestive of Muir-Torre syndrome and patients may be sent for genetic counseling and/or gene sequencing. Sometimes, IHC yields no clear aberrancy, an unusual pattern (PMS-2 loss only, for example), or is technically suboptimal. In these cases, if there is a strong clinical concern for Muir-Torre syndrome, MSI testing could be considered as there could be expression of nonfunctional (mutated) proteins or there could be a mutation in another gene in the mismatch repair pathway. In theory, MSI testing could be performed before IHC, but this is not common in practice, largely due to accessibility.

2.8 T-Cell Receptor (TCR) and Immunoglobulin (Ig) Gene Rearrangement Studies

Non-neoplastic T-cells are comprised of αβ and γδ T-cells. The majority of leukemias and lymphomas originate from αβ T-cells; however, a small subset come from γδ T-cells such as primary cutaneous γδ T-cell lymphoma. The T-cell receptor (TCR) is comprised of either αβ (95%) or γδ (5%) heterodimer. Each of the TCR chains (TCRα, TCRβ, TCRγ, and TCRδ) is made up of variable (V), diversity (D), joint (J), and constant (C) regions. V, J, and C segments are present within each TCR gene locus, while D segments are present in TRB and TRD loci. Rearrangement of beta, gamma, and delta chains may occur at the same time.[21–23]

(a)

(b)

(c)

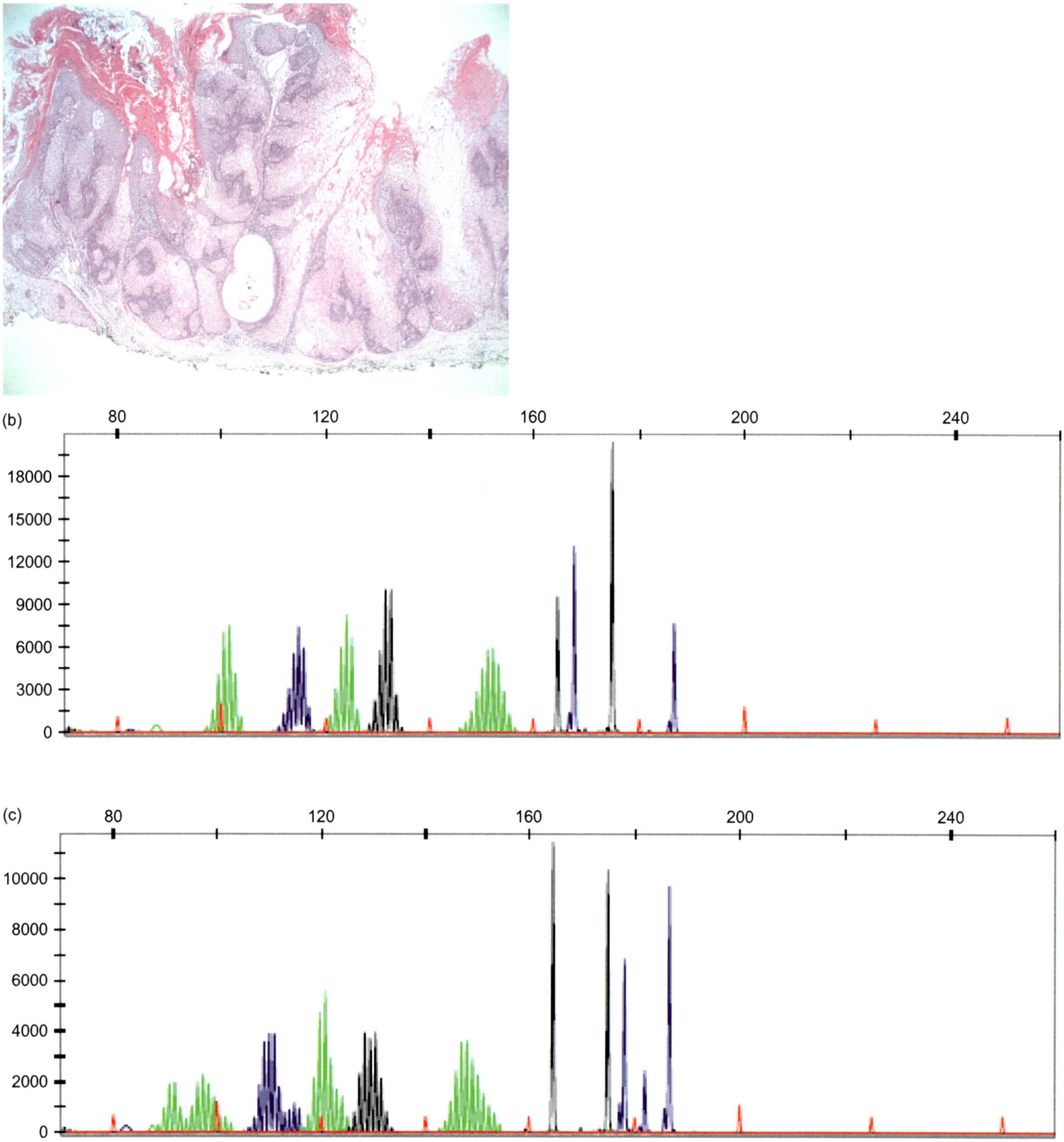

Figure 2.2 Microsatellite instability testing. A 40-year-old man presented with a papule on his cheek. On histopathology, there is a fairly symmetric sebaceous neoplasm diagnosed as sebaceous adenoma (A, H&E, X40). DNA was extracted from normal and lesional tissue. MSI testing of normal tissue shows fairly narrow peaks (fairly consistent PCR product sizes) from the various tested microsatellite regions (B, electropherogram). DNA from the sebaceous adenoma has peaks with more asymmetry and broader bases, indicating more variation in the PCR product sizes, i.e., microsatellite instability (C, electropherogram).

Principles

Since it is difficult to distinguish neoplastic T/B cells from reactive T/B cells in some cases, clonality testing such as immunoglobulin heavy chain (IgH) and T-cell receptor (TCR) gene rearrangement analyses facilitates the diagnosis of lymphoid malignancies. During the earliest stages of B-cell and T-cell development, a random combination of variable (V), diversity (D), and joining (J) genes results in a unique VDJ exon that encodes the variable domain or its antigen binding site. TCR gene rearrangement begins with TCRδ, then TCRγ, TCRβ, and finally TCRα.[24] As the result each lymphocyte possesses a unique antigen receptor molecule. TCRs recognize antigen together with the major histocompatibility complex molecule. Therefore, similar rearrangements support the clonal nature of a particular lymphoid infiltrate. Whether the Ig or TCR gene rearrangement is clonal or polyclonal forms the basis of clonality testing.

The most widely employed method is TCR gamma analysis since it is rearranged early in T-cell development in both αβ and γδ T-cells. With 12 variable segments the gene structure of TCRγ is the simplest. Current methods involve three steps: (1) DNA extraction, (2) multiplex PCR, and (3) electrophoresis. In brief, DNA is isolated from paraffin embedded skin biopsy and analyzed by a PCR technique using primers conjugated with fluorescent dyes that hybridize to TCR gamma chain gene V segment 1–8, 9, 10, 11 (Vg1-8, Vg9, Vg10, Vg11) and joining region (Jg1 and Jg2). The DNA is also amplified with control primers to multiple gene segments (64 to 600 bp in length) to assess the integrity and quality of the isolated DNA. The PCR products are analyzed by capillary gel electrophoresis. A clonal peak is typically greater than twofold over the background.

The European BIOMED-2 consortium was created to evaluate clonality in lymphoproliferations that are difficult to diagnose.[25] Multiplex PCR analyses have been standardized enabling routine diagnostic testing in the detection of clonality.[26] NGS method is more comprehensive and can be more quantitative than conventional assays; however, not many laboratories have access to this expensive and complex test. NGS analyses of IgH/TCR rearrangement facilitates clonality assessment, minimal residual disease detection, and repertoire analysis.[26,27]

Advantages and Disadvantages

The current PCR-based TCR gamma clonality testing has several limitations including false-negative and false-positive results. Since PCR-based techniques are subject to amplicon size restrictions, complete assay of the *TRA* gene is not possible. In addition, only part of the *TRB* locus is analyzed in the multiplex PCR assay.[28] TCR gene deletion can result in non-amplification.[29] False negative results can be due to paucity of clonal T-cells, DNA degradation, and employed primers might not cover all possible TCR gamma rearrangements. False positive results might be due to the detection of a dominant clone in reactive inflammatory diagnoses. Clonal T-cell proliferations have been documented in several benign conditions including pityriasis lichenoides et varioliformis acuta, lichen planus, and lichen sclerosus;[30,31] therefore, clonality does not equate to malignancy.

Applications

In the detection of early mycosis fungoides (MF), the sensitivity of TCR beta clonality test is 83% versus 43% of TCR gamma clonality test.[32] A combined use of both TCR beta and gamma tests can increased the detection rate of early MF (Schachter et al. 2020). NGS methods have been reported to have better sensitivity and can accurately identify recurrent MF.[26] The identification of identical clones from two different body sites is supportive of MF (**see Case Study 4**).[28]

EuroClonality-NGS DNA Capture (EuroClonality-NDC) assay was designed as an integrated tool to characterize these alterations by capturing IGH switch regions along with variable, diversity, and joining genes of all IG and TCR loci in addition to clinically relevant genes for translocations, copy number alterations, and sequence variants.[33]

Identification of TCR type is important for diagnosis and prognosis. Immunostains performed on FFPE tissues can readily identify the TCR type. BetaF1 immunostain detects αβ T-cells. Previously used TCR gamma-chain monoclonal antibody g3.20 is no longer available and TCR delta-chain H-41 antibody is currently used to detect γδ T-cells.[34] By flow cytometry, the T-cell receptor β constant region 1 (TRBC1) antibody has been reported to detect neoplastic T-cells.[35]

2.9 Case Studies

Case 2.1

Clinical history: An 85-year-old man presented with a polypoid lesion in his right thigh/groin region.

Microscopic description: Histologic sections show a condylomatous growth pattern with full-thickness atypia of keratinocytes (Figures 2.3 and 2.4). Diffuse block-like p16 staining is seen (Figures 2.5). *In situ* hybridization for HPV33 shows dot-like positivity (Figures 2.6 and 2.7) while negative for HPV6/11 and HPV16/18.

Diagnosis: High-grade squamous intraepithelial neoplasia, HPV-associated.

Discussion: HPV infection is the most common cause of squamous dysplasia in the anogenital sites.[36] HPV subtypes can be low-risk (HPV6/11), which has minimal risk of progression to SCC, or high-risk (HPV16/18, HPV33), which has a higher risk of progression to SCC. The availability of chromogenic mRNA *in situ* hybridization probes to these HPV subtypes has helped to diagnose and to risk stratify the patients with anogenital HPV infection.

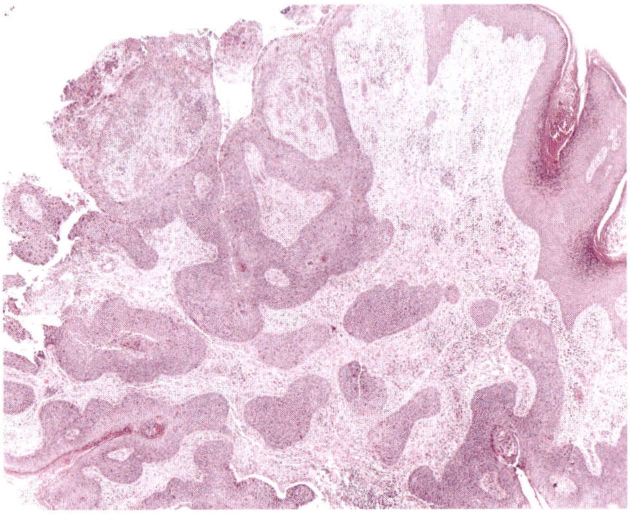

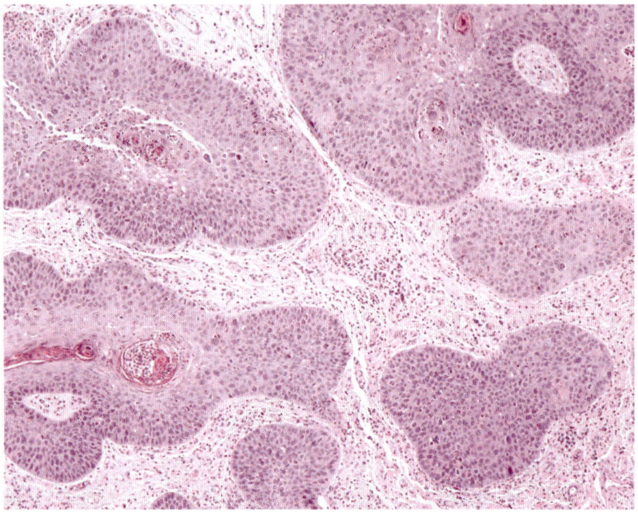

Figures 2.3 and 2.4 A polypoid growth with dysplastic squamous epidermis seen (X40 and X100).

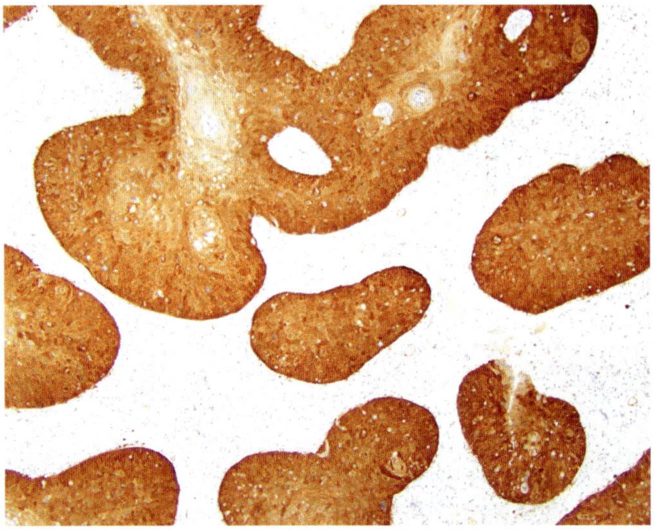

Figure 2.5 Block-like p16 positivity is noted within the squamous epithelium (X100).

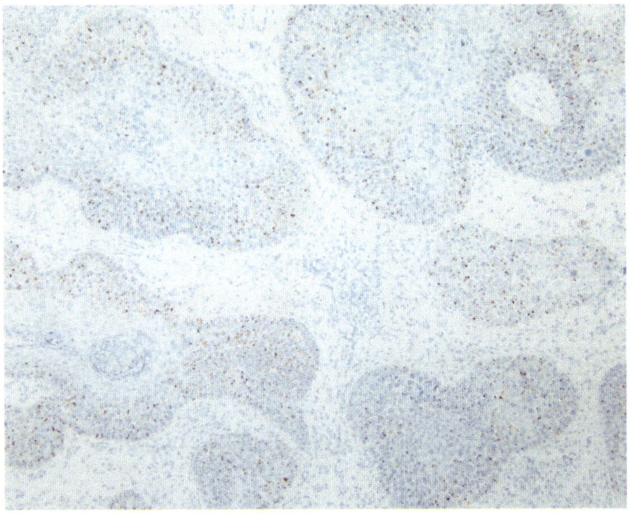

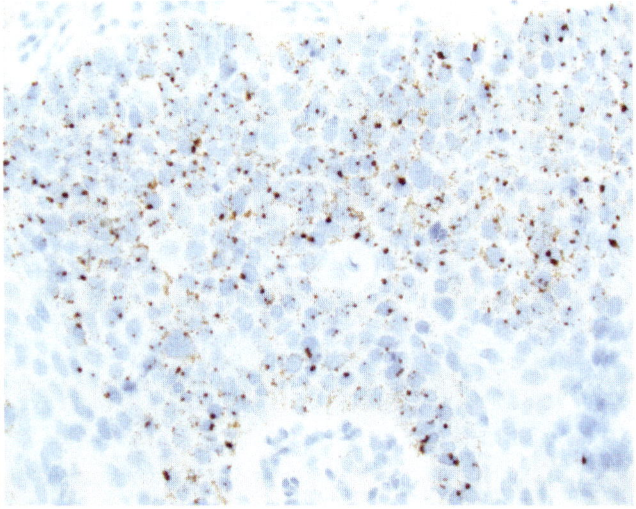

Figures 2.6 and 2.7 Dot-like positivity is seen on HPV33 mRNA *in situ* hybridization (X200 and X400).

Case 2.2

Clinical history: A 59-year-old woman presented to the emergency room with submassive pulmonary embolism and sepsis. At that time, a large and fungating basal cell carcinoma with involvement of her right proximal humerus was found. Multiple right axillary and subpectoral lymph nodes were found to be involved by metastatic tumor on positron emission tomography (PET) computed tomography (CT). Right lower lobe subpleural nodule measuring 7 mm was seen on chest CT. In order to salvage her limb, her tumor was sequenced for potential chemotherapeutic treatment. Targeted NGS assay of tumor DNA was positive for variants in *APC*, *SMO*, *TP53*, and *KRAS*. She was started on vismodegib.

Microscopic description: A proliferation of basaloid tumor nests with peripheral palisade and stromal clefting artifact is seen (Figures 2.8 and 2.9).

Diagnosis: Metastasizing basal cell carcinoma.

Discussion: Two months after chemotherapy, magnetic resonance imaging (MRI) of her humerus demonstrated tumor shrinkage. Segmental resection of the tumor was done instead of limb amputation. In 2012 and 2015 the U.S. Food and Drug Administration (FDA) approved vismodegib (Smoothened inhibitor) and sonidegib (Hedgehog/Smoothened antagonist) for treatment of advanced BCC, respectively.[37,38] Since then, multiple studies have shown treatment response in advanced BCC.[38] Our case illustrates the role of NGS assay in treatment decisions for patients with advanced tumors.

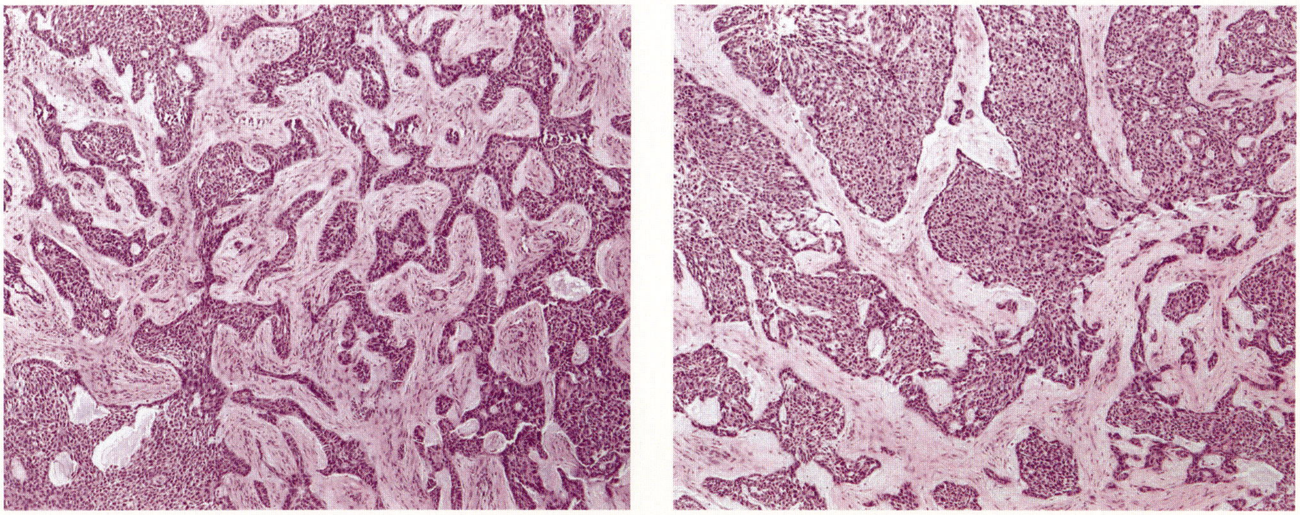

Figures 2.8 and 2.9 Infiltrative and nodular proliferation of basaloid tumor cells with peripheral palisade (X100, X100).

Case 2.3

Clinical history: A 65-year-old woman presented with a “keloid” on her back.

Microscopic description: A 3 mm skin biopsy was performed which extends only to deep dermis and the subcutaneous fat is not visualized (Figure 2.10). A storiform proliferation of slender spindle cells without prominent mitotic figures is seen (Figure 2.11). The tumor cells are strongly positive for CD34 (Figure 2.12), while they are negative for beta-catenin, Sox10, S100, and pan-TRK. A definitive diagnosis cannot be reached due to the superficial nature of biopsy and the patient was not amendable to further biopsy procedure. A molecular fusion assay was performed which revealed a *COL1A1::PDGFB* gene fusion (Figure 2.13).

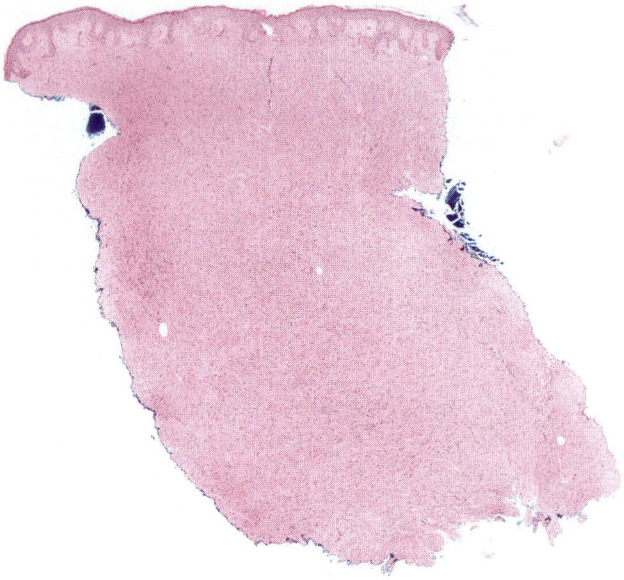

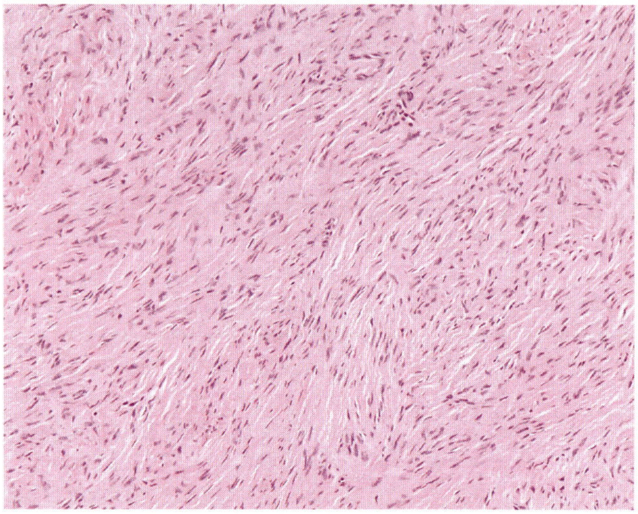

Figures 2.10 and 2.11 A proliferation of spindle cells is seen within the dermis (X40, X200).

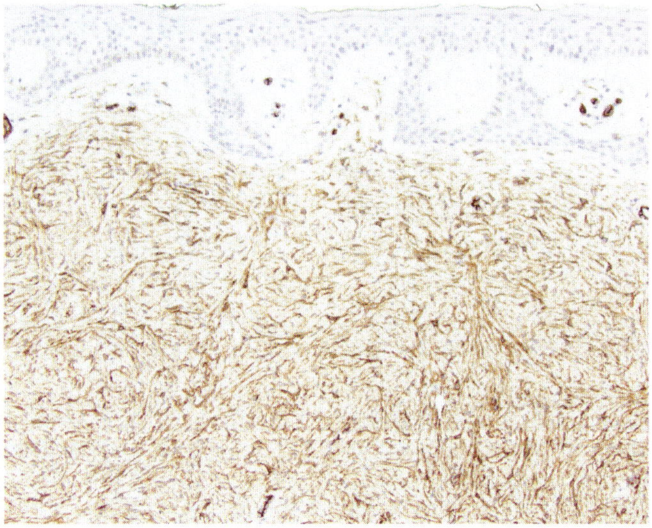

Figure 2.12 Diffuse CD34 expression is noted (X200).

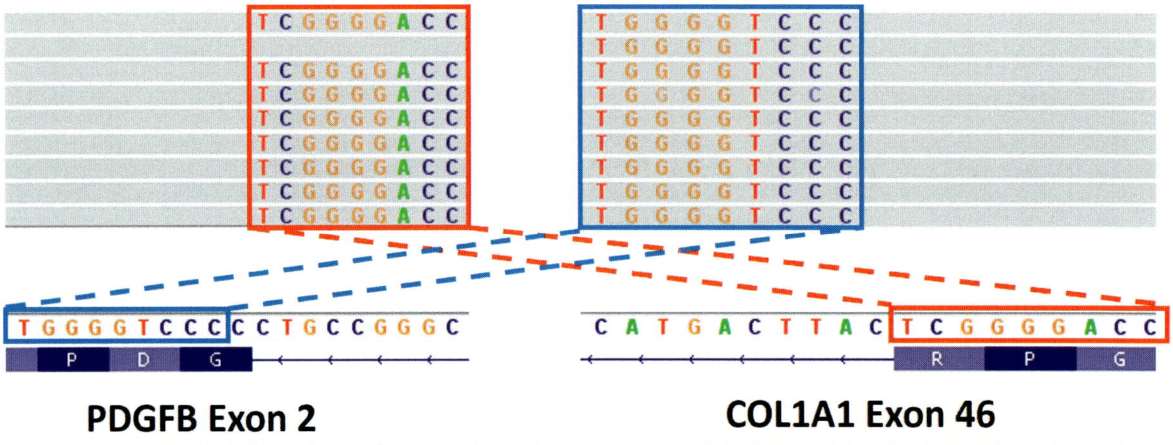

Figure 2.13 *COL1A1::PDGFB* gene rearrangement (Courtesy of Dr. Soma Jobbagy, Department of Pathology, Massachusetts General Hospital, Boston, MA).

Diagnosis: Dermatofibrosarcoma protuberans.

Discussion: IHC performed on the biopsy has helped excluding fibromatosis (beta-catenin), desmoplastic melanoma (Sox10 and S100), and NTRK-rearranged spindle cell neoplasm/lipofibromatosis-like neural tumor (pan-TRK). However, due to the strong CD34 expression, plaque-like CD34+ dermal fibroma/medallion-like dermal dendrocyte hamartoma, superficial CD34-positive fibroblastic tumor and dermatofibrosarcoma protuberans (DFSP) are still in the histologic differential diagnosis.[39] Ancillary molecular assay was helpful in reaching a definitive diagnosis which affected the treatment decision. It revealed a characteristic translocation of DFSP.[40] The excision specimen shows a honeycomb architecture characteristic of DFSP, confirming the diagnosis (Figures 2.14 and 2.15). This case illustrates that in challenging cases or in small biopsies, molecular studies to identify a *COL1A1::PDGFB* gene rearrangement can be of utility.

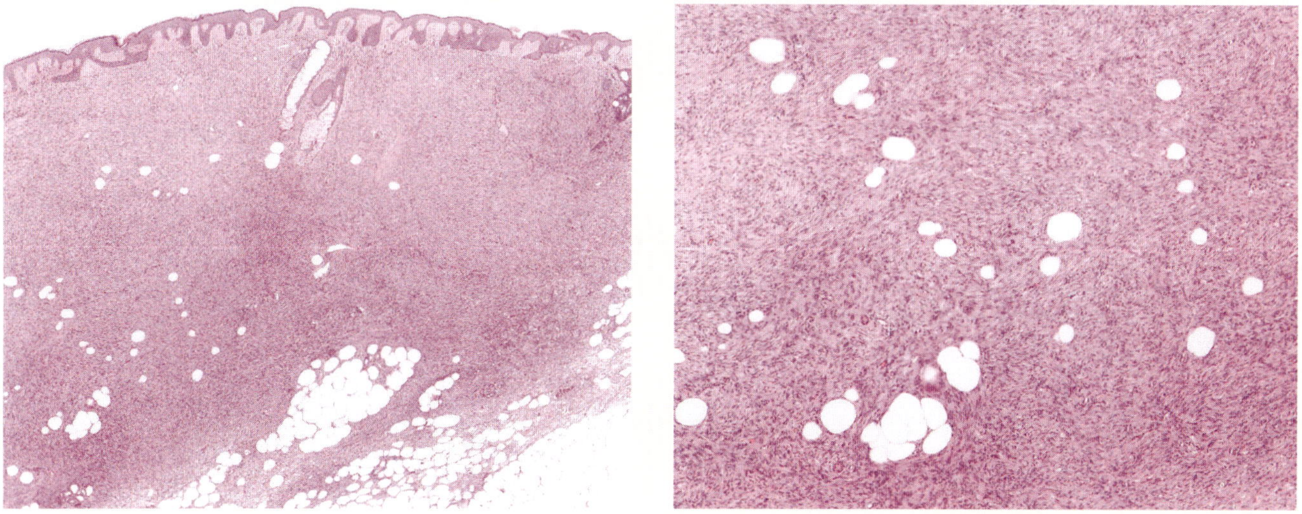

Figures 2.14 and 2.15 A tumor with subcutaneous honeycomb architecture is seen (X40, X100).

Lee et al.[40] performed *PDGFB*, *COL1A1*, *PDGFD*, *COL6A3*, and *EMILIN2* rearrangements by fluorescent *in situ* hybridization (FISH) on 188 DFSPs. The authors reported classic *PDGFB* rearrangement, cryptic *COL1A1::PDGFB* fusion, and *PDGFD* rearrangement were identified in 172 (91.4%), 8 (4.3%), and 8 (4.3%: 4 *COL6A3::PDFGD*, 4 *EMILIN2::PDGFD*) cases, respectively. Therefore, although the fusion can be detected by FISH, NGS fusion assay is better than FISH in detecting uncommon fusion and rearrangement.

Case 2.4

Clinical history: A 61-year-old man presented in 2018 for one-year history of rash. Faint pink scaly well-demarcated round thin plaques with some peripheral clearing were seen on bilateral thighs, right buttock, and right flank. Round scaly patches were also seen on bilateral cheeks and forehead. Skin biopsies of the right buttock and left forehead were performed.

Microscopic description: Both biopsies show an atypical lymphoid infiltrate comprised predominantly of small to medium-sized lymphoid cells with irregular nuclear contour, hyperchromasia, and scant cytoplasm (Figures 2.16 and 2.17). The majority of the lymphoid cells are CD3+ with no loss of CD2 or CD5 expression (Figures 2.18 and 2.19). CD4 and CD8 demonstrate an increased CD4:CD8 ratio (Figures 2.20 and 2.21). TCR gamma gene rearrangements show clonal population with identical peaks in both specimens, one from the buttocks and one from face. A biallelic clonal T cell receptor gamma chain gene rearrangement is identified with Vgamma1-8 primers (207 bp and 213 bp). The morphologic, immunophenotypic, and molecular findings are supportive of mycosis fungoides.

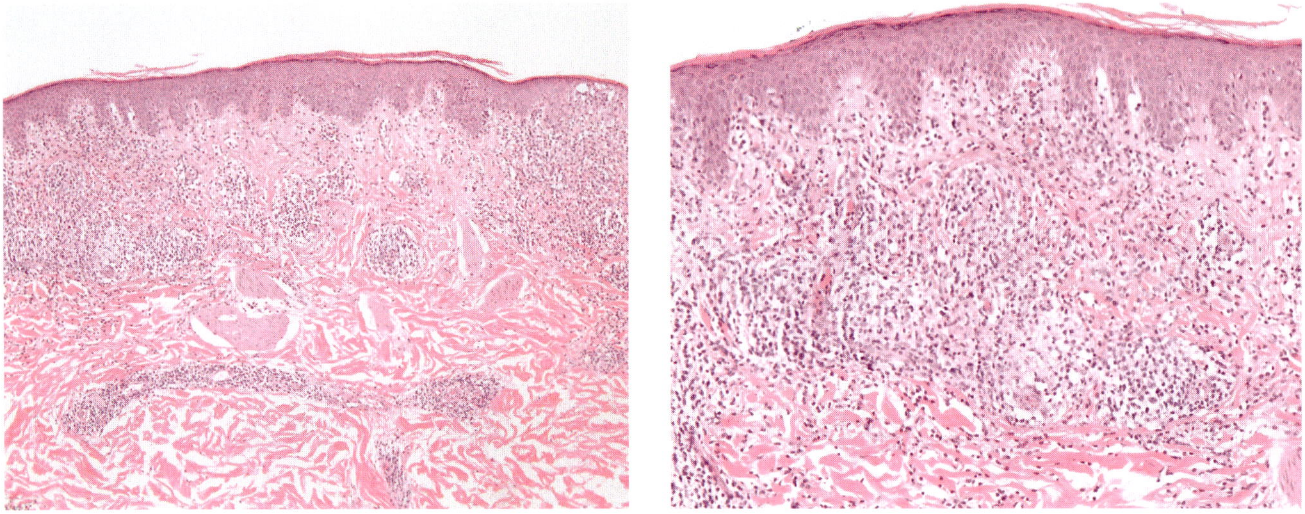

Figures 2.16 and 2.17 A patchy lichenoid infiltrate of atypical lymphoid cells extending into the overlying epidermis is seen (X100, X200).

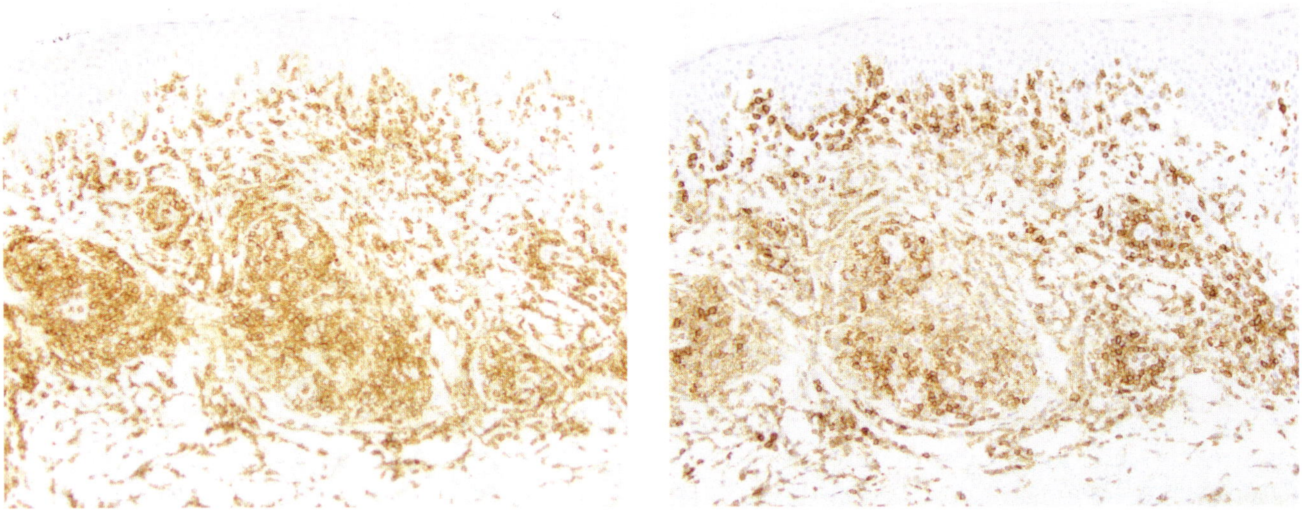

Figures 2.18 and 2.19 CD3 and CD5 highlight the lymphoid infiltrate. Note the "tagging" lymphoid cells at the dermal epidermal junction (X200, X200).

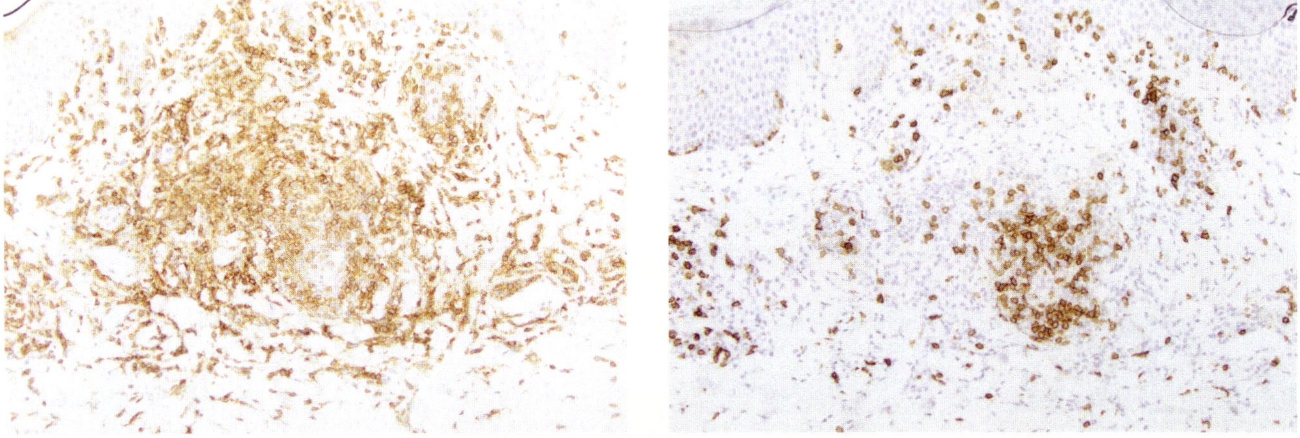

Figures 2.20 and 2.21 CD4 to CD8 ratio is increased (X200, X200).

Diagnosis: Mycosis fungoides/cutaneous T-cell lymphoma.

Discussion: The diagnosis of mycosis fungoides (MF), especially in early patch stage, can be clinically and histopathologically challenging. When there is aberrant immunophenotypic expression such as loss of CD2 and/or CD5 expression, the diagnosis of MF is in favor. However, loss of pan T-cell marker expression is not seen in all cases, as illustrated in the current case. In this setting ancillary studies such as TCR gamma gene rearrangement would be helpful. Identical clones were identified in two different anatomic sites in this study case, which has been reported to be supportive of MF.[28] Although a dominant T-cell clone can be seen in 40–90% of biopsies of MF, clonality does not equate to malignancy. Clonal T-cell population can be detected in a variety of inflammatory dermatoses including – pityriasis lichenoides et varioliformis acuta, lichen planus, and lichen sclerosus.[30,31] Therefore, the same clonal T-cell population is seen at different body sites is helpful in reaching the diagnosis of MF. Thurber and colleagues[28] reported the sensitivity and specificity of TCR gamma gene rearrangement in detecting an identical clone at different anatomic sites to be 82.6% and 95.7%, respectively.

Case 2.5

Clinical history: A 24-year-old female presented with an atypical pigmented lesion on the buttock.

Microscopic description: The lesion was fairly symmetric with a suggestion of maturation (Figure 2.22). There was pagetoid growth with enlarged melanocytes in the epidermis and superficial dermis and smaller cells with adnexotropism deeper (Figure 2.23). The histopathologic differential diagnosis at this point was atypical nevus versus superficially invasive melanoma arising in a nevus (pT1a) versus invasive nevoid melanoma (pT1b). Given the suggestion of maturation and adnexotropism, melanoma arising in a nevus was favored. However, PRAME immunostain was performed in an attempt to demonstrate two populations but was positive in the entire lesion (Figure 2.24). The PRAME positivity in the deeper nevus-appearing component is supportive of invasive melanoma and thus would upstage the lesion to pT1b. FISH analysis was performed and scored on the deeper component only. Copy number gains of *RREB1* are present (Figure 2.25).

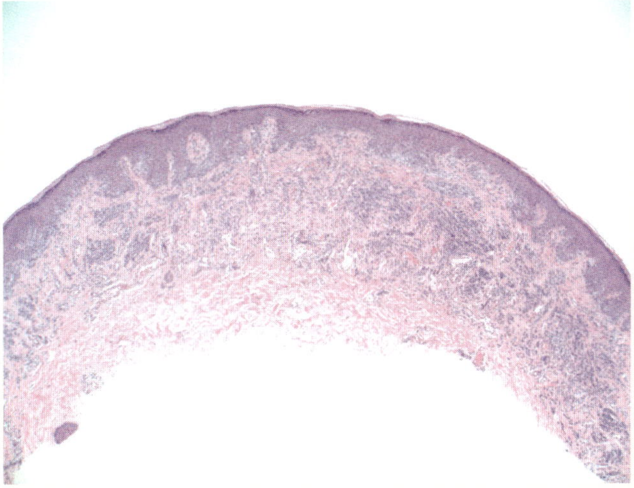

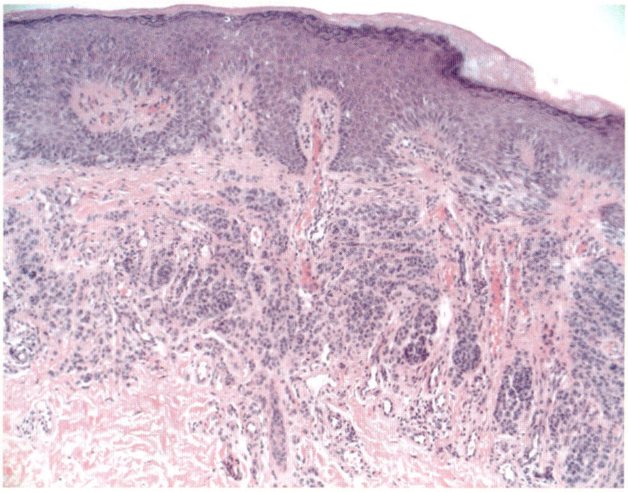

Figures 2.22 and 2.23 An atypical proliferation of melanocytes is seen within the epidermis and superficial dermis (X40, X100).

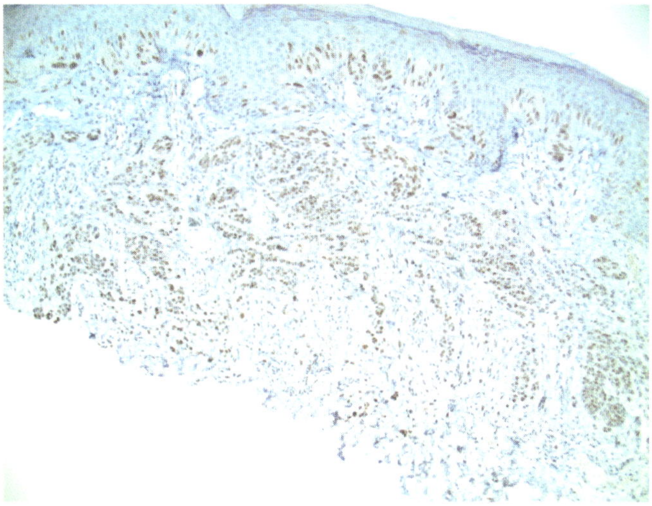

Figure 2.24 PRAME expression is seen in both epidermal and dermal component (X100).

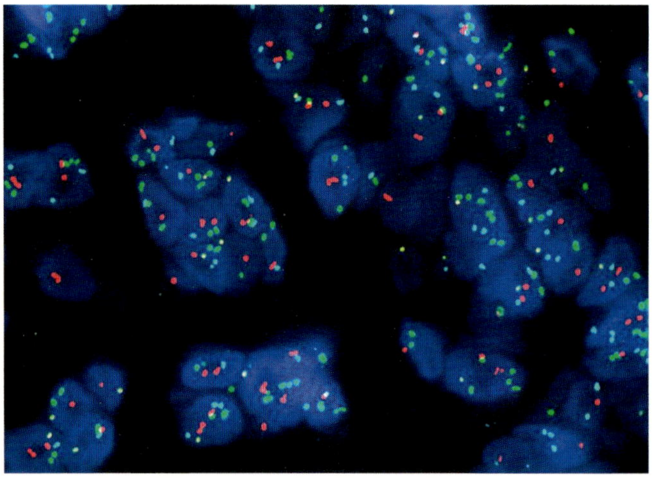

Figure 2.25 Fluorescence *in situ* hybridization. *RREB1* (green), *MYC* (aqua), *CDKN2A* (gold), *CCND1* (red) probes identified gains in *RREB1*.

Diagnosis: Invasive melanoma, pT1b.

Discussion: One of the main advantages of using FISH in the evaluation of melanocytic lesions is its ability to assess (score) specific cells of interest. This is not easily achieved using CGH or GEP. This particular case is an example of a heterogeneous lesion. The superficial aspect of the lesion is very atypical but the deeper portion contains smaller cells which are nevoid in appearance. Assessing the deeper component was important in this case as its characterization impacted staging (pT1a versus pT1b), which would likely determine whether or not this patient would be considered for sentinel lymph node biopsy.

References

1. Hosler GA, Murphy KM. *Molecular Diagnostics for Dermatology: Practical Applications of Molecular Testing for the Diagnosis and Management of the Dermatology Patient*. Berlin, Heidelberg: Springer Berlin Heidelberg; 2014. Available from: http://link.springer.com/10.1007/978-3-642-54066-0
2. Hosler GA, Murphy KM. Ancillary testing for melanoma: current trends and practical considerations. *Hum Pathol* 2023; **140**: 5–21.
3. Fung MA, Vidal CI, Armbrecht EA, et al. Appropriate use criteria for ancillary diagnostic testing in dermatopathology: New recommendations for 11 tests and 220 clinical scenarios from the American Society of Dermatopathology Appropriate Use Criteria Committee. *J Cutan Pathol* 2021; **49**: 231–45.
4. Vidal CI, Armbrect EA, Andea AA, et al. Appropriate use criteria in dermatopathology: Initial recommendations from the American Society of Dermatopathology. *J Cutan Pathol* 2018; **45**: 563–80.
5. Mirghani H, Casiraghi O, Amen F, et al. Diagnosis of HPV-driven head and

neck cancer with a single test in routine clinical practice. *Mod Pathol* 2015; **28**: 1518–27.

6. Mendez-Pena JE, Sadow PM, Nose V, Hoang MP. RNA chromogenic in situ hybridization assay with clinical automated platform is a sensitive method in detecting high-risk human papillomavirus in squamous cell carcinoma. *Hum Pathol* 2017; **63**: 184–9.
7. Rezk SA, Zhao X, Weiss LM. Epstein-Barr virus (EBV)-associated lymphoid proliferations, a 2018 update. *Hum Pathol* 2018; **79**: 18–41.
8. Poling JS, Yonescu R, Subhawong AP, Sharma R, Argani P, Ning Y, Cimino-Mathews A. MYB labeling by immunohistochemistry is more sensitive and specific for breast adenoid cystic carcinoma than MYB Labeling by FISH. *Am J Surg Pathol* 2017; **41**: 973–9.
9. Gerami P, Jewell SS, Morrison LE, et al. Fluorescence in situ hybridization (FISH) as an ancillary diagnostic tool in the diagnosis of melanoma. *Am J Surg Pathol* 2009; **33**: 1146–56.
10. Bastian BC, Olshen AB, LeBoit PE, Pinkel D. Classifying melanocytic tumors based on DNA copy number changes. *Am J Pathol* 2003; **163**: 1765–70.
11. Gerami P, Cook RW, Wilkinson J, et al. Development of a prognostic genetic signature to predict the metastatic risk associated with cutaneous melanoma. *Clin Cancer Res* 2015; **21**: 175–83.
12. Clarke LE, Warf MB, Flake DD 2nd, et al. Clinical validation of a gene expression signature that differentiates benign nevi from malignant melanoma. *J Cutan Pathol* 2015; **42**: 244–52.
13. Onken MD, Worley LA, Char DH, et al. Collaborative Ocular Oncology Group report number 1: prospective validation of a multi-gene prognostic assay in uveal melanoma. *Ophthalmology* 2012; **119**: 1596–603.
14. Huey RW, Shah AT, Reddi HV, et al. Feasibility and value of genomic profiling in cancer of unknown primary: real-world evidence from prospective profiling study. *J Natl Cancer Inst* 2023; **115**: 994–7.
15. Heerfordt IM, Philipsen PA, Andersen JD, et al. RNA analysis of tape strips to rule out melanoma in lesions clinically assessed as cutaneous malignant melanoma: a diagnostic study. *J Am Acad Dermatol* 2023; **89**: 537–43.
16. Gerami P, Alsobrook JP 2nd, Palmer TJ, Robin HS. Development of a novel noninvasive adhesive patch test for the evaluation of pigmented lesions of the skin. *J Am Acad Dermatol* 2014; **71**: 237–44.
17. He H, Bissonnette R, Wu J, et al. Tape strips detect distinct immune and barrier profiles in atopic dermatitis and psoriasis. *J Allergy Clin Immunol* 2021; **147**: 199–212.
18. Zarabi SK, Azzato EM, Tu ZJ, et al. Targeted next generation sequencing (NGS) to classify melanocytic neoplasms. *J Cutan Pathol* 2020; **47**: 691–704.
19. Roth A, Lampley N 3rd, Boutko A, et al. Next-generation sequencing improves agreement and accuracy in the diagnosis of Spitz and spitzoid melanocytic lesions. *J Cutan Pathol* 2022; **49**: 868–74.
20. Roth A, Boutko A, Lampley N 3rd, et al. Next-generation sequencing as a potential diagnostic adjunct in distinguishing between desmoplastic melanocytic neoplasms. *Am J Surg Pathol* 2023; **47**: 318–25.
21. Burtrum B, Kim S, Dudley E, et al. TCR gene recombination and alpha beta-gamma delta lineage divergence: productive TCR-beta rearrangement is neither exclusive nor preclusive of gamma/delta cell development. *J Immunol* 1996; **157**: 4293–6.
22. Krangel MS. Mechanics of T cell receptor gene rearrangement. *Curr Opin Immunol* 2009; **21**: 133–9.
23. Davis MM. The evolutionary and structural "logic" of antigen receptor diversity. *Semin Immunol* 2004; **16**: 239–43.
24. Blom B, Verschuren MC, Heemskerk MH, et al. TCR gene rearrangements and expression of the pre-T cell receptor complex during human T-cell differentiation. *Blood* 1999; **93**: 3033–43.
25. Langerak AW, Groenen PJ, Bruggemann M, et al. EuroClonality/BIOMED-2 guidelines for interpretation and reporting of Ig/TCR clonality testing in suspected lymphoproliferations. *Leukemia* 2012; **26**: 2159–71.
26. Sufficool KE, Lockwood CM, Abel HJ, et al. T-cell clonality assessment by next-generation sequencing improves detection sensitivity in mycosis fungoides. *J Am Acad Dermatol* 2015; **73**: 228–36.
27. Arcila ME, Yu W, Syed M, et al. Establishment of immunoglobulin heavy (IGH) chain clonality testing by next-generation sequencing for routine characterization of B-cell and plasma cell neoplasms. *J Mol Diagn* 2019; **21**: 330–42.
28. Thurber SE, Zhang B, Kim YH, et al. T-cell clonality analysis in biopsy specimens from two different skin sites shows high specificity in the diagnosis of patients with suggested mycosis fungoides. *J Am Acad Dermatol* 2007; **57**: 782–90.
29. Kandolf Sekulovic L, Cikota B, Stojadinovic O, et al. TCRgamma gene rearrangement analysis in skin samples and peripheral blood of mycosis fungoides patients. *Acta Dermatovenerol Alp Pannonica Adriat* 2007; **16**: 149–55.
30. Lukowsky A, Muche JM, Sterry W, Audring H. Detection of expanded T cell clones in skin biopsy samples of patients with lichen sclerosus et atrophicus by T cell receptor-gamma polymerase chain reaction assays. *J Invest Dermatol* 2000; **115**: 254–9.
31. Boer A, Tirumalae R, Bresch M, Falk TM. Pseudoclonality in cutaneous pseudolymphomas: a pitfall in interpretation of rearrangement studies. *Br J Dermatol* 2008; **159**: 394–402.
32. Schachter O, Tabibian-Keissar H, Debby A, Segal O, Baum S, Barzilai A. Evaluation of the polymerase chain reaction-based T-cell receptor β clonality test in the diagnosis of early mycosis fungoides. *J Am Acad Dermatol* 2020; **83**: 1400–05.
33. Stewart JP, Gazdova J, Darzentas N, et al.; EuroClonality-NGS Working Group. Validation of the EuroClonality-NGS DNA capture panel as an integrated genomic tool for lymphoproliferative disorders. *Blood Adv* 2021; **5**: 3188–98.
34. Jungbluth AA, Frosina D, Fayad M, et al. Immunohistochemical detection of γδ T lymphocytes in formalin-fixed paraffin-embedded tissues. *Appl Immunohistochem Mol Morphol* 2019; **27**: 581–3.
35. Waldron D, O'Brien D, Smyth L, Quinn F, Vandenberghe E. Reliable detection of T-cell clonality by flow cytometry in mature T-cell neoplasms using TRBC1: implementation as a reflex test and comparison with PCR-based clonality testing. *Lab Med* 2022; **53**: 417–25.
36. Li Z, Liu P, Wang Z, et al. Prevalence of human papillomavirus DNA and p16INK4a positivity in vulvar cancer and vulvar intraepithelial neoplasia: a

systematic review and meta-analysis. *Lancet Oncol* 2023; **24**: 403–14.

37. Sekulic A, Migden MR, Oro AE, et al. Efficacy and safety of vismodegib in advanced basal cell carcinoma. *N Engl J Med* 2012; **366**: 2171–9.
38. Chen L, Aria AB, Silapunt S, Lee HH, Migden MR. Treatment of advanced basal cell carcinoma with sonidegib: perspective from the 30-month update of the BOLT trial. *Future Oncol* 2018; **14**: 515–25.
39. Carter JM, Weiss SW, Linos K, DiCaudo DJ, Folpe AL. Superficial CD34-positive fibroblastic tumor: report of 18 cases of a distinctive low-grade mesenchymal neoplasm of intermediate (borderline) malignancy. *Mod Pathol* 2014; **27**: 294–302.
40. Lee PH, Huang SC, Wu PS, et al. Molecular characterization of dermatofibrosarcoma protuberans: the clinicopathologic significance of uncommon fusion gene rearrangements and their diagnostic importance in the exclusively subcutaneous and circumscribed lesions. *Am J Surg Pathol* 2022; **46**: 942–55.

Chapter

3 Epithelial or Squamous Neoplasms

Maria Teresa Fernandez Figueras, Mai P. Hoang, and Kristine M. Cornejo

3.1 Cutaneous Squamous Cell Carcinoma

Squamous cell carcinoma (SCC) and basal cell carcinoma (BCC) are the most common cutaneous epithelial neoplasms. The head and neck, trunk, and lower extremities are the most affected sites for ultraviolet (UV)-induced SCC.[1] The genitalia, hands, and feet are typical locations of verrucous carcinoma. Predisposed factors for developing SCC include chronic ulcer, burn scar, radiation, topical carcinogens, human papillomavirus infection, genetic predisposition (xeroderma pigmentosum), vitiligo, albinism, and others. Transplant patients often have multiple and aggressive SCC.

For risk stratification using histologic features, Cassarino et al.[2] have proposed a three-tier system: low (less than 2% metastatic risk), intermediate (3–10%), and high (> 10%). The low-risk group includes human papilloma virus (HPV)-associated SCC and trichilemmal carcinoma. Intermediate-risk group is comprised of acantholytic SCC, clear cell SCC, squamoid eccrine ductal carcinoma, and lymphoepithelioma-like carcinoma. High-risk group are adenosquamous SCC, SCC arising in transplant patients and in association with radiation and burn scars.[2]

Others have reported high-risk histologic features to include ear or lip location, tumor thickness greater than 2 mm, high histologic grade or poor differentiation, Clark level IV or V, and perineural invasion of peripheral nerves with > 0.1 mm diameter.[3]

Due to its diverse morphologic appearance including acantholytic, clear cell, adenosquamous, lymphoepithelioma-like, small cell, spindle cell, and sarcomatoid (carcinosarcoma), SCC can mimic a variety of epithelial, lymphoid, melanocytic as well as mesenchymal neoplasms of the skin.[2] All SCC would invariably express p40 and p63.[4] While the well-differentiated SCC expresses a spectrum of various keratins, the poorly differentiated tumors express focally the high molecular weight ones such as keratin 5/6, keratin MNF116, and keratin 903.[5] SCC can express low molecular weight keratins such as keratin 7, keratin 19, and keratin CAM5.2 that are typically seen in adnexal carcinomas.[6] Other epithelial markers which often mark glandular lesions such as epithelial membrane antigen (EMA) and carcinoembryonic antigen (CEA) can be positive in SCC.[6,7]

Squamous Cell Carcinoma versus Basal Cell Carcinoma

In the setting of a superficial or fragmented biopsy, it can be difficult to distinguish BCC from SCC and a panel of BerEP4 and EMA appear to be helpful (**Table 3.1**).[7–13] BerEP4 labels the majority of BCC and none of SCC (**Figures 3.1 and 3.2**).[8,9] On the other hand EMA labels 85–100% of SCC cases and only 2–8% of BCC cases.[7,8,10] While superficial BCC would be positive for BerEP4, actinic keratosis would be negative.[14] However, Yu et al.[15] have found in a recent study that BerEP4 labeling not to be reliable in superficial biopsies of BCC with squamoid features. In the skin, BerEP4 also labels Merkel cell carcinoma, Paget disease, and a subset of adnexal neoplasms.[11] When a BCC exhibits squamous differentiation, diffuse keratin 17 expression is helpful in distinguishing it from SCC which has patchy keratin 17 expression (**Figures 3.3 and 3.4**).[13] Bcl2 has been reported to be useful in distinguishing BCC from SCC with staining noted mainly in BCC.[11] Most subtypes of BCC, with the exception of the sclerosing variant, express CD10; while SCC only exhibit weak expression in the stroma.[12] CD10 was strongly expressed in the majority of 16 BCC cases but in none of 13 SCC.[16]

Table 3.1 Immunostaining of basal cell carcinoma versus squamous cell carcinoma [7-13]

	Basal cell carcinoma	Squamous cell carcinoma
BerEP4	100%	0%
EMA	0–8%	85–100%
Keratin 17	100% (diffuse staining)	68% (patchy staining)
Bcl2	100%	18%
CD10	60–88%	0–25%

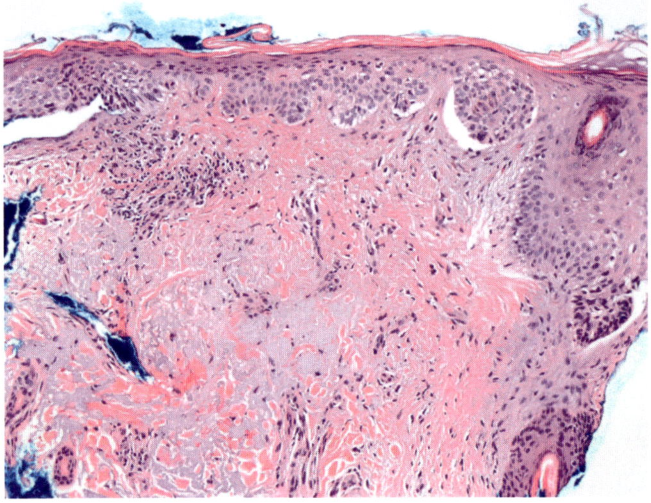

Figure 3.1 Basal cell carcinoma. Nests of epithelial cells with peripheral palisade and clefting for adjacent stroma characteristic of basal cell carcinoma.

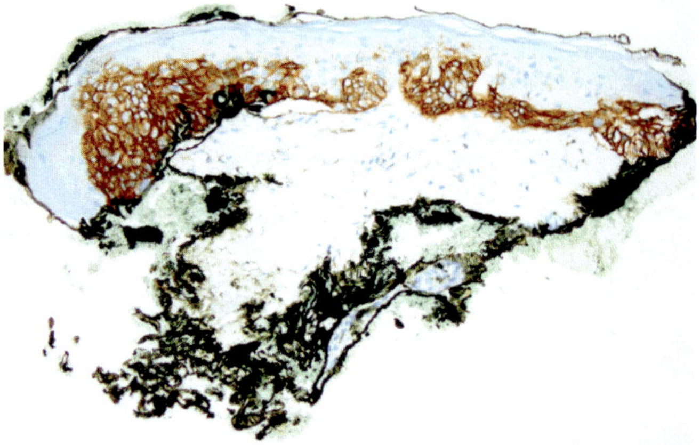

Figure 3.2 Basal cell carcinoma. Strong BerEP4 expression by the basaloid tumor cells is seen.

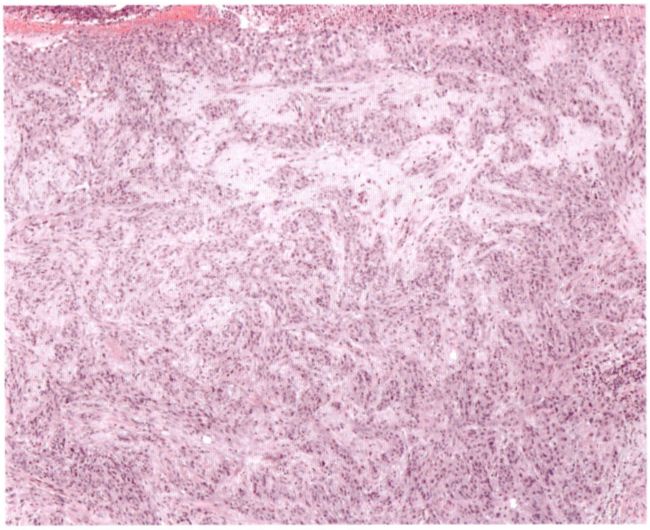

Figure 3.3 Metatypical basal cell carcinoma is characterized by squamous differentiation (X100).

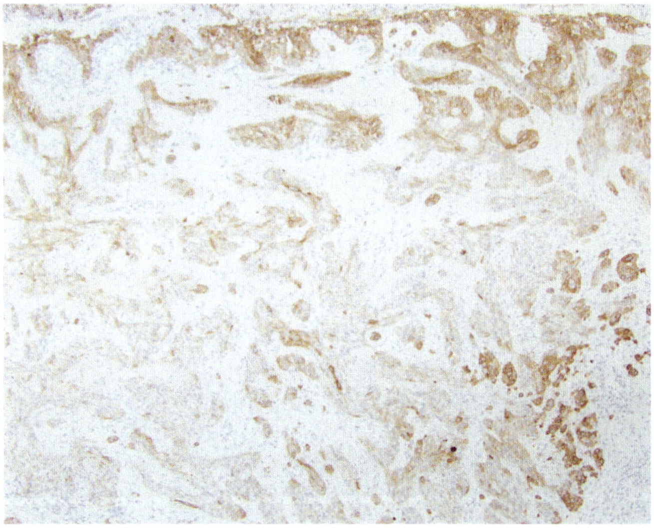

Figure 3.4 Metatypical basal cell carcinoma. Patchy keratin 17 expression is seen (X100).

Squamous cell carcinoma versus basal cell carcinoma

- Squamous cell carcinoma: EMA+BerEP4- keratin 17 + (patchy)
- Basal cell carcinoma: BerEP4+ EMA- keratin 17+ (diffuse)

Clear Cell Squamous Cell Carcinoma Versus Sebaceous Carcinomas

When SCC has a clear cell morphology, the differential diagnosis includes sebaceous carcinoma, especially the invasive and poorly differentiated ones. The cytoplasmic vacuoles of clear cell SCC are unilocular in contrast to microvesicular as observed in sebaceous carcinoma. They are periodic acid-Schiff (PAS) diastase-sensitive. Sebaceous carcinoma is an uncommon cutaneous malignancy, yet it is a common malignant eyelid tumor (2–4%).[17] A number of studies have shown that adipophilin, androgen receptor (AR), BerEP4, keratin CAM5.2, and GATA6 to be helpful in distinguishing sebaceous carcinoma from SCC (**Table 3.2**).[17–27] Adipophilin is one of the lipid droplet-associated proteins in the formation and maintenance of lipid droplets. Adipophilin has been shown to be more sensitive than Oil Red O in detecting intracellular lipids in sebaceous carcinoma;[19,20,23] however, its specificity is low due to its frequent expression in SCC (**Figures 3.5, 3.6 and 3.7**).[21] Published sensitivity and specificity for adipophilin were 88–100% and 25–100%, respectively.[19,20,23] Diffuse AR expression in sebaceous carcinomas is frequently seen with absence of AR expression in 12% of cases;[22] however, 20% sensitivity and 83% specificity for AR were reported in ocular sebaceous carcinoma.[20] Although Sramek et al.[20] reported BerEP4 expression in 80% of ocular sebaceous carcinomas, all 16 ocular sebaceous carcinoma were negative and only 2/19 of extra-ocular tumors were positive for

Table 3.2 Immunostaining of squamous cell carcinoma versus sebaceous carcinoma[17-27]

	Squamous cell carcinoma	Sebaceous carcinoma
AR	17%	20–100%
Adipophilin	0–10% (focal in 75%)	88–100%
GATA6	0%	91%
BerEP4	0%	10–80%*
CAM5.2	83%	73%
EMA	79–100%	80–100%
Keratin 7	68%	70–100%
CD10	Only stromal cells	40%
CD15	0%	43%
Perforin	0%	78%
PRAME	29%	37%
Gli–1	100%	36%

* Ocular carcinomas

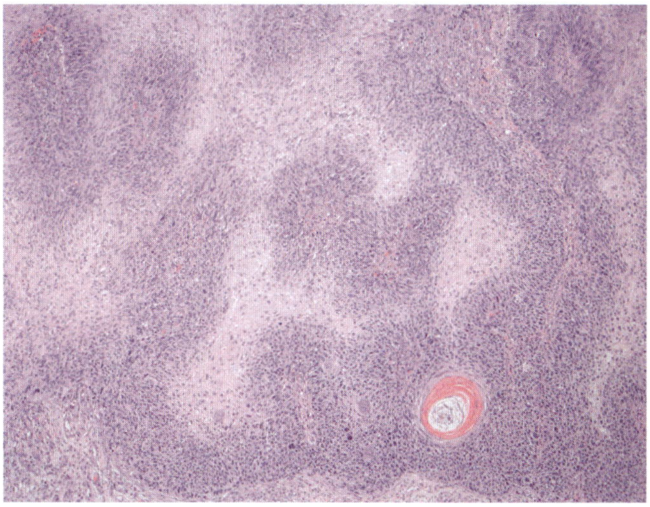

Figure 3.5 Squamous cell carcinoma is characterized by infiltrating nests of atypical keratinocytes (X100).

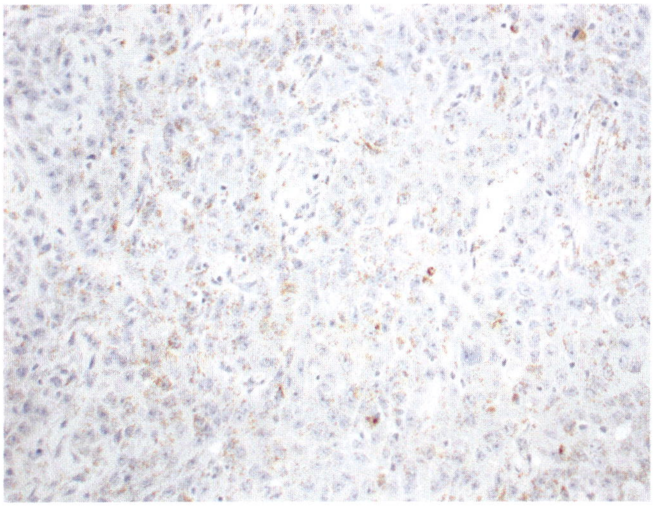

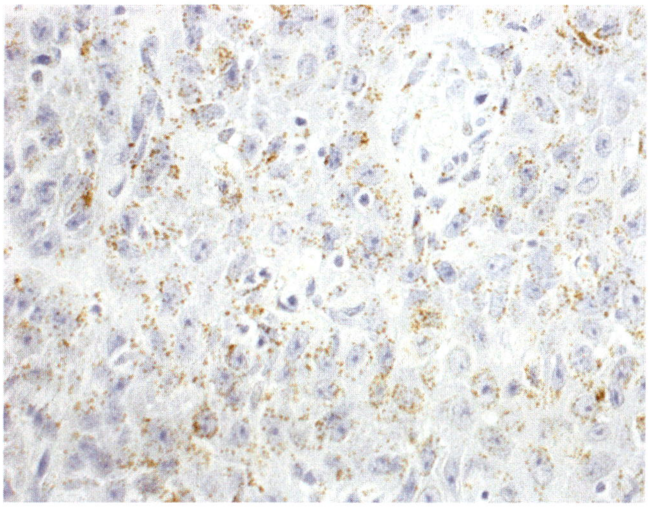

Figures 3.6 and 3.7 Squamous cell carcinoma. Adipophilin expression is typically granular in appearance (X200, X400).

BerEP4 in a series by Ansai et al.[23] Recently, GATA6 has been shown to have similar sensitivity yet better specificity than adipophilin in the distinction of sebaceous carcinoma versus SCC.[24] Perforin has exhibited strong sensitivity and specificity as well.[25] PRAME and Gli1 have not been shown to be good discriminating markers as well, with PRAME highlighting mature sebaceous differentiation yet invariably negative in high grade sebaceous carcinoma.[26,27] While 73–100% of sebaceous carcinomas can express keratin CAM5.2, its expression can be seen in 83% of SCC.[20] Staining with keratin 7, CD10, CD15, D2-40, EMA and p63 have not been shown to be helpful in distinguishing sebaceous carcinoma from SCC.

The main histologic differential diagnosis for sebaceous carcinoma *in situ* would be a clear cell SCC *in situ*. Others also include melanoma *in situ* and mammary or extramammary Paget disease. Including S100 and keratin 7 in the immunohistochemical panel would help to exclude melanoma and extramammary Paget disease, respectively.

Squamous cell carcinoma versus sebaceous carcinoma

- Squamous cell carcinoma: adipophilin-/+, AR-
- Sebaceous carcinoma: adipophilin+, AR+

Squamous Cell Carcinoma Versus Porocarcinoma

In SCCs that are not well differentiated, the presence of entrapped glands, pseudoglandular appearance, and acantholysis raise the possibility of porocarcinoma. On the other hand, extensive squamous differentiation can be seen in porocarcinoma. Distinguishing porocarcinoma from SCC is important since porocarcinoma has a greater propensity for lymph node metastases and poorer survival.[28]

A variety of markers has been reported in the diagnosis of porocarcinoma; however, there is overlapping staining pattern with SCC (**Table 3.3**).[5,7,8,28–41] Keratin 19 and keratin 7 have been found to be helpful markers in the distinction of porocarcinoma from SCC (**Figures 3.8 and 3.9**) (**Table 3.3**).[6] Although sensitivity of EN1 and keratin 19 for porocarcinoma are 81% and 69% respectively, a combination of EN1 and keratin 19 improves the specificity to 100% since none of SCC cases stained for both EN1 and keratin 19.[40] Carcinoembryonic antigen (CEA), highlighting foci of ductal differentiation, has been also shown to be positive in 30–80% of SCC cases.[7,8] In a series of 69 porocarcinomas by Robson et al.,[28] ducts were highlighted by periodic acid Schiff (PAS) and/or epithelial membrane antigen (EMA)/CEA in 49/69 cases, indicating that a third of tumors may be misdiagnosed if ductal differentiation is used as a major criterion

Table 3.3 Immunostaining of squamous cell carcinoma versus porocarcinoma [5,7,8,28-41]

	Squamous cell carcinoma	Porocarcinoma
Keratin 19	18–30%	50–67%
Keratin 7	13–26%	64–67%
YAP1-C loss	0%	58%
NUTM1	0%	11–29%
Nestin	37–45%	13–35%
Keratin 15	0–30%	41–49%
Keratin CAM5.2	58%	38–51%
CEA	30–80%	68–100% + ducts
EMA	85–100%	94–100%
CD10	25%	0%
p63	80–100%	100%
p40	100%	100%
Keratin 5/6	69%	100%
BerEP4	9%	57%
CD117	14%	79%
GATA3	73%	57%
EN1	16%	81%

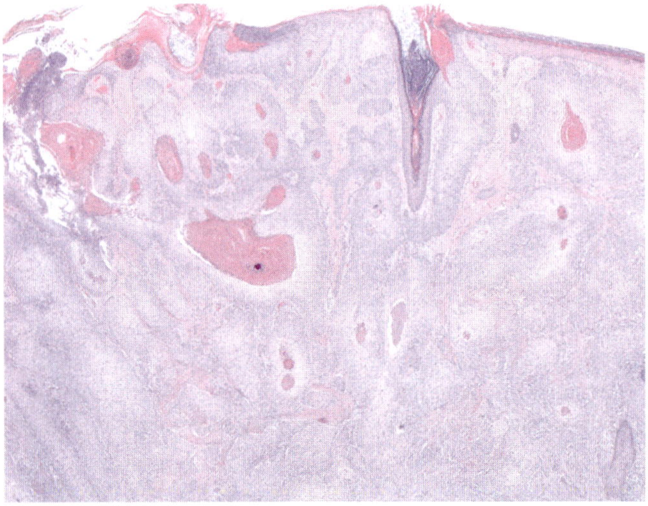

Figure 3.8 Squamous cell carcinoma. Infiltrative nests of keratinizing tumor cells (X100).

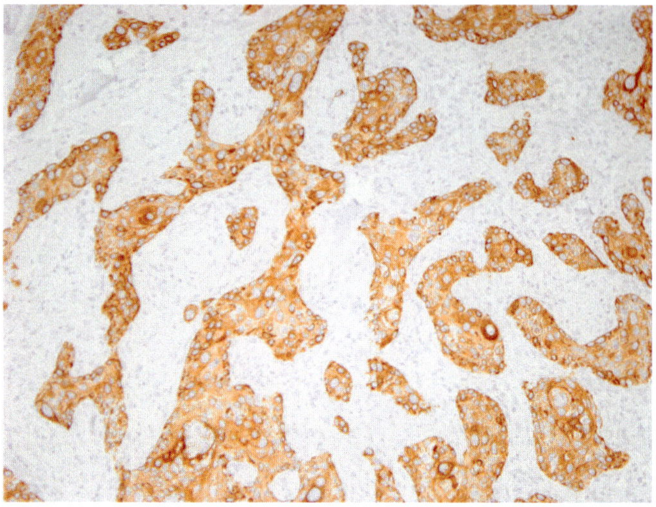

Figure 3.9 Squamous cell carcinoma. Keratin 7 expression can be seen (X100).

for diagnosis. In addition, both porocarcinoma[7,28,29] and SCC [7,8] can express EMA. While CD10 labels none of porocarcinoma, it labels only 25% of cases of SCC.[35] p63 and keratin 5/6 label most adnexal carcinomas including porocarcinoma and cutaneous SCC including the spindle cell variant.[5,32] BerEP4 can be seen in approximately 50% porocarcinoma.[37]

Since a subset of porocarcinoma harbor *YAP1* fusion, 64% porocarcinomas with *YAP1* fusions has been shown to exhibit loss of cytoplasmic YAP1-C expression. [42] Since all poromas and porocarcinomas with *YAP1::NUTM1* fusions exhibited YAP1 C-terminus loss and nuclear NUT expression, YAP1-C and NUT immunostains can be used to detect porocarcinomas harboring this fusion.[41,42]

Squamous cell carcinoma versus porocarcinoma

- Squamous cell carcinoma: keratin19-/+ keratin 7-/+
- Porocarcinoma: keratin 19+ keratin 7+ YAP1-C+/- NUT+/-

Spindle Cell/Sarcomatoid Squamous Cell Carcinoma versus Spindle Cell Lesions

Spindle cell squamous cell carcinoma is a poorly differentiated subtype that is comprised of pleomorphic and spindle tumor cells. The histologic differential diagnosis of a dermal spindle cell neoplasm would include sarcomatoid SCC, spindle cell or desmoplastic melanoma, atypical fibroxanthoma (AFX), and leiomyosarcoma (**Table 3.4**).[7,43-50] SCC would invariably be positive for keratin 903 (34BetaE12) and keratin 5/6.[43] Sarcomatoid SCC is often vimentin positive and may show only focal or weak expression with high molecular weight keratin such as keratin 903 and keratin 5/6 (Figures 3.10–12). Non-epithelial neoplasms, such as epithelioid sarcoma and epithelioid angiosarcoma, occasionally express keratin. Ko et al.[44] have reported that MNF116 and p63 stained poorly differentiated SCC and sarcomatoid SCC (**Figure 3.13**). Concordant staining for both

Table 3.4 Differential diagnosis of cutaneous spindle cell lesion[7,43-50]

	Spindle cell melanoma	Atypical fibroxanthoma	Sarcomatoid squamous carcinoma	Leiomyosarcoma
p40	-	-	+	-
p63	-	-/+	+	-/+
Keratin 903	-	-	+	-
Keratin 5/6	-	-	+	-
Sox10	+	-	-	-
S100	+	-	-	-
CD10	+/-	+	+/-	NR
Desmin	-	-	-	+
SATB2	-/+	+	-/+	+/-

NR: not reported

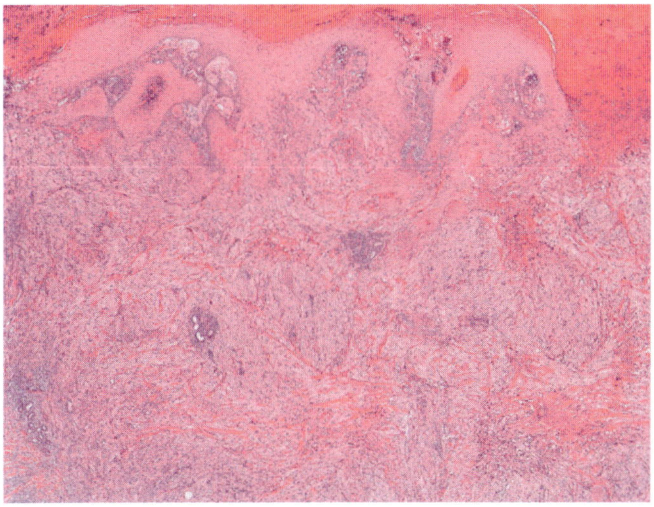

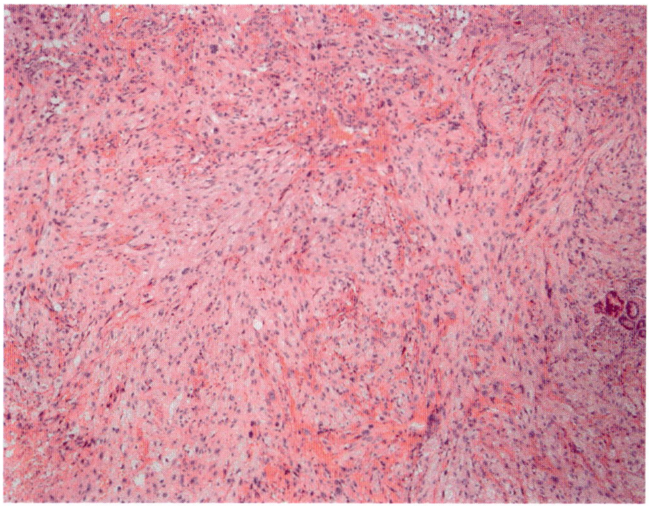

Figures 3.10 and 3.11 Sarcomatoid squamous cell carcinoma. Nests of strands of spindle epithelial cells seen dissecting the dermis (X40, X100).

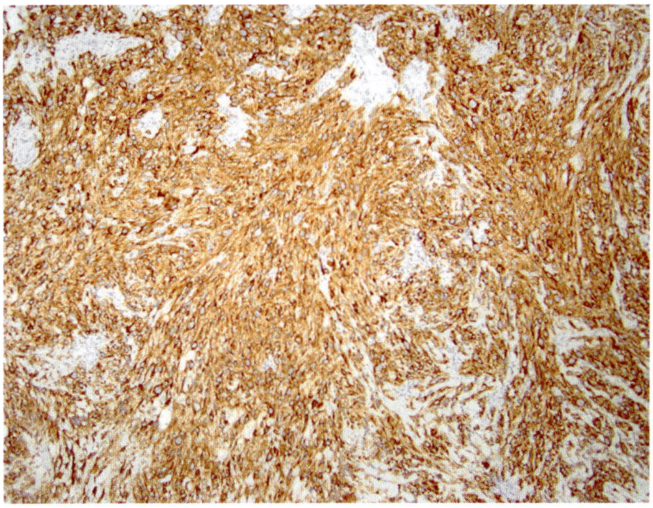

Figure 3.12 Sarcomatoid squamous cell carcinoma. Strong keratin 903 expression (X100).

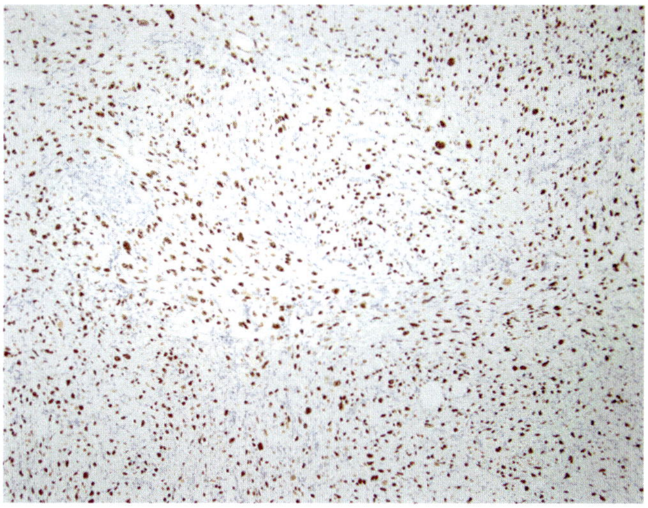

Figure 3.13 Sarcomatoid squamous cell carcinoma. Diffuse nuclear p63 expression (X100).

p63 and p40 were noted in 74% of sarcomatoid SCC.[51] p63 has been shown to be more sensitive than p40 in detecting sarcomatoid SCC.[51] However p40 has been shown to be more specific than p63 in the distinction of sarcomatoid carcinoma from other spindle cell neoplasms such as AFX and leiomyosarcoma.[7] While focal p63 expression has been reported in 20% of AFX and approximately half of leiomyosarcomas, p40 expression is absent in studied cases of AFX and leiomyosarcomas.[7,45]

Sox10 is a transcription factor that is expressed in melanocytic and schwannian tumors and its expression can be seen myoepitheliomas.[46] Spindle cell melanomas and desmoplastic melanomas consistently express Sox10 and S100, while only focal or absent staining for Melan-A, MiTF, and HMB45. Histiocytic markers such as CD68 and CD163 label AFX, a pleomorphic low-grade sarcoma; however, they are not specific and thus the diagnosis of AFX is generally one of exclusion. Although sensitive, CD10 is not a specific marker for AFX. CD10 expression has been documented in 94% of AFX, 33% in desmoplastic melanoma, and 50% of sarcomatoid SCC.[47] CD99 is not a sensitive marker since its expression has been reported in 35–75% of AFX.[48] Smooth muscle actin (SMA) expression can be seen in 45% of AFX but desmin is invariably negative.[49] Although SATB2 is positive in 45% of cutaneous sarcomatoid carcinoma, SATB2 expression is also seen in 78% of AFX, 53% of pleomorphic dermal sarcoma, 59% cutaneous leiomyosarcomas, and 36% of spindle cell melanoma.[50]

All sarcomas, even those with epithelioid features are positive for vimentin; however, the expression of this epithelial-mesenchymal transition marker can be observed not only in spindle cell SCC but also in the invasive front of any aggressive SCC.[52,53] Myoepithelial tumors and epithelioid sarcomas, both classical-type and proximal-type, are the soft tissue tumors that more closely resemble SCC. Most epithelioid sarcomas are positive for EMA and/or show widespread expression of the wide-spectrum keratin antibody AE1/AE3. In some cases, the high-molecular weight keratin marker 34βE12 and CD34 are also positive. Cutaneous myoepithelial tumors co-express epithelial and myogenic markers. In addition, they are often positive for S100 protein and glial fibrillary acidic protein (GFAP).[54] In a study of 101 myoepithelial tumors, 93% of cases expressed keratins (most often wide spectrum keratins such as AE1/AE3), 87% S100 protein, 86% calponin, 63% EMA, 46% GFAP, 36% smooth muscle actin (SMA), 23% p63, and 14% desmin.[55] However, in SMARCB1-deficient vulvar myoepithelial carcinomas EMA and SMA were the only markers consistently positive, while there was a limited expression of keratins, CD34, desmin, and S100 protein.[56]

Sarcomatoid squamous cell carcinoma versus sarcoma versus spindle cell lesions

- A helpful diagnostic immunohistochemical panel for a dermal spindle cell neoplasm includes p40, keratin 903, keratin 5/6, Sox10, S100 and CD10.
- Sarcomatoid squamous cell carcinoma: p40+, keratin 903+, keratin 5/6 +
- Spindle cell melanoma: Sox10+, S100+
- Atypical fibroxanthoma: CD10+

Poorly Differentiated Squamous Cell Carcinoma versus Mimics

The differential diagnosis of poorly differentiated SCC would include Merkel cell carcinoma (MCC), lymphoproliferative disorders, Langerhans cell histiocytosis, myoepithelial neoplasms, epithelioid sarcoma, and other sarcomas with round cell morphology such as those of the family of Ewing sarcoma/primitive neuroectodermal tumors (**see Chapter 9**).

MCC is characterized by a dual epithelial and neuroendocrine differentiation (**see Chapter 9**). The epithelial nature can be demonstrated using antibodies to low molecular weight keratins such as keratin CAM5.2 and keratin 20 that are also positive in SCC,[57] with the peculiarity in MCC that the staining often adopts a characteristic dot-like pattern, allowing its identification (**Figure 3.14**). Rare cases of MCC are keratin 20 negative but positive for keratin 7, simulating a metastatic small cell carcinoma from the lung.[58] For keratin 20-negative MCC, POU4F3 has recently reported to be a helpful marker in the distinction from small cell lung carcinoma (**Figure 3.15**).[59] MCC is consistently positive for neuroendocrine markers including INSM1, but the intensity of synaptophysin and chromogranin A expression varies from case to case and can be weak or focal.[60] In spite

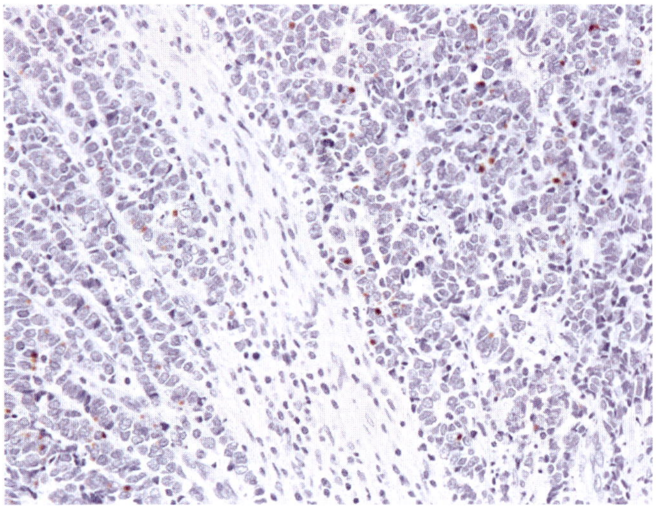

Figure 3.14 Keratin 20-positive Merkel cell carcinoma showing the characteristic dot-like pattern due to whorl of filaments. Whereas in this case not all tumor cells are positive, other tumors would show a diffuse cytoplasmic positivity.

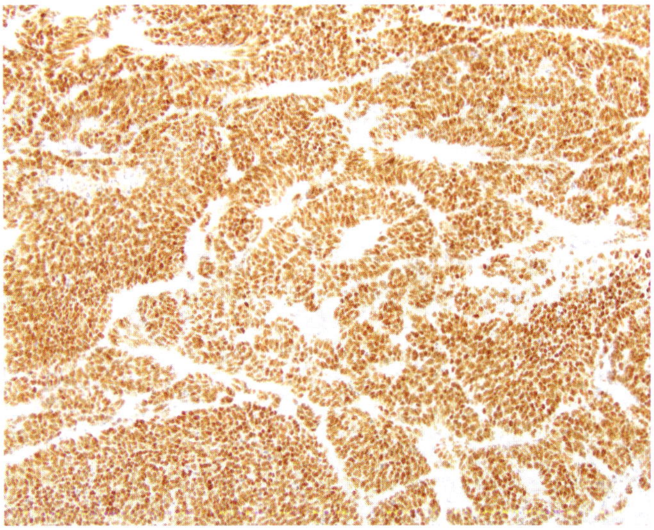

Figure 3.15 Merkel cell carcinoma. Strong nuclear POU4F3 expression in this keratin-20 negative tumor.

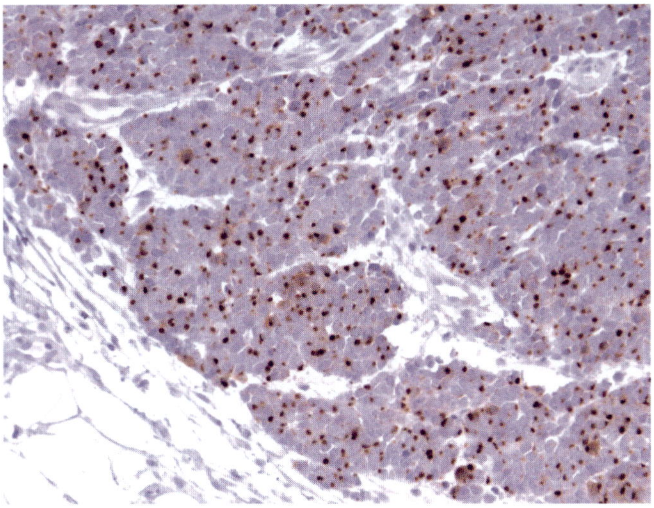

Figure 3.16 Merkel cell carcinoma. This dot-like staining for neurofilament is the most characteristic feature.

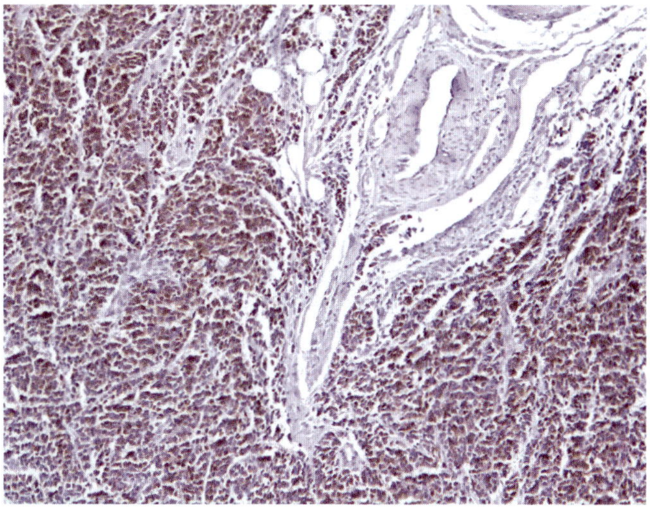

Figure 3.17 Merkel cell carcinoma. Positive staining with Merkel cell polyomavirus antibody confirms the diagnosis and allows distinction from non-viral related Merkel cell carcinoma.

of being less specific, CD56 has been found to be the most sensitive neuroendocrine marker for this neoplasm (**Figure 3.16**).[61] The expression of neurofilaments in a paranuclear dot pattern is another reliable marker of MCC and allows a clear cut distinction from SCC.[62] It is important to be aware that MCC can express EMA and p63 like SCC and BerEP4 similar to BCC.[8] Approximately 80% of MCC are positive for the Merkel cell polyomavirus, especially those from sun protected areas and its presence can be demonstrated using the antibodies CM2B4, CM5E1 or Ab3 with Ab3 being the most sensitive and specific (**Figure 3.17**).[63,64]

Primary or secondary involvement of the skin by lymphomas and malignant plasma cell proliferations can also simulate SCC. The immunohistochemical distinction is easy if this possibility is considered. All keratin antibodies are negative in lymphoproliferative disorders, but their use can highlight areas of epithelial invasion. Most lymphoid proliferations are positive for leukocyte common antigen (LCA). Additionally, specific lymphocytic markers such as CD3, CD4, CD8, or CD45RO (UCHL1) can be used for T-cell proliferations and CD20, CD79, or CD10 for B-cell proliferations. Plasma cell proliferations can be difficult to recognize because of their capacity to exhibit varied morphological appearances. They are characteristically CD79a, CD38, and CD138 positive. Additionally, it is possible to demonstrate kappa or lambda light chain restriction by immunostains or *in situ* hybridization.[65] Myeloid sarcomas stain characteristically for myeloperoxidase, lysozyme, CD68, CD43, and/or CD33. To avoid misinterpretation of the immunohistochemical results, it is important to keep in mind that some primary cutaneous lymphomas (usually large B cell lymphomas) can be p63 positive as in SCC.[66] In plasma cell proliferations, positive staining for EMA can be misinterpreted as indicative of epithelial differentiation and CD56 is a very important marker of natural killer cells, apart from being positive in tumor with neuroendocrine differentiation. Langerhans cell histiocytosis can involve selectively the genital area and its diagnosis can be confirmed by negativity for epithelial markers and expression of CD1a, langerin and S100. Tumors from the family Ewing sarcoma/primitive neuroectodermal are positive for CD99 in a membranous pattern and Fli-1 in a nuclear pattern and negative for S100, neuroendocrine, epithelial, lymphoid and myogenic markers. The demonstration of a *EWS/FLI-1* fusion transcript by reverse transcriptase polymerase chain reaction analysis can confirm the diagnosis.

Poorly differentiated small/medium sized cell squamous cell carcinoma versus mimics

- Squamous cell carcinoma: keratin19-/+ keratin 7-/+
- Merkel cell carcinoma: POU4F3+, CAM5.2+ and keratin 20+ (both often with a dot-like pattern), CD56+, synaptophysin+, chromogranin+, neurofilaments + (dot-like pattern), Merkel cell polyomavirus + in 80% of cases, keratin 7+ rarely

3.2 Anogenital Dysplasia and Squamous Cell Carcinoma

Anogenital Squamous Intraepithelial Neoplasia and Squamous Cell Carcinoma

Invasive SCC is the most common cancer involving the anogenital region. It may arise through two main pathways: the classical or usual pathway, associated with human papillomavirus (HPV) infection, and the differentiated or simplex pathway, which is HPV-independent and caused by *TP53* mutations.[67,68] In recent years, a third pathway has been described in the vulvar area, characterized by HPV-independence and p53 wild-type status. This pathway is often associated with mutations in *PIK3CA*, *NOTCH1*, and *HRAS*.[69,70]

These intraepithelial precursors of SCC present substantial differences in epidemiology, clinical presentation, and biological behavior, leading to specific nomenclatures for each process and location. Their diagnosis and differentiation from other pathologies are mainly based on histopathological characteristics. However, some cases may exhibit misleading patterns and overlapping features.[71–73] Immunohistochemistry emerges as the most rapid, effective, and cost-effective method for distinguishing among these different pathways and stratifying individual risk.

Basaloid (Cloacogenic) Squamous Cell Carcinoma of the Anus versus Mimics

The anal canal, lined with squamous epithelium with transitional features, is embryologically derived from the cloacal membrane and the origin site of a peculiar variant of SCCs known as cloacogenic carcinoma.[74–76] Cloacogenic carcinomas, which are often associated with high-risk HPV infection, can exhibit diverse histological patterns, including basaloid, transitional, adenoid cystic-like, and mucinous microcystic.[74,76,77] Basaloid SCCs are composed of small keratinocytes with scant eosinophilic cytoplasm, often arranged in a palisading configuration at the periphery. Nuclear features can include hyperchromasia, granular chromatin, and a high mitotic rate with atypical mitosis.[74,76,78]

The differential diagnosis of basaloid SCC includes poorly differentiated invasive SCC originated from HPV-associated anal intraepithelial neoplasia (AIN),[79] BCC, melanoma, mucoepidermoid carcinoma, neuroendocrine carcinomas, adenoid cystic carcinomas, mammary type tubulolobular carcinoma of the anogenital area, or papillary immature metaplasia of the anal canal.[74,80,81]

Basaloid SCC of the anus express keratins 5/6, p63 and in most cases p40 (**Figures 3.18**–3.21).[74,79] In addition, BerEP4 and Bcl2 can be positive, similar to BCC, which may pose a potential caveat. However, in BCC, the staining intensities are typically stronger, and they involve wider tumor areas.[74,78,82] The most useful marker for their differentiation is with p16 (CDKN2A) that shows continuous and intense nuclear and cytoplasmic staining, so-called "block-type", related to the high-risk HPV infection.[83] Conversely, the stain for p16 is either absent or much weaker in BCC. Although one study reported similar results

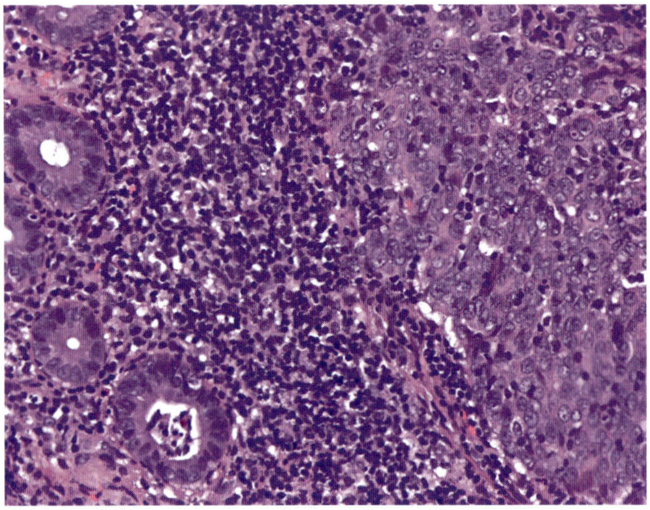

Figure 3.18 Basaloid squamous cell carcinoma of the anus.

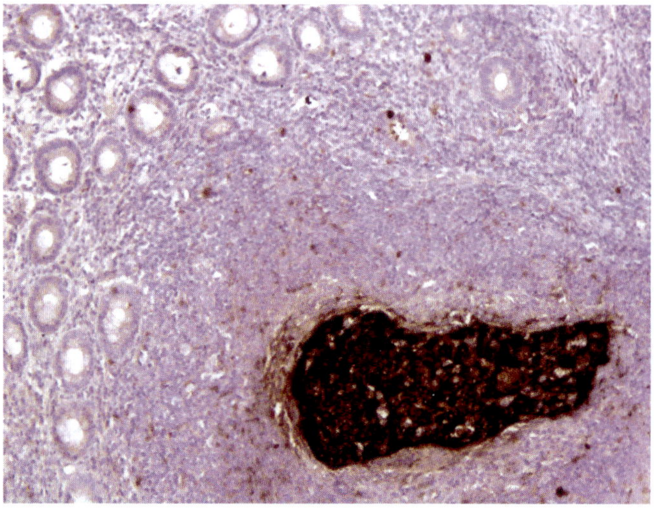

Figure 3.19 Basaloid squamous cell carcinoma of the anus. p16 overexpression is seen.

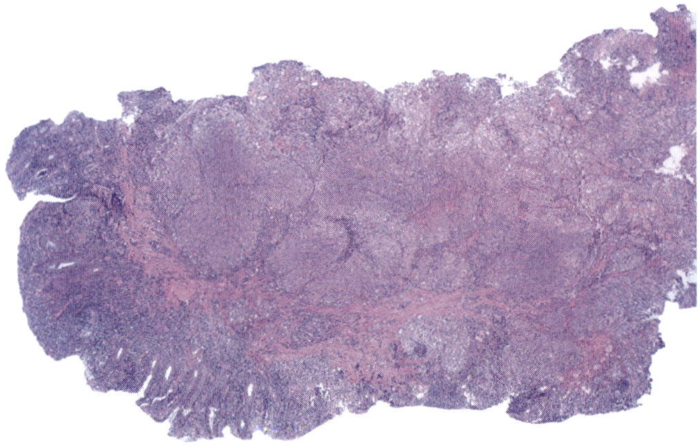

Figure 3.20 Basaloid squamous cell carcinoma of the anus.

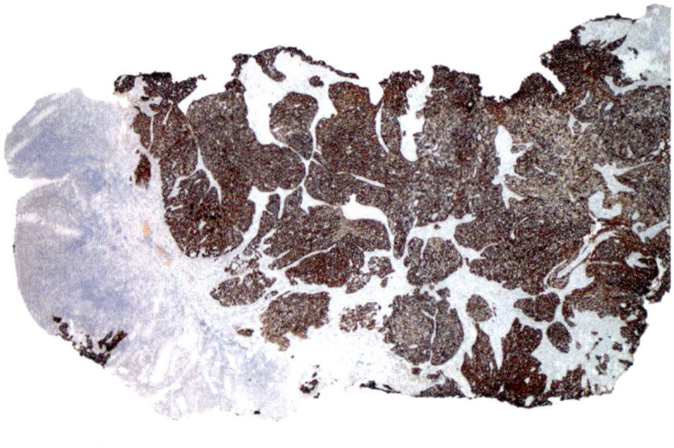

Figure 3.21 Basaloid squamous cell carcinoma of the anus. Keratin 5/6 is typically positive.

with Sox2,[78] subsequent research found that this expression was not consistent across all cases.[74] Proliferation rates, measurable with Ki67, are typically very high in basaloid SCC. However, the presence of atypical mitoses seems to be more relevant in supporting the diagnosis of basaloid SCC over BCC.[78]

Another important differential diagnosis to consider is MCC. The expression of CD56 has been documented in one case in basaloid SCC and can be also be present in BCCs making advisable the use of more specific markers such as synaptophysin, chromogranin or INSM1.[84–86] Additionally, MCC often presents dot-like positivity for low molecular weight keratins and neurofilaments.[87]

Basaloid SCCs with adenoid cystic-like pattern are CD117 negative while adenoid cystic carcinomas tend to be positive.[74] In addition, the expression of p63 is diffuse basaloid SCCs, but only present in the myoepithelial component of adenoid cystic carcinoma.[88] Some basaloid carcinomas with mucinous change have probably been reported in the literature as mucoepidermoid carcinomas, highlighting the complexity of differentiating both entities. Nevertheless, a widespread expression of p16 indicative of high-risk HPV infection clearly points towards basaloid SCC.[74] Papillary immature metaplasia of the anal canal is an exophytic lesion related to low-risk HPV and in these cases p16 is negative. Finally, the immunohistochemical profile, including S100 negativity, allows differentiation from melanoma.

It is worth mentioning that, according to the fifth edition of World Health Organization (WHO) classifications, the term 'basaloid SCC' is exclusively accepted for male genitalia.[89] In spite of the existence of several reports of basaloid SCC in the skin[90,91] and vulva,[92] the fifth edition of the WHO classifications does not recognize it in these locations.[93] Nonetheless, due to its misleading appearance, aggressive potential, and epidemiological significance, it is advisable to keep this entity in mind.[74,94]

Basaloid squamous cell carcinoma of the anus versus mimics

- Basaloid squamous cell carcinoma: p16+ block-type, CK5/6+, p63+, p40+
- Basaloid squamous cell carcinoma (potential caveats): BerEP4 and CD56 can be focally expressed
- Basal cell carcinoma: BerEP4+ keratin 17+
- Neuroendocrine carcinomas (including Merkel cell carcinoma): higher expression of neuroendocrine markers. Dot-like positivity for keratins and neurofilaments
- Adenoid cystic carcinoma: p63 stains only myoepithelial cells, p16 is negative

3.3 Vulva

Squamous Intraepithelial Lesions, HPV-Associated, of the Vulva

HPV infection stands as the most frequent cause of squamous intraepithelial lesions in the vulva, although its prevalence varies across different populations and is anticipated to decline following widespread HPV vaccination.[95] These lesions manifest in two distinct categories with significant biological and prognostic disparities: those associated with low-risk HPV, which predominantly cause warty proliferations and infrequent local aggressiveness, presenting a minimal risk of progressing to SCC; and those associated with high-risk HPV, with a higher risk of progression to *in situ* and invasive SCC. Of interest, despite its potential for progression, only a small percentage of high-risk HPV-associated SILs evolve to invasive SCC, which is most associated with non-HPV precursors. Remarkably, when invasive SCC does develop in the viral-associated cases, it generally carries a more favorable prognosis compared to its nonviral counterparts.[72,96]

The nomenclature for HPV-associated vulvar lesions has evolved over the years. The classical three-tiered classification of the vulvar intraepithelial neoplasia (VIN) in VIN I, VIN II and VIN III, according to the thickness of the transformed epithelium (lower third, two lower thirds or complete epithelium), has been progressively replaced or complemented by the "Lower Anogenital Squamous Terminology" (LAST) consensus classification for squamous intraepithelial lesion (SIL).[97] In the LAST terminology, low-risk HPV-associated flat or condylomatous VIN I lesions are predominantly low-grade SIL (LSIL), whereas high-grade SIL (HSIL) is the denomination for lesions involving the upper half of the epithelium, usually associated with high-risk HPV.[98] Histologically, features such as koilocytosis can contribute to identify lesions with viral etiology, but some cases may display overlapping features with those not related with HPV (**Figure 2.22**).[71,73] For this reason, immunohistochemistry plays a leading role in its diagnosis and classification.

The proliferative activity associated with HPV infection can be highlighted using Ki67.[97] HSIL cases can be identified by the presence of a high percentage of proliferating cells in the upper layers of the epithelium.[99] In the case of LSIL, Ki67 also can contribute to the diagnosis highlighting increased basal and parabasal staining and scattered cells in the upper rows of keratinocytes (**Figure 2.23**).[99] In an adequate clinicopathological setting, a cluster of at least two strongly stained epithelial nuclei in the upper two-thirds of the epithelial thickness has

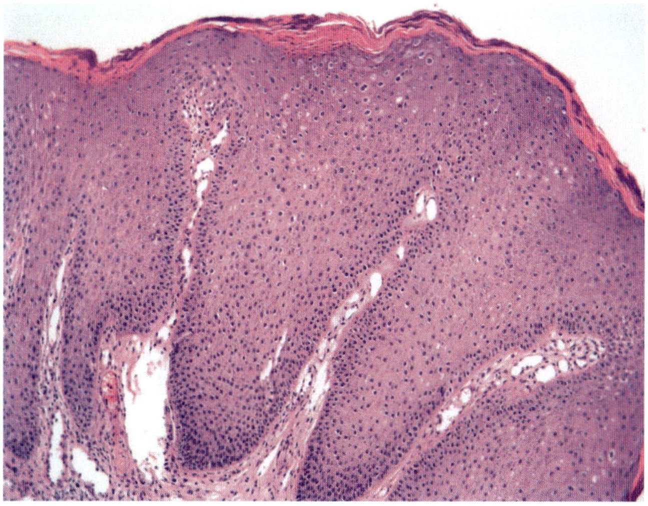

Figure 3.22 Low-grade intraepithelial neoplasia. Dysplasia (VIN I) is limited to the lower one third of the epidermis.

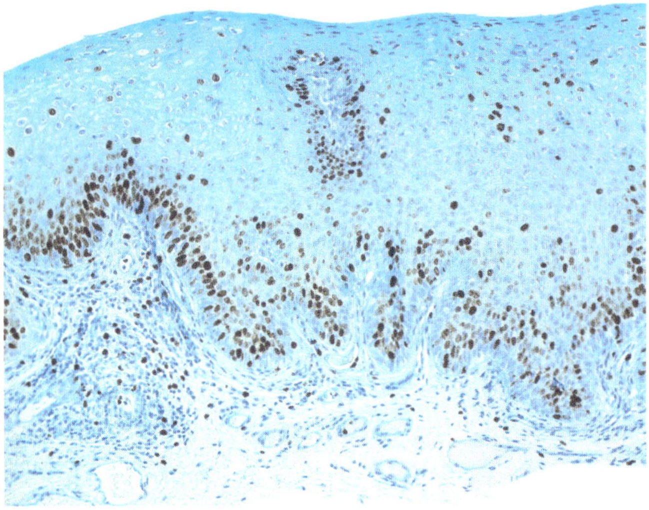

Figure 3.23 Low-grade intraepithelial neoplasia. Ki67 overexpressed in two contiguous cells in the upper two thirds of the epithelium.

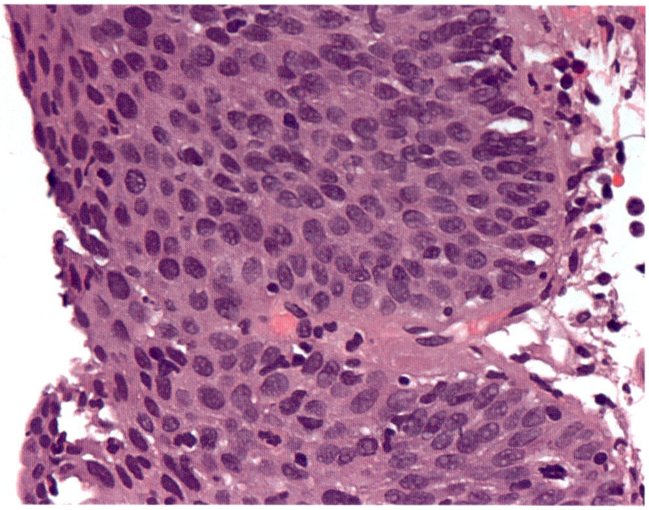

Figure 3.24 Squamous dysplasia involves the entire anal squamous epithelium in this HPV-related high-grade intraepithelial lesion (AIN III).

been considered the minimum requirement for the diagnosis of LSIL.[100] Similar results can be obtained using alternative proliferation markers, such as ProEx™ C.[101]

The aggressive behavior of high-risk-HPV is mainly related to the deregulatory effect of two early viral proteins E6 and E7 that can bind p53 protein promoting its ubiquination and degradation, escaping from its effect in cell cycle arrest and apoptosis. This mechanism explains the absence of p53 staining in areas of HSIL causing a pseudo-null-pattern that can be misinterpreted as indicative of *TP53* mutation.[102] In addition, E7 can bind phospho-Rb triggering a negative feedback loop that leads to increased expression of p16 (CDKN2A).[103] This mechanism has been exploited, making p16 the most accurate surrogate marker for high-risk HPV infection and aiding in the delineation of areas involved in high-grade squamous intraepithelial lesions (HSIL).

From a practical point of view, HPV-associated LSIL can be immunohistochemically diagnosed when Ki67 demonstrates overexpression in the basal layers and scattered superficial cells that often tend to form small groups and p16 shows only weak and patchy staining. Lesions of HPV-associated HSIL present a block-type (strong and diffuse) nuclear and/or cytoplasmic p16 overexpression within the mucosal epithelium (**Figures 2.24 and 2.25**), associated to a loss of p53. These results are reproducible, but slightly less consistent for high risk HPV-associated invasive SCC.[104] In the rare event of coexistence of a p53 mutational patterns and p16 block-type expression,[72,105] molecular studies can be conducted on the formalin-fixed paraffin-embedded tissue to elucidate the potential presence of HPV.[106]

The primary differential diagnosis of LSIL includes inflammatory or reactive processes that can induce pseudocarcinomatous changes in squamous cells, resulting in epithelial proliferation and an elevation in the proportion of Ki67-positive cells. However, this proliferative activity rarely extends to the upper layers of the epithelium.[97]

Finally, some cases of extramammary Paget disease can mimic histologically HSIL and exhibit p16 overexpression. However, the dispersed distribution of Paget cells in isolated elements or small groups contributes to recognizing this condition.[107]

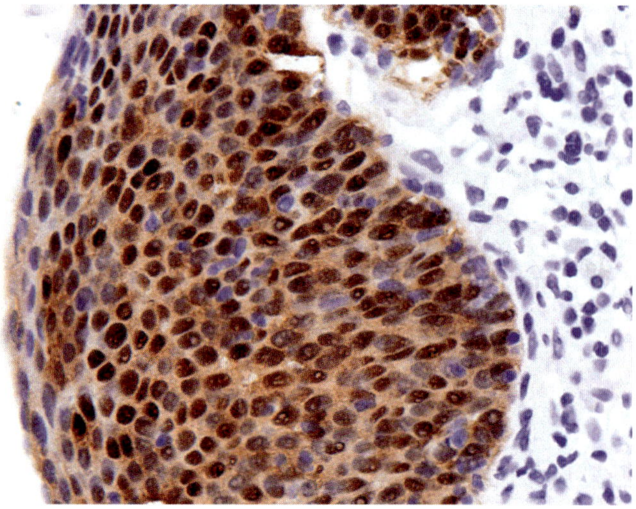

Figure 3.25 HPV-related high-grade intraepithelial lesion. The entire epithelium expresses p16 in a diffuse and block-like fashion.

HPV-associated low versus high grade squamous intraepithelial lesion

- Low grade squamous intraepithelial neoplasia (LSIL): Ki67 overexpression in the basal layer and scattered expression in the upper two thirds of the epithelium favors the diagnosis of condyloma or flat condylomatous lesion, especially when it involves at least two contiguous cells. In these cases, p16 shows only weak and patchy expression; p53 is negative.
- High grade squamous intraepithelial neoplasia (HSIL): Strong and diffuse nuclear and cytoplasmic ("block-type") expression of p16 that contributes to delineate the areas of involvement. The expression of Ki67+ is increased (25–50% of cells) including the upper layers of the epithelium; p53 is negative.

Differentiated Vulvar Intraepithelial Neoplasia (HPV-Independent)

The intraepithelial precursors of invasive SCC of the vulva developed through the differentiated pathway, are usually characterized by the deceptive absence of cytological atypia. Only the most basal epithelial layers may show some atypical features without a noticeable alteration in maturation. Conceptually, these lesions behave similarly to HSIL, as invasive tumors can emerge at any moment from this apparently minimally altered epithelium. Until recently, it was commonly believed that all these HPV-independent cases originated from *TP53* mutations. However, there is now a growing recognition of a third pathway, which is not only HPV-independent, but also presents a wild-type p53 status.

Differentiated Squamous Intraepithelial Neoplasia with Mutant p53

These cases are commonly referred to as differentiated VIN (dVIN) without further specification and often develop in association with a long-standing inflammatory process, such as lichen sclerosus (LS). Histologically, dVIN is characterized by the inconspicuous histologic atypia, often limited to mild pleomorphism, macronucleoli, and slight hyperchromasia in the basal layers of the epithelium. Other common features are acanthosis and altered cornification including parakeratosis and occasional keratin pearl formation. In most cases, there is a notable absence of atypia in the mid and upper layers of the epithelium. However, in this portion, keratinocytes may exhibit a polygonal shape, eosinophilic cytoplasm, and slight increase in the intercellular space in the absence of spongiosis, resulting in a characteristic cobblestone appearance.[67,108,109] Furthermore, a small subset of cases can present atypical changes involving most of the epithelial thickness resembling HSIL.[105]

Consequently, dVIN can be difficult to detect and diagnose, since it may be misinterpreted as a reactive benign epithelial change or as an HPV-related precursor of invasive SCC. The use of immunohistochemical studies with p16 and p53 antibodies has become a simple way to identify HSIL and dVIN cases, and it is highly advisable the use of this panel in all vulvar biopsies that may raise the slightest suspicion of this type of pathologies.

Most cases of dVIN harbor missense *TP53* mutations that produce an inactive p53 protein resistant to degradation that accumulates in the nucleus and can be demonstrated by the p53 immunostaining (**Figures 3.26**–3.28). Nevertheless, some invasive SCC are caused by deletions or nonsense *TP53* mutations leading to an identical neutralization of the p53 activity, but in the absence of mutated p53 accumulation (p53-null).[110] In this setting, p53 would be undetectable immunohistochemically (**Table 3.5**).

Recently, four p53 immunohistochemical patterns that correlate with *TP53* mutations have been described. These patterns, comprising continuous basal positivity, basal and parabasal expression, diffuse cytoplasmic expression, or complete absence ('null' pattern) of p53, indicate *TP53* mutation. Conversely, discontinuous basal positivity or mid-epithelial expression with basal sparing suggests the presence of wild-type

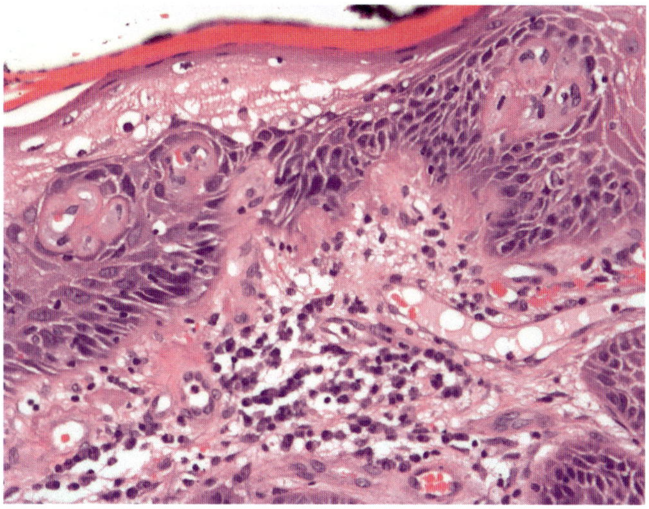

Figure 3.26 Histology of differentiated squamous intraepithelial neoplasia showing moderate pleomorphism and hyperchromasia in the basal layers of the epidermis that also show histological features of lichen sclerosus.

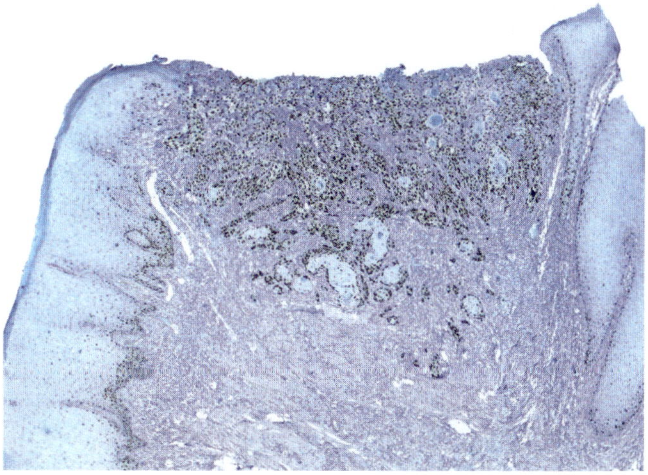

Figure 3.27 Overexpression of p53 in an invasive SCC originated from a non-HPV-related differentiated squamous intraepithelial neoplasia.

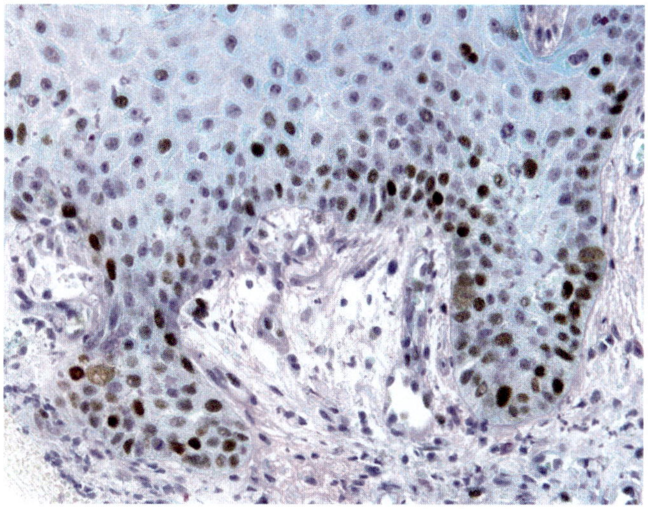

Figure 3.28 p53 positivity in differentiated squamous intraepithelial neoplasia differs from a reactive expression because it involves most basal keratinocytes as well as many suprabasal cells.

Table 3.5 Comparison of immunoprofiles between HPV-associated high grade intraepithelial neoplasia versus differentiated intraepithelial neoplasia associated with TP53 mutation

	HPV-associated high grade intraepithelial neoplasia	Differentiated intraepithelial neoplasia
p16	Diffuse block staining	Negative
p53	Two patterns:	Four patterns:
	Discontinuous basal	Continuous basal
	Mid-epithelial with basal sparing	Continuous basal and suprabasal
		Cytoplasmic
		Null (totally negative)
Ki67	25–50% of nuclei with involvement of the upper epithelial layers	Limited to the basal layers
GATA3	Expression loss in basal keratinocytes	Rare expression loss
Keratin 17	Overexpression	Overexpression
Sox2	Overexpression	Overexpression

p53.[111] The immunohistochemical testing with p53 can also contribute to identifying patchy areas of the cancer field that are histologically insufficient to make the diagnosis of dVIN. These areas, often located at the periphery of vulvectomies of invasive SCC originated from dVIN, are associated with an increased risk of local recurrence.[112]

The epithelial expression of keratin 17 or Sox2, especially when diffuse and intense, strongly supports the diagnosis of dVIN, but it must be associated with a p53 mutant pattern as these markers can also be overexpressed in HSIL.[113,114] Similarly, the loss of normal GATA3 staining in basal keratinocytes, even when it is focal, strongly favors dVIN allowing distinction from HSIL, which shows this loss less frequently.[115–117] Further studies are needed to confirm their utility and establish appropriate cut-off points.

The vast majority of HPV-independent dVIN cases are p16 negative. However, exceptional cases of p16 and p53 coexpression have been described, with the majority appearing to correspond to dVIN.[72,118] However, these cases warrant additional molecular studies to rule out the presence of HPV.

Differentiated Squamous Intraepithelial Neoplasia (dVIN)

- p53 mutational pattern (basal, basal and parabasal, diffuse cytoplasmic, and "null")
- p16 negative (PCR for HPV detection is advised if p16 coexpress with p53)
- Keratin 17 and Sox2 are overexpressed in dVIN (also in HSIL)
- Loss of GATA3 stain in the basal keratinocytes

Differentiated Squamous Intraepithelial Neoplasia with Wild-Type p53

This precursor of invasive SCC has been progressively acknowledged as a specific entity. Nonetheless, a consensus regarding its nomenclature and classification remains elusive. It is considered a subtype of differentiated dysplasia in the fifth edition of the WHO classification of Female Genital Tumours.[93] However, since its histologic appearance, molecular landscape and biological behavior differ from dVIN, the use of this acronym is not adequate.

These lesions were initially exhibited vulvar acanthosis with altered differentiation (VAAD) (Figures 3.29–32). In addition to epithelial acanthosis, they show hyperkeratosis with a variable amount of parakeratosis and contain squamous cells with cytoplasm wider and paler than usual. The granular layer tends to be lost and there is a variable degree of inflammation slightly resembling a lichen simplex chronicus.[119] The term differentiated exophytic vulvar intraepithelial lesion (DEVIL) (**Figure 3.33**) was coined for cases where the acanthosis displayed papillomatous features and the term verruciform lichen simplex chronicus (vLSC) (**Figure 3.34**) for cases with irregular acanthosis showing papillomatosis and hypergranulosis. This complex terminology is difficult to apply especially because many specimens show overlapping features and some patients developed in different areas lesions consistent with these three variants.[69,120]

The similarities among VAAD, DEVIL, and vLSC were confirmed by molecular studies demonstrating a common molecular landscape with somatic mutations that are frequently involved in *PIK3CA*, *NOTCH1*, and *HRAS* genes. Furthermore, the clinical analysis of a large cohort of cases confirmed that these lesions belong to a spectrum with similar risk of transformation to invasive SCC and overall survival.[120]

The denomination verruciform acanthotic vulvar intraepithelial neoplasia (vaVIN) has been suggested to encompass this group of HPV-independent, p53-wild-type pathologies.[69] The alternative umbrella term "vulvar aberrant maturation" (VAM), proposed by the international society of the study of vulvovaginal diseases,[83] is less mentioned in the literature because its histological description include lichenified lesions without a clear risk of malignant transformation. However, it has application in the clinical practice as a safe diagnosis for biopsies that do not seem to correspond clearly to precursors of SCC.

The immunohistochemical diagnosis of these lesions requires absence of p53 mutational pattern and lack of block-type p16 expression. In addition, recent studies suggest that likewise in dVIN, a combination of keratin 17 and Sox2 overexpression with loss of the GATA3 stain in basal keratinocytes can contribute to their identification.[116]

Verruciform acanthotic vulvar intraepithelial neoplasia (vaVIN)

- p53 non-mutant pattern and p16 negative
- Keratin 17 and Sox2 are overexpressed (also in dVIN and HSIL)
- Loss of GATA3 staining in the basal keratinocytes

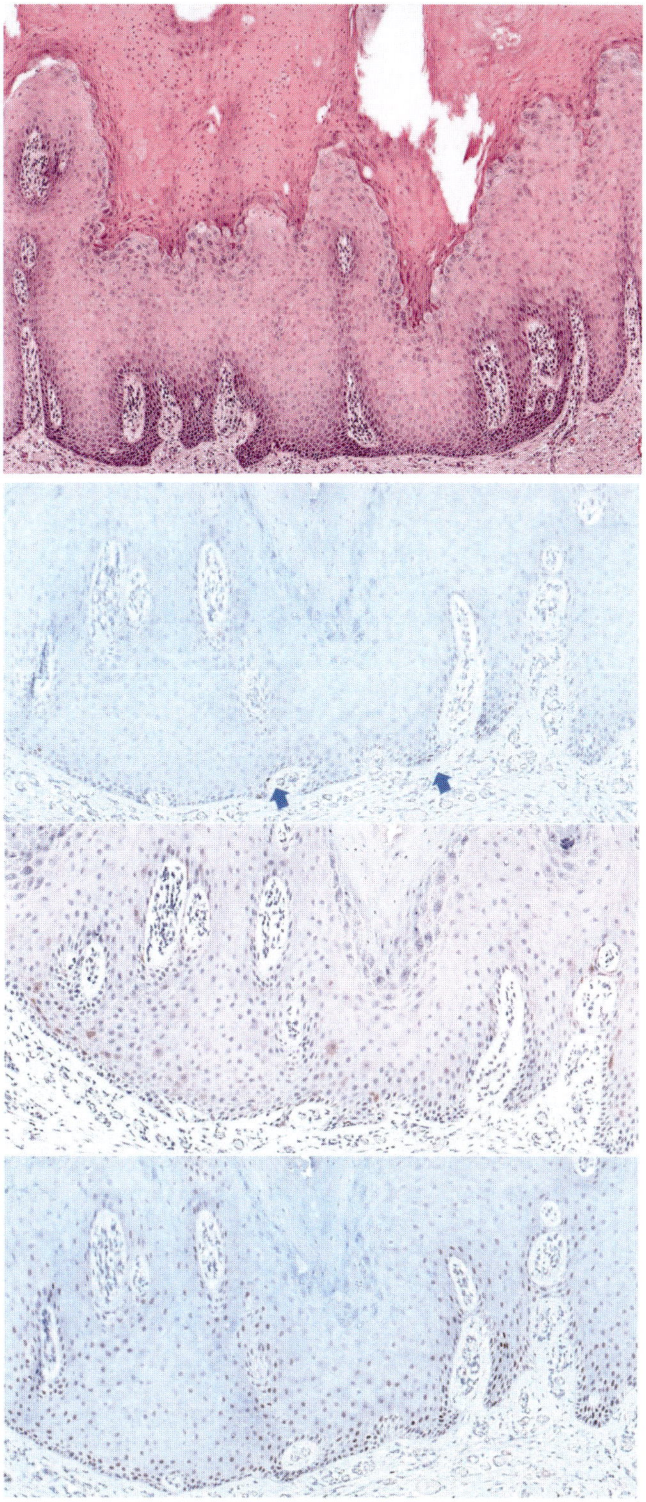

Figures 3.29–3.32 Vulvar acanthosis with altered differentiation (VAAD) is a variant of verruciform acanthotic vulvar intraepithelial neoplasia (vaVIN), characterized by epithelial acanthosis with hyperkeratosis, sometimes parakeratotic, containing pale squamous cells. The granular layer is focally lost, and there is a mild subepithelial lymphocytic infiltrate. The lesion shows a wildtype pattern of p53 (**Figure 3.30**), patchy expression of p16 (**Figure 3.31**), and focal loss of basal GATA3 expression (**Figure 3.32**).

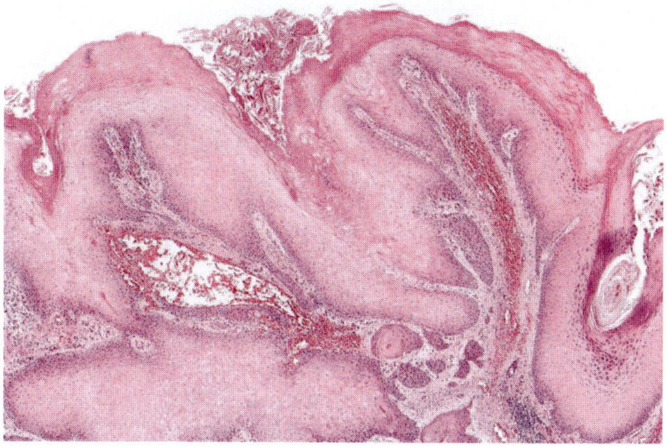

Figure 3.33 Differentiated exophytic vulvar intraepithelial lesion (DEVIL) is a variant of verruciform acanthotic vulvar intraepithelial neoplasia (vaVIN), similar to VAAD, but displays striking papillomatous features.

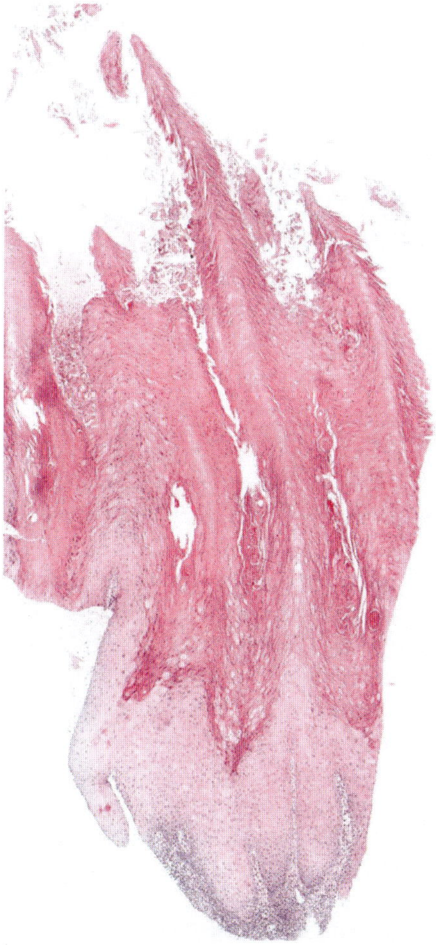

Figure 3.34 Verruciform lichen simplex chronicus (vLSC) is a variant of verruciform acanthotic vulvar intraepithelial neoplasia (vaVIN), similar to VAAD, but shows irregular acanthosis with papillomatosis and a thick granular layer, features that pose a differential diagnosis with lichen simplex chronicus.

Dedifferentiated Vulvar Intraepithelial Neoplasia versus Verruciform Acanthotic and Lichen Sclerosus

LS is an idiopathic inflammatory skin condition that predominantly affects postmenopausal women. Its pathogenesis is complex and includes genetic predisposition, an immune-mediated Th1- response, oxidative stress and alteration in the tissue remodeling associated genes and microRNAs. When compared to normal vulvar skin, LS overexpresses proteins related to the interferon-γ and antigen-presenting pathways.[121,122]

While the histological features of fully developed LS are highly characteristic, some cases can closely simulate dVIN, including an almost continuous basal expression of p53, which is secondary to inflammation and oxidative stress.[123,124] Similarly, the hypertrophic variant of LS may pose problems in the differential diagnosis with vaVIN.[125] A strict evaluation of the p53 mutational pattern, absent in LS[111] and clinicopathological correlation are of paramount importance to differentiate these processes, which carry very different prognoses and require completely different therapeutic approaches. Additionally, LS differs from dVIN and vaVIN in that it does not exhibit overexpression of CK17 and Sox2. Furthermore, in most cases, LS retains GATA3 expression at the basal layer of the epithelium.[113,116,117]

It is well known that women with vulvar LS are at a higher risk of developing dVIN and SCC.[121] Up to date, it is not possible to know which LS are at risk of developing dVIN. One study suggested that the early stages of progression can be identified by the development of a carcinogenic immunophenotype with alterations in the EIF2 translation pathway, characterized by CAV1 overexpression and AKAP12 underexpression.[122] Nevertheless, the study requires additional confirmation, and these markers are not commonly available in clinical practice.

Squamous Cell Carcinoma, HPV-Associated, of the Vulva

Vulvar squamous cell carcinoma (SCC) associated with HPV tends to affect younger patients compared to HPV-independent counterparts and its prevalence varies among different populations; for example, it is the most frequent variant in sub-Saharan Africa, but less common than HPV-independent SCCs in Europe.[126] It originates from intraepithelial areas of high-grade squamous intraepithelial lesions (HSIL) and the most frequent morphological appearances are basaloid or warty.[104,118]

Its identification is of major importance as these cases typically demonstrate lower aggressiveness and a more favorable response to radiation therapy compared to HPV-independent SCCs.[127] The most reliable diagnostic marker is p16 which stains diffusely the tumor. Of note, some of these cases may coexpress p53.[104,118] The main differential diagnosis of cases of vulvar SCCs displaying basaloid features is BCC and can be recognized by the lack of block-type p16 stain and expression of BerEP4.

Squamous Cell Carcinoma, HPV-Independent, of the Vulva

HPV-independent SCCs can originate from two types of intraepithelial precursors. Either dVIN, which is immunohistochemically characterized by p53 mutation patterns, or from the p53-wild type vaVIN, which is p53 negative. Morphologically, the former is characterized by the development of keratinizing SCC, while the latter is associated with a higher number of verrucous SCCs. Although cases arising from vaVIN demonstrated a higher tendency to recur, overall survival rates were higher than in cases associated with dVIN, though not as favorable as those associated with HPV.[118]

Immunohistochemically, HPV-independent SCCs are characterized by p16 negativity that is associated with mutational patterns of p53 in cases associated with dVIN.[128] However, it is important to be aware that some p53-mutated cases can exhibit p16 expression in the absence of HPV infection.[128] In addition, while the p53 immunohistochemical staining pattern typically remains consistent between invasive tumors and their precursors, cases where discordance occurs, such as wild-type invasive SCCs and p53-mutated dVIN, have been described.[128] Programmed cell death ligand-1 (PD-L1) expression, which may predict response to immunotherapy is frequently high in types of vulvar SCCs, but tends to be higher in HPV-independent cases.[129]

3.4 Penis

Squamous Intraepithelial Lesions, HPV-Associated

Condyloma Acuminatum

Penile carcinogenesis seems to parallel that of the vulva, the latter with a much more robust level of evidence and lesions similarly manifest into two different prognostic categories, those associated with (1) low-risk HPV, which results in anogenital warts and have minimal risk of malignant transformation and (2) high-risk HPV, which have a greater risk of progression to SCC.[130,131] Condyloma acuminatum which is synonymous with LSIL in the vulva, present as unifocal or more commonly multifocal warty exophytic lesions most frequently on the glans, followed by the prepuce and shaft.

Confluence of lesions can result in the formation of a giant condyloma acuminatum (Buschke-Lowenstein tumor), which can slowly enlarge into large cauliflower-like masses (up to 15 cm), which carries a risk of progression to SCC.[132,133] The most common etiological genotypes are HPV 6 and 11 and *in situ* hybridization can aid in confirming the diagnosis (Figures 3.35 and 3.36).[130] Since the oncoproteins of low-risk genotypes are not considered to result in significant alteration of tumor suppressor genes *P16*, *TP53*, and *RB1*, they contribute to a lesser extent in carcinogenesis.[134]

Histopathology of condylomata shows rounded fibrovascular cores covered by acanthotic epidermis with variable degrees of papillomatosis and hyperkeratosis displaying koilocytic changes. A subset of "atypical" condylomata demonstrates atypia above the basal layer due to co-infection or association with high-risk HPV which is supported by block-like p16 staining and/or positivity for *in situ* hybridization (ISH) for HPV 16/18.[135]

Verruciform genital-associated (VEGAS) xanthoma commonly occur on the penoscrotal region in men and are similarly acanthotic and papillomatous which can clinically

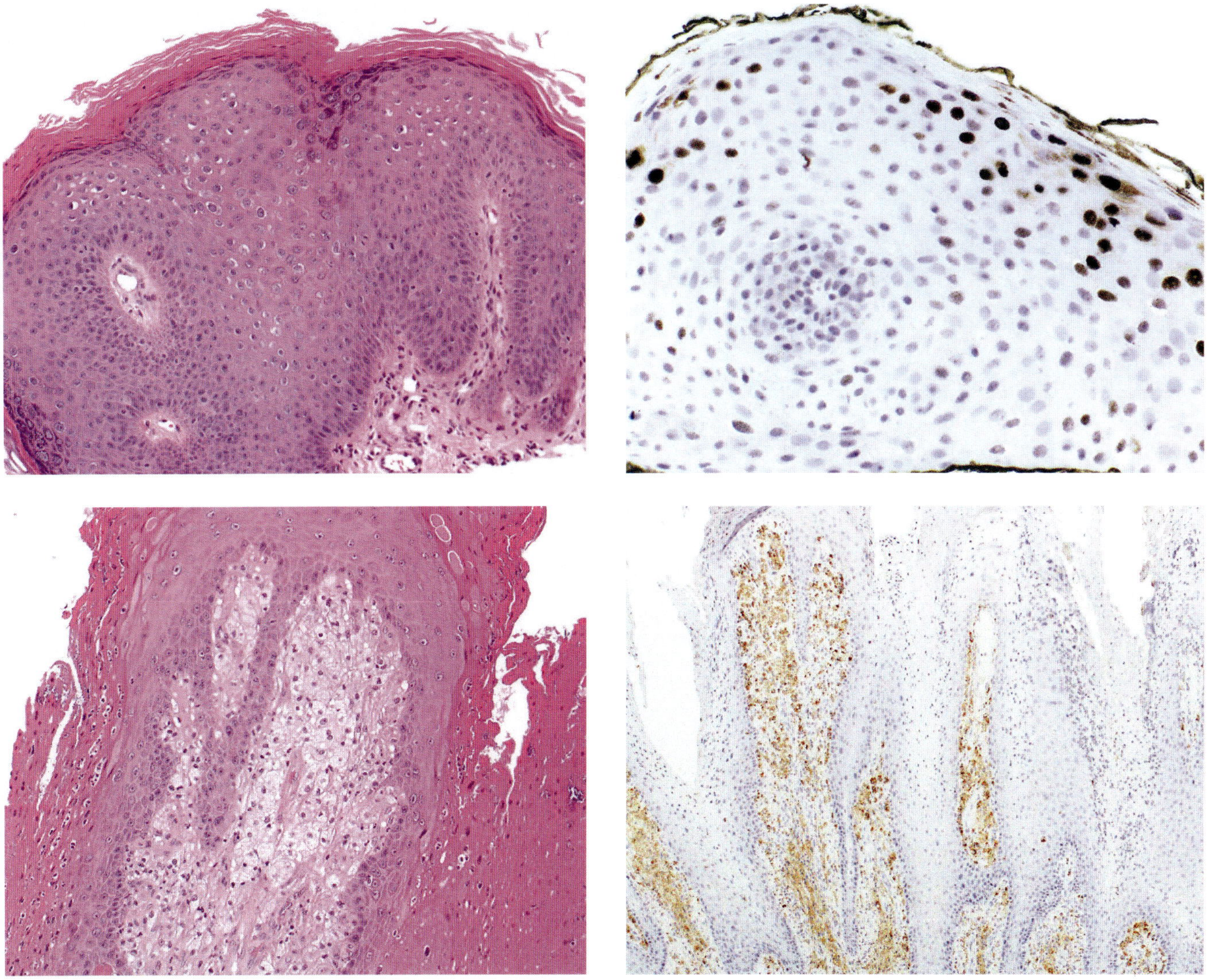

Figures 3.35–3.38 Penile condyloma acuminatum with epidermal acanthosis, papillomatosis and koilocytosis (**Figure 3.35**) which is positive for HPV 6/11 *in situ* hybridization (**Figure 3.36**). Penile verruciform xanthoma which similarly displays acanthosis and papillomatosis but with foamy histiocytes (xanthoma cells) in the papillary dermis (**Figure 3.37**) which are highlighted by a CD68 stain (**Figure 3.38**).

and morphologically mimic condyloma acuminatum.[136,137] However, they lack koilocytic change and display elongated rete ridges with foamy histiocytes (xanthoma cells) in the papillary dermis which can be highlighted by histiocytic markers such as CD68, CD163 or PU.1 (Figures 3.37 and 3.38).

Condyloma acuminatum

- p16 negative (high risk-HPV co-infection/associated if block-like p16+)
- HPV 6/11 ISH+

Penile Intraepithelial Neoplasia (PeIN), HPV-Associated

Penile intraepithelial neoplasia (PeIN) is similarly classified into two morphologic groups which are also molecularly distinct: (1) HPV-associated and (2) HPV-independent.[138] In the penis, HPV-associated neoplasia is separated into three main morphologic patterns: (1) basaloid, (2) warty, and (3) mixed warty-basaloid. The basaloid pattern is composed of a monotonous population of basaloid cells associated with numerous mitotic figures and apoptotic cells imparting a starry-sky appearance. The warty pattern shows verruciform acanthosis with pleomorphic cells showing koilocytic atypia and numerous mitoses. The warty-basaloid pattern displays overlapping features of both, usually of a verruciform surface with koilocytic change in the upper half and monotonous basaloid cells in the lower half of the epithelium. Most of these lesions are associated with a single genotype and HPV 16 is the most common, while on occasion multiple subtypes can occur, including a mixture of both low and high-risk variants, often in association with warty histology.[138–140]

Strong and diffuse block-like staining for p16 is widely accepted as positive and is typically seen in HPV-associated PeIN (**Figures 3.39 and 3.40**). A mosaic pattern in which there is more extensive, yet patchy and discontinuous staining may

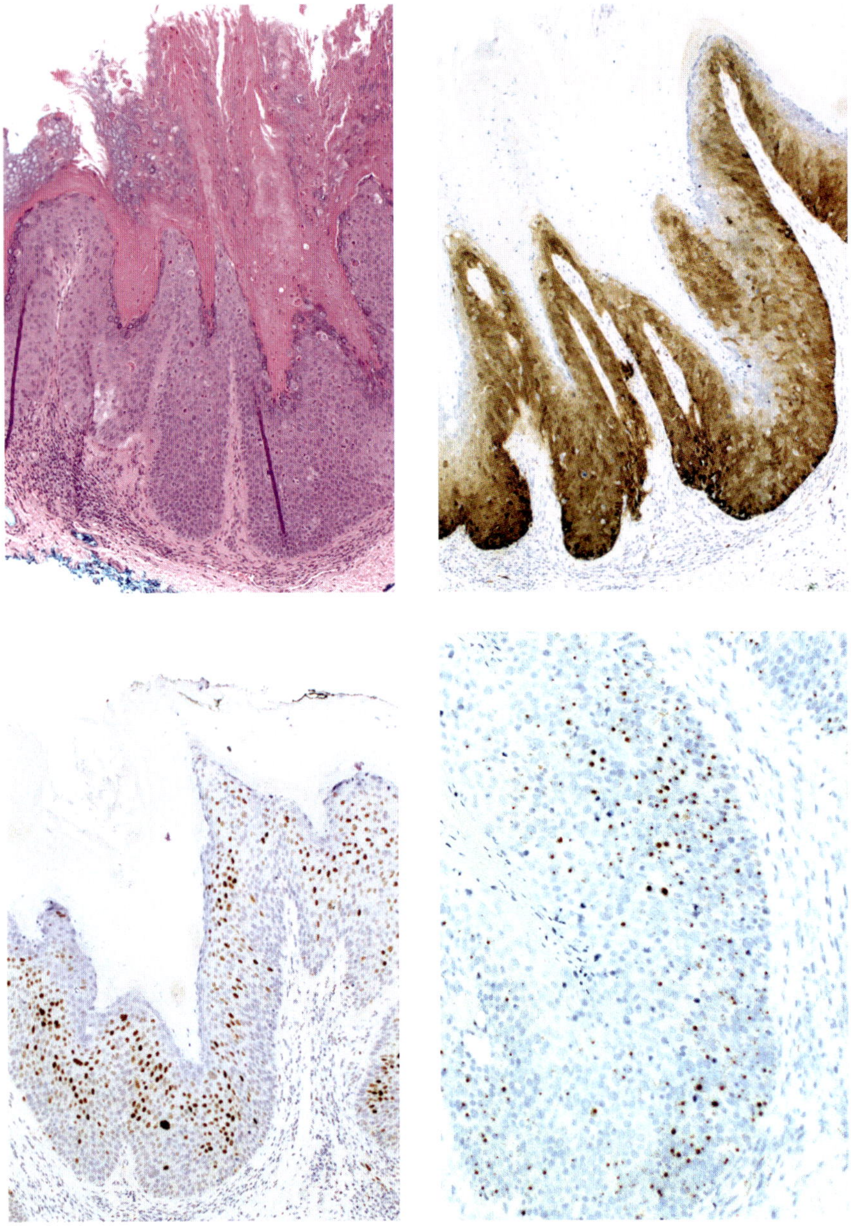

Figures 3.39–3.42 Warty penile intraepithelial neoplasia (PeIN) (**Figure 3.39**) showing verruciform acanthosis with pleomorphic cells showing koilocytic atypia and numerous mitoses, which is typically positive for p16 (**Figure 3.40**) and shows wild-type mid-epithelial p53 staining (**Figure 3.41**). *In situ* hybridization for HPV16/18 is strongly positive (**Figure 3.42**).

represent false negative cases and confirmation with PCR or ISH for high-risk HPV when available is recommended.[141] A helpful clue is the wild-type mid-epithelial (basal-sparing) pattern of p53 exclusively observed in HPV-associated lesions (**Figures 3.41 and 3.42**).[111] When identified, this helps inquire into the HPV-related nature of the lesion. Ki67 when performed is also elevated, often involving the upper third of the epithelium.[140]

HPV-associated intraepithelial neoplasia with concurrent lichen simplex chronicus (LSC) is a potential pitfall as it is a mimicker of differentiated intraepithelial neoplasia emphasizing the importance of performing immunohistochemistry.[142,143] Morphologically, there is significant overlap but when performing p16, there is diffuse, block-like positivity, often with more intense staining in the lower half of the epithelium and a mid-epithelial (basal-sparing) pattern with p53 (**Figures 3.43–3.45**).

Verruciform lesions enter the differential for warty or warty-basaloid PeIN, including condyloma acuminatum, giant condylomas and verrucous carcinoma. Verrucous carcinomas lack koilocytic change and are both p16 and HPV negative. Although condyloma acuminatum/giant condyloma will also display easily identifiable koilocytic change, there is much more nuclear pleomorphism, cytologic atypia and mitoses throughout the entire epithelium in PeIN. Positivity for P16 and the presence of high-risk-HPV will also support PeIN.[144]

HPV-Associated Penile Intraepithelial Neoplasia (PeIN) (Basaloid, Warty, Warty-Basaloid Patterns)

- p53 wild-type (mid-epithelial/basal-sparing pattern)
- p16 positive (diffuse block-like staining)
- Ki67 elevated (upper third of epithelium)

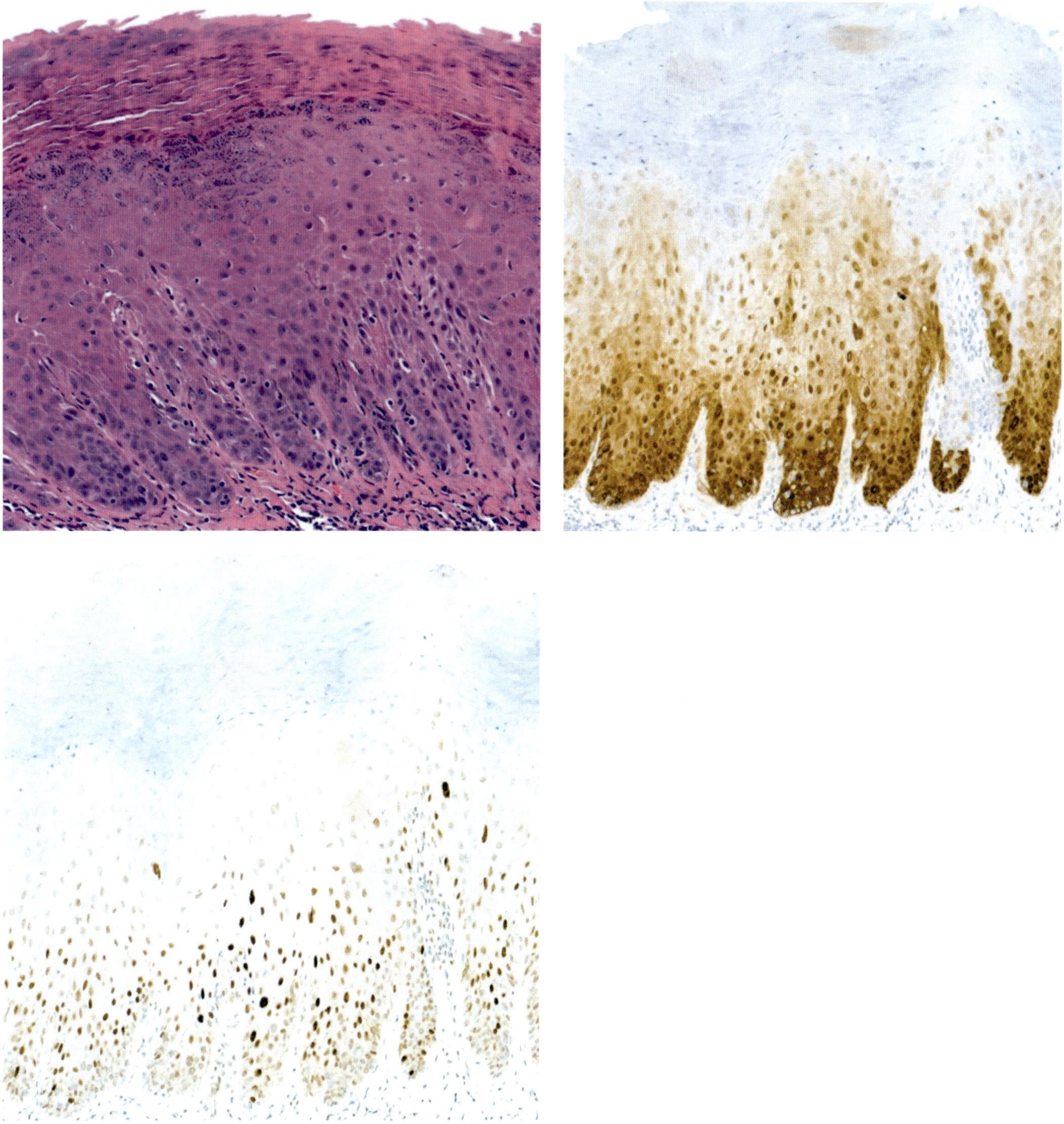

Figures 3.43–3.45 HPV-associated PeIN with lichen simplex chronicus (dPein-like) (**Figure 3.43**) showing morphologic overlap with differentiated PeIN (dPeIN) displaying epidermal acanthosis, abundant eosinophilic cytoplasm and hyperchromatic nuclei with atypia in basal/parabasal keratinocytes. In contrast to dPeIN, p16 shows strong, block-like positivity most prominent in the lower portion of the epithelium (**Figure 3.44**) with mid-epithelial p53 wild-type staining (**Figure 3.45**).

HPV-Negative Differentiated Penile Intraepithelial Neoplasia (dPeIN) with Basaloid Features (HSIL-like dPeIN)

- p53 mutational pattern (basal, basal/parabasal, absent/null and cytoplasmic)
- p16 negative

Squamous Intraepithelial Lesions, HPV-Independent

Similar to the vulva, HPV-independent intraepithelial neoplasia of the penis can be further subcategorized into those that are p53 mutant and p53 wild-type. However, the 2022 WHO classification of penile neoplasia only mentions HPV-independent p53 mutant or differentiated PeIN (dPeIN), likely due to the lack of published literature regarding the p53 wild-type lesions.[145]

Differentiated Penile Intraepithelial Neoplasia (dPeIN)/ (HPV-Independent p53 Mutant)

Differentiated penile intraepithelial neoplasia (dPeIN) often develop in association with chronic inflammatory dermatoses such as lichen sclerosus or lichen planus.[138,146] Histologically, there is epithelial hyperplasia, often associated with altered cornification (hyperkeratosis/parakeratosis) and elongating and anastomosing rete ridges. The keratinocytes display abnormal maturation with abundant eosinophilic cytoplasm and hyperchromatic nuclei most prominent within the basal and parabasal layers of the epithelium.[138,139,147] Similar to the vulva, most cases of dPeIN harbor *TP53* alterations resulting in mutant p53 expression and the same four patterns can be applied (**Figures 3.46–3.50**, mutant and wildtype p53 patterns) (**Table 3.6**).[111,146] P16 is typically negative, although it has been

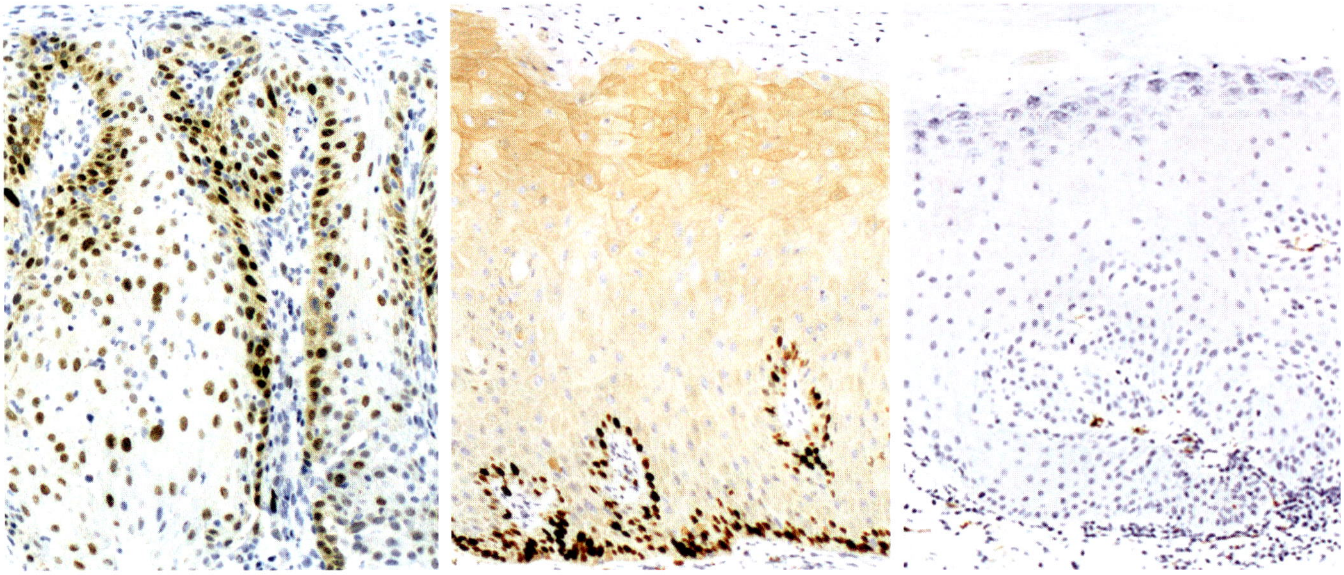

Figures 3.46–3.48 Parabasal/diffuse overexpression showing uniformly strong nuclear staining of >80% of basal cells and strong parabasal extension (**Figure 3.46**), p53 mutant pattern with basal overexpression showing uniformly strong nuclear staining in >80% of the basal cells without significant parabasal staining (**Figure 3.57**), and null/absent staining showing complete absence of immunoreactivity in the presence of a positive internal control (inflammatory/stromal cells) (**Figure 3.48**).

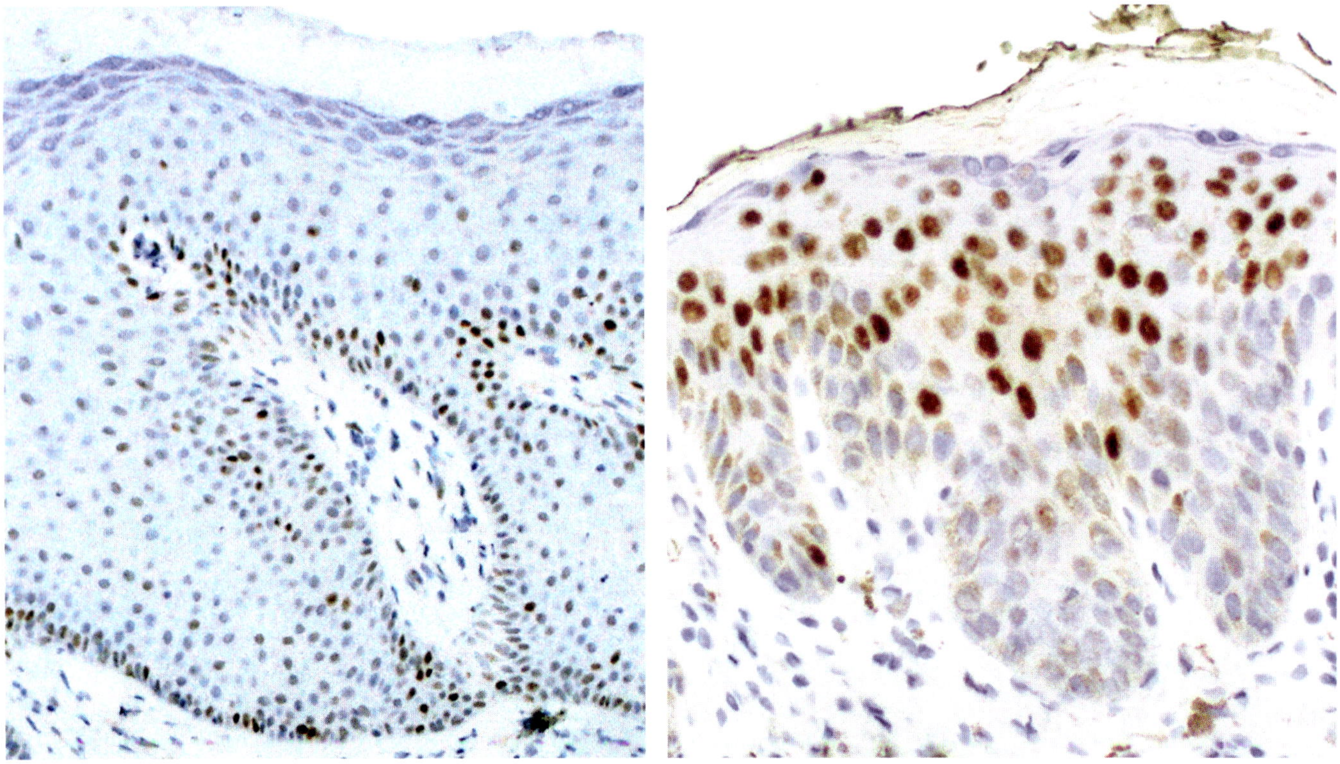

Figures 3.49–3.50 p53 wild-type patterns with scattered expression showing heterogeneous nuclear staining of variable intensities in basal and parabasal cells (**Figure 3.49**) and mid-epithelial (basal sparing) pattern showing heterogeneous but typically moderate to strong staining in mid-epithelial cells with sparing of basal cells and occasionally sparing the lower parabasal cells (**Figure 3.50**).

Table 3.6 Summary of p16 and p53 staining in vulvar and penile squamous intraepithelial neoplasia

	p16	p53
HPV-Associated Intraepithelial Neoplasia High-grade squamous intraepithelial lesion (HSIL)	Overexpressed/ block-like staining	Wild-type: - Mid-epithelial/ basal-sparing - Heterogeneous basal/parabasal staining
HPV-Independent p53 mutant Differentiated VIN (dVIN) and differentiated PeIN (d-PeIN)	Negative or patchy staining *Rare positive (due to *CDKN2A* mutation)	Mutant pattern: - Basal overexpression - Basal/parabasal diffuse expression - Absent/null - Cytoplasmic staining
HPV-independent p53 wildtype Verruciform/ acanthotic VIN (vaVIN) and PeIN (vaPeIN)	Negative or patchy staining	Wild-type - Heterogeneous basal/parabasal staining

reported to be positive in a subset of cases, with a number of cases attributed to *CDKN2A* mutations which can be concomitant with *TP53* alterations.[146]

An HSIL-like dPeIN with basaloid features which is HPV-negative by both p16 immunohistochemistry and testing for HPV DNA is a potential pitfall as it is a mimicker of the basaloid pattern of HPV-associated PeIN (**Figures 3.51–3.53**). These two lesions are morphologically indistinguishable but as mentioned p16 is negative and p53 will display a mutant pattern of staining.[148]

Differentiated Penile Intraepithelial Neoplasia (dPeIN)

- p53 mutational pattern (basal, basal/parabasal, absent/null and cytoplasmic)
- p16 negative

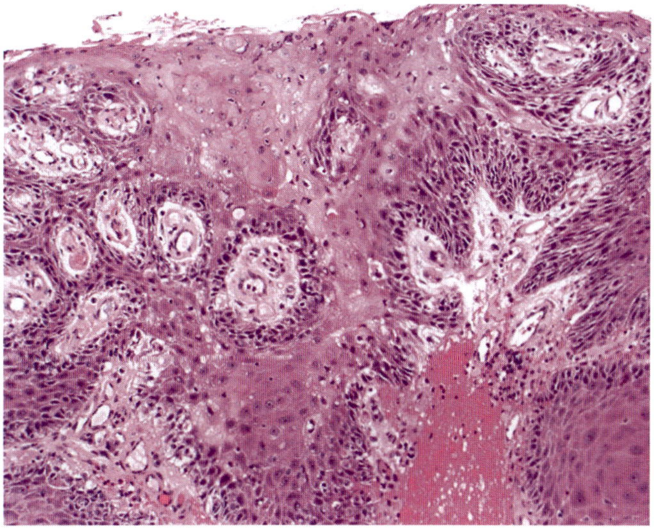

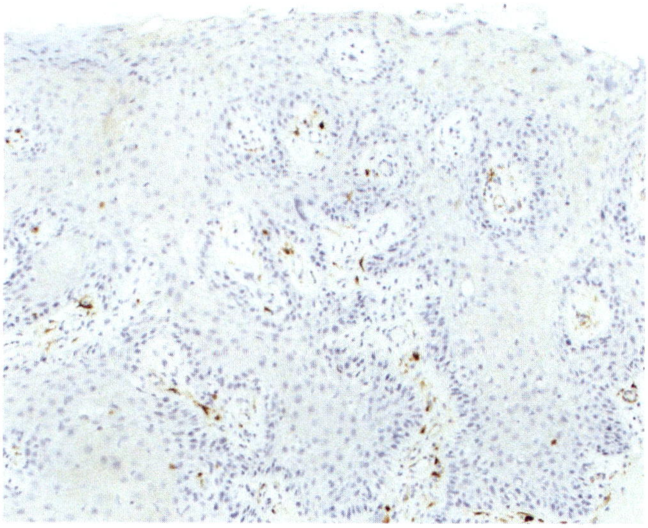

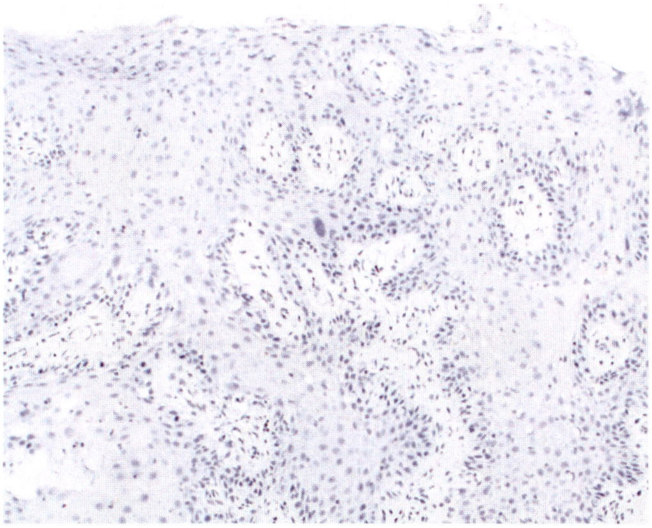

Figures 3.51–3.53 Differentiated penile intraepithelial neoplasia (dPeIN) showing epithelial hyperplasia with elongating and anastomosing rete ridges, abnormal maturation and hyperchromatic nuclei most prominent within the basal and parabasal layers of the epithelium (**Figure 3.49**), which is negative for p16 (**Figure 3.50**) and shows a mutant (null) pattern for p53 (**Figure 3.51**).

HPV-Associated Penile Intraepithelial Neoplasia (PeIN) with Concurrent Lichen Simplex Chronicus (dPeIN-like)

- p53 wild-type (mid-epithelial/basal-sparing pattern)
- p16 positive (diffuse block-like staining; often stronger in lower half of epithelium)

Penile Intraepithelial Neoplasia (HPV-Independent P53 Wild-Type)

Few studies have reported upon penile intraepithelial neoplasia that are HPV-independent p53 wild-type which do not appear to develop in association with chronic inflammatory dermatoses like dPeIN.[138,146] Histologically, there is variable acanthosis and verruciform hyperplasia often associated with altered cornification (hyperkeratosis/parakeratosis) and hypogranulosis. Unlike dPeIN, these lesions lack nuclear atypia and if present, are minimal typically in basal cells.[146] Akin to the vulva, these tumors lack *TP53* alterations resulting in wild-type p53 expression and are p16 negative (Figures 3.54–3.56).[111,146]

Squamous Cell Carcinoma, HPV-Associated of the Penis

Similar to PeIN, penile squamous cell carcinoma (PSCC) has two main etiologic pathways with respect to HPV. The most common HPV-associated PSCC variants are basaloid, warty and warty-basaloid subtypes, and often arise in the background of the same PeIN counterparts.[144,149,150] Basaloid carcinomas typically show a downward proliferation of islands/nests of basaloid cells that can have central areas of comedonecrosis or abrupt central keratinization (**Figures 3.57–3.60**). Basaloid PSCCs are associated with the worst prognosis with higher rates of regional lymph node metastases, which may relate to its associated high histologic grade, deeper extension correlating to advanced tumor (T) stage and presence of lymphovascular invasion.[144,150,151] Warty PSCC display an exophytic and endophytic growth pattern composed of condylomatous papillae lined by malignant koilocytosis and an invasive jagged interface between tumor and stroma. Amongst the HPV-associated PSCCs, these tumors have the most favorable outcome, likely related to the superficially invasive nature of the tumor and its associated low

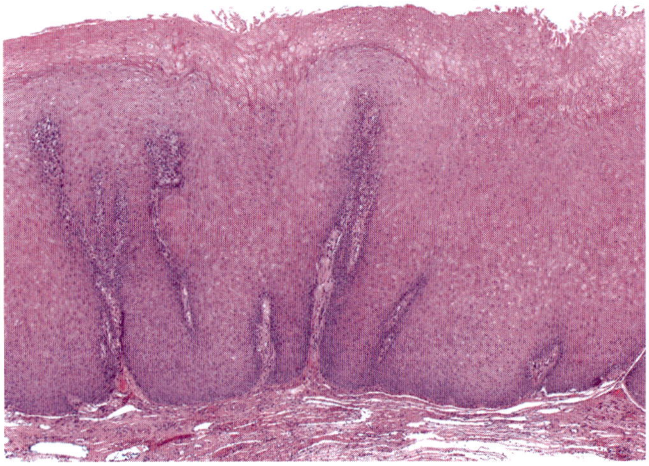

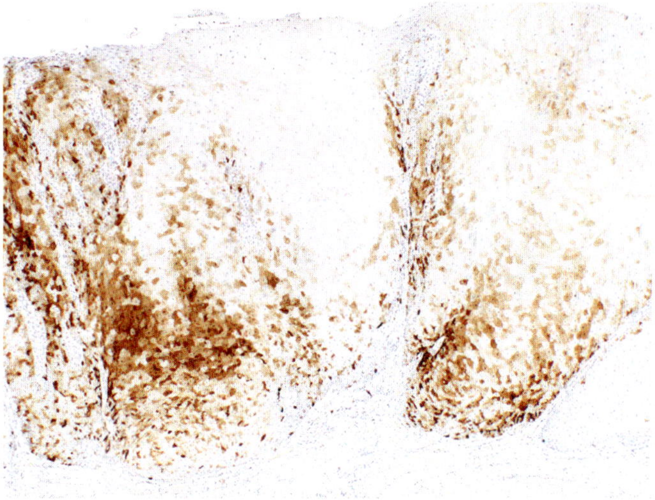

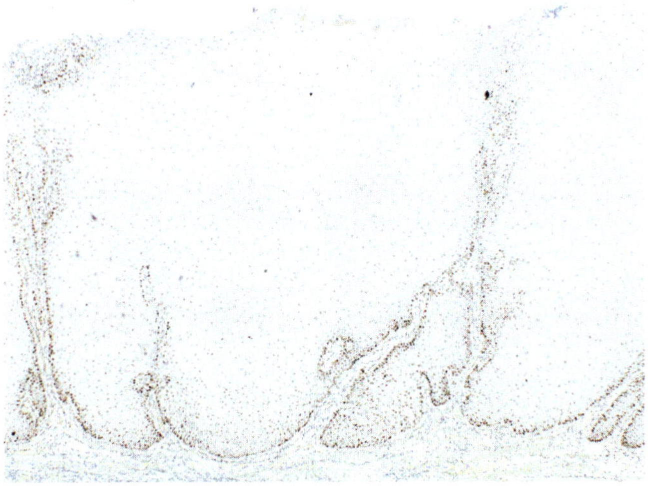

Figures 3.54–3.56 HPV-independent p53 WT PeIN (**Figure 3.54**) showing epidermal acanthosis with prominent hyper/parakeratosis and hypogranulosis, lacking significant cytologic atypia and showing negative staining for p16 (**Figure 3.55**) and wild-type p53 staining (**Figure 3.56**).

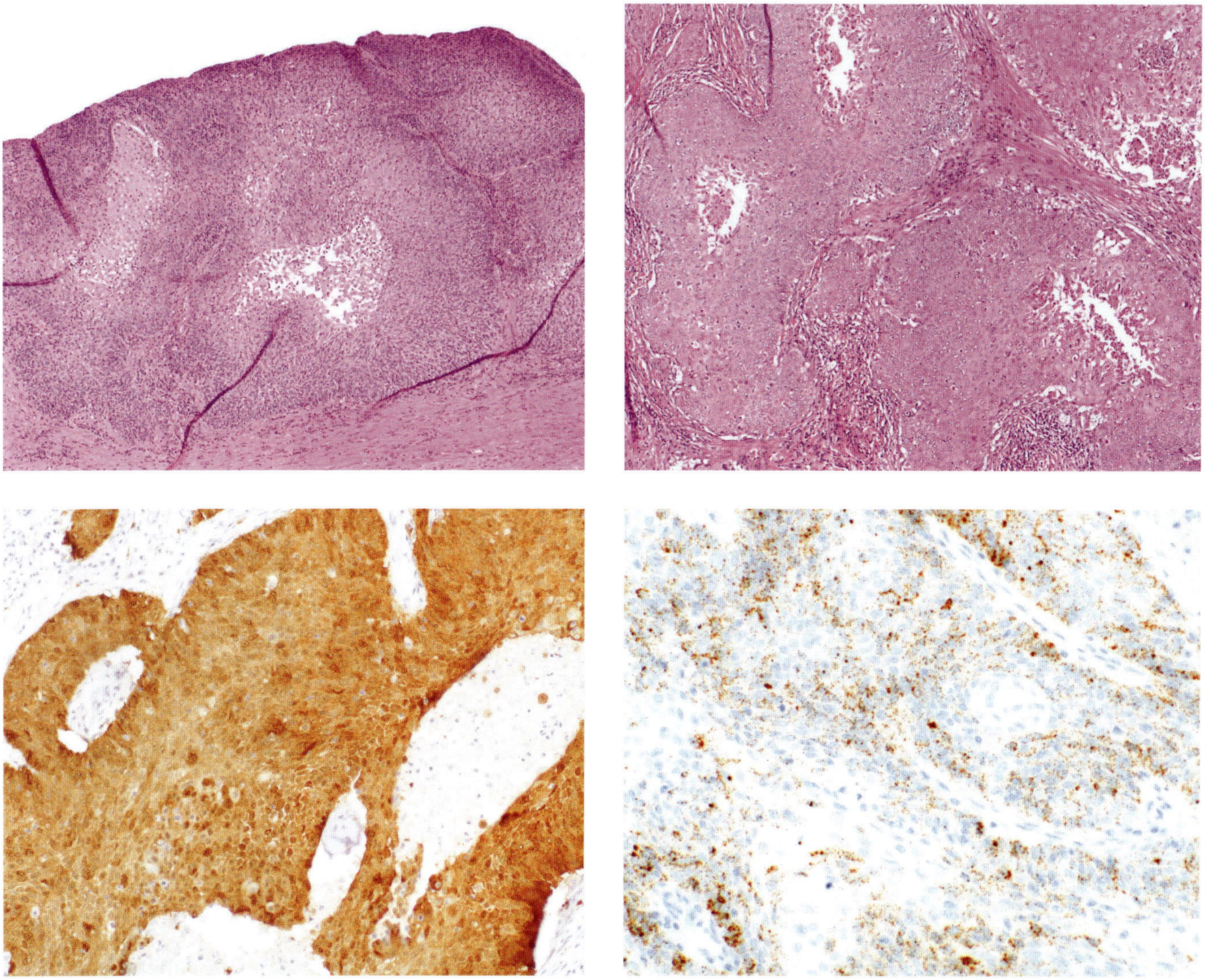

Figure 3.57–3.60 Basaloid penile squamous cell carcinoma (**Figure 3.57**, X40; **Figure 3.58**, X100), showing downward proliferation of islands/nests of basaloid cells that can have central areas of comedonecrosis or abrupt central keratinization, showing strong, block-like positivity for p16 (**Figure 3.59**, X100) and is positive for *in situ* hybridization for HPV 16/18 (**Figure 3.60**, X100).

histological grade.[144,150,152] Warty-basaloid PSCC display overlapping features, often with an exophytic papillomatous warty surface overlying invasive solid nests of basaloid cells and have an intermediate prognosis.[135,144,147,149,150]

P16 is the most helpful diagnostic immunohistochemical marker and will similarly show diffuse, block-like staining (**Figure 3.59**). Additional studies such as ISH and/or PCR can also be performed to identify high risk-HPV.[135,144,149] Basal cell carcinoma of the penoscrotal region is extremely rare, but if considered, can be recognized by diffuse positivity for keratin17.[13]

The proximity of the penile urethra may result in involvement of the adjacent penile glans which has significant morphologic overlap with basaloid PSCC (**Table 3.7**). Penile urethral carcinomas are typically negative for GATA3 and uroplakin and over half (63%) are positive for p16, with high-risk-HPV detected in a subset of cases.[153,154] In addition, similar to PSCC, the majority are positive for keratin 5/6 and p63. The presence of precursor neoplasia/carcinoma *in situ* and the main location of the mass centered on the penile urethra are therefore, the most helpful clues.[153]

Table 3.7 Comparison of basaloid penile squamous cell carcinoma (PSCC) and penile urethral carcinoma

	Basaloid PSCC	Penile urethral carcinoma
p16	Diffuse block-like staining	Diffuse block-like staining
GATA3	Negative	Negative
Uroplakin	Negative	Negative
CK5/6	Positive	Positive
p63	Positive	Positive
Location/precursor neoplasia	Penile (PeIN)	Urethral (CIS)

Squamous Cell Carcinoma, HPV-Independent of the Penis

HPV-independent PSCCs originate from two types of intraepithelial precursors, which relate to *TP53* mutation status and are immunohistochemically characterized by those with p53 mutant patterns (dPeIN) and those that are p53 wild-type.[146,155,156] Morphologically, PSCC that develop in the background of dPeIN often display usual type, typically low-grade, but can also be high-grade keratinizing SCC. [146,155,156] Those that arise in the background of p53 wild-type verruciform and acanthotic lesions are associated with adjacent verrucous carcinoma and harbor *HRAS* or *PIK3CA* mutations, similar to vaVIN.[146,155,157–159] Comparable to the vulva, p53 mutant cases can also co-express p16 in the absence of HPV infection, which is often due to *CDKN2A* missense mutations which alters the Rb pathway.[146]

3.5 Case Studies

Case 3.1

Case history: A 76-year-old man presented with a nodule on his right ear.

Description: Histologic sections show an infiltrative carcinoma in the dermis (**Figure 3.61**). Pagetoid growth of tumor cells in single cells and in nests is seen within the overlying epidermis (**Figure 3.62**). Central necrosis is seen in some of the superficial tumor nests. The tumor cells are strongly positive for keratin 903 (**Figure 3.63**). CEA, keratin 7 (**Figure 3.64**), and keratin 19 highlight only the entrapped eccrine ducts.

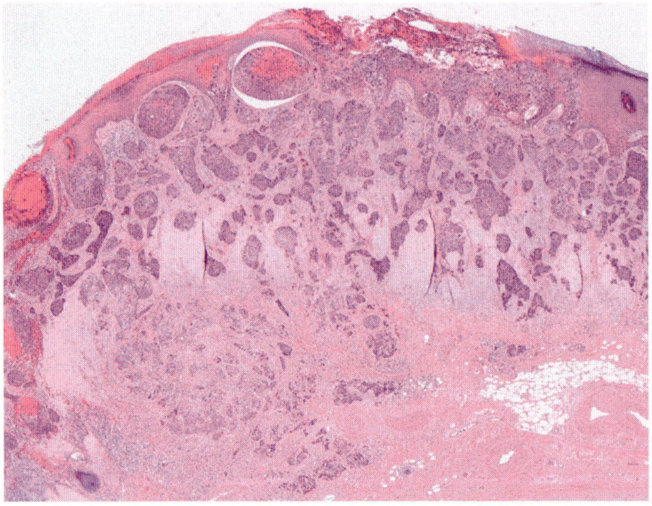

Figure 3.61 An infiltrative carcinoma is seen in the dermis (X40).

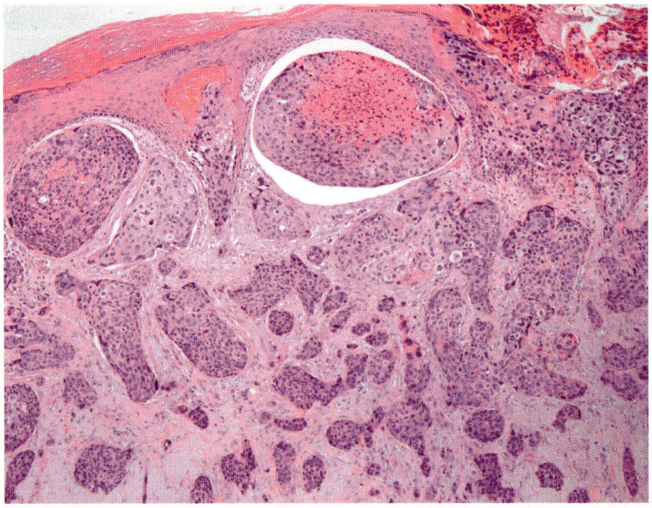

Figure 3.62 Large epithelial tumor nests with central necrosis as well as pagetoid growth pattern within the epidermis are seen (X100).

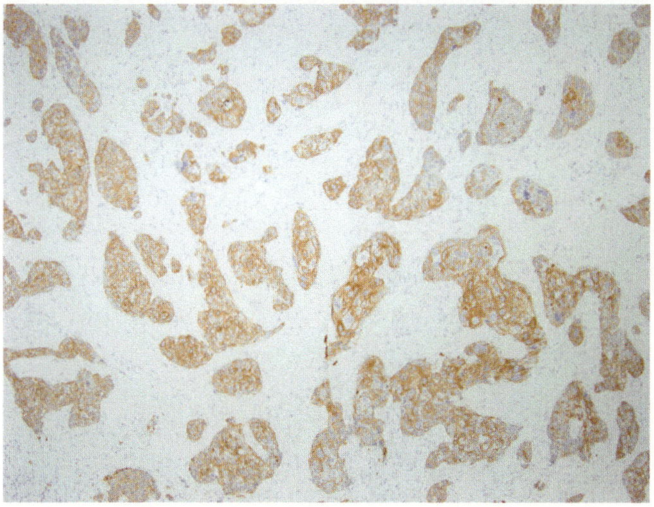

Figure 3.63 The tumor cells are strongly positive for keratin 903 (X100).

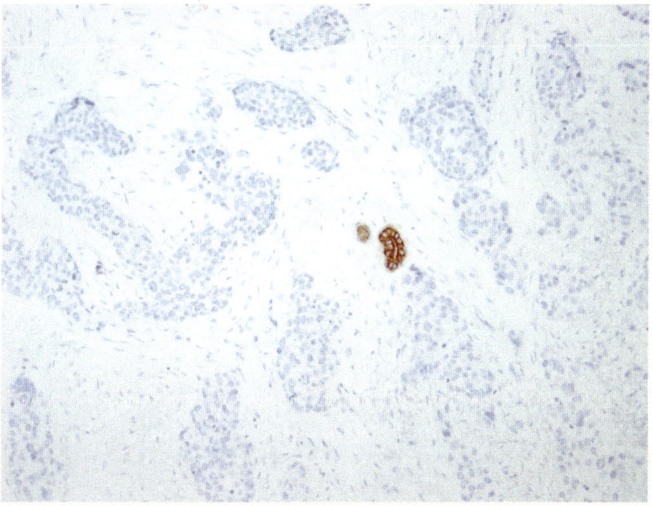

Figure 3.64 Only an entrapped eccrine duct is positive for keratin 7 (X200).

Diagnosis: Squamous cell carcinoma.

Discussion: Due to the central necrosis and pagetoid growth pattern porocarcinoma is the main differential diagnosis. The absence of keratin 7, keratin 19, and CEA is supportive of an SCC and excludes porocarcinoma.[6]

Case 3.2

Case history: An 89-year-old woman presented with a 7-year history of a growing and painful right lower leg lesion.

Description: The skin biopsy shows clusters as well as single atypical tumor cells with pale cytoplasm within the epidermis (**Figure 3.65**). The tumor cells exhibit prominent pagetoid spread (**Figure 3.66**). The intraepidermal tumor cells are positive for keratin 903 (**Figure 3.67**). They are negative for keratin 7 and S100 (**Figure 3.68**).

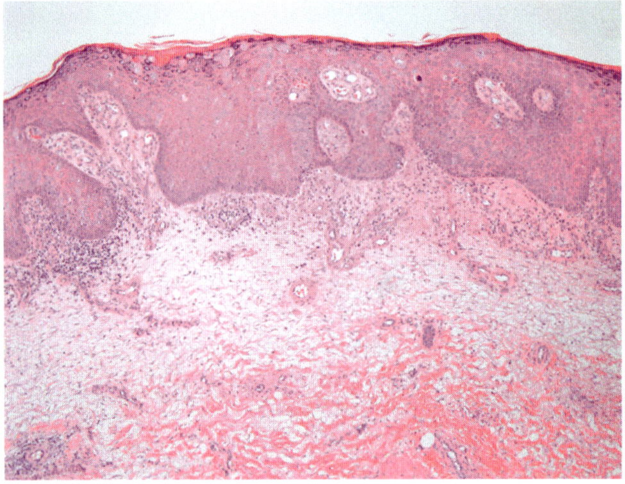

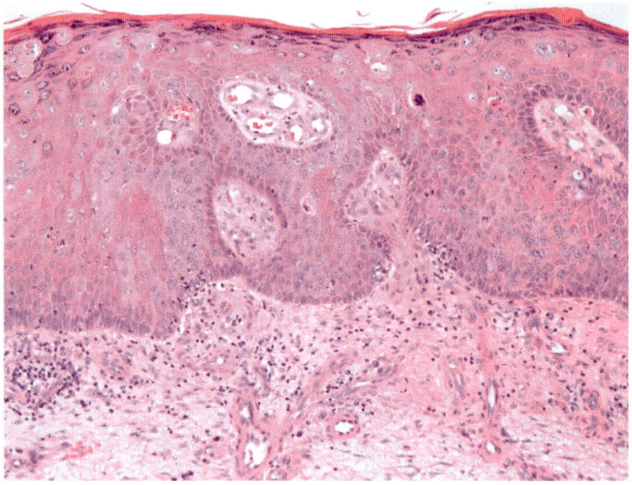

Figures 3.65 and 3.66 Nests and single intraepidermal tumor cells exhibit pagetoid growth pattern (X100, X200).

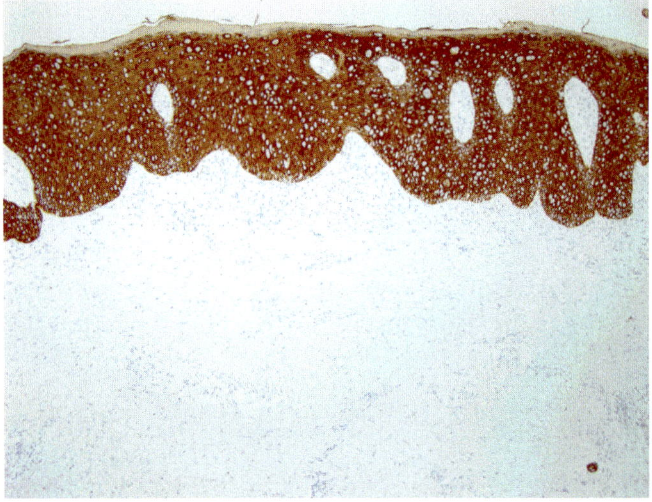

Figure 3.67 The tumor cells as well as the epidermis are positive for keratin 903 (X100).

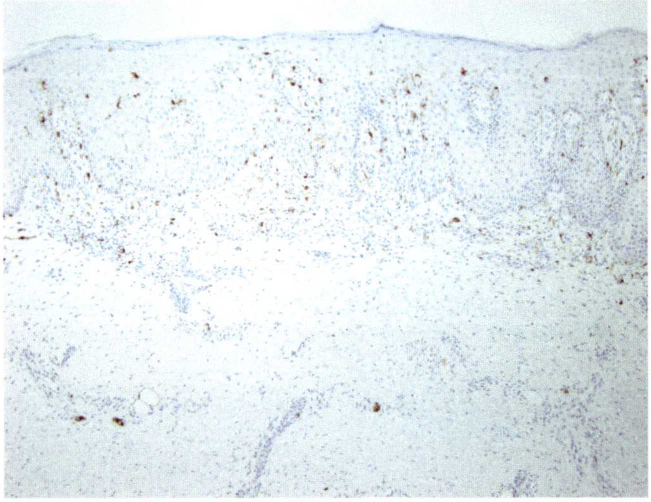

Figure 3.68 S100 immunostain highlights only the intraepidermal dendritic cells (X100).

Diagnosis: Pagetoid squamous cell carcinoma *in situ*.

Discussion: The differential diagnosis of a SCC *in situ* with pagetoid growth pattern would be melanoma *in situ*, extramammary Paget and sebaceous carcinoma *in situ*. Melanoma *in situ* would express melanocytic markers such as S100, MelanA, HMB45 and MiTF. Primary extramammary Paget and sebaceous carcinoma *in situ* would express keratin 7. The lack of both keratin 7 and S100 expression in this case supports the diagnosis of SCC *in situ*. In addition, cytoplasmic mucin and dyskeratotic cells would be seen in extramammary Paget and SCC *in situ* on histologic sections, respectively.

Case 3.3

Case history: A 74-year-old woman with long-standing "atrophy" on her vulvar mucosa and recent development of verrucous lesions.

Description: The biopsy contains an invasive keratinizing squamous cell carcinoma. The edges of the tumor show epidermal dysmaturation and cytological hyperchromasia involving the lower third of the epithelium (**Figure 3.69**).

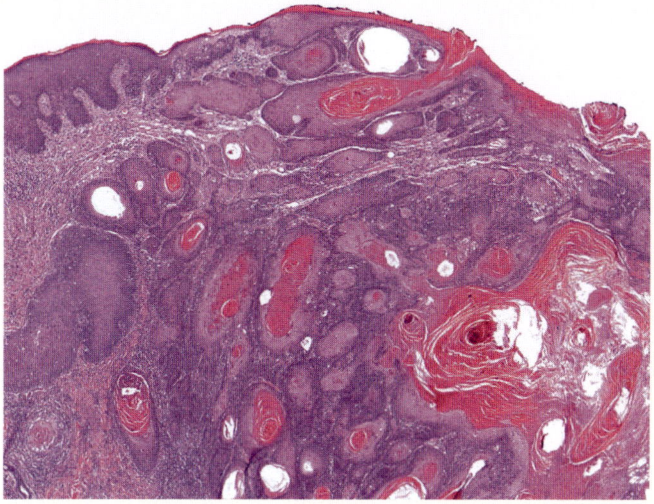

Figure 3.69 Invasive SCC showing basal membrane thickening and keratinocyte atypia in the lower third of the epidermis.

Diagnosis: Keratinizing squamous cell carcinoma.

Discussion: This keratinizing squamous cell carcinoma (SCC) is originated from a squamous epithelium with atypia limited to the basal layers. The mucosa at its edges contains areas with basal membrane thickening and lymphocytic infiltrate with inflammatory cells. All these findings are highly suggestive of a SCC developed through the differentiated pathway in a patient suffering lichen sclerosus. These tumors typically present mutational patterns of p53 (**Figure 3.70**) while p16 is negative.

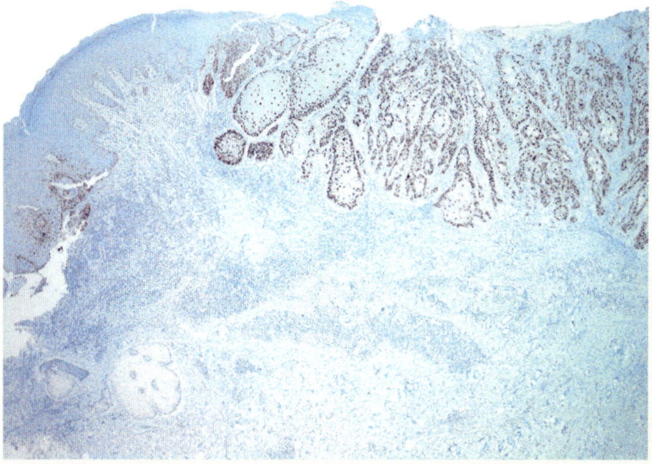

Figure 3.70 p53 positivity in an invasive SCC originated through the differentiated pathway. This immunohistochemical marker also highlights the areas of differentiated dysplasia present at the edges.

Case 3.4

Case history: A 35-year-old woman with verrucous vulvar lesions.

Description: The biopsy corresponds to an invasive squamous cell carcinoma that focally displays a papillomatous silhouette. The image corresponding to the intraepidermal neoplasm shows complete substitution of the normal epidermal cells by hyperchromatic keratinocytes that often display basaloid appearance. There is lack of maturation, and many mitoses are noted in the upper epithelial layers. Additional findings are multinucleated keratinocytes, koilocytosis and parakeratosis (**Figure 3.71**).

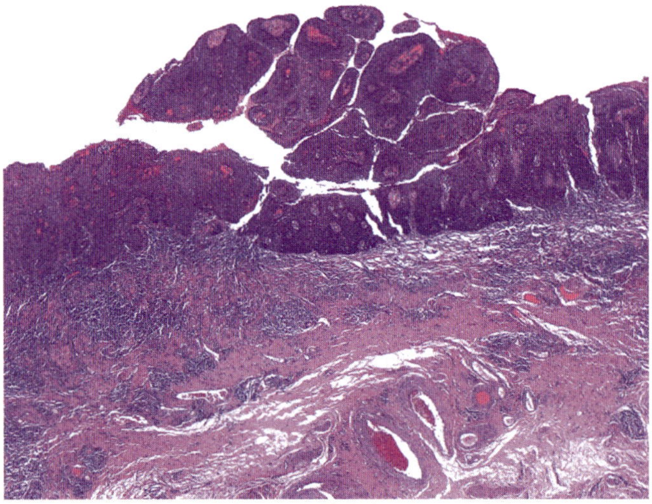

Figure 3.71 This invasive squamous cell carcinoma presents a papillomatous silhouette and complete effacement of the normal keratinocytes by hyperchromatic basaloid cells without evidence of maturation.

Diagnosis: HPV-related vulvar squamous cell carcinoma.

Discussion: This SCC shows basaloid morphology with papillomatous silhouette typical of HPV-related vulvar SCC. This is the second most common pathway of vulvar SCC development accounting for approximately 40% of cases. It is known as usual or classical pathway and it is associated with high-risk human papilloma virus (HPV) infection, often HPV-16. This form of vulvar intraepithelial lesion differs immunohistochemically from the differentiated pathway due to the absence of p53 overexpression. Conversely, p16 is characteristically diffuse and strongly expressed in basal and parabasal layers of the squamous epithelium (**Figure 3.72**). Discontinuous or patchy nuclear and cytoplasmic staining is considered non-specific.

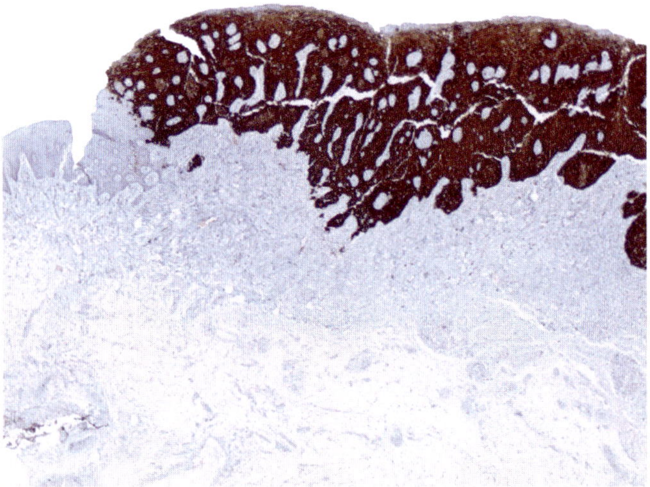

Figure 3.72 Widespread p16 overexpression in the invasive HPV-related squamous cell carcinoma and in the adjacent areas of high-grade intraepithelial neoplasia.

Case 3.5

Case history: A 75-year-old woman presented with an indurated verrucous lesion on her vulva. The surrounding tissue exhibited a lichenified appearance with thickening and hyperkeratosis. Focally, there were slightly papillomatous changes.

Description: The biopsy shows (**Figure 3.73**) different degrees of epithelial acanthosis with a pale hue, prominent hyperkeratosis and focal papillomatosis. The thickest area has tumoral aspect and endophytic growth with bulbous silhouette. A second sample (**Figure 3.74**) from a separate area of involvement presented similar features in the epithelium but lacked the endophytic component. In both specimens there was a lack of cytological atypia, p16 was negative and p53 showed mild expression in scattered cells consistent with a wild-type pattern (**Figure 3.75**).

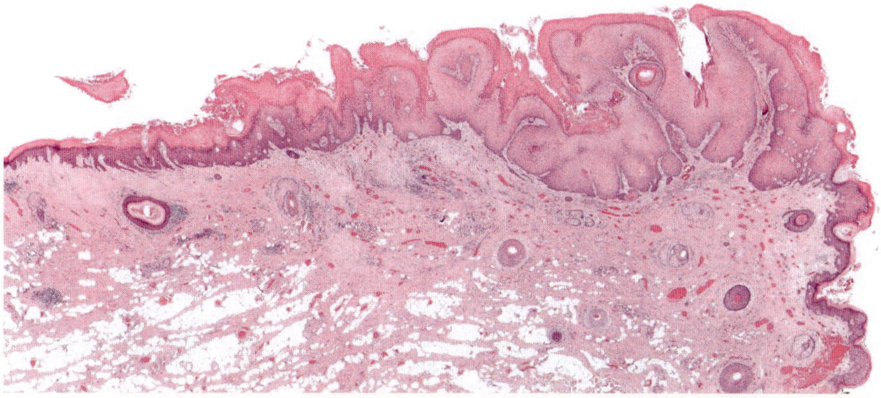

Figure 3.73 A well-differentiated squamous proliferation consistent with a verrucous squamous cell carcinoma.

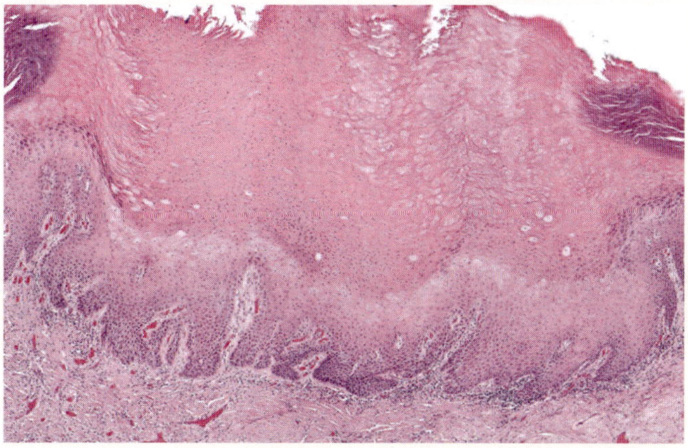

Figure 3.74 Area exhibiting features of verruciform acanthotic vulvar intraepithelial neoplasia.

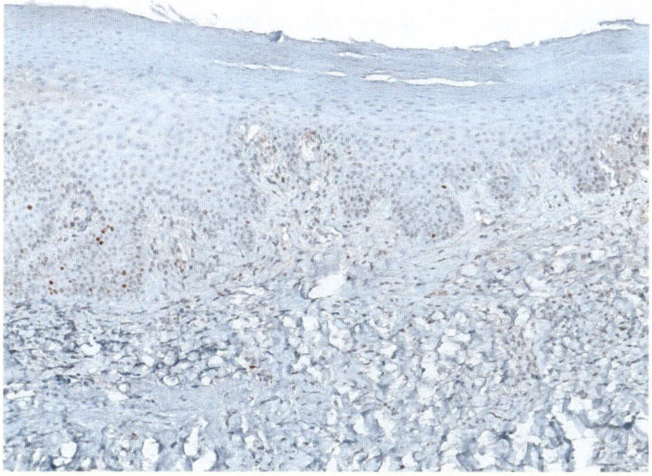

Figure 3.75 Only occasional basal keratinocytes express p53 supportive of a wildtype p53 staining pattern.

Diagnosis: Verrucous carcinoma developed in verruciform acanthotic VIN (vaVIN).

Discussion: This highly differentiated squamous proliferation with endophytic bulbous growth corresponds to the periphery of a verrucous SCC (**Figure 3.73**). The mucosal surface at the tumor edges and a second specimen from a distant area (**Figure 3.74**) exhibit acanthosis with a thick layer of hyperkeratosis large and pale keratinocytes lacking nuclear atypia. Immunohistochemically, these areas tested negative for p16 and showed mild p53 expression in scattered cells, indicative of a wild-type pattern (**Figure 3.75**). These features together support the diagnosis of verrucous SCC developed on vulvar intraepithelial neoplasia (vaVIN), which displays an increased propensity for this SCC variant compared to other SCC precursors.

Case 3.6

Case history: An 80-year-old man presented with a 3.9 cm exophytic mass on the penile foreskin and glans (**Figure 3.76**).

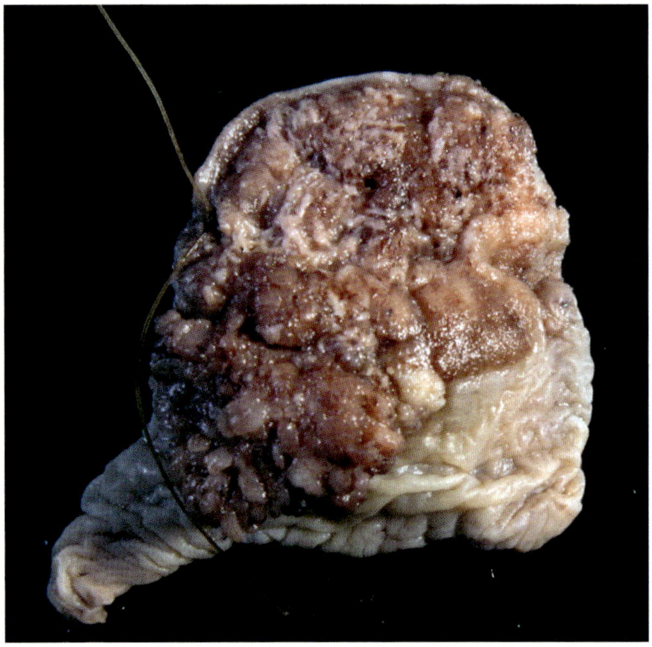

Figure 3.76 Gross photo showing a penile excision/circumcision containing a 3.9 cm × 3.5 cm tan-red exophytic and papillary tumor with ulceration located on the foreskin and penile glans.

Description: Histologic sections show an exophytic and superficially infiltrative carcinoma (**Figure 3.77**). The surface is predominantly verruciform with malignant koilocytosis (**Figure 3.78**). There is a jagged interface between the tumor and stroma with areas displaying more nuclear pleomorphism and malignant koilocytosis (top-left), islands with basaloid morphology (top-right) and infiltrating nests of tumor cells (center) (**Figure 3.79**). The tumor cells are strongly positive for p16 (**Figure 3.80**) and HPV 16/18 by *in situ* hybridization (**Figure 3.81**).

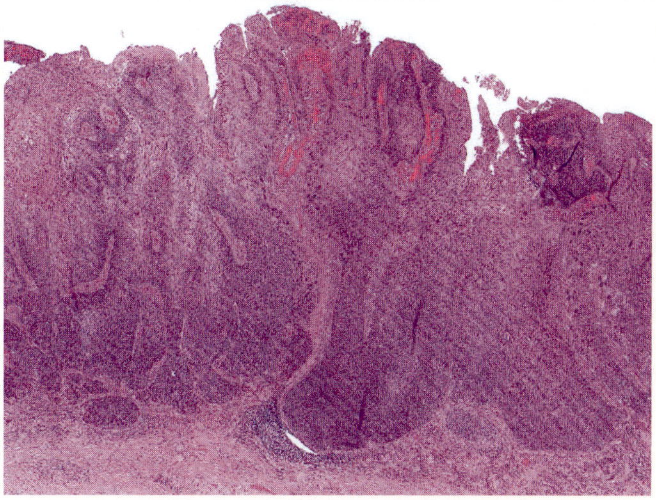

Figure 3.77 A verruciform and exophytic carcinoma is seen with superficial involvement of the subepithelial tissue (X40).

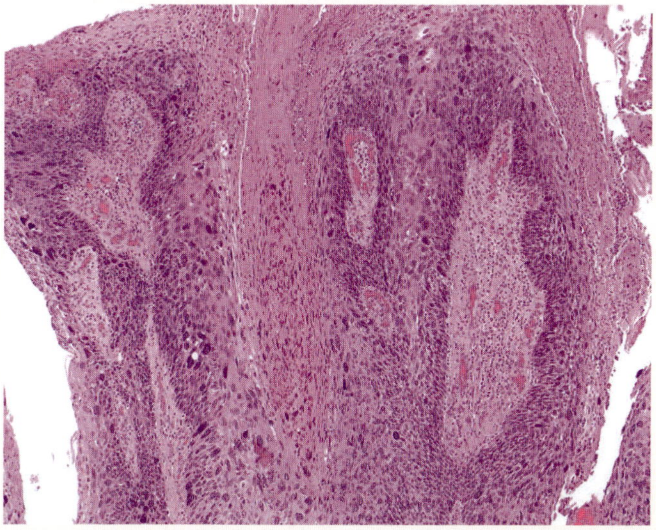

Figure 3.78 Condylomatous papillae lined by malignant koilocytosis (X100).

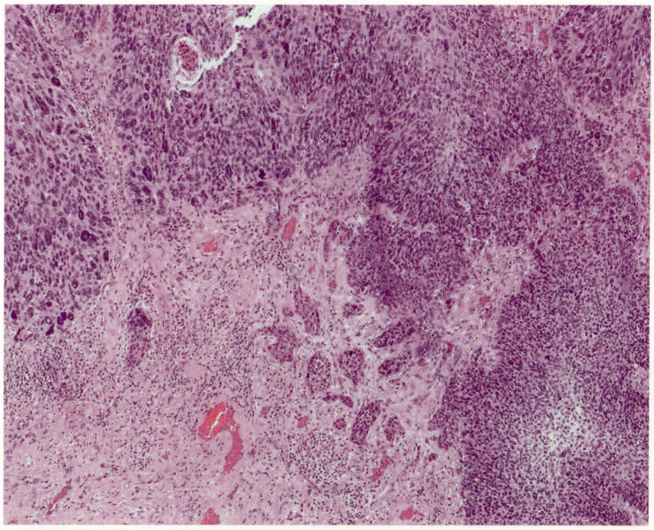

Figure 3.79 An invasive jagged interface between tumor and stroma showing foci of superficial invasion in the center, a warty component with easily identifiable malignant koilocytosis on the top left and a basaloid component with islands of monotonous tumor cells on the top right, supporting a mixed warty-basaloid subtype.

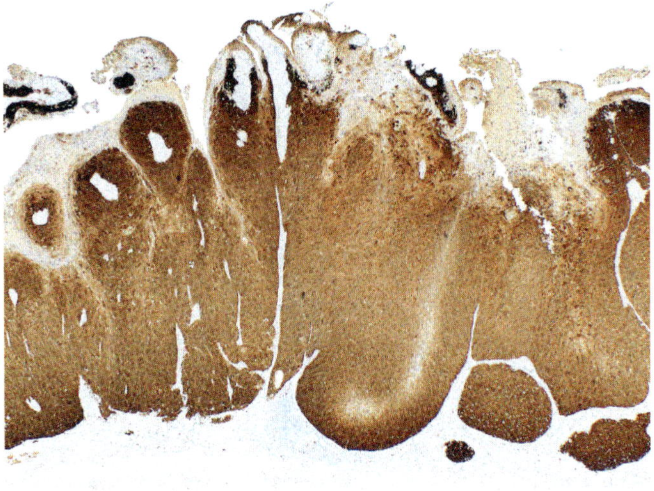

Figure 3.80 Strong diffuse, block-like positivity for p16 (X40).

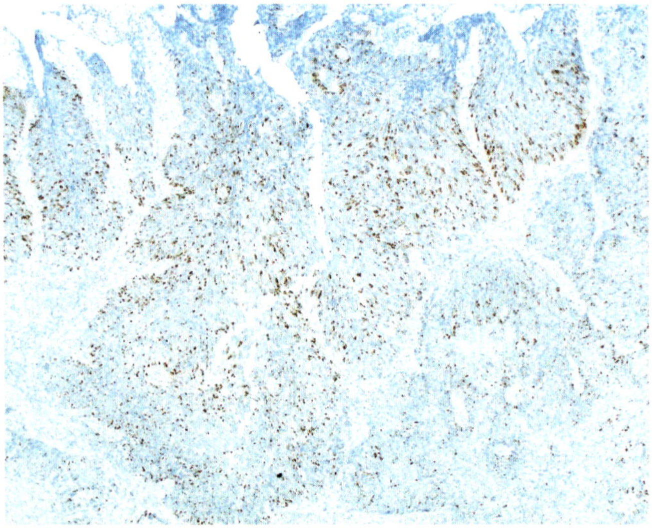

Figure 3.81 High-risk-HPV (16/18) positivity by *in situ* hybridization (X100).

Diagnosis: Penile squamous cell carcinoma, HPV-associated, warty-basaloid subtype.

Discussion: Due to the mixed patterns of verruciform areas with malignant koilocytosis and islands of more monotonous basaloid cells with superficial invasion, this is most consistent with a warty-basaloid PSCC. The presence of diffuse, block-like staining for p16 and presence of HR-HPV by ISH confirms the diagnosis of an HPV-associated PSCC.

References

1. Kim K, Kim JW, Santos I, Oakley A. Body site locations of basal cell carcinoma, squamous cell carcinoma and actinic keratosis in patients referred to the Waikato District Health Board teledermoscopy clinic. *J Prim Health Care* 2022; **14**: 80–6.
2. Cassarino DS, Derienzo DP, Barr RJ. Cutaneous squamous cell carcinoma: a comprehensive clinicopathologic classification. Part one. *J Cutan Pathol* 2006; **33**: 191–206.
3. Ross AS, Whalen FM, Elenitsas R, Xu X, Troxel AB, Schmults CD. Diameter of involved nerves predicts outcomes in cutaneous squamous cell carcinoma with perineural invasion: an investigator-blinded retrospective cohort study. *Dermatol Surg* 2009; **35**: 1859–66.
4. Henderson SA, Torres-Cabala CA, Curry JL, et al. p40 is more specific than p63 for the distinction of atypical

fibroxanthoma from other cutaneous spindle cell malignancies. *Am J Surg Pathol* 2014; **38**: 1102–10.

5. Sigel JE, Skacel M, Bergfeld WF, House NS, Rabkin MS, Goldblum JR. The utility of cytokeratin 5/6 in the recognition of cutaneous spindle cell squamous cell carcinoma. *J Cutan Pathol* 2001; **28**: 520–4.
6. Mahalingam M, Richards JE, Selim MA, Muzikansky A, Hoang MP. An immunohistochemical comparison of cytokeratin 7, cytokeratin 15, cytokeratin 19, CAM5.2, carcinoembryonic antigen, and nestin in differentiating porocarcinoma from squamous cell carcinoma. *Hum Pathol* 2012; **43**: 1265–72.
7. Heyderman E, Graham RM, Chapman DV, Richardson TC, McKee PH. Epithelial markers in primary skin cancer: an immunoperoxidase study of the distribution of epithelial membrane antigen (EMA) and carcinoembryonic antigen (CEA) in 65 primary skin carcinomas. *Histopathology* 1984; **8**: 423–34.
8. Beer TW, Shepherd P, Theaker JM. Ber-EP4 and epithelial membrane antigen aid distinction of basal cell, squamous cell and basosquamous carcinomas of the skin. *Histopathology* 2000; **37**: 218–23.
9. Hoang MP, Dresser KA, Kapur P, High WA, Mahalingam M. Microcystic adnexal carcinoma: an immunohistochemical reappraisal. *Mod Pathol* 2008; **21**: 178–85.
10. Fan YS, Carr RA, Sanders DS, Smith AP, Lazar AJ, Calonje E. Characteristic Ber-EP4 and EMA expression in sebaceoma is immunohistochemically distinct from basal cell carcinoma. *Histopathology* 2007; **51**: 80–6.
11. Swanson PE, Fitzpatrick MM, Ritter JH, Glusac EJ, Wick MR. Immunohistologic differential diagnosis of basal cell carcinoma, squamous cell carcinoma, and trichoepithelioma in small cutaneous biopsy specimens. *J Cutan Pathol* 1998; **25**: 153–9.
12. Pham TT, Selim MA, Burchette JL Jr, Madden J, Turner J, Herman C. CD10 expression in trichoepithelioma and basal cell carcinoma. *J Cutan Pathol* 2006; **33**: 123–8.
13. Linskey KR, Gimbel DC, Zukerberg LR, Duncan LM, Sadow PM, Nazarian RM. BerEp4, cytokeratin 14, and cytokeratin 17 immunohistochemical staining aid in differentiation of basaloid squamous cell carcinoma from basal cell carcinoma with squamous metaplasia. *Arch Pathol Lab Med* 2013; **137**: 1591–8.
14. Tope WD, Nowfar-Rad M, Kist DA. Ber-EP4-positive phenotype differentiates actinic keratosis from superficial basal cell carcinoma. *Dermatol Surg* 2000; **26**: 415–18.
15. Yu L, Galan A, McNiff JM. Caveats in BerEP4 staining to differentiate basal and squamous cell carcinoma. *J Cutan Pathol* 2009; **36**: 1074–6.
16. Wagnoner J, Keehn C, Morgan MB. CD-10 immunostaining differentiates superficial basal cell carcinoma from cutaneous squamous cell carcinoma. *Am J Dermatopathol* 2007; **29**: 555–8.
17. Shields JA, Demirici H, Marr BP, Eagle RC Jr, Shields CL. Sebaceous carcinoma of the ocular region: a review. *Surv Ophthalmol* 2005; **50**: 103–22.
18. Asadi-Amoli F, Khoshnevis F, Haeri H, Jahanzad I, Pazira R, Shahsiah R. Comparative examination of androgen receptor reactivity for differential diagnosis of sebaceous carcinoma from squamous cell and basal cell carcinoma. *Am J Clin Pathol* 2010; **134**: 22–6.
19. Ostler DA, Prieto VG, Reed JA, Deavers MT, Lazar AJ, Ivan D. Adipophilin expression in sebaceous tumors and other cutaneous lesions with clear cell histology: an immunohistochemical study of 117 cases. *Mod Pathol* 2010; **23**: 567–73.
20. Sramek B, Lisle A, Loy T. Immunohistochemistry in ocular carcinomas. *J Cutan Pathol* 2008; **35**: 641–6.
21. Boussahmain C, Mochel MC, Hoang MP. Perilipin and adipophilin expression in sebaceous carcinoma and mimics. *Hum Pathol* 2013; **44**: 1811–16.
22. Bourlond F, Velter C, Cribier B. Androgen receptor expression in epidermal and adnexal tumours. *Ann Dermatol Venereol* 2021; **148**: 116–21.
23. Ansai S, Arase S, Kawana S, Kimura T. Immunohistochemical findings of sebaceous carcinoma and sebaceoma: retrieval of cytokeratin expression by a panel of anti-cytokeratin monoclonal antibodies. *J Dermatol* 2011; **38**: 951–8.
24. Oules B, Deschamps L, Sohier P, et al. Diagnostic accuracy of GATA6 immunostaining in sebaceous tumors of the skin. *Mod Pathol* 2023; **36**: 100101. doi: 10.1016/j.modpat.2023.100101.
25. Mittal R, Araujo I, Czanner G, Coupland SE. Perforin expression in eyelid sebaceous carcinomas: a useful and specific immunomarker for the differential diagnosis of eyelid carcinomas. *Acta Opthalmol* 2016; **94**: e325-30. doi: 10.1111/aos.12972.
26. Ng JKM, Choi PCL, Chow C, et al. PRAME immunostain expression in sebaceous lesions, cutaneous carcinomas and adnexal structures. *Pathology* 2022; 54: 721–8.
27. Gradecki SE, Eid MV, Pramoonjago P, Wick MR. Glioma-associated oncogene-1 expression in basal cell carcinoma and its histologic mimics. *Am J Dermatopathol* 2021; **43**: 637–41.
28. Robson A, Greene J, Ansari N, et al. Eccrine porocarcinoma (malignant eccrine poroma): a clinicopathologic study of 69 cases. *Am J Surg Pathol* 2001; **25**: 710–20.
29. Goh SGN, Dayrit JF, Calonje E. Sarcomatoid eccrine porocarcinoma: report of two cases and a review of the literature. *J Cutan Pathol* 2007; **34**: 55–60.
30. Qureshi HS, Ormsby A, Lee MW, Zarbo RJ, Ma CK. The diagnostic utility of p63, CK5/6, CK7 and CK20 in distinguishing primary cutaneous adnexal neoplasms from metastatic carcinomas. *J Cutan Pathol* 2004; **31**: 145–52.
31. Pulitzer M, Desman G, Busam KJ. CK7 expression in primary cutaneous squamous cell carcinoma. *J Cutan Pathol* 2010; **37**: 966–72.
32. Mahalingam M, Nguyen LP, Richards JE, Muzikansky A, Hoang MP. The diagnostic utility of immunohistochemistry in distinguishing primary skin adnexal carcinomas from metastatic adenocarcinoma to skin: an immunohistochemical reappraisal using cytokeratin 15, nestin, p63, D2-40, and calretinin. *Mod Pathol* 2010; **23**: 713–19.
33. Kurokawa I, Urakawa Y, Senba Y, et al. Keratin profiles may differ between intraepidermal and intradermal invasive eccrine porocarcinoma. *Oncol Rep* 2006; **16**: 473–7.
34. Chen S, Takahara M, Kido M, et al. Increased expression of an epidermal stem cell marker, cytokeratin 19, in cutaneous squamous cell carcinoma. *Br J Dermatol* 2008; **159**: 952–5.

35. Yada K, Kashima K, Daa T, Kitano S, Fujiwara S, Yokoyama S. Expression of CD10 in basal cell carcinoma. *Am J Dermatopathol* 2004; **26**: 463–71.
36. Lee JJ, Mochel MC, Piris A, Boussahmain C, Mahalingam M, Hoang MP. p40 exhibits better specificity than p63 in distinguishing primary skin adnexal carcinomas from cutaneous metastases. *Hum Pathol* 2014; **45**: 1078–83.
37. Afshar M, Deroide F, Robson A. BerEP4 is widely expressed in tumors of the sweat apparatus: a source of potential diagnostic error. *J Cutan Pathol* 2013; **40**: 259–64.
38. Goto K, Ishikawa M, Hamada K, et al. Comparison of immunohistochemical expression of cytokeratin 19, c-KIT, BerEP4, GATA3, and NUTM1 between porocarcinoma and squamous cell carcinoma. *Am J Dermatopathol* 2021; **43**: 781–7.
39. Macagno N, Kervarrec T, Sohier P, et al. NUT is a specific immunohistochemical marker for the diagnosis of YAP1-NUTM1-rearranged cutaneous poroid neoplasms. *Am J Surg Pathol* 2021; **45**: 1221–7.
40. Miura K, Akashi T, Namiki T, et al. Engrailed homeobox 1 and cytokeratin 19 are independent diagnostic markers of eccrine porocarcinoma and distinguish it from squamous cell carcinoma. *Am J Clin Pathol* 2020; **154**: 499–509.
41. Russell-Goldman E, Hornick JL, Hanna J. Utility of YAP1 and NUT immunohistochemistry in the diagnosis of porocarcinoma. *J Cutan Pathol* 2021; **48**: 403–10.
42. Sekine S, Kiyono T, Ryo E, et al. Recurrent YAP1-MAML2 and YAP1-NUTM1 fusions in poroma and porocarcinoma. *J Clin Invest* 2019; **129**: 3827–32.
43. Folpe AL, Cooper K. Best practices in diagnostic immunohistochemistry: pleomorphic cutaneous spindle cell tumors. *Arch Pathol Lab Med* 2007; **131**: 1517–24.
44. Ko CJ, McNiff JM, Glusac EJ. Squamous cell carcinoma with single cell infiltration: a potential diagnostic pitfall and the utility of MNF116 and p63. *J Cutan Pathol* 2008; **35**: 353–7.
45. Bishop JA, Montgomery EA, Westra WH. Use of p40 and p63 immunohistochemistry and human papillomavirus testing as ancillary tools for the recognition of head and neck sarcomatoid carcinoma and its distinction from benign and malignant mesenchymal processes. *Am J Surg Pathol* 2014; **38**: 257–64.
46. Miettinen M, McCue PA, Sariomo-Rikala M, et al. Sox-10 – a marker for not only schwannian and melanocytic neoplasms but also myoepithelial cell tumors of soft tissue: a systematic analysis of 5134 tumors. *Am J Surg Pathol* 2015; **39**: 826–35.
47. Hultgren TL, DiMaio DJ. Immunohistochemical staining of CD10 in atypical fibroxanthomas. *J Cutan Pathol* 2007; **34**: 415–19.
48. Mirza B, Weedon D. Atypical fibroxanthoma: a clinicopathological study of 89 cases. *Australas J Dermatol* 2005; **46**: 235–8.
49. Luzar B, Calonje E. Morphological and immunohistochemical characteristics of atypical fibroxanthoma with a special emphasis on potential diagnostic pitfalls: a review. *J Cutan Pathol* 2010; **37**: 301–9.
50. Szczepanski JM, Siddiqui J, Patel RM, Harms PW, Hrycaj SM, Chan MP. Expression of SATB2 in primary cutaneous sarcomatoid neoplasms: a potential diagnostic pitfall. *Pathology* 2023; **55**: 350–4.
51. Ha Lan TT, Chen SJT, Arps DP, et al. Expression of the p40 isoform of p63 has high specificity for cutaneous sarcomatoid squamous cell carcinoma. *J Cutan Pathol* 2014; **41**: 831–8.
52. Chokoeva AA, Tchernev G, Cardoso JC, et al. Vulvar sarcomas: Short guideline for histopathological recognition and clinical management. Part 1. *Int J Immunopathol Pharmacol* 2015; **28**: 168–77.
53. Costa LC, Leite C, Cardoso S, et al. Expression of epithelial-mesenchymal transition markers at the invasive front of oral squamous cell carcinoma. *J Appl Oral Sci* 2015; **23**: 169–78.
54. Mentzel T, Requena L, Kaddu S, et al. Cutaneous myoepithelial neoplasms: clinicopathologic and immunohistochemical study of 20 cases suggesting a continuous spectrum ranging from benign mixed tumor of the skin to cutaneous myoepithelioma and myoepithelial carcinoma. *J Cutan Pathol* 2003; **30**: 294–302.
55. Hornick JL, Fletcher CD. Myoepithelial tumors of soft tissue: a clinicopathologic and immunohistochemical study of 101 cases with evaluation of prognostic parameters. *Am J Surg Pathol* 2003; **27**: 1183–96.
56. Folpe AL, Schoolmeester JK, McCluggage WG, et al. SMARCB1-deficient vulvar neoplasms: a clinicopathologic, immunohistochemical, and molecular genetic study of 14 cases. *Am J Surg Pathol* 2015; **39**: 836–49.
57. Watanabe S, Ichikawa E, Takahashi H, Otsuka F. Changes of cytokeratin and involucrin expression in squamous cell carcinomas of the skin during progression to malignancy. *Br J Dermatol* 1995; **132**: 730–9.
58. Reddi DM, Puri PK. Expression of focal TTF-1 expression in a case of CK7/CK20-positive Merkel cell carcinoma. *J Cutan Pathol* 2013; **40**: 431–3.
59. Karpinski P, Mendez-Pena JE, Wu C-L, et al. POU4F3 is a sensitive and specific marker of Merkel cell carcinoma. *Mod Pathol* 2025; 38: 100627. doi: 10.1016/j.modpat.2024.100627 .
60. Kurokawa M, Nabeshima K, Akiyama Y, et al. CD56: a useful marker for diagnosing Merkel cell carcinoma. *J Dermatol Sci* 2003; **31**: 219–24.
61. Fernández-Figueras MT, Puig L, Musulén E, et al. Expression profiles associated with aggressive behavior in Merkel cell carcinoma. *Mod Pathol* 2007; **20**: 90–101.
62. McCalmont TH. Paranuclear dots of neurofilament reliably identify Merkel cell carcinoma. *J Cutan Pathol* 2010; **37**: 821–3.
63. Wong SQ, Waldeck K, Vergara IA, et al. UV-associated mutations underlie the etiology of MCV-negative Merkel cell carcinomas. *Cancer Res* 2015; **75**: 5228–34.
64. Molina-Ruiz AM, Santonja C, Rütten A, Cerroni L, Kutzner H, Requena L. Immunohistochemistry in the diagnosis of cutaneous viral infections- part II: cutaneous viral infections by parvoviruses, poxviruses, paramyxoviridae, picornaviridae, retroviruses and filoviruses. *Am J Dermatopathol* 2015; **37**: 93–106.
65. Requena L, Kutzner H, Palmedo G, et al. Cutaneous involvement in multiple myeloma: a clinicopathologic, immunohistochemical, and cytogenetic study of 8 cases. *Arch Dermatol* 2003; **139**: 475–86.

66. Robson A, Shukur Z, Ally M, et al. Immunocytochemical p63 expression discriminates between primary cutaneous follicle centre cell and diffuse large B-cell lymphoma-leg type, and is of the TAp63 isoform. *Histopathology* 2016; **69**: 11–19.

67. Schneider M, Crimmins J, Selim A. An etiology-focused overview of vulvar and penile squamous cell carcinoma and its precursors: similarities, differences and emerging concepts. *Diagn Histopathol* 2024; **30**: 1–14.

68. Jenkins TM, Mills AM. Putative precancerous lesions of vulvar squamous cell carcinoma. *Semin Diagn Pathol* 2021; **38**: 27–36.

69. Parra-Herran C, Nucci MR, Singh N, et al. HPV-independent, p53-wild-type vulvar intraepithelial neoplasia: a review of nomenclature and the journey to characterize verruciform and acanthotic precursor lesions of the vulva. *Mod Pathol* 2022; **35**: 1317–26.

70. Akbari A, Pinto A, Amemiya Y, Seth A, Mirkovic J, Parra-Herran C. Differentiated exophytic vulvar intraepithelial lesion: Clinicopathologic and molecular analysis documenting its relationship with verrucous carcinoma of the vulva. *Mod Pathol* 2020; **33**: 2011–18.

71. Rakislova N, Alemany L, Clavero O, et al. HPV independent precursors mimicking high-grade squamous intraepithelial lesions (HSIL) of the vulva. *Am J Surg Pathol* 2020; **44**: 1506–14.

72. Yang H, Almadani N, Thompson EF, et al. Classification of vulvar squamous cell carcinoma and precursor lesions by p16 and p53 immunohistochemistry: considerations, caveats, and an algorithmic approach. *Mod Pathol* 2023; **36**: 100–45.

73. Rakislova N, Alemany L, Clavero O, et al. Differentiated vulvar intraepithelial neoplasia-like and lichen sclerosus-like lesions in HPV-associated squamous cell carcinomas of the vulva. *Am J Surg Pathol* 2018; **42**: 828–35.

74. Graham RP, Arnold CA, Naini BV, Lam-Himlin DM. Basaloid squamous cell carcinoma of the anus revisited. *Am J Surg Pathol* 2016; **40**: 354–60.

75. Gillespie JJ, MacKay B. Histogenesis of cloacogenic carcinoma. Fine structure of anal transitional epithelium and cloacogenic carcinoma. *Hum Pathol* 1978; **9**: 579–87.

76. WHO Classification of Tumours Editorial Board. Digestive system tumours. Lyon (France): International Agency for Research on Cancer; 2019. (WHO classification of tumours series, 5th ed.; vol. 1). https://publications.iarc.fr/579.

77. Zhu X, Jamshed S, Zou J, et al. Molecular and immunophenotypic characterization of anal squamous cell carcinoma reveals distinct clinicopathologic groups associated with HPV and TP53 mutation status. *Mod Pathol* 2021; **34**: 1017–30.

78. Patil DT, Goldblum JR, Billings SD. Clinicopathological analysis of basal cell carcinoma of the anal region and its distinction from basaloid squamous cell carcinoma. *Mod Pathol* 2013; **26**: 1382–9.

79. Patil DT, Yang B. Utility of human papillomavirus capsid protein L1 and p16 in the assessment and accurate classification of anal squamous intraepithelial lesions. *Am J Clin Pathol* 2015; **144**: 113–21.

80. Kazakov DV, Spagnolo DV, Kacerovska D, Michal M. Lesions of anogenital mammary-like glands: an update. *Adv Anat Pathol* 2011; **18**: 1–28.

81. Roberts JM, Cornall AM, Ekman D, et al. Papillary immature metaplasia of the anal canal: a low-grade lesion that can mimic a high-grade lesion. *Am J Surg Pathol* 2016; **40**: 348–53.

82. Bartoš V. Expression of p16 protein in cutaneous basal cell carcinoma: still far from being clearly understood. *Acta Dermatovenerol Croat* 2020; **28**: 43–4.

83. Heller DS, Day T, Allbritton JI, et al. Diagnostic criteria for differentiated vulvar intraepithelial neoplasia and vulvar aberrant maturation. *J Low Genit Tract Dis* 2021; **25**: 57–70.

84. Madahian S, Judelson R, Zhu X, et al. CD56 expression in basaloid anal squamous cell carcinoma – A potential diagnostic pitfall. *Ann Diagn Pathol* 2021; **53**: 151758. doi: 10.1016/j.anndiagpath.2021.151758.

85. George E, Swanson PE, Wick MR. Neuroendocrine differentiation in basal cell carcinoma: an immunohistochemical study. *Am J Dermatopathol* 1989; **11**: 131–5.

86. Lilo MT, Chen Y, LeBlanc RE. INSM1 is more sensitive and interpretable than conventional immunohistochemical stains used to diagnose Merkel cell carcinoma. *Am J Surg Pathol* 2018; **42**: 1541–8.

87. van Wyk AC, Moolla Z, Motala AI, et al. Merkel cell carcinoma of the anorectum: a case report and review of the literature. *Clin J Gastroenterol* 2022; **15**: 740–5.

88. Chetty R, Serra S, Hsieh E. Basaloid squamous carcinoma of the anal canal with an adenoid cystic pattern: histologic and immunohistochemical reappraisal of an unusual variant. *Am J Surg Pathol* 2005; **29**: 1668–72.

89. WHO Classification of Tumours Editorial Board. Skin tumours [Internet; beta version ahead of print]. Lyon (France): International Agency for Research on Cancer; 2023. (WHO classification of tumours series, 5th ed.; vol. 12). Available from: https://tumourclassification.iarc.who.int/chapters/64.

90. Boyd AS, Stasko TS, Tang YW. Basaloid squamous cell carcinoma of the skin. *J Am Acad Dermatol* 2011; **64**: 144–51.

91. Vu TT, Soong L, Hung T, Fiorillo L, Joseph K. Cutaneous HPV16 and p16 positive basaloid squamous cell carcinoma with brain metastasis: a case report. *SAGE Open Med Case Rep* 2020; **8**: 2050313X20935260.

92. Kurman RJ, Toki T, Schiffman MH. Basaloid and warty carcinomas of the vulva. Distinctive types of squamous cell carcinoma frequently associated with human papillomaviruses. *Am J Surg Pathol* 1993; **17**: 133–45.

93. McCluggage WG, editor. Chapter XI. Tumours of the vulva. In: WHO Classification of Tumours Editorial Board. Female genital tumours. Lyon (France): International Agency for Research on Cancer; 2020. pp.419-434(WHO classification of tumours series, 5th ed.; vol. 4).

94. Serota AI, Weil M, Williams RA, Wollman JS, Wilson SE. Anal cloacogenic carcinoma: classification and clinical behavior. *Arch Surg* 1981; **116**: 456–9.

95. Bigby SM, Eva LJ, Tous S, et al. Prevaccine human papillomavirus status in invasive and intraepithelial lesions of the vulva in New Zealand women. *J Low Genit Tract Dis* 2022; **26**: 323–7.

96. Quick CM. 2 – Squamous Neoplasms of the Vulva. In: Nucci MR, Parra-Herran C, editors. Gynecologic Pathology (Second Edition) [Internet]. Philadelphia: Elsevier; 2020 [cited

2024 Apr 27]. p. 47–70. (Foundations in Diagnostic Pathology). Available from: www.sciencedirect.com/science/article/pii/B9780323359092000023

97. Maniar KP, Nayar R. HPV-related squamous neoplasia of the lower anogenital tract: an update and review of recent guidelines. *Adv Anat Pathol* 2014; **21**: 341–58.

98. Darragh TM, Colgan TJ, Thomas Cox J, et al. The lower anogenital squamous terminology standardization project for HPV-associated lesions: background and consensus recommendations from the College of American Pathologists and the American Society for Colposcopy and Cervical Pathology. *Int J Gynecol Pathol* 2013; **32**: 76–115.

99. Stewart CJR, Crook ML. Fascin and cyclin D1 immunoreactivity in non-neoplastic vulvar squamous epithelium, vulvar intraepithelial neoplasia and invasive squamous carcinoma: correlation with Ki67 and p16 protein expression. *J Clin Pathol* 2014; **67**: 319–25.

100. Pirog EC. Immunohistochemistry and in situ hybridization for the diagnosis and classification of squamous lesions of the anogenital region. *Semin Diagn Pathol* 2015; **32**: 409–18.

101. Ungureanu C, Socolov DG, Anton G, et al. Role of ProEx C immunocytochemistry in cervical high-grade squamous intraepithelial lesions detection. *Rom J Morphol Embryol* 2021; **62**: 1029–34.

102. Travé G, Zanier K. HPV-mediated inactivation of tumor suppressor p53. *Cell Cycle* 2016; **15**: 2231–2.

103. Maniar KP, Sanchez B, Paintal A, Gursel DB, Nayar R. Role of the biomarker p16 in downgrading -IN2 diagnoses and predicting higher-grade lesions. *Am J Surg Pathol* 2015; **39**: 1708–18.

104. Dong F, Kojiro S, Borger DR, Growdon WB, Oliva E. Squamous cell carcinoma of the vulva: a subclassification of 97 cases by clinicopathologic, immunohistochemical, and molecular features (p16, p53, and EGFR). *Am J Surg Pathol* 2015; **39**: 1045–53.

105. Carreras-Dieguez N, Saco A, Del Pino M, et al. Vulvar squamous cell carcinoma arising on human papillomavirus-independent precursors mimicking high-grade squamous intra-epithelial lesion: a distinct and highly recurrent subtype of vulvar cancer. *Histopathology* 2023; **82**: 731–44.

106. Dongre HN, Elnour R, Tornaas S, et al. TP53 mutation and human papilloma virus status as independent prognostic factors in a Norwegian cohort of vulva squamous cell carcinoma. *Acta Obstet Gynecol Scand* 2024; **103**: 165–75.

107. Sah SP, McCluggage WG. Florid vulval Paget disease exhibiting p16 immunoreactivity and mimicking classic VIN. *Int J Gynecol Pathol* 2013; **32**: 221–7.

108. Dasgupta S, Ewing-Graham PC, van Kemenade FJ, van Doorn HC, Noordhoek Hegt V, Koljenović S. Differentiated vulvar intraepithelial neoplasia (dVIN): the most helpful histological features and the utility of cytokeratins 13 and 17. *Virchows Arch* 2018; **473**: 739–47.

109. Dasgupta S, Ewing-Graham PC, Swagemakers SMA, et al. Precursor lesions of vulvar squamous cell carcinoma – histology and biomarkers: A systematic review. *Crit Rev Oncol Hematol* 2020; **147**: 102866. doi: 10.1016/j.critrevonc.2020.102866.

110. Singh N, Leen SL, Han G, et al. Expanding the morphologic spectrum of differentiated VIN (dVIN) through detailed mapping of cases with p53 loss. *Am J Surg Pathol* 2015; **39**: 52–60.

111. Tessier-Cloutier B, Kortekaas KE, Thompson E, et al. Major p53 immunohistochemical patterns in in situ and invasive squamous cell carcinomas of the vulva and correlation with TP53 mutation status. *Mod Pathol* 2020; **33**: 1595–605.

112. Thompson EF, Wong RWC, Trevisan G, et al. p53-abnormal "fields of dysplasia" in human papillomavirus-independent vulvar squamous cell carcinoma impacts margins and recurrence risk. *Mod Pathol* 2023 Feb; **36**(2): 100010. doi: 10.1016/j.modpat.2022.100010.

113. McMullen-Tabry ER, Schechter SA, Wang GY, et al. p53/CK17 dual stain improves accuracy of distinction between differentiated vulvar intraepithelial neoplasia and its mimics. *Int J Gynecol Pathol* 2022; **41**: 298–306.

114. Dasgupta S, Koljenović S, van den Bosch TPP, et al. Evaluation of immunohistochemical markers, CK17 and SOX2, as adjuncts to p53 for the diagnosis of differentiated vulvar intraepithelial neoplasia (dVIN). *Pharmaceuticals* 2021; **14**: 324. doi: 10.3390/ph14040324.

115. Roberts JNT, Bentz JL, LeBlanc RE, Cass I. Correlation of histopathologic findings with clinical predictors of disease recurrence and progression to vulvar carcinoma in patients with differentiated vulvar intraepithelial neoplasia (dVIN). *Gynecol Oncol Rep* 2024; **52**: 101358. doi: 10.1016/j.gore.2024.101358.

116. Cook E, Van de Vijver K, Parra-Herran C. Diagnosis of verruciform acanthotic vulvar intra-epithelial neoplasia (vaVIN) using CK17, SOX2 and GATA3 immunohistochemistry. *Histopathology* 2024; **84**: 1212–23.

117. Zare SY, Fard EV, Fadare O. GATA3 immunohistochemistry as a diagnostic adjunct for differentiated vulvar intraepithelial neoplasia: utility and limitations. *Hum Pathol* 2023; **139**: 55–64.

118. Carreras-Dieguez N, Saco A, Del Pino M, et al. Human papillomavirus and p53 status define three types of vulvar squamous cell carcinomas with distinct clinical, pathological, and prognostic features. *Histopathology* 2023; **83**: 17–30.

119. Nascimento AF, Granter SR, Cviko A, Yuan L, Hecht JL, Crum CP. Vulvar acanthosis with altered differentiation: a precursor to verrucous carcinoma? *Am J Surg Pathol* 2004; **28**: 638–43.

120. Roy SF, Wong J, Le Page C, et al. DEVIL, VAAD and vLSC constitute a spectrum of HPV-independent, p53-independent intra-epithelial neoplasia of the vulva. *Histopathology* 2021; **79**: 975–88.

121. De Luca DA, Papara C, Vorobyev A, et al. Lichen sclerosus: The 2023 update. *Front Med* 2023; **10**: 1106318. doi: 10.3389/fmed.2023.1106318.

122. Gleue CA, Xie F, Deschaine M, et al. Differential proteomic expression in indolent vulvar lichen sclerosus, transforming vulvar lichen sclerosus and normal vulvar tissue. *Exp Dermatol* 2022; **31**: 1920–6.

123. Chaudhari AS, McFadden JR, Bentz J, Evans RH, Selim MA, Sriharan A. A mimicker of differentiated vulvar intraepithelial neoplasia: reactive atypia from noncompliance with lichen sclerosus therapy. *Am J Dermatopathol* 2024; **46**: 519–22.

124. Liegl B, Regauer S. p53 immunostaining in lichen sclerosus is related to ischaemic stress and is

not a marker of differentiated vulvar intraepithelial neoplasia (d-VIN). *Histopathology* 2006; **48**: 268–74.

125. Lee ES, Allen D, Scurry J. Pseudoepitheliomatous hyperplasia in lichen sclerosus of the vulva. *Int J Gynecol Pathol* 2003; **22**: 57–62.

126. Rakislova N, Carreras-Dieguez N, Manzotti C, et al. Differential etiopathogenic features of vulvar squamous cell carcinomas in sub-Saharan Africa and Europe. *Int J Cancer* 2023; **152**: 496–503.

127. Proctor L, Hoang L, Moore J, et al. Association of human papilloma virus status and response to radiotherapy in vulvar squamous cell carcinoma. *Int J Gynecol Cancer* 2020; **30**: 100–6.

128. Rakislova N, Alemany L, Clavero O, et al. p53 immunohistochemical patterns in HPV-independent squamous cell carcinomas of the vulva and the associated skin lesions: a study of 779 cases. *Int J Mol Sci* 2020; **21**: 8091. doi: 10.3390/ijms21218091.

129. Baandrup L, Sand FL, Aalborg GL, Nøttrup TJ, Fiehn AMK, Kjaer SK. PD-L1 expression in vulvar cancer: a systematic review and meta-analysis. *Histopathology* 2024; **84**: 742–52.

130. Anic GM, Lee JH, Stockwell H, et al. Incidence and human papillomavirus (HPV) type distribution of genital warts in a multinational cohort of men: the HPV in men study. *J Infect Dis* 2011; **204**: 1886–92.

131. Olesen TB, Sand FL, Rasmussen CL, et al. Prevalence of human papillomavirus DNA and p16(INK4a) in penile cancer and penile intraepithelial neoplasia: a systematic review and meta-analysis. *Lancet Oncol* 2019; **20**: 145–58.

132. Shabbir M, Minhas S, Muneer A. Diagnosis and management of premalignant penile lesions. *Ther Adv Urol* 2011; **3**: 151–8.

133. Irshad U, Puckett Y. Giant condylomata acuminata of Buschke and Lowenstein. In: StatPearls [www.ncbi.nlm.nih.gov/books/NBK560714/]. Treasure Island (FL): StatPearls Publishing. 2024.

134. Shabbir M, Barod R, Hegarty PK, Minhas S. Primary prevention and vaccination for penile cancer. *Ther Adv Urol* 2013; **5**: 161–9.

135. Canete-Portillo S, Velazquez EF, Kristiansen G, et al. Report from the International Society of Urological Pathology (ISUP) consultation conference on Molecular Pathology of Urogenital Cancers V: Recommendations on the use of immunohistochemical and molecular biomarkers in penile cancer. *Am J Surg Pathol* 2020; **44**: e80–e6.

136. Stiff KM, Cohen PR. Vegas (verruciform genital-associated) xanthoma: a comprehensive literature review. *Dermatol Ther* 2017; **7**: 65–79.

137. Trinh NB, Tran GH. Penile verruciform xanthoma mimicking large genital wart. *Int J Dermatol* 2022; **61**: e43–e4.

138. Fernandez-Nestosa MJ, Clavero O, Sanchez DF, et al. Penile intraepithelial neoplasia: Distribution of subtypes, HPV genotypes and p16(INK4a) in 84 international cases. *Hum Pathol* 2023; **131**: 1–8.

139. Straub Hogan MM, Spieker AJ, Orejudos M, et al. Pathological characterization and clinical outcome of penile intraepithelial neoplasia variants: a North American series. *Mod Pathol* 2022; **35**: 1101–9.

140. Velazquez EF, Chaux A, Cubilla AL. Histologic classification of penile intraepithelial neoplasia. *Semin Diagn Pathol* 2012; **29**: 96–102.

141. Chaux A, Pfannl R, Lloveras B, et al. Distinctive association of p16INK4a overexpression with penile intraepithelial neoplasia depicting warty and/or basaloid features: a study of 141 cases evaluating a new nomenclature. *Am J Surg Pathol* 2010; **34**: 385–92.

142. Watkins JC, Yang E, Crum CP, et al. Classic vulvar intraepithelial neoplasia with superimposed lichen simplex chronicus: a unique variant mimicking differentiated vulvar intraepithelial neoplasia. *Int J Gynecol Pathol* 2019; **38**: 175–82.

143. Griesinger LM, Walline H, Wang GY, et al. Expanding the morphologic, immunohistochemical, and HPV genotypic features of high-grade squamous intraepithelial lesions of the vulva with morphology mimicking differentiated vulvar intraepithelial neoplasia and/or lichen sclerosus. *Int J Gynecol Pathol* 2021; **40**: 205–13.

144. Chaux A, Sanchez DF, Fernandez-Nestosa MJ, et al. The dual pathogenesis of penile neoplasia: the heterogeneous morphology of human papillomavirus-related tumors. *Asian J Urol* 2022; **9**: 349–58.

145. Cornejo KM, Hutchinson L, O'Donnell P, et al. Molecular profiling of syringocystadenocarcinoma papilliferum reveals RAS-activating mutations. *Arch Pathol Lab Med* 2024; **148**: 215–22.

146. Regauer S, Ermakov M, Kashofer K. The spectrum of HPV-independent penile intraepithelial neoplasia: a proposal for subclassification. *Am J Surg Pathol* 2023; **47**: 1449–60.

147. Canete-Portillo S, Sanchez DF, Cubilla AL. Pathology of invasive and intraepithelial penile neoplasia. *Eur Urol Focus* 2019; **5**: 713–17.

148. Guerrero J, Trias I, Veloza L, et al. HPV-negative penile intraepithelial neoplasia (PeIN) with basaloid features. *Am J Surg Pathol* 2022; **46**: 1071–7.

149. Eich ML, Del Carmen Rodriguez Pena M, Schwartz L, et al. Morphology, p16, HPV, and outcomes in squamous cell carcinoma of the penis: a multi-institutional study. *Hum Pathol* 2020; **96**: 79–86.

150. Chaux A, Tamboli P, Ayala A, et al. Warty-basaloid carcinoma: clinicopathological features of a distinctive penile neoplasm. Report of 45 cases. *Mod Pathol* 2010; **23**: 896–904.

151. Cubilla AL, Reuter VE, Gregoire L, et al. Basaloid squamous cell carcinoma: a distinctive human papilloma virus-related penile neoplasm: a report of 20 cases. *Am J Surg Pathol* 1998; **22**: 755–61.

152. Cubilla AL, Velazques EF, Reuter VE, Oliva E, Mihm MC, Jr., Young RH. Warty (condylomatous) squamous cell carcinoma of the penis: a report of 11 cases and proposed classification of 'verruciform' penile tumors. *Am J Surg Pathol* 2000; **24**: 505–12.

153. Zhang M, Adeniran AJ, Vikram R, et al. Carcinoma of the urethra. *Hum Pathol* 2018; **72**: 35–44.

154. Chaux A, Han JS, Lee S, et al. Immunohistochemical profile of the penile urethra and differential expression of GATA3 in urothelial versus squamous cell carcinomas of the penile urethra. Hum Pathol 2013; **44**: 2760–7.

155. Ermakov MS, Kashofer K, Regauer S. Different mutational landscapes in human papillomavirus-induced and human papillomavirus-independent invasive penile squamous cell cancers. *Mod Pathol* 2023; **36**: 100250. doi: 10.1016/j.modpat.2023.100250.

156. Kashofer K, Winter E, Halbwedl I, et al. HPV-negative penile squamous cell carcinoma: disruptive mutations in the TP53 gene are common. *Mod Pathol* 2017; **30**: 1013–20.

157. Tessier-Cloutier B, Pors J, Thompson E, et al. Molecular characterization of invasive and in situ squamous neoplasia of the vulva and implications for morphologic diagnosis and outcome. *Mod Pathol* 2021; **34**: 508–18.

158. Akbari A, Pinto A, Amemiya Y, Seth A, Mirkovic J, Parra-Herran C. Differentiated exophytic vulvar intraepithelial lesion: Clinicopathologic and molecular analysis documenting its relationship with verrucous carcinoma of the vulva. *Mod Pathol* 2020; **33**: 2011–18.

159. Watkins JC, Howitt BE, Horowitz NS, et al. Differentiated exophytic vulvar intraepithelial lesions are genetically distinct from keratinizing squamous cell carcinomas and contain mutations in PIK3CA. *Mod Pathol* 2017; **30**: 448–58.

Chapter 4

Neoplasms of Cutaneous Appendages

Mai P. Hoang

Introduction

Tumors derived from the cutaneous appendages can differentiate toward hair follicle, sebaceous gland, apocrine gland, or eccrine gland. Their biologic behavior ranges from benign to low-grade to high-grade carcinoma. In a retrospective review of 9646 cutaneous adnexal tumors in the Surveillance, Epidemiology, and End Results registry database from 2000 to 2018 in the United States, the median age was 64 years.[1] Males and females were affected in 57% and 43% of cases, respectively.[1] Most tumor types exhibited higher incidence in non-Hispanic Whites. Mucinous carcinoma incidence was greater than two-fold in non-Hispanic Blacks.[1] From 2014 to 2019 in France, 2573 cutaneous adnexal carcinomas were reviewed by expert pathologists via the national network and changes in diagnosis from benign to malignant and vice versa were observed in 117 cases (5%).[2] This highlights the diagnostic challenge in diagnosing cutaneous adnexal neoplasms.

Traditionally tumors derived from the cutaneous appendages are classified according to their lines of differentiation: either follicular, sebaceous, eccrine, or apocrine. However, there are overlapping histologic features and the classification is far from being straight forward. Often a tumor would exhibit multiple lines of differentiation with features of both eccrine and apocrine and even sebaceous differentiation. In many instances, immunohistochemistry can be of help in distinguishing epidermal from adnexal origin, benign from malignant adnexal neoplasms, and primary adnexal carcinoma from cutaneous metastases (**Table 4.1**). Recently, several adnexal neoplasms have been shown to harbor characteristic fusions. Their molecular signatures also serve as diagnostic clues.

Table 4.1 Commonly used diagnostic epithelial markers

Antibody	Commonly used clones	Staining pattern	Normal structures
Adipophilin	AP125	cytoplasmic	Sebaceous glands
Androgen receptor	AR441, SP107	nuclear	Sebaceous glands, apocrine glands
BerEP4	Ber-EP4	membranous	Hair follicle bulge
BRAFV600E	VE1	cytoplasmic	Pilar muscle
Carcinoembryonic antigen (CEA)	CEA31, COL–1, II–7	cytoplasmic	Eccrine glands
CD117	EP10	membranous	Mast cells, squamous epithelium
CDX2	EPR2764Y, DAK-CDX2, CDX2–88	nuclear	Colonic epithelium
Chromogranin	LK2H10, DAK-A3	cytoplasmic	Islets of pancreas
DOG1	K9	membranous	Interstitial cells of Cajal
Epithelial membrane antigen (EMA)	E29	cytoplasmic	Eccrine glands
Estrogen receptor (ER)	SP1, 6F11, EP1, 1D5	nuclear	Breast epithelium
GATA3	L50–823	nuclear	Epidermis, hair follicle
GATA6	D61E4	nuclear	Sebaceous glands
Gross cystic disease fluid protein–15 (GCDFP–15)	23A3, D6	cytoplasmic	Eccrine glands, apocrine glands
Her2	4B5, CB11	membranous	
INSM1	Bsb–123	nuclear	Islets of pancreas
Keratin 5	XM26, EP1601Y	cytoplasmic	Epidermis, hair follicles
Keratin 5 and 6	D5/16B4	cytoplasmic	Epidermis, hair follicles

Table 4.1 (cont.)

Antibody	Commonly used clones	Staining pattern	Normal structures
Keratin 7	OV-TL 12/30, SP52	cytoplasmic	Eccrine glands
Keratin 8	35BH11	cytoplasmic	Eccrine glands
Keratin 14	LL002	cytoplasmic	Epidermis, hair follicles
Keratin 15	LHK15	cytoplasmic	Hair follicle bulge
Keratin 17	E3, SP95	cytoplasmic	Normal epithelium
Keratin 18	DC10	cytoplasmic	Eccrine glands
Keratin 19	RCK108, A53-B/A2.26	cytoplasmic	Eccrine glands
Keratin 20	Ks–20.8, SP33	cytoplasmic	Merkel cells
Keratin 903/ high molecular weight keratin	34betaE12	cytoplasmic	Normal epithelium
Pan keratin (Cocktail of keratins 1–8, 10, 14–16, 19)	AE1/AE3, AE1/AE3/5D3	cytoplasmic	Normal epithelium
Keratin, low molecular weight (cocktail of keratins 8 and 18)	5D3, CAM5.2	cytoplasmic	Eccrine glands
Keratin MNF116	5D3	cytoplasmic	Normal epithelium
Laminin gamma 2			
Mammaglobin	304–1A5, 31A5	cytoplasmic	Apocrine glands
MLH1	ES05, M1, G168–15	nuclear	Normal epithelium, lymphocytes
MSH2	G219–1129, FE11	nuclear	Normal epithelium, lymphocytes
MSH6	EP49, SP93, EPR3945, BC/44	nuclear	Normal epithelium, lymphocytes
MUC2	Ccp58, MRQ–18	cytoplasmic	Intestinal epithelium
MUC5AC	MRQ–19	cytoplasmic	Gastric epithelium
MUC6	MRQ–20	cytoplasmic	Gastric epithelium
MYB	EP769Y	nuclear	lymphocytes
NUT	C52B1	nuclear	Testes
Pan-TRK	EPR17341	cytoplasmic	
p40	BC28	nuclear	Epidermis, myoepithelial cells
p63	4A4, DAK-p63	nuclear	Epidermis, myoepithelial cells
p75/ CD271	MLR2	cytoplasmic	Peripheral nerves
PHLDA1 (TDAG51)	RN–6E2	cytoplasmic	Normal melanocytes
PLAG1	3B7	nuclear	
Progesterone receptor (PR)	PgR 636, 16, PgR 1294	nuclear	Breast epithelium
PMS2	EP51, EPR3947, A16–4	nuclear	Normal epithelium, lymphocytes
S100	Polyclonal, 4C4.9	cytoplasmic	Peripheral nerves, dendritic cells
Sox10	N–20	nuclear	Eccrine glands
Synaptophysin	27G12, SP11, DAK-SYNAP	cytoplasmic	Islet cells
TTF–1	8G7G3/1, SPT24	nuclear	pneumocytes
YAP1	D8H1X	cytoplasmic	Intestinal epithelium

4.1 Follicular Neoplasms

Basal Cell Carcinoma

Basal cell carcinoma (BCC) is the most common malignant cutaneous neoplasm that typically is present on sun-exposed sites but can involve any part of the skin of adults. When occurring in a child, genetic syndromes such as nevoid basal cell carcinoma syndrome (Gorlin-Goltz syndrome), xeroderma pigmentosum, and Bazex-Dupre-Christol syndrome should be considered. BCC has a low recurrence rate of 5–10% and can rarely metastasize to regional lymph nodes and lungs.[3] BCC can have many histopathologic subtypes including superficial, nodular, morpheaform/infiltrative, basosquamous/metatypical, metaplastic/sarcomatoid, and others. BerEP4 is invariably expressed in BCC and a panel of BerEP4 and EMA is helpful in the distinction from squamous cell carcinoma (SCC) (**see Chapter 3**).[4] BCC exhibits strong and diffuse keratin 17 expression which is helpful in distinguishing it from SCC which has patchy keratin 17 expression (**Figures 4.1–4.3**).[5]

Trichoepithelioma/Trichoblastoma

In the latest WHO classification trichoblastoma is defined as a benign cutaneous tumor composed of follicular germinative cells. Trichoblastoma most commonly presents as a solitary

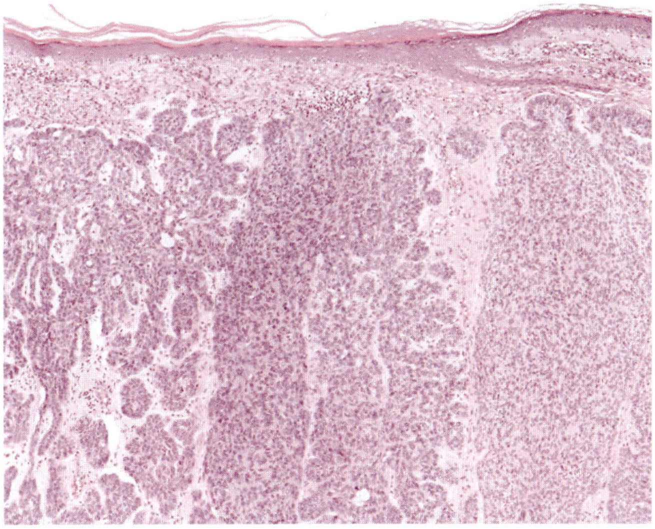

Figure 4.1 Basal cell carcinoma is characterized by nests of basaloid cells with peripheral palisade and retraction artifact (X100).

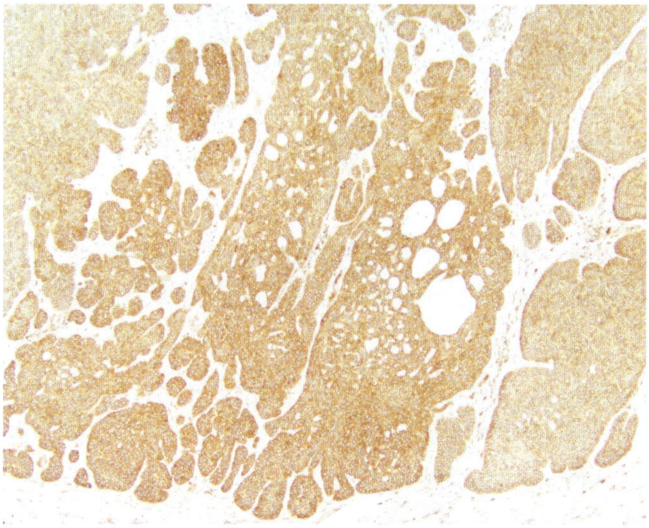

Figure 4.2 Basal cell carcinoma. Diffuse and strong Bcl2 expression is seen (X100).

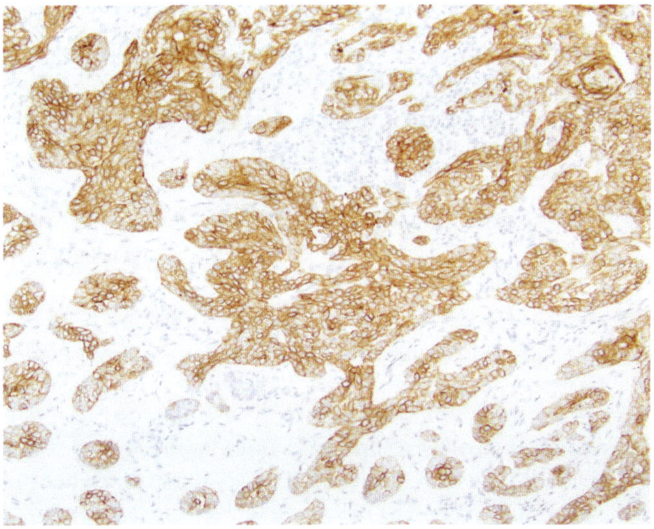

Figure 4.3 Basal cell carcinoma. Keratin 17 expression is invariably seen (X100).

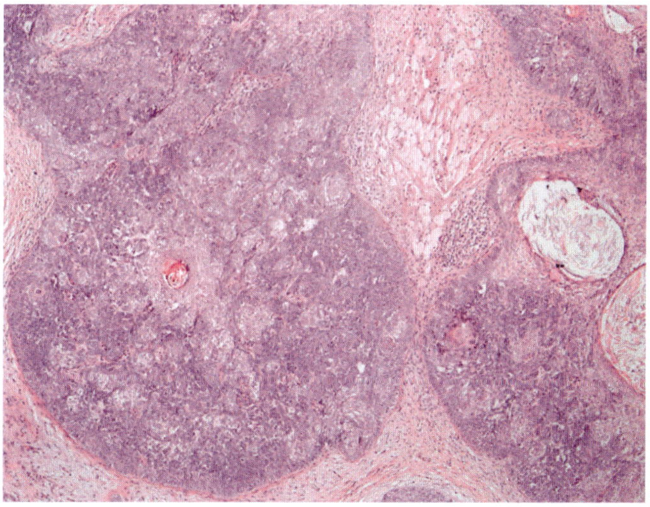

Figure 4.4 Trichoblastoma. Keratocysts, follicular and mesenchymal cells are seen within a cellular stroma (X100).

asymptomatic nodule on the head and neck area. On histologic sections a well-circumscribed dermal tumor comprised of follicular and mesenchymal cells is seen within an abundant cellular stroma. The epithelial cells of trichoblastoma express keratins 14, 15, 17, and 19.[6]

Trichoepithelioma/trichoblastoma versus basal cell carcinoma

Desmoplastic trichoepithelioma (dTE) is a benign follicular neoplasm frequently occurring on the cheek of a young person. Distinction from BCC would have treatment and subsequent cosmetic implication. The combined keratin 20-positive intratumoral Merkel cells and androgen receptor (AR)-negative tumor cells) immunophenotype has been found to be a great discriminator in diagnosing trichoepithelioma, trichoblastoma, and desmoplastic trichoepithelioma (dTE) versus other sclerosing adnexal neoplasms including morpheaform BCC. Merkel cells highlighted by keratin 20 can be seen in trichoepithelioma/ trichoblastoma versus rare cells or none in BCC (**Figures 4.4 and 4.5**).[7–9] A combination of AR and Bcl2 has been

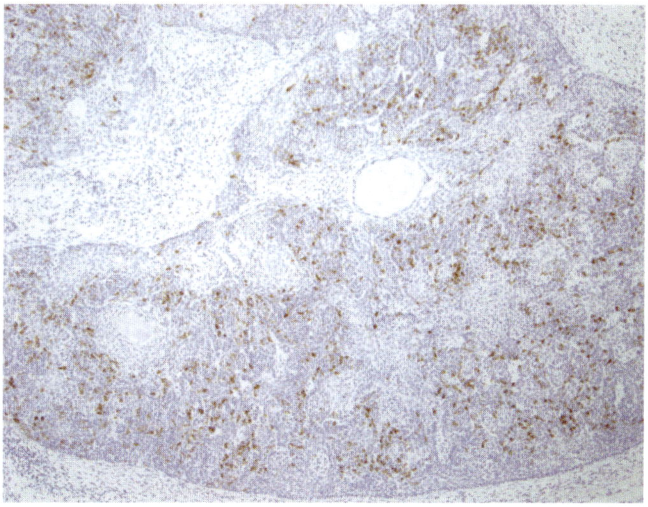

Figure 4.5 Trichoblastoma. Keratin 20 highlights many intratumoral Merkel cells (X100).

Table 4.2 Immunoprofiles of trichoepithelioma, trichoblastoma and basal cell carcinoma[6,7–9,11–14]

	Trichoepithelioma	Trichoblastoma	Basal cell carcinoma
Keratin 20+ Merkel cells	100%	42–100%	0–9%
Androgen receptor	0%	0%	60–78%
P75	100%		14%
PHLDA1 (TDAG51)	94–100%		0–44%
CD34	100% (stromal cells)		0%
BerEP4	57–75%		100%
Bcl2	73% peripheral staining		100%
CD10	15% (92%, stromal cells)	80%	60–87%
Laminin gamma 2	0%		96%

reported to exhibit high specificity (100%) in the distinction between BCC and TE.[10]

Recently p75 has been reported to label 17/17 cases of desmoplastic trichoepithelioma (dTE) in contrast to only 2/14 morpheaform BCC.[11] PHLDA1 (pleckstrin homology-like domain, family A, member 1 protein) or TDAG51 (T-cell death-associated gene 51), a follicular stem cell marker, stains the majority of trichoepitheliomas, both conventional and desmoplastic types, in contrast to 44% of the studied BCC.[12] While Laminin (Ln)-gamma 2 expression is seen in BCC and microcystic adnexal carcinoma (MAC), its expression is absent in trichoepithelioma.[13] Although p75, laminin-gamma 2, and PHLDA1 appear to be helpful markers, these markers are not readily available in most clinical laboratories.

CD34 has been reported to label the peritumoral stroma in cases of trichoepithelioma in contrast to negative staining in BCC cases; however, it is not helpful in the distinction of dTE versus BCC.[8] Pham et al.[14] reported that CD10 labels the basaloid cells in BCC while it highlights the peritumoral stroma in trichoepithelioma. Keratin 17 and keratin 19 expression have been reported in both BCC and trichoepithelioma or trichoblastoma.[6] In summary, the distinction of trichoepithelioma/trichoblastoma versus BCC, a panel of keratin 20 and AR would be most helpful **(Table 4.2)**.[6,7–9,11–14]

Trichoepithelioma/trichoblastoma versus basal cell carcinoma

- Trichoepithelioma/trichoblastoma: keratin 20+ Merkel cells, AR-
- Basal cell carcinoma: keratin 20-, AR+

Trichilemmoma

Trichilemmoma is a solitary lesion that commonly occurs on the central face of adults. Multiple lesions can be observed in the setting of PTEN hamartoma tumor syndrome (Cowden syndrome). Histopathologically, trichilemmoma appears as an exophytic and well-circumscribed proliferation of clear neoplastic cells surrounded by a thick basement membrane. A desmoplastic and hyalinized stroma is seen in desmoplastic trichilemmoma. CD34 expression in trichilemmoma is a helpful marker in distinguishing desmoplastic trichilemmoma from other cutaneous desmoplastic neoplasm.[15] The main differential diagnosis of trichilemmal carcinoma would be clear cell squamous cell carcinoma which is typically negative for CD34 and p75, and positive for keratin 17.[16] However some authors believe that both may represent the same entity. Clear cell BCC would be positive for keratin 17 and negative for CD34.[5] Diffuse and strong keratin 17 is seen in BCC (3+, 97%) whereas absent staining of peripheral basaloid rim in desmoplastic trichilemmoma (3+, 18%).[17] PTEN immunostain can be a helpful screening test for trichilemmomas associated with PTEN hamartoma tumor syndrome (Cowden syndrome) **(Figures 4.6–4.8)** **(see Chapter 10)**.

4.2 Sebaceous Neoplasms

Cutaneous sebaceous neoplasms typically affect the head and neck region.[18] Sebaceoma presents as a solitary smooth nodule mainly on the head and neck area. The association of sebaceoma with Muir-Torre syndrome is not as common as sebaceous adenoma and sebaceous carcinoma **(see Chapter 10)**. A multinodular dermal lesion comprised of basaloid cells and sebocytes is seen in the dermis. The mature sebocytes express EMA and adipophilin.

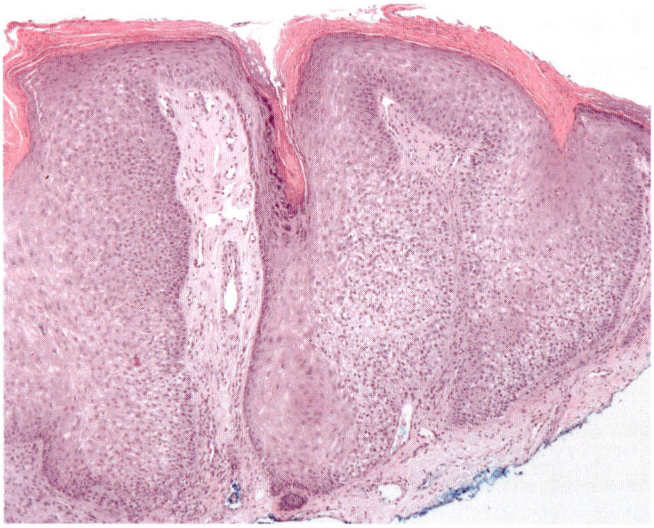

Figure 4.6 Trichilemmoma is characterized by keratinocytic cells with clear cytoplasm (X100).

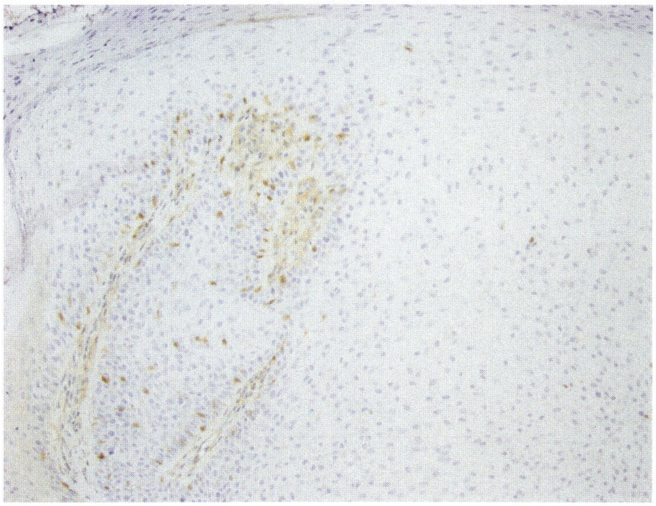

Figure 4.7 Lack of PTEN expression in a Cowden syndrome-associated trichilemmoma (X100).

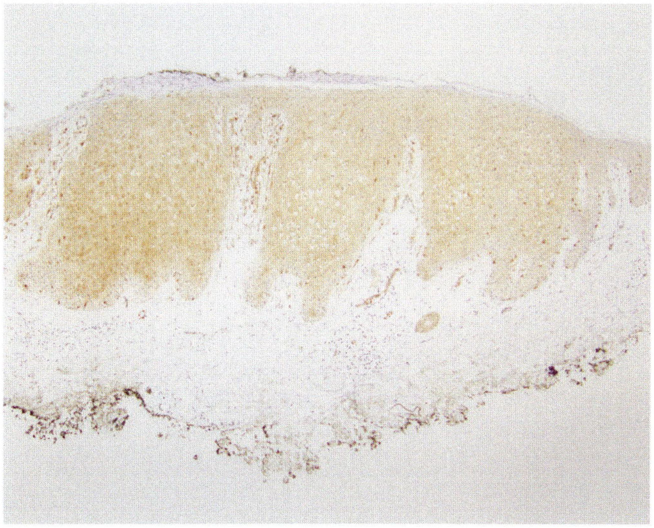

Figure 4.8 PTEN expression is seen in a sporadic trichilemmoma (X100).

Sebaceous carcinoma most frequently occurs as a yellow nodule on the head and neck area of elderly individuals. Nodules of tumors composed of atypical basaloid cells exhibiting variable degrees of sebaceous differentiation are seen in the dermis. EMA and adipophilin are typically used to determine sebaceous differentiation. Including mismatched repair (MMR) screening into clinical practice guidelines has been recommended for detection of Muir-Torre syndrome/Lynch syndrome (MTS/LS).[19] In patients with Lynch syndrome, sebaceous adenomas (43%), sebaceous carcinomas (27%), keratoacanthoma (16%), sebaceoma (13%), squamous cell carcinomas (23%), and basal cell carcinomas (10%) are seen.[20] Human papillomavirus (HPV) can be detected in approximately 8% of sebaceous carcinoma.[21]

Sebaceous Neoplasms versus Basal Cell Carcinoma and Squamous Cell Carcinoma

It can be a diagnostic challenge to distinguish sebaceous carcinoma from cutaneous tumors that exhibit focal clear cell change.

Table 4.3 Immunostaining of squamous cell carcinoma versus sebaceous carcinoma [22–29]

	Sebaceous carcinoma	Squamous cell carcinoma
AR	20–100%	17%
Adipophilin	88–100%	0–10% (focal in 75%)
BerEP4	10–80% *	0%
CAM5.2	73%	83%
EMA	80–100%	79–100%
Keratin 7	70–100%	68%
CD10	40%	Only stromal cells
CD15	43%	0%
GATA6	91%	0%
Perforin	78%	0%
PRAME	37%	29%
Gli1	36%	100%

* Ocular carcinomas

Immunohistochemical staining with adipophilin, androgen receptor (AR), BerEP4, GATA6, and perforin has been found to be helpful in distinguishing sebaceous carcinoma from SCC (**Table 4.3**).[22–29] Whereas keratin 7, CD10, CD15, D2-40, epithelial membrane antigen, and p63 have not been shown to be helpful.

Adipophilin has been reported to be the most sensitive marker for sebaceous carcinoma and useful in the distinction from SCC.[22,23] Although sensitive, its specificity has been reported in 25–100% of cases. [22,23] Adipophilin stained the rim of cytoplasmic lipid droplets in various tumor types, including sebaceous carcinomas, eccrine-apocrine carcinomas, and SCC.[23] Some authors have reported four staining patterns: foamy, reticular, granular, and punctate.[24] Since "granular" adipophilin staining is often noted in SCC and a variety of carcinoma, it is not a good marker for distinguishing SCCIS with clear cell change from sebaceous carcinoma *in situ* (**Figures 4.9–4.13**).[22,23] Recently, GATA6 has been shown to have similar sensitivity yet better specificity than adipophilin in the distinction of sebaceous carcinoma versus SCC.[26] Perforin has exhibited strong sensitivity and specificity as well.[27]

In normal skin, AR nuclear expression has been documented in sebocytes of sebaceous glands and, less often, within the luminal epithelial cells of the secretory apparatus of eccrine and apocrine glands. Ansai et al.[22] performed an immunohistochemical study using 7 antibodies (CEA, EMA, CA15-3, CA19-9, AR, BerEP4, adipophilin) on 35 cases of sebaceous carcinomas (16 ocular and 19 extraocular) and 10 SCC. The authors concluded that AR and adipophilin were helpful in differentiating sebaceous carcinoma from SCC. On the contrary, Sramek et al.[25] reported only 20% sensitivity and 83% specificity for AR in sebaceous carcinoma.

BerEP4 is the most specific marker for sebaceous carcinomas; however, its sensitivity is quite low. In the series by Ansai et al.,[22] only 2/19 extraocular sebaceous carcinomas expressed

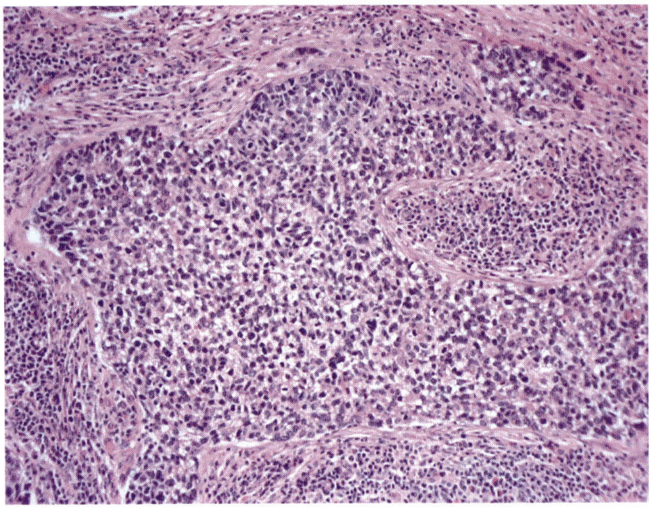

Figure 4.9 Sebaceous carcinoma. Neoplastic cells with clear and bubbly cytoplasm is seen (X200).

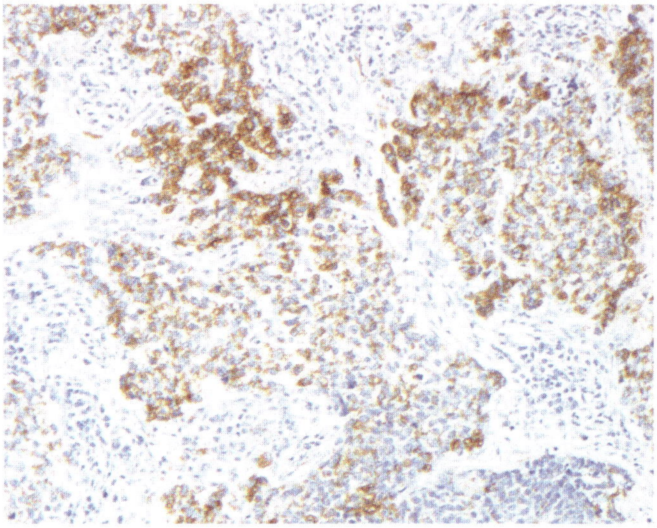

Figure 4.10 Sebaceous carcinoma. Membranous staining of lipid vacuoles noted with adipophilin (X200).

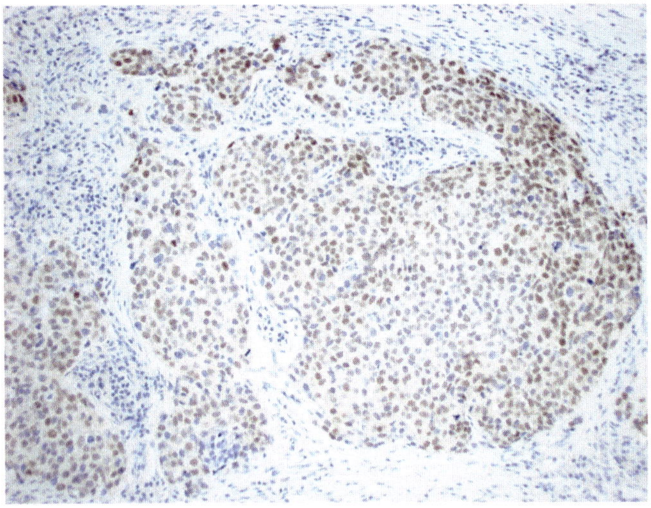

Figure 4.11 Sebaceous carcinoma. Diffuse nuclear staining with androgen receptor (X200).

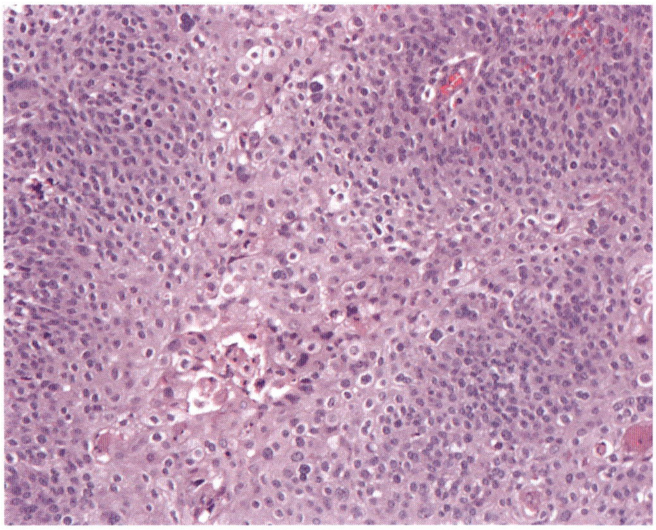

Figure 4.12 Squamous cell carcinoma. Atypical keratinocytes with keratin pearl formation (X200).

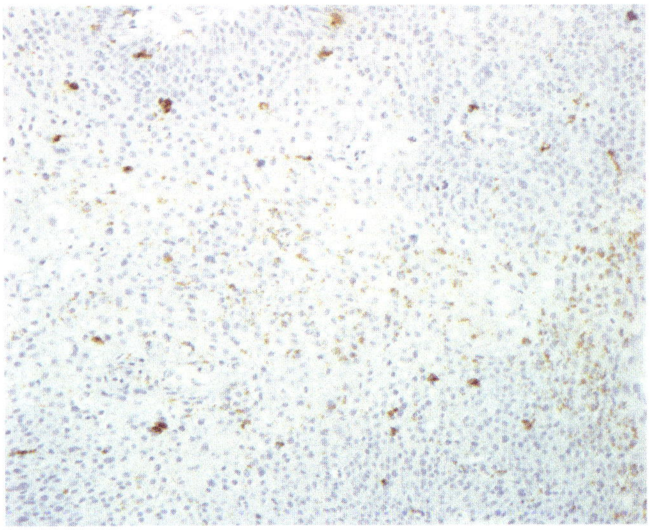

Figure 4.13 Squamous cell carcinoma. Granular adipophilin positivity is seen (X200).

BerEP4 (6%) and none of 10 SCC expressed BerEP4. On the contrary, 80% of 6 ocular sebaceous carcinomas and none of the SCC in the series by Sramek et al.[25] expressed BerEP4. Since all BCC are invariably positive for BerEP4, this would not be a good marker to distinguish BCC from sebaceous carcinoma. PRAME and Gli1 have not been shown to be good discriminating markers as well, with PRAME highlighting mature sebaceous differentiation yet invariably negative in high-grade sebaceous carcinoma.[28,29]

Squamous cell carcinoma versus sebaceous carcinoma

Sebaceous carcinoma: adipophilin +, AR +/-

Squamous cell carcinoma: adipophilin -/+, AR –

4.3 Eccrine and Apocrine Neoplasms

Currently there is overlap in classifying tumors into eccrine versus apocrine in origin. Therefore, the carcinomas of cutaneous appendages are separated into those with low-grade and high-grade biologic behavior (**Table 4.4**).

Syringoma

Syringoma is a common adnexal neoplasm that presents as numerous asymptomatic, skin-colored papules on the face, especially eyelids, and anogenital region of mainly women.[30] Up to 76% of cases can be multiple syringomas and 29% as eruptive syringomas.[30] The involved sites in decreasing order include face, chest, and neck.[30] On histologic sections a well-circumscribed tumor composed of small ductal structures distributed in a collagenous stroma. Cuboidal cells surrounded by myoepithelial cells are seen. Deep extension can rarely be seen in cases in the vulva.

Syringoma has been reported to express a number of keratins including keratin 5, keratin 6, keratin 7, keratin 11, keratin 14, and keratin 19. SMA highlights the myoepithelial cells.[31] However, these markers are not routinely used in clinical practice. The lesions on the vulva have been reported to express estrogen receptor and progesterone receptor.

Mixed Tumor (Chondroid Syringoma) and Malignant Mixed Tumor

Mixed tumor or pleomorphic adenoma/chondroid syringoma is tumor that can occur in the salivary gland, breast, and skin. It is the most common benign salivary gland tumors.

Histology Features

It is characterized morphologically by a biphasic pattern: epithelial/glandular component and mesenchymal one (**Figure 4.14**).[32,33] Benign lesions exhibit circumscription and absence of hypercellularity. Tumors with infiltrative border, satellite tumor nodules, and tumor necrosis are classified as atypical mixed tumor.[32]

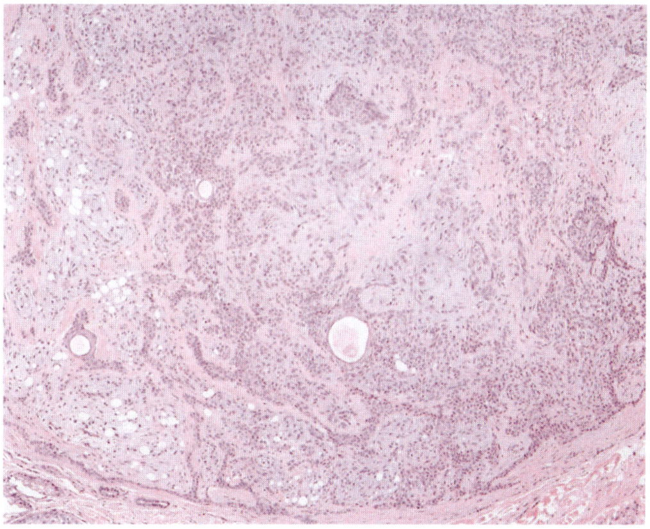

Figure 4.14 Chondroid syringoma. A biphasic morphology is seen: glandular component and chondroid matrix (X100).

In cutaneous apocrine mixed tumors, a variety of metaplastic changes can be seen in the epithelial component which include squamous, oxyphilic, columnar, and hobnail metaplasia.[32] Clear cell change and cytoplasmic vacuolization can be present.[32] The myoepithelial component can be clear, hyalinized, plasmacytoid, and spindled.[32] Chondroid, osseous, and adipocytic metaplasia can be seen in the stroma.[32] On the other hand, cutaneous eccrine mixed tumors do not exhibit decapitation secretion nor follicular/sebaceous differentiation.[33]

Table 4.4 Sweat gland tumors with low-grade and high-grade biologic behavior

Low-grade biologic behavior
Adenoid cystic carcinoma
Cribriform carcinoma
Endocrine mucin producing sweat gland carcinoma
Mucinous carcinoma
Secretory carcinoma
Microsecretory carcinoma
Malignant proliferating pilar tumor
Microcystic adnexal carcinoma
Squamoid eccrine ductal carcinoma
Low-grade carcinoma arising in pre-existing spiradenoma, cylindroma, and spiradenocylindroma
High-grade biologic behavior
Adnexal carcinoma, not otherwise specified
Apocrine carcinoma
Digital papillary adenocarcinoma
Extramammary Paget disease
Hidradenocarcinoma
Porocarcinoma
Signet-ring cell/histiocytoid carcinoma
Syringocystadenocarcinoma papilliferum
High-grade carcinoma arising in pre-existing spiradenoma, cylindroma, and spiradenocylindroma

Molecular Findings

In approximately 70% of pleomorphic adenomas there are recurrent translocations mostly involving *PLAG1* (pleomorphic adenoma gene 1) which result in overexpression of PLAG1 protein.[34] Recurrent gene fusions involving pleomorphic adenoma gene 1 (*PLAG1*) on 8q12 (>50%) or *HMGA2* on 12q14.3 (10–15%) are seen in pleomorphic adenomas of salivary gland.[35] A subset of breast, and skin tumors harbors *PLAG1* rearrangement including beta-catenin gene (*CTNNB1::PLAG1*, t(3;8)(p21;q12)), leukemia inhibitory factor receptor gene (*LIFR::PLAG1*, t(5;8)(p13;q12)), and coiled-coil-helix-coiled-coil-helix domain containing 7 gene (*CHCHD7::PLAG1*).[36–38] *PLAG1* fuses with one of seven recurrent partner genes: *CTNNB1*, *FGFR1*, *LIFR*, *CHCHD7*, *TCEA1*, *NFIB*, and *BOC*; whereas *HMGA2* fuses with one of four recurrent partner genes: *FHIT*, *NFIB*, *TMTC2*, and *WIF1*.[39–46] Concurrent or isolated *HMGA2* amplification have also been reported.[42,46]

In a series of 105 pleomorphic adenomas and 11 carcinoma ex pleomorphic adenomas, *PLAG1* fusions were detected in 40/116 cases (34%): 22 (19%) with *CTNNB1::PLAG1*, 14 (12%) with *CHCHD7::PLAG1*, 4 (3%) with *LIFR::PLAG1*. Two cases (2%) harbored *HMGA2* fusions and *CTNNB1::PLAG1* was detected in 4 carcinoma ex pleomorphic adenomas.[37] Fusions with *HMGA2* have been reported: *HMGA2::NFIB*,[41] *HMGA2::FHIT*,[47] and *HMGA2::WIF1*.[42] *NDRG1::PLAG1* and *TRPS1::PLAG1* have been reported in cutaneous chondroid syringoma,[38] and *PHF1::TFE3* in a malignant chondroid syringoma.[48]

Immunohistochemical Findings

PLAG1 expression has been reported in all 45 studied pleomorphic adenomas in this same series and in all 16 cutaneous mixed tumors in a subsequent series (**Figure 4.15**).[49,50] Thus, PLAG1 overexpression is invariably seen in pleomorphic adenoma regardless of the *PLAG1* status. In a series of 243 mesenchymal tumors, the specificity of PLAG1 was 94% with its expression seen in 8/10 lipoblastomas, 2/7 gastrointestinal stromal tumors, 1/2 angiomyofibroblastomas, and 1/12 myxofibrosarcomas (Matsuyama 2012).[50] In summary, PLAG1 immunostain exhibits 100% sensitivity and 93–100% specificity for pleomorphic adenoma. However, its sensitivity decreases to 77–100% for carcinoma ex pleomorphic adenoma (**Table 4.5**).[49–52]

Low-Grade Carcinoma

Adenoid Cystic Carcinoma

Adenoid cystic carcinoma (ACC) can occur in the skin, salivary gland, breast, prostate, gastrointestinal tract, as well as lung. A rare cutaneous neoplasm, adenoid cystic carcinoma often presents as a slow growing solitary nodule on the scalp, trunk and abdomen. The tumor exhibits a high propensity for recurrence and distant metastases to lung, liver, and bones are frequently observed.[53]

Histology Features

On histologic sections the tumor displays three main growth patterns – cribriform, tubular, and solid and with frequent perineural invasion. In the most common cribriform pattern, microcystic-like spaces filled with eosinophilic hyaline materials or basophilic mucinous materials are seen. It is comprised of two types of cells, inner epithelial/luminal and outer myoepithelial cells (**Figure 4.16**). Immunohistochemical stain shows expression of keratin 5/6, keratin 7, keratin 15, and CD117 (**Figure 4.17**) in the epithelial component while p63 (**Figure 4.18**), p40, SMA, and calponin staining in the myoepithelial component. Diffuse CD117, Sox10, and keratin 7 expression is noted in the majority of cases.[54] The main differential diagnosis is adenoid BCC which has a nodular growth pattern, peripheral palisade, and retraction artifact. While diffuse CD117 expression is invariably seen in adenoid cystic carcinoma, only a small subset of adenoid basal cell carcinoma would exhibit CD117 positivity.

Molecular findings

The genomic hallmark of ACC is t(6;9) or t(8;9) translocations, resulting in *MYB::NFIB* and *MYBL1::NFIB* fusions, respectively.[55] A recurrent specific translocation t(6;9) (*MYB* gene

Table 4.5 PLAG1 expression in pleomorphic adenoma and carcinoma ex pleomorphic adenoma

References	N	Pleomorphic adenoma	Carcinoma ex pleomorphic adenoma	Other tumors	Sensitivity	Specificity
Matsuyama 2011[49]	91	45/45 *	4/4	3/42	100%	93%
Matsuyama 2011[49]	24	16/16 **	ND	0/8	100%	100%
Matsuyama 2012[50]	243	ND	ND	14/243	ND	94%
Bahrami 2012[51]	61	ND	17/22	0/39	77%	100%
Mendoza 2013[52]	7	7/7 ***	ND	ND	100%	ND

ND: not done; * salivary gland tumor, ** cutaneous tumor, *** lacrimal gland tumor

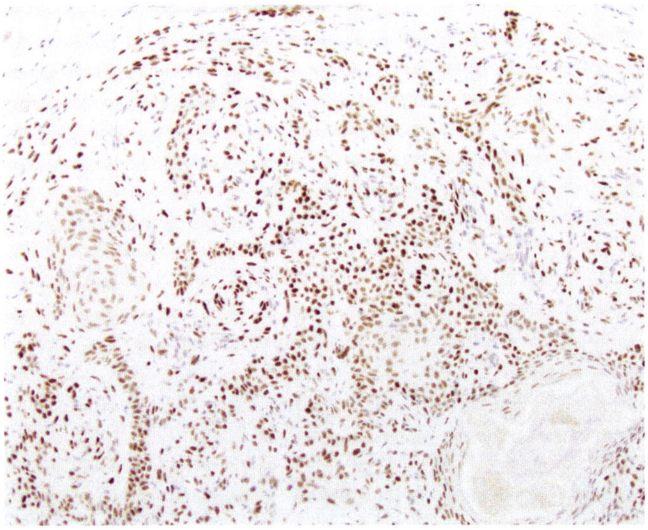

Figure 4.15 Chondroid syringoma. Nuclear PLAG1 expression is seen (X100).

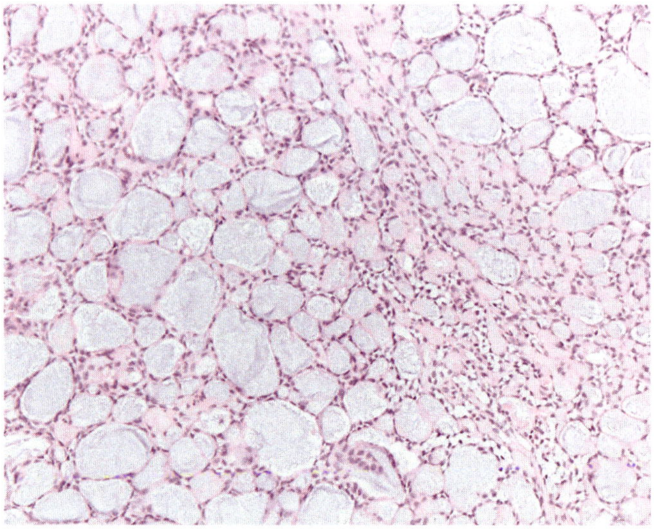

Figure 4.16 Cribriform architecture of an adenoid cystic carcinoma (X200).

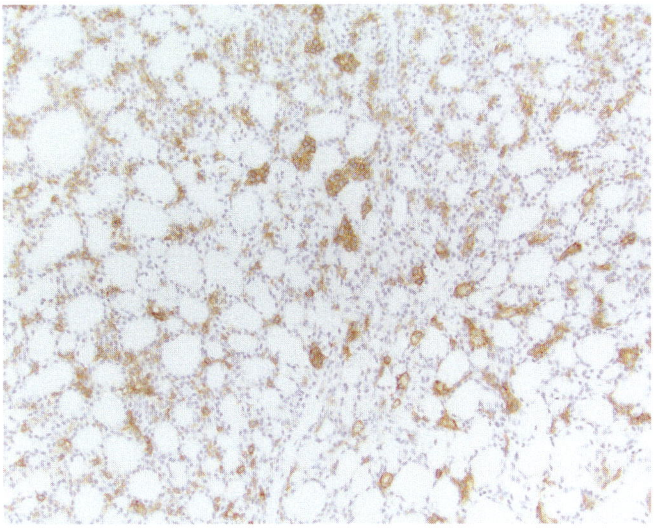

Figure 4.17 Adenoid cystic carcinoma. CD117 highlights a subset of the tumor cells (X200).

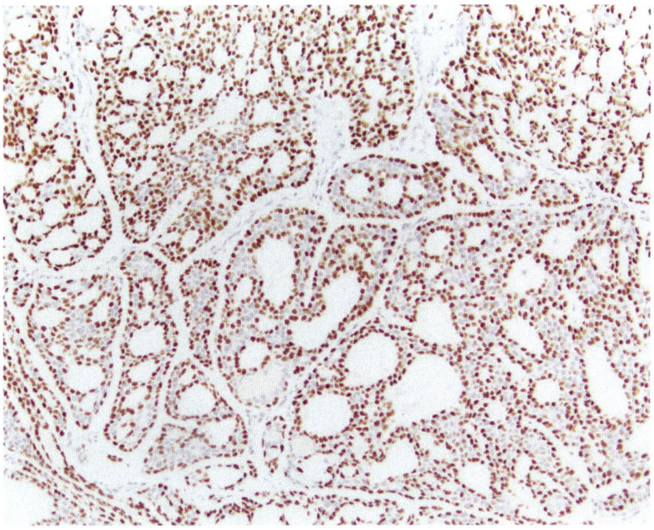

Figure 4.18 Adenoid cystic carcinoma. p63 highlights the myoepithelial cells (X200).

on 6q22-23 and transcription factor *NFIB* gene on chromosome 9p23-24) has been documented in ACC of salivary gland, breast, larynx, skin, and lacrimal and ceruminous glands.[54] *MYB* transcription factor has been shown to affect downstream target genes of neoplastic processes including cyclooxygenase-2 (COX-2), Bcl-2, Bclx, and c-kit.[55] In a large series of 37 ACC, 112 other salivary gland carcinomas, and 409 nonsalivary gland tumors; the *MYB*::*NFIB* translocation was seen in 49% (18/37) of ACC and abnormal *MYB* fluorescence *in situ* hybridization (FISH) was present in an additional 16% (6/37) of ACC cases.[56] *MYB*::*NFIB* fusion was documented in 28% primary and 35% metastatic ACCs, but not in other salivary gland carcinomas;[55] and this gene fusion contributes to MYB overexpression. Rare cases *EWSR1*::*MYB* and *FUS*::*MYB* have been reported.[57]

Immunohistochemical Findings

Although specific, the sensitivity of MYB immunostain is not high with its nuclear expression seen in 55% of 156 ACCs [58] to

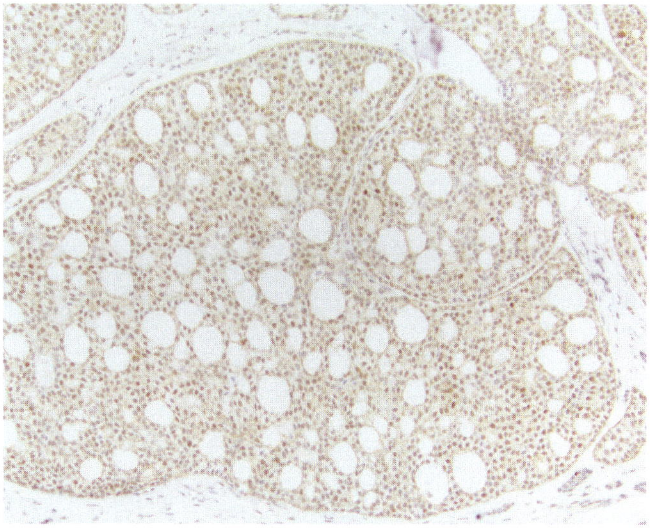

Figure 4.19 Adenoid cystic carcinoma. Diffuse nuclear MYB expression is noted (X200).

82% of 68 ACCs (**Figure 4.19**).[59] MYB expression can be seen in ACCs without documented *MYB*::*NFIB* fusion.[54] MYB *in situ* hybridization is an alternative ancillary test to detect *MYB* fusion.[60]

Cribriform Carcinoma

Primary cutaneous cribriform carcinoma was first reported as an apocrine neoplasm by Requena et al. in 1998.[61] Review of the literature showed a female predominance (67% versus 33%) and lower (47%) and upper (34%) extremities site preference.[62] Recurrences occurred in rare cases due to incomplete excision.[62] Otherwise, no metastases have been reported.[62]

Histologic Findings

An un-encapsulated dermal nodule comprised of epithelial nests with cystic spaces and luminal formation within a fibrotic/desmoplastic stroma. Intraluminal bridges, cuboidal or flattened, are seen. Myoepithelial layers are not appreciated. Focal presence of decapitation secretion suggests the apocrine derivation of this tumor.[62]

Immunohistochemical Findings

Cutaneous cribriform apocrine carcinomas typically express keratin 7 and keratin CAM5.2.[63]

Differential Diagnosis

The differential diagnosis includes tubular adenoma, adenoid cystic carcinoma, and metastatic mammary adenocarcinoma (**Table 4.6**). Adenoid cystic carcinoma would exhibit intraluminal basophilic mucinous materials. Metastatic adenocarcinoma with cribriform architecture from breast, salivary gland, colon, prostate, uterus, and ovaries is also in the histologic differential diagnosis. BRST-2, ER, PR, keratin 20, CDX2, PSA, and PAX8 immunostains would be helpful.

Endocrine Mucin-Producing Sweat Gland Carcinoma

Endocrine mucin-producing sweat gland carcinoma is a rare tumor that commonly presents as a solitary and slow-growing papule on the eyelid of women.[64] The average age at presentation

Table 4.6 Differential diagnosis of cutaneous cribriform carcinoma[61,62]

	Primary cutaneous cribriform carcinoma	Tubular adenoma	Adenoid cystic carcinoma	Cutaneous secretory carcinoma
Keratin AE1/3	+			
Keratin MNF116	+			
Keratin 5/6	+	+		
Keratin 7	+	+		
Keratin 20	-	-	-	
EMA	+			
CD117	+			
BRST–2/ GCDFP–15	-	-	-	
ER/PR	-	-	-	
S100	-	-	+	+
Calponin	+ stroma	+ myoepithelial		
Smooth muscle actin	+ stroma	+ myoepithelial		
p63	+ stroma	+ myoepithelial		
Gene fusion	-	-	*MYB::NFIB*	*ETV6::NTRK3*

EMA: epithelial membrane antigen, ER: estrogen receptor, PR: progesterone receptor

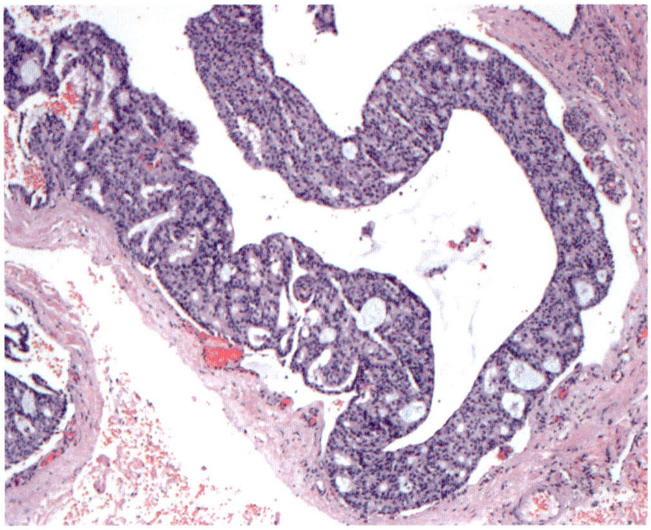

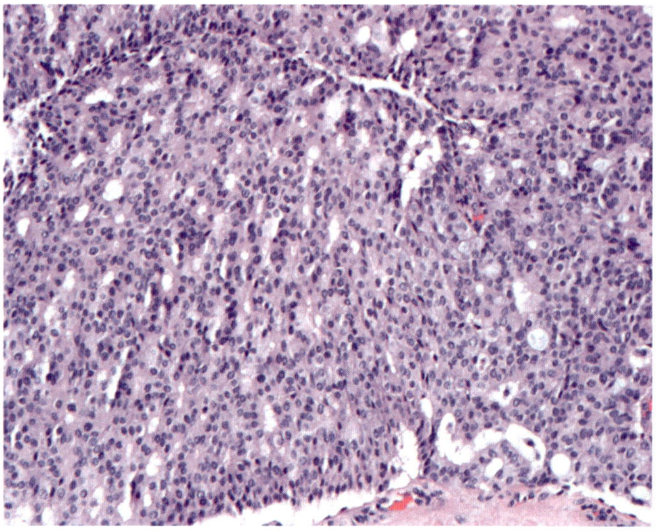

Figures 4.20 and 4.21 Endocrine mucin-producing sweat gland carcinoma. A solid and cystic tumor exhibiting cribriform and glandular architecture (X100, X200).

is 64 years.[64] Association with mucinous carcinoma is seen in 33% of cases.[64] Recurrence is documented in 21% and 30% for the neuroendocrine type and non-neuroendocrine mucinous carcinoma, respectively.[64] The tumor can rarely metastasize.[65]

A multinodular, solid and cystic tumor with papillary and cribriform architecture is seen in the dermis (**Figures 4.20 and 4.21**). In half of the cases reported by Zembowicz et al.[66] an invasive mucinous carcinoma was observed and the authors suggested that endocrine mucin-producing sweat gland carcinoma is a precursor of some cutaneous invasive mucinous carcinomas. The tumor cells are polygonal and eosinophilic. They are invariably positive for EMA, keratin 7, CAM5.2, estrogen receptor, progesterone receptor (**Figures 4.22, 4.23 and 4.24**). Positivity with at least one neuroendocrine markers especially chromogranin, synaptophysin, and INSM1 is seen (**Figure 4.25**). Calponin, SMA, and p63 would highlight the myoepithelial cells around the ducts involved by carcinoma *in situ*.[66]

Mucinous Carcinoma

Primary cutaneous mucinous carcinoma is a rare neoplasm that presents as a solitary and slow-growing nodule on the scalp, face, and eyelids.[67] The histologic features are similar to those of mammary mucinous carcinoma (**Figure 4.26**). In the pure variant small cellular nests are seen amidst an abundant mucinous stroma that comprised greater than 90% of the tumor. An invasive ductal carcinoma is seen in addition to the mucinous component in the mixed variant.

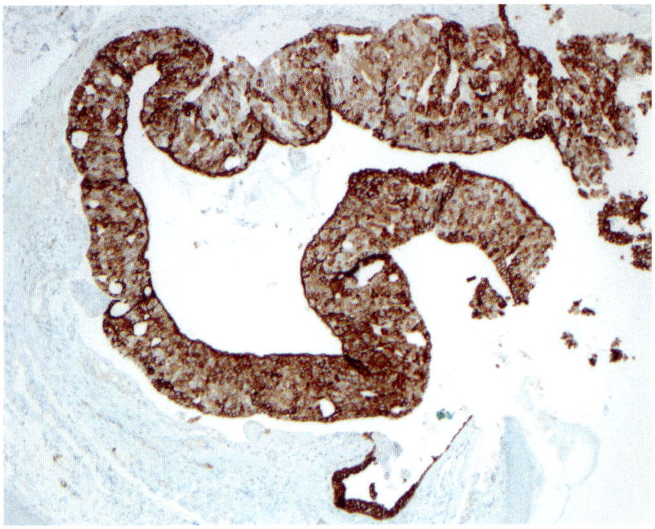

Figure 4.22 Endocrine mucin-producing sweat gland carcinoma. Diffuse keratin 7 expression (X100).

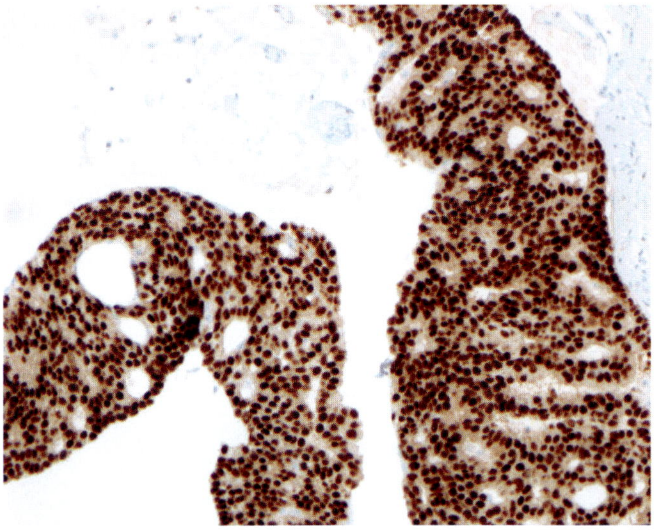

Figure 4.23 Endocrine mucin-producing sweat gland carcinoma. Diffuse estrogen receptor expression (X200).

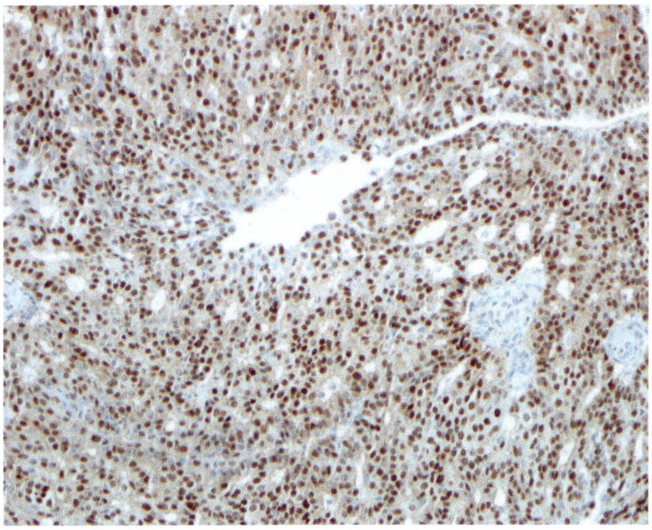

Figure 4.24 Endocrine mucin-producing sweat gland carcinoma. Diffuse progesterone receptor expression (X100).

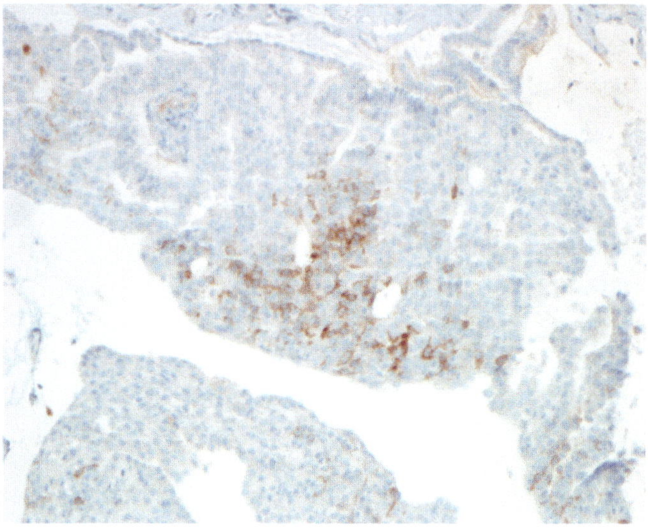

Figure 4.25 Endocrine mucin-producing sweat gland carcinoma. Focal synaptophysin expression (X200).

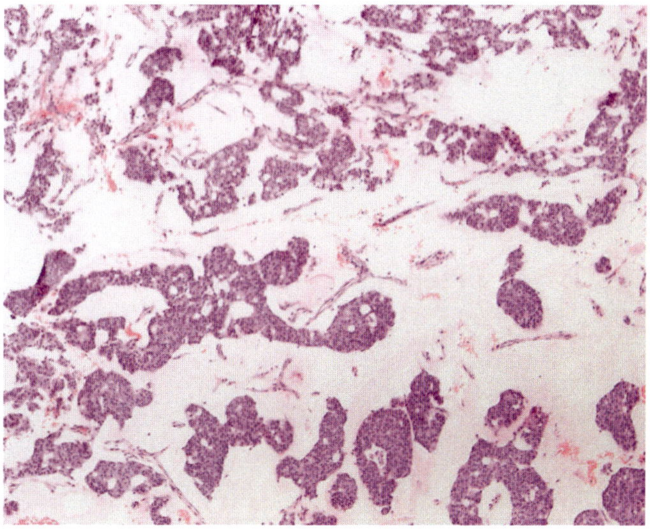

Figure 4.26 Primary cutaneous mucinous carcinoma. Epithelial tumor nests are seen associated with abundant extracellular mucin (X100).

p63, calponin, and SMA would highlight the myoepithelial cells. ER and PR can be seen in some cases (**Figure 4.27**). Expression of S100, BerEP4, CEA, EMA, GCDFP15, and MUC2 (**Figure 4.28**); and neuroendocrine differentiation with positivity for chromogranin A, synaptophysin, and neuron specific enolase can be seen (**Figure 4.29**) (**Table 4.7**).[68,69,70] The tumor would express keratin 7 similar to mammary mucinous carcinoma but not keratin 20 as seen in colonic mucinous carcinoma.[69] Focal keratin 5/6 is seen in primary cutaneous but not mammary mucinous carcinoma.[69] Although additional cases need to be studied, the co-expression of MYB and GATA3 is supportive of a primary cutaneous mucinous carcinoma (**Figures 4.30 and 4.31**).[71] Careful clinical work up must be done to exclude the possibility of metastases from breast, gastrointestinal tract, ovary and lung. The diagnosis can be made if (1) a metastatic mucinous carcinoma is excluded and/or (2) an *in situ* component is present which is rarely identified.

Table 4.7 Immunoprofile of primary cutaneous mucinous carcinoma versus metastases from breast and gastrointestinal site[68,69]

Immunostains	Primary cutaneous mucinous carcinoma	Breast	Gastrointestinal site
Keratin 7	+	+	-
Keratin 20	-	-	+
CDX2	-	-	+
MUC2	+	+	+
MUC5AC	-	-	+
p40	-	-	-
Estrogen receptor	+	+	-
Progesterone receptor	+	+	-

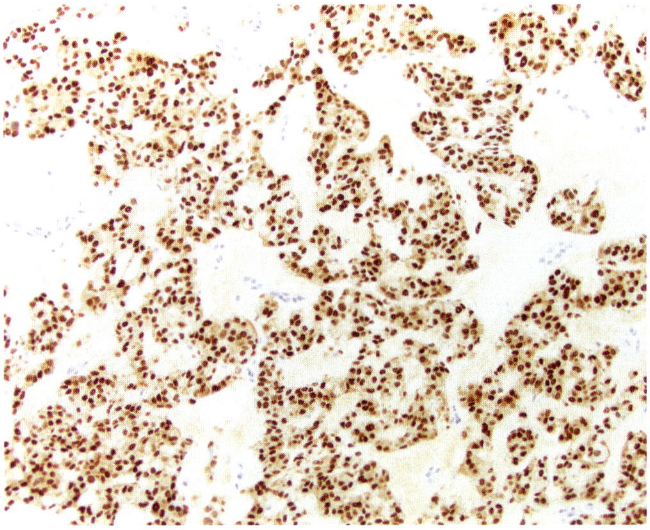

Figure 4.27 Primary cutaneous mucinous carcinoma. Diffuse progesterone receptor expression is noted (X200).

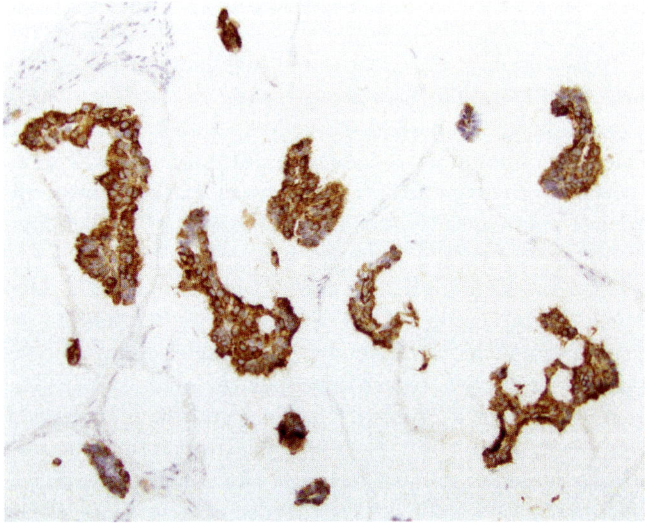

Figure 4.28 Primary cutaneous mucinous carcinoma. MUC2 expression is seen (X200).

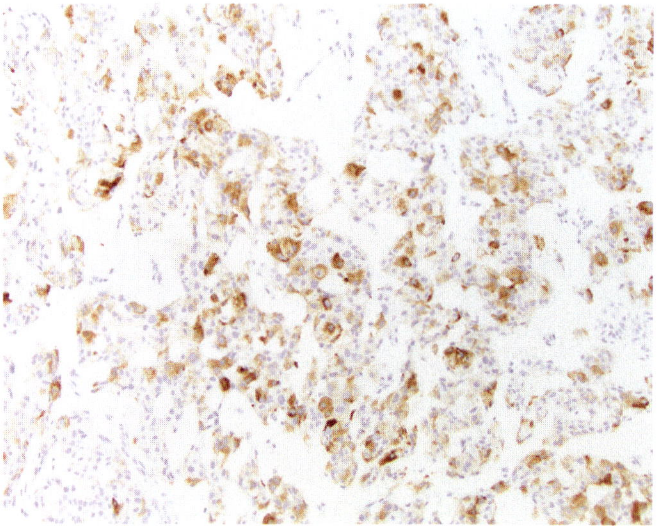

Figure 4.29 Primary cutaneous mucinous carcinoma. Synaptophysin is partly positive (X200).

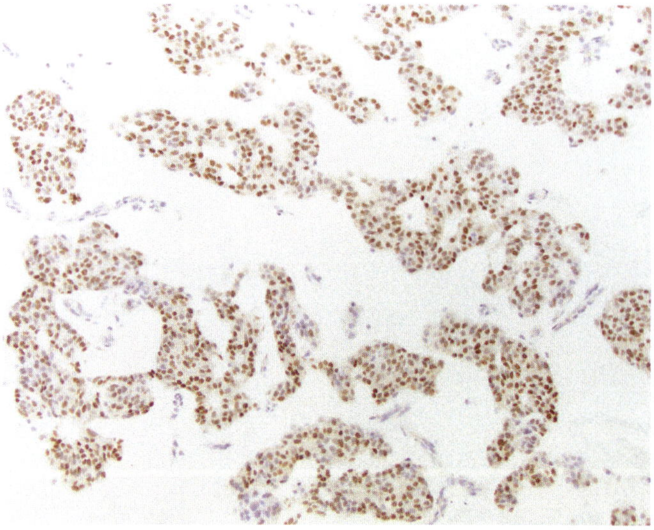

Figure 4.30 Primary cutaneous mucinous carcinoma. Diffuse nuclear GATA3 expression (X200).

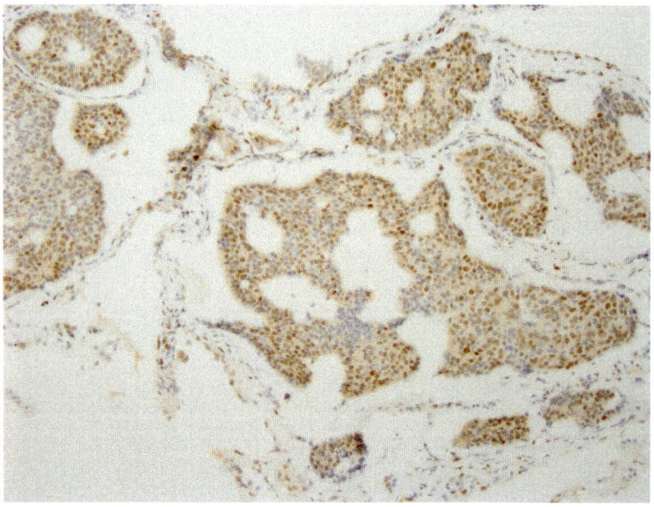

Figure 4.31 Primary cutaneous mucinous carcinoma. Nuclear MYB expression (X100).

Secretory Carcinoma

Though rare, secretory carcinoma is the most common mammary carcinoma in the pediatric population.[72] Secretory carcinoma with similar histologic and molecular features have been reported in the salivary gland (most commonly in the parotid)[73] and rarely in the skin.[72,74–76] The cutaneous tumors follow an indolent biologic course.[74]

Histology Features

On histology, a well-circumscribed tumor comprised of bland neoplastic cells with pale pink vacuolated and foamy cytoplasm, exhibiting several histologic patterns including solid, tubular, microcystic, and papillary (**Figure 4.32**). Abundant eosinophilic and bubbly secretion within the lumens, diastase-resistant PAS, is a characteristic histologic feature. Rare mitotic figures and perineural invasion can be seen.[72,73]

Immunohistochemical Findings

By immunohistochemistry, the tumor cells are typically positive for S100, Sox10, and mammaglobin.[77] Although the tumors cells are negative for p40 and p63, these markers can highlight the myoepithelial cells.[75] They can express GATA3, cytokeratin 7, cytokeratin 5/6, cytokeratin 8/18, estrogen receptor (ER), progesterone receptor (PR), Her2/neu, epithelial membrane antigen (EMA), carcinoembryonic antigen (CEA), mammaglobin, D2-40, smooth muscle actin, paired box 8 (PAX8), thyroid transcription factor 1 (TTF1), and STAT5 (**Figure 4.33**).[72,73,75] Variable staining with epidermal growth factor receptor (EGFR), cytokeratin CAM5.2, cytokeratin 19, MUC1, MUC4, gross cystic disease fluid protein-15 (GCDFP-15), has been reported.[73] Pan-TRK immunostain detects *NTRK*1/2/3 gene fusions with high sensitivity and specificity ranging from 95% to 100% and 92% to 100% in secretory carcinoma, respectively.[76,78]

Molecular Findings

A balanced t(12;15)(p13;q25) translocation resulted in *ETV6::NTRK3* fusion detected in majority (approximately 90%) of the cases from salivary gland, breast, and skin.[72–74,77]

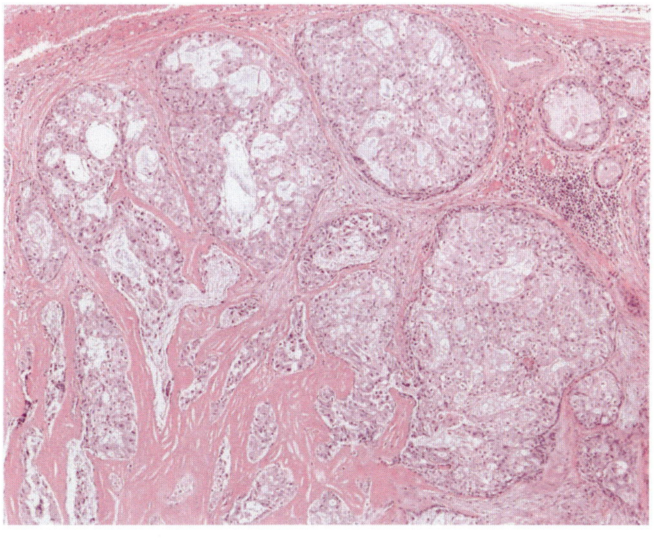

Figure 4.32 Secretory carcinoma. A proliferation of tumor cells with pale eosinophilic, vacuolated, and foamy cytoplasm is seen (X100).

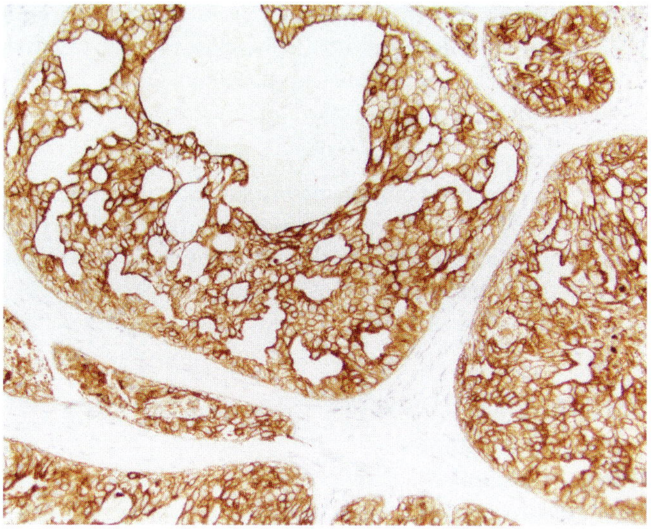

Figure 4.33 Secretory carcinoma. Strong keratin 7 expression by the tumor cells is seen (X200).

NFIX::PKN1 translocation has been reported in rare cutaneous secretory carcinoma.[76] *ETV6::X* fusion has been reported in six salivary gland secretory carcinomas.[77,79] *ETV6::MET* [80], *ETV6::RET*,[81] and *VIM::RET*[82] fusions have been reported in 1, 10, and 1 salivary secretory carcinoma, respectively. Dual *ETV6*, *NTRK3*, *MAML3*[83] fusion has been reported. *ETV6::NTRK3* fusion has been reported in infantile fibrosarcoma, congenital mesoblastic nephroma, and acute myelogenous leukemia.[72]

Differential Diagnosis

Immunostaining and fusion study would be helpful in the distinction of secretory carcinoma from mucoepidermoid carcinoma which is negative for S100 and associated with t(11;19) translocation, *CRTCR::MAML2* fusion.[84] Secretory carcinomas would be negative for DOG1 (positive in acinic cell carcinoma) and p63.[85]

Microsecretory Adenocarcinoma

Previously classified as adenocarcinoma, not otherwise specified, microsecretory adenocarcinoma of salivary glands is now diagnosed with characteristic *MEF2C::SS18* fusion.[86] Most tumors have arisen in the oral cavity, affecting most frequently the palate and buccal mucosal. Rare cases of cutaneous microsecretory adenocarcinoma have been reported.[87–90] Microsecretory adenocarcinoma is an indolent tumor without documented local recurrence or metastasis status post excision.[86,88,89]

Histology Features

At low power the tumor is nodular, well-circumscribed yet unencapsulated, with infiltrative borders invading into skeletal muscle, collagen, and adipose tissue.[86] At high power, microcysts, small tubules, and cords of tumor cells with basophilic luminal secretion are seen embedded in a fibromyxoid stroma.

The tumor cells of both salivary gland[86] and cutaneous tumors[87–89] are positive for Sox10, S100, p63, and TLE1; and negative for p40, calponin, and mammoglobin. The myoepithelial component is positive for p40.[87]

Molecular Findings

MEF2C::SS18 fusion was detected in five salivary microsecretory adenocarcinoma[86] and three cutaneous tumors.[87] *SS18::ZBTB7A* fusion was detected in a rare case.[86]

Differential Diagnosis

While the secretion of microsecretory adenocarcinoma is basophilic, it is eosinophilic in secretory carcinoma. The p63 expression seen in microsecretory adenocarcinoma is negative in secretory carcinoma. In addition, secretory carcinoma is characterized by fusion of *ETV6* and *NTRK3* as well as other partner genes.[90]

Carcinoma Arising in Preexisting Spiradenoma, Cylindroma, and Spiradenocylindroma

Multiple cylindromas, spiradenomas, trichoepitheliomas, and basal cell salivary gland tumors are seen in Brooke-Spiegler syndrome, an autosomal dominant disorder with a germline *CYLD* mutation. Carcinomas arising in preexisting spiradenoma, cylindroma, and spiradenocylindroma can exhibit four histology patterns: (1) low-grade salivary gland basal cell adenocarcinoma-like pattern, (2) high-grade salivary gland basal cell adenocarcinoma-like pattern, (3) infiltrating adenocarcinoma, not otherwise specified, and (4) sarcomatoid or metaplastic carcinoma.[91]

While the benign cylindroma, spiradenoma, and spiradenocylindroma are focally (5–20% of the tumor cells) highlighted by MYB immunostain, the carcinoma component of all 16 low-grade spiradenocarcinoma is MYB negative.[92] p53 expression has not been found to be helpful in separating the benign from malignant component.[93]

Malignant Proliferating Pilar Tumor

Malignant proliferating pilar tumors (MPPT) are rare tumors that have an indolent biologic behavior and rarely can metastasize.[94] The histologic features associated with MPPT include size greater than 2.5 cm, adjacent desmoplastic stroma, small nests or cords of atypical epithelium in surrounding stroma, irregular infiltration or borders, abnormal keratinization, large hyperchromatic nuclei, prominent nucleoli, severe cytologic atypia, nuclear pleomorphism, necrosis, and increased mitotic figures (Figures 4.34 **and** 4.35). MPPT harbors copy number gains of 15q and losses of 6p and 6q, findings previously reported in benign PPT.[95] However, different from cutaneous squamous cell carcinoma (SCC), MPPT possesses low tumor mutational burden and typically lacks a UV signature, suggestive of a different etiologic pathway than SCC.

In a comparison of 10 MPPT versus 13 benign PPT by Moran et al[94], p53 expression pattern (**Figure 4.36**) and Ki67 proliferation index were not helpful in distinguishing MPPT from benign PPT. Positivity for calretinin and CD34 has been reported to support an outer root sheath origin, favoring benign PPT/MPPT over SCC; however, CD34 can be also negative in MPPT.[96] Keratin 15 has been reported to be positive in the proliferative areas of PPT and negative in SCC, and keratin 7 and keratin 19 are reported to demonstrate single cell positivity in PPT and negativity in SCC.[97]

Sweat-Gland Carcinoma with Neuroendocrine Differentiation

Low-grade neuroendocrine carcinoma of the skin (LGNECS) was proposed in 2017 as a new primary cutaneous neoplasm with neuroendocrine differentiation.[98] *PTEN* c.165-1G>A splice site mutation was detected in one case, and *GATA3* P409fs*99 and *SETD2* R1708fs*4 in another case. All 8 cases with tumor size larger than 2cm experienced lymph node metastasis while only in 1/5 cases whose size was less than 2cm.[98] The tumor size appears to be a better prognostic factor than nuclear atypia, mitotic count, and Ki67 proliferation index, contrary to neuroendocrine tumors.[98]

Histologic and Immunohistochemical Features

Histology shows a well-differentiated neuroendocrine tumor with intraepidermal pagetoid spread in 60% and stromal mucin deposition in 30% of cases.[98] Keratin 7, keratin 19, EMA, BerEP4, CEA, chromogranin A, synaptophysin, INSM1, GCDFP15, GATA3, ER, and bcl-2 expression were variably present.[98]

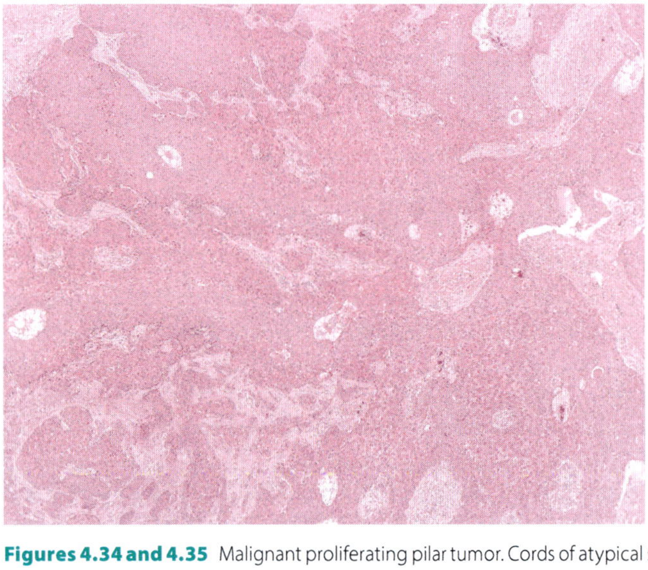

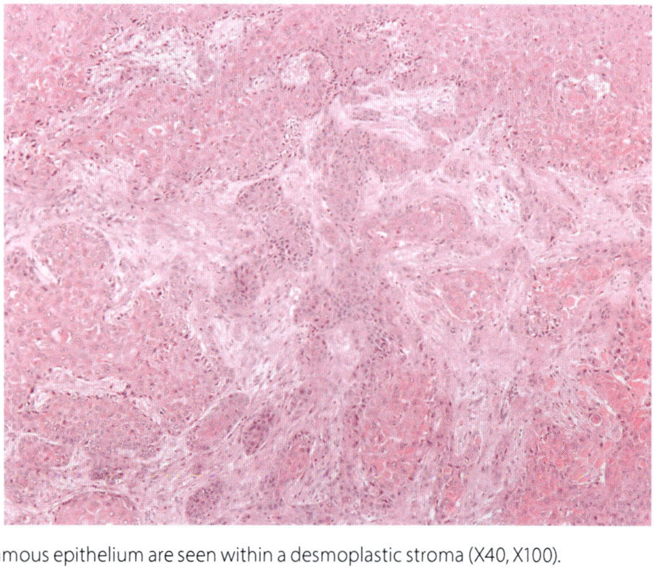

Figures 4.34 and 4.35 Malignant proliferating pilar tumor. Cords of atypical squamous epithelium are seen within a desmoplastic stroma (X40, X100).

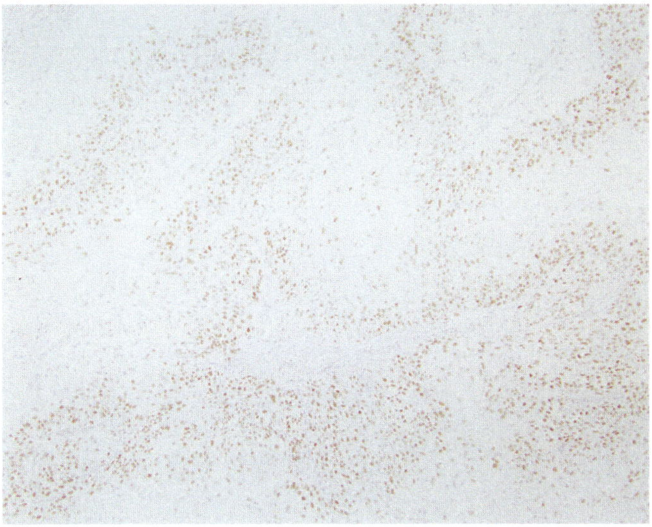

Figure 4.36 Malignant proliferating pilar tumor. p53 overexpression is seen (X100).

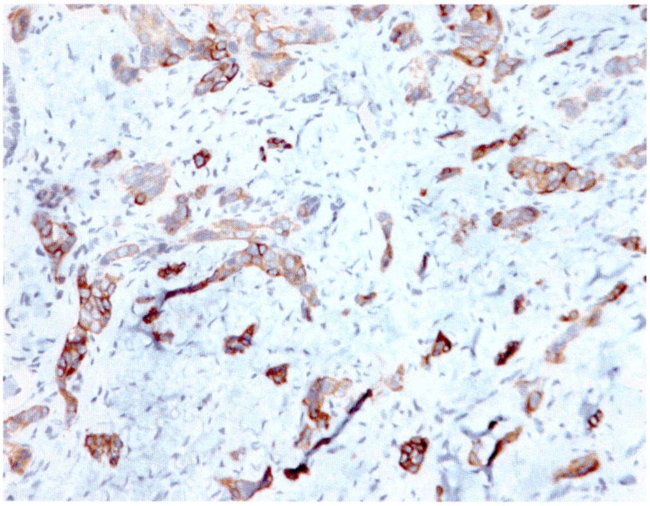

Figure 4.38 Microcystic adnexal carcinoma. The tumor cells strongly express keratin 19 (X100).

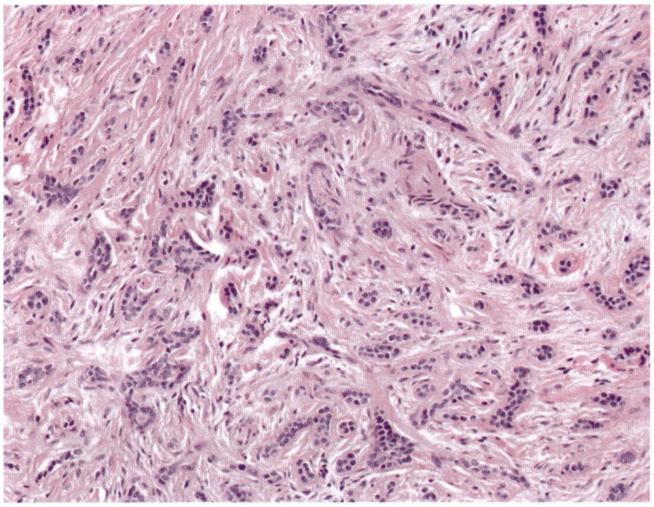

Figure 4.37 Microcystic adnexal carcinoma. Infiltrative strands of tumor cells are seen in the dermis (X200).

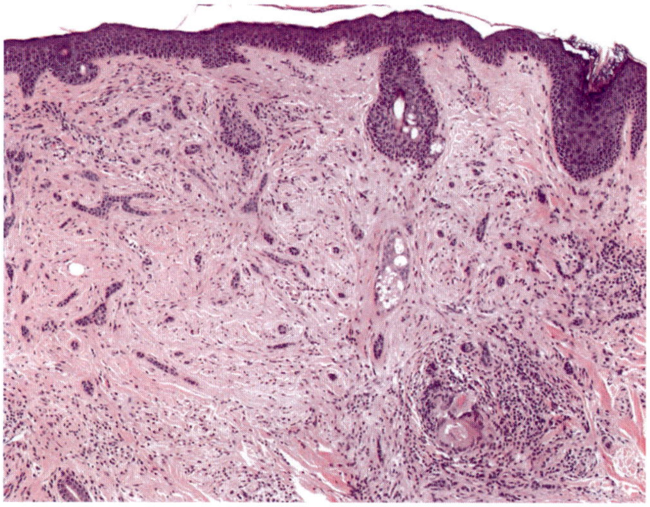

Figure 4.39 Desmoplastic trichoepithelioma is characterized by infiltrative basaloid nests and ruptured keratocysts (X100).

Microcystic Adnexal Carcinoma

Microcystic adnexal carcinoma (MAC) is a locally aggressive tumor with a predilection for the central face, especially upper lip and nasolabial fold, of adults.[99] On histologic sections it is characterized by an infiltrative architecture and three zones: superficial keratocysts, nests and strands of tumor cells in the middle portion, and duct-like structures in the deep aspect. Perineural and skeletal muscle invasion is frequently seen. Solid carcinoma is thought to be a variant of MAC.[100]

Microcystic Adnexal Carcinoma versus Other Sclerosing Neoplasms

Due to the location of the tumor the biopsy is often superficial; thus, it is difficult to recognize the characteristic stratified appearance of MAC and perineural invasion in the deep aspect of the tumor. Its histologic mimics include dTE, infiltrative or morpheaform BCC, and even SCC. Expression of keratin 19 favors MAC over dTE and iBCC (**Figures 4.37–4.40**).[101] Keratin

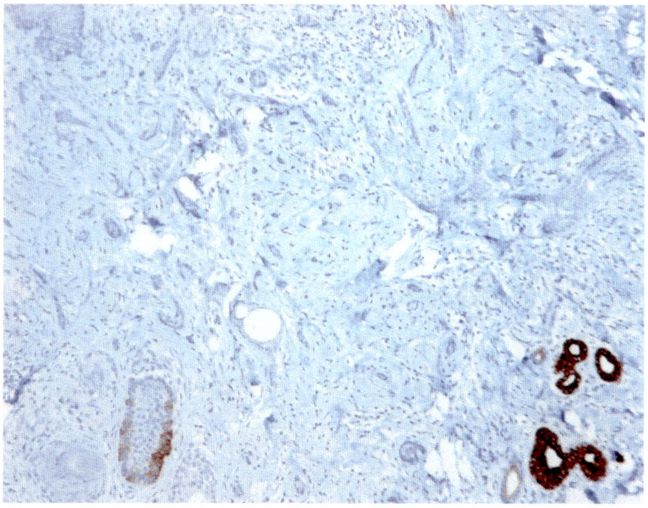

Figure 4.40 Desmoplastic trichoepithelioma. The tumor cells are negative for keratin 19 while the eccrine glands and hair bulge region are positive (X100).

Table 4.8 Immunoprofiles of desmoplastic trichoepithelioma, microcystic adnexal carcinoma and basal cell carcinoma[12,101,102,104–107]

	Desmoplastic trichoepithelioma	Syringoma	Microcystic adnexal carcinoma	Basal cell carcinoma
Keratin 19	22–57%	0%	70–100%	41%
Keratin 15	95–100%		44–92%	0–47%
BerEP4	57–76%		0–38%	100%
Keratin 20+ Merkel cells	100%		0%	0–9%
CEA			3–100% (ducts)	0%
Keratin 7	0%		15%	40%
PHLDA1	100%		67%	0–6%
P75 (>90%)	94% (100%)		44% (100%)	36% (100%)
Ki67	3%		8%	
Laminin gamma 2	0%	0%	90%	96%
GLI1 RNA ish	50%		0%	95%

15, a specific marker of hair follicle stem cells, can be expressed in 92% of MAC and 100% of dTE, but in none of the infiltrating BCC or SCC.[102]

Although Ber-EP4 has been shown to be negative in MAC cases, BerEP4 expression can be seen in 38% of cases in other series.[102] CEA has been traditionally the marker of choice in demonstrating ductal differentiation in MAC whose expression can be seen from 31% (4/13) to 100% (7/7).[102] Recently, p63 has been reported by Vidal and colleagues to label the peripheral neoplastic cells only in the deep aspect of MAC; however, this is not useful since we often receive superficial biopsies.[103] Sixty-seven percent of MAC cases can express PHLDA1 thus it is of limited value in distinguish a benign versus a malignant sclerosing neoplasm.[12] p75 has not been found to be a helpful distinguishing marker (**Table 4.8**). [12,101,102,104–107] The mean Ki67 proliferation index has been reported to be higher in MAC (8%) versus dTE (3%).[105]

Deep syringoma can be misdiagnosed as MAC, reportedly in 30% of cases.[108] Lack of keratin 19 expression, p63 staining of only the outer myoepithelial layer, lack of follicular differentiation, and marked ductal proliferation are supportive of deep syringoma over MAC.[108] Syringoid eccrine carcinoma typically expresses keratin 5/6/8/19; therefore, its immunoprofile is overlapping with MAC.[109]

Microcystic adnexal carcinoma versus other sclerosing neoplasms

- Microcystic adnexal carcinoma: keratin 15+ keratin 19+ BerEP4-/+
- Desmoplastic trichoepithelioma: keratin 15+ keratin 19- BerEP4-/+
- Basal cell carcinoma: keratin 15-/+ keratin 19- BerEP4+

Squamoid Eccrine Ductal Carcinoma

Squamoid eccrine ductal carcinoma (SEDC) is a rare tumor that affects the head, neck, or extremities of elderly patients, likely under-recognized.[109,110] Local recurrence in 25% of cases, lymph node metastasis in 12.5% [109] and rare cases with widespread metastasis have been reported.[109,111] Wide local excision is the treatment of choice.[109,112]

Histology and Immunohistochemical Findings

An infiltrative tumor, highlighted by keratin 5/6 and p63, is seen in the dermis and sometimes subcutaneous tissue. Nests, cords, and strands of epithelial cells with severe cytologic atypia and frequent mitoses are seen within a desmoplastic stroma. Van der Horst et al.[109] documented necrosis, perineural invasion, and lymphovascular invasion in 23%, 26%, and 6% of cases. The superficial aspect of the tumor resembles a well to moderately differentiated SCC. The presence of keratocysts and squamous eddies also raises the possibility of MAC in the differential diagnosis; however, mild cytologic atypia would be seen in MAC (**Figure 4.41**). CEA and EMA highlight the ductal differentiation in the deep aspect of tumor, distinguishing SEDC from SCC (**Figure 4.42**).

The histologic differential diagnosis also includes porocarcinoma with squamous differentiation and eccrine carcinoma (**Table 4.9**). YAP1-C and NUT immunostains to document

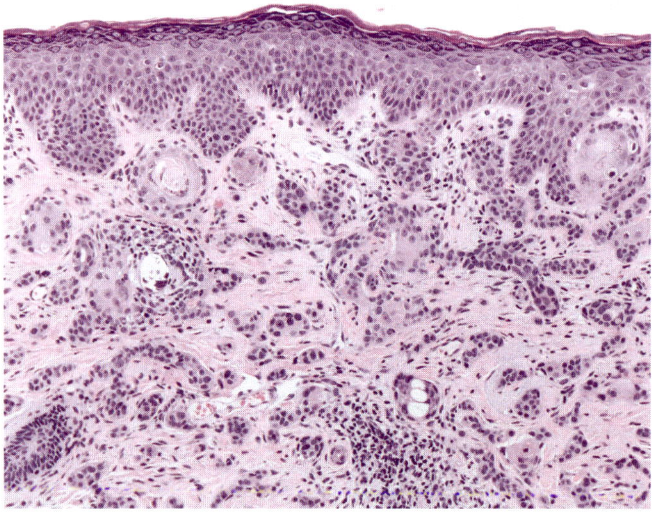

Figure 4.41 Squamoid eccrine ductal carcinoma. Nests, cords, and strands of atypical epithelial cells are seen within a desmoplastic stroma (X200).

Table 4.9 Differential diagnosis of squamoid eccrine ductal carcinoma

Histologic features	Squamoid eccrine ductal carcinoma	Microcystic adnexal carcinoma	Squamous cell carcinoma	Porocarcinoma	Syringoid eccrine carcinoma
Anatomic location	Head and neck	Head and neck	Sun-exposed skin	Extremities	Face or scalp
Zonal pattern	+	+	–	–	–
Infiltrative growth	+	+	+/–	+	+
Subcutaneous invasion	+	+/–	+/–	+	+
Epidermal connection	+	–	+	+	–
Keratocysts	+	+	+	–	–
Squamous eddies	+	–	+/–	+/–	–
Squamous differentiation	superficial	–	+	+	–
Desmoplastic stroma	+	+	+/–	+/–	–
Marked cytologic atypia	+	–	+	+	–
Necrosis	+/–	–	+/–	+	+/–
Perineural invasion	+	+	+/–	+/–	+
Lymphovascular invasion	+/–	–	+/–	+/–	–
Keratin 5/6	+	+	+	+	+/–
p63	+	+	+	+	+/–
EMA	+ lumen	–	+	+	+
CEA	+ lumen	+ lumen	–	+	+

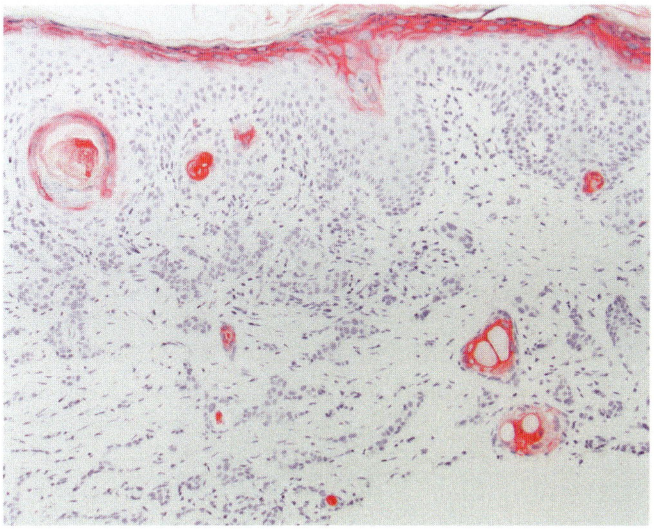

Figure 4.42 Squamoid eccrine ductal carcinoma. CEA highlights foci of ductal differentiation (X200).

possible *YAP1* and *NUT* fusions would be helpful in ruling in porocarcinoma; however, fusions are seen in only 64% of porocarcinomas.[113,114] Syringoid eccrine carcinoma would typically lacks squamous differentiation. Overall, immunohistochemistry has a limited role, and the diagnosis relies mainly on histopathologic findings.

High-Grade Carcinoma

Cutaneous Apocrine Carcinoma

Primary cutaneous apocrine carcinoma is rare and most often involves the axillae, but also the scalp, eyelid, extremities, and anogenital areas. It frequently metastasizes to the regional lymph nodes and is associated with a poor prognosis.[115] A non-encapsulated tumor is seen in the dermis exhibiting papillary, tubular, cord-like and solid growth patterns. The neoplastic cells have abundant eosinophilic cytoplasm (**Figures 4.43 and 4.44**). The tumor cells express keratin 7 and GCDFP15. Peripheral myoepithelial cells staining with p63, calponin and SMA are seen at the peripheral of the tumor nests in an *in situ* component. Cribriform carcinoma and digital papillary adenocarcinoma are considered by some to be variants of apocrine carcinoma. Currently there is no distinctive immunoprofile reported for these variants.

Cutaneous Apocrine Carcinoma versus Metastatic Mammary Apocrine Carcinoma

The main differential diagnosis of cutaneous apocrine carcinoma would be metastatic mammary apocrine carcinoma to the skin since both tumors exhibit similar histologic features and overlapping immunohistochemical profile. The distinction is important since treatment options are available for metastatic mammary apocrine carcinoma while there is no consensus in treatment guideline for cutaneous apocrine carcinoma. Apocrine carcinoma of the breast is defined as a carcinoma in which the majority of the tumor cells have apocrine morphology characterized by abundant eosinophilic cytoplasm, vesicular nucleus and prominent nucleoli. Pure infiltrating apocrine carcinoma may be less aggressive than high-grade infiltrating ductal carcinomas and might respond differently to therapeutic agents. By immunohistochemistry, mammary apocrine carcinoma is frequently androgen receptor (AR) positive, estrogen receptor (ER) negative, and progesterone receptor (PR) negative.[116]

Cutaneous apocrine carcinomas show consistent strong AR expression similar to its mammary counterpart.[115,117]

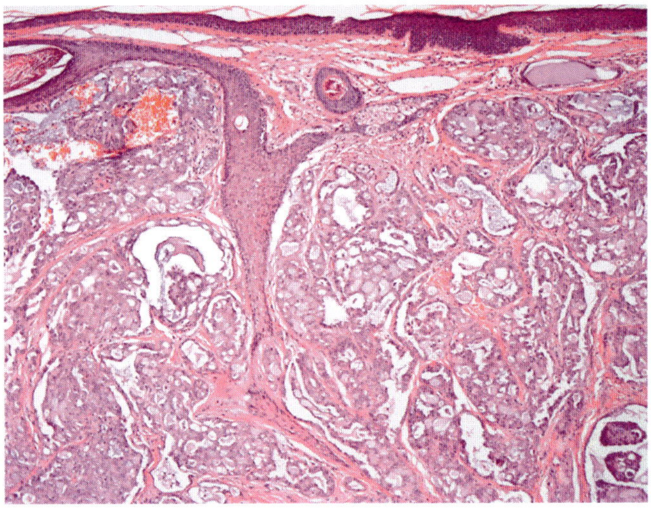

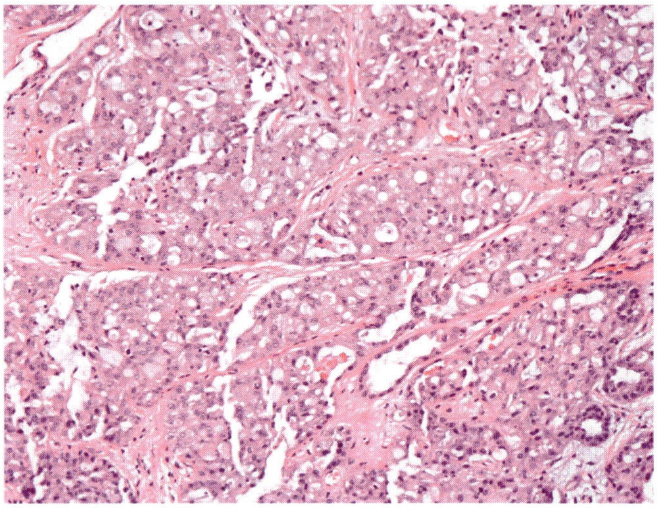

Figures 4.43 and 4.44 Cutaneous apocrine carcinoma. Glandular and cribriform proliferation of epithelial tumor cells with abundant eosinophilic cytoplasm is seen (X100, X200).

Adipophilin expression is seen significantly more frequent in mammary apocrine carcinomas than in the cutaneous counterpart, with strong expression seen only in mammary apocrine carcinoma in up to 40% of the studied cases.[118] ER and PR expression is seen more frequently in cutaneous apocrine carcinoma than in the mammary counterpart. Thus, an immunoprofile of AR+ ER+ PR+/- favors a cutaneous apocrine carcinoma. 3+ Her2 overexpression with *HER2* gene amplification were only seen in mammary apocrine carcinomas **(Figure 4.45)**.[118] In a large series by Plumb et al.[119] of 228 benign and malignant adnexal neoplasms and 27 cutaneous metastases (17 from breast primary), diffuse keratin 5/6 would favor a primary cutaneous tumor **(Figure 4.46)**, while negative or focal/weak expression would favor a metastasis. Although mammaglobin can be seen in both mammary and cutaneous apocrine carcinomas, diffuse and strong mammaglobin staining was noted only in cutaneous apocrine carcinomas **(Figure 4.47)**.[118]

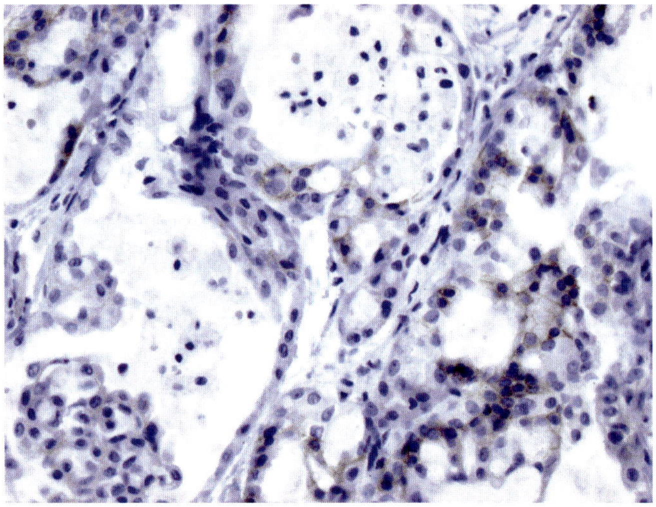

Figure 4.45 Cutaneous apocrine carcinoma. Weak 1+ Her2 expression (X400).

Cutaneous apocrine carcinoma versus metastatic mammary apocrine carcinoma

- Cutaneous apocrine carcinoma: adipophilin- ER+PR+/- Her2- and can exhibit strong and diffuse keratin 5/6 and/or mammaglobin expression
- Mammary apocrine carcinoma: adipophilin+ ER-PR- and often exhibit 3+ Her2 with corresponding *HER2* gene amplification

Aggressive Digital Papillary Adenocarcinoma

Digital papillary adenocarcinoma (DPAC) is an adnexal carcinoma that preferentially affects the acral sites, especially the fingers and toes, of men more frequently than women.[120] Clinically the lesion is often diagnosed as a cyst. Although rare, tumors at non-acral sites such as anogenital sites have been reported.[121] Due to frequent recurrence, partial amputation is often the treatment of choice and metastasis has been documented in 26% to 50% in the literature.[122]

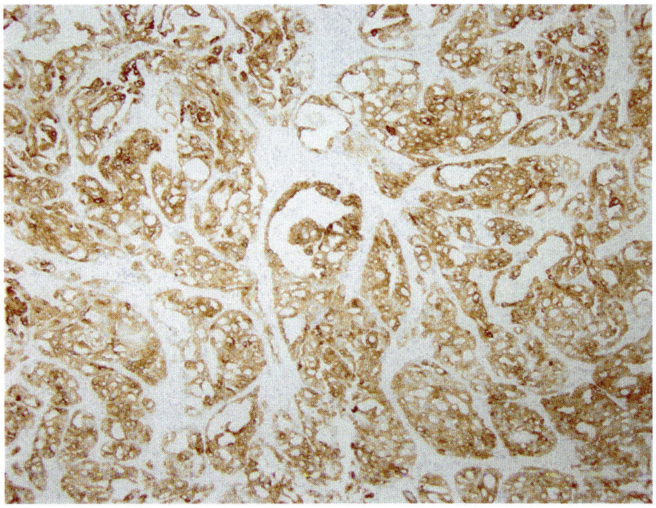

Figure 4.46 Cutaneous apocrine carcinoma. Diffuse keratin 5/6 expression (X200).

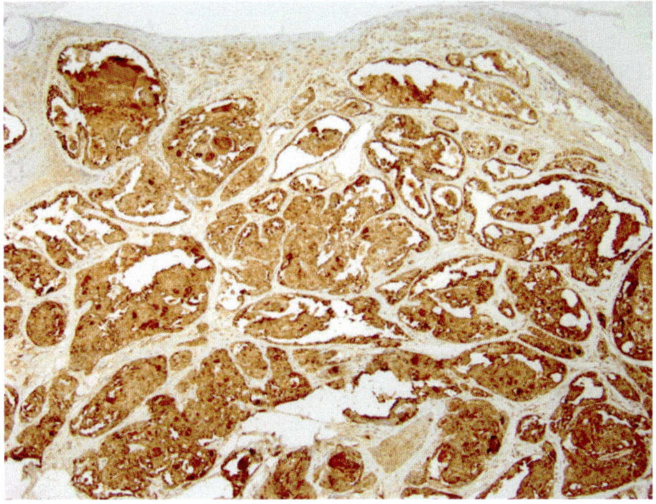

Figure 4.47 Cutaneous apocrine carcinoma. Diffuse mammaglobin expression (X200).

Histologic Findings

A non-encapsulated and multinodular proliferation of epithelial cells with solid, papillary and/or cystic architecture is seen in the dermis and subcutaneous tissue. Back-to-back glands formed by inner epithelial cells with apocrine differentiation and outer myoepithelial cells are seen (**Figure 4.48**). Hyalinized stroma, variable cytologic atypia and mitotic figures are seen. Necrosis can be present. Clear cells, spindle cells, mucus-secreting cells, and sebaceous differentiation can be seen (**Figure 4.49**).

Immunohistochemical Findings

The tumor is positive for S100, keratin 7, PHLDA1, and EMA.[120] Ki67 proliferation index can range from 2% to 30%.[120] The main differential diagnosis is acral hidradenoma.[120] p63 and p40 highlight only the myoepithelial layer of DPAC (**Figure 4.50**). In contrast, diffuse p63 and p40 expression is noted in acral hidradenoma (**Figures 4.51**–4.53).[122] *CRTC1::MAML2* fusion can be seen in approximately 50% of hidradenoma.[123] Recently, HPV42 DNA was detected in DPAC by molecular analyses.[124] *In situ* hybridization for HPV42 has been shown in all 10 tested DPAC, and absent in 30 other adnexal tumors including 8 acral hidradenomas.[124] In a study by Bui and colleagues,[125] BRAFV600E immunostain was positive in four DPAC while HPV *in situ* hybridization was negative.

Extramammary Paget Disease

EMPD is a rare cutaneous malignancy that affects elderly individuals (60–80 years), especially postmenopausal women and Asian men.[126] EMPD typically affects anatomic regions with high concentration of apocrine glands such as axillae and anogenital region.[126] Mohs micrographic surgery has been shown to be more superior than wide excision for primary EMPD.[127] Other treatment modalities for EMPD includes topical imiquimod for noninvasive vulvar Paget disease, radiotherapy, and Her2-targeted therapy for advanced tumor with *HER2* amplification.

Extramammary Paget Disease (EMPD) can be either primary or secondary. Primary EMPD presents as well-demarcated, erythematous plaque which can mimic various dermatitis such as eczema, intertrigo, psoriasis, and fungal infections. Occasionally, EMPD can present synchronously in both axillary and anogenital regions.[128] Primary EMPD has a high recurrence rate yet rarely metastasizes, contrary to the secondary form. Primary EMPD can be either an intraepithelial neoplasm with or without invasion, or as a manifestation of an underlying primary adenocarcinoma. Chanda et al.[129] identified that 29% of 197 EMPD cases were associated with an underlying malignancy. Through a mechanism reminiscent of mammary Paget's disease, secondary EMPD is thought to originate from epidermotropic spread of malignant cells or within contiguous epithelium. Many cases of vulvar secondary EMPD have been described in association with other gynecologic and genitourinary (bladder) neoplasms. Perianal Paget's disease is strongly associated with adenocarcinoma of the anus and colorectum.

Primary versus Secondary Extramammary Paget Disease

The tumor cells in EMPD are usually positive for mucicarmine, Alcian blue and periodic-acid Schiff with diastase stains. Primary EMPD lesions would typically exhibit a sweat gland phenotype (keratin 7+/ keratin 20-/ gross cystic disease fluid protein

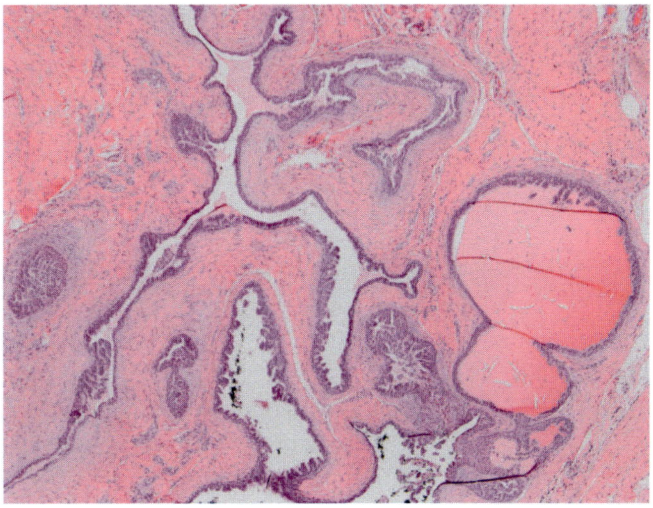

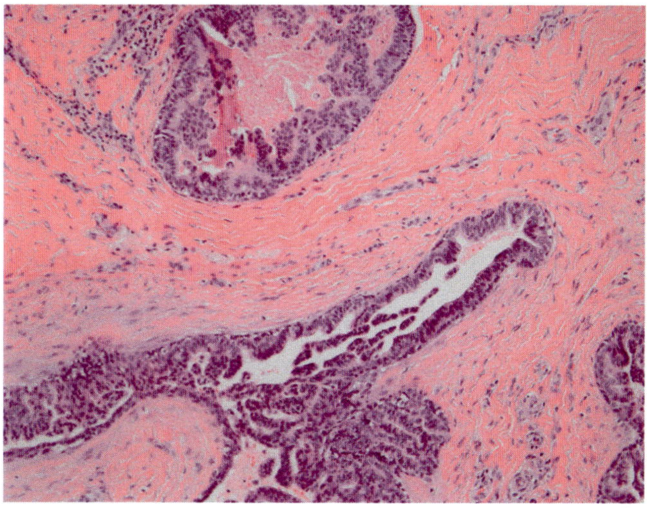

Figures 4.48 and 4.49 Aggressive digital papillary adenocarcinoma. A proliferation of epithelial cells with papillary and cystic architecture is seen (X40, X100).

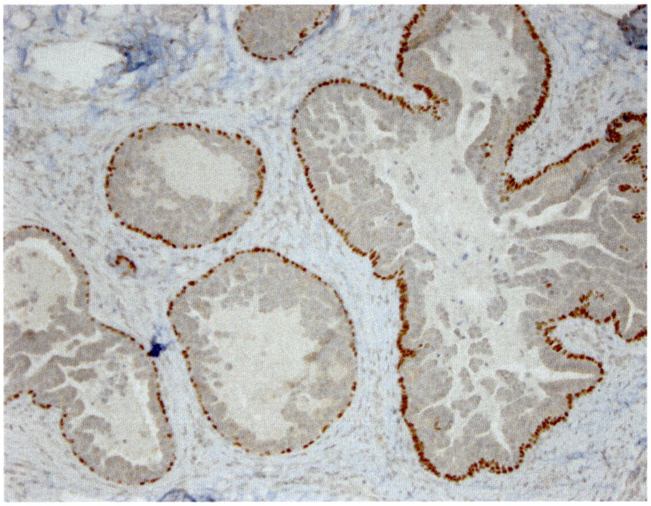

Figure 4.50 Aggressive digital papillary adenocarcinoma. p63 highlights the outer myoepithelial layer (X100).

(GCDFP)-15-), whereas secondary EMPD lesions would exhibit an endodermal phenotype (keratin 7+/keratin 20+/GCDFP-15-) (**Figures 4.54 and 4.55**).[130] Co-expression of keratin 20 and CDX2 is indicative of secondary EMPD of colorectal origin.[131] HER-2/neu and CDX2 have been found to be useful in distinguishing primary EMPD from secondary EMPD of anorectal adenocarcinoma.[131] It should be emphasized however that the burden of delineation between primary and secondary EMPD lies on the clinician.

Our understanding of the genetic basis for extramammary Paget's disease (EMPD) is currently limited. The expression of Her2/neu and androgen receptor indicates potential benefit from targeted therapy.[132,133] However, fluorescence *in situ* hybridization demonstrates no evidence of *HER2* gene amplification.[134]

The differential diagnosis of EMPD includes both benign conditions such as vulvar Toker cells, mucinous metaplasia, vulva intraepithelial neoplasia with pagetoid spread of malignant cells and malignant melanoma (**Table 4.10**). The

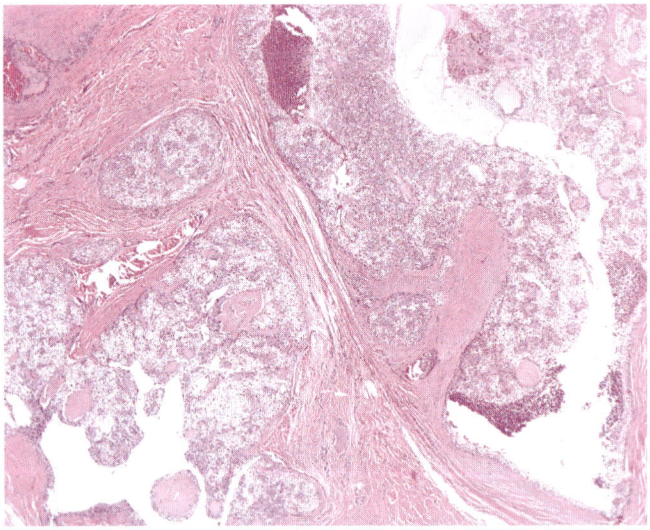

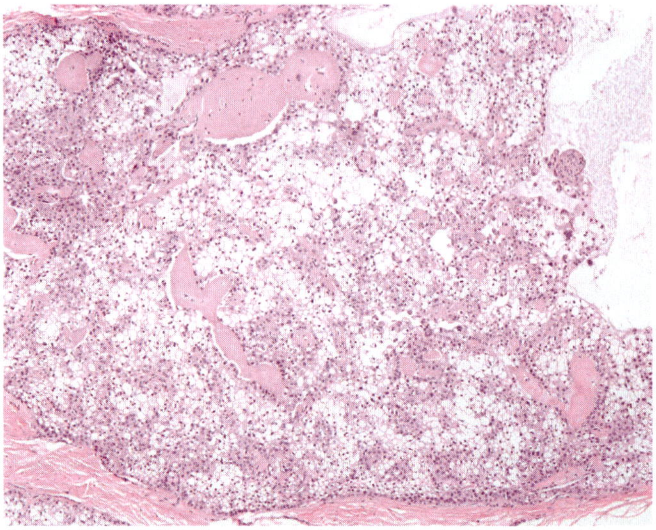

Figures 4.51 and 4.52 Hidradenoma of digit. A solid and cystic proliferation of epithelial cells with clear cytoplasm is noted. (X40, X100).

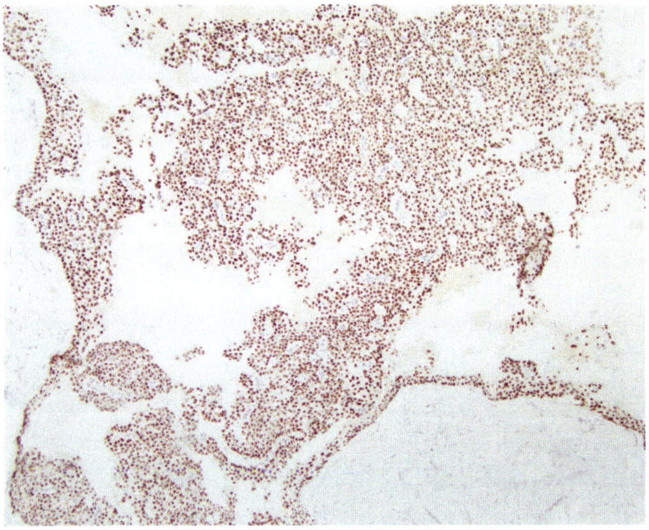

Figure 4.53 Hidradenoma of digit. Diffuse p63 expression is seen (X100).

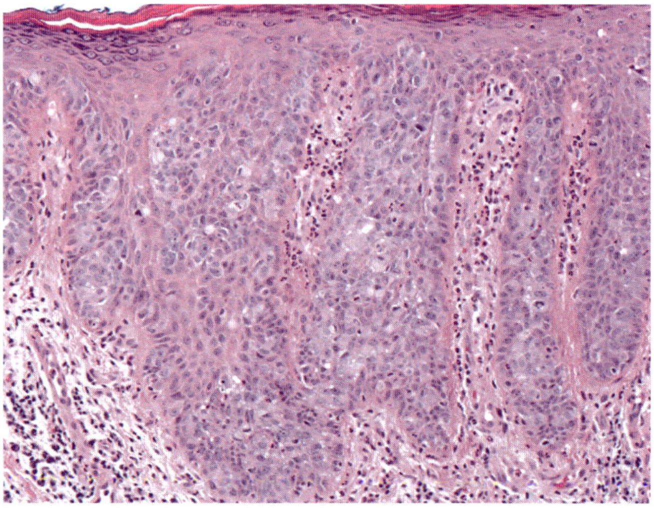

Figure 4.54 Extramammary Paget disease. Intraepidermal neoplastic cells with pagetoid growth and cytoplasmic mucin are seen (X200).

Table 4.10 Differential diagnoses of extramammary Paget disease[136–138]

Immunostain	Primary	Secondary colorectal	Secondary urothelial	Squamous cell carcinoma *in situ*	Melanoma *in situ*
Keratin 7	+	-/+	-/+	+/-	-
Keratin 20	-	+	+	-	-
GCDFP–15	+	-	-	-	-
Her2/neu	+	-	-	-	-
CDX2	-	+	-	-	-
MUC2	-	+	-	-	-
MUC5AC	+	-	-	-	-
Uroplakin III	-	-	+	-	-
p63	-	-	+	+	-
Keratin 903	-	-	-	+	-
S100	-	-	-	-	+
Melan A	-	-	-	-	+
TRSP1	+	ND	ND	-	-

GCDFP-15: gross cystic disease fluid protein-15, SCCIS: squamous cell carcinoma *in situ*, MIS: melanoma *in situ*, ND: not done

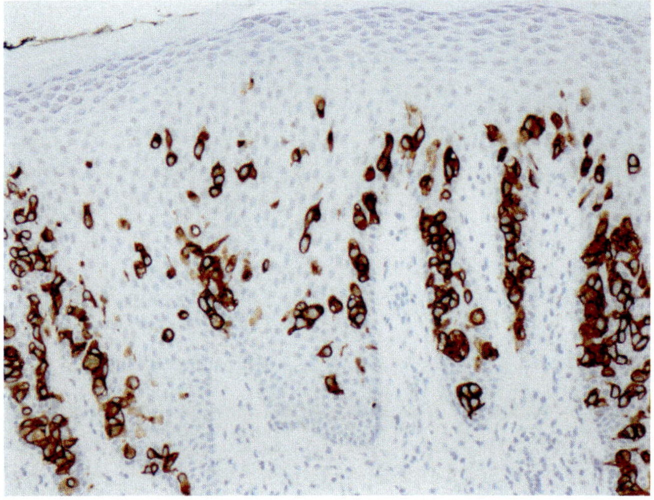

Figure 4.55 Extramammary Paget disease. The neoplastic cells express keratin 7 (X200).

profile of mucin expression of EMPD would be MUC1+ MUC2- MUC5AC+ while that of mammary Paget is MUC1+ MUC2- MUC5AC-.[135] In a recent study of 56 patients, Shaco-Levy et al.[136] reported that a panel of pan-keratin, keratin 7, CEA and EMA labels 100% of primary EMPD cases, while no cases stained with S100, HMB-45 and MART-1 distinguishing EMPD from malignant melanoma. SCC *in situ* would be positive for p63 and keratin 903.[137] EMPD would strongly express TRPS1, a breast marker.[138]

Extramammary Paget disease

Primary versus secondary EMPD: keratin 7, keratin 20, CDX2 and p63

Primary EMPD versus squamous cell carcinoma *in situ* versus melanoma: keratin 7, keratin 903, S100 and Melan A

Hidradenocarcinoma and Hidradenoma

Clear cell hidradenomas are relatively frequent benign adnexal tumors. The lesion typically presents as a solitary, asymptomatic, slow growing and well-circumscribed nodule on the trunk, head and neck areas, and extremities.[139]

Histology Features

In the majority of cases a solid and/or cystic growth pattern is seen on the histologic sections. A variety of cell types can be seen including clear cells, eosinophilic cells, squamoid or epidermoid cells, and mucinous cells (Figures 4.51 and 4.52). The tumor can be low-grade in histologic appearance mimicking benign hidradenoma.[183] The tumor would stain for keratin 7, keratin MNF116, and CAM5.2.[139] EMA and CEA would highlight the luminal border of the ductal structures.[140]

Atypical Hidradenoma versus Hidradenocarcinoma

The malignant counterpart of hidradenoma, malignant hidradenoma or hidradenocarcinoma, is a very rare tumor that has been reported mostly as case reports and isolated small case series.[140,141] Accepted histologic criteria for diagnosing a malignant hidradenoma or hidradenocarcinoma include the lack of circumscription, an infiltrative growth pattern, deep extension, nuclear pleomorphism, necrosis, vascular invasion, perineural invasion, and presence of increased number of mitoses.[141] However, rendering a diagnosis of hidradenocarcinoma can be challenging since some of the lesions do not possess all of the above-mentioned criteria. Occasionally, benign-appearing tumors show focal atypical features including lack of circumscription, nuclear pleomorphism, focal necrosis or prominent mitotic activity.[141] They have been designated as atypical hidradenoma by pathologists (**Figure 4.56**). Histologic features of malignant hidradenomas that significantly differ from atypical hidradenomas include infiltrative growth pattern, deep extension, necrosis, nuclear pleomorphism, and four or more mitoses per 10 high power fields. Atypical hidradenoma has a significantly lower Ki-67 and PHH3 expression than the malignant

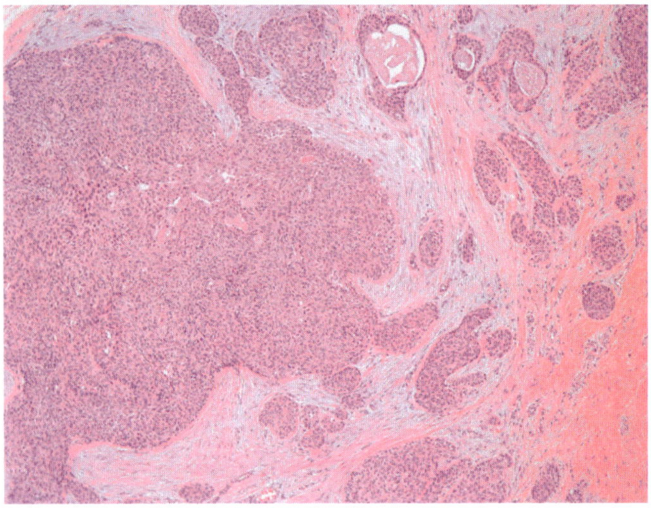

Figure 4.56 Atypical hidradenoma is characterized by an infiltrative growth pattern yet possessing bland cytologic features (X100).

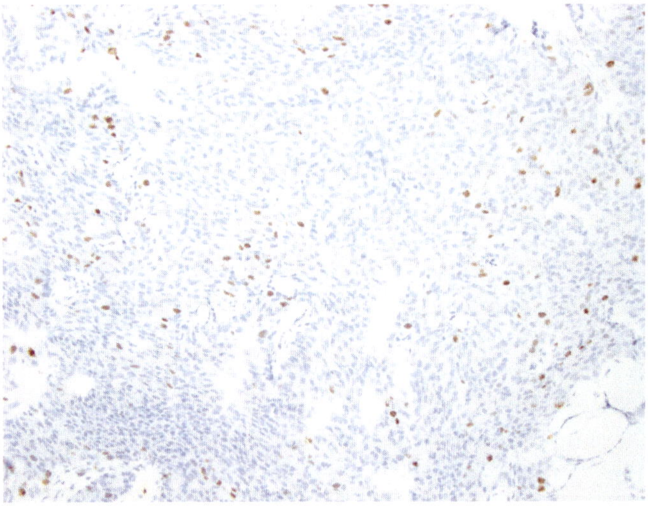

Figure 4.57 Atypical hidradenoma. Ki-67 demonstrates a low proliferation index (X200).

counterpart and the metastasizing adnexal carcinoma. A tumor with Ki-67 > 11% and/or PHH3 > 0.7% would likely be a malignant rather than an atypical hidradenoma (**Figure 4.57**).[141] Ki-67 and PHH3 may be helpful diagnostic adjuncts in classifying hidradenoma in the setting of small or partial biopsy specimen.

Molecular Findings

The majority of hidradenomas harbors *MAML2* gene rearrangement.[142] *TORC1/ CTRC1::MAML2* and *CTRC3::MAML2* fusions have been detected in cutaneous clear cell hidradenoma.[143–146] In a series of 36 clear cell hidradenomas and 3 poroid hidradenomas, *CTRC1::MAML2* fusion was detected in 10 cases (26%) and *CTRC3::MAML2* fusion was detected in 2 cases (5%).[145] All 12 cases had clear cell morphology. *EWSR1::FOU5F1* was detected in hidradenoma.[147] *CTRC1::MAML2*, *CTRC3::MAML2*, and *EWSR1::FOU5F1* fusions have been reported in both hidradenoma and mucoepidermoid carcinoma.[147]

Porocarcinoma

In a series of 453 cases,[148] the mean age was 68 years. Head and neck are the most commonly affected site, followed by the lower extremity. Metastases, most commonly to regional lymph node, were documented in 31% of cases. Surgery was the main treatment modality.[148] Porocarcinoma is an uncommon cutaneous carcinoma that present as an ulcerated nodule or tumor or verrucous plaque with sizes ranging from 1 to 20 cm. The common sites include the lower extremities, then trunk, upper extremities and head and neck; whereas its benign counterpart, poroma, is commonly seen on the palms and soles. In the largest series of porocarcinoma (69 cases) studied to date, Robson et al.[149] report that 17% and 19% of cases experienced local recurrence and lymph node metastases, respectively. More recurrences (7% versus none) and nodal metastases (10% versus 4%) were observed for porocarcinoma in comparison to the moderately differentiated SCC cases, with similar median follow-up for porocarcinomas and SCC cases.[150]

On histologic sections the *in situ* component is intraepidermal and the invasive component is comprised of infiltrative nests surrounded by desmoplasia. Large zones of necrosis, ductal differentiation, clear cell change, pigmentation, perineural invasion, and intravascular tumor can be seen.[149] High-grade tumors can exhibit squamous differentiation.

Molecular Findings

YAP1::MAML2 and *YAP1::NUTM1* fusions in poroid tumors were first reported by Sekine et al.,[113] with *YAP1* fusions detected in 88% (92/104) of poromas and 64% (7/11) of porocarcinomas.[113] *YAP1::MAML2, MAML2::YAP1, YAP1::NUTM1*, and *WWTR1::NUTM1* fusions were detected in 71 (68%), 48 (46%), 21 (20%), and 1 (1%) poromas, respectively.[113] *YAP1::NUTM1* fusion was seen in 54.5% of porocarcinomas.[113] *WWTR1::NUTM1* was identified only in rare poroma.[113]

Differential Diagnosis: Porocarcinoma versus Squamous Cell Carcinoma

Since porocarcinomas have a higher incidence of nodal metastases and poorer survival, distinction from SCC can have treatment implication.[149,151] However, the lack of defined diagnostic criteria together with overlapping immunostaining pattern can make the distinction of porocarcinoma and SCC difficult. Keratin 19 with a sensitivity of 67% and specificity of 82% can be a helpful marker when use together with keratin 7 in the distinction of porocarcinoma from SCC (**Figures 4.58 and 4.59**).[150] Carcinoembryonic antigen (CEA), highlighting foci of ductal differentiation, has been also shown to be positive in 30–80% of SCC cases.[4,152] Both porocarcinomas and SCC can express EMA, CAM5.2, CD10, p63, keratin 5/6, and BerEP4. Although sensitivity of EN1 and keratin 19 for porocarcinoma are 81% and 69%, respectively; a combination of EN1 and keratin 19 improves the specificity to 100% since none of SCC cases stained for both EN1 and keratin 19 (**Table 4.11**).[4,114,149,150,152–154]

100/104 (96%) poromas and 7/11 (64%) porocarcinomas with *YAP1* fusions exhibited diffuse nuclear expression of N terminal portion of YAP1 (7/11).[113] NUT has been reported to be a specific marker for cutaneous poroid tumors harboring *YAP1::NUTM1* fusions,[114] though sensitivity is low (11–29%).[154] None of the cases showed any expression of the C-terminus antibody.[113] Since all poromas and porocarcinomas with

Table 4.11 Immunostaining of squamous cell carcinoma versus porocarcinoma[4,114,149,150,152–154]

	Porocarcinoma	Squamous cell carcinoma
Keratin 19	50–93%	18–30%
Keratin 7	64–67%	13–26%
Nestin	13–35%	37–45%
Keratin 15	41–49%	0–30%
CAM5.2	38–51%	58%
CEA	68–100% + ducts	30–80%
EMA	94–100%	85–100%
CD10	0%	25%
CD15	10%	0%
p63	100%	80–100%
p40	100%	100%
Keratin 5/6	100%	69%
CD117	79%	14%
BerEP4	57%	9%
GATA3	57%	73%
NUTM1	11–29%	0%
YAP1-C loss	58%	0%
EN1	81%	16%

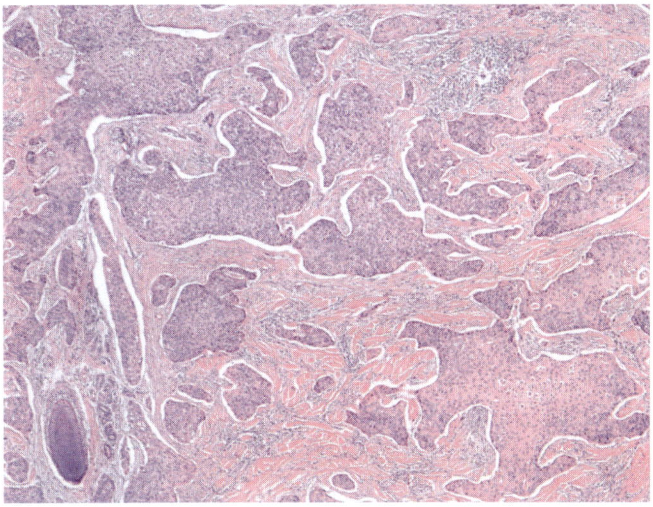

Figure 4.58 Porocarcinoma. Infiltrating nests of carcinoma are seen in the dermis (X40).

YAP1::NUTM1 fusions exhibited YAP1 C-terminus loss and nuclear NUT expression, YAP1-C and NUT immunostains can be used as screening tests.[113,114]

NUTM1 rearrangements have been well described in NUT carcinoma, various sarcomas including subsets of spindle cell and round cell sarcomas (*CIC::NUTM1*, *MGA::NUTM1*, *MXD4::NUTM1*), and pediatric/infant acute lymphoblastic leukemias.[155,156]

Squamous cell carcinoma versus porocarcinoma

Porocarcinoma: Keratin 19+ keratin 7+

Squamous cell carcinoma: Keratin19-/+ keratin 7-/+

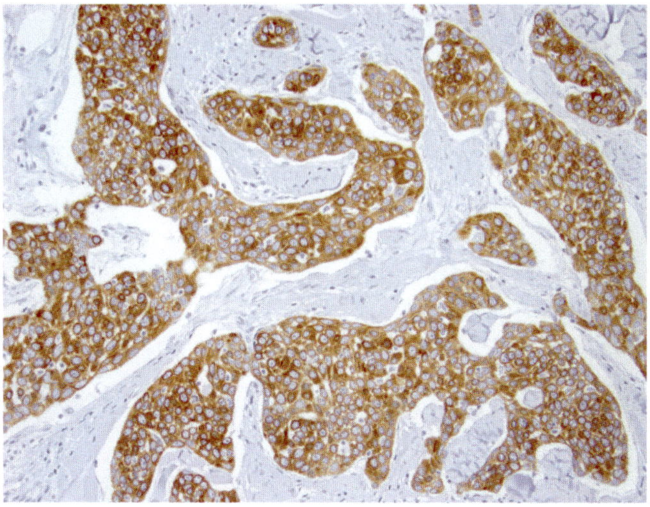

Figure 4.59 Porocarcinoma. Diffuse keratin 19 expression is seen (X200).

Signet-Ring Cell Histiocytoid Carcinoma

A rare and aggressive tumor of mainly the eyelid and seldom the axillae, signet-ring cell or histiocytoid carcinoma most commonly affect older men.[157] Metastasis is common and has been reported to be more frequently in axillary than eyelid cases.[157,158]

Sheets and cords of tumor cell are seen infiltrating the dermal collagen bundles and underlying structures on histologic sections. The neoplastic cells resemble histiocytes in the histiocytoid variant. They express diffuse reactivity for CAM5.2, keratin 7, AE1/AE3 and MNF16 keratins, CEA, EMA, GCDFP-15, mucin-1 (MUC-1), MUC5AC, GCDFP15,[157] androgen receptor, BerEP4 and E-cadherin (**Figures 4.60**–4.62). There is variable expression for estrogen receptor and progesterone receptor, MUC6.[157,159] Keratin 20, p63, MUC2, CD117, Sox10, TTF1, and CDX2 were negative.[157] The immunoprofile is similar for eyelid and axillary signet-ring cell/histiocytoid carcinoma and cutaneous apocrine carcinoma.[157]

PIK3CA mutation is a recurrent abnormality.[157,160] *CDH1* mutation detected in signet ring cell carcinoma.[160] The main differential diagnosis would be metastatic breast carcinoma. In contrast to cutaneous metastases, signet-ring cell carcinomas express p63 and D2-40.[159]

Syringocystadenocarcinoma Papilliferum and Syringocystadenoma Papilliferum

Syringocystadenocarcinoma papilliferum (SCACP) is the rare malignant counterpart of syringocystadenoma papilliferum. Head and neck are the most common location; however, the trunk, extremities, and anogenital region can be affected.[161] It can arise as a sporadic tumor or in association with a nevus sebaceus.[161] The tumor can rarely metastasize.

The carcinoma component is seen arising from areas with histologic features of syringocystadenoma papilliferum. The *in situ* carcinoma can be either adenocarcinoma *in situ* or squamous cell carcinoma *in situ*.[162] In these settings, p63 and smooth muscle actin immunostains would highlight the intact myoepithelial layer around the *in situ* carcinoma and their absence in the invasive component.

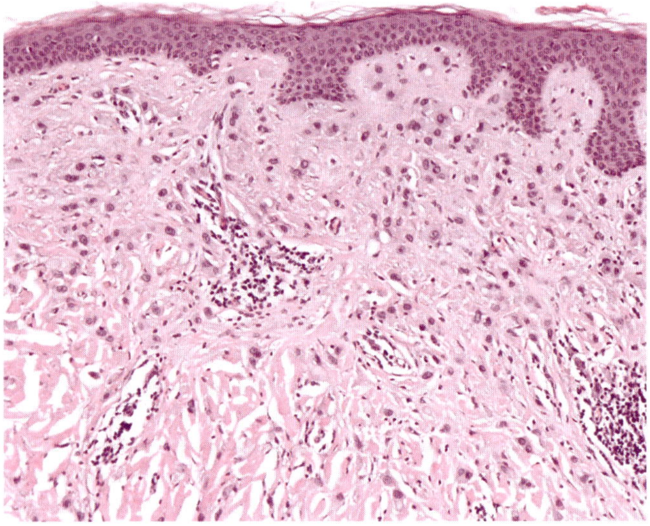

Figure 4.60 Signet-ring cell histiocytoid carcinoma. Cords of single tumor cells with histocytoid appearance (X200).

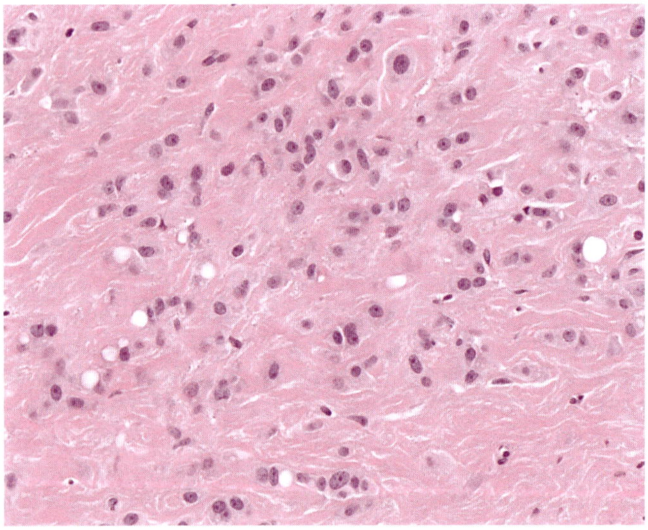

Figure 4.61 Signet-ring cell histiocytoid carcinoma. Signet-ring cell morphology is seen (X400).

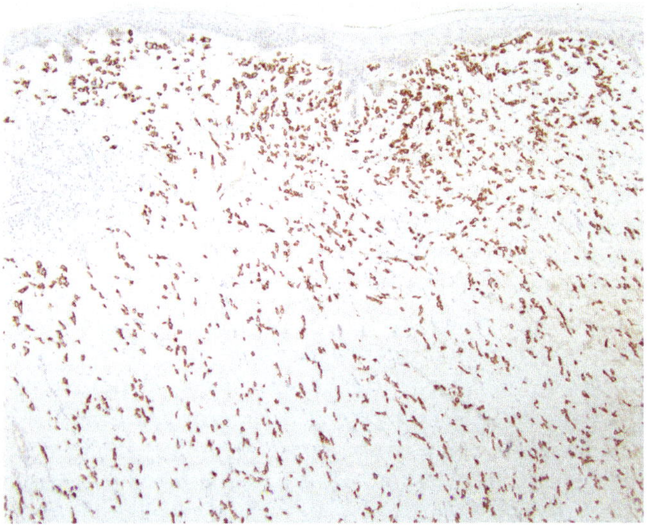

Figure 4.62 Signet-ring cell histiocytoid carcinoma. Diffuse keratin 7 expression is noted (X100).

Activating mutations in the RAS/MAPK signaling pathway have been identified in both SCAP and nevus sebaceous. Molecular analyses performed on 11 cases of SCACP revealed RAS-activating mutations in 50% of cases (*HRAS*, *KRAS*, and *BRAF* mutations).[162] Head and neck cases harbored *HRAS* mutation, while a case from the extremity harbored *KRAS* mutation.[162]

Primary Adnexal Carcinoma versus Cutaneous Metastases

Cutaneous metastasis of an internal malignancy is often indicative of a poor prognosis and most commonly associated with malignancies of the breast, lung, gastrointestinal system, and kidney. Currently p40, p63, and keratin 5/6 are the most helpful markers in the distinction of primary adnexal carcinoma from cutaneous metastases with p40 being the most specific marker (**Figures 4.63–4.65**) (**Table 4.12**).[163–165] p40, an isoform of p63, shows better specificity than p63 for excluding cutaneous metastases, especially from tumors of the breast, lung, endometrium, stomach, and thyroid.[163] Primary cutaneous adnexal neoplasms, SCC of various sites, BCC, as well as urothelial carcinomas express p63, a transcription factor belonging to the p53 family. The sensitivity and specificity of p63 has been reported to

Table 4.12 A primary adnexal carcinoma would invariable be positive for p40 and p63, while a cutaneous metastasis would likely be negative for these 2 markers[163–165]

	Primary adnexal carcinomas	Cutaneous metastases
p40	80%	8%
p63	89–100%	0–22%
Keratin 5/6	91–100%	27–56%
Keratin 15	40%	2%
D2–40	44–95%	0–4%
GATA3	47%	40%
Calretinin	14–64%	10–28%
Nestin	37%	8%

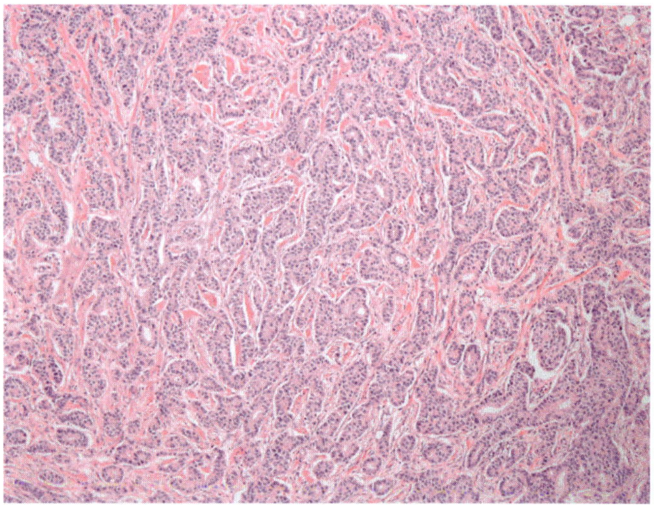

Figure 4.63 Infiltrating neoplastic ductal structures in the dermis in metastatic breast ductal carcinoma to the skin (X100).

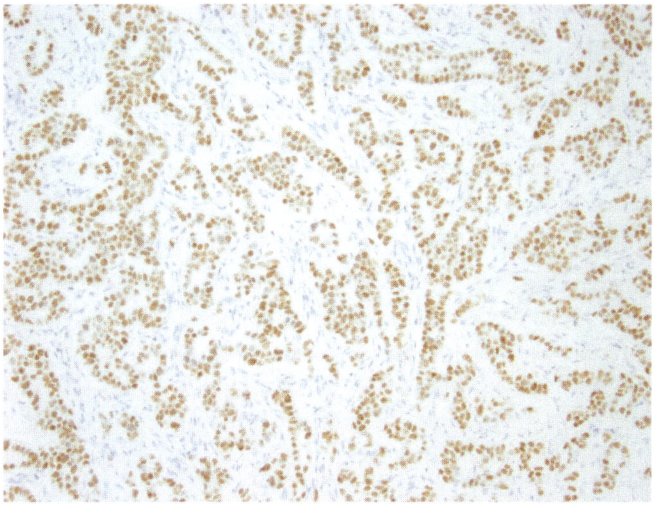

Figure 4.64 Mammary ductal carcinoma. Strong nuclear GATA3 expression by the tumor cells (X200).

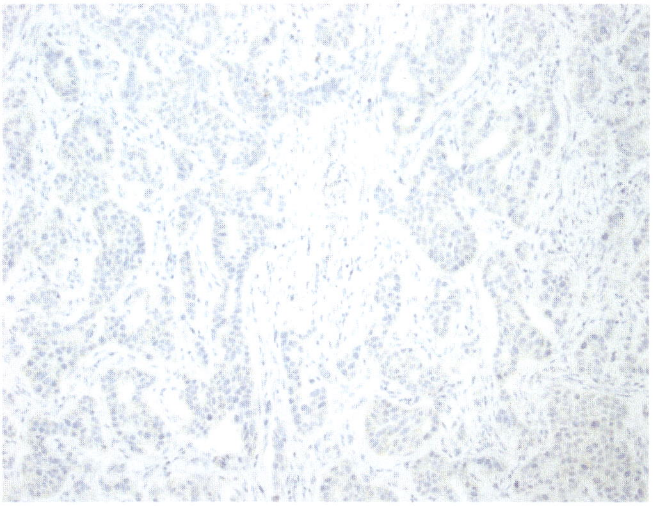

Figure 4.65 Mammary ductal carcinoma. Absent p40 expression (X200).

range from 89–100% and 89–100%, respectively.[164] Keratin 5/6 is a basic, high molecular weight cytokeratin with an expression profile similar to that of p63. p63 can be expressed in 11–22% of cutaneous metastases and keratin 5/6 expression can also be seen in 9–27% of adenocarcinomas of various primary sites.[163] GATA3 is not specific for carcinomas of the breast, bladder and salivary gland, since it can stain up 47% of cutaneous adnexal carcinomas.[163] In their comparative study of cutaneous metastases from breast carcinomas and primary sweat gland neoplasms, Rollins-Raval et al.[165] reported an overall sensitivity of 100% and specificity of 91% when using a panel of stains including p63, keratin 5/6, keratin 14, keratin 17, and mammaglobin. Therefore, the overall sensitivity and specificity may be better when a panel of immunostains is used.

Primary adnexal carcinoma versus cutaneous metastases

Primary adnexal carcinoma: p40+ p63+

Cutaneous metastases: p40- p63-

Primary Adnexal Carcinomas versus Salivary Gland Primary

Cutaneous, salivary and mammary tumors can display similar morphologic, immunohistochemical and molecular findings, reflecting their common embryologic origins.[166] Many cutaneous adnexal tumors share morphologic and molecular features with tumors arising in the salivary glands and breast. Fusions have become increasingly important in classifying these tumors (**Table 4.13**).[167]

Table 4.13 Summary of fusions reported in breast, salivary gland, and skin tumors

Tumor type	Fusion		References
Poroma	*YAP1::MAML2* *YAP1::NUTM1* *WWTR1::NUTM1*	68% 20–66% Rare case	Sekine 2019[113]
Porocarcinoma	*YAP1::NUTM1* *YAP1::MAML2* *EMC7::NUTM1*	54–60% 9% Rare case	
Hidradenoma	*CRTC1::MAML2* *CRTC3::MAML2* *EWSR1::FOU5F1*	48–50% Rare case Rare case	Behboudi 2005[144] Kuma 2017[145] Moller 2008[147]
Hidradenocarcinoma	*CRTC1::MAML2*	18%	
Adenoid cystic carcinoma	*MYB::NFIB* *MYBL1::NFIB* *EWSR1::MYB* *FUS::MYB*	40%	Weinreb 2023[57] Weinreb 2023[57]
Chondroid syringoma	*CTNNB1::PLAG1* *CHCHD7::PLAG1* *LIFR::PLAG1* *NDRG1::PLAG1* *TRPS1::PLAG1* *HMGA2::NFIB* *HMGA2::FHIT* *HMGA2::WIF1* *PHF1::TFE3*	19% 12% 3% skin skin Rare case	Asahina 2019[37] Panagopoulos 2020[38] Panagopoulos 2020[38] Astrom 1999[41] Geurts 1997[47] Persson 2009, Agaimy 2022[42,46] Panagopoulos 2019[48]
Soft tissue myoepithelioma	*EWSR1::PBX3* *EWSR1::POU5F1* *EWSR1::PBX1* *EWSR1::PBX3* *EWSR1::ZNF444* *EWSR1-ATF1* *EWSR1::KLF17* *FUS::KLF17* *EWSR1::KLF15*		Agaram 2015[183] Antonescu 2010[188] Brandal 2008[184] Jo 2019[178] Brandal 2009[186] Flulcke 2012[187] Huang 2015[189] Huang 2015[189] Bodis 2021[190]
Secretory carcinoma	*ETV6::NTRK3* *ETV6::X* *ETV6::MET* *ETV6::RET* *NFIX::PKN1* Dual *ETV6, NTRK3, MAML3* *VIM::RET*	Rare case Rare case	Bishop 2017,[74] Amin 2016,[72] Skalova 2016[77] Skalova 2016[77] Rooper 2018[80] Skalova 2018[81] Guilmette 2019[83] Guilmette 2019[83] Skalova 2020[82]
Microsecretory adenocarcinoma	*MEF2C::SS18* *SS18::ZBTB7A*		Bishop 2019[86]

Table 4.13 (cont.)

Tumor type	Fusion		References
Mucoepidermoid carcinoma	*CRTC1::MAML2* *CRTC3::MAML2* *EWSR1::FOU5F1*	34% salivary Rare case	Nakayama 2009,[173] Lennerz 2009[171] Nakayama 2009[173] Moller 2008[174]
NUT adnexal carcinoma	*BRD3::NUTM1* *NSD3::NUTM1*	2 cases	French 2014[192]
Unclassified adnexal carcinoma	*BRD3::NUTM2B* *BRD3::NUTM1*	3 cases	Rubio Gonzalez 2021[196]

Mucoepidermoid carcinoma

Mucoepidermoid carcinoma (MEC) is the most common salivary gland carcinoma, affecting mainly the parotid gland, then the submandibular gland and sublingual gland.[168] MEC can rarely be seen in the skin[169] and even in association with nevus sebaceus. A retrospective review of Surveillance, Epidemiology, and End Results (SEER) database from 1973 to 2016 yielded 89 patients with cutaneous MEC.[170] There is a predominance of Caucasian male and face location.[170] Surgery (82%), radiation (16%), and chemotherapy (7%) were the treatment for these patients.[170]

Histology Features

The tumor is usually solid but can be mainly cystic. The tumor is characteristically comprised of mucous (mucin producing/mucinous) goblet cells, squamoid cells, and intermediate cells.[168] Clear or oncocytic tumor cells can be the predominant cell type.

The tumor cells typically express p63, p40, and keratin 7; while they are negative for S100 and Sox10.[171] DOG1 and Sox10 expression is supportive of a distal intercalated duct/acinar phenotype.[85,172]

Molecular Findings

One third of salivary MECs have a t(11;19)(q21;p13) translocation involving *MECT1* or *CRTC1/TORC1/WAMTP1* (CREB-regulated transcription coactivator 1) and *MAML2* genes.[168,173] *CRTC1::MAML2* and *CRTC3::MAML2* were detected in 34% and 6% of 101 salivary MECs.[173] Rare case harbors t(6;22)(p21;q12) translocation with *EWSR1::POU5F1* fusion.[174] MECs with *CRTC3::MAML2* fusion are associated with more favorable clinicopathologic features and younger than those with *CRTC1::MAML2* fusion.[173] In another series of 71 MECs by Okabe et al.,[175] *CRTC1::MAML2* fusion was reported to be associated with favorable prognosis. *CRTC1* rearrangement was seen in all 8 analyzed cutaneous MECs.[171]

Differential Diagnosis

Although *CRTC1/3::MAML2* fusions can be seen in hidradenoma, mucoepidermoid carcinoma is rarely seen in the skin but mainly a tumor of salivary glands. Clinical correlation is needed to distinguish primary cutaneous MEC from salivary gland tumor.

Soft Tissue Myoepithelial Tumors

Myoepithelial tumors (ME) of soft tissue are comprised of a heterogeneous group of tumors including parachordomas. They involve the skin and subcutis and have similar morphologic features to those of salivary glands.[176] Myoepithelial tumors of soft tissue are classified as benign (myoepithelioma and mixed tumor/chondroid syringoma) and malignant (myoepithelial carcinoma). The thigh is the most common location, followed by the calf, arms, and head and neck.[176] It has been proposed that cutaneous myoepitheliomas, cutaneous myoepithelial carcinomas, and chondroid syringomas are within a spectrum of tumors.[177]

Histology Features

Myoepitheliomas have a wide morphologic appearance with linear, cords, nested, solid to trabecular architecture.[176] Malignant tumors have an infiltrative growth pattern and with larger size. The tumor cells can be epithelioid, ovoid, polygonal, clear, plasmacytoid, or spindled. The stroma is commonly either myxoid or hyalinized with fatty, chondroid, squamous or osseous metaplasia seen in rare instances.[176] Cutaneous syncytial myoepithelioma, a rare variant of cutaneous myoepithelioma,[178] shows a syncytial proliferation of spindled, histiocytoid, or epithelioid cells in a chondromyxoid or collagenous stroma. Currently cytologic atypia is the single predictor of aggressive biologic behavior in soft tissue myoepithelial tumors.[177] 1–5 mitoses can be seen per 10 high power fields in majority of cases. Atypical mitoses are typically absent.

Immunohistochemical Findings

Myoepithelial neoplasms exhibit dual differentiation with characteristic expression of myoid (S100, Sox10, p63, GFAP, calponin, smooth muscle actin) and epithelial (pan-keratin, AE1/AE3, CAM5.2, keratin 7, EMA) markers.[177,179] One exception is cutaneous syncytial myoepithelioma which infrequently expresses keratin.[178] 80% of cases express Sox10.[180] CAM5.2 (16%), AE1/AE3 (44%), EMA expression is variable (19–79%).[179] GFAP (27–54%).[179] p63 expression is seen in 17–70% and 7–40% of myoepithelioma and myoepithelial carcinoma, respectively.[179] Expression of muscle markers is variable: calponin (22–90%), SMA (34–64%), and desmin (0–20%).[179] Loss of SMARCB1/INI1 expression can be seen in a subset of myoepithelial carcinomas, corresponding to SMARCB1 inactivation.[181] Acral myoepitheliomas express Sox10, S100, keratin 5/6, and PLAG1.[182]

Molecular Findings

Soft tissue myoepithelial tumors are characterized by fusions involving *EWSR1* including *EWSR1::PBX3*,[183] *EWSR1::PBX1*,[184] *EWSR1::PBX3*,[185] *EWSR1::ZNF444*,[186] *EWSR1::ATF1*,[187] *EWSR1::POU5F1*,[188] *EWSR1::KLF17*, *FUS::KLF17*,[189] and *EWSR1::KLF15*.[190]

Differential Diagnosis

Spitz nevi would be in the differential diagnosis of cutaneous syncytial myoepithelioma; however, Spitz nevi would exhibit an intraepidermal component and melanin pigment. Although both cutaneous syncytial myoepithelioma and epithelioid sarcoma express EMA and keratin, S100 and myoepithelial markers are negative in epithelioid sarcoma. Myoepithelioma-like tumors of the vulvar region would express actin, EMA, and estrogen receptor; yet are negative for SMARCB1/INI1, S100, GFAP, CD34 (**Table 4.14**).[191]

Table 4.14 Differential diagnosis of soft tissue myoepithelioma[177–179,191]

	Sox10	S100	keratin	EMA	GFAP	Desmin	CD34	INI1	other
Soft tissue myoepithelioma	+ (80%)	+	+	+	+	-/+	-	+	p63 (70%)
Soft tissue myoepithelial carcinoma	+ (30%)	+	+	+	+	-/+	-	loss (10%)	p63 (30%)
Cutaneous syncytial myoepithelioma		+	-/+ (86%)	+	+/-				
Chondroid syringoma	+	+	+	+	+	-	-	+	PLAG1
Myoepithelioma-like tumors of the vulvar region	ND	-	-/+	+	-	-	-	loss	ER
Proximal-type epithelioid sarcoma	-	-	+	+	-	-	+ (50%)	loss	p53 (55%)
NUT carcinoma	-	-	+	+	-	-	-	+	NUT, p63
Melanoma	+	+	-	-	-	-	-	+	Melan-A

NUT Carcinoma

NUT carcinomas typically have an undifferentiated or poorly differentiated SCC histologic appearance and harbor fusions of *NUTM1* with bromodomain-containing 4 (*BRD4*) on 19p13.1, most common partner, or bromodomain-containing 3 (*BRD3*) on 9q34.[192] NUT carcinomas mainly affect young adults, ages 16–22, and exhibit and aggressive clinical course with median survival of 6.7 to 9.7 months.[192]

Rare additional fusion partners including *NSD3::NUT*,[192] *CIC::NUTM1*,[193] *MXD4::NUTM1*,[194] and *MGA::NUTM1*.[195] Rarely, an unclassified adnexal carcinoma with follicular and ductal differentiation harboring *BRD3::NUTM2B* fusion has been reported.[196] NUTM1 immunostain can serve as a surrogate for NUTM1 rearrangement (**Figures 4.66–4.68**).[197]

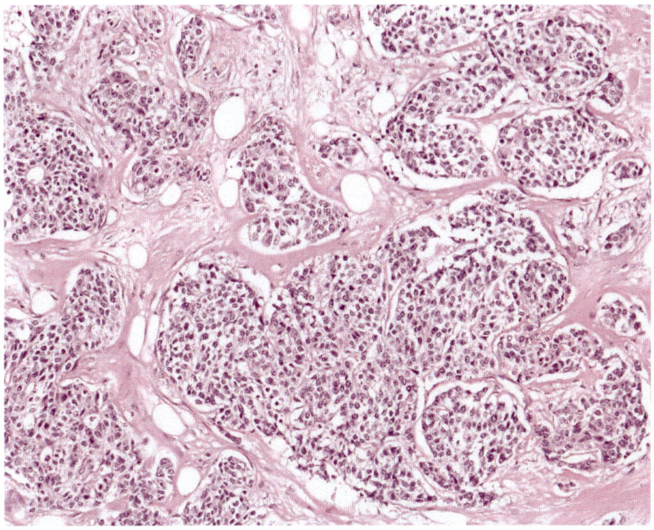

Figure 4.66 NUT carcinoma. A poorly differentiated carcinoma is seen in the dermis (X100).

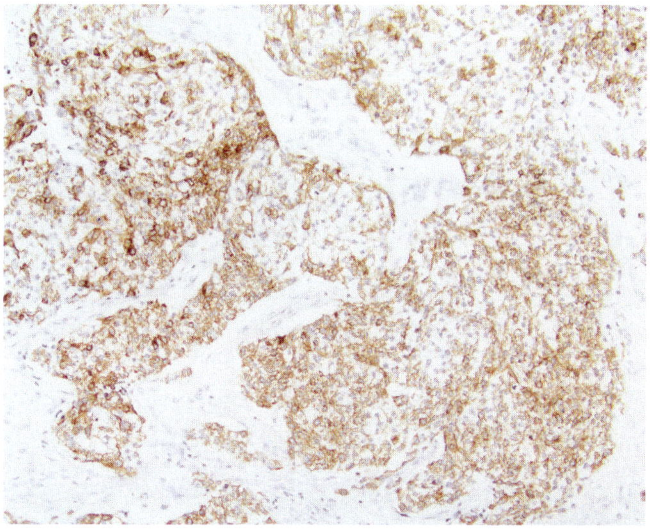

Figure 4.67 NUT carcinoma. The tumor cells are positive for keratin MNF116 (X200).

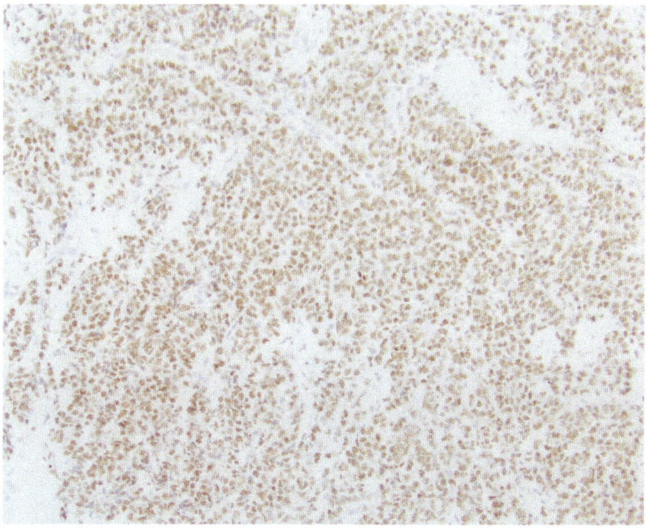

Figure 4.68 NUT carcinoma. NUT nuclear expression is seen (X200).

4.4 Case Studies

Case 4.1

Case history: A 52-year-old man presented with an abdominal wall mass.

Description: Cross-section of the resection specimen shows a tumor with gelatinous cut surface involving the skin and subcutaneous tissue (**Figure 4.69**). Histologic sections show a proliferation of atypical epithelial nests amid abundant extracellular mucin (**Figures 4.70 and 4.71**). The tumor cells are positive for keratin 7 (**Figure 4.72**), keratin 5/6, estrogen receptor (**Figure 4.73**), progesterone receptor, GATA3, MYB, and MUC2. They are negative for p63, keratin 20, CDX2, and CA19.9.

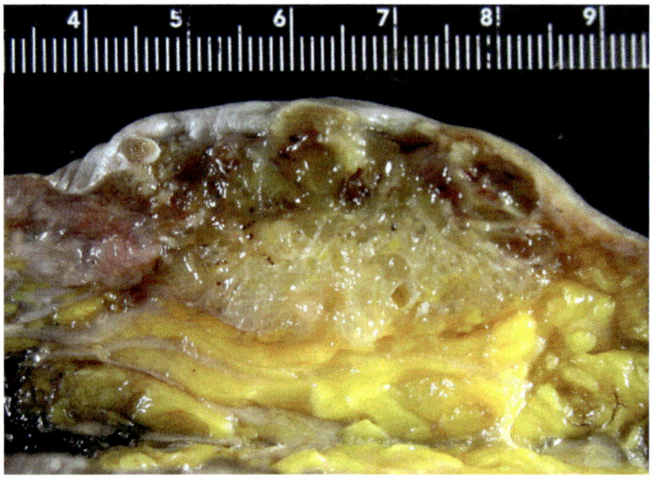

Figure 4.69 Gelatinous cut surface of a mucinous carcinoma.

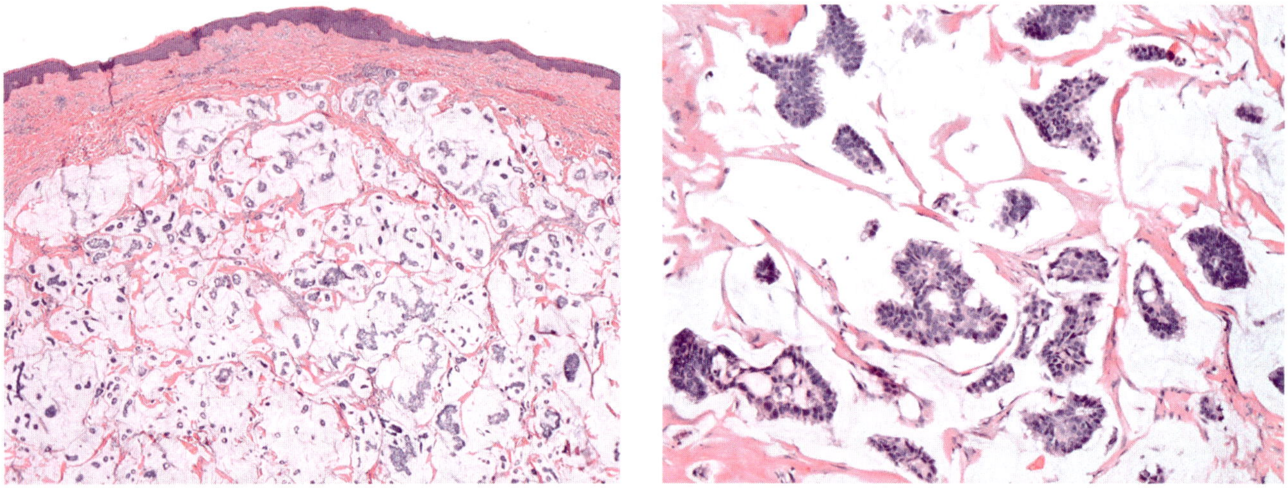

Figures 4.70 and 4.71 Mucinous carcinoma. Nests of epithelial tumor cells are seen among extracellular mucin (X40, X100).

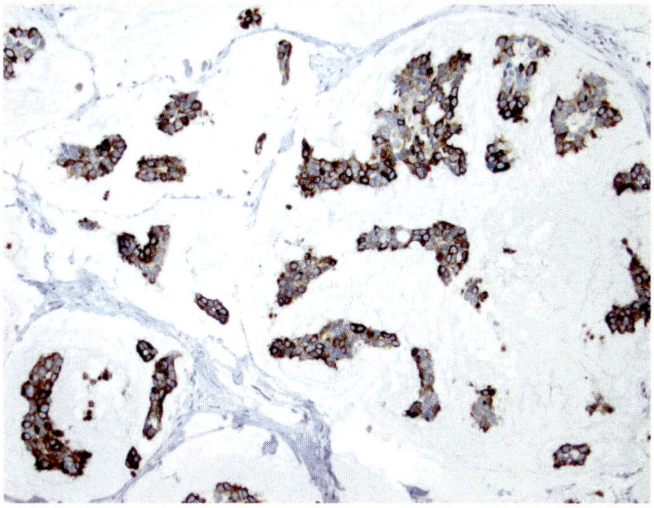

Figure 4.72 Mucinous carcinoma. The tumor cells express keratin 7 (X200).

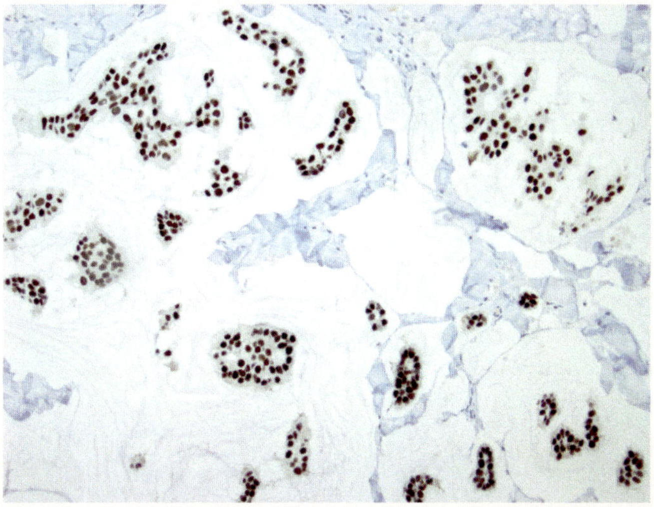

Figure 4.73 Mucinous carcinoma. Diffuse nuclear estrogen receptor is noted (X200).

Diagnosis: Primary cutaneous mucinous carcinoma.

Discussion: Primary cutaneous mucinous carcinoma is a rare tumor. Although it is still of dispute whether the origin is eccrine or apocrine, the expression of S100 favors eccrine origin by some.[67] The tumor is invariably positive for keratin 7, GCDFP-15, ER, and PR.[68,69] When an *in situ* component is present, the myoepithelial cells are highlighted by p63, keratin 5/6, calponin, and smooth muscle actin.[68] Expression of S100, BerEP4, and EMA; and neuroendocrine differentiation with positivity for chromogranin A and neuron specific enolase can be seen (**Table 4.7**). In this case, the negative expression for keratin 20 and CDX2 is most helpful in excluding a colorectal origin. One histologic consideration would be endocrine mucin-producing sweat gland carcinoma;[66] however, these lesions typically occur near the eyes and the mucinous component is a minor one. Although additional cases need to be studied, the co-expression of MYB and GATA3 is supportive of a primary cutaneous mucinous carcinoma.[71]

Case 4.2

Case history: A 65-year-old woman presented with 6.5 × 4.2 cm ulcerated mass on her right thigh. The mass has a mottled gray-white to tan-pink and focally glistening gray cut surface (**Figure 4.74**). The mass appears to be encapsulated with focal cystic areas.

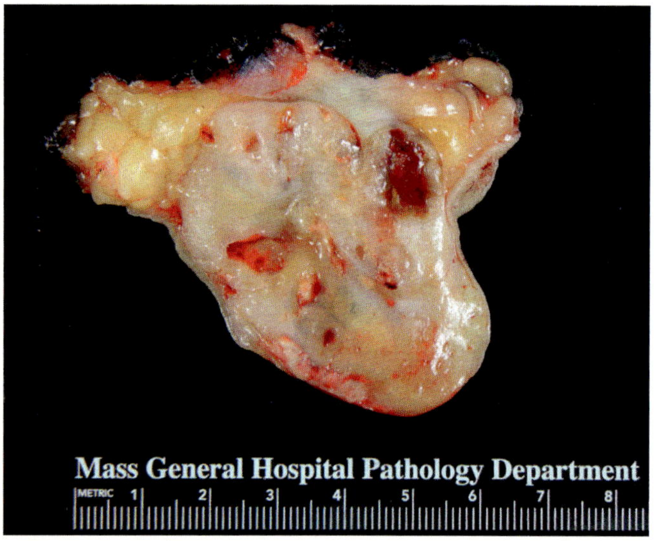

Figure 4.74 A multinodular tumor with tan as well as hemorrhagic cut surface is seen.

Description: Histologic sections show the tumor to have a biphasic appearance. Irregular epithelial nests are surrounded by spindle neoplastic cells (**Figure 4.75**). At higher magnification the epithelial nests exhibit comedo necrosis (**Figure 4.76**) and focal clear cell change. The epithelial component is positive for keratin7 (**Figure 4.77**) while the spindle cell component is positive for SMA (**Figure 4.78**). Both components exhibit a high Ki-67 proliferation index (**Figure 4.79**).

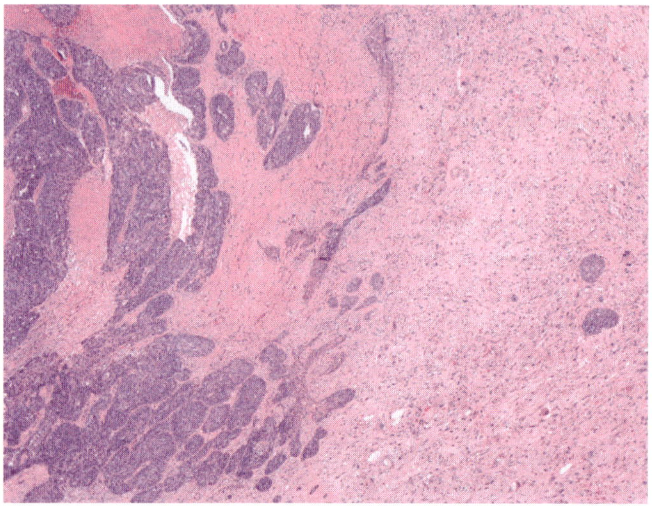

Figure 4.75 A biphasic tumor characterized by irregular epithelial nests surrounded by spindle neoplastic cells (X40).

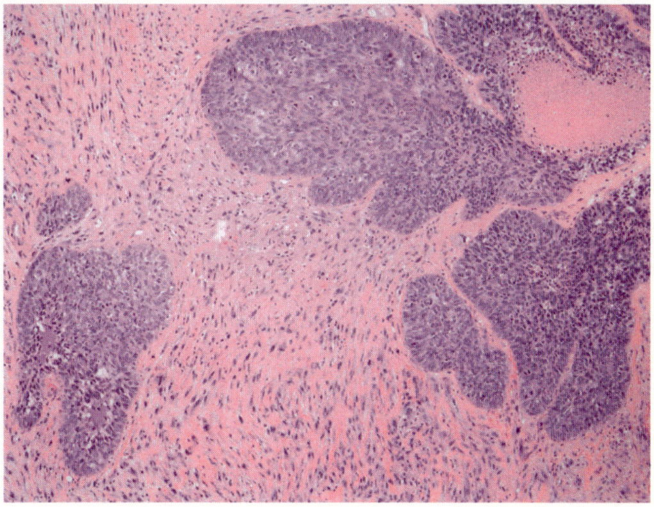

Figure 4.76 Epithelial nests exhibit comedo necrosis while pleomorphic spindle cells are seen in the sarcomatous component (X100).

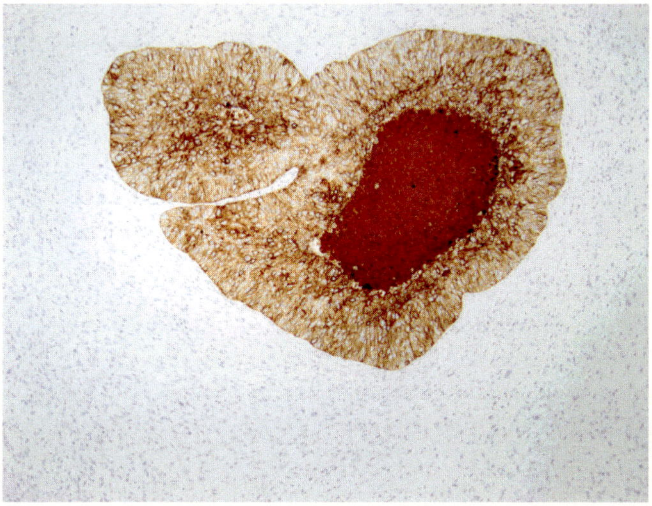

Figure 4.77 Keratin 7 labels the epithelial component but not the stromal component (X100).

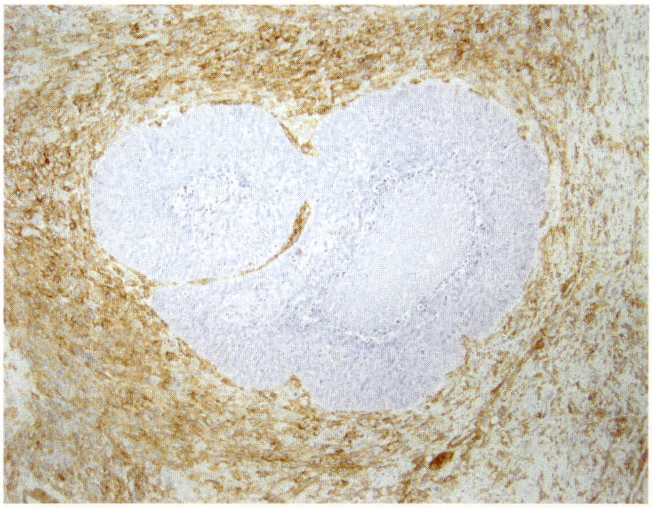

Figure 4.78 The stromal component expresses smooth muscle actin while the epithelial component is negative (X100).

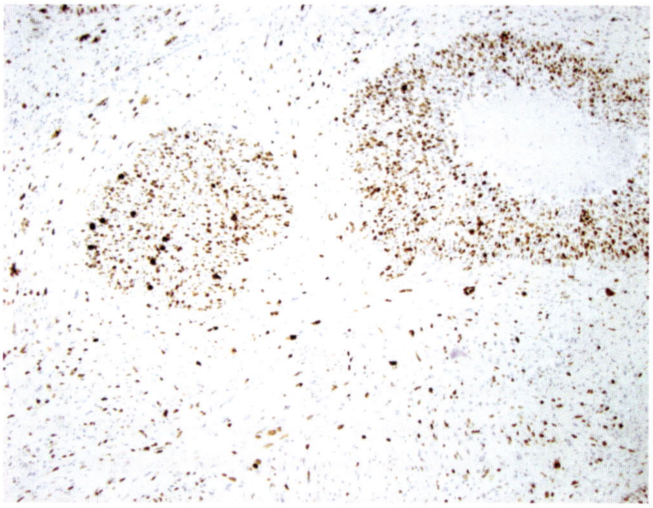

Figure 4.79 High nuclear Ki-67 proliferation index is noted in both the epithelial and sarcomatous components (X100).

Diagnosis: Eccrine carcinoma with sarcomatoid differentiation.

Discussion: Cutaneous carcinosarcomas are often SCC or BCC.[198] Rarely cutaneous adnexal neoplasms have a sarcomatous component including spiradenocarcinoma, porocarcinoma, malignant cylindroma, and malignant proliferating trichilemmal tumor.[94] It has been suggested that tumors with a neoplastic epithelial component of the adnexal type are more aggressive than those with the epidermal type.[94] The epithelial component may show transition to the sarcomatous stroma. The epithelial component is typically positive for cytokeratins while the sarcomatous component is positive for vimentin, alpha smooth muscle actin and even focally for cytokeratins.[198]

There have been three proposed theories about the origin of the sarcomatous component in sarcomatoid carcinomas in the literature: (1) monoclonal/ divergence, (2) multiclonal, and (3) convergence hypotheses. The monoclonal or divergence theory proposed that the epithelial and sarcomatous components arise from a single totipotent stem cell. In the multiclonal theory, the epithelial and sarcomatous components are hypothesized to independently arise from two or more stem cells. In the convergence theory the carcinoma component undergoes metaplasia to give rise to the sarcomatous component. Recent molecular studies appear to support the first theory since similar genetic abnormalities are found in both components.

Case 4.3

Case history: An 89-year-old woman presented with a 5-year history of a growing mass behind her left ear. The lesion has become increasingly protuberant and foul smelling. There is a history of an existing lesion since birth from which this has arisen from.

Description: A nodular tumor comprised of basaloid neoplastic cells is seen in the dermis (**Figure 4.80**). Marked necrosis is seen. In part of the tumor, prominent melanin pigment is seen within the cytoplasm of the tumor cells (**Figure 4.81**). The majority of the tumor cells stain for BerEP4 (**Figure 4.82**). Sox10 immunostain demonstrates scattered melanocytes within these basaloid tumor nests (**Figure 4.83**).

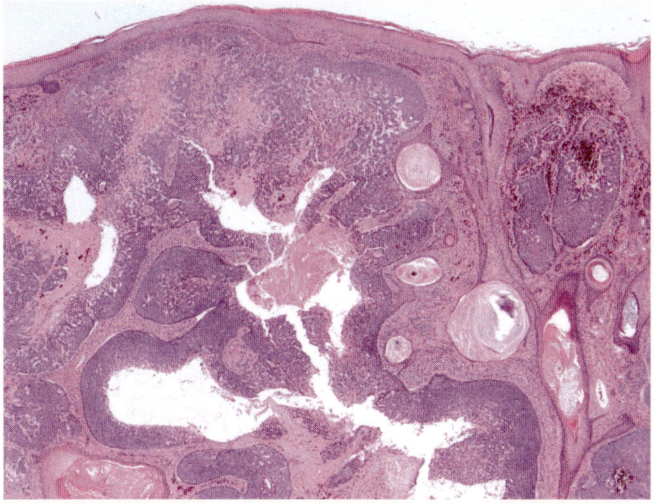

Figure 4.80 A multinodular tumor comprising of basaloid neoplastic cells seen in the dermis (X40).

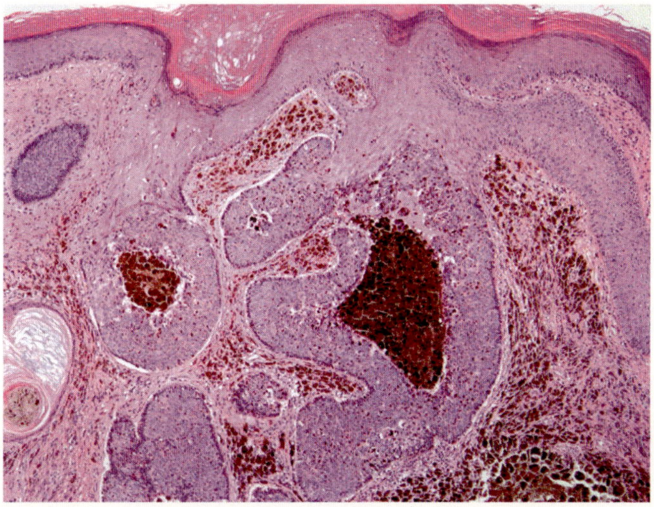

Figure 4.81 Although peripheral palisade and retraction artifact are noted at the periphery of these basaloid nests, prominent cytoplasmic pigment within the tumor cells and surrounding melanophages is also noted (X100).

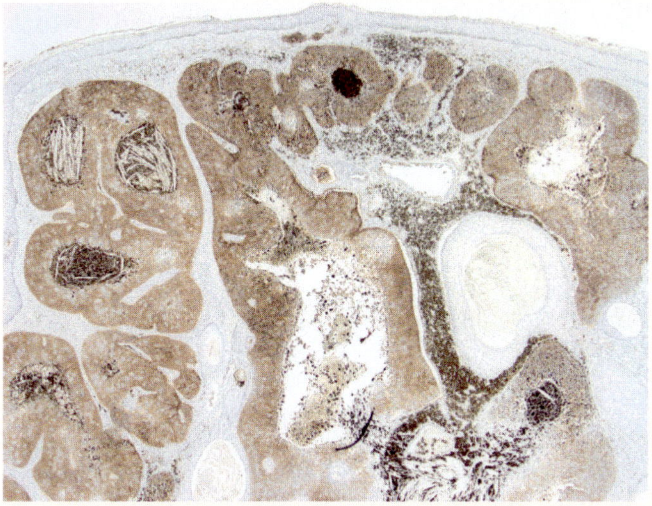

Figure 4.82 BerEP4 highlights all the epithelial nests (X40).

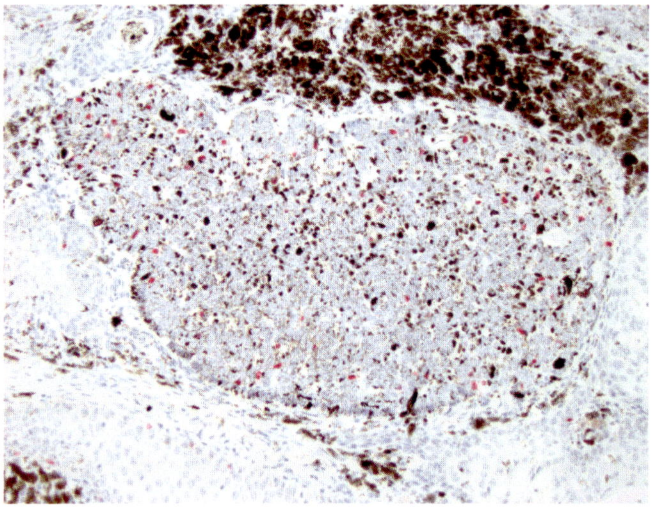

Figure 4.83 Sox10 highlights occasional melanocytes within the pigmented epithelial nests (X200).

Diagnosis: Basomelanocytic tumor.

Discussion: In a series of 69 cutaneous collision tumors Boyd and Rapini[199] reported the combination of BCC and melanocytic nevus to be one of the most common. The combination of BCC and melanoma is exceedingly rare. Contrary to collision tumors, there is intermingling of epithelial cells and melanocytes in combined tumors. The epithelial cells express keratin AE1/AE3 and keratin 903 while the melanocytes express S100, Melan-A, Mart-1, and HMB-45 in basomelanocytic tumors.[200]

The differential diagnosis would include either a melanoma *in situ* or a metastatic melanoma that colonizes a BCC. A rare case of malignant basomelanocytic tumor on the scalp has been reported in which only the melanoma component metastasized to the cervical lymph node fourteen months later. The epithelial component was immunoreactive for wide-spectrum keratin and BerEP4. The colonizing melanocytes were positive for Melan-A, HMB-45, tyrosinase and focally for S100.[200] The authors postulated that perhaps the melanoma component was obliterated by the associated basal cell carcinoma.[200]

One possibility is non-neoplastic proliferation of melanocytes within a BCC. Absence of cytologic atypia, prominent pigmentation, even distribution, and dendritic morphology have been described to represent non-neoplastic colonization, whereas clustering of two or more cells, high density and presence of cytologic atypia are in favor of a neoplastic process. In pigmented SCC, pigmented BCC, melanocytic matricoma, melanotrichoblastoma, and pigmented eccrine porocarcinoma, the melanocytes are very pigmented, dendritic in appearance, and not atypical.

Case 4.4

Case history: and description A 79-year-old man presented with bleeding lesion on his left anus. A biopsy of the anal skin shows an intraepidermal proliferation of atypical cells with intracytoplasmic mucin (**Figure 4.84**). The tumor cells are positive for keratin 7 (**Figure 4.85**) and keratin 20 (**Figure 4.86**). Subsequent workup reveals a mucin producing adenocarcinoma involving the rectum (**Figure 4.87**). The carcinoma exhibits strong keratin 20 (**Figure 4.88**) and nuclear CDX2 (**Figure 4.89**) expression.

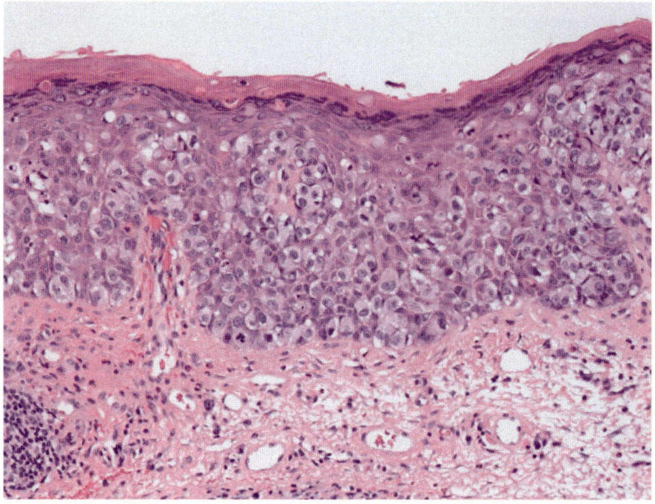

Figure 4.84 Intraepidermal neoplastic cells in secondary extramammary Paget disease (X200).

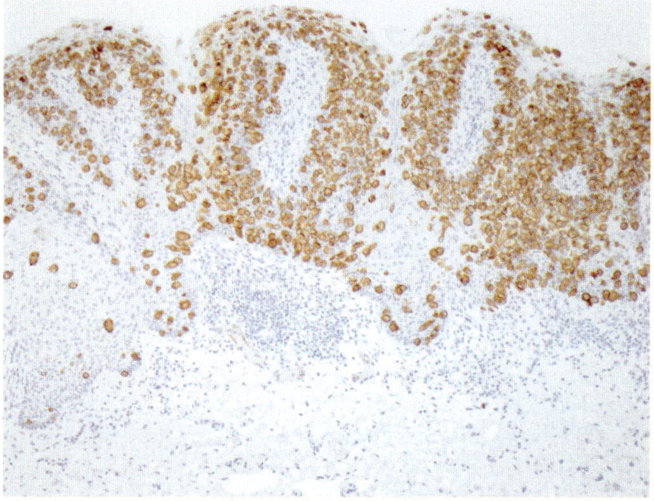

Figure 4.85 Diffuse keratin 7 expression (X100).

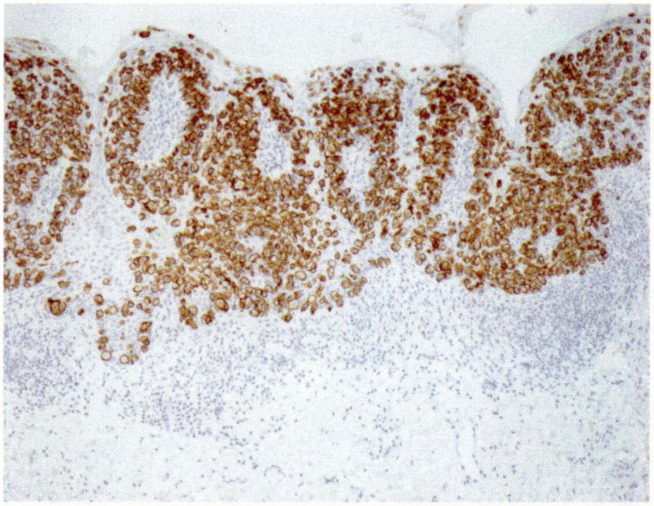

Figure 4.86 Diffuse keratin 20 expression (X100).

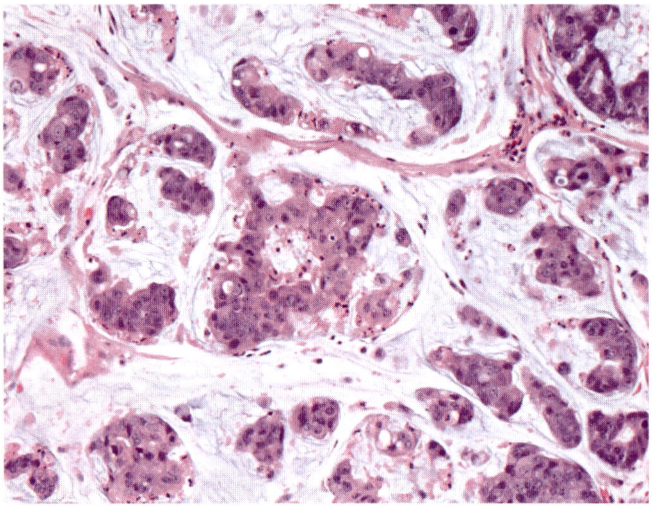

Figure 4.87 Clusters of epithelial nests with abundant extracellular mucin in mucinous carcinoma (X200).

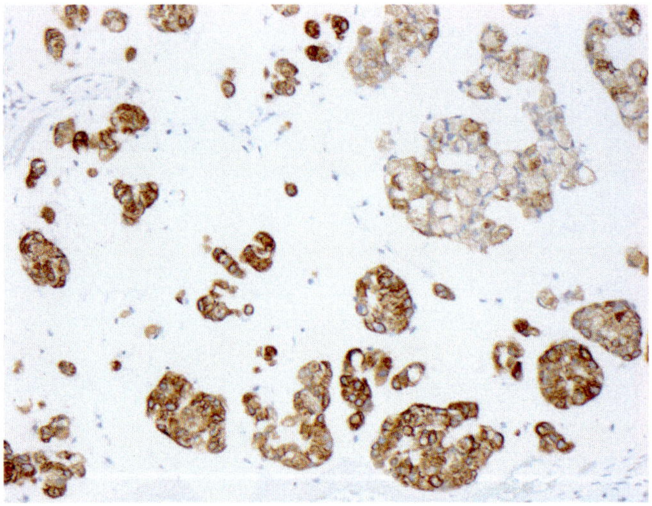

Figure 4.88 Diffuse keratin 20 expression (X200).

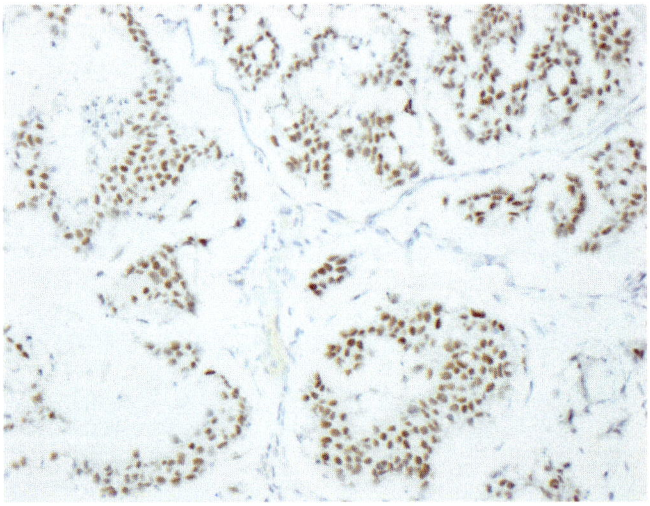

Figure 4.89 Diffuse nuclear CDX2 expression (X200).

Diagnosis: Secondary extramammary Paget disease.

Discussion: Secondary EMPD arises from an underlying gastrointestinal origin, distal colon or rectum, carcinoma of genitourinary origin, bladder, or prostate (**Table 4.7**). Perianal EMPD accounts for approximately 20% of EMPD cases. As illustrated in this case, it is strongly associated with adenocarcinoma of the anus and colorectum. EMPD from colorectal origin expresses keratin 20, CDX2, and MUC2, while EMPD from urothelial carcinoma expresses p63 and uroplakin.

Case 4.5

Case history: A 32-year-old pregnant woman presented with a growing pedunculated lesion on her left posterior scalp (**Figure 4.90**). Areas of pigmentation were noted and a clinical concern for pigmented basal cell carcinoma or melanoma was raised.

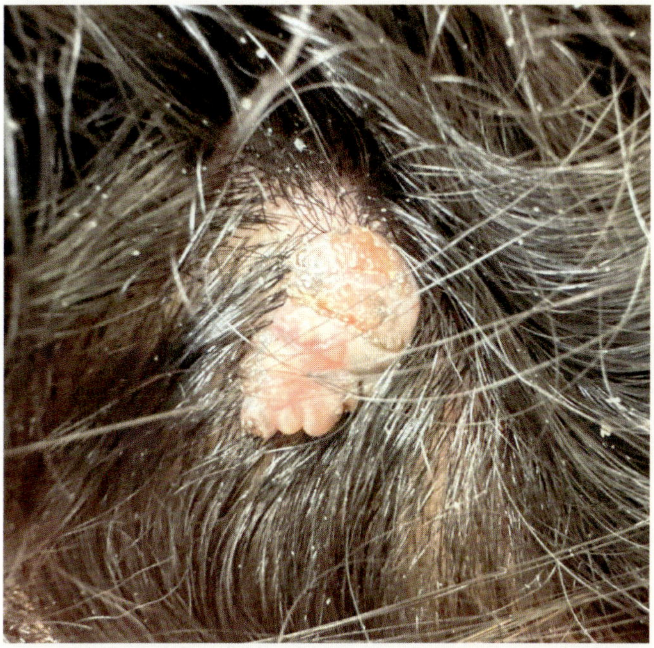

Figure 4.90 A polypoid and pedunculated mass seen on the patient's scalp.

Description: Histologic sections show a proliferation of uniform basaloid cells in broad and anastomosing cords in the dermis (**Figures 4.91 and 4.92**). Duct formation is highlighted by keratin 7 and keratin 19. The tumor exhibits NUT nuclear expression (**Figure 4.93**) and loss of YAP1 cytoplasmic expression (**Figure 4.94**).

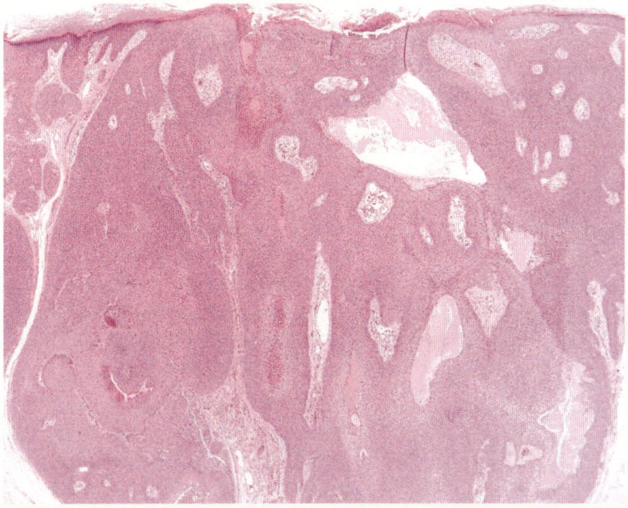

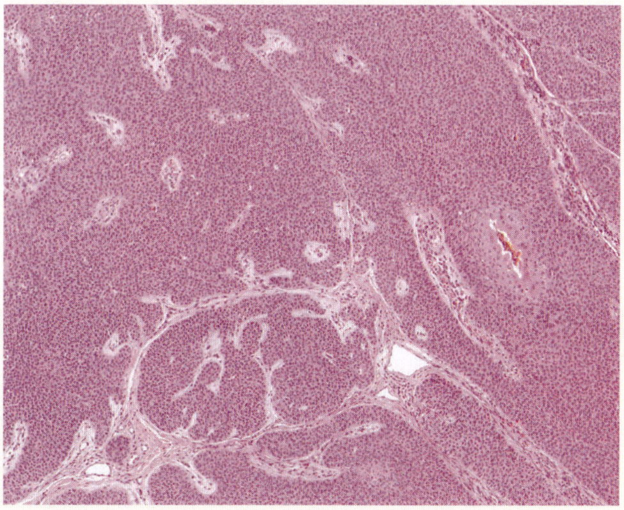

Figures 4.91 and 4.92 Cords of uniform tumor cells with focal duct differentiation are seen in the dermis (X40, X100).

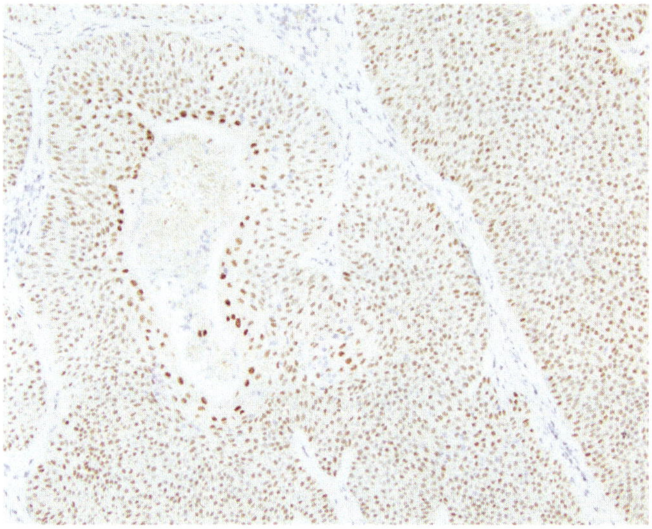

Figure 4.93 Nuclear NUT expression (X200).

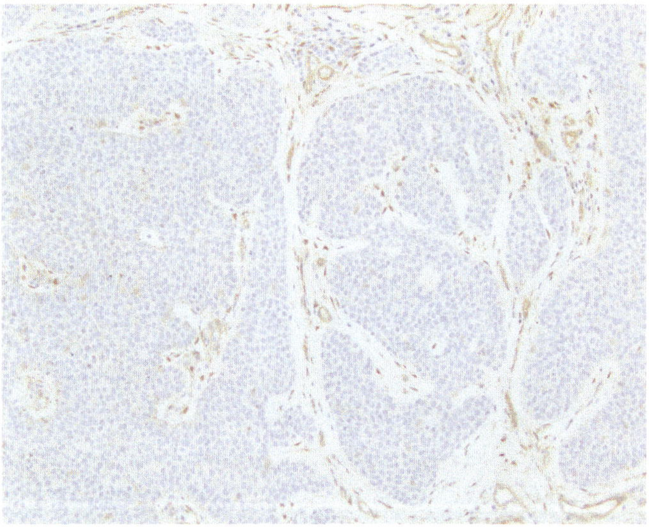

Figure 4.94 Loss of YAP1 cytoplasmic expression (X200).

Diagnosis: Poroma.

Discussion: *YAP1::MAML2* and *YAP1::NUTM1* fusions have been reported in poroid tumors with *YAP1* fusions detected in 88% of poromas and 64% of porocarcinomas.[113] The NUT nuclear expression and loss of YAP1 cytoplasmic expression has been reported as cost-effective surrogate in detecting *YAP1::NUTM1* fusion (Russell-Goldman 2021).[114] The immunohistochemical results of the current case are helpful in rendering the diagnosis of poroma.

References

1. Gibbs DC, Yeung H, Blalock TW. Incidence and trends of cutaneous adnexal tumors in the United States in 2000–2018: a population-based study. *J Am Acad Dermatol* 2023; **88**: 226–8.
2. Battistella M, Balme B, Jullie ML, et al. Impact of expert pathology review in skin adnexal carcinoma diagnosis: analysis of 2573 patients from the French CARADERM network. *Eur J Cancer* 2022; **163**: 211–21.
3. Wysong A, Aasi SZ, Tang JY. Update on metastatic basal cell carcinoma: a summary of published cases from 1981 through 2011. *JAMA Dermatol* 2013; **149**: 615–16.
4. Beer TW, Shepherd P, Theaker JM. BerEP4 and epithelial membrane antigen aid distinction of basal cell, squamous cell and basosquamous carcinomas of the skin. *Histopathology* 2000; **37**: 218–23.
5. Linskey KR, Gimbel DC, Zukerberg LR, Duncan LM, Sadow PM, Nazarian RM. BerEp4, cytokeratin 14, and cytokeratin 17 immunohistochemical staining aid in differentiation of basaloid squamous cell carcinoma from basal cell carcinoma with squamous metaplasia. *Arch Pathol Lab Med* 2013; **137**: 1591–8.
6. Kurzen H, Esposito L, Langbein L, Hartschuh W. Cytokeratins as markers of follicular differentiation: an immunohistochemical study of trichoblastoma and basal cell carcinoma. *Am J Dermatopathol* 2001; **23**: 501–9.

7. Evangelista MT, North JP. Comparative analysis of cytokeratin 15, TDAG51, cytokeratin 20 and androgen receptor in sclerosing adnexal neoplasms and variants of basal cell carcinoma. *J Cutan Pathol* 2015; **42**: 824–31.
8. Costache M, Bresch M, Boer A. Desmoplastic trichoepithelioma versus morphoeic basal cell carcinoma: a critical reappraisal of histomorphological and immunohistochemical criteria for differentiation. *Histopathology* 2008; **52**: 865–76.
9. Katona TM, Perkins SM, Billings SD. Does the panel of cytokeratin 20 and androgen receptor antibodies differentiate desmoplastic trichoepithelioma from morpheaform/ infiltrative basal cell carcinoma? *J Cutan Pathol* 2008; **35**: 174–9.
10. Carrasquillo OY, Cruzval-O'Reilly E, Sanchez JE, Valentin-Nogueras SM. Differentiation of basal cell carcinoma and trichoepithelioma: an immunohistochemical study. *Am J Dermatopathol* 2021; **43**: 191–7.
11. Krahl D, Sellheyer K. p75 neurotrophin receptor differentiates between morphoeic basal cell carcinoma and desmoplastic trichoepithelioma: insights into the histogenesis of adnexal tumours based on embryology and hair follicle biology. *Br J Dermatol* 2010; **163**: 138–45.
12. Yeh I, McCalmont TH, LeBoit PE. Differential expression of PHLDA1 (TDAG51) in basal cell carcinoma and trichoepithelioma. *Br J Dermatol* 2012; **167**: 1106–10.
13. Koga K, Anan T, Fukumoto T, Fujimoto M, Nabeshima K. Ln-gamma 2 chain of laminin-332 is a useful marker in differentiating between benign and malignant sclerosing adnexal neoplasms. *Histopathology* 2022; **76**: 318–24.
14. Pham TTN, Selim MA, Burchette JL, Madden J, Turner J, Herman C. CD10 expression in trichoepithelioma and basal cell carcinoma. *J Cutan Pathol* 2006; **33**: 123–8.
15. Illueca C, Monteagudo C, Revert A, et al. Diagnostic value of CD34 immunostaining in desmoplastic trichilemmoma. *J Cutan Pathol* 1998; **25**: 435–9.
16. Dalton SR, LeBoit PE. Squamous cell carcinoma with clear cells: how often is there evidence of tricholemmal differentiation? *Am J Dermatopathol* 2008; **30**: 333–9.
17. Chaudet KM, Stagner AM, Nazarian RM. Use of cytokeratin 17 in the differentiation between desmoplastic trichilemmoma and cutaneous basal cell carcinoma. *Am J Dermatopathol* 2022; **44**: 886–90.
18. Ferreira I, Wiedemeyer K, Demetter P, Adams DJ, Arends MJ, Brenn T. Update on pathology, genetics and somatic landscape of sebaceous tumours. *Histopathology* 2020; **76**: 640–9.
19. Cook S, Pethick J, Kibbi N, et al. Sebaceous carcinoma epidemiology, associated malignancies and Lynch/ Muir-Torre syndrome screening in England from 2008 to 2018. *J Am Acad Dermatol* 2023; S0190-9622(23)00536-4. doi: 10.1016/j.jaad.2023.03.046.
20. Ariz S, O'Sullivan H, Heelan K, Alam A, McVeigh TP. Characterization of sebaceous and non-sebaceous cutaneous manifestations in patients with lynch syndrome: a systematic review. *Fam Cancer* 2023; **22**: 167–75.
21. Saliba M, Shaheen M, Hajj RE, et al. Sebaceous neoplasms: prevalence of HPV infection and relation to immunohistochemical surrogate markers. *Eur J Dermatol* 2021; **31**: 170–5.
22. Ansai S, Arase S, Kawana S, Kimura T. Immunohistochemical findings of sebaceous carcinoma and sebaceoma: retrieval of cytokeratin expression by a panel of anti-cytokeratin monoclonal antibodies. *J Dermatol* 2011; **38**: 951–8.
23. Boussahmain C, Mochel MC, Hoang MP. Perilipin and adipophilin expression in sebaceous carcinoma and mimics. *Hum Pathol* 2013; **44**: 1811–16.
24. Li FZ, Ye Q, Ran LW, Fang S. Adipophilin expression in skin lesions with clear cell histology. *J Clin Pathol* 2022; **75**: 627–31.
25. Sramek B, Lisle A, Loy T. Immunohistochemistry in ocular carcinomas. *J Cutan Pathol* 2008; **35**: 641–6.
26. Oules B, Deschamps L, Sohier P, et al. Diagnostic accuracy of GATA6 immunostaining in sebaceous tumors of the skin. *Mod Pathol* 2023; **36**: 100101. doi: 10.1016/j.modpat.2023.100101.
27. Mittal R, Araujo I, Czanner G, Coupland SE. Perforin expression in eyelid sebaceous carcinomas: a useful and specific immunomarker for the differential diagnosis of eyelid carcinomas. *Acta Opthalmol* 2016; **94**: e325-30. doi: 10.1111/aos.12972.
28. Ng JKM, Choi PCL, Chow C, et al. PRAME immunostain expression in sebaceous lesions, cutaneous carcinomas and adnexal structures. *Pathology* 2022; **54**: 721–8.
29. Gradecki SE, Eid MV, Pramoonjago P, Wick MR. Glioma-associated oncogene-1 expression in basal cell carcinoma and its histologic mimics. *Am J Dermatopathol* 2021; **43**: 637–41.
30. Ciarloni L, Frouin E, Bodin F, Cribier B. Syringoma: a clinicopathological study of 244 cases. *Ann Dermatol Venereol* 2016; **143**: 521–8.
31. Missall TA, Burkemper NM, Jensen SL, Hurley MY. Immunohistochemical differentiation of four benign eccrine tumors. *J Cutan Pathol* 2009; **36**: 190–6.
32. Kazakov DV, Belousova IE, Bisceglia M, et al. Apocrine mixed tumor of the skin ("mixed tumor of the folliculosebaceous-apocrine complex"). Spectrum of differentiations and metaplastic changes in the epithelial, myoepithelial, and stromal components based on a histopathologic study of 244 cases. *J Am Acad Dermatol* 2007; **57**: 467–83.
33. Kazakov DV, Kacerovska D, Hantschke M, et al. Cutaneous mixed tumor, eccrine variant: a clinicopathologic and immunohistochemical study of 50 cases, with emphasis on unusual histopathologic features. *Am J Dermatopathol* 2011; **33**: 557–68.
34. Bullerdiek J, Wobst G, Meyer-Bolte K, et al. Cytogenetic subtyping of 220 salivary gland pleomorphic adenomas: correlation to occurrence, histological subtype, and in vitro cellular behavior. *Cancer Genet Cytogenet* 1993; 65: 27–32.
35. Stenman G. Fusion oncogenes in salivary gland tumors: molecular and clinical consequences. *Head Neck Pathol* 2013; 7 **Suppl**: S12-9. doi: 10.1007/ s12105-013-0462-z.
36. Ma S, Zhao D, Liu Y, et al. Some pleomorphic adenomas of the breast share PLAG1 rearrangements with the analogous tumour of the salivary glands. *Histopathology* 2021; **79**: 1030–9.
37. Asahina M, Saito T, Hayashi T, Fukumura Y, Mitani K, Yao T. Clinicopathological effect of PLAG1 fusion genes in pleomorphic adenoma and carcinoma ex pleomorphic adenoma with special emphasis on histological features. *Histopathology* 2019; **74**: 514–25.
38. Panagopoulos I, Gorunova L, Andersen K, et al. NDRG1-PLAG1 and TRPS1-PLAG1 fusion genes in chondroid syringoma. *Cancer Genomics Proteomics* 2020; **17**: 237–48.
39. Kas K, Voz ML, Roijer E, et al. Promoter swapping between the genes for a novel zinc finger protein and beta-catenin

in pleiomorphic adenomas with t(3;8)(p21;q12) translocation. *Nat Genet* 1997; **15**: 170–4.

40. Voz ML, Astrom AK, Kas K, Mark J, Stenman G, van de Ven WJ. The recurrent translocation t(5;8)(;13;q12) in pleomorphic adenomas results in upregulation of PLAG1 gene expression under control of the LIFR promoter. *Oncogene* 1998; **16**: 1409–16.
41. Astrom AK, Voz ML, Kas K, et al. Conserved mechanism of PLAG1 activation in salivary gland tumors with and without chromosome 8q12 abnormalities: identification of SII as a new fusion partner gene. *Cancer Res* 1999; **59**: 918–23.
42. Persson F, Andren Y, Winnes M et al. High-resolution genomic profiling of adenomas and carcinomas of the salivary glands reveals amplification, rearrangement, and fusion of HMGA2. *Genes Chromosom Cancer* 2009; **48**; 69–82.
43. Wasserman JK, Dickson BC, Smith A, Swanson D, Purgina BM, Weinreb I. Metastasizing pleomorphic adenoma: recurrent PLAG1/HMGA2 rearrangements and identification of a novel HMGA2-TMTC2 fusion. *Am J Surg Pathol* 2019; **43**: 1145–51.
44. Afshari MK, Fehr A, Nevado PT, Andersson MK, Stenman G. Activation of PLAG1 and HMGA2 by gene fusions involving the transcriptional regulator gene NFIB. *Genes Chromosomes Cancer* 2020; **59**: 652–60.
45. Pei J, Liu JC, Ehya H, et al. BOC-PLAG1, a new fusion gene of pleomorphic adenoma: Identified in a fine-needle aspirate by RNA next-generation sequencing. *Diagn Cytopathol* 2021; **49**: 790–2.
46. Agaimy A, Ihrler S, Baněčková M, et al. HMGA2-WIF1 rearrangements characterize a distinctive subset of salivary pleomorphic adenomas with prominent trabecular (canalicular adenoma-like) morphology. *Am J Surg Pathol* 2022; **46**: 190–9.
47. Geurts JM, Schoenmakers EF, R€oijer E, Stenman G, Van de Ven WJ. Expression of reciprocal hybrid transcripts of HMGIC and FHIT in a pleomorphic adenoma of the parotid gland. *Cancer Res* 1997; **57**; 13–17.
48. Panagopoulos I, Gorunova L, Lund-Iversen M, Bassarova A, Heim S. Fusion of the genes PHF1 and TFE3 in malignant chondroid syringoma. *Cancer Genomics Proteomics* 2019; **16**: 345–51.
49. Matsuyama A, Hisaoka M, Hashimoto H. PLAG1 expression in cutaneous mixed tumors: an immunohistochemical and molecular genetic study. *Virchows Arch* 2011; **459**: 539–45.
50. Matsuyama A, Hisaoka M, Hashimoto H. PLAG1 expression in mesenchymal tumors: an immunohistochemical study with special emphasis on the pathogenetical distinction between soft tissue myoepithelioma and pleomorphic adenoma of the salivary gland. *Pathol Int* 2012; **62**: 1–7.
51. Bahrami A, Dalton JD, Shivakumar B, Krane JF. PLAG1 alteration in carcinoma ex pleomorphic adenoma: immunohistochemical and fluorescence in situ hybridization studies of 22 cases. *Head Neck Pathol* 2012; **6**: 328–35.
52. Mendoza PR, Jakobiec FA, Krane JF. Immunohistochemical features of lacrimal gland epithelial tumors. *Am J Ophthalmol* 2013; **156**: 1147–58.
53. Von Holstein SL, Fehr A, Persson M, et al. Adenoid cystic carcinoma of the lacrimal gland: MYB gene activation, genomic imbalances, and clinical characteristics. *Ophthalmology* 2013; 210: 2130–8.
54. North JP, McCalmont TH, Fehr A, van Zante A, Stenman G, LeBoit PE. Detection of MYB alterations and other immunohistochemical markers in primary cutaneous adenoid cystic carcinoma. *Am J Surg Pathol* 2015; **39**: 1347–56.
55. Mitani Y, Li J, Rao PH, Zhao YJ, et al. Comprehensive analysis of the MYB-NFIB gene fusion in salivary adenoid cystic carcinoma: incidence, variability and clinicopathologic significance. *Clin Cancer Res* 2010; **16**: 4722–31.
56. West RB, Kong C, Clarke N, et al. MYB expression and translocation in adenoid cystic carcinomas and other salivary gland tumors with clinicopathologic correlation. *Am J Surg Pathol* 2011; **35**: 92–9.
57. Weinreb I, Rooper LM, Dickson BC, et al. Adenoid cystic carcinoma with striking tubular hypereosinophilia: a unique pattern associated with nonparotid location and both canonical and novel EWSR1::MYB and FUS::MYB fusions. *Am J Surg Pathol* 2023; **47**: 497–503.
58. Bell D, Roberts D, Karpowicz M, et al. Clinical significance of Myb protein and downstream target genes in salivary adenoid cystic carcinoma. *Cancer Biol Ther* 2011; **12**: 569–73.
59. Brill LB, Kanner WA, Fehr A, et al. Analysis of MYB expression and MYB-NFIB gene fusions in adenoid cystic carcinoma and other salivary neoplasms. *Mod Pathol* 2011; **24**: 1169–76.
60. Tadi S, Ka-Yan Cheung V, Lee CS, et al. MYB RNA detection by in situ hybridisation has high sensitivity and specificity for the diagnosis of adenoid cystic carcinoma. *Pathology* 2023: S0031-3025(23)00084–3. doi: 10.1016/j.pathol.2023.01.007.
61. Rütten A, Kutzner H, Mentzel T, et al. Primary cutaneous cribriform apocrine carcinoma: a clinicopathologic and immunohistochemical study of 26 cases of an under-recognized cutaneous adnexal neoplasm. *J Am Acad Dermatol* 2009; **61**: 644–51.
62. Arps DP, Chan MP, Patel RM, Andea AA. Primary cutaneous cribriform carcinoma: report of six cases with clinicopathologic data and immunohistochemical profile. *J Cutan Pathol* 2015; **42**: 379–87.
63. Davis A, Khachemoune A. Reappraisal and literature review of primary cutaneous cribriform apocrine carcinoma. *Arch Dermatol Res* 2023; **315**: 7–16.
64. Agni M, Raven M, Bowen RC, et al. An update on endocrine mucin-producing sweat gland carcinoma: clinicopathologic study of 63 cases and comparative analysis. *Am J Surg Pathol* 2020; **44**: 1005–16.
65. Hadi R, Xu H, Barber BR, Shinohara MM, Moshiri AS. A case of endocrine mucin-producing sweat gland carcinoma with distant metastasis. *J Cutan Pathol* 2021; **48**: 937–42.
66. Zembowicz A, Garcia CF, Tannous ZS, et al. Endocrine mucin-producing sweat gland carcinoma. Twelve new cases suggest that it is a precursor of some invasive mucinous carcinomas. *Am J Surg Pathol* 2005; **29**: 1330–9.
67. Rismiller KP, Crowe DR, Knackstedt TJ. Prognostic factors, treatment, and survival in primary cutaneous mucinous carcinoma. A SEER database analysis. *Dermatol Surg* 2020; **46**: 1141–7.
68. Qureshi HS, Salama ME, Chitale D, et al. Primary cutaneous mucinous carcinoma: presence of myoepithelial cells as a clue to the cutaneous origin. *Am J Dermatopathol* 2004; **26**: 353–8.
69. Levy G, Finkelstein A, McNiff JM. Immunohistochemical techniques to compare primary vs. metastatic mucinous carcinoma of the skin. *J Cutan Pathol* 2010; **37**: 411–15.

70. Adkins KE, Busam K, Pulitzer M. Cutaneous neuroendocrine mucinous carcinomas are low-grade but may be associated with other cancers. *Am J Surg Pathol* 2023; **47**: 1186–91.

71. Pardal J, Sundram U, Selim MA, Hoang MP. GATA3 and MYB expression in cutaneous adnexal neoplasms. Am J Dermatopathol 2017; **39**: 279–86.

72. Amin SM, Beattie A, Ling X, Jennings LJ, Guitart J. Primary cutaneous mammary analog secretory carcinoma with ETV6-NTRK3 translocation. *Am J Dermatopathol* 2016; **38**: 842–5.

73. Skalova A, Vanecek T, Sima R, et al. Mammary analogue secretory carcinoma of salivary glands, containing the ETV6-NTRK3 fusion gene: a hitherto undescribed salivary gland tumor entity. *Am J Surg Pathol* 2010; **34**: 599–608.

74. Bishop JA, Taube JM, Su A, et al. Secretory carcinoma of the skin harboring ETV6 gene fusions: a cutaneous analogue to secretory carcinomas of the breast and salivary glands. *Am J Surg Pathol* 2017; **41**: 62–6.

75. Huang S, Liu Y, Su J, et al. "Secretory" carcinoma of the skin mimicking secretory carcinoma of the breast: case report and literature review. *Am J Dermatopathol* 2016; **38**: 698–703.

76. Kastnerova L, Luzar B, Goto K, et al. Secretory carcinoma of the skin: report of 6 cases, including a case with a novel NFIX-PKN1 translocation. *Am J Surg Pathol* 2019; **43**: 1092–8.

77. Skálová A, Vanecek T, Simpson RH, et al. Mammary analogue secretory carcinoma of salivary glands: molecular analysis of 25 ETV6 gene rearranged tumors with lack of detection of classical ETV6-NTRK3 fusion transcript by standard RT-PCR: report of 4 cases harboring ETV6-X gene fusion. *Am J Surg Pathol* 2016; **40**: 3–13.

78. Ye Q, Chen H, Han C, et al. Nuclear staining of pan-Trk by immunohistochemistry is highly specific for secretory carcinoma of breast: pant-Trk in various subtypes of breast carcinoma. *J Clin Pathol* 2023. Aug 16:jcp-2023–208989. doi: 10.1136/jcp-2023-208989.

79. Ito Y, Ishibashi K, Masaki A, et al. Mammary analogue secretory carcinoma of salivary glands: a clinicopathologic and molecular study including 2 cases harboring ETV6-X fusion. *Am J Surg Pathol* 2015; **39**: 602–10.

80. Rooper LM, Karantanos T, Ning Y, Bishop JA, Gordon SW, Kang H. Salivary secretory carcinoma with a novel ETV6-MET fusion: expanding the molecular spectrum of a recently described entity. *Am J Surg Pathol* 2018; **42**: 1121–6.

81. Skálová A, Vanecek T, Martinek P, et al. Molecular profiling of mammary analog secretory carcinoma revealed a subset of tumors harboring a novel ETV6-RET translocation: report of 10 cases. *Am J Surg Pathol* 2018; **42**: 234–46.

82. Skálová A, Banečkova M, Thompson LDR, et al. Expanding the molecular spectrum of secretory carcinoma of salivary glands with a novel VIM-RET fusion. *Am J Surg Pathol* 2020; **44**: 1295–307.

83. Guilmette J, Dias-Santagata D, Nosé V, Lennerz JK, Sadow PM. Novel gene fusions in secretory carcinoma of the salivary glands: enlarging the ETV6 family. *Hum Pathol* 2019; **83**: 50–8.

84. Nakayama T, Miyabe S, Okabe M, et al. Clinicopathological significance of the CRTC3-MAML2 fusion transcript in mucoepidermoid carcinoma. *Mod Pathol* 2009; **22**: 1575–81.

85. Chenevert J, Duvvuri U, Chiosea S, et al. DOG1: a novel marker of salivary acinar and intercalated duct differentiation. *Mod Pathol* 2012; **25**: 919–29.

86. Bishop JA, Weinreb I, Swanson D, et al. Microsecretory adenocarcinoma: a novel salivary gland tumor characterized by a recurrent MEF2C-SS18 fusion. *Am J Surg Pathol* 2019; **43**: 1023–32.

87. Bishop JA, Williams EA, McLean AC, et al. Microsecretory adenocarcinoma of the skin harboring recurrent SS18 fusions: a cutaneous analog to a newly described salivary gland tumor. *J Cutan Pathol* 2022; **50**: 134–9.

88. Panse G. Microsecretory adenocarcinoma: cutaneous counterpart of a newly described salivary gland tumor with recurrent MEF2C::SS18 fusion. *J Cutan Pathol* 2023; **50**: 188–90.

89. Dibbern ME, Gru AA, Stelow EB. Microsecretory adenocarcinoma of the external ear canal. *J Cutan Pathol* 2023; **50**: 106–9.

90. Skalova A, Vanecek T, Sima R, et al. Mammary analogue secretory carcinoma of salivary glands, containing the ETV6-NTRK3 fusion gene: a hitherto undescribed salivary gland tumor entity. *Am J Surg Pathol* 2010; **34**: 599–608.

91. Kazakov DV, Zelger B, Rütten A, et al. Morphologic diversity of malignant neoplasms arising in preexisting spiradenoma, cylindroma, and spiradenocylindroma based on the study of 24 cases, sporadic or occurring in the setting of Brooke-Spiegler syndrome. *Am J Surg Pathol* 2009; **33**: 705–19.

92. van der Horst MP, Marusic Z, Hornick JL, Luzar B, Brenn T. Morphologically low-grade spiradenocarcinoma: a clinicopathologic study of 19 cases with emphasis on outcome and MYB expression. *Mod Pathol* 2015; **28**: 944–53.

93. Kazakov DV, Grossmann P, Spagnolo DV, et al. Expression of p53 and TP53 mutational analysis in malignant neoplasms arising in preexisting spiradenoma, cylindroma, and spiradenocylindroma, sporadic or associated with Brooke-Spiegler syndrome. *Am J Dermatopathol* 2010; **32**: 215–21.

94. Moran JMT, DeSimone MS, Mariño-Enríquez A, et al. Malignant proliferating pilar tumor. Clinicopathologic, immunohistochemical, and molecular study of 17 cases. *Am J Surg Pathol* 2023; **47**: 1151–9.

95. Moran JMT, Hoang MP, Mariño-Enríquez A, DeSimone MS. Malignant proliferating pilar tumor with sarcomatous transformation ("carcinosarcoma"): case report with molecular profile. *Am J Dermatopathol* 2025; 47:65-69.

96. Chaichamnan K, Satayasoontorn K, Puttanupaab S, Attainsee A. Malignant proliferating trichilemmal tumors with CD34 expression. *J Med Assoc Thai* 2010; **93** Suppl 6: S28–34.

97. Haas N, Audring H, Sterry W. Carcinoma arising in a proliferating trichilemmal cyst expresses fetal and trichilemmal hair phenotype. *Am J Dermatopathol* 2002; **24**: 340–4.

98. Goto K, Kukita Y, Honma K, et al. Sweat-gland carcinoma with neuroendocrine differentiation (SCAND): a clinicopathologic study of 13 cases with genetic analysis. *Mod Pathol* 2022; **35**: 33–43.

99. Chiller K, Passaro D, Scheuller M, Singer M, McCalmont T, Grekin RC. Microcystic adnexal carcinoma: forty-eight cases, their treatment, and their outcome. *Arch Dermatol* 2000; **136**: 1355–9.

100. Llamas-Velasco M, Perez-Gonzalez YC, Bosch-Princep R, Fernandez-Figueras MT, Rutten A. Solid carcinoma is a variant of microcystic adnexal carcinoma: a 14-case series. *J Cutan Pathol* 2018; 45: 897–904.
101. Tse JY, Nguyen AT, Le LP, Hoang MP. Microcystic adnexal carcinoma versus desmoplastic trichoepithelioma: a comparative study. *Am J Dermatopathol* 2013; **35**: 50–5.
102. Hoang MP, Dresser KA, Kapur P, High WA, Mahalingam M. Microcystic adnexal carcinoma: an immunohistochemical reappraisal. *Mod Pathol* 2008; **21**: 178–85.
103. Vidal CI, Goldberg M, Burstein DE, Emanuel HJ, Emanuel PO. P63 immunohistochemistry is a useful adjunct in distinguishing sclerosing cutaneous tumors. *Am J Dermatopathol* 2010; **32**: 257–61.
104. Jedrych J, McNiff JM. Expression of p75 neurotrophin receptor in desmoplastic trichoepithelioma, infiltrative basal cell carcinoma, and microcystic adnexal carcinoma. *Am J Dermatopathol* 2013; **35**: 308–15.
105. Mohanty SK, Sardana R, McFall M, et al. Does immunohistochemistry add to morphology in differentiating trichoepithelioma, desmoplastic trichoepithelioma, morpheaform basal cell carcinoma, and microcystic adnexal carcinoma? *Appl Immunohistochem Mol Morphol* 2022; **30**: 273–7.
106. Koga K, Anan T, Fukumoto T, Fujimoto M, Nabeshima K. Ln-gamma 2 chain of laminin-332 is a useful marker in differentiating between benign and malignant sclerosing adnexal neoplasms. *Histopathology* 2020; **76**: 318–24.
107. Menge TD, Durgin JS, Hrycaj SM, et al. Utility of GLI1 RNA chromogenic in situ hybridization in distinguishing basal cell carcinoma from histopathologic mimics. *Mod Pathol* 2023; **36**: 100265. doi: 10.1016/j.modpat.2023.100265.
108. Regmi A, Zelman B, Mudaliar KM, Speiser JJ. Solitary vulvar syringoma with deep extension; potential for misdiagnosis as the microcystic adnexal carcinoma (MAC). *Am J Dermatopathol* 2023; **45**: 180–4.
109. Van der Horst M, Garcia-Herrera A, Markiewicz D, Martin B, Eduardo C, Brenn T. Squamoid eccrine ductal carcinoma: a clinicopathologic study of 30 cases. *Am J Surg Pathol* 2016; **40**: 755–60.
110. Wong TY, Suster S, Mihm MC. Squamoid eccrine ductal carcinoma. *Histopathology* 1997; **30**: 288–93.
111. Mckissack SS, Wohltmann W, Dalton SR, Miletta NR. Squamoid eccrine ductal carcinoma: an aggressive mimicker of squamous cell carcinoma. *Am J Dermatopathol* 2019; **41**: 140–3.
112. Lim MM, Macdonald JA. Squamoid eccrine ductal carcinoma: treatment and outcomes. *Am J Dermatopathol* 2022; **44**: 249–53.
113. Sekine S, Kiyono T, Ryo E, et al. Recurrent YAP1-MAML2 and YAP1-NUTM1 fusions in poroma and porocarcinoma. *J Clin Invest* 2019; **129**: 3827–32.
114. Russell-Goldman E, Hornick JL, Hanna J. Utility of YAP1 and NUT immunohistochemistry in the diagnosis of porocarcinoma. *J Cutan Pathol* 2021; **48**; 403–10.
115. Robson A, Lazar AJ, Ben Nagi J, et al. Primary cutaneous apocrine carcinoma: a clinicopathologic analysis of 24 cases. *Am J Surg Pathol* 2008; **32**: 682–90.
116. Niemeier LA, Dabbs DJ, Beriwal S, Striebel JM, Bhargava R. Androgen receptor in breast cancer: expression in estrogen receptor-positive tumors and in estrogen receptor-negative tumors with apocrine differentiation. *Mod Pathol* 2010; **23**: 205–12.
117. Le LP, Dias-Santagata D, Pawlak AC, et al. Apocrine-eccrine carcinomas: molecular and immunohistochemical analyses. *PLoS One* 2012; **7**: e47290. doi: 10.1371/journal.pone.0047290.
118. Piris A, Peng Y, Boussahmain C, Essary LR, Gudewicz TM, Hoang MP. Cutaneous and mammary apocrine carcinomas have different immunoprofiles. *Hum Pathol* 2014; 45: 320–6.
119. Plumb SJ, Argenyi ZB, Stone MS, De Young BR. Cytokeratin 5/6 immunostaining in cutaneous adnexal neoplasms and metastatic adenocarcinoma. *Am J Dermatopathol* 2004; **26**: 447–51.
120. Weingertner N, Gressel A, Battistella M, Cribier B. Aggressive digital papillary adenocarcinoma: a clinicopathological study of 19 cases. *J Am Acad Dermatol* 2017; **77**: 549–58.
121. Kervarrec T, Imbeaud S, Veyer D, et al. Digital papillary adenocarcinoma in nonacral skin: clinicopathologic and genetic characterization of 5 cases. *Am J Surg Pathol* 2023; **47**: 1077–84.
122. Xavier-Junior JCC, Camilo-Junior DJ, Carneiro Dias AL, et al. Value of immunohistochemistry to differentiate digital papillary adenocarcinoma from acral hidradenoma with papillary structures. *Am J Dermatopathol* 2022; **44**: 843–5.
123. Winnes M, Mölne L, Suurküla M, et al. Frequent fusion of the CRTC1 and MAML2 genes in clear cell variants of cutaneous hidradenomas. *Genes Chromosomes Cancer* 2007; **46**: 559–63.
124. Vanderbilt C, Brenn T, Mo AP, et al. Association of HPV42 with digital papillary adenocarcinoma and the use of in situ hybridization for its distinction from acral hidradenoma and diagnosis at non-acral sites. *Mod Pathol* 2022; **35**: 1405–10.
125. Bui CM, Pukhalskaya T, Smoller BR, et al. Two distinct pathways of digital papillary adenocarcinoma – BRAF mutation or low-risk HPV infection. *J Cutan Pathol* 2023; **50**: 568–76.
126. Simonds RM, Segal RJ, Sharma A. Extramammary Paget's disease: a review of the literature. *Int J Dermatol* 2019; **58**: 871–9.
127. Kim SJ, Thompson AK, Zubair AS, et al. Surgical treatment and outcomes of patients with extramammary Paget disease: a cohort study. *Dermatol Surg* 2017; **43**: 708–14.
128. Inui S, Fukuhara S, Asada H, et al. Double involvement of extramammary Paget's disease in the genitalia and axilla. *J Dermatol* 2000; **27**: 409–12.
129. Chanda JJ. Extramammary Paget's disease: prognosis and relationship to internal malignancy. *J Am Acad Dermatol* 1985; 13: 1009–14.
130. Goldblum JR, Hart WR. Perianal Paget's disease: a histologic and immunohistochemical study of 11 cases with and without associated rectal adenocarcinoma. *Am J Surg Pathol* 1998; **22**: 170–9.
131. Perrotto J, Abbott JJ, Ceilley RI, Ahmed I. The role of immunohistochemistry in discriminating primary from secondary extramammary Paget's disease. *Am J Dermatopathol* 2010; **32**: 137–43.
132. Plaza JA, Torres-Cabala C, Ivan D, Prieto VG. HER-2/neu expression in extramammary Paget disease: a clinicopathologic and immunohistochemistry study of 47 cases with and without underlying malignancy. *J Cutan Pathol* 2009; **36**: 729–33.

133. Liegl B, Horn HC. Moinfar F. Androgen receptors are frequently expressed in mammary and extramammary Paget's disease. *Mod Pathol* 2005; **18**: 1283–8.

134. Hikita T, Ohtsuki Y, Maeda T, Furihata M. Immunohistochemical and fluorescence studies on noninvasive and invasive extramammary Paget's disease. *Int J Surg Pathol* 2012; **20**: 441–8.

135. Kuan S-F, Montag AG, Hart J, Krausz T, Recant W. Differential expression of mucin genes in mammary and extramammary Paget's disease. *Am J Surg Pathol* 2001; **25**: 1469–77.

136. Shaco-Levy R, Bean SM, Vollmer RT, et al. Paget disease of the vulva: a histologic study of 56 cases correlating pathologic features and disease course. *Int J Gynecol Pathol* 2010; **29**: 69–78.

137. Wieland R, Adhikari P, North J. The utility of p63, CK7, and CAM5.2 staining in differentiating pagetoid intraepidermal carcinomas. *J Cutan Pathol* 2023; **50**: 1110–15.

138. Cook EE, Harrison BT, Hirsch MS. TRPS1 expression is sensitive and specific for primary extramammary Paget disease. *Histopathology* 2023; **83**: 104–8.

139. Plaza JA, Wakely P, Roman J, et al. Low-grade hidradenocarcinomas: a clinicopathologic study of an unusual carcinoma that can mimic its benign counterpart. *Am J Surg Pathol* 2023; **47**: 907–14.

140. Hernandez-Parez E, Cestoni-Parducci R. Nodular hidradenoma and hidradenocarcinoma. A 10-year review. *J Am Acad Dermatol* 1985; **12**: 15–20.

141. Nazarian RM, Kapur P, Rakheja D, et al. Atypical and malignant hidradenomas: a histologic and immunohistochemical study. *Mod Pathol* 2009; **22**: 600–10.

142. Russell-Goldman E, Hanna J. MAML2 gene rearrangement occurs in nearly all hidradenomas: a reappraisal in a series of 20 cases. *Am J Dermatopathol* 2022; **44**: 806–11.

143. Winnes M, Molne L, Suurkula M, et al. Frequent fusion of the CRTC1 and MAML2 genes in clear cell variants of cutaneous hidradenomas. *Genes Chromosomes Cancer* 2007; **46**: 559–63.

144. Behboudi A, Winnes M, Gorunova L, et al. Clear cell hidradenoma of the skin–a third tumor type with a t(11;19)-associated TORC1-MAML2 gene fusion: *Genes Chromosomes Cancer* 2005; **43**: 202–5.

145. Kuma Y, Yamada Y, Yamamoto H, et al. A novel fusion gene CRTC3-MAML2 in hidradenoma: histopathological significance. *Hum Pathol* 2017; **70**: 55–61.

146. Kyrpychova L, Kacerovska D, Vanecek T, et al. Cutaneous hidradenoma: a study of 21 neoplasms revealing neither correlation between the cellular composition and CRTC1-MAML2 fusions nor presence of CRTC3-MAML2 fusions. *Ann Diagn Pathol* 2016; **23**: 8–13.

147. Moller E, Stenman G, Mandahl N, et al. POU5F1, encoding a key regulator of stem cell pluripotency, is fused to EWSR1 in hidradenoma of the skin and mucoepidermoid carcinoma of the salivary glands. *J Pathol* 2008; **215**: 78–86.

148. Salih AM, Kakamad FH, Baba HO, et al. Porocarcinoma: presentation and management, a meta-analysis of 453 cases. *Ann Med Surg* 2017; **20**: 74–9.

149. Robson A, Greene J, Ansari N, et al. Eccrine porocarcinoma (malignant eccrine poroma): a clinicopathologic study of 69 cases. *Am J Surg Pathol* 2001; **25**: 710–20.

150. Mahalingam M, Richards JE, Selim MA, Muzikansky A, Hoang MP. An immunohistochemical comparison of cytokeratin 7, cytokeratin 15, cytokeratin 19, CAM5.2, carcinoembryonic antigen, and nestin in differentiating porocarcinoma from squamous cell carcinoma. *Hum Pathol* 2012; **43**: 1265–72.

151. Mahomed F, Blok J, Grayson W. The squamous variant of eccrine porocarcinoma: a clinicopathological study of 21 cases. *J Clin Pathol* 2008; **61**: 361–5.

152. Heyderman E, Graham RM, Chapman DV, Richardson TC, McKee PH. Epithelial markers in primary skin cancer: an immunoperoxidase study of the distribution of epithelial membrane antigen (EMA) and carcinoembryonic antigen (CEA) in 65 primary skin carcinomas. *Histopathology* 1984; **8**: 423–34.

153. Miura K, Akashi T, Namiki T, et al. Engrailed homeobox 1 and cytokeratin 19 are independent diagnostic markers of eccrine porocarcinoma and distinguish it from squamous cell carcinoma. *Am J Clin Pathol* 2020; **154**: 499–509.

154. Goto K, Ishikawa M, Hamada K, et al. Comparison of immunohistochemical expression of cytokeratin 19, c-KIT, BerEP4, GATA3, and NUTM1 between porocarcinoma and squamous cell carcinoma. *Am J Dermatopathol* 2021; **43**: 781–7.

155. Stevens TM, Morlote D, Xiu J, et al. NUTM1-rearranged neoplasia: a multi-institution experience yields novel fusion partners and expands the histologic spectrum. *Mod Pathol* 2019; **32**: 764–73.

156. McEvoy CR, Fox SB, Prall OWJ. Emerging entities in NUTM1-rearranged neoplasms. *Genes Chromosomes Cancer* 2020; **59**: 375–85.

157. Goto K, Kukita Y, Honma K, et al. Signet-ring cell/histiocytoid carcinoma of the axilla: a clinicopathological and genetic analysis of 11 cases, review of the literature, and comparison with potentially related tumours. *Histopathology* 2021; 79: 926–39.

158. Philips R, Langston L, Hwang H, et al. Primary cutaneous histiocytoid carcinoma with distant metastasis. *J Cutan Pathol* 2017; **44**: 376–80.

159. Requena L, Prieto VG, Requena C, et al. Primary signet-ring cell/histiocytoid carcinoma of the eyelid: a clinicopathologic study of 5 cases and review of the literature. *Am J Surg Pathol* 2011; **35**: 378–91.

160. Raghavan SS, Clark M, Louie CY, et al. Molecular profiling of a primary cutaneous signet-ring cell/histiocytoid carcinoma of the eyelid. *J Cutan Pathol* 2020; **47**: 860–4.

161. Konstantinova AM, Kacerovska D, Stewart CJR, et al. Syringocystadenocarcinoma papilliferum in situ-like changes in extramammary Paget disease: a report of 11 cases. *Am J Dermatopathol* 2016; **38**: 882–6.

162. Cornejo KM, Hutchinson L, O'Donnell P, et al. Molecular profiling of syringocystadenocarcinoma papilliferum reveals RAS-activating mutations. *Arch Pathol Lab Med* 2024; **148**: 215–22.

163. Lee JJ, Mochel MC, Piris A, Boussahmain C, Mahalingam M, Hoang MP. p40 exhibits better specificity than p63 in distinguishing primary skin adnexal carcinomas from cutaneous metastases. *Hum Pathol* 2014; **45**: 1078–83.

164. Mahalingam M, Nguyen LP, Richards JE, Muzikansky A, Hoang MP. The diagnostic utility of immunohistochemistry in

distinguishing primary skin adnexal carcinomas from metastatic adenocarcinoma to skin: an immunohistochemical reappraisal using cytokeratin 15, nestin, p63, D2-40, and calretinin. *Mod Pathol* 2010; **23**: 713–19.

165. Rollins-Raval M, Chivukula M, Tseng GC, Jukic D, Dabbs DJ. An immunohistochemical panel to differentiate metastatic breast carcinoma to skin from primary sweat gland carcinomas with a review of the literature. *Arch Pathol Lab Med* 2011; **135**: 975–83.

166. Macagno N, Sohier P, Kervarrec T, et al. Recent advances on immunohistochemistry and molecular biology for the diagnosis of adnexal sweat gland tumors. *Cancers* 2022; **14**: 476. doi: 10.3390/cancers14030476.

167. Agaimy A. Fusion-positive skin/ adnexal carcinomas. *Genes Chromosomes Cancer* 2022; **61**: 274–84.

168. Behboudi A, Enlund F, Winnes M, et al. Molecular classification of mucoepidermoid carcinomas-prognostic significance of the MECT1-MAML2 fusion oncogene. *Genes Chromosomes Cancer* 2006; **45**: 470–81.

169. Riedlinger W, Hurley M, Dehner L, Lind A. Mucoepidermoid carcinoma of the skin: a distinct entity from adenosquamous carcinoma: a case study with a review of the literature. *Am J Surg Pathology* 2005; **29**: 131–5.

170. Mirza FN, Yumeen S, Zogg CK, Mirza HN, Leventhal JS. Epidemiology, treatment, survival, and prognostic factors of cutaneous mucoepidermoid carcinoma: a distinct entity with an indolent clinical course. *J Am Acad Dermatol* 2020; **83**: 1827–30.

171. Lennerz JK, Perry A, Dehner LP, et al. CRTC1 rearrangements in the absence of t(11;19) in primary cutaneous mucoepidermoid carcinoma. *Br J Dermatol* 2009; **161**: 925–9.

172. Ohtomo R, Mori T, Shibata S, et al. Sox10 is a novel marker of acinus and intercalated duct differentiation in salivary gland tumors: a clue to the histogenesis for tumor diagnosis. *Mod Pathol* 2013; **26**: 1041–50.

173. Nakayama T, Miyabe S, Okabe M, et al. Clinicopathological significance of the CRTC3-MAML2 fusion transcript in mucoepidermoid carcinoma. *Mod Pathol* 2009; **22**: 1575–81.

174. Möller E, Stenman G, Mandahl N, et al. POU5F1, encoding a key regulator of stem cell pluripotency, is fused to EWSR1 in hidradenoma of the skin and mucoepidermoid carcinoma of the salivary glands. *J Pathol* 2008; **215**: 78–86.

175. Okabe M, Miyabe S, Nagatsuka H, et al. MECT1-MAML2 fusion transcript defines a favorable subset of mucoepidermoid carcinoma. *Clin Cancer Res* 2006; **12**: 3902–7.

176. Okorie CL, Yan S, Kerr DA, Tafe LJ, Sriharan A. Cutaneous myoepithelioma with EWSR1 gene rearrangement and its differentials: A diagnostic challenge. *J Cutan Pathol* 2023; **50**: 632–6.

177. Mentzel T, Requena L, Kaddu S, et al. Cutaneous myoepithelial neoplasms: clinicopathologic and immunohistochemical study of 20 cases suggesting a continuous spectrum ranging from benign mixed tumor of the skin to cutaneous myoepithelioma and myoepithelial carcinoma. *J Cutan Pathol* 2003; **30**: 294–302.

178. Jo VY, Antonescu CR, Zhang L, Dal Cin P, Hornick JL, Fletcher CD. Cutaneous syncytial myoepithelioma: clinicopathologic characterization in a series of 38 cases. *Am J Surg Pathol* 2013; **37**: 710–18.

179. Plaza JA, Brenn T, Chung S, et al. Histomorphological and immunophenotypical spectrum of cutaneous myoepitheliomas: a series of 35 cases. *J Cutan Pathol* 2021; **48**: 847–55.

180. Miettinen M, McCue PA, Sarlomo-Rikala M, et al. SOX10—a marker for not only schwannian and melanocytic neoplasms but also myoepithelial cell tumors of soft tissue: a systematic analysis of 5134 tumors. *Am J Surg Pathol* 2015; **39**: 826–35.

181. Le Loarer F, Zhang L, Fletcher CD, et al. Consistent SMARCB1 homozygous deletions in epithelioid sarcoma and in a subset of myoepithelial carcinomas can be reliably detected by FISH in archival material. *Genes Chromosomes Cancer* 2014; **53**: 475–86.

182. Mehta A, Davey J, Gharpuray-Pandit D, et al. Cutaneous myoepithelial neoplasms on acral sites show distinctive and reproducible histopathologic and immunohistochemical features. *Am J Surg Pathol* 2022; **46**: 1241–9.

183. Agaram NP, Chen HW, Zhang L, et al. EWSR1-PBX3: a novel gene fusion in myoepithelial tumors. *Genes Chromosomes Cancer* 2015; **54**: 63–71.

184. Brandal P, Panagopoulos I, Bjerkehagen B, et al. Detection of a t(1;22)(q23;q12) translocation leading to an EWSR1-PBX1 fusion gene in a myoepithelioma. *Genes Chromosomes Cancer* 2008; **47**: 558–64.

185. Jo VY, Antonescu CR, Dickson BC, et al. Cutaneous syncytial myoepithelioma is characterized by recurrent EWSR1-PBX3 fusions. *Am J Surg Pathol* 2019; **43**: 1349–54.

186. Brandal P, Panagopoulos I, Bjerkehagen B, Heim S. t(19;22)(q13;q12) Translocation leading to the novel fusion gene EWSR1-ZNF444 in soft tissue myoepithelial carcinoma. *Genes Chromosomes Cancer* 2009; **48**: 1051–6.

187. Flucke U, Mentzel T, Verdijk MA, et al. EWSR1-ATF1 chimeric transcript in a myoepithelial tumor of soft tissue: a case report. *Hum Pathol* 2012; **43**: 764–8.

188. Antonescu CR, Zhang L, Chang NE, et al. EWSR1-POU5F1 fusion in soft tissue myoepithelial tumors. A molecular analysis of sixty-six cases, including soft tissue, bone, and visceral lesions, showing common involvement of the EWSR1 gene. *Genes Chromosomes Cancer* 2010; **49**: 1114–24.

189. Huang SC, Chen HW, Zhang L, et al. Novel FUS-KLF17 and EWSR1-KLF17 fusions in myoepithelial tumors. *Genes Chromosomes Cancer* 2015; **54**: 267–75.

190. Bodis S, Kroiss S, Tchinda J, Fritz C, Wagner U, Bode PK. Myoepithelial carcinoma of soft tissue with an EWSR1-KLF15 gene fusion in an infant. *Pediatr Dev Pathol* 2021; **24**: 371–7.

191. Yoshida A, Yoshida H, Yoshida M, et al. Myoepithelioma-like tumors of the vulvar region: a distinctive group of SMARCB1-deficient neoplasms. *Am J Surg Pathol* 2015; **39**: 1102–13.

192. French CA, Rahman S, Walsh EM, et al. NSD3-NUT fusion oncoprotein in NUT midline carcinoma: implications for a novel oncogenic mechanism. *Cancer Discov* 2014; **4**: 928–41.

193. Schaefer IM, Dal Cin P, Landry LM, Fletcher CDM, Hanna GJ, French CA. CIC-NUTM1 fusion: a case which expands the spectrum of NUT-rearranged epithelioid malignancies. *Genes Chromosomes Cancer* 2018; **57**: 446–51.

194. Tamura R, Nakaoka H, Yoshihara K, et al. Novel MXD4-NUTM1 fusion transcript identified in primary ovarian undifferentiated small round cell sarcoma. *Genes Chromosomes Cancer* 2018; **57**: 557–63.

195. Diolaiti D, Dela Cruz FS, Gundem G, et al. A recurrent novel MGA-NUTM1

fusionidentifies a new subtype of high-grade spindle cell sarcoma. *Cold Spring Harb Mol Case Stud* 2018; **4**: a003194.

196. Rubio Gonzalez B, Ortiz MV, Ross DS, Busam KJ. Skin adnexal carcinoma with BRD3-NUTM2B fusion. *J Cutan Pathol* 2021; **48**: 1508–13.

197. Haack H, Johnson LA, Fry CJ, et al. Diagnosis of NUT midline carcinoma using a NUT-specific monoclonal antibody. *Am J Surg Pathol* 2009; **33**: 984–91.

198. Bigby SM, Charlton A, Miller MV, et al. Biphasic sarcomatoid basal cell carcinoma (carcinosarcoma): four cases with immunohistochemistry and review of the literature. *J Cutan Pathol* 2005; **32**: 141–7.

199. Boyd AS, Rapini RP. Cutaneous collision tumors: an analysis of 69 cases and review of the literature. *Am J Dermatopathol* 1994; **16**: 253–7.

200. Erickson LA, Myers JL, Mihm MC, Markovic SN, Pittelkow MR. Malignant basomelanocytic tumor manifesting as metastatic melanoma. *Am J Surg Pathol* 2004; **28**: 1393–6.

Chapter 5

Inflammatory Dermatoses Mimicking Lymphomas

Emily M. Hartsough, M. Angelica Selim, and Mai P. Hoang

Introduction

The skin provides the interface between the outside environment and the rest of the body, and its constant exposure to a variety of antigens has led to the development of a complex innate and adaptive immune microenvironment. Normally, the epidermal infiltrate is comprised predominantly of CD8+ T cells and CD4+ CD1a+ Langerhans cells. The dermis contains a diversity of immunologic cell types, including CD4+ T cells, natural killer (NK) T cells, various dendritic cell (DC) subtypes, a small number of B cells, among others.[1] The T cells of the epidermis are predominantly αβ T cells, whereas the T cells in the dermis are a mixture of αβ- and γδ-T cells.[2]

Cutaneous lymphoid hyperplasia (CLH) comprise a group of benign reactive lymphoproliferative disorders characterized by a robust proliferation of B cells and/or T cells, with variable other inflammatory cells such as plasma cells or histiocytes, which can mimic the clinical and histopathologic appearance of cutaneous lymphomas. This hyperplasia may be idiopathic or arise in response to antigens such as drugs, arthropod bites (e.g. *Borrelia burgdorferi*), trauma, vaccinations, tattoos (cinnabar, red tattoo pigment), drugs, among others.[3-6] A solitary nodule on the head and neck is the most frequent clinical presentation; however, clusters or widely distributed papules and plaques can also be seen.[3]

Classically, CLH was divided into three categories, 1) B-cell rich CLH, 2) T-cell rich CLH, and 3) B-cell/T-cell CLH.[3,7] Mitteldorf and Kempf recently proposed a novel classification of CLH based on clinicopathologic characteristics as 1) nodular pseudolymphoma, 2) pseudo-mycosis fungoides and simulators of other CTCLs, 3) other pseudolymphoma (representing distinct clinical entities), and 4) intravascular pseudolymphoma.[6] The most recent edition of the WHO 5th edition delineates reactive B-cell rich (rB-LPs) and reactive T-cell rich lymphoid proliferations (rT-LPs).[8]

In some cases, B lymphocytes can accumulate and resemble primary cutaneous follicle-center lymphoma (PCFCL) and primary cutaneous marginal zone lymphoma (PCMZL) histopathologically. T-cell pseudolymphomas include several inflammatory dermatoses that exhibit various degrees of epidermotropism and can mimic T-cell lymphoproliferative disorders such as mycosis fungoides (MF). These include lymphomatoid contact dermatitis, lymphomatoid drug eruption, follicular mucinosis, lupus erythematosus panniculitis, pigmented purpuric dermatosis, pityriasis lichenoides chronica (PLC)/pityriasis lichenoides et varioliformis acuta (PLEVA), and pseudolymphomatous folliculitis, among others. In some instances, the infiltrate is rich in plasma cells, as in IgG4-related disease in the skin. In these settings, ancillary testing, such as gene rearrangement studies and immunohistochemistry (IHC), plays an important role in excluding cutaneous lymphoma. A list of commonly used markers in the clinical laboratory for the diagnosis of hematolymphoid lesions is outlined in **Table 5.1**. Ultimately, however, ancillary studies must be used in conjunction with clinicopathologic correlation, as T-cell markers such as CD7 can be lost in both neoplastic and inflammatory dermatoses,[9] and T-cell gene rearrangements may be present in reactive/inflammatory skin conditions[10] and absent in early cutaneous lymphomas (**Table 5.2**).[11] While most pseudolymphomas exhibit an indolent clinical course, a small subset may progress to lymphoma.[12]

Table 5.1 Common hematolymphoid markers

Antibody	Commonly used clones	Staining pattern	Normal structures
ALK1 (CD246)	5A4, ALK1	cytoplasmic	tumors with NPM-ALK translocation*
Bcl–2	124, 100/D5	membranous cytoplasmic	T cells
Bcl–6	GI191E/A8, LN22, PG-B6p	nuclear	follicle center cells
Beta F1	8A3	membranous	alpha-beta T-cells
BOB.1	SP92	nuclear	follicle center cells
CD1a	MTB1, O10, EP3622	membranous	Langerhans cells, dendritic cells, cortical thymocytes
CD2	AB75, MT910	membranous cytoplasmic	pan T-cell marker, Langerhans cells, mast cells
CD3	2GV6, PS1, LN10	membranous cytoplasmic	pan T-cell marker, cytoplasmic staining of NK cells
CD4	4B12, 1F6, SP35	membranous	T-cell helper subset, monocytes, histiocytes
CD5	4C7, SP19	membranous	pan T-cell marker
CD7	CBC.37, SP94	membranous	pan T-cell marker, NK cells
CD8	C8/144B, 4B11	membranous	T-cell cytotoxic subset
CD10	56C6, SP67	membranous	mature and precursor B-cells
CD15	Carb–3, MMA	membranous	neutrophils, myeloid precursor cells
CD19	LE-CD19	membranous	B cells
CD20	L26	membranous	B cells
CD21	IF8, 2G9, EP3093	membranous	follicular dendritic cells, B cells
CD23	1B12, SP23	membranous, dendrites	follicular dendritic cells, activated B-cells
CD25	4C9, SP176	membranous cytoplasmic	interleukin–2 receptor
CD30	Ber-H2, 1G12	membranous cytoplasmic	activated T- and B- cell marker
CD34	QBEnd10, My10	membranous cytoplasmic	myeloblasts, endothelial cells
CD43	L60, SP55	membranous	T cells, myeloid cells
CD45	2B11+PD7/26	membranous	both T- and B-cells
CD45RA	4KB5,	membranous	naive T-cells
CD45RO	UCHL1	membranous	activated or memory T-cells
CD56	1B6, 123C3, MRQ–42	membranous	natural killer cell marker, myeloid cells
CD57	NK–1, TB01	membranous	natural killer cells, T cells
CD68	KP1, PG-M1	cytoplasmic	histiocytes, monocytes
CD79a	JCB117, SP18, 11E3	membranous	B cells, plasma cells
CD99	12E7, H036–1.1, O13	membranous	lymphocytes, endothelial cells
CD117	Polyclonal A4502, YR145, 9.7	membranous	mast cells
CD123	7G3	cytoplasmic	plasmacytoid dendritic cells, blastic plasmacytoid dendritic cell neoplasm*
CD138	B-A38, M115	membranous	plasma cells, squamous epithelial cells
CD163	10D6, MRQ–26	cytoplasmic	histiocytes, monocytes
CD303	124B3.13	cytoplasmic	plasmacytoid dendritic cell type II
CXCL13	53610	cytoplasmic	follicular T-helper lymphocytes
D2–40	D2–40	cytoplasmic	lymphatic spaces
EBER ISH	*In situ* hybridization probe	nuclear	EBV-encoded RNA in infected cells
Granzyme B	polyclonal	cytoplasmic granular	cytotoxic T-cells, natural killer cells
ICOS/ CD278	ISA–3	cytoplasmic	follicular T-helper lymphocytes
IgG4	MRQ–44, EP138	cytoplasmic	IgG4-positive plasma cells

Table 5.1 (cont.)

Antibody	Commonly used clones	Staining pattern	Normal structures
Kappa light chain	L1C1	cytoplasmic	kappa-positive plasma cells
Ki–67	MIB–1, SP6	nuclear	cells in active phases of cell cycle (G1, S, G2, mitosis) but not resting cells (G0)
Lambda light chain	Lamb14	cytoplasmic	lambda-positive plasma cells
Langerin (CD207)	12D6	cytoplasmic	Langerhans cells
LEF1	EP310, EPR2029Y	nuclear	T cells, pre B-cells
Latent membrane protein 1 (LMP1)	MRQ–47	cytoplasmic/membranous	expressed by EBV-infected cells
Lysozyme	polyclonal	cytoplasmic	myeloid cells, histocytes, macrophages and monocytes
Myeloperoxidase (MPO)	Polyclonal, SP72	cytoplasmic	granulocytes, monocytes
MUM1	MRQ–43, EAU32	nuclear	plasma cells, fraction of B-cells, activated T-cells
OCT2	Oct–207	nuclear	B-cell transcription factor
PAX5	SP34	nuclear	pan B-cells, pre-B-cells
PD1 (CD279)	MRQ–22	cytoplasmic	activated T-cells, B-cells and myeloid cells
Perforin	MRQ–23, 5B10	cytoplasmic	cytotoxic T-cells, natural killer cells
TCL1	SP263, MRQ–7	cytoplasmic and nuclear	T cells, plasmacytoid dendritic cells type II
TRBC1	E6Z3S	membranous and cytoplasmic	T-cell receptor constant beta chainre
TCR delta	H–41	cytoplasmic	gamma-delta T-cells
TCR gamma	Gamma 3.20	cytoplasmic	gamma-delta T-cells
TdT	SEN28	nuclear	cortical thymocytes, pre-B-acute lymphoblastic leukemia *
TOX	HPH018322	nuclear	T-cells
TIA–1	EP243, MRQ–59	cytoplasmic and granular	cytotoxic T-cells, natural killer cells
Tryptase	AA1, G3	cytoplasmic	mast cells

* Staining in tumors

5.1 Reactive B-Cell Rich Lymphoid Proliferations That Mimic B-Cell Lymphomas (rB-LPs)

The histopathologic appearance of a rB-LPs is variable, often presenting as a nodular or diffuse dermal (classically "top heavy") proliferation B cells, often with associated germinal centers containing tingible body macrophages. RB-LPs commonly exhibit reactive CD20+, PAX-5+, CD79a+ B cells with CD10+, Bcl-6+ and Bcl-2- germinal centers and polytypic plasma cells (**Figures 5.1, 5.2, 5.3, and 5.4**).[4] Mantle zones may be present or absent.[13] Other features highlighting the reactive nature of the follicles include normal (high) Ki-67 proliferative index of the germinal centers and associated polarization. CD21+, CD23+ follicular dendritic cell (FDC) meshworks should be encompassing germinal centers. Expression of CD20 and CD79a should be nearly equal in the reactive B cells, loss of CD79a may be suggestive of an aberrant B-cell phenotype seen in B-cell neoplasm.[14]

The main differential diagnosis of rB-LP includes low-grade B-cell lymphoma (see **Chapter 6**) (**Table 5.3**).[15,16] Overall, the presence of eosinophils and granulomas are in favor of CLH over a low-grade B-cell lymphoma. PCMZL is characterized by peri- and interfollicular proliferation of CD20+, CD79a+, Bcl-2+, Bcl-6-, CD5-, and CD10- marginal zone cells.[15,17,18] Commonly, aggregates of plasma cells seen at the periphery of the tumor exhibit kappa or lambda light chain restriction.[15,18] Light-chain restriction has diagnostic significance when the kappa to lambda ratios are >10:1 or <0.5:1.[19] CD21 often highlights a disrupted FDC meshwork due to the neoplastic marginal zone or plasmacytoid cells mixing with reactive follicular cells.[15] PCFCL characteristically appears as a nodular to diffuse lymphoid proliferation with CD20+, CD79a+, Bcl-6+, and Bcl-2- neoplastic follicle center B cells.[17]

Reactive B-cell rich lymphoid proliferations

- Reactive CD20+, CD79a+, CD10+ B cells and Bcl–6+ and Bcl–2- germinal centers with preserved CD21+, CD23+ FDC meshworks.
- A panel to exclude low-grade B-cell lymphoma would include CD3, CD20, Bcl–2, Bcl–6, CD21, kappa and lambda light chains.

Borrelia-Associated Reactive B-Cell Rich Lymphoid Proliferation

Borrelia infection is a common cause of B-cell pseudolymphoma (previously known as lymphadenosis cutis benigna) in endemic areas such as the Northeastern part of the United

Table 5.2 Flow chart of pseudolymphoma work-up

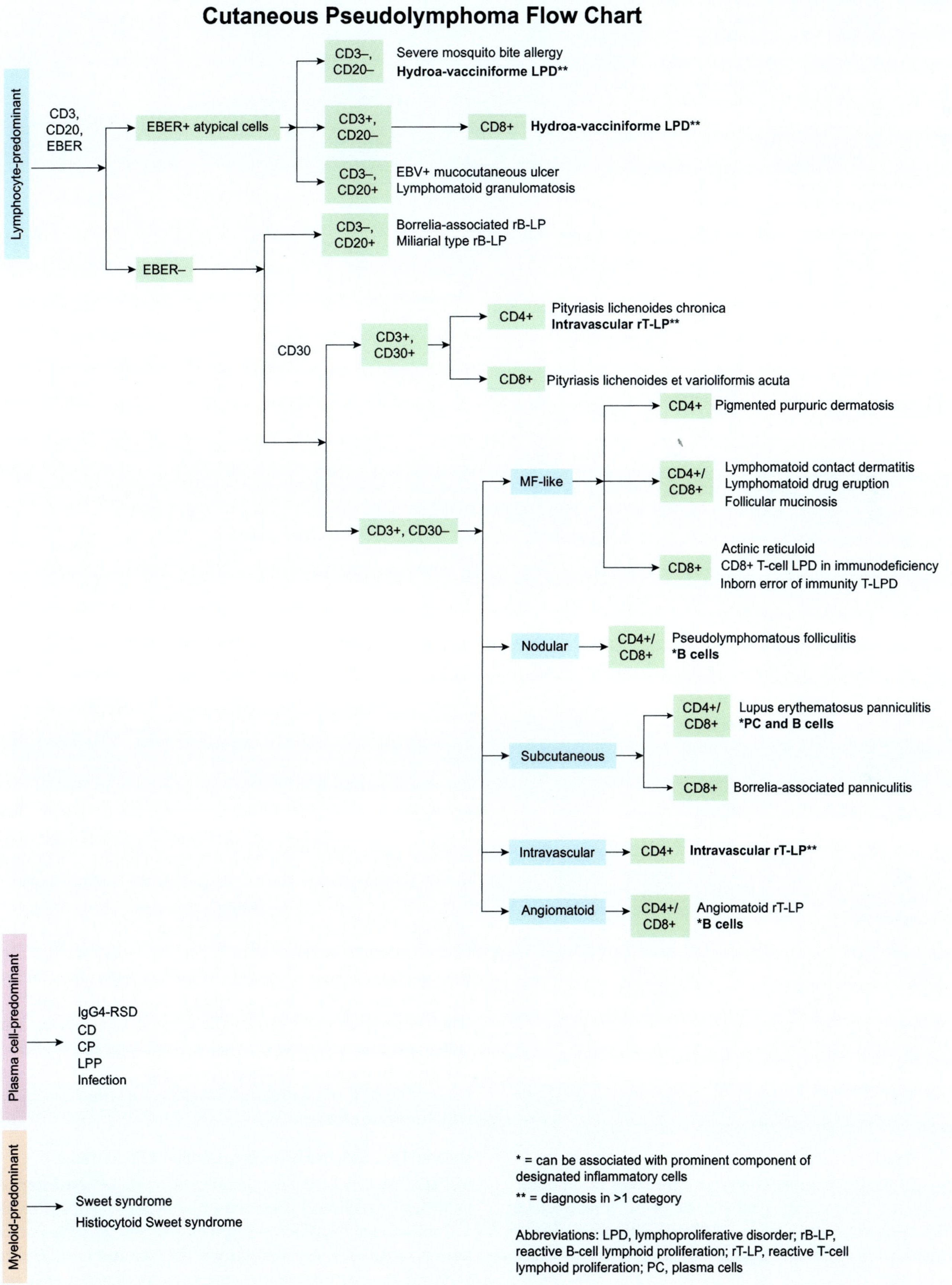

Table 5.3 Immunoprofile of reactive lymphoid hyperplasia versus low-grade B-cell lymphoma[15,16]

	Reactive lymphoid hyperplasia	Primary cutaneous marginal zone lymphoma	Primary cutaneous follicle center lymphoma
CD20	Germinal center +	+	+
Bcl–2	Mantle zone + Germinal center -	+	-/+
Bcl–6	Germinal center +	-	+
CD21	Intact follicular dendritic cell meshworks	Disrupted follicular dendritic cell meshworks	Expanded follicular dendritic cell meshworks
Kappa and lambda	Mixed expression	Light chain restriction	Light chain restriction

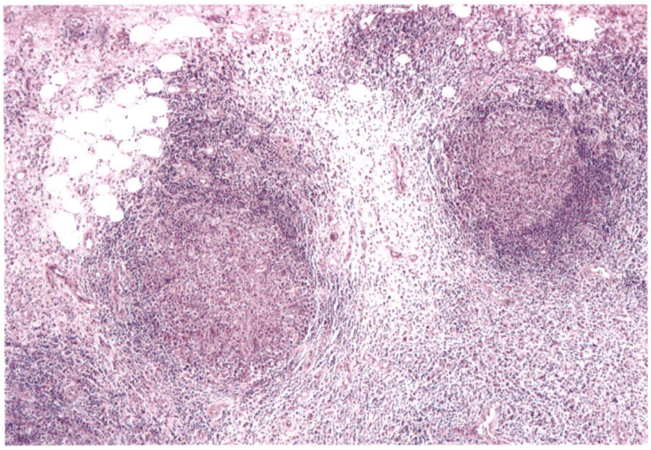

Figure 5.1 Prominent germinal centers are seen in this example of persistent arthropod bite reaction (X100).

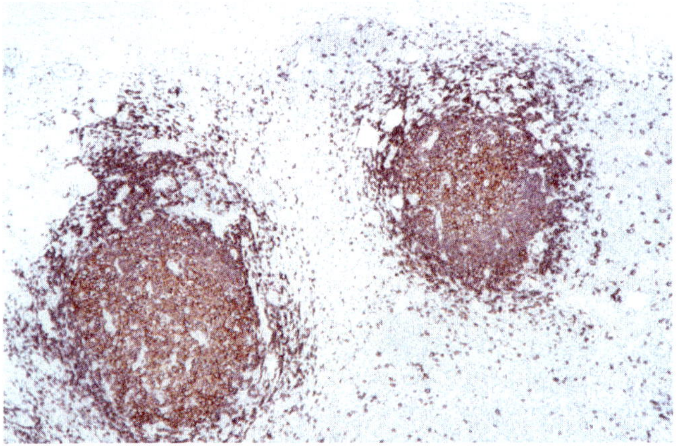

Figure 5.2 CD20 highlights the reactive germinal centers (X100).

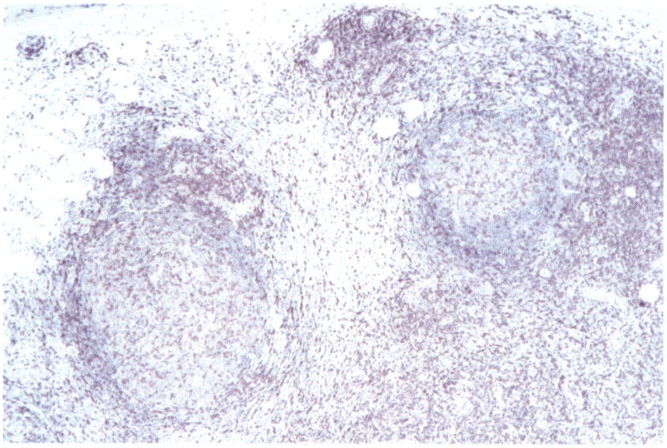

Figure 5.3 CD3 highlights the reactive T lymphocytes (X100).

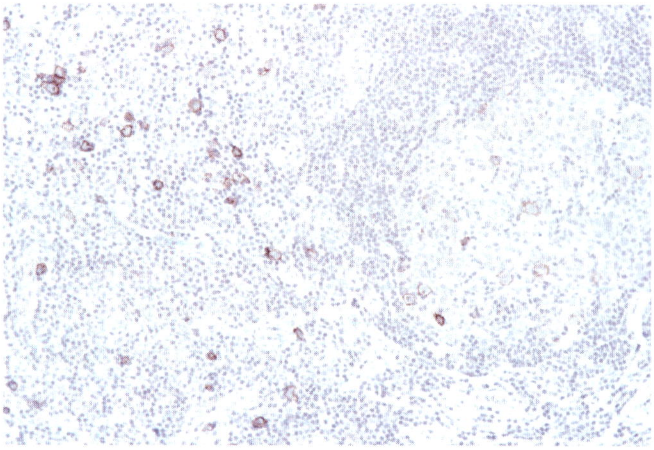

Figure 5.4 CD30 highlights occasional immunoblasts (X100).

States.[4] Clinically, it most commonly presents as a solitary lesion often on the nipple, genital area, or ear lobe weeks or months following transmission of the microorganism,[4,7] associated with erythema migrans in a minority of cases.[4] *B. burgdorferi* DNA is found in approximately 68% (54/80) of formalin-fixed paraffin embedded tissue samples, with one study demonstrating serologic positivity in 96% of cases tested (45/47).[4] In one study, immunoglobulin heavy chain (IgH) gene rearrangements showed polyclonal pattern in the majority of cases (31/33), with a monoclonal band in 2 cases (6%).[4] Histologically, classic presentations include a mixed inflammatory infiltrate including plasma cells and eosinophils associated with large confluent lymphoid follicles with polarized germinal centers containing tingible body macrophages. Interestingly, a lack of mantle zone has been described as characteristic of Borrelia-induced rB-LP at typical sites.[4] It is important to note that Borrelia infection can be associated with cutaneous B-cell lymphomas, but this is less often reported in North America in comparison to Europe.[20] There have also been cases of T-cell lymphoproliferative disorders associated with Borrelia infection.[12,21]

Miliarial Type Reactive B-Cell Rich Lymphoid Proliferation

Miliarial type rB-LP is a rare manifestation rB-LP characterized by its unusual clinical presentation of multiple asymptomatic, 1–2 millimeter, translucent-skin-colored papules with a predilection for the sun-exposed skin of the face and neck.[22,23] This variant has a predominantly superficial localization of B cells with nodular, folliculitis-like, and diffuse patterns described.[23]

It is important to differentiate this variant from miliarial follicle center lymphoma, which will demonstrate atypical lymphoid follicles with clonal IgH.[24]

5.2 Reactive T-Cell Rich Lymphoid Proliferations That Mimic T-Cell Lymphomas (rT-LPs)

Mycosis Fungoides-Like T-Cell Rich Lymphoid Proliferation (MF-like rT-LP)

Lymphomatoid Contact Dermatitis

Lymphomatoid contact dermatitis occurs in the setting of exposure to a contact allergen and clinically and histologically can resemble MF. Clinically, lymphomatoid contact dermatitis can exhibit the "bathing trunk" distribution commonly seen in early MF.[25] Pruritic, discrete or confluent, erythematous, scaly papules, and plaques are seen commonly at the site of contactant exposure.[7,26] Orbaneja and colleagues were the first to describe this entity and proposed four diagnostic criteria: 1) a localized eruption compatible with the clinical impression of contact dermatitis, 2) histologic features mimicking MF, 3) positive patch-test results, and 4) clinical response to avoidance of allergen and corticosteroids.[27] In a meta-analysis of 23 patients from 19 publications by Knackstedt and Zug, men are more commonly affected.[25] A variety of contact allergens, including rubber, dyes, metals, and preservatives, among others have been reported in the literature.[25,26]

The primary histologic finding is a superficial band-like infiltrate of T cells with exocytosis and some cytologic atypia, resembling MF.[7,12,26,27] Focal epidermal spongiosis and microvesiculation can help to distinguish lymphomatoid contact dermatitis from MF.[25] CD4+ or CD8+ T cells can predominate, with CD30+ lymphocytes being described.[12,25] Although the infiltrate is often comprised primarily of CD4+ T-cells, IHC can be helpful in highlighting the prominent infiltration of CD1a+ dendritic cells within the epidermis (**Figures 5.5, 5.6, 5.7, 5.8 and 5.9**).[28,29] Clonal T-cell populations have only rarely been described.[25,30]

Lymphomatoid contact dermatitis

- Epidermal spongiosis and microvesicles are seen in contrast to mycosis fungoides.
- Prominent CD1a+ dendritic cells within the epidermis.

Lymphomatoid Drug Eruption

Lymphomatoid drug reaction is a delayed-type hypersensitivity reaction that exhibits infiltration of the epidermis by lymphocytes mimicking MF.[31] It is most commonly caused by anticonvulsants, calcium-channel blockers, angiotensin-converting enzyme (ACE) inhibitors, antidepressants, and other drugs that alter lymphocyte function.[7,32] It has been more frequently observed in people with atopy or autoimmune disease.[32,33] It

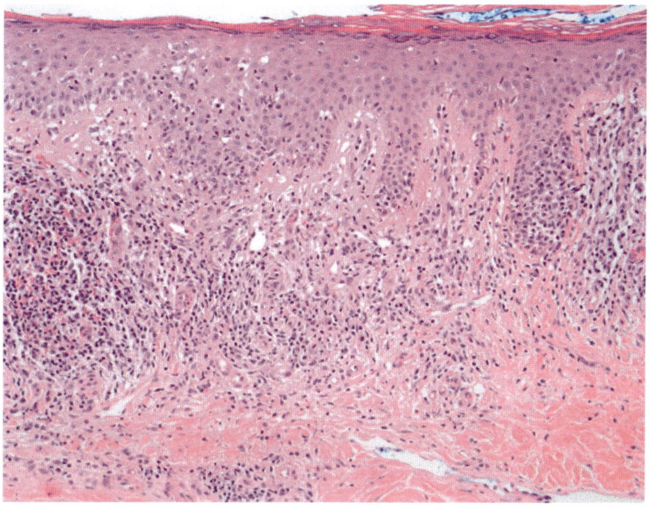

Figure 5.5 A dense and band-like inflammatory infiltrate is seen below a spongiotic epidermis (X200).

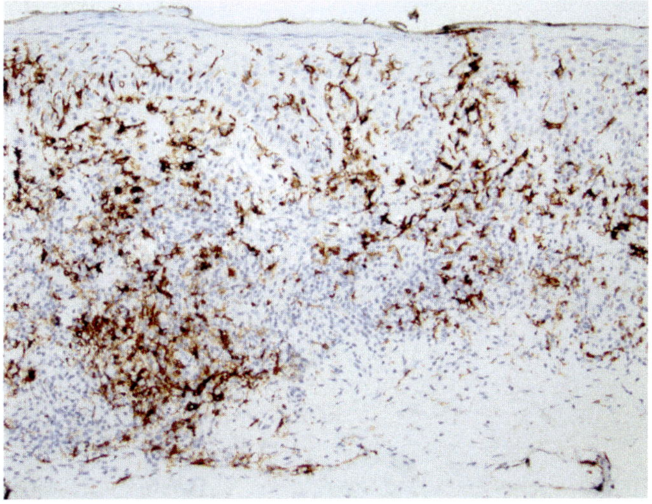

Figure 5.6 CD1a demonstrates prominent dendritic cells within the epidermis and in the dermal infiltrate (X200).

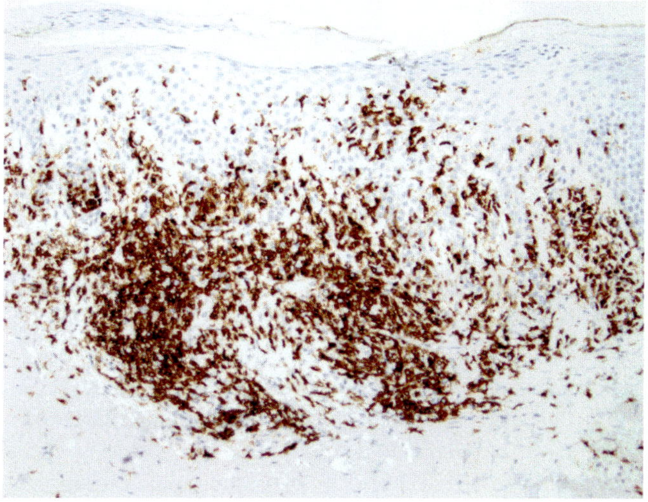

Figure 5.7 CD3 highlights the T lymphocytes with some being within the epidermis (X200).

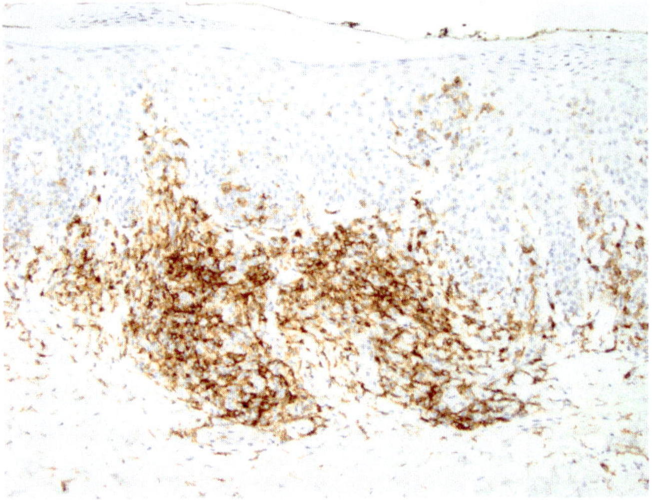

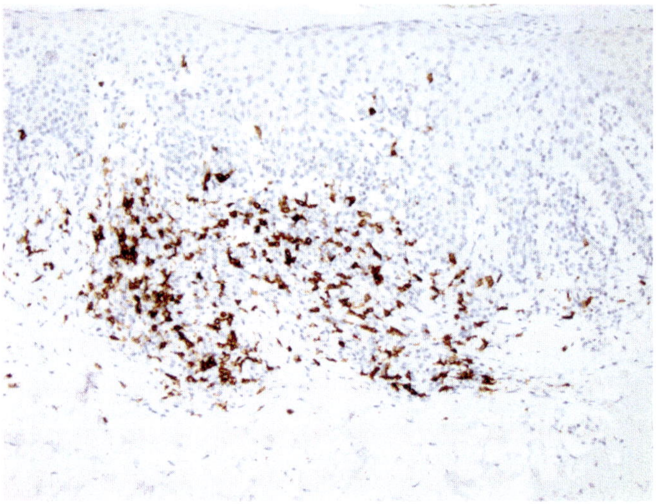

Figures 5.8 and 5.9 The majority of the intraepidermal lymphoid cells are negative for CD4 and CD8 (X200, X200).

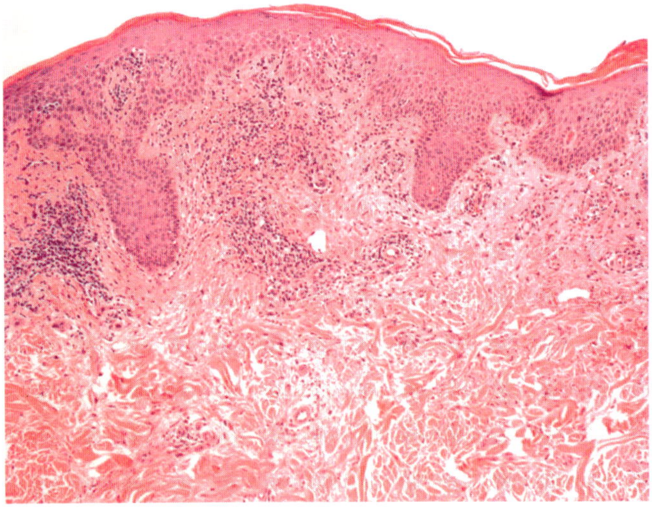

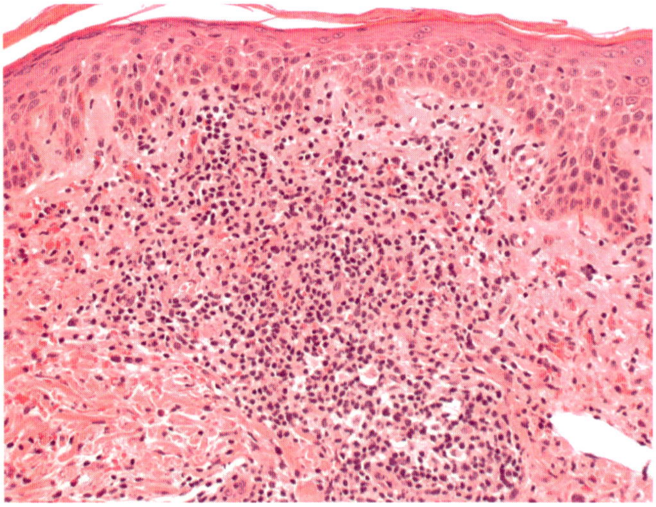

Figures 5.10 and 5.11 A patchy band-like infiltrate of lymphocytes with associated infiltration into the overlying epidermis is noted in the superficial dermis.

typically presents with a single lesion or photodistributed rash that develops within weeks to months of starting the medication and classically resolves with cessation of the drug.[26,32,33]

Histologically, there are two patterns of lymphomatoid drug eruption: 1) lymphocytoma cutis (dense nodular infiltrates resembling a low-grade T- or B-cell lymphoma) or 2) an infiltrate that resembles T-cell lymphoproliferative disease, particularly MF; however, mimickers of lymphomatoid papulosis (LyP), pityriasis lichenoides chronica (PLC), and pigmented purpuric dermatosis (PPD) have also been described.[26] Classic features of a delayed-type hypersensitivity reaction including vacuolar, interface, and/or spongiotic dermatitis with erythrocyte extravasation, keratinocyte necrosis, eosinophils, and only mild exocytosis into the epidermis are a helpful histologic clue for the diagnosis.[32,33] While less commonly present, decreased CD7 expression and even clonal TCR gene rearrangements have been observed in lymphomatoid drug eruption.[9,34] Striking loss of CD7, partial loss of CD2 or CD5, loss of multiple T-cell antigens, elevated CD4:CD8, and/or a low CD8:CD3 ratio can be helpful in favoring MF over a reactive inflammatory condition.[9,26,35,36] In MF, more CD4+ lymphoid cells are seen in the epidermis. On the contrary, more CD8+ lymphoid cells are seen in the epidermis in the setting of lymphomatoid drug reaction[26] (**Figures 5.10, 5.11, 5.12 and 5.13**). CD30+ immunoblasts comprising up to 30% of the dermal infiltrate or angiocentric transformed CD30+ lymphocytes have also been reported in lymphomatoid drug eruption.[26,33]

Lymphomatoid drug eruption

- CD8+ lymphoid cells are more prominent than CD4+ cells within the epidermis.
- Eosinophils are common.
- The combination of high grade cytologic atypia and high Ki-67 proliferation index would favor mycosis fungoides.

Follicular mucinosis

Follicular mucinosis (FM) can be primary/idiopathic or a secondary epiphenomenon in a variety of conditions such as

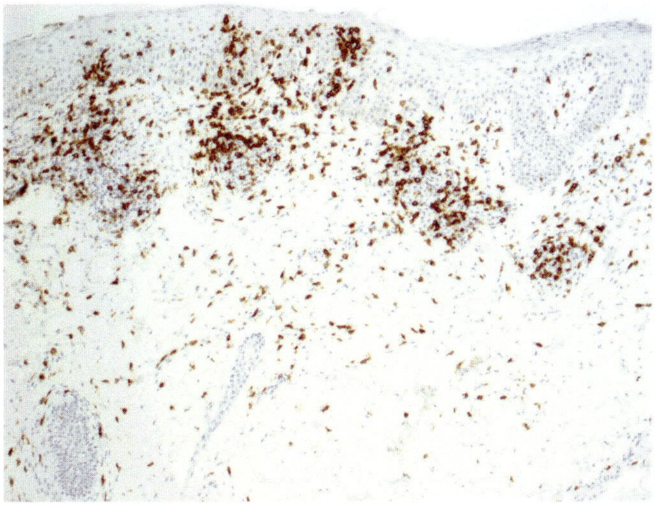

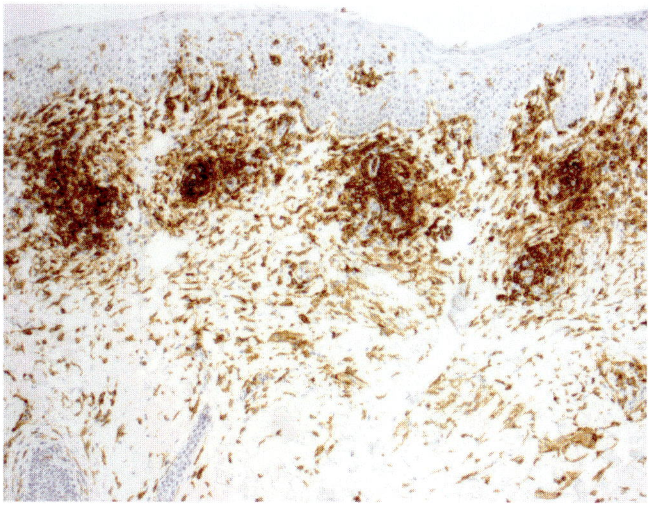

Figures 5.12 and 5.13 A greater number of intraepidermal lymphoid cells are CD8-positive in comparison to CD4 (X100, X100).

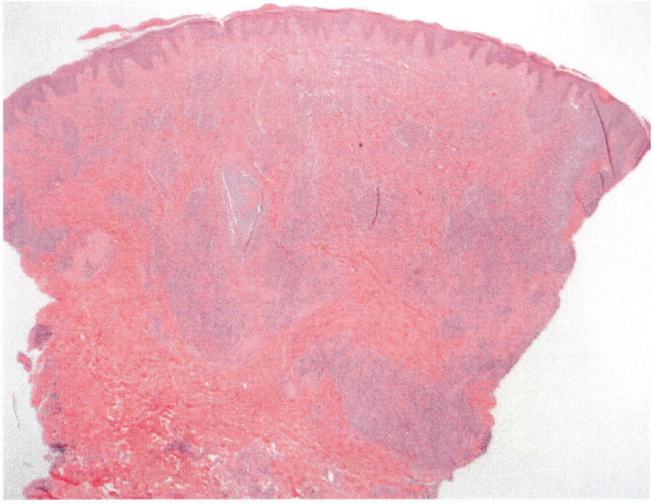

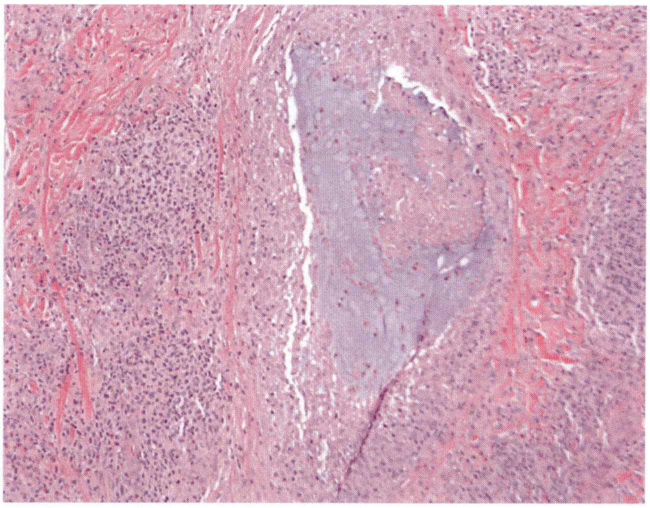

Figures 5.14 and 5.15 Lymphoma-associated follicular mucinosis. Prominent mucin deposition is noted within a hair follicle associated with dense lymphoid infiltrate (X20, X100).

arthropod bite reaction, lupus erythematosus, eosinophilic folliculitis, or, most importantly, folliculotropic MF and other lymphoproliferative disorders (see **Chapter 6**).[37–40] Typically, primary FM affects younger patients than folliculotropic MF and FM is typically localized as a single lesion on the head and neck that spontaneously regress, though some cases may remain persistent.[37,40] In some instances, follicular mucinosis may be the first presentation of folliculotropic MF.[37]

Histologically, FM is associated with dense folliculotropic lymphocytic infiltrate and large, cystic mucin-filled spaces. The lymphocytes usually lack significant atypia, there is no significant epidermotropism, and the infiltrate exhibits an equivalent CD4+:CD8+ ratio [40]. In comparison, cases of lymphoma-associated FM exhibit CD4+ predominance (CD4:CD8 ratio of at least 4:1) (**Figures 5.14, 5.15, 5.16, 5.17 and 5.18**) and often loss of pan-T-cell markers (e.g. CD2, CD5).[41] The typical immunoprofile of folliculotropic MF is similar to that of conventional MF: CD3+, CD4+, CD8-, CD45RO+, CD5+/-, CD7+/-,

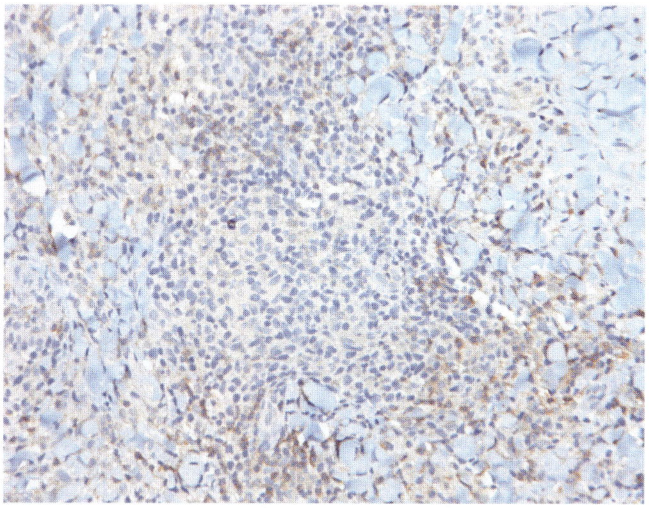

Figure 5.16 Loss of CD5 expression by T-lymphocytes is noted (X200).

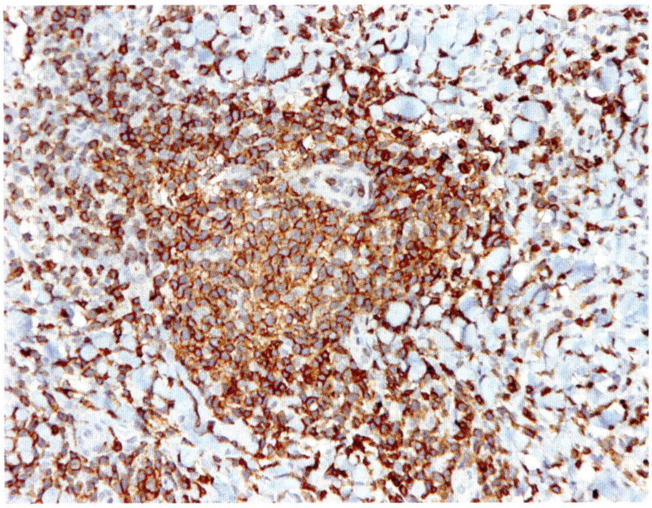

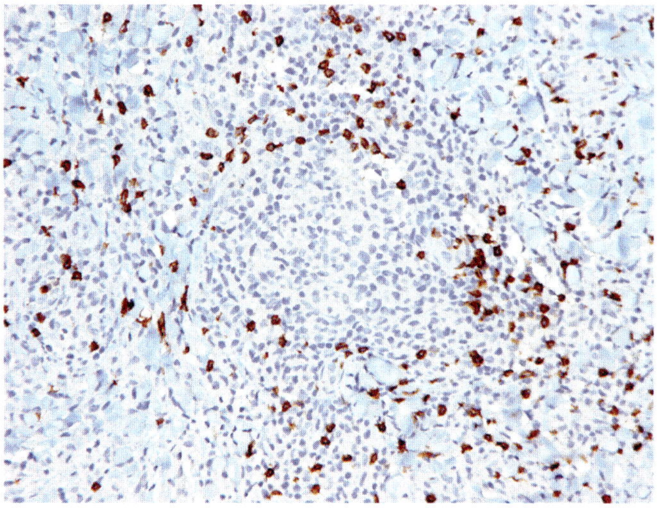

Figures 5.17 and 5.18 Lymphoma-associated follicular mucinosis. An elevated ratio of CD4 to CD8 T-lymphocytes of CD4 and CD8 T-lymphocytes is noted (X200, X200).

CD30-/+.[38,42,43] A recent study found that CD103 expression may be useful in distinguishing primary from lymphoma-associated FM.[44] The presence of clonal TCR gene rearrangement does not allow for definitive distinction between primary FM and lymphoma-associated FM since clonality has been reported in a subset of primary FM.[37,40,45] Ultimately, at this time there are no reliable clinical, histopathologic, or molecular markers to distinguish primary versus secondary FM, and the diagnosis requires careful clinicopathologic correlation and close patient follow-up.

Follicular mucinosis

- CD4:CD8 ratio is approximately 1:1 in primary follicular mucinosis, versus CD4+ predominant in mycosis fungoides-associated follicular mucinosis.
- Lymphocyte atypia is more conspicuous in mycosis fungoides-associated follicular mucinosis.

Pigmented Purpuric Dermatosis

Pigmented purpuric dermatosis (PPD) describes a group of cutaneous lesions most often confined to the lower extremities that display a purpuric clinical appearance due to the presence of extravasated erythrocytes. Histologic features can range from superficial perivascular to lichenoid dermatitis with associated red blood cell extravasation, hemosiderin deposition, and occasionally epidermal changes (e.g. spongiosis). PPD is commonly associated with venous stasis, autoimmune diseases, and/or medications. The primary differential diagnosis is PPD-like MF, with a small subset of PPD progressing to CTCL.[46]

IHC is not helpful in differentiating benign PPD from PPD-like MF, since the infiltrate is comprised predominantly of CD4+ T-cells.[46] However, the presence of dermal hemosiderin deposition seen with an iron stain can be helpful in distinguishing pigmented purpuric dermatosis from pigmented purpuric dermatosis-like MF. The detection of decreased expression of CD7 is of limited use, as it has been also described in benign PPD.[46] While PPD can also demonstrate clonal TCR, in one study, only cases with restricted TCR clonality progressed to MF.[46] Close follow-up is warranted particularly in individuals with clonal TCR and clinically widespread disease.[46] The presence of lesions outside the extremities (persistent and/or generalized) is clinically more supportive of MF.[47]

Actinic reticuloid

Actinic reticuloid (otherwise known as chronic actinic dermatitis) is characterized by a photosensitive rash composed of erythematous lichenified papules and plaques commonly in older men, mimicking MF in severe cases.[12,48] The skin lesions are intensely pruritic and can progress to erythroderma.[12] On biopsy, there is epidermal psoriasiform hyperplasia/acanthosis, spongiosis, compact orthokeratosis, and focal parakeratosis, with histologic features similar to atopic dermatitis.[12,48] Within the dermis, there is a superficial perivascular infiltrate composed of small, slightly atypical lymphocytes with focal exocytosis admixed with eosinophils, plasma cells, and Langerhans cells.[12,48] The lymphocytes are predominantly composed of CD8+ T-cells (low CD4:CD8) with polyclonal TCR, in contrast to conventional MF.[48] Prominent dermal dendritic cells and XIIIa and S100+ multinucleated giant cells can be seen.[48]

Actinic reticuloid

- In comparison to CTCL, more epidermal changes are seen, it is composed predominantly of CD8+ T cells, and TCR is polyclonal.

CD8+ T-Cell Pseudolymphoma in Immunodeficiency/Human Immunodeficiency Virus (HIV)-Related CD8+ Atypical Infiltrate

Development of CD8+ LPD have been described in the setting of acquired immunodeficiency. Most commonly, it has been described in the setting of human immunodeficiency virus infection (HIV), but there also have been reports of CD8+ LPD in transplant recipients.[12,49,50]

It is well-known that some patients with HIV infection develop polyclonal cutaneous infiltrates that histologically mimic MF, often associated with a late stage of HIV/AIDS.[51–53] Clinically, these patients can present with patches, plaques, nodules, or erythroderma, occasionally in a photodistributed pattern. Involvement of bone marrow and lymph nodes may be seen.[52] Histologically, there is a band-like, interface dermatitis composed of mildly atypical lymphocytes with focal exocytosis into the epidermis. The infiltrate can involve adnexal structures such as the hair follicles and eccrine glands, and eosinophils are often conspicuous.[52]

The infiltrate is predominantly composed of CD3+, CD8+, αβ+ T cells, unlike most dermatoses seen in HIV+ patients which are composed primarily of CD4+ T cells[51,52] (**Figures 5.19–5.22**). The lesional cells have been shown to be HIV-specific and express cytotoxic markers TIA-1 and granzyme-B.[6,54] CD30 is negative in the lesional cells.[50] Loss of CD7 expression has been described, although it is typically less pronounced than seen in MF.[51–53] TCR gene rearrangement studies are frequently polyclonal.[51,52]

CD8+ T-cell pseudolymphoma in immunodeficiency

- In contrast to typical mycosis fungoides, CD8+ T-cell pseudolymphoma in immunodeficiency is predominantly composed of CD8+ T cells with preserved pan-T cell markers and polyclonal TCR.

Inborn Error of Immunity-Associated Lymphoproliferative Disorders

The most recent version of the WHO Blue Book includes this category of diseases characterized by CD8-predominant T-cell LPD associated with inborn immunodeficiencies and not associated with EBV infection.[8,50] Granulomatous infiltrates have been described in patients with common variable immunodeficiency, severe combined immunodeficiency, ataxia-telangiectasia, Bruton X-linked agammaglobulinemia, IgA deficiency, and

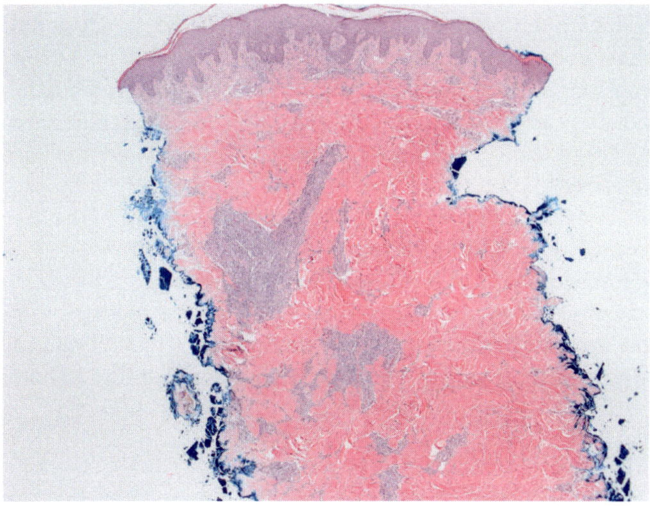
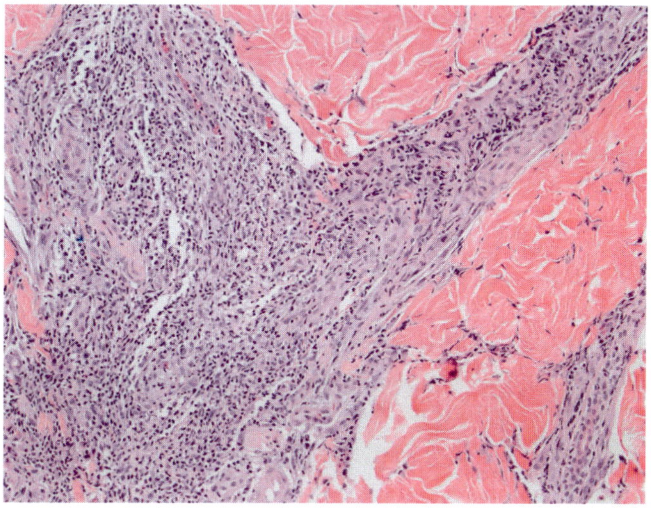

Figures 5.19 and 5.20 CD8+ dermatitis in the setting of HIV infection (X40, X200).

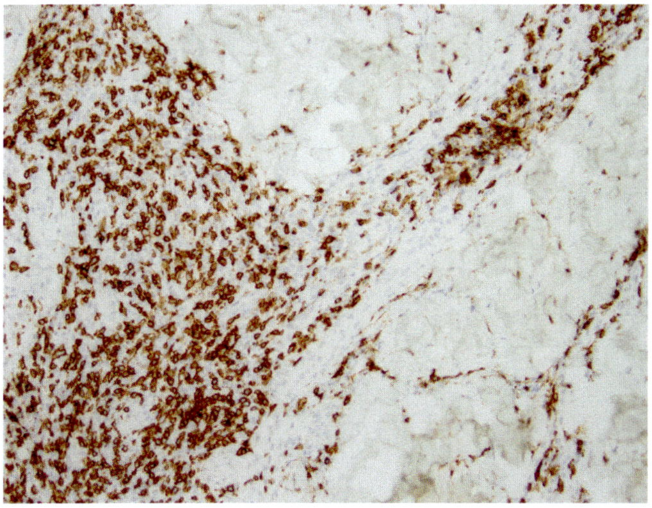
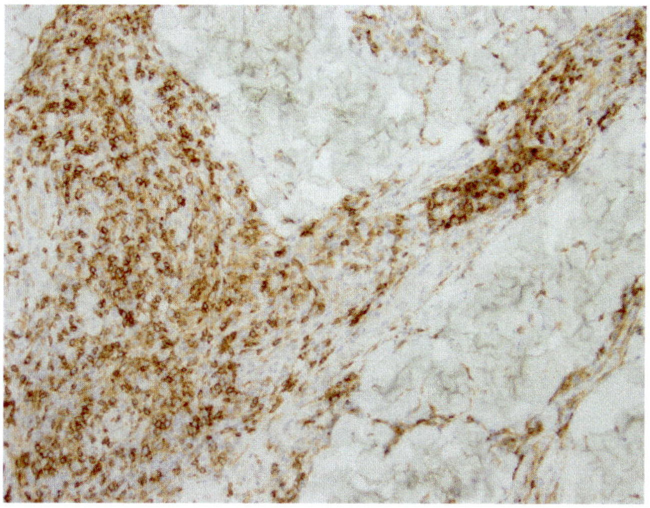

Figures 5.21 and 5.22 Prominent CD8+ lymphoid cells are seen (5.21) in comparison to CD4 (5.22) (X200, X200).

familial hemophagocytic lymphohistiocytosis.[50,55] Defective T-cell immune surveillance is implicated in the development of granulomatous reactions, which can lead to uncontrolled viral replication, classically in the case of Rubella virus.[8] Clinically, these cases present with a generalized erythematous-violaceous papulonodular rash.[55]

Histologically, this condition is characterized by a dermal-based proliferation of small–medium-sized mildly atypical CD8+ T cells with numerous admixed histiocytes and multinucleated giant cells forming small granulomas.[50] The T cells are positive for cytotoxic markers TIA-1 and granzyme-B, and negative for CD30.[50] EBER *in situ* hybridization (ISH) negativity is a requirement for the diagnosis.[8,50] The histiocytic infiltrate is CD68+, CD163+, CD1a-, and S100-.[8] TCR gene rearrangements have been observed.[50,55] Clinical course is variable, with some exhibiting a self-limiting course and others developing long-standing disease with low-grade malignant potential.[50] Due to the granulomatous nature of the infiltrate, infectious etiologies must be excluded in addition to other lymphoproliferative disorders such as granulomatous CD8+ MF (**Table 5.4**).

Inborn error of immunity-associated lymphoproliferative disorders

- Clinical context and numerous admixed histiocytes and granulomas can help differentiate from mycosis fungoides.

Nodular T-Cell Rich Lymphoid Proliferations (Nodular rT-LP)

Nodular rT-LP (otherwise known as nodular T-cell rich or mixed pseudolymphoma) has an indistinguishable clinical presentation from rB-LP (nodular B-cell pseudolymphomas) with solitary or multiple nodules.[12] Histologically, it presents as a dermal-based nodular or diffuse infiltrate of T cells often admixed with B cells, plasma cells, eosinophils, and histiocytes.[12] There can be focal exocytosis of T cells into the epidermis and predominant follicular involvement can be seen in some cases (see **Pseudolymphomatous folliculitis** section below). By IHC, the infiltrate is predominantly composed of CD3+, CD4+, CD8-, CD30- T-helper cells. CD20+ B cells should not exceed 30% of the infiltrate.[12] Variable numbers of medium-to-large CD4+ T cells with T-follicular helper (TFH) phenotype can be seen (PD-1, Bcl-6, CXCL13). There is significant overlap with primary cutaneous CD4-positive small or medium T-cell lymphoproliferative disorder (CD4+ PCSM-LPD), which has a characteristically benign clinical course, and some argue that rT-LP and CD4+ PCSM-LPD represent the same disease process.[12,57] While the absence of clonality can be supportive of rT-LP, it is not entirely specific.[8]

Pseudolymphomatous Folliculitis

Pseudolymphomatous folliculitis was first coined by McNutt and colleagues in 1986 then established as a pseudolymphoma variant by Arai and colleagues in 1999.[58,59] Clinically these lesions often present as solitary dome-shaped or flat nodule most commonly on the face, but scalp, neck or upper trunk can be affected.[59,61] Uncommonly, pseudolymphomatous folliculitis can present as multiple lesions.[62] Although it followed a benign clinical course, a rare case with recurrence has been reported.[60]

A dense and nodular lymphoid infiltrate is seen in the deep dermis surrounding enlarged or distorted hair follicles or pilosebaceous units (**see Case Study 1**). The presence of an activated or distorted pilosebaceous unit has been reported to be the most helpful histopathological feature.[61] The infiltrate can consist of a mixture of T and B cells, predominantly T cells, or

Table 5.4 Comparison of clinical histologic, and immunophenotypic features of cutaneous CD8+ predominant lymphoproliferative disorders[8,50,56]

	IEI-associated T-LPD	CD8+ LPD in acquired immunodeficiency	Primary cutaneous Acral CD8+ LPD	Primary cutaneous CD8+ PTCL, NOS	PAETCL	CD8+ Mycosis fungoides
Clinical	Papulonodular rash in setting of congenital immunodeficiency	Multiple papules/patches commonly in HIV, rarely in solid organ transplant	Non-ulcerated acral nodule	Ulcerated tumors	Ulcerated tumors	Non-erosive erythematous/ hypopigmented patches
Epidermotropism	-/+	-/+	-	-	++	++
Histopathology/ Immunophenotype	Small CD8+ T cells (+)TIA–1, granzyme Background histiocytic and granulomatous inflammation	Small CD8+ T cells (+)TIA–1, granzyme	Medium CD8+ T cells (+)TIA–1, CD68(dot-like) (-)granzyme, perforin	Medium-large CD8+ T cells (+)TIA–1 (+)granzyme, perforin (-)CD68	Medium-large CD8+ T cells (+)CD45RA (+)TIA–1 (+)granzyme, perforin (-)CD68 (-)CD2, CD5 (+/-)CD7	Medium-large atypical CD8+ T cells (-)CD45RA (-)CD2, CD5, CD7
Molecular studies	Typically polyclonal	Typically polyclonal	Typically clonal	Typically clonal	Typically clonal	Typically clonal

IEI-associated T-LPD: inborn error of immunity T-cell lymphoproliferative disease, LPD: lymphoproliferative disorder, PTCL, NOS: Peripheral T-cell lymphoma, not otherwise specified, PAETCL: PAETCL, Primary cutaneous CD8+ aggressive epidermotropic cytotoxic T-cell lymphoma predominantly B cells.[59] Plasma cells, eosinophils, and granulomas can be seen.[61] Marked CD1a+ and S100+ dendritic cell infiltration of hair follicles is characteristic.[14,59,63] An interstitial distribution of CD1a+ dendritic cells can also be seen.[64] However, subsequent study has not found the distribution of CD1a+ cells to be diagnostically helpful.[61] Goyal et al. also showed a significant increase in PD-1+ T-cells can be helpful in the differentiation from marginal cell lymphoma.[64] Although MF and lymphomatoid papulosis can involve the hair follicles, the absence of cytologic atypia and heterogeneous nature of the infiltrate are supportive of pseudolymphomatous folliculitis.[65] Others classify pseudolymphomatous folliculitis as a follicular manifestation of CD4+ PCSM-LPD.[12] This is supported by studies that have demonstrated that approximately 50% of cases have T-cell clonality.[63] IgH clonal rearrangements are less commonly reported.[63]

Pseudolymphomatous folliculitis

- Marked infiltration of hyperplastic follicular epithelium by CD1a+ and S100+ dendritic cells.
- Heterogeneous nature of the inflammatory infiltrate helps differentiate from CTCL.

CD30+ T-Cell Rich Lymphoid Proliferations (CD30+ rT-LP)

CD30+ rT-LP is characterized by a medium CD30+ lymphocytic infiltrate scattered or in small clusters.[8,66] The primary diagnoses of exclusion are lymphomatoid papulosis (LyP), anaplastic large-cell lymphoma (ALCL), and transformed MF. CD30+ rT-LP has been reported in association with a variety of medications (antiepileptics, antibiotics, anti-hypertensives, anti-depressants, antihistamines, gold acupuncture), infection-related inflammatory processes (HSV, VZV, molluscum, scabies), and non-infectious inflammatory processes such as PLEVA[33,66–68] (**Table 5.5**).

Pityriasis Lichenoides Chronica (PLC)/Pityriasis Lichenoides et Varioliformis Acuta (PLEVA)

Pityriasis lichenoides chronica (PLC) and pityriasis lichenoides et varioliformis acuta (PLEVA) represent two ends of a spectrum of the papulosquamous dermatoses known as pityriasis lichenoides, with PLEVA representing the acute phase and PLC representing the chronic phase of the disease.[69] PLC/PLEVA typically occur in children and young adults, with an uncertain etiology. Leading theories include an inflammatory response to infection, vaccination, medication, an immune-complex mediated hypersensitivity vasculitis or hypersensitivity reaction, or lymphoproliferative disorder.[69,70] PLC and PLEVA have overlapping clinical as well as histologic features. While both are characterized by a lichenoid interface dermatitis with lymphocyte exocytosis, dyskeratosis, acanthosis, parakeratosis, and perivascular, often wedge-shaped, inflammation with associated extravasated erythrocytes, PLEVA has a deeper and denser dermal infiltrate with associated epidermal ulceration (**Figure 5.23**).[70]

The infiltrate has been reported to be composed of either CD4+ or CD8+ T cells, with CD8+ T-cells predominating in PLEVA and CD4+ T-cells in PLC (**Figures 5.24, 5.25 and 5.26**).[71] Intraepithelial CD1a+ Langerhans cell collections can be seen.[71] Loss of CD5 or CD7 should not be considered alarming as it has been reported in a subset of these cases (**Figure 5.27**).[71] Large and CD30+ atypical cells can be seen within the infiltrate of PLEVA, mimicking LyP.[72] While PLEVA and LyP can have

Table 5.5 Comparison of CD30+ lymphoproliferative disorders[8]

	PLC/PLEVA	CD30+ rT-LP	LyP/ALCL
Clinical presentation	Papulosquamous rash that occurs in children and young adults	Drug-associated: Symptoms begin and resolve temporally with medication. Infection-associated: Symptoms resolve after treatment of infection.	LyP: Waxing and waning popular rash. ALCL: Typically single lesion with spontaneous regression
Helpful histologic features	Intraepithelial Langerhans cell collections can be seen	Drug-associated: – Eosinophils – Plasma cells – RBC extravasation – Apoptotic keratinocytes – Urticarial edema – Endothelial swelling Infection: Viral inclusions	LyP: Broad histopathologic appearance, often wedge-shaped all with medium-sized atypical cells in a polymorphous background. ALCL: Anaplastic large cells predominant
Immunophenotype	CD8+ or CD4+ with occasional small-medium CD30+ cells	CD30+ small-medium sized cells (rarely large) Scattered cells or small clusters	CD30+ atypical, large pleomorphic cells in clusters
Molecular studies	Clonal/non-clonal	Typically non-clonal Infection-associated: Viral DNA extracted from lesions	Often clonal

PLC: Pityriasis lichenoides chronica, PLEVA: pityriasis lichenoides et varioliformis acuta (PLEVA), rT-LP: T-cell rich lymphoid proliferation, LyP: lymphomatoid papulosis, ALCL: anaplastic large cell lymphoma

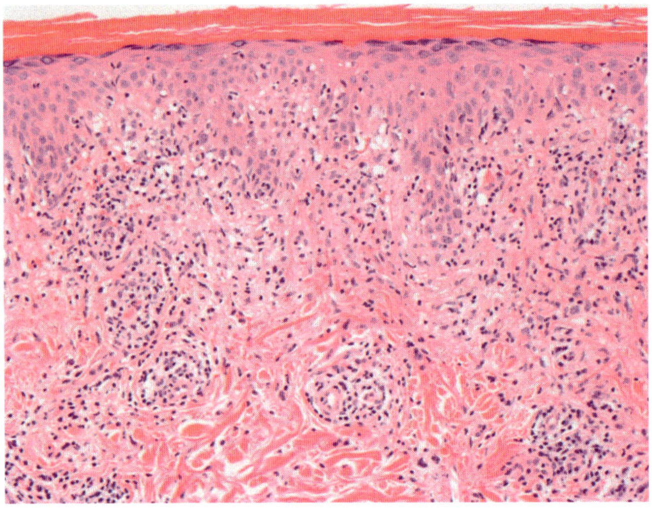

Figure 5.23 An interface and lichenoid dermatitis with associated extravasated erythrocytes is noted in this example of pityriasis lichenoides chronica.

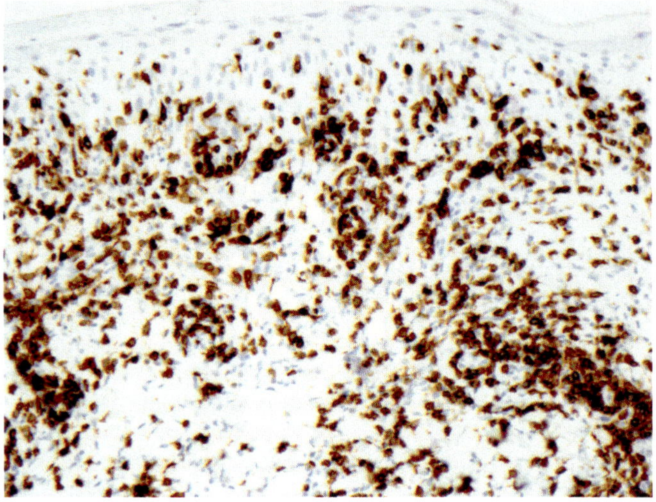

Figure 5.24 CD3 highlights the majority of the dermal infiltrate (X200).

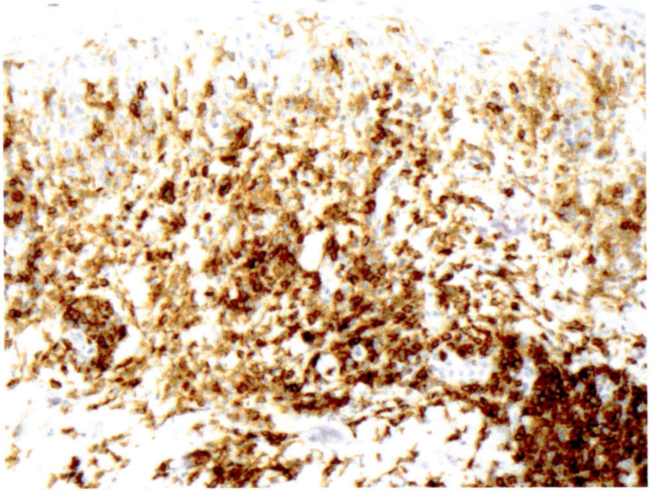

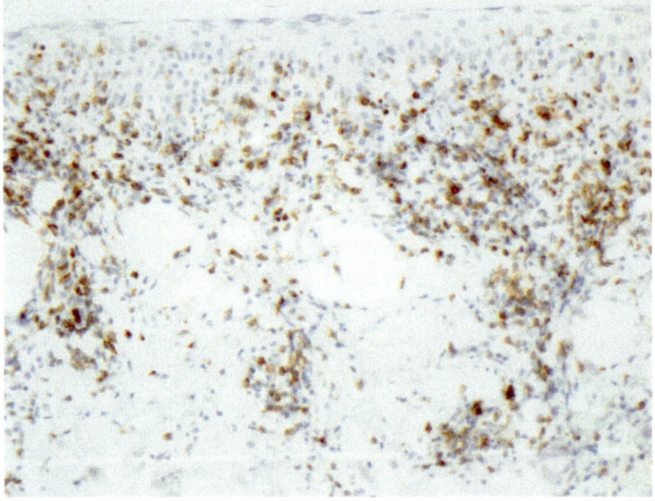

Figures 5.25 and 5.26 There appears to be more CD4- than CD8-positive T-lymphocytes within the infiltrate (X200, X200).

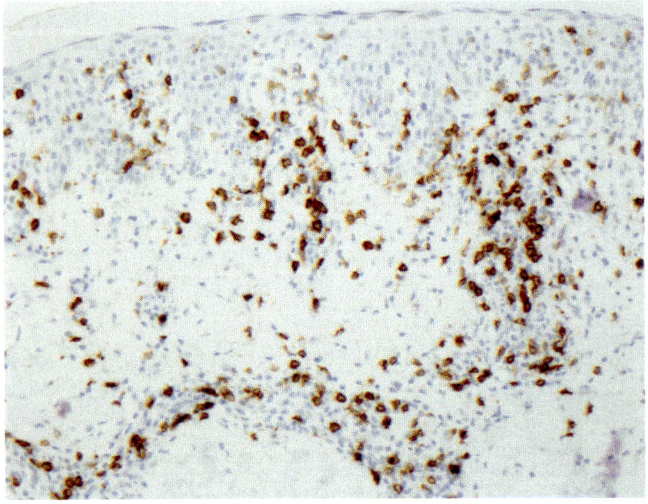

Figure 5.27 Focal loss of CD7 expression is noted (X200).

histologic overlap, PLEVA lacks the clinical waxing and waning course of LyP and the CD30+ cells are small to medium in size.[72] In addition, γδ T cells can be prominent in pityriasis lichenoides, raising the possibility of aggressive cutaneous γ/δ T-cell lymphoma.[73] Notably, clonal TCR rearrangements have also been described in pityriasis lichenoides.[71,72]

Pityriasis lichenoides chronica (PLC)/pityriasis lichenoides et varioliformis acuta (PLEVA)

- CD4+ or CD8+ lichenoid dermatitis with scattered, small-to-medium sized cells (often less conspicuous component and less atypical than the CD30+ cells of lymphomatoid papulosis).
- Wedge-shaped inflammation, extravasated erythrocytes, and epidermal changes can be helpful from differentiating from cutaneous T-cell lymphoma.

Subcutaneous T-Cell Rich Lymphoid Proliferation (Subcutaneous rT-LP)

Subcutaneous rT-LP display a dense pattern of lobular panniculitis composed of atypical small T lymphocytes. Examples include Borrelia infection and lupus erythematosus panniculitis.

Lupus Erythematosus Panniculitis

Lymphocytic lobular panniculitis (LEP) is a subcutaneous inflammatory disorder observed in a subset of patients with lupus erythematosus.[74,75] Epidermal and dermal changes of lupus erythematosus, such as vacuolar interface dermatitis and dermal mucinosis, are described in 50–75% of cases of LEP.[74,76] Characteristically, LEP displays prominent lobular lymphoplasmacytic panniculitis with germinal center formation and occasional lymphocytic rimming of adipocytes; lymphocytic nuclear dust and hyaline fat necrosis have also been described.[74,75] Therefore, it can mimic the subcutaneous lymphomas, including subcutaneous panniculitis-like T-cell lymphoma (SPTCL) and primary cutaneous γ/δ T-cell lymphoma (PCGD-TCL).[74,77]

The lymphoid infiltrate of lupus erythematosus panniculitis usually comprises a mixture of CD20+ B and CD3+, αβ T cells, although a minority of cases show exclusively T cell infiltrates.[75,76] While immunohistochemical studies often demonstrate a predominant CD4+ T-cell infiltrate,[75,76] others have shown a CD8+ T-cell predominance (**see Case Study 2**) (**Table 5.6**).[74] Diminished expression of CD7, CD3, and/or CD5 can be seen in LEP.[74] B-cell follicles and plasma cell clusters favor LEP over lymphoma, which can be highlighted by CD20 or CD138.[78] Aggregates of CD123+ plasmacytoid dendritic cells (pDC) comprising ≥20% of the infiltrate can also help differentiate LEP from lymphomas.[79] TCR-γ gene rearrangement studies are often polyclonal in most LEP cases, although a small minority of cases can exhibit a monoclonal TCR-γ gene rearrangement.[74,75]

Histologically, PCGD-TCL expresses a mature γδ T-cell phenotype: CD3+, CD4-, CD8-, βF1-, TIA-1+, perforin+, granzyme B+, and CD56+/-.[8,80,81] On the contrary, SPTCL expresses an αβ, cytotoxic T-cell phenotype: CD3+, CD4-, CD8+, βF1+, TIA-1+, perforin+, granzyme B+, and CD56-.[8,81] The presence of "Ki-67 hot spots," defined as aggregates of CD8+ subcutaneous lymphocytes with >30% Ki-67 staining, appears to be a reliable diagnostic clue to separate SPTCL from LEP.[78] Reports of cases showing histopathologic features of both LEP and SPTCL suggest that there may be a spectrum of disease between these two conditions.[74,82] TCR-γ gene rearrangement analysis has demonstrated clonality in the majority cases for both types of lymphoma.[80] A recent study by Manchan and colleagues found that LEP and SPTCL have distinct gene expression profiles and the molecular background of cases with histologic overlap between the two entities more closely resemble LEP.[83] The integration of clinical, histopathologic and immunohistochemical features, and molecular studies are essential in classifying these entities (**Table 5.7**).

Lupus erythematosus panniculitis

- A panel to exclude subcutaneous lymphoma would include CD3, CD4, CD8, CD20, CD56, granzyme B, TIA–1, Ki–67, BetaF1, and TCR γ.
- CD123+ plasmacytoid dendritic cell aggregates can help differentiate from lymphoma.
- Classic epidermal changes and dermal mucinosis favors lupus erythematosus panniculitis.

Borrelia-Associated Panniculitis

Panniculitis is a rare manifestation of Borreliosis.[88] In a case report by Kempf et al, there was a predominance of CD8+, TIA-1+, Beta F1+ T cells that lacked CD56 and CD30. Only occasional TCR γδ cells were present and scattered CD68+ histiocytes, CD138+ plasma cells, and CD123+ pDCs were seen in the background.[88] Similar to LEP, it is necessary to exclude subcutaneous panniculitis-like T-cell lymphoma (SPTCL) and primary cutaneous γ/δ T-cell lymphoma (PCGD-TCL) by using IHC and molecular methods to establish the polyclonal nature of the lesion. In some cases, *Borrelia sp.* DNA can be extracted from the cutaneous lesion by PCR.[88]

Table 5.6 Typical immunoprofile of lupus panniculitis versus subcutaneous lymphoma[76,77,84–87]

	Lupus panniculitis	Subcutaneous panniculitis-like T-cell lymphoma	Cutaneous γ/δ T-cell lymphoma
CD20	germinal centers +	–	–
CD3	+	+	+
CD4	+	frequently -	–
CD8	-/focally +	+	–
CD56	–	-	+
Granzyme B	–	+	+
TIA–1	-/focally +	+	+
CD123	clusters in superficial dermis and subcutis	single cells only	–
βF1	+	+	–
TCRγ	–	–	+

Table 5.7 Comparison of lupus erythematosus panniculitis from subcutaneous lymphomas[8,81]

	Lupus erythematosus panniculitis	SPTCL	PCGD-TCL
Histopathology	Lymphoplasmacytic lobular panniculitis with adipocyte rimming, often associated with: • Hyaline fat necrosis and lymphocytic nuclear dust • B cell follicles; aggregates of plasma cells and plasmacytoid dendritic cells Other features of lupus erythematosus can be seen. • Dermal mucinosis • Vacuolar interface dermatitis	Subcutaneous infiltrate of atypical lymphocytes with prominent rimming of adipocytes • +/- Hemophagocytosis	Proliferation of atypical lymphocytes in the epidermis, dermis, and subcutaneous tissues, with rimming of adipocytes
Immunophenotype	Predominantly CD3+, CD4+ αβ T cells CD20, CD138, and CD123 highlight admixed B cell follicles, plasma cells, and plasmacytoid dendritic cells, respectively.	CD3+, CD4-, CD8+, βF1+ T cells that express cytotoxic markers (TIA–1+, perforin+, granzyme B+) • CD56- "Ki–67 hotspots" of CD8+ lymphocytes rimming adipocytes are characteristic.	CD3+, CD4-, CD8-, βF1-, TCR-γ/TCR-δ+ T cells that express cytotoxic markers (TIA–1+, perforin+, granzyme B+) • CD56+/-
Molecular studies	Typically polyclonal	Typically clonal	Typically clonal

SPTCL: subcutaneous panniculitis-like T-cell lymphoma, PCGD-TCL: primary cutaneous γ/δ T-cell lymphoma

Intravascular T-Cell Rich Lymphoid Proliferation (Intravascular rT-LP)

Intravascular T-cell rich lymphoid proliferation (intravascular rT-LP) is a rare condition defined by large atypical blastoid cells in and around lymphatic vessels, often associated with a dense mixed inflammatory component.[8,89] This condition can raise concern for intravascular lymphoma, but it is benign and self-limiting. The etiology is uncertain, but there appears to be a disruption in immune trafficking, and it has been reported to be associated with trauma, benign cutaneous vascular lesions, oral and cutaneous ulcers, ulcerated lichen sclerosus, hidradenitis suppurativa, and drug rash with eosinophilia and systemic symptoms (DRESS).[89–97]

The atypical cells are CD2+, CD3+, CD4+ T cells and they are typically negative for CD56.[94] CD7 can be diminished but pan-T cell markers should overall demonstrate preserved expression.[89,94] They are often CD30+, but CD30- cases have been reported.[91,94] A subset of cases has been described as having an activated T-regulatory phenotype (CD45RO+, CD25+, FOXP3+, MUM-1/IRF4+),[91,97] possibly responding to an inflammatory trigger.[89] Some studies have shown that the intravascular T cells can be highlighted by Ki67 and CCR7 (chemokine involved in T-cell homing), implying local activation and migration to lymph nodes.[91] These proliferations are typically polyclonal by TCR.[89,94]

The primary differential diagnosis is intravascular lymphoma (IVL), which often portends poor prognosis (**Table 5.8**). Most cases of IVL represent a form of diffuse large B-cell lymphoma, but there have been reports of rare T-cell intravascular lymphomas, NK-cell intravascular lymphomas (EBER+), intralymphatic ALCL, and even angioinvasive LyP (type E).[94] Notably, the aggressive lymphomas, in addition to LyP type E, largely involve blood vasculature rather than lymphatics.[93] D2-40 may be helpful in highlighting the lymphatic spaces and an inflammatory background may be suggestive of intravascular rT-LP.[89] Kempf et al. and Calamaro and Cerroni both proposed histopathologic criteria for the diagnosis of intravascular rT-LP: 1) presence of a background inflammatory skin disorder, trauma, and/or ulceration 2) clusters of medium-to-large T lymphocytes within D2-40+ lymphatics, often CD30+, 3) lack of aberrant T-cell phenotype (except CD7) and absence of EBV, 4) no evidence of cutaneous or systemic lymphoma, and 5) indolent course with regression of ulceration or inflammation.[89,94]

Intravascular T-cell rich lymphoid proliferation

- Pan-T-cell markers, CD20, CD4, CD8, CD56, CD30, and EBER ISH can be useful in differentiating intravascular rT-LP from intravascular lymphomas.
- D2–40 can be useful in highlighting the intra-lymphatic nature of the atypical cells.

Angiomatoid T-Cell Rich Lymphoid Proliferation (Angiomatoid rT-LP)

Angiomatoid rT-LP is characterized by a benign nodular lymphocytic infiltrate admixed a proliferation of small vessels, also known as acral pseudolymphomatous angiokeratoma.[12] The etiology is unclear, possibly related to a persistent arthropod bite reaction or a benign vascular process.[12] Clinically, the first description of this spectrum of lesions was of multiple erythematous-violaceous keratotic papules at acral sites in children, otherwise known as acral pseudolymphomatous angiokeratoma of children (APACHE).[98] However, more recently, there have been other presentations described, including solitary nodules and plaques, lesions in non-acral sites, and similar

Table 5.8 Comparison of intralymphatic/intravascular lymphoid proliferations[8,89,94]

	Intravascular T-cell rich lymphoid proliferation	Lymphomatoid papulosis type E	Intralymphatic anaplastic large cell lymphoma	NK/T-cell intravascular lymphoma	Intravascular B-cell lymphoma
Clinical features	Often associated with inflammatory skin disorder	Waxing and waning ulcerative lesions	Lack of associated inflammatory skin disorder	Large indurated area	Large indurated area
Histologic features	Atypical cells predominantly within lymphatics; Scattered inflammation outside of lymphatics	Destruction of vessel walls with associated hemorrhage; Associated with inflammatory infiltrate outside vessels	Atypical cells predominantly within lymphatics; No extra-lymphatic inflammation	Atypical cells confined to blood vessels; Lack of inflammation outside vessels	Atypical cells confined to blood vessels; Lack of inflammation outside vessels
Immunophenotype	CD2+, CD3+, CD4+, CD5+ CD7+/- EBER+/- D2–40+ lymphatic spaces	CD30+ CD8+ TIA–1+, SATB1+	CD30+ ALK–1-, EMA- D2–40+ lymphatic spaces	CD2+, CD3+/-, CD8+, CD56+/- EBER+ CD30-	CD20+, CD79a+ MUM1+/-, CD5+/-, PD-L1+/-
Molecular studies	Typically polyclonal	Variable	Typically clonal	Typically clonal	Typically clonal

presentations in adults.[99] The lesions commonly occur on the head and neck and trunk, often clinically mimicking pyogenic granulomas.[99]

Histologically, there is a dense dermal-based polypoid proliferation of mildly atypical T lymphocytes with admixed histiocytes and plasma cells associated with prominent vessels lined by plump endothelial cells.[99] Occasionally, an epidermal collarette, Grenz zone, or eosinophils can be seen.[99] The lymphocytic infiltrate is composed of admixed CD4+ and CD8+ T cells, with cases of APACHE having admixed CD20+ B cells.[99] The majority of cases are polyclonal.[99] Scattered CD30+ cells may be seen.[99]

Angiolymphoid hyperplasia with eosinophilia (ALHE) also is characterized by a prominent dermal proliferation of bizarre-shaped vessels with plump endothelial cells with characteristic cytoplasmic vacuoles, possibly arising in response to tissue damage.[12] Clinically, it most commonly presents as a red-brown papulonodular eruption on the head and neck.[12] The vascular proliferation is CD31+, ERG+ and negative for the lymphatic marker D2-40. There is an associated dense infiltrate of predominantly CD3+ T lymphocytes and admixed CD20+ B cells forming follicles with reactive germinal centers.[12] Eosinophils and plasma cells can be present. Clonal TCR have been reported.[12]

5.3 Reactive Plasma-Cell Rich Lymphoid Proliferations

Benign cutaneous reactive infiltrates with numerous plasma cells can occasionally mimic plasma cell neoplasms or plasma-cell rich lymphomas. Importantly, with any plasma-cell rich proliferation, infectious causes must be excluded (**Table 5.9**).

IgG4-Related Disease in the Skin

IgG4-related disease (IgG4-RD) is a systemic syndrome characterized by mass-forming fibroinflammatory lesions with lymphoplasmacytic infiltration, tissue fibrosis, increased number of IgG4-positive plasma cells, and elevated serum IgG4 levels.[101] The disease can involve either one or more of the following organs: lacrimal gland, salivary gland, lymph node, breast, mediastinum, soft tissue, retroperitoneum, pancreas, hepatobiliary tree, prostate, lung, kidney, and central nervous system.[101]

Three major histologic features associated with IgG4-related disease include: 1) dense lymphoplasmacytic infiltrate, 2) fibrosis being focally storiform-type, and 3) obliterative phlebitis.[102] A consensus statement proposed that the diagnosis of IgG4-related disease be based primarily on morphology, and that tissue IgG4 cell counts and IgG4/IgG ratios are of secondary importance. IgG4+ cell counts for different organs have been proposed to account for varied levels of fibrosis and cellularity, with the proposed the IgG4 density should be above 200 cells per high power field for cutaneous biopsies.[102] An IgG4/IgG ratio exceeding 0.40 is considered supportive of IgG4-related disease in all organs;[102] however, an elevated ratio is not diagnostic. The IgG4/IgG ratio has been shown by meta-analysis to be effective in diagnosing IgG-related disease.[103]

IgG4-RD involving the skin is exceedingly rare.[104–108] It typically is associated with extracutaneous disease, but skin-limited disease has been documented and may precede development of systemic disease.[108] Tokura and colleagues categorized the skin lesions of IgG4-RD into seven subtypes: 1) cutaneous plasmacytosis, 2) pseudolymphoma and angiolymphoid hyperplasia with eosinophilia, 3) Mikulicz disease, 4) psoriasis-like eruption, 5) unspecified maculopapular or erythematous eruptions, 6) hypergammaglobulinemia purpura and urticarial vasculitis, and 7) ischemic digit.[107] They further categorized types 1–3 as primary lesions caused by direct infiltration of IgG4+ plasma cells forming plaques, nodules, or tumors with direct infiltration of IgG4+ plasma cells and secondary non-specific lesions (types 4–7).[107] Sato and colleagues reported a series of 10 patients that presented with erythematous plaques or subcutaneous pseudolymphomas on the head and neck.[104] In addition to prominent, mass-forming polyclonal plasma cells admixed with CD3+ T lymphocytes and CD20+ B lymphocytes forming germinal centers, eosinophils were readily identified.[104,107]

Table 5.9 Differential diagnosis of cutaneous plasma cell-rich proliferations[8,12,100]

	Infection	IgG4-related skin disease	Cutaneous Castleman disease	Cutaneous plasmacytosis	Lymphoplasmacytic plaque	Primary cutaneous marginal zone lymphoma
Epidemiology	N/A	N/A	N/A	Typically adults	Typically children	Typically adults
Clinical	Variable	Often associated with systemic IgG–4 RD	Multiple erythematous nodules	Multiple plaques +/- systemic symptoms	Solitary plaque or linear	Non-ulcerated plaques/nodules
Histology	Dermal-based lymphoplasmacytic inflammation	Lymphoplasmacytic inflammation with GC formation, storiform fibrosis and obliterative phlebitis +/- eosinophils	Lymphoplasmacytic inflammation with regressed GC, hyalinized vessels	Perivascular dermal inflammation	Lichenoid interface or deep inflammation	Dense dermal lymphoplasmacytic infiltrate with follicles with reactive germinal centers, with peripheral accentuation of plasma cells
Clonality	Polyclonal plasma cells	Polyclonal plasma cells	Polyclonal plasma cells	Polyclonal plasma cells	Polyclonal plasma cells	Clonal plasma cells
Additional studies	Infection-specific special studies/ cultures	IgG4 >200/high power field IgG4/IgG >0.40	IgG4 <200/high power field IgG4/IgG >0.40	N/A	N/A	Neoplastic B cells Bcl–2 positive; variable IgG4

N/A: not available

Caution should be taken when interpreting increased numbers of IgG4+ plasma cells in skin biopsies. The presence of an elevated number of IgG4+ plasma cells in cases of Zoon balanitis and a variety of inflammatory cutaneous lesions has been observed.[109,110] In a recent study by Skopec and colleagues studying IgG4 levels in cutaneous disorders with prominent lymphoplasmacytic infiltrates, none of these IgG4-RD mimics demonstrated ≥200 IgG4+/HPF, but a subset demonstrated an IgG4/IgG ratio of >0.4 and/or a mean IgG4+ count of >10/HPF, particularly autoimmune blistering diseases.[108] Therefore, characteristic histopathologic features of IgG4-RD need to be seen before further screening with IHC.[108]

IgG4-related skin disease

- IgG4 density should be above 200 cells per high power field for a cutaneous biopsy.
- An IgG4/IgG ratio exceeding 0.40 is considered supportive of IgG4-related disease.

Cutaneous Castleman's Disease

Castleman's disease (CD) is an uncommon lymphoproliferative disorder that is characterized by lymphadenopathy, systemic symptoms, laboratory abnormalities, and rare involvement of extranodal sites including the skin.[111] It clinically presents as a multinodular erythematous rash.[112] There are three histologic variants, including hyaline-vascular type, plasma cell type, or mixed type. It can be associated with HIV or idiopathic, with dysregulation of IL-6 and/or HHV-8 playing an important role in the pathogenesis of the disease.[111] Biopsy reveals a multinodular dermal infiltrate of lymphocytes forming follicles with regressed germinal centers and distinct mantle zones, often penetrated by hyalinized vessels.[112] In contrast, IgG4-RSD often has normal-appearing germinal centers often with associated eosinophils.[112] Plasma cells are prominent in the interfollicular zones, many of which are IgG4+. The IgG/IgG4 ratio can be >0.40; however, cutaneous CD does not have >200 IgG4 plasma cells/HPF in comparison to IgG4-RSD.[112] There is no light chain restriction and immunoglobulin heavy-chain rearrangements are not seen.[112]

Cutaneous Plasmacytosis

Cutaneous plasmacytosis is a rare disorder characterized by multiple red-brown cutaneous nodules primarily involving the trunk of adults, predominantly in people of Asian descent.[12,113] Systemic involvement has been described.[12] Biopsy of the lesions demonstrates a perivascular dermal infiltrate of mature plasma cells and B lymphocytes, with admixed mast cells seen by chloroacetate esterase.[113] Associated findings include increased dermal vascularity, epidermal hyperplasia, and an increase in basal layer melanin pigmentation.[113] The plasma cells are polytypic for kappa and lambda and the B-cell infiltrate is polyclonal by IgH rearrangement studies.[113]

Lymphoplasmacytic Plaque

Lymphoplasmacytic plaque is a recently described rare disorder characterized by a longstanding plaque or well-circumscribed linear red-brown papules and plaques of uncertain etiology, often in children with a predilection for the lower leg.[12,100] Histologically, there is a lichenoid to deep nodular lymphoplasmacytic infiltrate in a peri-adnexal and peri-vascular distribution.[12] Interface dermatitis and acanthosis are prominent in cases with a lichenoid inflammation pattern.[100]

Associated histiocytic inflammation highlighted by CD163 may aggregate to granulomas around "free floating" sclerotic collagen bundles ("pseudorosettes").[100] Prominent CD31+ vascularity can be seen, possibly representing a spectrum of angiomatoid rT-LP.[12] Plasma cells are polyclonal for kappa and lambda.[100] IgG4 expression has been described in 5–30% of the plasma cells, lower than that typically seen in IgG4 related disease.[100]

Infection-Associated Plasma Cell Proliferations

Various infections can induce a pseudolymphomatous lymphocyte-rich infiltrate, often with numerous admixed polytypic CD138+ plasma cells, including cutaneous leishmaniasis, syphilis, mycobacterial, and fungal infections.[12] Borrelia-associated reactive B-cell rich lymphoid proliferations also can have prominent plasma cell proliferations (see above section). Various stains (PAS, GMS, AFB, microbe-specific IHC), tissue-based PCR, and/or correlation with microbiology studies is critical for diagnosis of these cases.

5.4 EBV-Positive Lymphoproliferative Diseases

EBV-Positive Lymphoproliferative Diseases of Childhood

Both severe mosquito bite allergy and hydroa vacciniforme lymphoproliferative disorder (LPD) are cutaneous forms of chronic active Epstein-Barr virus (EBV) infection caused by the persistent presence of EBV-infected cytotoxic NK or T cells that are recruited cutaneously due to sun exposure or mosquito bite stimuli and create tissue damage, with additional genetic, immunologic, and/or environmental events leading to a subset with a more aggressive clinical course.[114] Both predominantly affect children and adolescents in East Asia and Latin America.[115]

Severe Mosquito Bite Allergy

Severe mosquito bite allergy is a rare, transient, EBV-associated natural killer (NK) cell LPD, most often occurring in children, most prevalent in East Asia and Latin America.[116,117] It presents as a blister or bullae at the site of mosquito bite that subsequently ulcerates and scars, in addition to systemic symptoms such as fever, lymphadenopathy, and hepatosplenomegaly.[116] The symptoms typically resolve after several weeks, until a subsequent mosquito bite.[116] It is thought to be induced by local CD4+ T-cell activation triggered at the site of mosquito bite that induces EBV reactivation and proliferation of EBV-infected NK cells.[116,118] While typically transient, due to its association with EBV, it may progress to chronic active EBV disease, hemophagocytic lymphohistiocytosis (HLH), or EBV-associated malignancies such as aggressive NK-cell leukemia and extranodal NK/T-cell lymphoma.[116]

On histopathology, there is a dense perivascular infiltration of small to focally large atypical lymphocytic inflammation. The epidermis may show intraepidermal bullae acutely that subsequently becomes necrotic and ulcerated in the recovery phase.[116] The majority of the infiltrate is composed of surface CD3-, CD56+, TIA-1+, granzyme-B+, NK cells positive by EBER *in situ* hybridization and admixed CD68+ histiocytes.[8,116,119] Few, admixed CD4+ and CD8+ T cells and CD20+ B cells can be seen.[119] Clonal expansion of NK cells has been demonstrated by monoclonal or oligoclonal DNA in infected cells.[116,117,120] Interestingly, monoclonal expansion can be seen in progression towards malignancy.[116,120]

Severe mosquito bite allergy

- In a classic presentation, a panel of CD3, CD56, TIA–1, granzyme-B, and EBER can assist in the diagnosis.

Hydroa Vacciniforme Lymphoproliferative Disorder

Hydroa vacciniforme lymphoproliferative disorder (HV-LPD) is a rare EBV-mediated T-cell or NK-cell LPD that carries a risk of progression to lymphoma, with classic and systemic subtypes.[8] Similar to severe mosquito bite allergy, it is more common in the pediatric population, with most cases reported in East Asia and Latin America.[121] Clinically, it is characterized by a papulovesicular photodermatosis leading to ulceration and scarring, with seasonal recurrences in the spring and summer.[115] In classic hydroa vacciniforme, the photodermatosis remits after adolescence; however, it was subsequently discovered that there was an association between HV-LPD and clonal T-cell proliferations and progression to lymphoma or more aggressive systemic disease such as hemophagocytic syndrome (HLH), particularly in patients of Eastern Asian and Latin American descent.[121–123] Due to the inability to predict which cases will behave in an indolent or malignant manner, the term HV-LPD has been adopted in the most recent versions of the WHO Blue Book.[8]

Biopsy of the cutaneous lesions demonstrates a small–medium perivascular and periadnexal lymphocytic infiltrate associated with epidermal vesiculation and necrosis. Additional epidermal changes ("reticulated epidermal degeneration"), such as spongiosis and exocytosis can be seen.[124] Angiodestruction and involvement of the subcutis may be prominent in severe cases and can histologically mimic subcutaneous panniculitis-like T-cell lymphoma.[123,124] The culprit cells are typically cytotoxic T-cells (CD3+, CD45RO+, CD8+, TIA-1+, granzyme-B+, perforin+) or, less commonly, NK cells (CD56+, surface CD3-, surface TCR-), with variable expression of CD5, CD7, CD43, and CD25.[122,124] CD20+ B cells, reactive CD4+ T cells, and eosinophils can be scattered within the cytotoxic T-cell infiltrate.[123] EBER ISH highlights a subset of the infiltrate, with only a limited number of cells staining positively for LMP-1.[123] There is no correlation between number of EBER+ cells and severity of disease, the severity does not differ among T- or NK-cell phenotypes.[123,124] CD30 staining is variably seen, more frequently in the NK-cell phenotype.[123] T cells can be αβ or γδ.[122,123] Clonal TCR rearrangements are observed in cases of the T-cell phenotype.[123]

Hydroa vacciniforme lymphoproliferative disorder

- In a classic presentation, a panel of CD3, CD4, CD8, CD56, TIA–1, granzyme-B, and EBER can assist in the diagnosis.

EBV-Positive Mucocutaneous Ulcer

EBV-positive mucocutaneous ulcer is a rare disorder that typically presents as a single, sharply demarcated ulcer in elderly and immunosuppressed patients that follows an indolent clinical course.[122] It typically presents in the oropharyngeal mucosa, but other sites may be involved, including the perioral skin or skin of acral sites or the trunk.[125] Biopsy of the lesions shows ulcerated epithelium with surrounding reactive epidermal changes, such as acanthosis and pseudoepitheliomatous hyperplasia. Undermining the ulcer is a mixed inflammatory infiltrate composed of lymphocytes, large apoptotic plasmacytoid immunoblasts, "Reed-Sternberg-like" cells, plasma cells, histiocytes, and eosinophils. Vascular invasion and necrosis can be prominent.[125]

By IHC, the atypical B-immunoblasts and Reed-Sternberg-like cells are PAX5+, OCT2+, BOB1+, MUM1+, CD45+/-, CD20-/+, and CD79a-/+. CD30 is uniformly positive, and CD15 expression can be variable.[122,125,126] EBER ISH is uniformly positive, with the majority of cases staining positively for LMP-1.[127] There is often a rim of small CD3+ T cells (CD4+ > CD8+) at the base of the lesion.[122,127] In approximately 1/3 of cases, clonal T-cell receptor or IgH rearrangements can be seen.[122,125]

EBV-positive mucocutaneous ulcer

- B-cell markers (PAX5, OCT2, BOB1, CD20, CD79a), CD30, CD15, EBER ISH can be useful in highlighting the atypical cells.

5.5 Sweet Syndrome

Sweet syndrome (SS; acute febrile neutrophilic dermatosis) is characterized by fever, neutrophilia, and abrupt onset of tender erythematous skin lesions.[128] It can be idiopathic (classical), drug-induced, or malignancy-associated, with the majority of these being myeloid neoplasms such as acute myeloid leukemia (AML) or myelodysplastic syndrome/myeloproliferative neoplasm (MDS/MPN).[129] A diagnosis of SS may be the first manifestation of hematologic malignancy and can also signal recurrence.[130]

It is characterized by a dense neutrophilic infiltrate in the superficial dermis associated with leukocytoclasia and marked papillary dermal edema but without leukocytoclastic vasculitis.[129] Rare cases can involve the epidermis or subcutaneous tissue.[130] Recent studies have demonstrated clonality between the cells within the cutaneous lesions of SS and bone marrow by molecular methods, implying that the neutrophils in the skin have a common progenitor, suggestive of either a hematologic malignancy differentiating into mature neutrophils in the skin or cutaneous involvement of a non-malignant neutrophil arising from a dysfunctional progenitor.[129,131,132]

Histiocytoid Sweet Syndrome

Histiocytoid Sweet syndrome is a rare variant of the disorder first described by Requena and colleagues.[133] It is predominantly composed of mononuclear "histiocytoid" immature cells of myeloid lineage, rather than neutrophils. Typically, it presents with a dermal-based band-like infiltrate of mononuclear cells with associated dermal edema. The mononuclear cells are characterized by large, elongated, kidney-shaped nuclei with inconspicuous nucleoli and scant eosinophilic cytoplasm.[134] The majority of the mononuclear cells in the infiltrate are positive for myeloperoxidase (MPO) and myeloid cell nuclear differentiation antigen (MNDA), demonstrating their myeloid lineage, with CD163+ histiocytic cells in a peripheral arrangement, and was typically not coexpressed with MNDA or MPO. MPO highlights immature and mature myeloid cells.[134] Histiocytoid Sweet syndrome is associated with malignancy or MDS/MPN in 30–61% of cases,[132] and may represent MDS-cutis[135] (**see Case Study 4**).

Sweet Syndrome

- The histiocytoid variant of Sweet syndrome can be confirmed by MPO and CD163 immunostains.

5.6 Case Studies

Case 1

Case history: A 42-year-old man presented with a nodule on his right nasal ala.

Description: A dense and nodular lymphoid infiltrate is seen in the deep dermis surrounding enlarged or distorted hair follicles or pilosebaceous units (**Figure 5.28**). CD1a demonstrates many dendritic cells within hair follicular epithelium as well as interstitially within the dermis (**Figure 5.29**). The infiltrate is comprised of predominantly CD3+ T lymphocytes (**Figure 5.30**) in comparison to CD20+ B-lymphocytes (**Figure 5.31**) There is an approximately equal ratio of CD4+ (**Figure 5.32**) to CD8+ cells (**Figure 5.33**) lymphocytes. CD21 highlights intact FDC meshworks surrounding reactive germinal centers. Bcl-6 highlights scattered cells. Kappa and lambda *in situ* hybridization demonstrate no evidence of light chain restriction.

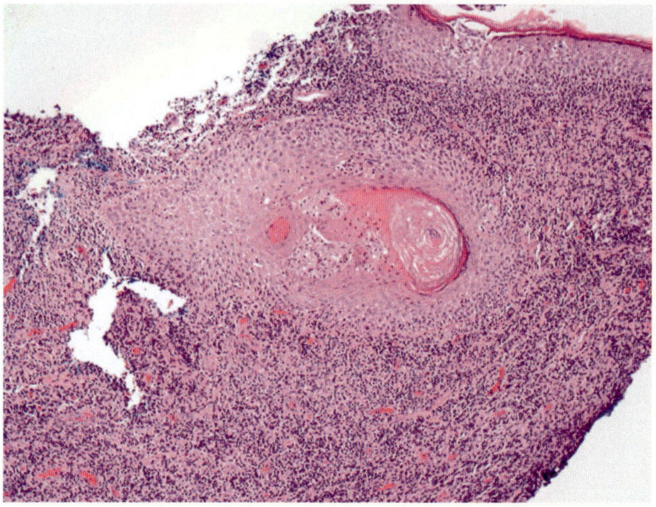

Figure 5.28 A dense inflammatory infiltrate is noted surrounding a distorted hair follicle (X100).

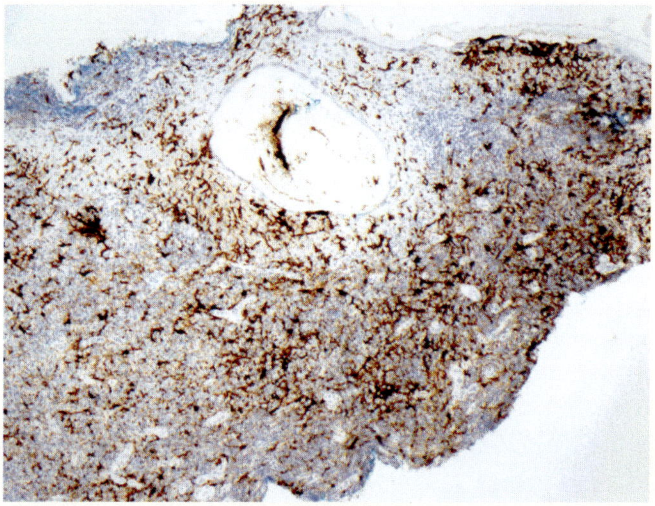

Figure 5.29 A prominent infiltrate of CD1a-positive dendritic cells (X100).

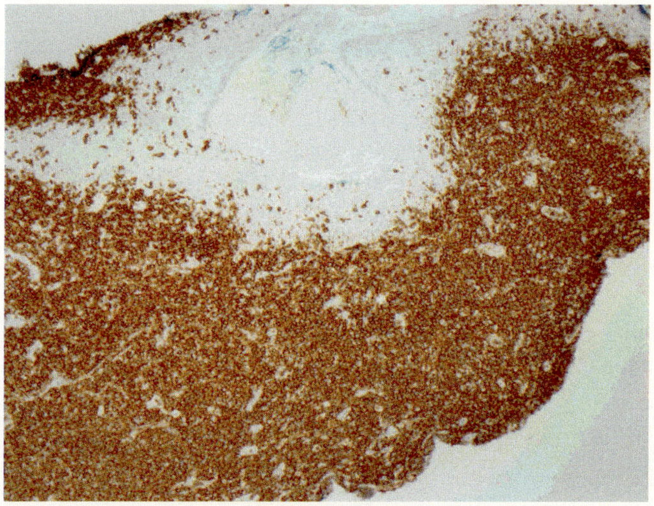

Figure 5.30 CD3 highlights the majority of the infiltrate (X100).

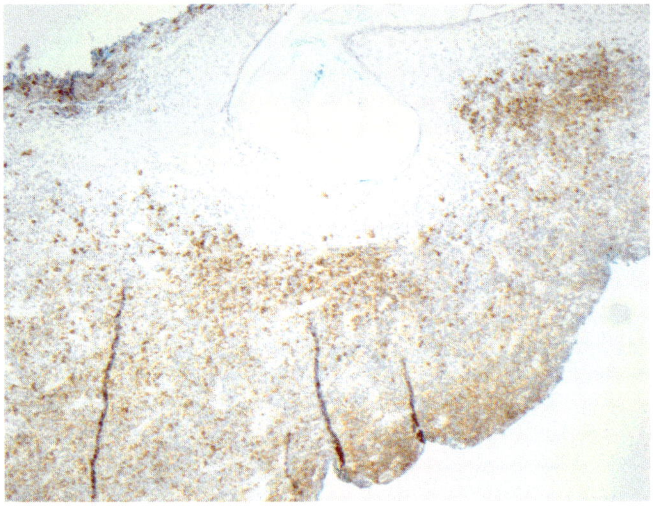

Figure 5.31 CD20 highlights only occasional B-cells within the infiltrate (X100).

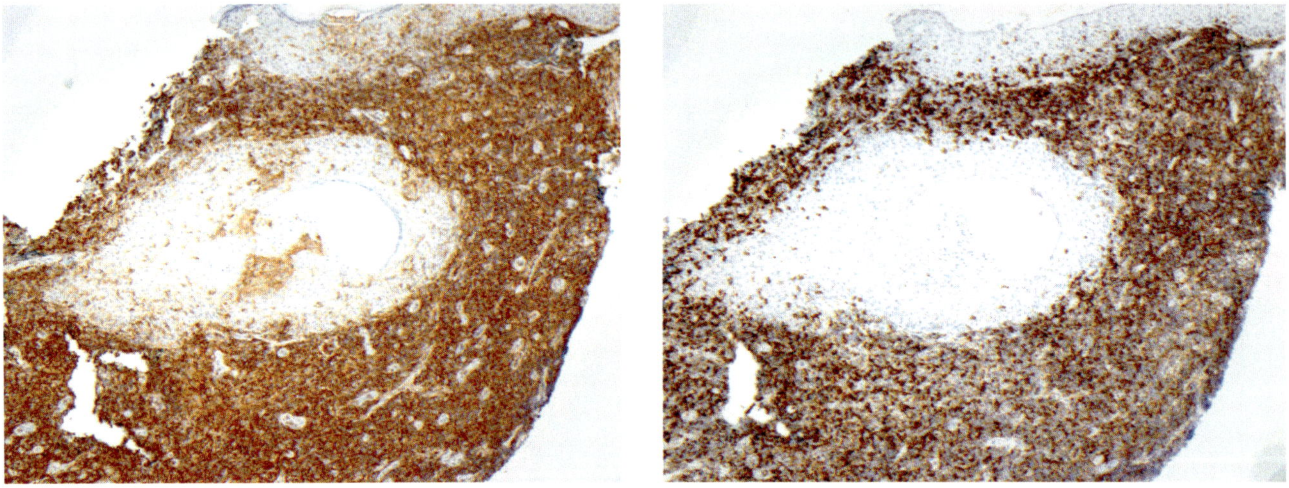

Figures 5.32 and 5.33 An equal proportion of CD4 and CD8 (X100, X100).

Diagnosis: Pseudolymphomatous folliculitis.

Discussion: Pseudolymphomatous folliculitis presents as a dense lymphoid infiltration around hyperplastic hair follicles. Clinically, it is characterized by a single or eruptive, erythematous to violaceous, firm, nodule(s) on the face, especially nose, cheek, eyelid, or forehead. Rapid growth can be seen over several weeks or months making MF a clinical possibility.[62] The clinical differential diagnosis for pseudolymphomatous folliculitis includes a wide range of diseases including epidermoid cyst, chronic folliculitis, sarcoidosis, and arthropod assault. Rarely pseudolymphomatous folliculitis can present with multiple[62] and even recurrent lesions.[60]

This case highlights the diagnostic criteria proposed by Arai and colleagues as it shows activated and distorted hair follicles and a predominantly CD3+ T-cell diffuse infiltrate with aggregates of CD1a and S-100 T-cell associated dendritic cells.[59] The absence of lymphocytic atypia and a predominantly polyclonal CD4+ T-cell population makes folliculotropic mycosis fungoides unlikely. As a predominantly B-cell type pseudolymphomatous folliculitis, cutaneous marginal zone lymphoma is the main differential diagnosis. The latter can be differentiated by the presence of a clonal CD20-positive centrocyte-like cell proliferation with monotypic plasma cell population and the presence of lymphoepithelial lesions involving the adnexal and sebaceous glands.

Case 2

Case history: The patient is a 45-year-old female with multiple indurated nodules and plaques without ulceration on her left upper arm.

Description: There is a dense inflammatory infiltrate in the dermis and subcutaneous tissue (**Figure 5.34**). A mixed infiltrate of lymphocytes, histiocytes, and plasma cells with germinal center formation is seen in the subcutaneous tissue (**Figures 5.35, 5.36 and 5.37**). There is a predominance of CD4+ lymphocytes (**Figure 5.38**) in comparison to CD8+ lymphocytes rimming the adipocytes (**Figure 5.39**).

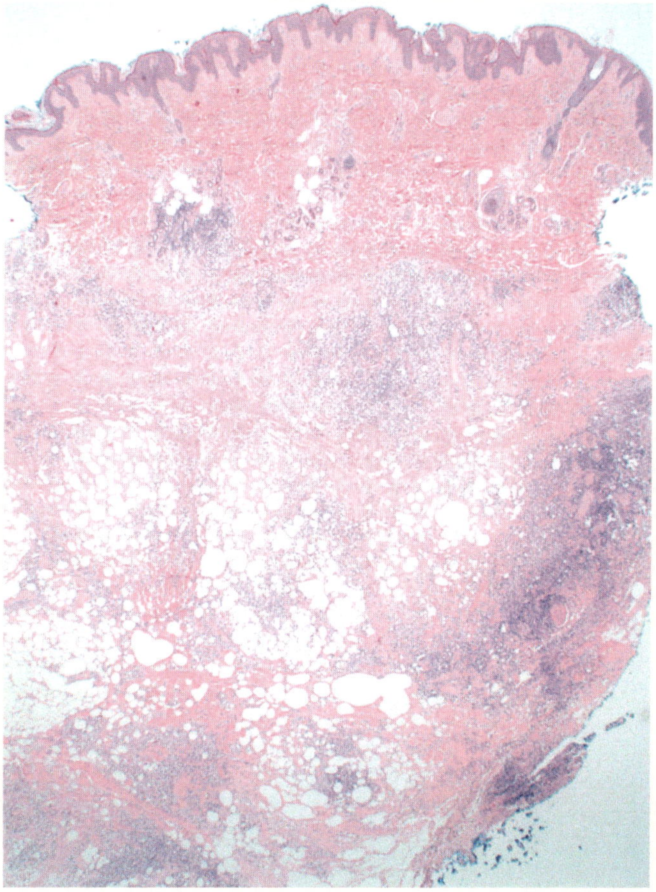

Figure 5.34 A prominent inflammatory infiltrate is seen in the dermis and subcutaneous tissue (X40).

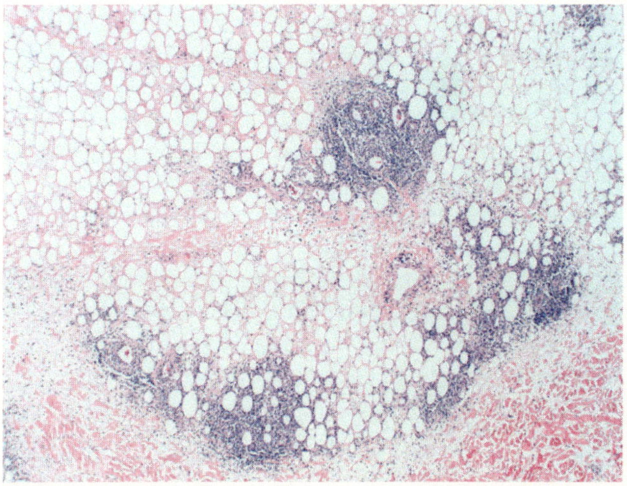

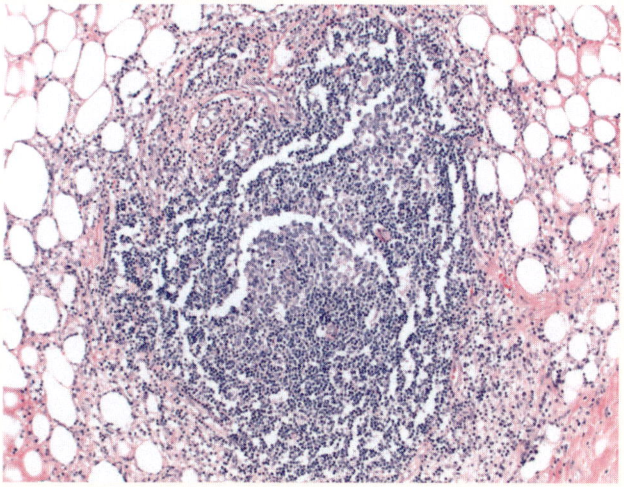

Figures 5.35 and 5.36 Germinal formation is noted (X100, X200).

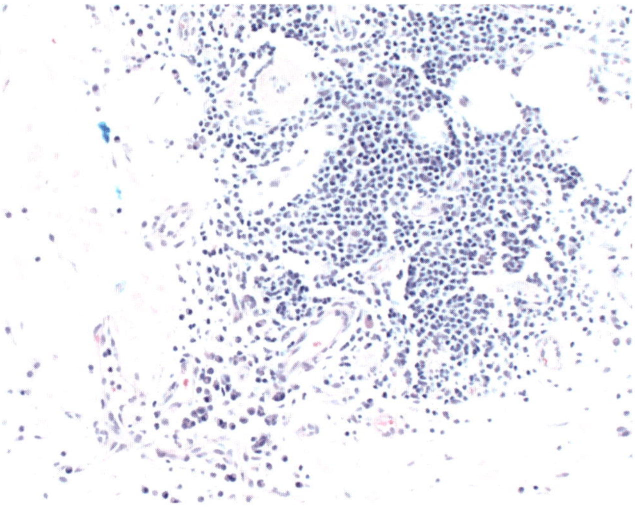

Figure 5.37 A mixed infiltrate of lymphocytes and plasma cells (X200).

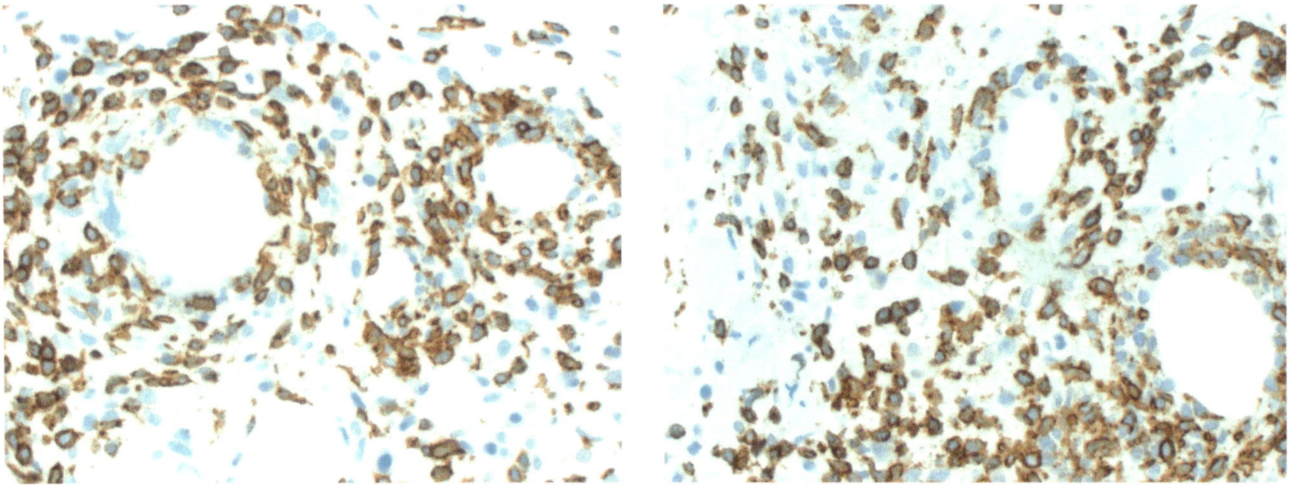

Figures 5.38 and 5.39 The infiltrate is comprised of mainly CD4-positive T-lymphocytes in comparison to CD8-positive T-lymphocytes (X200, X200).

Diagnosis: Lupus erythematosus panniculitis.

Discussion: The sections show a panniculitic lesion with a predominant lymphocytic infiltrate. The differential diagnoses include lupus panniculitis versus subcutaneous panniculitis-like T-cell lymphoma (SPTCL). Clinically, both diseases overlap as they present as nodules or plaques affecting limbs. Even more, patients suffering from lupus erythematosus have subsequently developed SPTCL.[136] This event underscores that the diagnosis of one disease does not rule out the other. The clinical overlap parallels the absence of significant number of distinguishing histologic features. Features that can be seen more frequently in lupus panniculitis than in SPTCL are nodular aggregates of B-cells at the periphery of the lesion and collection of plasma cells occasionally forming germinal centers.[137] Other features more commonly in lupus panniculitis, but not necessarily present in all cases are the presence of interface changes, dermal mucin deposition and periadnexal infiltration. Adipocyte rimming can be seen in both disorders; however the lymphocytes in lupus panniculitis are a mixture of CD4 > CD8 positive cells. CD123 plasmacytoid dendritic cells in aggregates also supports the diagnosis of lupus panniculitis (**Table 5.5**).[137,138] TCR gene rearrangement in lupus panniculitis is commonly polyclonal, rarely monoclonal.

Case 3

Case history: A 46-year-old man with no significant past medical history presented to the emergency room with a three-week history of worsening and diffuse cutaneous eruption, joint pain, sore throat and cough. On physical examination nodules with some being ulcerated seen on his back (**Figure 5.40**) and his lower extremity (**Figure 5.41**).

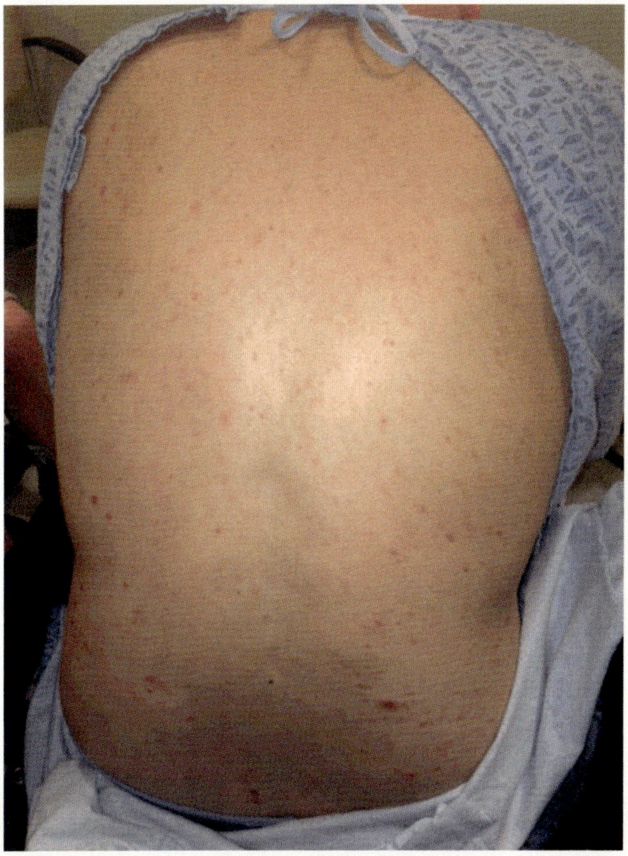

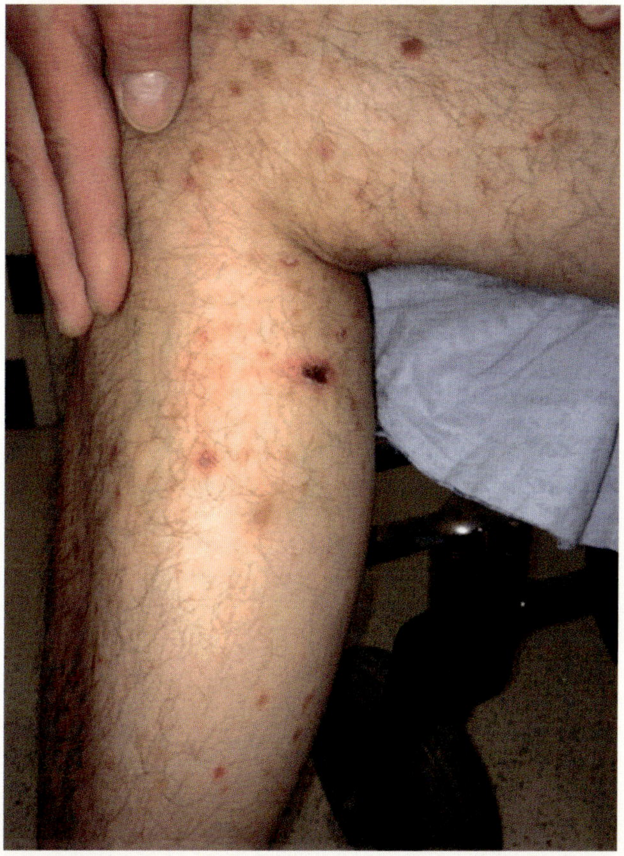

Figures 5.40 and 5.41 Ulcerated nodules are seen on the patient's back and lower extremity (Courtesy of Avery H. Lachance M.D, Department of Dermatology, Massachusetts General Hospital, Boston, MA).

Description: A wedge-shaped infiltrate of inflammatory cells is seen in the dermis (**Figure 5.42**). A band-like infiltrate obscuring the dermal epidermal junction is seen (**Figure 5.43**). CD3 and CD68 show the majority of the infiltrate to be T-lymphocytes and histiocytes, respectively (**Figure 5.44 and Figure 5.45**). CD20 highlights occasional B-lymphocytes. CD30 highlights occasional immunoblasts (**Figure 5.46**).

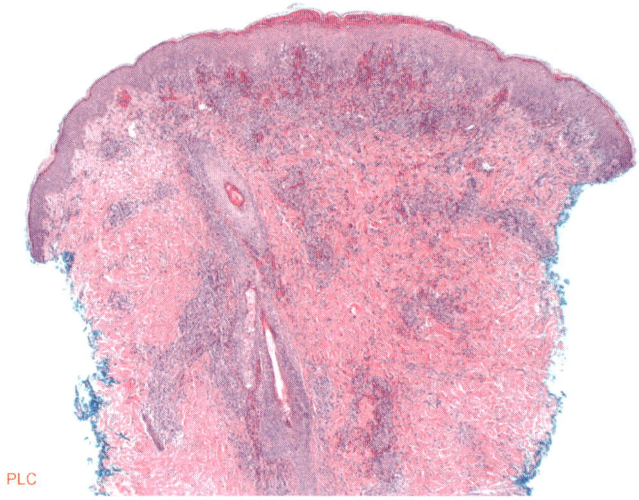

Figure 5.42 A wedge-shaped dermal inflammatory infiltrate (X40).

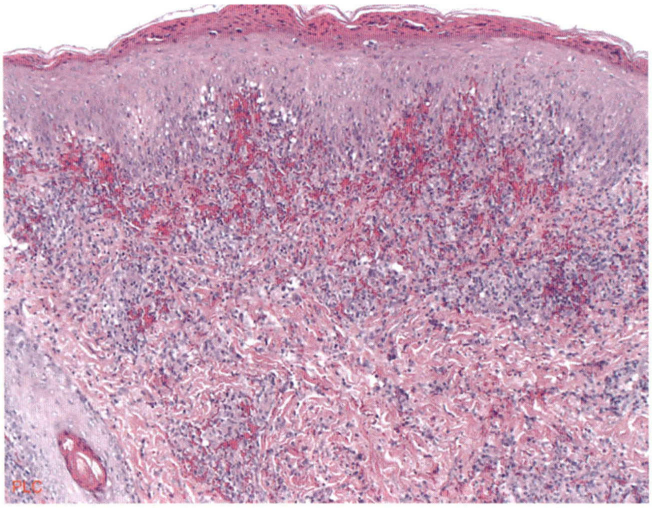

Figure 5.43 A band-like inflammatory infiltrate obscuring the dermal epidermal junction (X100).

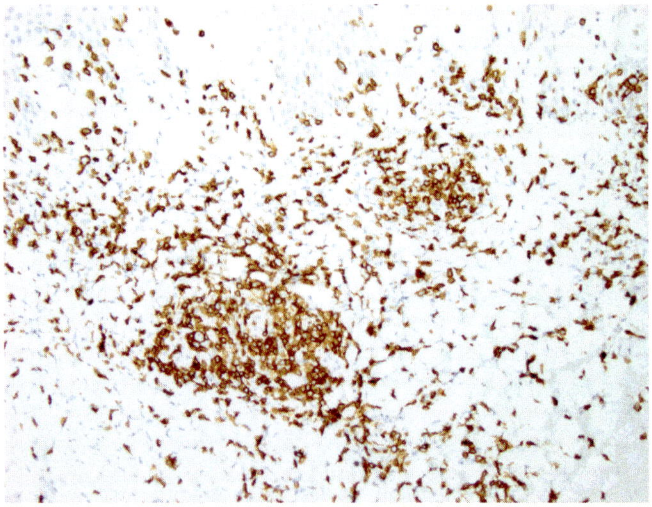

Figure 5.44 CD3 labels the T-lymphocytes (X200).

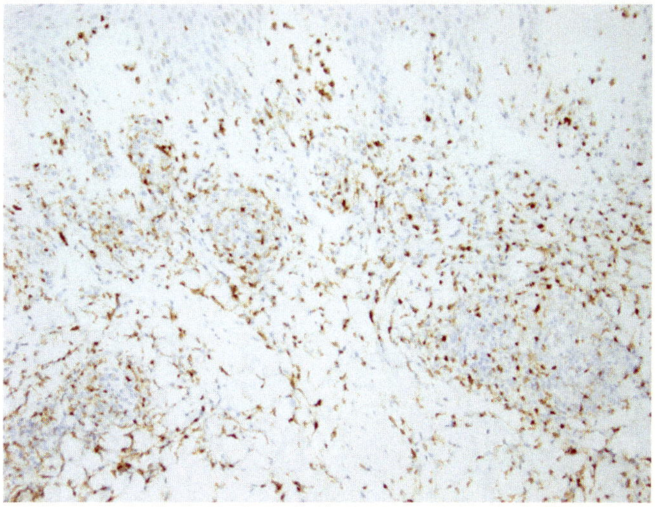

Figure 5.45 CD68 labels the histiocytes (X200).

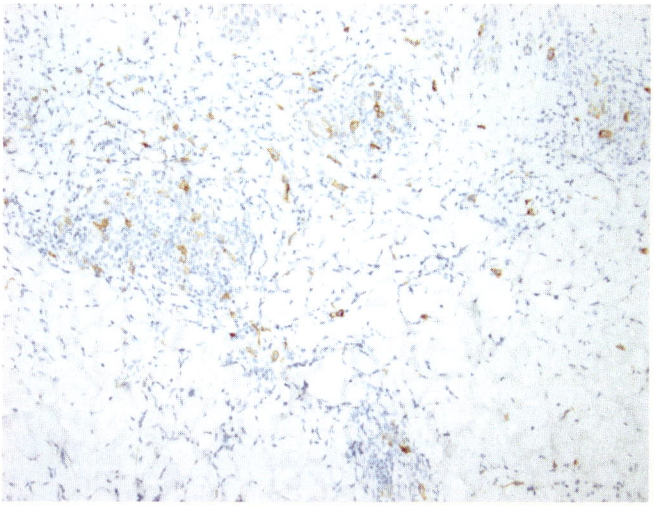

Figure 5.46 CD30 highlights occasional immunoblasts within the dermal infiltrate (X200).

Diagnosis: Pityriasis lichenoides et varioliformis acuta.

Discussion: The differential diagnosis of pityriasis lichenoides et varioliformis acuta (PLEVA) includes secondary syphilis, lymphomatoid papulosis, and arthropod bite reaction. The infiltrate can be CD4 as well as CD8 predominant.[71] The loss of CD5 or CD7 can be seen in a subset of these cases. In addition, PLEVA can have a prominent infiltrate of CD30-positive cells as observed in this case.[72]

Case 4

Case history: A 54-year-old woman presented with multiple, polymorphous and targetoid erythematous patches and plaques on her left medial trapezial neck and right posterior shoulder. The clinical impression was erythema multiforme.

Description: Histologic sections of both biopsies showed a dense perivascular and interstitial infiltrate in the dermis (**Figure 5.47**). Prominent papillary dermal edema is noted (**Figure 5.48**). CD3 highlights the T cells within the dermal infiltrate (**Figure 5.49**). A high proportion of the dermal inflammatory cells is stained with CD4 (**Figure 5.50**) and CD68 (**Figure 5.51**), consistent with histiocytes. Myeloperoxidase highlights occasional cells within the dermal infiltrate (**Figure 5.52**).

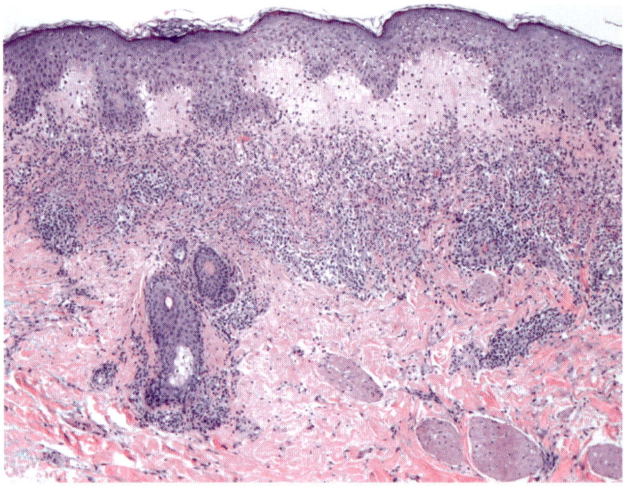

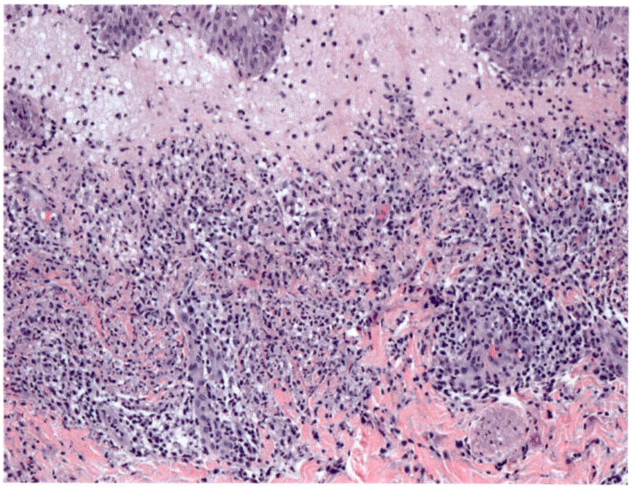

Figures 5.47 and 5.48 Prominent superficial dermal edema and dense band-like inflammatory infiltrate (X100, X200).

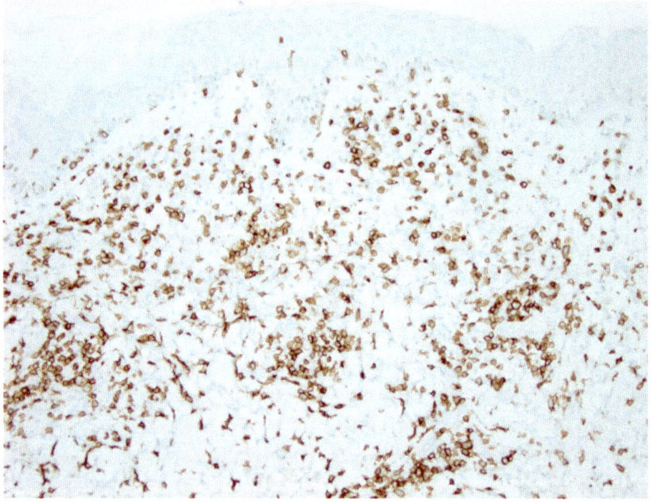

Figure 5.49 CD3 highlights the T-lymphocytes within the infiltrate (X200).

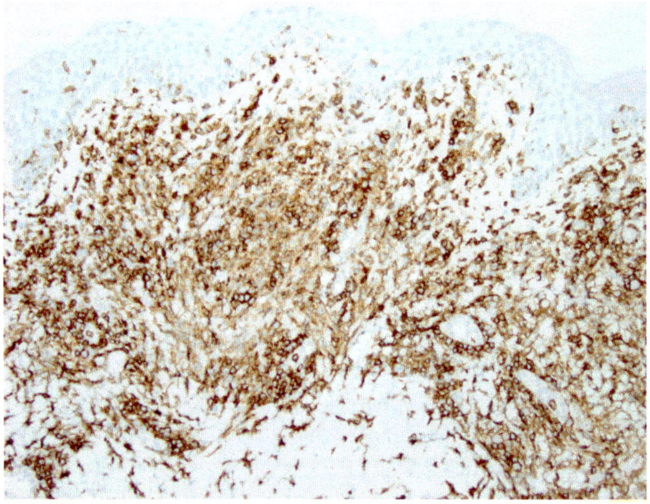

Figure 5.50 CD4 highlights the T-lymphocytes as well as the histiocytes (X200).

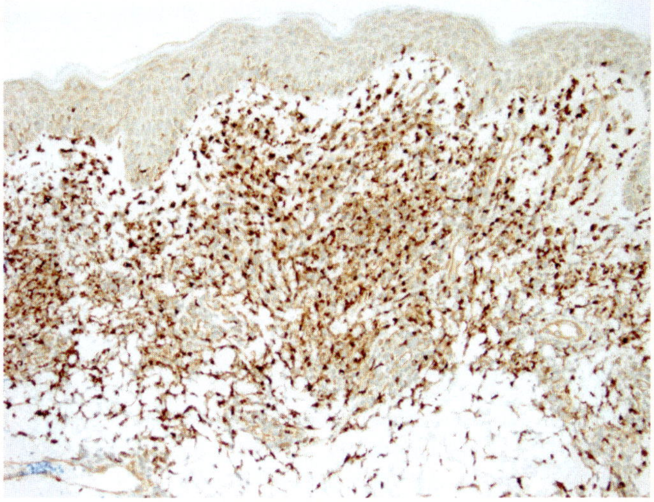

Figure 5.51 CD68 highlights the histiocytes (X200).

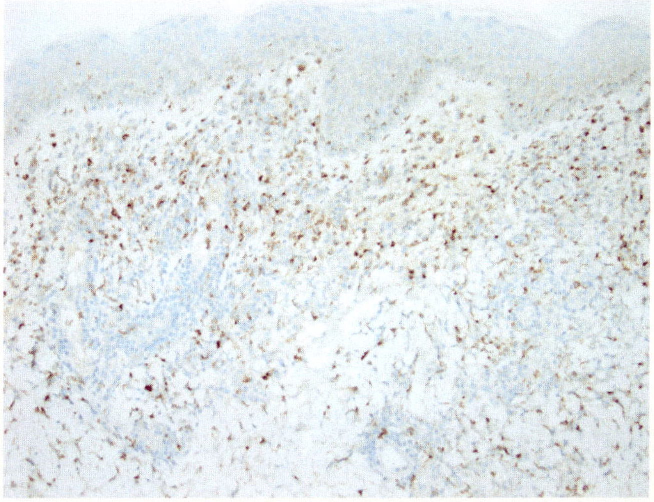

Figure 5.52 Myeloperoxidase highlights the neutrophils within the dermal inflammatory infiltrate (X200).

Diagnosis: Histiocytoid Sweet syndrome.

Discussion: Sweet syndrome or acute febrile neutrophilic dermatosis can be idiopathic, drug-induced or associated with malignancy. Requena and colleagues reported the presence of immature myeloid cells in Sweet syndrome and introduced the term "histiocytoid" Sweet syndrome in 2005.[133] An association with myelogenous leukemia or myelodysplastic syndromes has been reported in histiocytoid Sweet syndrome. One third of patients with histiocytoid Sweet syndrome can be associated with myelodysplastic syndromes which is higher than that observed in patients with conventional Sweet syndrome.[139] Histiocytoid Sweet syndrome is a rare variant of Sweet syndrome in which the mononuclear cells are predominant over neutrophils. The mononuclear cells within the dermal infiltrate of histiocytoid Sweet syndrome express CD68, CD163 or myeloperoxidase.[133,139] CD34 and CD117 are typically negative. Due to overlapping immunoprofiles and frequent association with myelodysplastic syndrome, correlation with clinical findings and laboratory studies is necessary to differentiate from leukemia cutis.

References

1. Nestle FO, Di Meglio P, Qin JZ et al. Skin immune sentinels in health and disease. *Nat Rev Immunol* 2009; 9: 679–91.
2. Heath WR, Carbone FR. The skin-resident and migratory immune system in steady state and memory: innate lymphocytes, dendritic cells and T cells. *Nat Immunol* 2013; 14: 978–85.
3. Nihal M, Mikkola D, Horvath N, et al. Cutaneous lymphoid hyperplasia: a lymphoproliferative continuum with lymphomatous potential. *Hum Pathol* 2003; 34: 617–22.
4. Colli C, Leinweber B, Müllegger R, et al. Borrelia burgdorferi-associated lymphocytoma cutis: clinicopathologic, immunophenotypic, and molecular study of 106 cases. *J Cutan Pathol* 2004; 31: 232–40.
5. Miguel D, Peckruhn M, Elsner P. Treatment of cutaneous pseudolymphoma: a systematic review. *Acta Derm Venereol.* 2018; 98: 310–17.
6. Mitteldorf C, Kempf W. Cutaneous pseudolymphoma—a review on the spectrum and a proposal for a new classification. *J Cutan Pathol* 2020; 47: 76–97.
7. Ploysangam T, Breneman DL, Mutasim DF. Cutaneous pseudolymphomas. *J Am Acad Dermatol* 1998; 38: 877–98.
8. WHO Classification of Tumours Editorial Board. Skin Tumours [Internet; beta version ahead of print] (WHO classification of tumours series). 5th ed. Vol. 12. Lyon (France): International Agency for Research on Cancer; 2023.
9. Murphy M, Fullen D, Carlson JA. Low CD7 expression in benign and malignant cutaneous lymphocytic infiltrates experience with an antibody reactive with paraffin-embedded tissue. *Am J Dermatopathol* 2002; 24: 6–16.
10. Ponti R, Quaglino P, Novelli M, et al. T-cell receptor γ gene rearrangement by multiplex polymerase chain reaction/heteroduplex analysis in patients with cutaneous T-cell lymphoma (mycosis fungoides/Sézary syndrome) and benign inflammatory disease: correlation with clinical, histological and immunophenotypical findings. *Br J Dermatol* 2005; 153: 565–73.
11. Erős N, Károlyi Z, Marschalkó M, et al. Clinical, histopathological, immunophenotypic and molecular analysis of 60 patients with cutaneous T-cell infiltrates with follow up of indeterminate cases to identify T-cell lymphoma. *Path Oncol Res* 2008; 14: 63–7.
12. Mitteldorf C, Kempf W. Cutaneous pseudolymphoma. *Surg Pathol Clin.* 2017; 10: 455–76.
13. Bergman R, Khamaysi K, Khamaysi Z, et al. A study of histologic and immunophenotypical staining patterns in cutaneous lymphoid hyperplasia. *J Am Acad Dermatol* 2011; 65: 112–24.
14. Arai E, Shimizu M, Hirose T. A review of 55 cases of cutaneous lymphoid hyperplasia: Reassessment of the histopathologic findings leading to reclassification of 4 lesions as cutaneous marginal zone lymphoma and 19 as pseudolymphomatous folliculitis. *Hum Pathol* 2005; 36: 505–11.
15. De Leval L, Harris NL, Longtine J, Ferry JA, Duncan LM. Cutaneous B-cell lymphomas of follicular and marginal zone types use of Bcl-6, CD10, Bcl-2, and CD21 in differential diagnosis and classification. *Am J Surg Pathol* 2001; 25: 732–41.
16. Goodlad JR, Krajewski AS, Batstone PJ, et al. Primary cutaneous follicular lymphoma: A clinicopathologic and molecular study of 16 cases in support of a distinct entity. *Am J Surg Pathol* 2002; 26: 733–41.
17. Cerroni L, Arzberger E, Pü Tz B et al. Primary cutaneous follicle center cell lymphoma with follicular growth pattern. *Blood* 2000; 95: 3922–8.
18. Servitje O, Gallardo F, Estrach T, et al. Primary cutaneous marginal zone B-cell lymphoma: a clinical, histopathological, immunophenotypic and molecular genetic study of 22 cases. *Br J Dermatol* 2002; 147: 1147–58.
19. LeBoit PE, McNutt NS, Reed JA, Jacobson M, Weiss LM. Primary cutaneous immunocytoma: a B-cell lymphoma that can easily be mistaken for cutaneous lymphoid hyperplasia. *Am J Surg Pathol* 1994; 18: 969–78.
20. Wood GS, Kamath N V., Guitart J, et al. Absence of Borrelia burgdorferi DNA in cutaneous B-cell lymphomas from the United States. *J Cutan Pathol* 2001; 28: 502–7.
21. Cho WC, Gill P, Nagarajan P, et al. Cutaneous lymphoid hyperplasia with T-cell clonality and monotypic plasma cells secondary to a tick bite: a hidden critter and the power of deeper levels. *Am J Dermatopathol* 2021; 44: 226–9.
22. Moreno A, Curco N, Serrano T, Garcia J, Llistosella E, Bordas X. Disseminated, miliarial type lymphocytoma cutis. *Acta Derm Venerol* 1991; 71: 334–6.
23. Villalobos-Ayala RA, Espinoza-Gurrola AA, Guevara-Gutiérrez E, et al. Lymphocytoma cutis (cutaneous B-cell pseudolymphoma): study of 102 cases with emphasis on the histological characteristics and immunohistochemistry of the miliarial type. *Int J Dermatol* 2022; 61: 316–23.
24. Moulonguet I, Ghnassia M, Molina T, et al. Miliarial-type perifollicular B-cell pseudolymphoma (lymphocytoma cutis): a misleading eruption in two women. *J Cutan Pathol* 2012; 39: 1016–21.
25. Knackstedt TJ, Zug KA. T cell lymphomatoid contact dermatitis: a challenging case and review of the literature. *Contact Dermatitis.* 2015; 72: 65–74.
26. Magro CM, Daniels BH, Crowson AN. Drug induced pseudolymphoma. *Semin Diagn Pathol* 2018; 35: 247–59.
27. Gómez Orbaneja J, Iglesias Diez L, Sánchez Lozano JL, et al. Lymphomatoid contact dermatitis A syndrome produced by epicutaneous hypersensitivity with clinical features and a histopathologic picture similar to that of mycosis fungoides. *Contact Dermatitis* 1976; 2: 139–43.
28. Smolle J, Torne R, Soyer HP, et al. Immunohistochemical classification of cutaneous pseudolymphomas: delineation of distinct patterns. *J Cutan Pathol* 1990; 17: 149–59.
29. Haynes BF, Hensley LL, Jegasothy B V. Phenotypic characterization of skin-infiltrating T cells in cutaneous T-cell lymphoma: comparison with benign cutaneous T-cell infiltrates. *Blood* 1982; 60: 463–73.
30. Marliere V, Beylot-Barry M, Doutre M-S, et al. Lymphomatoid contact dermatitis caused by isopropyl-diphenylenediamine: two cases. *J Allergy Clin Immunol* 1998; 102: 152–3.
31. Souteyrand P, d'Incan M. Drug induced mycosis fungoides like lesions. *Curr Probl Dermatol* 1990; 19: 176–82.
32. Magro CM, Crowson AN. Drug-induced immune dysregulation as a cause of atypical cutaneous lymphoid

infiltrates: a hypothesis. *Hum Pathol* 1996; 27: 125–32.

33. Pulitzer MP, Nolan KA, Oshman RG, Phelps RG. CD30+ lymphomatoid drug reactions. *Am J Dermatopathol* 2013; 35: 343–50.

34. Brady SP, Magro CM, Diaz-Cano SJ, Wolfe HJ. Analysis of clonality of atypical cutaneous lymphoid infiltrates associated with drug therapy by PCR/DGGE. *Hum Pathol* 1999; 30: 130–6.

35. Ortonne N, Buyukbabani N, Delfau-Larue MH, et al. Value of the CD8-CD3 ratio for the diagnosis of mycosis fungoides. *Mod Pathol* 2003; 16: 857–62.

36. Florell SR, Cessna M, Lundell RB, et al. Usefulness (or lack thereof) of immunophenotyping in atypical cutaneous T-cell infiltrates. *Am J Clin Pathol* 2006; 125: 727–36.

37. Cerroni L, Fink-Puches R, Bä Ck; B, Kerl H. Follicular mucinosis: a critical reappraisal of clinicopathologic features and association with mycosis fungoides and Sézary syndrome. *Arch Dermatol* 2002; 138: 182–9.

38. Gerami P, Rosen S, Kuzel T, Boone SL, Guitart J. Folliculotropic mycosis fungoides: an aggressive variant of cutaneous T-cell lymphoma. *Arch Dermatol* 2008; 144: 738–46.

39. Burg G, Kempf W, Cozzio A, et al. WHO/EORTC classification of cutaneous lymphomas 2005: histological and molecular aspects. *J Cutan Pathol* 2005; 32: 647–74.

40. Rongioletti F, De Lucchi S, Meyes D, et al. Follicular mucinosis: a clinicopathologic, histochemical, immunohistochemical and molecular study comparing the primary benign form and the mycosis fungoides-associated follicular mucinosis. *J Cutan Pathol* 2010; 37: 15–19.

41. Demirkesen C, Esirgen G, Engin B, et al. The clinical features and histopathologic patterns of folliculotropic mycosis fungoides in a series of 38 cases. *J Cutan Pathol* 2015; 42: 22–31.

42. van Doorn R, Scheffer E, Willemze R. Follicular mycosis fungoides, a distinct disease entity with or without associated follicular mucinosis. *Arch Dermatol* 2002; 138: 191–8.

43. Flaig MJ, Cerroni L, Schuhmann K, et al. Follicular mycosis fungoides: a histopathologic analysis of nine cases. *J Cutan Pathol* 2001; 28: 525–30.

44. Wang J, Wang Y, Zhou H, et al. Clinicopathological features, therapeutic options, and significance of CD103 expression in 15 patients with follicular mucinosis. *Front Med (Lausanne)* 2023; 10. doi:10.3389/fmed.2023.1032072.

45. Brown HA, Gibson LE, Pujol RM, et al. Primary follicular mucinosis: long-term follow-up of patients younger than 40 years with and without clonal T-cell receptor gene rearrangement. *J Am Acad Dermatol* 2002; 47: 856–62.

46. Magro CM, Schaefer JT, Crowson AN, et al. Pigmented purpuric dermatosis: classification by phenotypic and molecular profiles. *Am J Clin Pathol* 2007; 128: 218–29.

47. Sun J, Liu K, Dang J, Xiong S, Pan H, Wang Y. Pigmented purpura dermatosis-like mycosis fungoides: four case reports and a review of published cases. *Eur J Dermatol* 2023; 33: 635–41.

48. Sidiropoulos M, Deonizio J, Estela Martinez-Escala M, Gerami P, Guitart J. Chronic actinic dermatitis/actinic reticuloid: a clinicopathologic and immunohistochemical analysis of 37 cases. *Am J Dermatopathol* 2014; 36: 875–81.

49. Baykal C, Büyükbabani N, Seçkin D, et al. Cutaneous atypical papular CD8+ lymphoproliferative disorder at acral sites in a renal transplant patient. *Clin Exp Dermatol* 2017; 42: 902–5.

50. Kempf W, Petrella T, Willemze R, et al. Clinical, histopathological and prognostic features of primary cutaneous acral CD8+ T-cell lymphoma and other dermal CD8+ cutaneous lymphoproliferations: results of an EORTC Cutaneous Lymphoma Group workshop. *Br J Dermatol* 2022; 186: 887–97.

51. Zhang P, Chiriboga L, Jacobson M, et al. Mycosis fungoides like T-cell cutaneous lymphoid infiltrates in patients with HIV infection. *Am J Dermatopathol* 1995; 17: 29–35.

52. Guitart J, Variakojis D, Kuzel T, et al. Cutaneous CD8+ T cell infiltrates in advanced HIV Infection. *J Am Acad Dermatol* 1999; 41: 722–7.

53. Friedler S, Parisi MT, Waldo E, et al. Atypical cutaneous lymphoproliferative disorder in patients with HIV infection. *Int J Dermatol* 1999; 38: 111–18.

54. Bachelez H, Hadida F. Massive infiltration of the skin by HIV-specific cytotoxic CD8+ T cells. *NEJM* 1996; 335: 61–2.

55. Gammon B, Robson A, Deonizio J, et al. CD8+ granulomatous cutaneous T-cell lymphoma: a potential association with immunodeficiency. *J Am Acad Dermatol* 2014; 71: 555–60.

56. Kempf W, Mitteldorf C, Cerroni L, et al. Classifications of cutaneous lymphomas and lymphoproliferative disorders: an update from the EORTC cutaneous lymphoma histopathology group. *J Eur Acad Dermatol Venerol* 2024; 28: 1491–1503.

57. Cetinozman FC, Jansen PM, Willemze R. Expression of programmed death-1 in primary cutaneous CD4-positive small/medium-sized pleomorphic T-cell lymphoma, cutaneous pseudo-T-cell lymphoma, and other types of cutaneous T-cell lymphoma. *Am J Surg Pathol* 2012; 36: 109–16.

58. McNutt N. Cutaneous lymphohistiocytic infiltrates simulating malignant lymphoma. In: Murphy G, Mihm M, editors. *Lymphoproliferative Disorders of the Skin*. Boston, MA: Butterworths, 1986; 356–385.

59. Arai E, Okubo H, Tsuchida T, et al. Pseudolymphomatous folliculitis. *Am J Surg Pathol* 1999; 23: 1313–9.

60. Kwon EJ, Kristjansson AK, Meyerson HJ, et al. A case of recurrent pseudolymphomatous folliculitis: A mimic of cutaneous lymphoma. *J Am Acad Dermatol* 2009; 60: 994–1000.

61. Shojiguchi N, Arai E, Anan T, et al. Distribution of CD1a-positive cells is not different between pseudolymphomatous folliculitis and primary cutaneous marginal zone lymphoma. *J Dermatol* 2021; 48: 464–9.

62. Horikiri M, Abe N, Ueda K. Multiple nodules on the left cheek represented pseudolymphomatous folliculitis. *Clin Case Rep* 2016; 4: 568–71.

63. Kazakov D V, Belousova IE, Kacerovska D, et al. Hyperplasia of hair follicles and other adnexal structures in cutaneous lymphoproliferative disorders: a study of 53 cases, including so-called pseudolymphomatous folliculitis and overt lymphomas. *Am J Surg Pathol* 2008; 32: 1468–78.

64. Goyal A, Moore JB, Gimbel D, et al. PD-1, S-100 and CD1a expression in pseudolymphomatous folliculitis,

primary cutaneous marginal zone B-cell lymphoma (MALT lymphoma) and cutaneous lymphoid hyperplasia. *J Cutan Pathol* 2015; 42: 6–15.

65. Kempf W, Kazakov D V., Baumgartner HP, et al. Follicular lymphomatoid papulosis revisited: a study of 11 cases, with new histopathological findings. *J Am Acad Dermatol* 2013; 68: 809–16.
66. Kempf W. CD30+ lymphoproliferative disorders: histopathology, differential diagnosis, new variants, and simulators. *J Cutan Pathol.* 2006; 33: 58–70.
67. Werner B, Massone C, Kerl H, et al. Large CD30-positive cells in benign, atypical lymphoid infiltrates of the skin. *J Cutan Pathol* 2008; 35: 1100–7.
68. Magro CM, Guo R, Nguyen GH, et al. Pityriasis lichenoides-like drug reaction: a clinical histopathologic study of 10 cases. *Dermatol Online J* 2017; 23: 13030/qt7xd8j71z.
69. Geller L, Antonov NK, Lauren CT, Morel KD, Garzon MC. Pityriasis lichenoides in childhood: review of clinical presentation and treatment options. *Pediatr Dermatol* 2015; 32: 579–92.
70. Bowers S, Warshaw EM. Pityriasis lichenoides and its subtypes. *J Am Acad Dermatol.* 2006; 55: 557–72.
71. Magro C, Crowson AN, Kovatich A, et al. Pityriasis lichenoides: a clonal T-cell lymphoproliferative disorder. *Hum Pathol* 2002; 33: 788–95.
72. Kempf W, Kazakov D V, Palmedo G, et al. Pityriasis lichenoides et varioliformis acuta with numerous CD30 + cells: a variant mimicking lymphomatoid papulosis and other cutaneous lymphomas: a clinicopathologic, immunohistochemical, and molecular biological study of 13 cases. *Am J Surg Pathol* 2012; 36: 1021–9.
73. Martinez-Escala ME, Sidiropoulos M, Deonizio J, et al. γδ T-cell-rich variants of pityriasis lichenoides and lymphomatoid papulosis: benign cutaneous disorders to be distinguished from aggressive cutaneous γδ T-cell lymphomas. *Br J Dermatol* 2015; 172: 372–9.
74. Magro CM, Crowson AN, Kovatich AJ, et al. Lupus profundus, indeterminate lymphocytic lobular panniculitis and subcutaneous T-cell lymphoma: a spectrum of subcuticular T-cell lymphoid dyscrasia. *J Cutan Pathol* 2001; 28: 235–47.
75. Park HS, Choi JW, Kim BK, Cho KH. Lupus erythematosus panniculitis: clinicopathological, immunophenotypic, and molecular studies. *Am J Dermatopathol* 2010; 32: 24–30.
76. Massone C, Kodama K, Salmhofer W, *et al.* Lupus erythematosus panniculitis (lupus profundus): clinical, histopathological, and molecular analysis of nine cases. *J Cutan Pathol* 2005; 32: 396–404.
77. Aguilera P, Mascaró JM, Martinez A, et al. Cutaneous γ/δ T-cell lymphoma: a histopathologic mimicker of lupus erythematosus profundus (lupus panniculitis). *J Am Acad Dermatol* 2007; 56: 643–7.
78. Leblanc RE, Tavallaee M, Kim YH, Kim J. Useful parameters for distinguishing subcutaneous panniculitis-like T-cell lymphoma from lupus erythematosus panniculitis. *Am J Surg Pathol* 2016; 40: 745–54.
79. Chen SJT, Tse JY, Harms PW, et al. Utility of CD123 immunohistochemistry in differentiating lupus erythematosus from cutaneous T cell lymphoma. *Histopathology* 2019; 74: 908–16.
80. Willemze R, Jaffe ES, Nter Burg G et al. WHO-EORTC classification for cutaneous lymphomas. *Blood* 2005; 105: 3768–85.
81. Willemze R, Jansen PM, Cerroni L, et al. Subcutaneous panniculitis-like T-cell lymphoma: definition, classification, and prognostic factors: an EORTC Cutaneous Lymphoma Group Study of 83 cases. *Blood* 2008; 111: 838–45.
82. Magro CM, Schaefer JT, Morrison C, et al. Atypical lymphocytic lobular panniculitis: a clonal subcutaneous T-cell dyscrasia. *J Cutan Pathol* 2008; 35: 947–54.
83. Machan S, Rodríguez M, Alonso-Alonso R, et al. Subcutaneous panniculitis-like T-cell lymphoma, lupus erythematosus profundus, and overlapping cases: molecular characterization through the study of 208 genes. *Leuk Lymphoma* 2021; 62: 2130–40.
84. Massone C, Chott A, Metze D, et al. Subcutaneous, blastic natural killer (NK), NK/T-cell, and other cytotoxic lymphomas of the skin: a morphologic, immunophenotypic, and molecular study of 50 patients. *Am J Surg Pathol* 2004; 28: 719–35.
85. Hoque SR, Child FJ, Whittaker SJ, et al. Subcutaneous panniculitis-like T-cell lymphoma: a clinicopathological, immunophenotypic and molecular analysis of six patients. *Br J Dermatol* 2003; 148: 516–25.
86. Go RS, Wester SM. Immunophenotypic and molecular features, clinical outcomes, treatments, and prognostic factors associated with subcutaneous panniculitis-like T-cell lymphoma: a systematic analysis of 156 patients reported in the literature. *Cancer* 2004; 101: 1404–13.
87. Garcia-Herrera A, Song JY, Chuang SS, et al. Nonhepatosplenic gamma-delta T-cell lymphomas represent a spectrum of aggressive cytotoxic T-cell lymphomas with a mainly extranodal presentation. *Am J Surg Pathol* 2011; 35: 1214–25.
88. Kempf W, Kazakov D V., Kutzner H. Lobular panniculitis due to Borrelia burgdorferi infection mimicking subcutaneous panniculitis-like T-cell lymphoma. *Am J Dermatopathol* 2013; 35. doi:10.1097/DAD.0b013e31827132cb.
89. Calamaro P, Cerroni L. Intralymphatic proliferation of T-cell lymphoid blasts in the setting of hidradenitis suppurativa. *Am J Dermatopathol* 2016; 38: 536–40.
90. Baum CL, Stone MS, Liu V. Atypical intravascular CD30+ T-cell proliferation following trauma in a healthy 17-year-old male: first reported case of a potential diagnostic pitfall and literature review. *J Cutan Pathol* 2009; 36: 350–4.
91. Ardighieri L, Lonardi S, Vermi W, et al. Intralymphatic atypical T-cell proliferation in a cutaneous hemangioma. *J Cutan Pathol* 2010; 37: 497–503.
92. Riveiro-Falkenbach E, Fernández-Figueras MT, Luis Rodríguez-Peralto J. Benign atypical intravascular CD30 + T-cell proliferation: a reactive condition mimicking intravascular lymphoma. *Am J Dermatopathol* 2013; 35: 143–50.
93. Samols MA, Su A, Ra S, et al. Intralymphatic cutaneous anaplastic large cell lymphoma/lymphomatoid papulosis expanding the spectrum of CD30-positive lymphoproliferative disorders. *Am J Surg Pathol* 2014; 38: 1203–11.
94. Kempf W, Keller K, John H, et al. Benign atypical intravascular CD30+ T-cell proliferation: a recently described reactive lymphoproliferative process and simulator of intravascular

lymphoma: report of a Case Associated with Lichen Sclerosus and Review of the Literature. *Am J Clin Pathol* 2014; 142: 694–9.

95. Jang NR, Kim MK, Shin DH, et al. Benign atypical intralymphatic CD30+ T-Cell proliferation: a case report and literature review. *Ann Dermatol*; 2019; 31: 108–10.
96. Weingertner N, Mitcov M, Chenard MP, et al. Intralymphatic CD30+ T-cell proliferation during DRESS: a mimic of intravascular lymphoma. *J Cutan Pathol* 2016; 43: 1036–40.
97. Ferrisse TM, Almeida LY, Silveira HA, et al. Benign atypical intralymphatic CD30+ lymphoid proliferation with activated regulatory T-cell phenotype in the oral cavity. *J Cutan Pathol* 2019; 46: 891–4.
98. Ramsay B, Dahl M, Malcolm A. Acral pseudolymphomatous angiokeratoma of children. *Arch Dermatol* 1990; 126: 1524–5.
99. Dayrit JF, Wang WL, Goh SGN, et al. T-cell-rich angiomatoid polypoid pseudolymphoma of the skin: a clinicopathologic study of 17 cases and a proposed nomenclature. *J Cutan Pathol* 2011; 38: 475–82.
100. Mitteldorf C, Palmedo G, Kutzner H, et al. Diagnostic approach in lymphoplasmacytic plaque. *J Eur Acad Dermatol Venereol*; 2015; 29: 2206–15.
101. Lin W, Lu S, Chen H, et al. Clinical characteristics of immunoglobulin G4-related disease: a prospective study of 118 Chinese patients. *Rheumatology (United Kingdom)* 2015; 54: 1982–90.
102. Deshpande V, Zen Y, Chan JKC, et al. Consensus statement on the pathology of IgG4-related disease. *Mod Pathol* 2012; 25: 1181–92.
103. Deng C, Li W, Chen S, et al. Histopathological diagnostic value of the IgG4 +/IgG + ratio of plasmacytic infiltration for IgG4-related diseases. *Medicine (United States)* 2015; 94: e579.
104. Sato Y, Takeuchi M, Takata K, et al. Clinicopathologic analysis of IgG4-related skin disease. *Mod Pathol* 2013; 26: 523–32.
105. Cheuk W, Lee KC, Chong LY, Yuen ST, Chan JKC. IgG4-related sclerosing disease: a potential new etiology of cutaneous pseudolymphoma. *Am J Surg Pathol* 2009; 33: 1713–19.
106. Hattori T, Miyanaga T, Tago O, et al. Isolated cutaneous manifestation of IgG4-related disease. *J Clin Pathol* 2012; 65: 815–18.
107. Tokura Y, Yagi H, Yanaguchi H, et al. IgG4-related skin disease. *Br J Dermatol* 2014; 171: 959–67.
108. Skopec Z, Alsawas M, Maxwell T, et al. Assessment of specificity of dermatopathologic criteria for IgG4-related skin disease. *J Cutan Pathol* 2024; 51: 163–9.
109. Aggarwal N, Parwani A V, Ho J, Cook JR, Swerdlow SH. Plasma cell (Zoon) balanitis: another inflammatory disorder that can be rich in IgG4 + plasma cells. *Am J Surg Pathol* 2014; 38: 1437–43.
110. Lehman JS, Smyrk TC, Pittelkow MR. Increased immunoglobulin (Ig) G4-positive plasma cell density and IgG4/IgG ratio are not specific for IgG4-related disease in the skin. *Am J Clin Pathol* 2014; 141: 234–8.
111. Walsh NM, Kutzner H, Requena L, et al. Plasmacytic cutaneous pathology: a review. *J Cutan Pathol* 2019; 46: 698–708.
112. Takeuchi M, Sato Y, Takata K, et al. Cutaneous multicentric Castleman's disease mimicking IgG4-related disease. *Pathol Res Pract* 2012; 208: 746–9.
113. Han XD, Lee SSJ, Tan SH, et al. Cutaneous plasmacytosis: a clinicopathologic study of a series of cases and their treatment outcomes. *Am J Dermatopathol* 2018; 40: 36–42.
114. Quintanilla-Martinez L, Fend F. Deciphering hydroa vacciniforme. *Blood* 2019; 133: 2735–7.
115. Montes-Mojarro IA, Kim WY, Fend F, et al. Epstein-Barr virus positive T and NK-cell lymphoproliferations: morphological features and differential diagnosis. *Semin Diagn Pathol* 2020; 37: 32–46.
116. Yamada M, Ishikawa Y, Imadome KI. Hypersensitivity to mosquito bites: a versatile Epstein–Barr virus disease with allergy, inflammation, and malignancy. *Allergol Int* 2021; 70: 430–8.
117. Tokura Y, Ishihara S, Tagawa S, et al. Hypersensitivity to mosquito bites as the primary clinical manifestation of a juvenile type of Epstein-Barr virus-associated natural killer cell leukemia/lymphoma. *J Am Acad Dermatol* 2001; 45: 569–78.
118. Asada H. Hypersensitivity to mosquito bites: a unique pathogenic mechanism linking Epstein-Barr virus infection, allergy and oncogenesis. *J Dermatol Sci* 2007; 45: 153–60.
119. Kanno H, Onodera H, Endo M, et al. Vascular lesion in a patient of chronic active Epstein-Barr virus infection with hypersensitivity to mosquito bites: vasculitis induced by mosquito bite with the infiltration of nonneoplastic Epstein-Barr virus-positive cells and subsequent development of natural killer/T-cell lymphoma with angiodestruction. *Hum Pathol* 2005; 36: 212–18.
120. Ishihara S, Ohshima K, Tokura Y, et al. Hypersensitivity to mosquito bites conceals clonal lymphoproliferation of Epstein-Barr viral DNA-positive natural killer cells. *Jpn J Cancer Res* 1997; 88: 82–7.
121. Cohen JI, Manoli I, Dowdell K, et al. Hydroa vacciniforme-like lymphoproliferative disorder: an EBV disease with a low risk of systemic illness in whites. *Blood* 2019; 133: 2753–64.
122. Gru AA, Jaffe ES. Cutaneous EBV-related lymphoproliferative disorders. *Semin Diagn Pathol* 2017; 34: 60–75.
123. Quintanilla-Martinez L, Ridaura C, Nagl F, et al. Hydroa vacciniforme-like lymphoma: a chronic EBV+ lymphoproliferative disorder with risk to develop a systemic lymphoma. *Blood* 2013; 122: 3101–10.
124. Iwatsuki K, Satoh M, Yamamoto T, et al. Pathogenic link between hydroa vacciniforme and Epstein-Barr virus-associated hematologic disorders. *Arch Dermatol* 2006; 142: 587–95.
125. Natkunam Y, Goodlad JR, Chadburn A, et al. EBV-Positive B-cell proliferations of varied malignant potential. *Am J Clin Pathol* 2017; 147: 129–52.
126. Ikeda T, Gion Y, Nishimura Y, et al. Epstein–barr virus-positive mucocutaneous ulcer: a unique and curious disease entity. *Int J Mol Sci* 2021; 22: 1–14.
127. Dojcinov SD, Venkataraman G, Raffeld M, et al. EBV positive mucocutaneous ulcer-A study of 26 cases associated with various sources of immunosuppression. *Ame J Surg Pathol* 2010; 34: 405–17.
128. Sweet R. An acute febrile neutrophilic dermatosis. *Br J Dermatol* 1964; 76: 349–56.
129. Heath MS, Ortega-Loayza AG. Insights into the pathogenesis of Sweet's syndrome. *Front Immunol.* 2019; 10. doi:10.3389/fimmu.2019.00414.
130. Cohen PR. Sweet's syndrome: a comprehensive review of an acute

febrile neutrophilic dermatosis. *Orphanet J Rare Dis*. 2007; 2. doi:10.1186/1750-1172-2-34.

131. Passet M, Lepelletier C, Vignon-Pennamen MD, et al. Next-generation sequencing in myeloid neoplasm-associated Sweet's syndrome demonstrates clonal relation between malignant cells and skin-infiltrating neutrophils. *J Invest Dermatol* 2020; 140: 1873–6. e5. doi: 10.1016/j.jid.2019.12.040

132. Prieto-Torres L, Requena L, Rodríguez-Pinilla SM. Clinical, histopathological and molecular spectrum of cutaneous lesions in myelodysplastic syndrome and myeloproliferative neoplasms (MDS/MPN): an integrative review. *Cancers* 2023; 15. doi:10.3390/cancers15245888.

133. Requena L, Kutzner H, Palmedo G, et al. Histiocytoid Sweet syndrome: a dermal infiltration of immature neutrophilic granulocytes. *Arch Dermatol* 2005; 141: 834–42.

134. Alegría-Landa V, Rodríguez-Pinilla SM, Santos-Briz A, et al. Clinicopathologic, immunohistochemical, and molecular features of histiocytoid sweet syndrome. *JAMA Dermatol* 2017; 153: 651–9.

135. Delaleu J, Kim R, Zhao LP, et al. Clinical, pathological, and molecular features of myelodysplasia cutis. *Blood* 2022; 139: 1251–3.

136. Pincus LB, Leboit PE, Mccalmont TH, et al. Subcutaneous panniculitis-like T-cell lymphoma with overlapping clinicopathologic features of lupus erythematosus: coexistence of 2 entities? *Am J Dermatopathol* 2009; 31: 520–6.

137. Shiau CJ, Daoud MSA, Wong SM, et al. Lymphocytic panniculitis: an algorithmic approach to lymphocytes in subcutaneous tissue. *J Clin Pathol* 2015; 68: 954–62.

138. Lozzi GP, Massone C, Citarella L, et al. Rimming of adipocytes by neoplastic lymphocytes: a histopathologic feature not restricted to subcutaneous T-cell lymphoma. *Am J Dermatopathol* 2006; 28: 9–12.

139. Ghoufi L, Ortonne N, Ingen-Housz-Oro S, et al. Histiocytoid Sweet syndrome is more frequently associated with myelodysplastic syndromes than the classical neutrophilic variant. *Medicine* 2016; 95. e3033. doi:10.1097/MD.0000000000003033.

Chapter 6

Cutaneous Lymphoid Neoplasms

Mai P. Hoang and M. Angelica Selim

Introduction

Primary cutaneous lymphomas are comprised of a group of B- and T-cell lymphomas that do not have extracutaneous involvement at the time of diagnosis. They are the second most common group of extranodal lymphomas. Prior to the 1980s only mycosis fungoides was recognized as a cutaneous lymphoma and any other types of lymphoma was thought to be cutaneous involvement of a systemic lymphoma. In 2005 a classification of primary cutaneous lymphomas established jointly by the European Organization for Research and Treatment of Cancer (EORTC) and the World Health Organization (WHO) acknowledged that cutaneous B- and T-cell lymphomas possess distinct clinical presentation and different biologic behavior than their nodal counterparts.[1,2] Despite this awareness among dermatologists and dermatopathologists, these guidelines were not incorporated into the World Health Organization (WHO) classification of tumors of hematopoietic and lymphoid tissues until 2008.[1] The nomenclature of the recent 2018 WHO classification contains some changes concerning cutaneous lymphomas (**Table 6.1**).[3,4] These include the provisional entities cutaneous acral CD8+ lymphoproliferative disorder and cutaneous CD4+ small/medium T-cell lymphoproliferative disorder. In addition, hydroa vacciniforme-like lymphoma is currently classified as hydroa vacciniforme-like lymphoproliferative disorder.

Table 6.1 Differences in the 2008, 2016, and 2018 World Health Organization classifications for some mature T and NK neoplasms[1,3,4]

2008	2016	2018
Indolent CD8+ proliferation of acral sites	Primary cutaneous acral CD8+ T-cell lymphoma (provisional entity)	Primary cutaneous acral CD8+ T-cell lymphoproliferative disorder (provisional entity)
Primary cutaneous CD4+ small/medium T-cell lymphoma (provisional entity)	Primary cutaneous CD4+ small/ medium T-cell lymphoproliferative disorder (provisional entity)	Primary cutaneous CD4+ small/ medium T-cell lymphoproliferative disorder (provisional entity)
Hydroa vacciniforme-like lymphoma	Hydroa vacciniforme-like lymphoproliferative disorder	Hydroa vacciniforme lymphoproliferative disorder

Immunohistochemistry plays an important role in the classification of B- and T-cell lymphoid lesions. A number of immunostains have recently become commercially available. They include lymphoid enhancer-binding factor 1 (LEF1), CD160, and CD200 in diagnosing chronic lymphocytic lymphoma/ small lymphocytic leukemia; sex-determining region Y box 11 (Sox11) for mantle cell lymphoma; human germinal center-associated lymphoma (HGAL), LIM-only transcription factor 2 (LMO2), and germinal center B-cell expressed transcript 1 (GCET1) for follicle center lymphoma; and immunoglobulin superfamily receptor translocation-associated 1 (IRTA1) for marginal zone lymphoma. They can serve as alternative markers in cases without characteristic immunohistochemical staining in defining the cutaneous atypical lymphoid infiltrate.

6.1 Cutaneous B-Cell Lymphomas

Cutaneous B-cell lymphomas include a group of B-cell lymphomas that involve only the skin without extra-cutaneous disease at the time of diagnosis. They are generally classified into three main subgroups: cutaneous marginal zone B-cell lymphoma, cutaneous follicle center lymphoma, and cutaneous large B-cell lymphoma, leg type in the World Health Organization (WHO)-European Organization for Research and Treatment of Cancer (EORTC) joint classification.[1–4] The different subtypes of cutaneous B-cell lymphomas are outlined in **Table 6.2**.

Table 6.2 Subtypes of cutaneous B-cell lymphomas

- Cutaneous marginal zone B-cell lymphoma
- Cutaneous follicle center lymphoma
- Cutaneous diffuse large B-cell lymphoma, leg type
- Cutaneous EBV+ diffuse large B-cell lymphoma
- Intravascular large B-cell lymphoma
- Cutaneous plasmablastic lymphoma
- Cutaneous T-cell/histiocyte-rich B-cell lymphoma

Cutaneous Marginal Zone B-Cell Lymphoma

Primary cutaneous marginal zone B-cell lymphomas (PCMZLs) is a low-grade lymphoma commonly with recurrence but rarely with systemic or bone marrow involvement.[5] Accounting for 35–40% of all cutaneous B-cell lymphomas, PCMZL affects mainly adult males in the fifth or sixth decades.[2] Although the etiology is unknown in majority of cases, chronic antigen stimulation such as tattoos, vaccination sites, and *Borrelia burgdorferi* infection have been proposed as etiologic factors.[6] The prognosis of this lymphoma is excellent, five-year survival of the conventional type is 98%. PCMZLs can present as solitary or multiple violaceous plaques or nodules on the trunk or extremities.

PCMZL is divided into two groups: (1) more common heavy chain class-switched cases (90%, Th2 cytokine background) and (2) less common IgM-positive cases (10%, Th1 cytokine background) which often express IgG4.[7] Peripherally located monotypic plasma cells are seen in heavy chain class-switched cases in comparison to scattered plasma cells in non-class switched cases.[8] The heavy chain class-switched PCMZL have frequent relapses but without extracutaneous spread and 99–100% five-year disease-specific survival.[8]

PCMZL typically involves the dermis in a nodular growth pattern with reactive germinal centers noted (**Figures 6.1 and 6.2**). PCMZL is characterized by dense dermal infiltrate of lymphoid cells often with scattered germinal center below an uninvolved epidermis. The tumor cells are small- to medium-sized with indented nuclei and pale cytoplasm. They are CD20+, CD79a+, Bcl2+, Bcl6-, CD5-, and CD10- (**Figures 6.3–6.6**).[9,10] Commonly, aggregates of plasma cells are seen at the periphery of the tumor exhibiting monotypic light chain expression in 75% of cases (**Figures 6.7 and 6.8**).[9] A light chain ratio of 5:1 to 10:1 would be considered by most to be monotypic. The plasma cells of PCMZL often express IgG4.[11] Reactive T-cells can be prominent in the class-switched cases.[12] IgM-positive cases have features similar to other non-cutaneous MALT lymphomas including greater proportion of neoplastic B-cells and frequent CXCR4 expression.[8] Clusters of CD123+ plasmacytoid dendritic cells can be seen at the periphery of the lesion.[13] PCMZL, but not other low grade B-cell lymphomas, show reactivity with immunoglobulin receptor translocation associated 1 (IRTA1); however, this antibody currently is not widely used in clinical laboratories.[14] CD21, a marker of follicular dendritic cells (FDC), often highlights an expanded follicular dendritic meshwork due to colonized neoplastic marginal zone or plasmacytoid cells admixed with reactive follicular cells.[9] This pattern of CD21 staining, highlighting the colonized germinal centers with distorted architecture, can be helpful in establishing the diagnosis of PCMZL.

The differential diagnosis of PCMZL includes cutaneous lymphoid hyperplasia/pseudolymphomatous folliculitis, IgG4-related sclerosing disease, primary cutaneous follicle center lymphoma, and cutaneous involvement by a non-cutaneous MZL. The presence of Bcl2+, Bcl6-, and CD10- infiltrating lymphocytes strongly supports the diagnosis of PCMZL over PCFCL

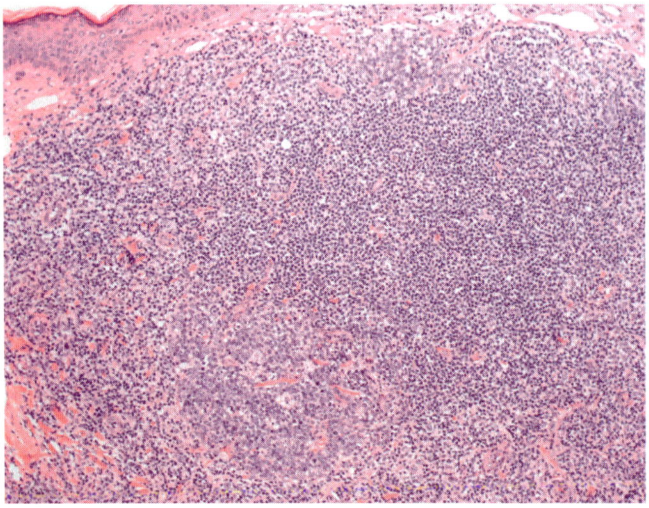

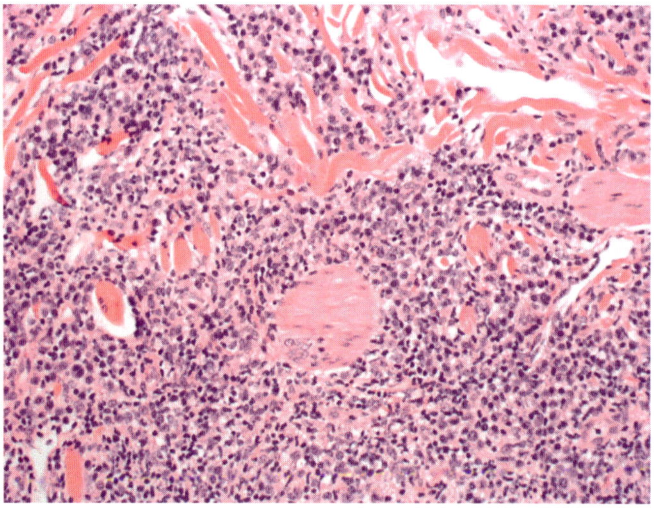

Figures 6.1 and 6.2 A nodular lymphoid infiltrate with prominent plasma cells is seen in the dermis in cutaneous marginal zone B-cell lymphoma (X100 and X200).

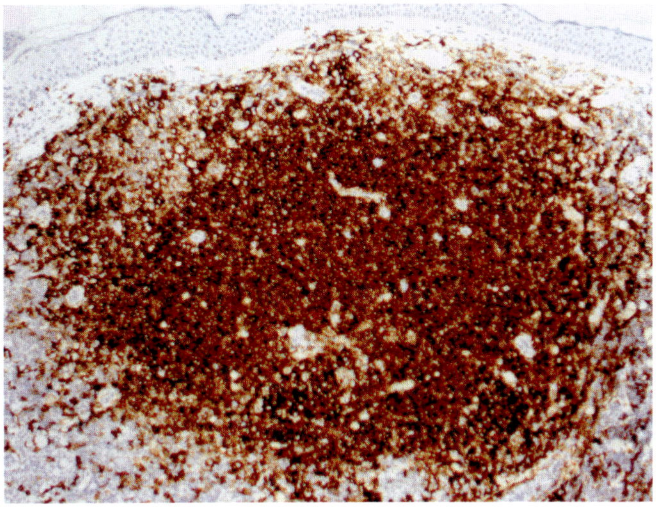

Figure 6.3 Cutaneous marginal zone B-cell lymphoma. The lymphoid nodule is positive for CD20 (X200).

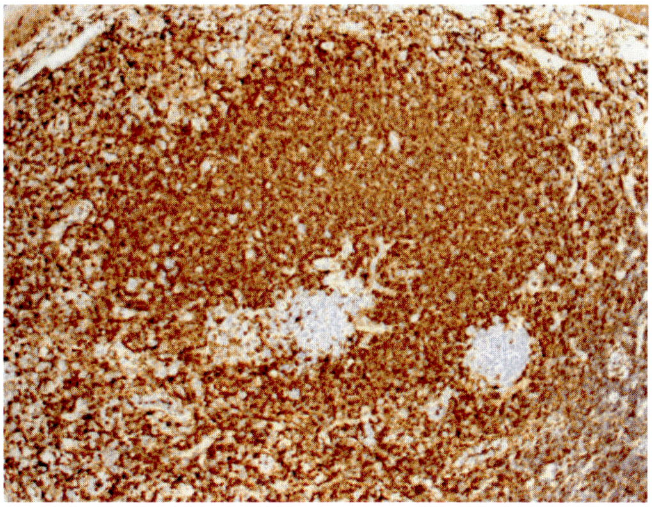

Figure 6.4 Cutaneous marginal zone B-cell lymphoma. Bcl2 highlights the neoplastic cells as well as the reactive T-lymphocytes (X200).

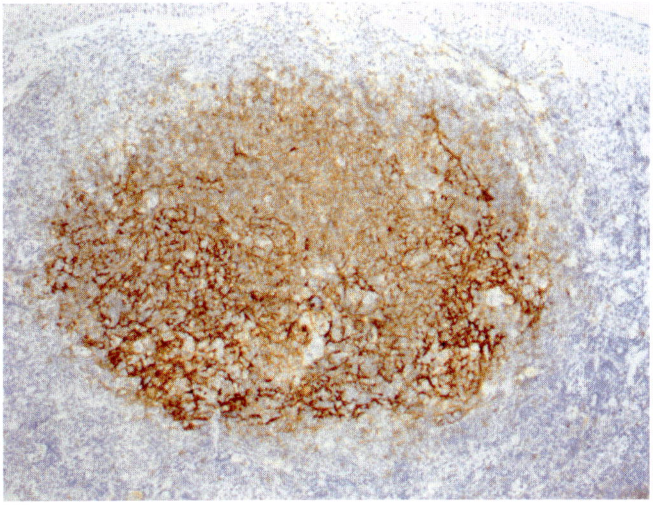

Figure 6.5 Cutaneous marginal zone B-cell lymphoma. CD21 demonstrates an expanded dendritic meshwork (X200).

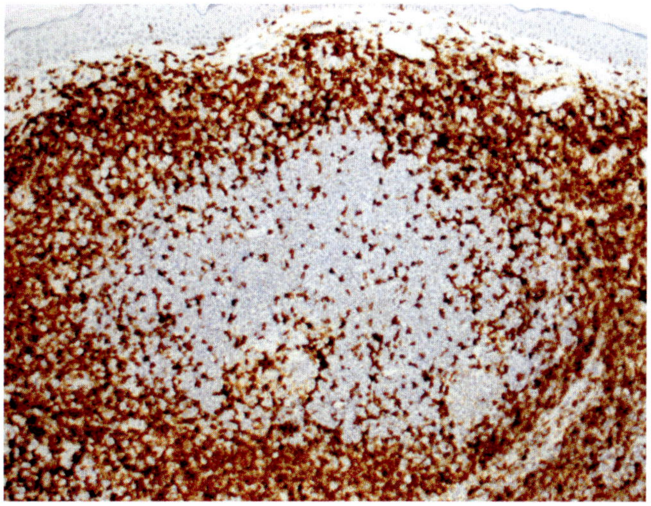

Figure 6.6 Cutaneous marginal zone B-cell lymphoma. CD3 highlights only the reactive T-lymphocytes (X200).

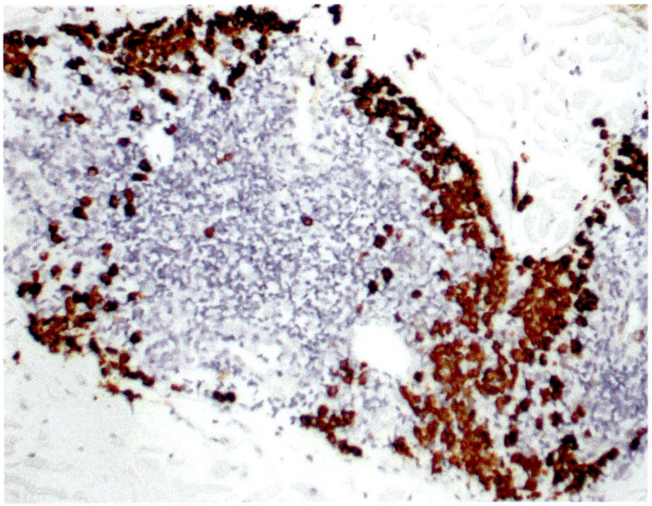

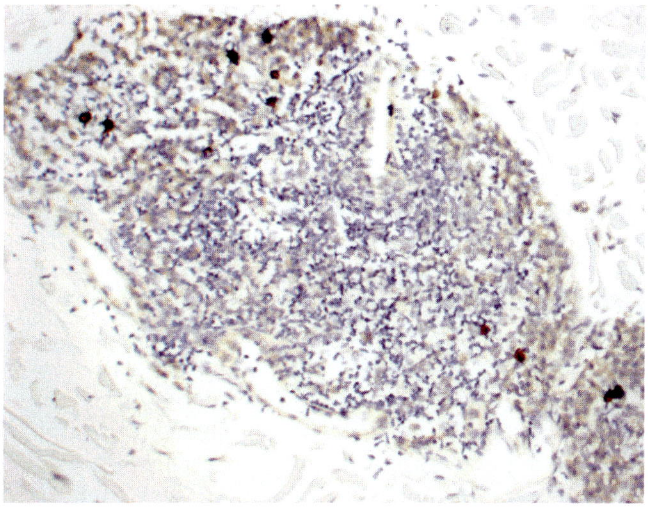

Figures 6.7 and 6.8 Cutaneous marginal zone B-cell lymphoma. Lambda and kappa *in situ* hybridization demonstrate lambda light chain restriction (X200).

or reactive lymphoid hyperplasia;[15] however, one must be aware that reactive interfollicular T-cells can also demonstrate this pattern of staining. PCMZL is often associated with reactive follicles showing the CD10+ Bcl2- Bcl6+ immunophenotype which may represent a diagnostic pitfall if is not recognized.[9,15] In contrast to cells of PCFCLs, cells of PCMZL are CD5-, CD10-, and Bcl6-.[15] PCMZL express IgG4 in 39% of cases in contrast to less than 1% in non-cutaneous MZL.[11] PCMZL more often express IgG, IgA, or IgE in contrast to IgM in non-cutaneous MZL.[11] Clonal Ig heavy and light chain gene rearrangements are supportive of PCMZL.

As discussed in **Chapter 5**, a panel of CD3, CD20, Bcl2, Bcl6, CD21, kappa, and lambda light chain would be helpful in the differential diagnosis of reactive lymphoid hyperplasia versus a low-grade B-cell lymphoma.

Cutaneous marginal zone B-cell lymphoma

- CD20+, CD79a+, Bcl2+, and monotypic light chain
- Bcl6-, CD5-, and CD10-
- CD21 highlighting the colonized germinal centers with distorted architecture

Cutaneous Follicle Center Lymphoma

Primary cutaneous follicle center lymphoma (PCFCL) consists of a neoplastic proliferation of germinal center cells confined to the skin associated with excellent prognosis. PCFCL is comprised of 50% of cutaneous B-cell lymphomas and 10% of all primary cutaneous lymphomas.[2] Cutaneous relapses can be seen in a third of the patients; however, the prognosis of PCFCL is excellent with a five-year survival of 95%.[2,16] Solitary or grouped papules, plaques and tumors typically present on the scalp, forehead or trunk.[2] Leg lesions are seen in 5% and multiple lesions in 15%.[2] However, PCFCL with diffuse pattern affecting the leg may have a less favorable behavior than those arising on the head and neck areas.[2] Plaques of tumors surrounded by erythematous macules and papules is a distinct clinical presentation also called in the past as "Crosti's lymphoma." Miliary and agminated-type and macular lesions on the head have been reported.[17,18]

PCFCL characteristically appears as a nodular to diffuse lymphoid proliferation in the dermis and subcutaneous tissue with neoplastic follicle center B-cells (**Figure 6.9**). The tumor is consisted of proliferation of small, medium and large cleaved cells (centrocytes) admixed with variable number of large and round cells with 1–3 peripheral nucleoli (centroblasts) in a follicular and/or diffuse pattern (**Figure 6.10**).[1] The follicular growth pattern is characterized by monomorphic neoplastic follicles due to the absence of light and dark areas, reduction of the mantle zone, and rarity or absence of tingible body macrophages. In the diffuse growth pattern, uniform proliferation of large centrocytes and admixed centroblasts is seen. A rare presentation of PCFCL with predominance of spindle and bizarre cells is called "cutaneous spindle cell B-cell lymphoma," with centrocytes acquiring different size and shapes.[19]

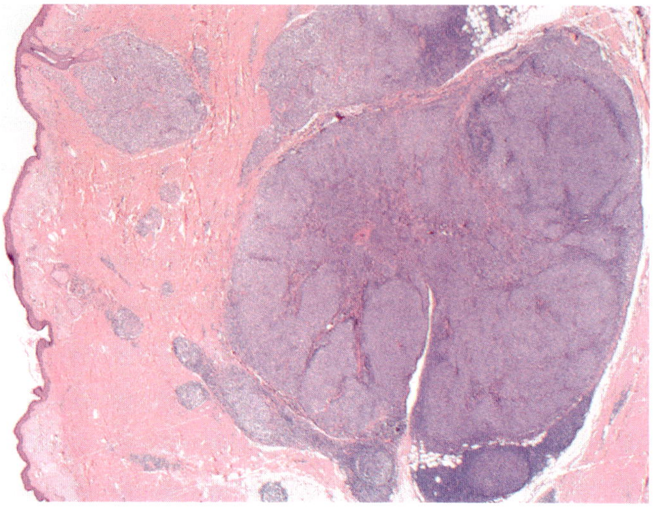

Figure 6.9 A nodular lymphoid proliferation is seen in the dermis in this example of cutaneous follicle center lymphoma (X20).

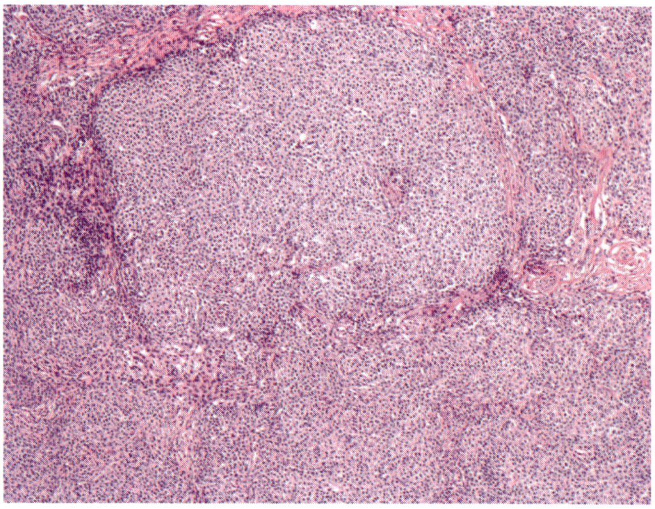

Figure 6.10 Cutaneous follicle center lymphoma. A mixture of centrocytes and variable number of centroblasts is seen in a follicular pattern (X100).

The tumor cells are CD20+, CD79a+, Bcl6+, CD10+/-, Bcl2-, and Ig- (**Figures 6.11 and 6.12**).[10,15] CD10 is frequently lost in the diffuse form of this lymphoma. Although Bcl2 is absent in the majority of PCFCLs, in 10–25% of the cases Bcl2 and MUM1/IRF4 can be detected.[20] The Bcl2 expression may represent the presence of 1p36 deletion or *BCL2* translocation.[21] The neoplastic follicles of PCFCL often show less than 50% positivity for Ki-67; however, greater than 90% of the reactive follicle cells are Ki-67 positive.[10] In PCFCL with a prominent nodular arrangement, CD21+ follicular dendritic cells are present as a sharply-defined and thick rim surrounding neoplastic follicles.[9,10] This CD21+ follicular dendritic cell meshwork is likely absent in the cases with diffuse growth pattern. The presence of small clusters of CD10+ and Bcl6+ neoplastic follicular cells in the interfollicular area is called "migration." This event is not commonly seen in reactive lymphoid hyperplasia. Kappa and lambda light chain stains might demonstrate monotypic light chain expression.

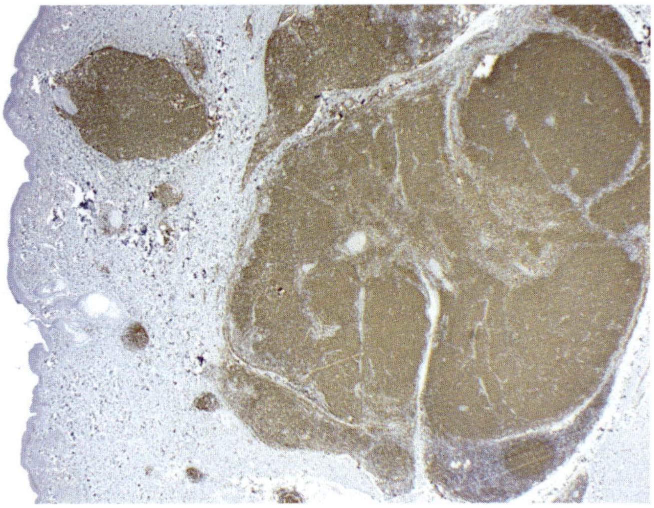

Figure 6.11 Cutaneous follicle center lymphoma. The tumor cells express CD20 (X20).

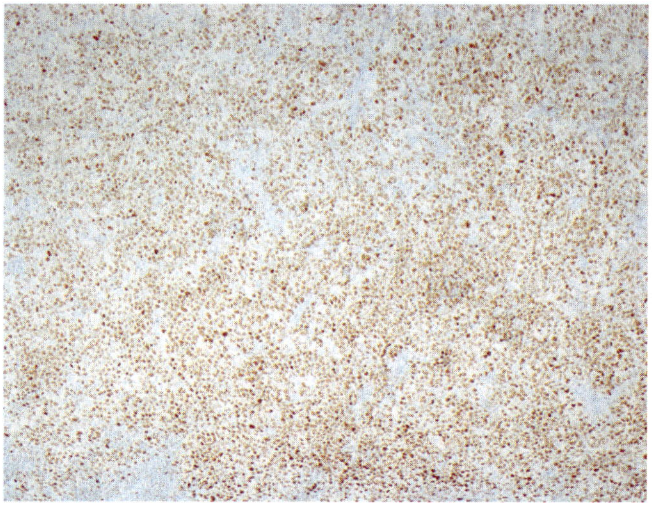

Figure 6.12 Cutaneous follicle center lymphoma. They are positive for Bcl6 (X100).

While the neoplastic cells of PCFCL are typically Bcl2- in contrast to the Bcl2 positivity demonstrated by nodal follicular lymphoma which harbor the t(14;18) translocation.[9,15] Strong and diffuse Bcl2 and CD10 expression is typically seen in cutaneous involvement by nodal follicular lymphoma. The absence of reactivity to Bcl2, IgM, p63, and MUM1 can differentiate diffuse PCFCL from cutaneous diffuse large B-cell lymphoma, leg type.[22,23] A panel of CD20, Bcl2, Bcl6, MUM1, and IgM is helpful in the distinction of diffuse PCFCL from cutaneous diffuse large B-cell lymphoma, leg type. Of note, classically the neoplastic follicle center cells are typically positive for the B-cell marker CD20. However, recurrent lymphoma after treatment with anti-CD20 monoclonal antibody (rituximab) may no longer express CD20[24]; therefore, other B-cell-associated markers such as CD79a, CD19, and PAX5 would be helpful in this setting. Rarely diffuse CD30 expression can be seen in PCFCL.[25]

Cutaneous follicle center lymphoma

- CD20+, CD79a+, PAX5+, Bcl6+, CD10+/-
- IgM-, MUM1-, Bcl2-, p63- and reduced Ki–67 proliferation index
- Loss of CD20 expression after rituximab (anti-CD20) therapy
- Bcl2 expression raises the possibility of skin involvement by nodal follicular lymphoma; however, this does not rule out primary cutaneous follicle center lymphoma
- Negative Bcl–2, MUM1, and IgM differentiates PCFCL from diffuse large B-cell lymphoma, leg type

Cutaneous Diffuse Large B-Cell Lymphoma, Leg Type

Primary cutaneous large B-cell lymphoma, leg type (PCLBCL-LT) comprises 10–20% of cutaneous B-cell lymphomas and 3–4% of all primary cutaneous lymphoma.[2] PCLBCL-LT often present as rapidly growing and ulcerated, red or bluish-red tumors on one or both lower legs of elderly women with a median age of 75 years.[26] 10–25% of cases can arise in the trunk or upper extremities.[16,27] PCLBCL-LT has an estimated disease-specific five-year survival of 40–50%. Relapses are frequent with extracutaneous spread occurring a few years after diagnosis despite treatment.[16,26,27]

A diffuse proliferation of uniform and large centroblasts or immunoblasts is seen in the dermis and frequently in the subcutaneous tissue (**Figure 6.13**). Background reactive T-cells are sparse. The neoplastic B cells are typically CD20+, CD79a+, Bcl2+, MUM1+, PAX5+, Bcl6+, Fox-P1+, MYC+. IgM+, CD10-, and with high Ki-67 proliferation index (**Figures 6.14 and 6.15**).[28] The main differential diagnosis of PCLBCL-LT is the diffuse variant of PCFCL. Bcl2 strong expression and higher expression of transcription factors multiple myeloma-1/interferon regulatory factor 4 (*MUM1/IRF4*) are seen in PCDLBL in comparison to PCFCL.[28] However, Bcl2 expression can be negative in 10% of PCLBCL cases. Recently, IgM has been reported as an additional marker in the distinction of PCDLBC from PCFCL.[22] In the study by Koens and colleagues,[22] IgM expression was seen in all 40 PCBCL-LT in contrast to only 5 of 53 PCFCL (**Figure 6.16**). Recently p63 expression was demonstrated in the majority of PCBCL-LT while only in few cases of PCFCL.[23] PCLBCL-LT typically lacks follicular dendritic cell network. Cutaneous involvement of systemic large B-cell lymphomas and transformed lymphomas are also in the differential diagnosis. Expression of EBER would exclude EBV-positive lymphoproliferative disorders and plasmablastic lymphomas.[29] Highly recurrent mutations (>40%) involving *MYD88*, *PIM1*, and *CD79B* have been reported in PCBCL-LT.[30] In challenging cases, the presence of *MYD88* and/or *CD79B* is supportive of PCBCL-LT.[30]

Primary cutaneous large B-cell lymphoma, leg type

- CD20+, CD79a+, PAX5+, Bcl6+, IgM+, Bcl2+, MUM1+, p63+
- CD10-
- Bcl2+, MUM1+, IgM+: helpful in distinguishing PCBCL-LT from PCFCL

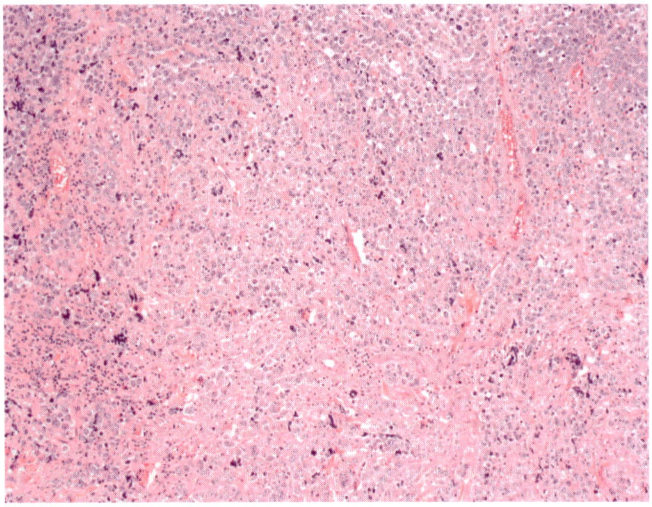

Figure 6.13 A diffuse proliferation of large lymphoid cells is seen in the dermis in cutaneous diffuse large B-cell lymphoma (X100).

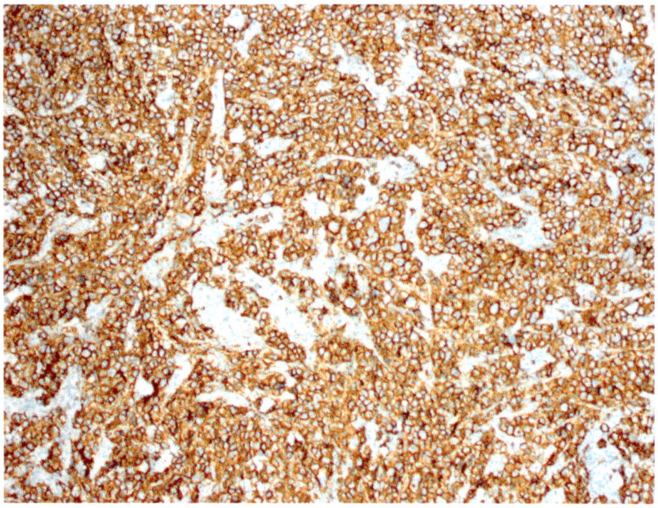

Figure 6.14 Cutaneous diffuse large B-cell lymphoma. The tumor cells are strongly positive for CD20 (X100).

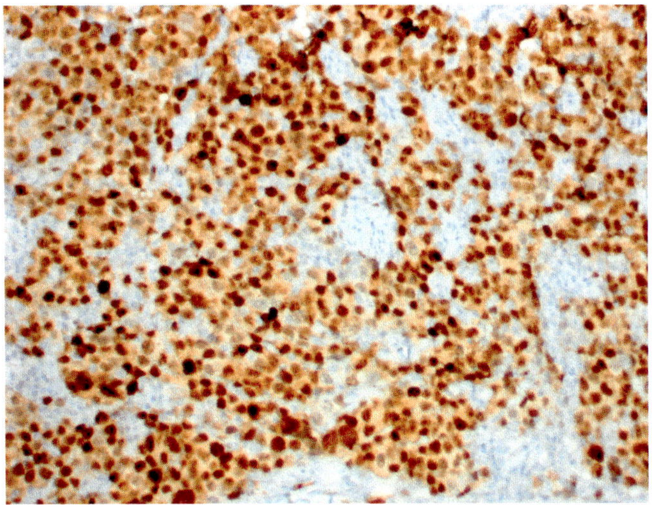

Figure 6.15 Cutaneous diffuse large B-cell lymphoma. Diffuse nuclear MUM1 expression is noted (X200).

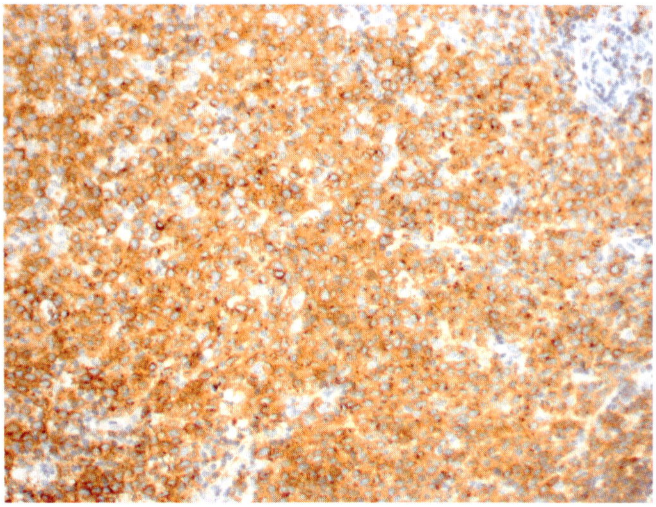

Figure 6.16 Cutaneous diffuse large B-cell lymphoma. They are positive for IgM (X200).

Intravascular Large B-Cell Lymphoma

Intravascular B-cell lymphoma (IVBL), characterized by large neoplastic B-cells within lumina of small to medium-sized blood vessels, is a rare subtype of B-cell lymphoma with poor prognosis. This lymphoma subtype can involve any organ but not typically the lymph nodes. IVBL exhibits three subtypes: (1) the "classical"/Western variant which affecting skin and central nervous system, (2) the hemophagocytic syndrome-associated form /Asian variant which involving multiple organs, associated with hemophagocytic lymphohistiocytosis,[31] and (3) isolated cutaneous form which is associated with better prognosis attributing to timely diagnosis.[32] A leukemic phase of the disease has rarely been reported.[33]

The incidence of IVBL was reported by SEER data to be 0.095 (case/1,000,000) in 2000–2013.[34] The median age at diagnosis was 70 years. The median three-year and five-year overall survival rates were 51.8% and 46.3%, respectively.[34] On multivariate analyses older age, higher stage, and male gender correlated with worse overall survival.[34]

In a meta-analysis of over 300 cases, Han et al.[35] reported the ages of the patients ranging from 32 to 92 years (median 67) and with no gender predilection. The clinical presentation is variable including cutaneous lesions, B-symptoms (fever, night sweats, and weight loss), anemia, thrombocytopenia, hypoxemia, impaired consciousness, very low serum albumin level, high serum lactate dehydrogenase (LDH), soluble interleukin-2 receptor (sIL2 R), and ferritin.[35] Hemophagocytosis has been reported predominantly in the Asian population.

Cutaneous involvement occurs in approximately half of the "classical" form including maculopapular eruption, violaceous plaques, nodules, purpura, and ulcers.[36] Biopsy hemangiomas has been shown to increase the likelihood of capturing the involved vessels.[37] While cutaneous involvement can be seen up to 39% of the classic variant, it is seen in only 5% of the hemophagocytic syndrome-associated variant. In contrast, bone marrow involvement is seen in 75% of the hemophagocytic syndrome-associated variant versus 32% of the classic variant.[38]

Random biopsy of normal skin and capillary hemangioma has been shown to be a good diagnostic approach.[37] A scoring system based on three laboratory results (LDH > 256IU/L, serum sIL-2 R > 2011U/mL, and platelet count < 107 x109/L) has been shown to correlate with IVBL: 18% and 86% for score 2 and 3, respectively.[39]

On histologic sections large pleomorphic tumor cells with vesicular nuclei and prominent nucleoli distend the intravascular spaces of capillaries and small venules in the dermis and often the subcutaneous tissue (**Figure 6.17**). In the hemophagocytic variant, histiocytes with hemophagocytosis are seen in biopsies from liver, spleen, and bone marrow. Histologic sections show the tumor cells expressing CD20 (**Figure 6.18**), CD79a, Pax5, MUM1, and Bcl6 (22–52% in contrast to 5% of DLBCL); Bcl2, CD5, and CD10 (13%) in a subset; 20–100% Ki67 proliferation index. CD3 is negative.[33] There is variable expression of CD5 and the tumor cells are typically negative for EBV.[40] The differential diagnosis includes intravascular NK/T-cell lymphoma and KSHV/HHV8+.[41]

Intravascular large B-cell lymphoma

- CD20+, CD79a+, Bcl2+, MUM1+, CD5+/-
- CD3-, Bcl6-, CD10-, EBER-

Cutaneous T-Cell/Histiocyte-Rich Large B-Cell Lymphoma

T-cell/histiocyte-rich B-cell lymphoma is a rare variant of B-cell lymphoma that typically presents clinically as solitary lesions on the head, trunk or extremities. The lesion is comprised of neoplastic B-cells and greater than 90% by reactive T-cells and/or histiocytes. Primary cutaneous cases are rare.[42] The disease commonly presents at diagnosis as advanced systemic disease with spleen, liver, and bone marrow diagnosis.[43] The neoplastic B-cells are CD20+, CD79a+, Bcl6+, CD30-, and EBER-; while the background reactive T-lymphocytes are CD3+, CD4+, and CD8- (**Figures 6.19–6.22**).[42,44]

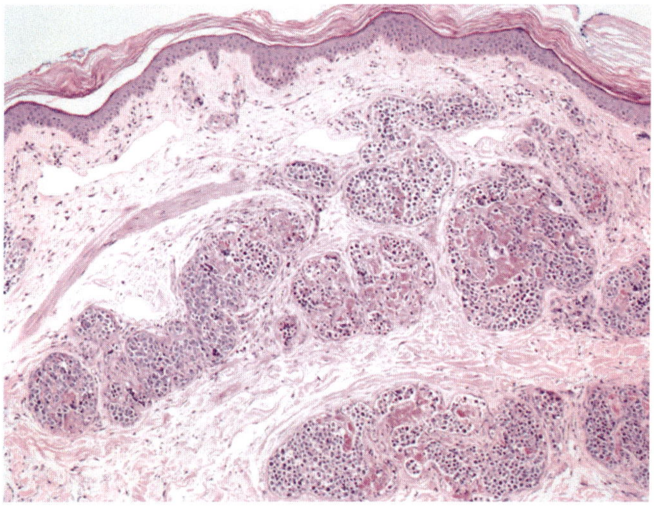

Figure 6.17 Large tumor cells are present within the vascular spaces in the dermis in intravascular large B-cell lymphoma (X100).

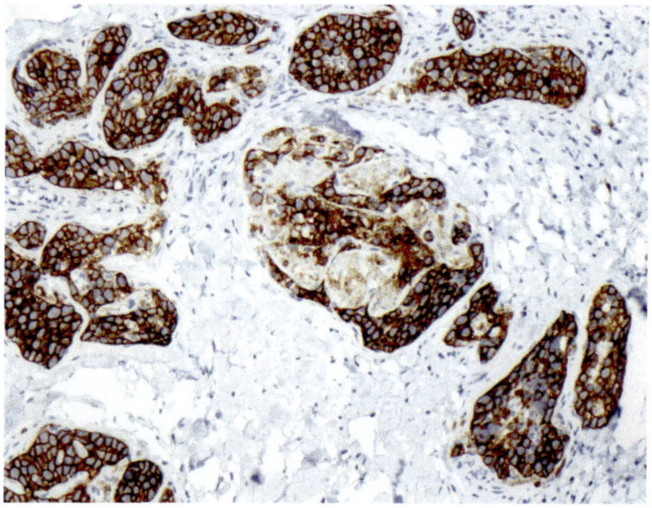

Figure 6.18 *Intravascular large B-cell lymphoma*. The tumor cells are strongly positive for CD20 (X200).

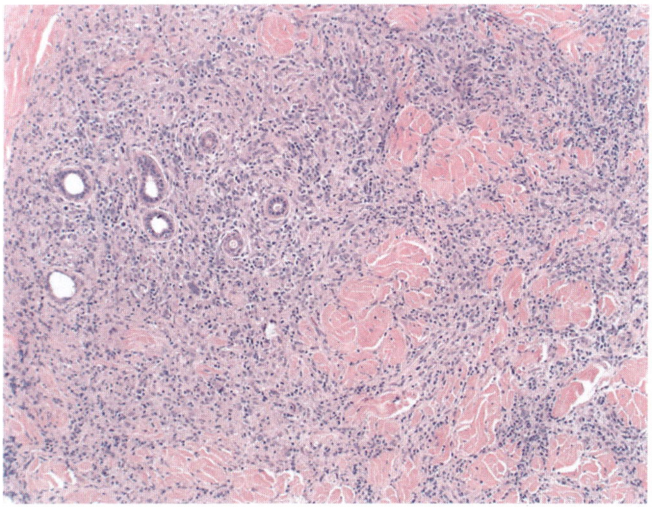

Figure 6.19 A dense infiltrate of small to large cells is seen in the dermis in cutaneous T-cell/histiocyte-rich B-cell lymphoma (X100).

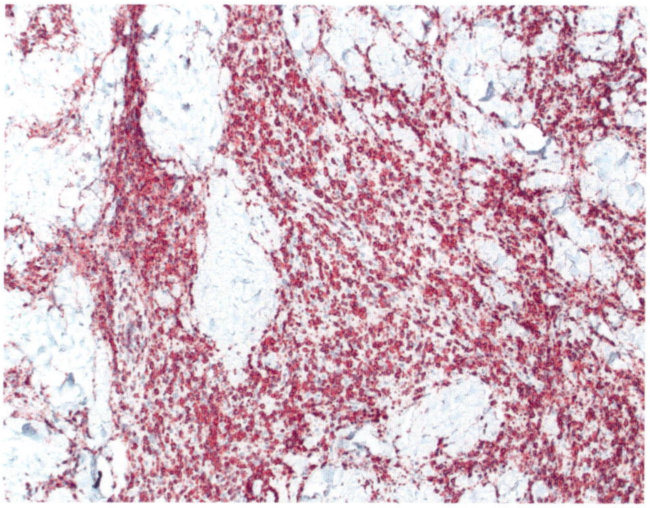

Figure 6.20 Cutaneous T-cell/histiocyte-rich B-cell lymphoma. CD163 decorates an exuberant histiocytic infiltrate (X100).

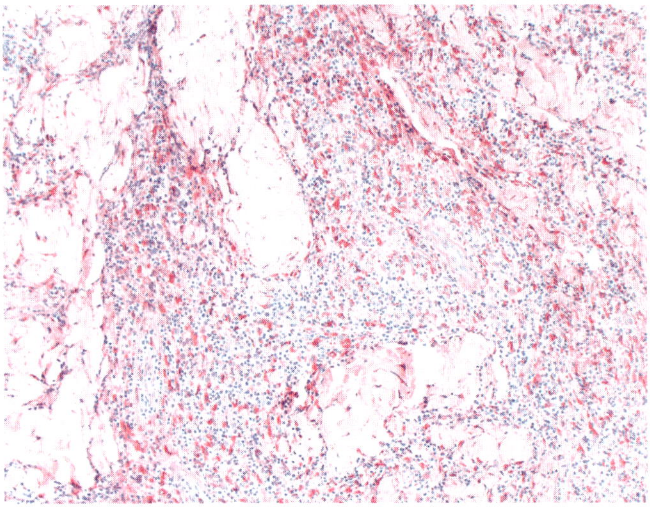

Figure 6.21 Cutaneous T-cell/histiocyte-rich B-cell lymphoma. A small population of reactive T-cell lymphocytes is decorated by CD3 (X100).

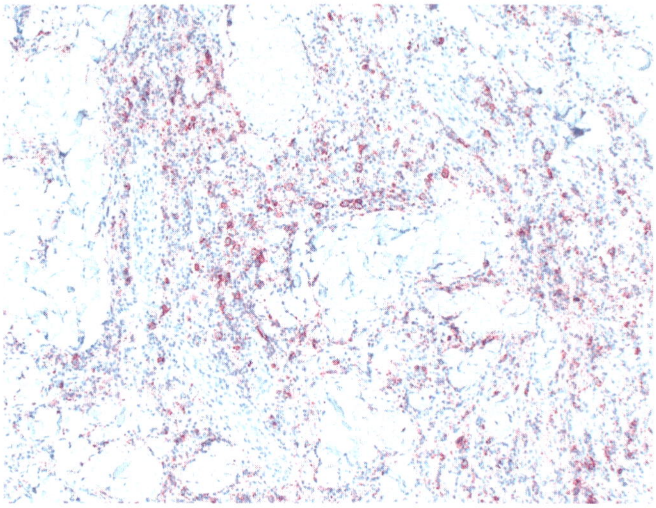

Figures 6.22 Cutaneous T-cell/histiocyte-rich B-cell lymphoma. The large cells in the infiltrate are CD20 positive (X100).

Cutaneous T-cell/histiocyte-rich B-cell lymphoma

- Neoplastic cells: CD20+, CD79a+, Bcl6+, CD30-, EBER-
- Reactive lymphocytes: CD3+, CD4+, CD8-

6.2 Cutaneous Involvement by Extracutaneous B-Cell Lymphoma

Cutaneous EBV+ Diffuse Large B-Cell Lymphoma

Epstein Barr virus (EBV)-positive diffuse large B-cell lymphoma is a distinct entity from EBV-positive lymphoproliferative disorders and lymphomas in the setting of in-born or acquired immune deficiency. EBV-positive DLBCL is more common in Asia, Africa, and Latin America than in Western countries.[45] This type of diffuse large B-cell lymphoma is EBV-associated, involves immunocompetent individuals older than 50 years without prior history of lymphoma.[46] This is a very aggressive lymphoma with a median survival of approximately 2 years. Although the lymph nodes and internal organs are more commonly involved in patients younger than 45 years, cutaneous cases have been reported.[46,47]

The histologic appearance can be either polymorphic showing a mixture of Reed-Sternberg-like cells, immunoblasts, and plasmablasts; or monomorphic with mainly immunoblasts (**Figures 6.23 and 6.24**).[46,48] Large immunoblasts and Reed-Sternberg cells are seen in a background of lymphocytes, plasma cells, and histiocytes in the polymorphic type. On the other hand, diffuse infiltrate of large and atypical lymphoid cells is seen in the monomorphic type, indistinguishable from EBV-negative DLBCL. Angiocentric growth pattern and geographic necrosis can be seen in some cases. While expressing CD79a, PAX5, BOB1, and OCT2, EBV+ diffuse large B-cell lymphoma may show loss of CD20 expression. EBER, LMP1, CD30, and MUM1 are invariably positive (**Figures 6.25– 6.28**).[46–48] Most cases express EBV-LMP1 and only a subset expresses EBNA2.[49] While Reed-Sternberg cells of classic Hodgkin lymphoma express CD200, the tumor cells of EBV-positive diffuse large B-cell lymphoma are negative.[50] The differential diagnosis includes EBV-positive mucocutaneous ulcer and lymphomatoid granulomatosis.

Cutaneous EBV+ diffuse large B-cell lymphoma

- EBER+, LMP1+, CD79a+, PAX5+, MUM1+, CD20+/-, Bcl2+/-, CD30+/-
- CD3-, CD5-, CD56-, Bcl6-

Cutaneous Plasmablastic Lymphoma

Plasmablastic lymphoma (PBL) is a rare subtype of diffuse large B-cell lymphoma often associated with Epstein-Barr virus that is seen in the setting of HIV infection, immunocompromised individuals and also elderly individuals without known immunodeficiency.[51,52] PBL comprises 2% of HIV-related lymphomas and 1% of large B-cell lymphomas.[53] PBL affects nasal/oral cavity, digestive system, bone and soft tissues, and skin in decreasing frequency. This is an extremely aggressive lymphoma; survival is commonly less than one year.

A dense infiltrate of plasmablastic and immunoblasts is typically seen in submucosa and less commonly in the dermis and often the subcutaneous tissue (**Figure 6.29**). The tumor cells express plasma cell differentiation markers including CD38, CD138, VS38c, BLIMP1, and XBP1. They are also CD43+, CD45+, MUM1+, and monotypic light chain (**Figures 6.30–6.32**).[54] They are typically negative for B-cell (CD20, PAX5) and T-cell (CD3, CD4, CD5, CD8) markers, CD15, Bcl2, Bcl6, CD57, TIA1, CD34, and myeloperoxidase.[52,55] CD79a expression can be seen in 40% of cases. CD10, CD56, and CD30 can be positive in a subset of cases. MYC expression is seen, especially in cases with MYC translocation or amplification.[56] Ki67 proliferation index is high.[57] In cases associated with HHV8, immunostain

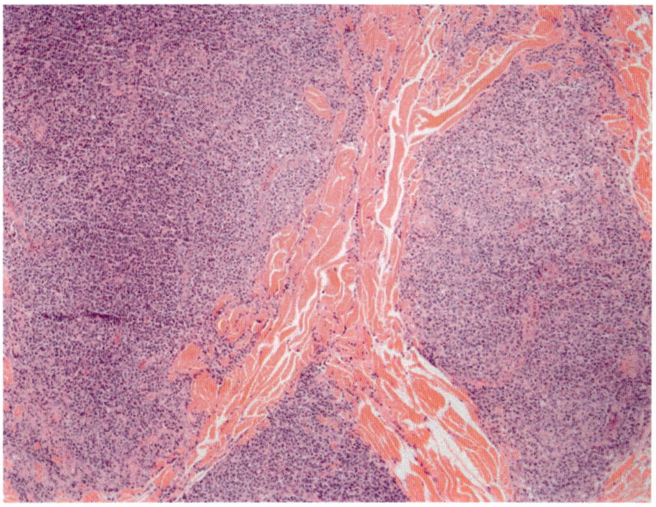

Figure 6.23 In this example of EBV-associated diffuse large B-cell lymphoma a multinodular proliferation of lymphoid cells is noted in the dermis (X100).

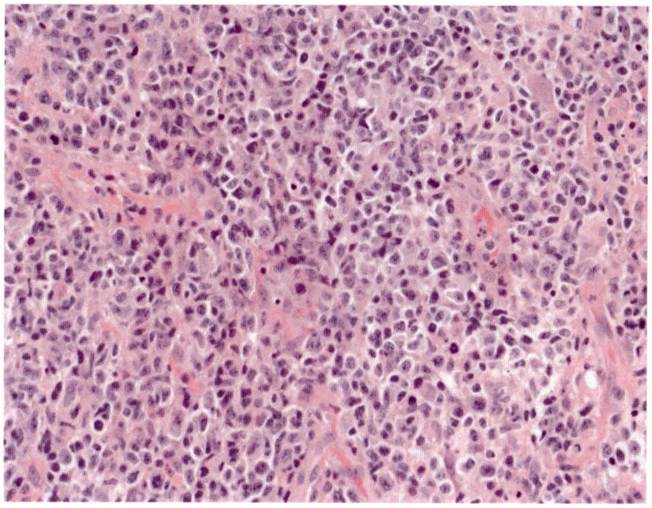

Figure 6.24 EBV-associated diffuse large B-cell lymphoma. The tumor cells are large and resemble immunoblasts (X400).

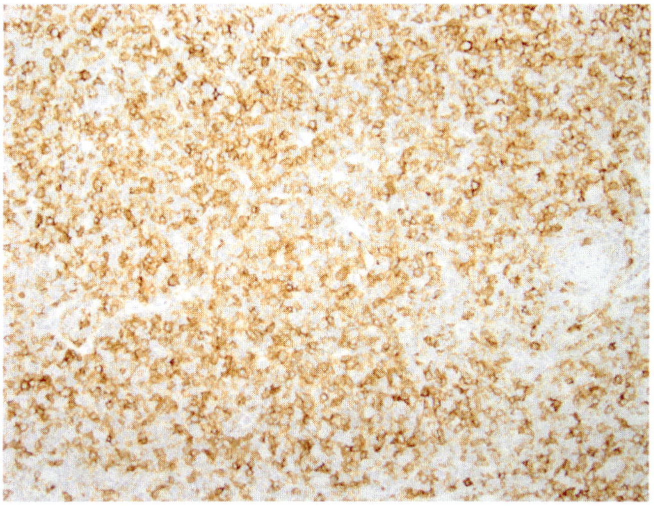

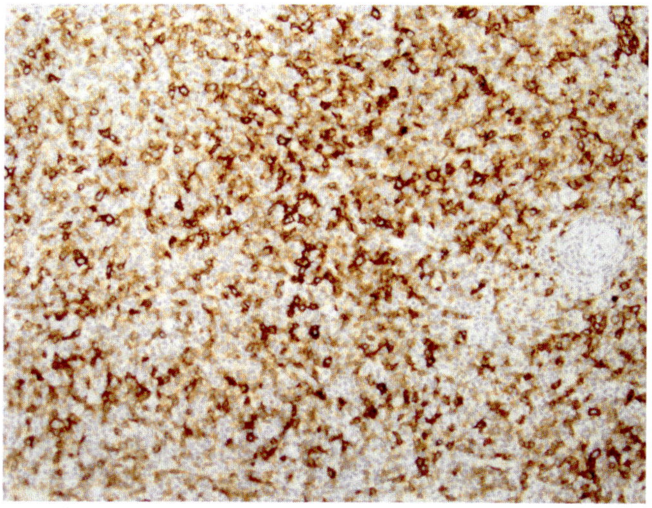

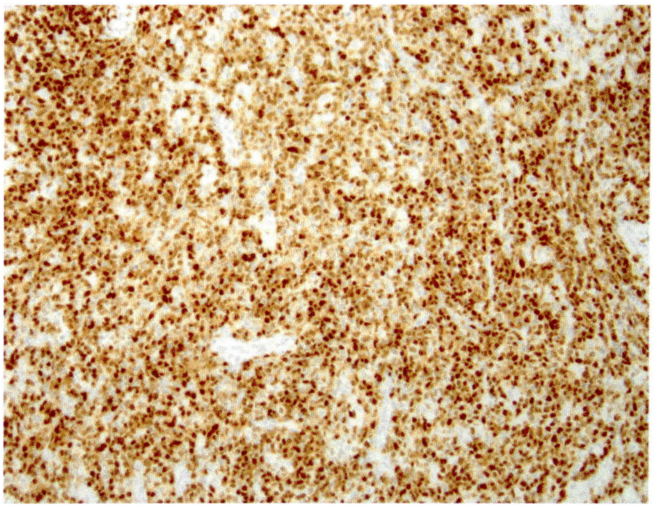

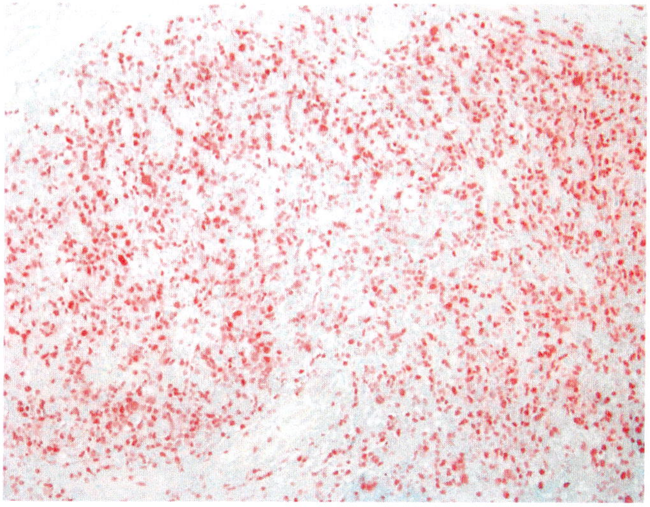

Figures 6.25–6.28 EBV-associated diffuse large B-cell lymphoma. The tumor is strongly positive for CD20 (6.25, X200), CD30 (6.26, X200), MUM1 (6.27, X200) and EBV (6.28, X200).

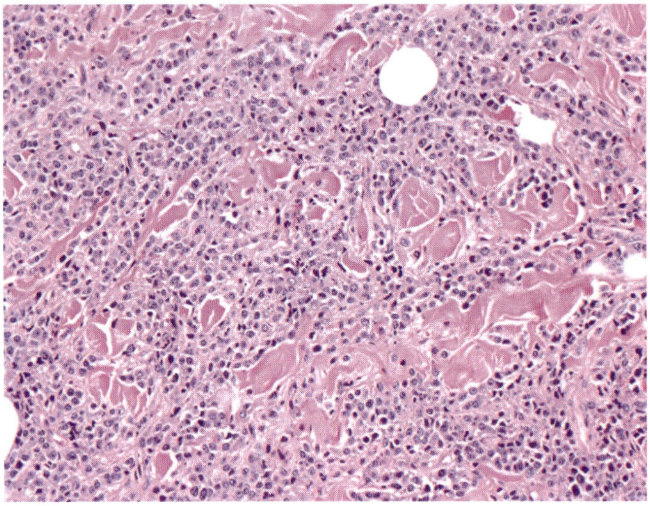

Figure 6.29 A dense infiltrate of small lymphocytes and histiocytes admixed with scattered large cells is seen in the dermis in cutaneous plasmablastic lymphoma (X100).

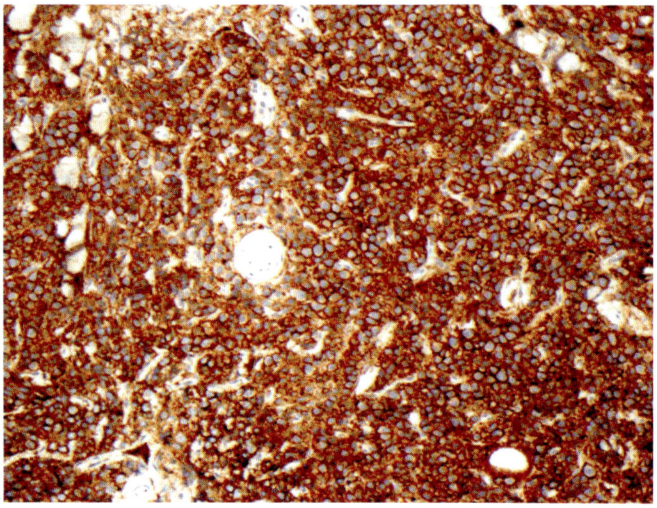

Figure 6.30 Cutaneous plasmablastic lymphoma. The tumor cells are strongly positive for CD138 (X200).

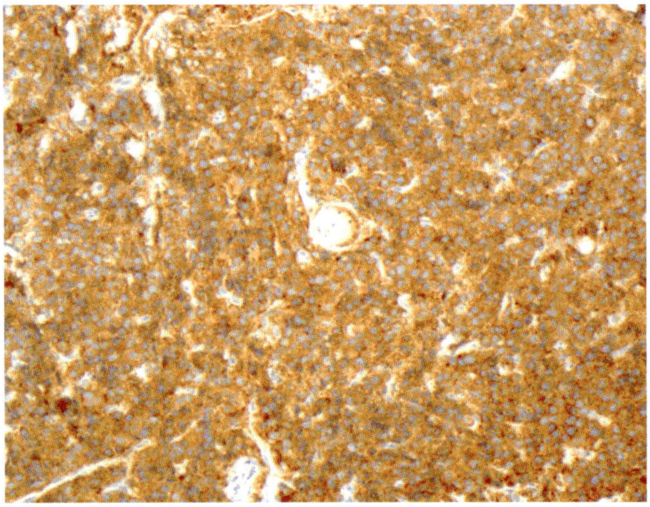

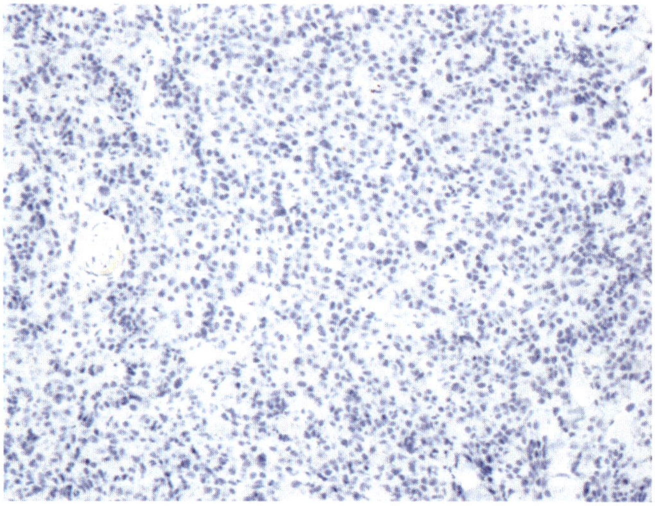

Figures 6.31 and 6.32 Cutaneous plasmablastic lymphoma. Kappa and lambda immunostains demonstrate kappa light chain restriction (X200, X200).

for HHV8 latency-associated nuclear antigen would be positive.[55] EBV is identified in about 60% of cases, especially in HIV patients.[58]

The main differential diagnosis of PBL is DLBCL. The strong expression of B-cell markers such as CD20 and PAX5 is in support of DLBCL; while expression of CD138, CD38, XBP1, and BLIMP1 is supportive of PBL.

Cutaneous plasmablastic lymphoma

- CD38+, CD138+, CD43+, CD45+, MUM1+, EBER+, and monotypic light chain
- CD20-, CD79a-, PAX5-, CD3-, CD4-, CD8-

Mantle Cell Lymphoma

Deriving from the inner mantle zone of lymphoid follicles mantle cell lymphoma is rare and cutaneous manifestation can be the first presentation of the disease.[59] Mantle cell lymphoma is a B-cell lymphoma that expresses CD20 and CD5, and not CD23. It harbors a characteristic translocation t(11;14)(q13;q32) and the lymphoma is classified as cyclin D1-positive mantle cell lymphoma and cyclin D1-negative mantle cell lymphoma.[59] Mantle cell lymphoma expresses B-cell markers including CD19, CD20, and CD79a. CD5 is positive while CD10 and Bcl6 are negative. Cyclin D1 expression is seen in greater than 95% of cases due to *CCDN1* rearrangement.[59] For cases that are negative for CD5 or cyclin D1, Sox11 is helpful since its expression can be seen in greater than 90% of cases.[60]

B-Cell Chronic Lymphocytic Leukemia/Small Lymphocytic Lymphoma

B-cell chronic lymphocytic leukemia/ small lymphocytic lymphoma (CLL/SLL) is characterized by an infiltrate of mature B-cells with coexpression of CD5 and CD23 in the blood and bone marrow, and frequently the lymph node, spleen, and tonsils.[61] Cutaneous lesions can be seen in 25–45% of CLL/SLL patients. They can be (1) "specific" such as leukemic infiltrate and Richter's syndrome, or (2) "nonspecific" such as eosinophilic dermatosis of hematologic malignancy (EDHM).

A dense perivascular and periadnexal infiltrate of CD20+ and CD5+ is seen in the dermis. In addition to co-expression of CD5 and CD23, CLL/SLL cells express B-cell markers (CD19, CD20, CD79a, and PAX5). Expression of LEF1 is seen in approximately 95% of cases.[62] CD10, cyclin D1, and Sox11 are negative.

6.3 Cutaneous T-Cell and NK-Cell Lymphomas

The different subtypes of cutaneous T-cell and NK-cell lymphomas are outlined in the **Table 6.3**. Mycosis fungoides (MF) represent the majority of the T-cell and NK-cell lymphoma category. The majority of mature T-cells possess alpha beta heterodimers and only approximately 5% possess gamma delta heterodimers; currently there are BetaF1 and TCR gamma immunostains directed against these subsets, respectively.[63,64] These tumors can derive from the helper T-cells (CD4+), cytotoxic T-cells (CD8+) and gamma-delta T-cells (CD56+), or follicle helper T-cells (CD279/PD1+).

Mycosis Fungoides

Mycosis fungoides (MF) is a mature T-cell lymphoma whose clinical presentation ranges from patches to plaques to tumors on non-sun-exposed skin. The localized lesions are located on sun protected or "bathing trunk" distribution such as skin of axillae, groins, and buttocks. In the later stage of the disease, lymph nodes and internal organs and peripheral blood can be involved. In general, MF is a lymphoma of low-grade malignant potential, with only 15–20% of patients dying from their diseases.[65] Furthermore, only 1–2% of patients with stage IA/IB MF will annually progress to the tumor stage.[66]

A proliferation of small to medium pleomorphic lymphocytes with cerebriform nuclei is seen, with frequent infiltration into the overlying epidermis. They may form aggregates of atypical lymphocytes and Langerhans cells, known as "Pautrier's microabscess." When these aggregates are large (>10 lymphocytes), they are associated with the worst prognosis.[67,68] The tumor cells initially line up at the dermal-epidermal junction, and they may display perinuclear halos (**Figures 6.33**). As the tumor progresses, the dermal infiltrate will become denser with a band-like nodular growth pattern and less epidermotropism.

Derived from CD45RO+ memory T-cells, the atypical lymphocytes of MF are often CD4+ CD8- and TCRbeta-1+ with a CD4:CD8 ratio greater than or equal to 6 in the majority of cases (**Figures 6.34–6.36**). A subset of cases exhibits the CD8+CD4- phenotype, with rare reports of CD4+CD8+ or CD4-CD8- phenotypes. A third of cases exhibit loss of CD7 expression in the early stages (**Figure 6.37**). As the tumor progresses, loss of CD2, CD3 and/or CD5 expression is frequently noted. Rarely, MF may exhibit a gamma-delta immunophenotype. Although some cases in the literature support no impact on clinical evolution, others report patients having an indolent start with a classic MF clinical presentation that eventually and sometimes abruptly evolves into an aggressive lymphoma. Furthermore, recent publications propose the classification of this type of lymphoma alongside primary cutaneous gamma delta T-cell lymphomas due to their shared genetic abnormalities. At present, there is an ongoing debate regarding the most appropriate categorization of these epidermotropic T-cell lymphomas with a gamma/delta phenotype. It is widely accepted that careful observation of these patients is essential, with a specific emphasis on indicators of disease progression such as erosive lesions, tumor growth, necrotic keratinocytes, hemorrhage, adnexotropism, and extension to the subcutis. Based on these indicators, we may classify these lymphomas as cutaneous gamma/delta T-cell lymphomas instead of MF.[69–71] Clonal T-cell receptor gene (TCR) rearrangements tested by standard polymerase chain reaction (PCR) or next generation sequencing is positive in most cases of MF. Clonal TCR gene rearrangement can be seen in some elderly individuals and those with chronic dermatoses or autoimmune

Table 6.3 Subtypes of cutaneous T-cell and NK-cell lymphomas

Mycosis fungoides
Folliculotropic
Syringotropic
Pagetoid reticulosis
Hypopigmented
Large cell transformation
Sezary syndrome
CD30 lymphoproliferative disorders
Lymphomatoid papulosis
Anaplastic large cell lymphoma
Cutaneous peripheral T-cell lymphoma, not otherwise specified.
Cutaneous HTLV–1 adult T-cell leukemia/lymphoma
Subcutaneous panniculitis-like T-cell lymphoma
Cutaneous gamma delta T-cell lymphoma
Cutaneous CD8+ aggressive epidermotropic cytotoxic T-cell lymphoma
Cutaneous extranodal NK/T-cell lymphoma, nasal type
Cutaneous acral CD8+ T-cell lymphoproliferative disorder (provisional entity)
Cutaneous CD4+ small/medium T-cell lymphoproliferative disorder (provisional entity)
Hydroa vacciniforme-like lymphoproliferative disorder

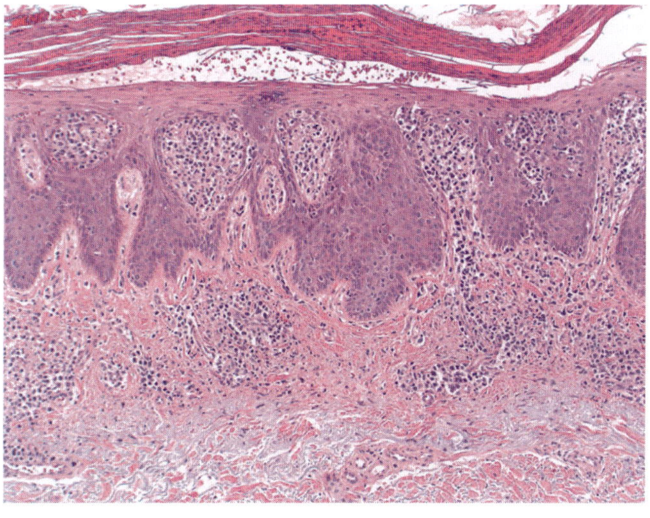

Figure 6.33 Epidermotropic atypical lymphocytic infiltrate with Pautrier microabscess formation and halo artifact as well as lining along the basal layer in mycosis fungoides (X100).

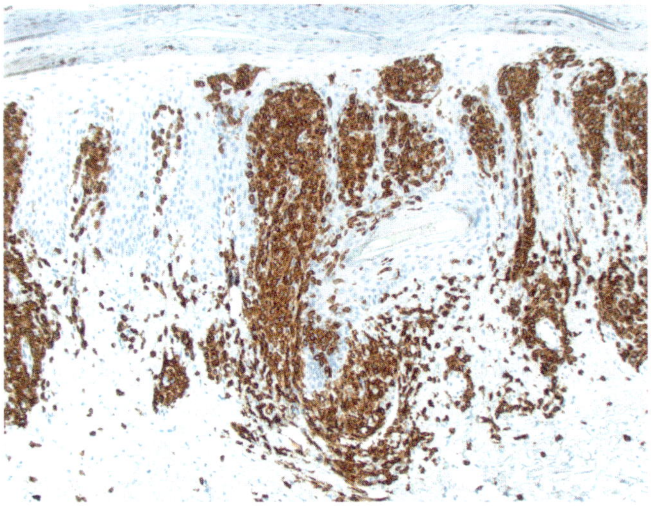

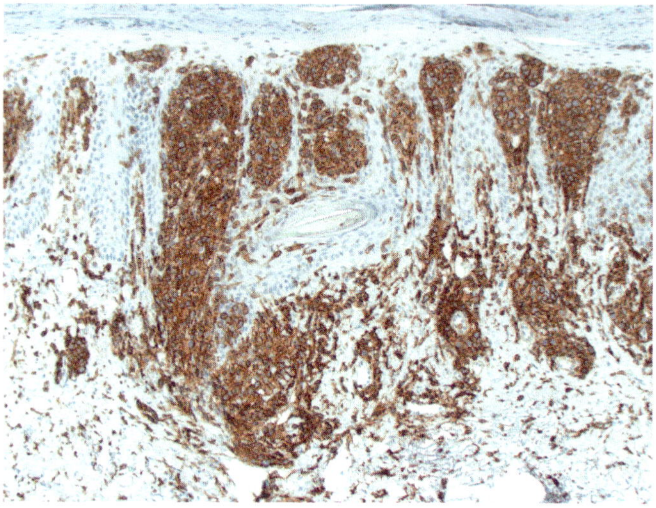

Figures 6.34 and 6.35 Mycosis fungoides. The majority of the infiltrate reacts with CD3 and CD4 (X100, X100).

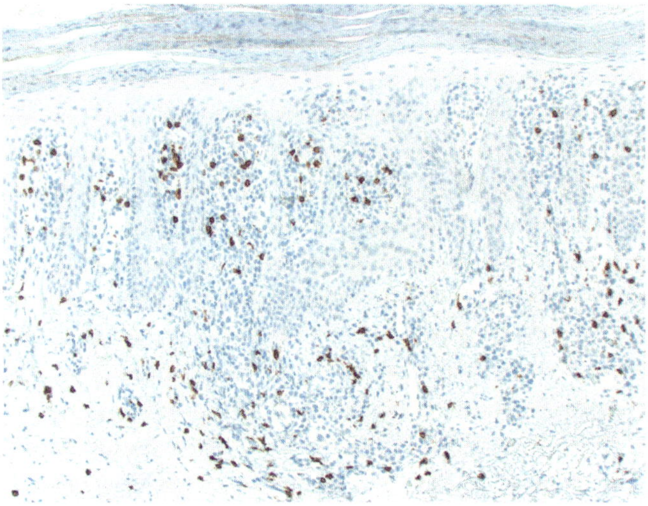

Figure 6.36 Mycosis fungoides. Scattered reactive CD8 positive cells are noted (X100).

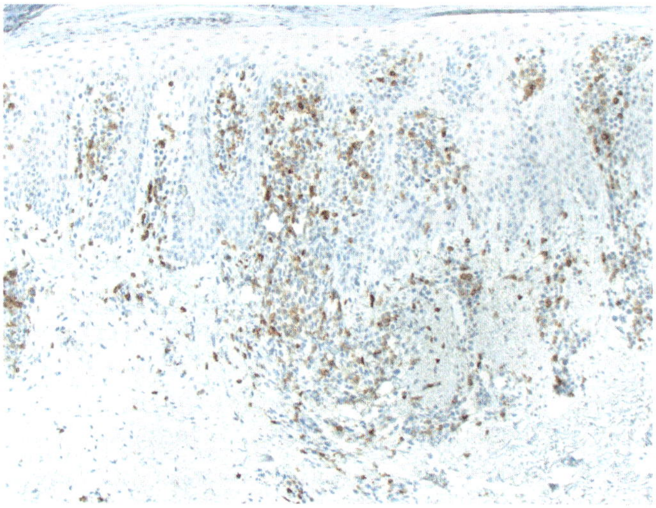

Figure 6.37 Mycosis fungoides. Significant decreased expression of CD7 (X100)

diseases.[72,73] On the other hand, negative TCR gene rearrangement results can be seen in early MF cases. Matching clones identified at different sites over time are diagnostically helpful.[74]

Folliculotropic MF is the most common type. It can present in many different ways in the skin, such as plaques or tumors with follicular accentuation, follicular papules, acneiform or rosacea-like lesions, alopecia, and comedones. Histologic sections are characterized by peri and intrafollicular atypical lymphoid infiltrate, sometimes associated with follicular mucinosis (**Figures 6.38–6.41**).[75] Biopsies may also show cysts, granulomatous inflammation, follicular hyperplasia, and eosinophilic folliculitis-like changes. The immunoprofile is typically CD4+ alpha/beta TCR+. The presence of follicular mucinosis has been associated with reduced disease progression and therefore a better prognosis; on the other hand, interfollicular epidermotropism, a proliferation index above 10%, predominantly medium to large lymphocytes, or more than 10% large cells, have been seen as associated with a worse prognosis.[76] Recent studies have proposed to separate folliculotropic MF into early and late stages, as they differ in prognosis and treatment recommendations.[77] Patients who have erythematous plaques, papules, keratosis pilaris-like, or acneiform-like lesions are in the early stages and have a favorable clinical evolution. Patients who have plaques, nodules, tumors, erythroderma, or involvement outside of the skin are in the advanced stages. Plaque stage lesions have been separated into early stages with superficial to mid dermal intra- or perifollicular few mainly small lymphoid cells associated with a good prognosis, whereas dense, confluent deep follicular infiltrates of medium to large lymphocytes are late stages.[77] Charli-Joseph and colleagues[77] demonstrated that the 5-, 10-, and 15-year overall survival rates for early-stage disease are 96%, 82%, and 65%, while for advanced stage disease, they are 70%, 70%, and 53%, respectively. In the syringotropic variant of MF, the atypical lymphoid infiltrate is seen concentrated around hyperplastic eccrine glands (**Figures 6.42–6.44**).[78]

Also known as Woringer-Kolopp disease, pagetoid reticulosis is a distinct localized variant of MF that typically involves the distal extremities and has an excellent prognosis.[79]

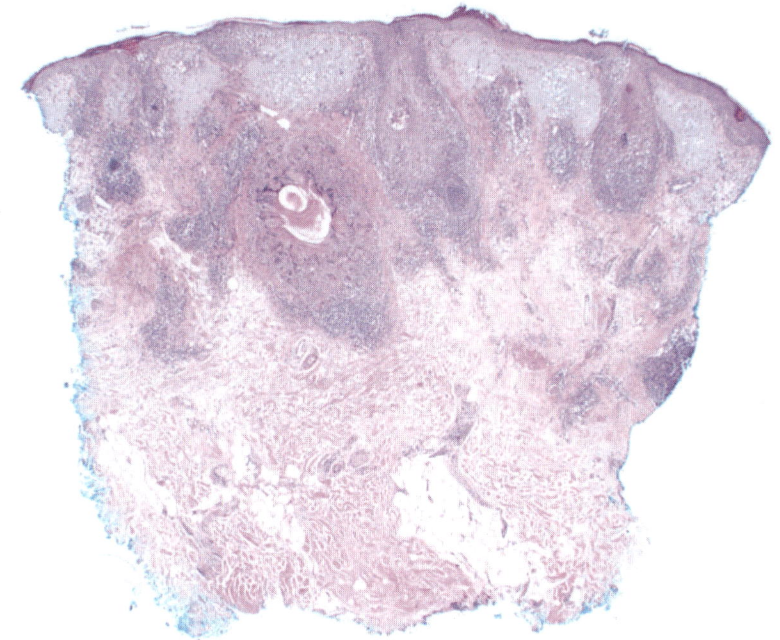
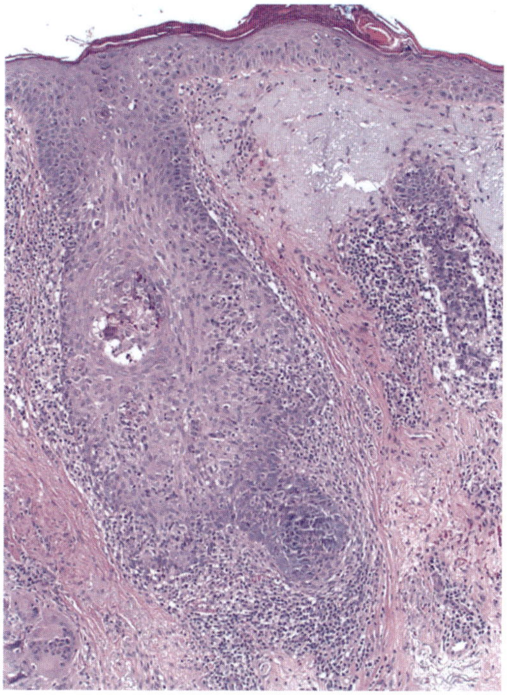

Figures 6.38 and 6.39 A dense lymphocytic infiltrate affects hair follicles leading to destruction with giant cell reaction in folliculotropic mycosis fungoides (X40, X100).

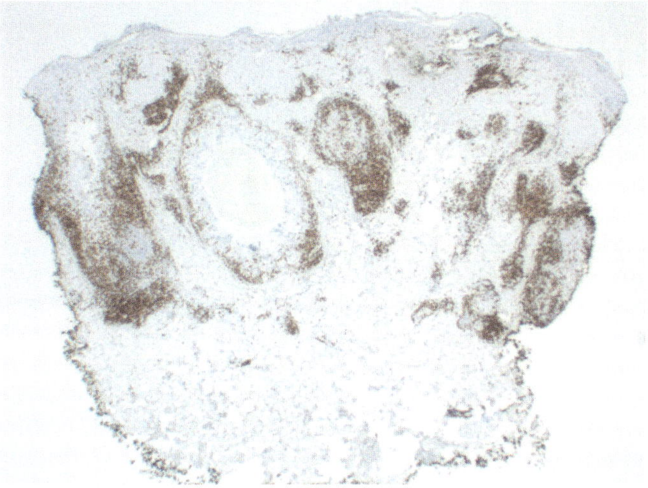
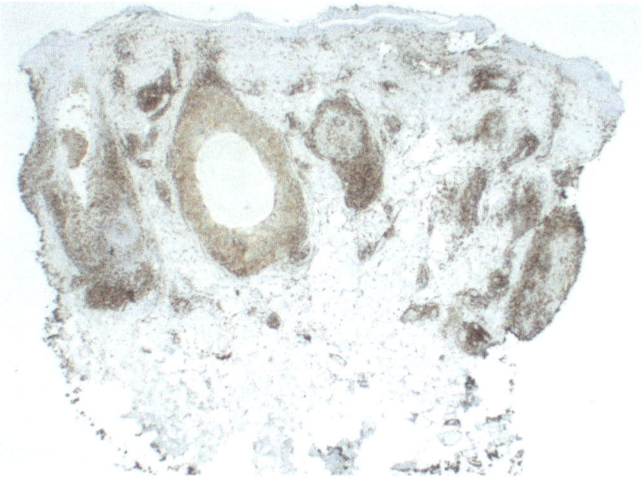

Figures 6.40 and 6.41 Folliculotropic mycosis fungoides. CD3 decorates the majority of the lymphocytes with a predominance of CD4 expression (X100, X100).

Well-circumscribed psoriasiform or keratotic plaques affect the distal extremities or trunk. Histologically, epidermal acanthosis or verrucous hyperplasia is noted with a marked epidermotropic infiltrate of medium- to large, atypical T-cells involving all levels of the epidermis. The tumor cells are most often CD8+; however, CD4+ and CD4-CD8- phenotypes have been reported.[79] The predominant phenotype can be CD8+ in the hypopigmented variant, poikilodermatous presentation, and pediatric cases (**Figures 6.45–6.48**).[80]

Granulomatous slack skin is a rare variant of MF characterized by slow growing pendulous skin folds on intertriginous and flexural regions due to the destruction of elastic fibers.[81] These cases show a granulomatous histiocytic infiltrate with elastophagocytosis, multinucleated giant cells, and lymphocytic infiltrate with a variable degree of atypia.[82] Epidermotropism may not be prominent. The atypical lymphocytes are CD3+, CD4+, CD45RO+, and CD8-. The lesion is associated with elastic fibers loss, elastophagocytosis, and multinucleated CD14+CD68+ histiocytes.[81] Similar to other variants of MF, CD8+ cases have been reported. Most of the cases exhibit a monoclonal T-cell population.[83]

A large cell transformation occurs when cells in at least 25% of the dermal infiltrate are more than four times the size of small lymphocytes and/or form microscopic nodules.[84,85] The neoplastic cells in the setting of transformation can be CD30 positive or negative. However, a negative CD30 antibody in large

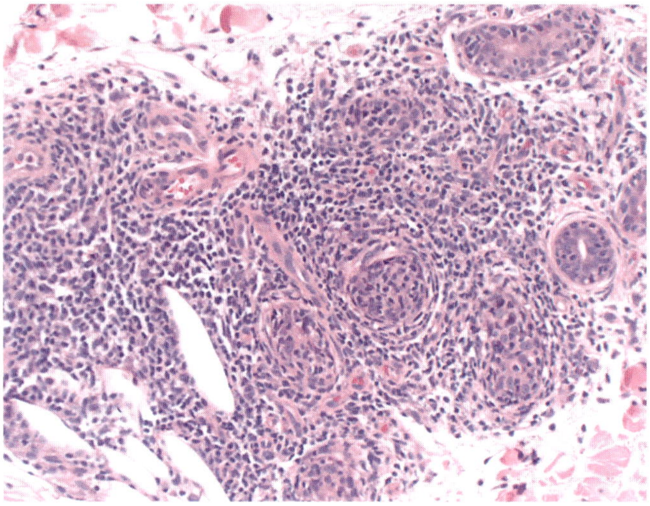

Figure 6.42 The eccrine glands are infiltrated by atypical lymphocytes altering their normal architecture in eccrinotropic mycosis fungoides (X200).

cell transformation has been associated with a poor prognosis.[84] Aberrant expressions of B-cell markers like CD20 can also occur in transformed MF.[86] Researchers have recently found pathways involved in MF that could be used as therapeutic targets. These include the NFkappaB signaling, JAK3/STAT3, and MAPK pathways, among others.

Mycosis fungoides

- CD2+, CD3+, CD4+, CD5+, BetaF1+, CD45RO+
- CD8-, TCR gamma-, TIA1-
- Often exhibits loss of pan T-cell markers CD2 and CD5
- A subset of mycosis fungoides: CD3+, CD4-, CD5+, CD8+, BetaF1+, TIA–1+
- Hypopigmented mycosis fungoides: CD8+
- Large cell transformation: CD30+/-

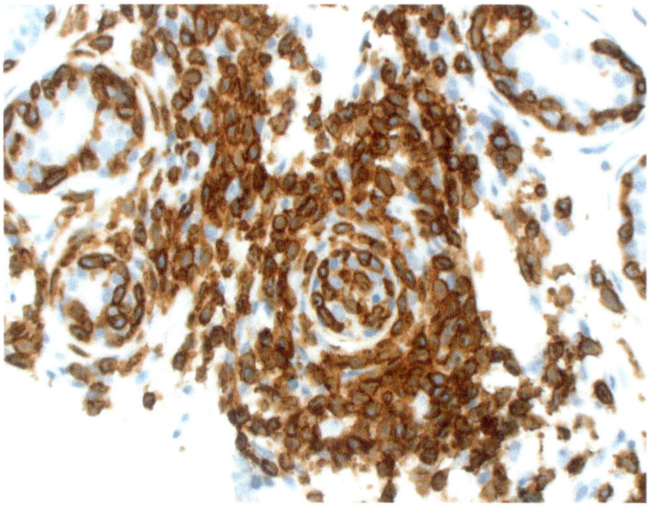

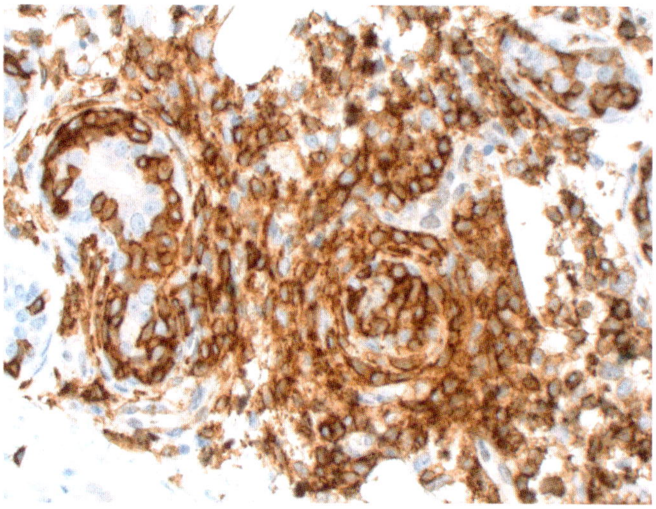

Figures 6.43 and 6.44 Eccrinotropic mycosis fungoides. The infiltrate is predominantly CD3 and CD4 positive (X200, X200).

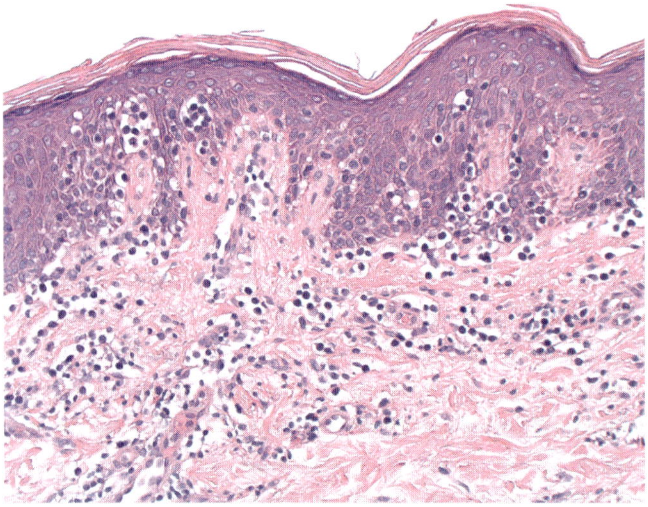

Figure 6.45 A predominantly epidermotropic atypical lymphocytic infiltrate seen in CD8+ mycosis fungoides (X200).

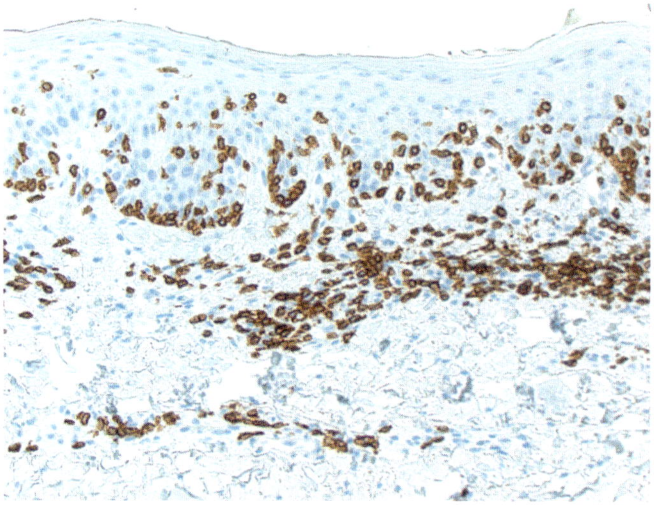

Figure 6.46 CD8+ mycosis fungoides. The intraepidermal and dermal component express CD3 (X200).

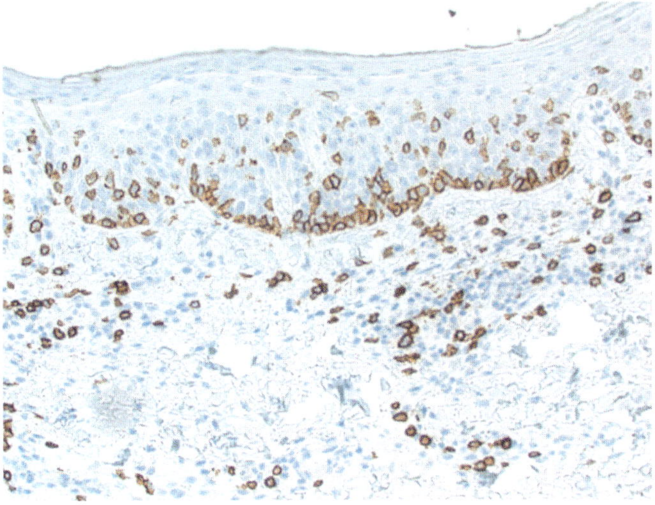

Figure 6.47 CD8+ mycosis fungoides. The majority of the intraepidermal component and scattered dermal lymphocytes are CD8 positive (X200).

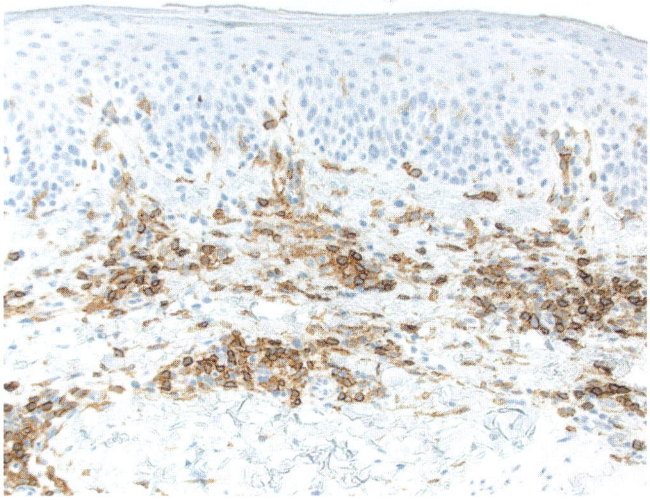

Figure 6.48 CD8+ mycosis fungoides. CD4 decorates predominantly the dermal lymphocytes (X200).

Sezary Syndrome

Sezary syndrome affects elderly individuals who present with a triad of erythroderma, lymphadenopathy, and clonally related neoplastic T-cells in the skin, lymph nodes, and peripheral blood.[2] The patients present with lymphadenopathy and erythroderma, but also diffuse alopecia, ectropion, palmar and plantar hyperkeratosis, and onychodystrophy. Absence of erythroderma can rarely be seen. The patients have an increased association with secondary skin tumors and non-cutaneous malignancies. Sezary syndrome has a poor prognosis, the disease specific five-year survival in The Dutch and Austrian registries was 24%.[2]

Epidermotropism can be either absent or minimal, thus making the distinction between Sezary syndrome, mycosis fungoides, and inflammatory erythrodermic conditions difficult.[87] The neoplastic cells typically express CD2, CD3, CD4, and CD5; and are negative for CD7, CD8, and CD26 with a CD4:CD8 ratio of 10:1 or greater (**Figures 6.49–6.52**).[87] A lack of CD7 expression, a low number of CD8+ intraepidermal lymphocytes, TOX expression, and higher Ki-67 proliferation are all signs that point to Sezary syndrome instead of inflammatory erythrodermic conditions.[87] While the neoplastic cells of Sezary syndrome express PD1, the tumor cells of mycosis fungoides are mainly negative.[88] Sezary cells also express TCR beta, CD25, ICOS/CD278. In addition, some also express CXCL13 and Bcl6, suggesting a T-follicular helper phenotype.[88] T regulatory (reg) phenotype (FOXP3+/CD25-) has also been detected in these patients and associated with the worst prognosis in one study.[89] Peripheral blood and flow cytometric analyses are necessary for a definitive diagnosis and staging, as the skin biopsy can reveal non-specific findings in up to 40% of cases. *TP53* mutations and/or deletions are detected in a large percentage of SS patients, providing an additional diagnostic tool to separate this disease from erythrodermic inflammatory dermatoses.[90] Although the genetic landscape of SS is complex, pathways with potential targetable mutations have been described in JAK-STAT signalling, TCR-NFkB signalling, and MAP kinase signalling.[91]

Sezary syndrome

- CD2+, CD3+, CD4+, CD5+, PD1+
- CD7-, CD8-, CD26-
- Distinction from mycosis fungoides: PD1+, CD26-
- Distinction from erythrodermic skin diseases: PD1+, CD7-, CD8-, increased Ki–67 proliferation index

Cutaneous CD30-Positive T-Cell Lymphoproliferative Disorders

Cutaneous anaplastic large cell lymphoma (cALCL) and lymphomatoid papulosis (LyP) are both classified as CD30 lymphoproliferative disorders, which constitute the second most common type of cutaneous T-cell lymphoma (CTCL), accounting for around 20% of cases.[92] In the 5th edition of the WHO classification, LyP and cALCL are categorized as distinct entities. However, it is explained in the chapters dedicated to these two entities that they are part of the CD30+ lymphoproliferative diseases.

Lymphomatoid Papulosis

Lymphomatoid papulosis (LyP) is a chronic and recurring cutaneous lymphoproliferative disorder that presents as multiple waxing and waning papulonodular eruption. Adult males with 35–45 years of median age of onset are commonly affected.[93] The trunk and extremities are frequently involved sites.[93] The oral mucosa can rarely be affected.[94] The lesions spontaneously regress within weeks or months. There is a 15–50% risk of developing a second lymphoma such as MF and cutaneous ALCL which can develop before, during, or after LyP diagnosis.[93,95] Therefore, long-term follow-up is recommended.

At present, there are six histologic subtypes of LyP and the histopathologic appearance together with immunoprofile can help in classifying these subtypes. LyP type A is CD30+CD4+ and the most common type with a significant subset expressing

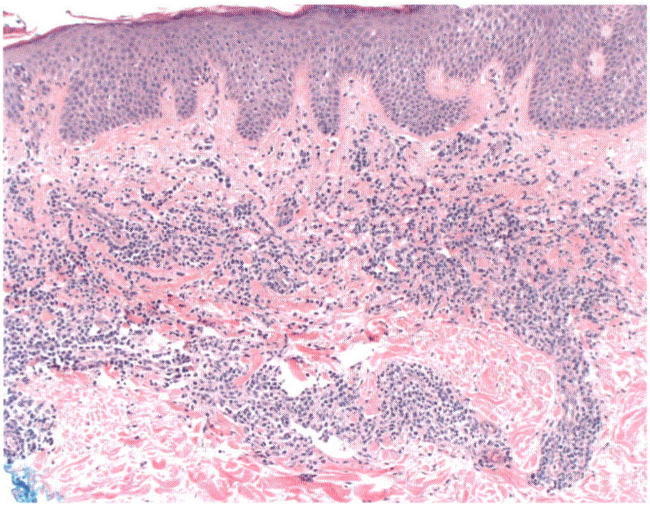

Figure 6.49 Atypical lymphocytes are arranged around vessels with focal epidermotropism in Sezary syndrome (X100).

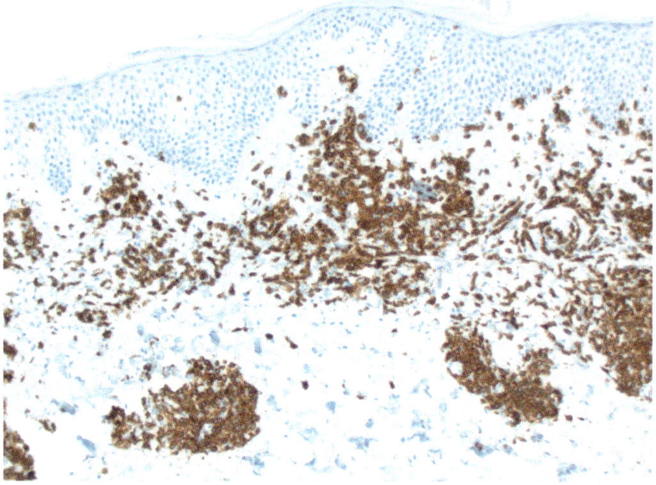

Figure 6.50 Sezary syndrome. CD3 decorates the majority of the lymphocytes (X100).

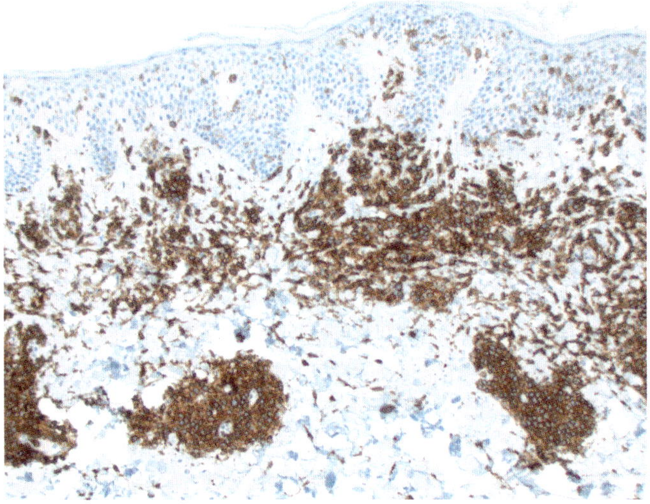

Figure 6.51 Sezary syndrome. The T-cell lymphocytes are predominantly CD4 positive (X100).

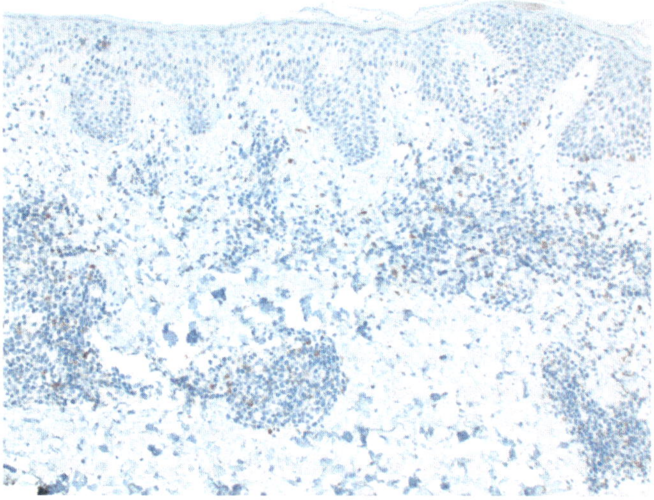

Figure 6.52 Sezary syndrome. Marked decrease of CD7 is noted (X100).

cytotoxic markers like TIA-1.[96] The CD30+CD4+ cells of LyP type B infiltrate the epidermis mimicking patch stage mycosis fungoides; can be distinguished from MF based on clinical history of resolving lesions.[96] This variant often fails to show CD30 expression. LyP type C is characterized by a diffuse proliferation of CD30+CD4+ atypical cells resembling ALCL (**Figures 6.53–6.55**).[96] The CD30+CD8+ cells of LyP type D infiltrate the epidermis in a pagetoid pattern with expression of cytotoxic markers and loss of pan T-cell markers.[97] Type E is characterized by CD30+CD8+ tumor cells that have the ability of angioinvasion and angiodestruction.[98] The recently described LyP with *DUSP::IRF4* rearrangement has a biphasic pattern, characterized by the presence of small to medium sized atypical lymphocytes in the epidermis and dense infiltrate of medium to large cells in the dermis with stronger CD30 staining than the epidermotropic component.[99] Most cases are CD4-/CD8- and TCR-beta positive, while CD4 and CD8 positive cases occur. LEF1+ combined with absence of TIA-1

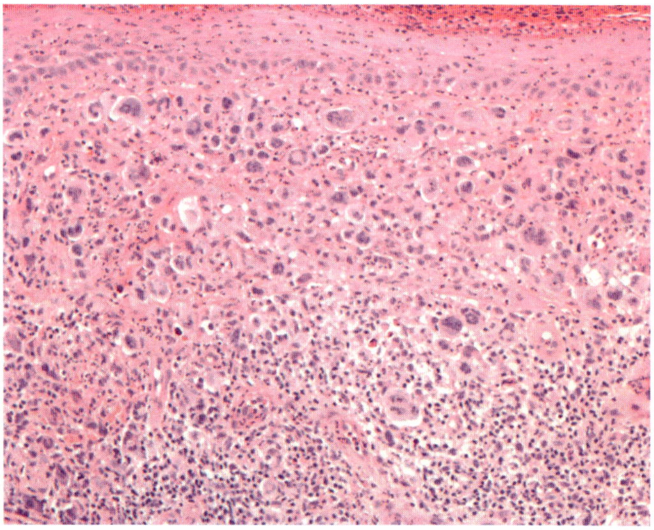

Figure 6.53 An infiltrate of pleomorphic cells is seen in the superficial dermis in lymphomatoid papulosis (X200).

Table 6.4 The histologic and immunohistologic features of lymphomatoid papulosis subtypes

Subtype	Histology	Immunoprofile	Molecular finding
A	Wedge shaped	CD30+ CD4+	
B	Epidermotropic	CD30-/+ CD4+	
C	Dense dermal infiltrate	CD30+ CD4+	
D	Pagetoid and perivascular	CD30+ CD8+	
E	Angioinvasive	CD30+ CD8+	
F	Epidermotropic, folliculotropic and eccrinotropic	CD30+ CD4- CD8-	*DUSP22* locus on 6p25.3 rearrangement

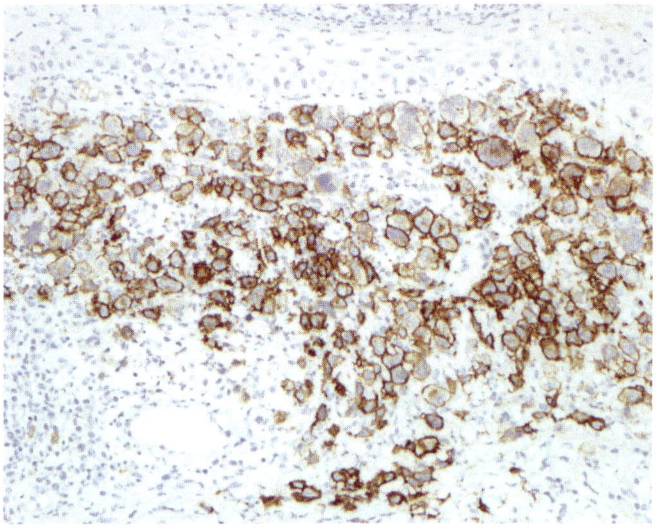

Figure 6.54 Lymphomatoid papulosis. The tumor cells are positive for CD30 (X200).

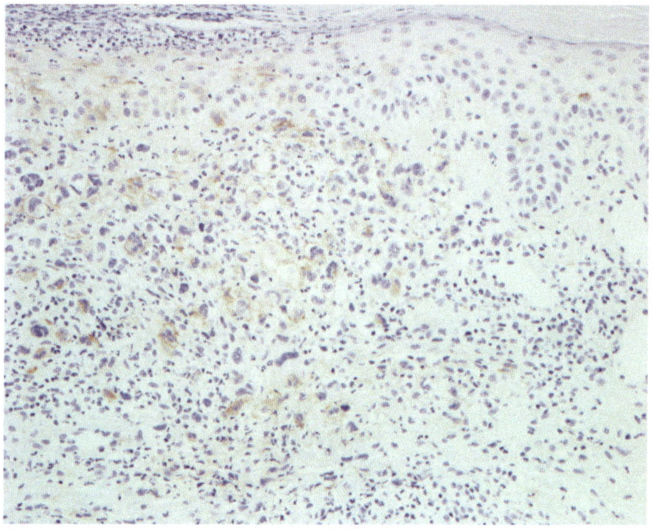

Figure 6.55 Lymphomatoid papulosis. They are weakly positive for EMA (X200).

or STAT3 are surrogate markers for *DUSP22* rearrangement.[100] This rearrangement can also be seen in ALCL cutaneous or systemic as well as MF. The differential expression of CD4 and CD8 together with the histology can be of help in classifying the subtypes of LyP (**Table 6.4**). Additional variants, including folliculotropic, syringotropic, granulomatous, mainly intralymphatic and those with TCR gamma/delta expression, have been documented. The subtypes may co-exist and do not have significant impact on behavior, but it does emphasize the histopathologic diversity.[101] Around 40–100% of LyP cases show clonal TCR rearrangement.

Due to advances in antigen retrieval techniques in immunohistochemistry, it is now possible to identified CD30 positivity in several non-neoplastic processes in the skin. Scattered CD30+ cells can be seen in several conditions such as insect and spider bites;[102] infections including milker's nodule, Herpes simplex virus infection, molluscum contagiosum, scabies infestation, leishmaniasis, and syphilis; lymphomatoid drug eruption;[103] hidradenitis; pityriasis lichenoides et varioliformis et acuta (PLEVA); and various other type of lesions.[104] Some authors report that the CD30+ cells of LyP and ALCL tend to be large, atypical, and sometimes arranged in nests or sheets, in contrast the CD30+ cells observed in reactive processes are generally smaller, less atypical, and scattered mostly as single cells.[105] Whereas other authors reported clusters of CD30-positive large cells with perinuclear staining in reactive processes – a pattern observed in CD30+ lymphoproliferative disorders.[106] Cases of PLEVA with CD30-positive cells and monoclonality can be very difficult to distinguish from LyP types B and D.[104] Multiple biopsies from lesions with different clinical appearances might be helpful.

Cutaneous Anaplastic Large Cell Lymphoma

Cutaneous anaplastic large cell lymphoma (cALCL) is a CD30+ large T-cell lymphoma that mostly affects the skin and possesses a good prognosis.[107] Despite the high-grade lymphoma morphology of cALCL, the prognosis is favorable with a five-year survival rate above 90%. The prognosis is much worse when cALCL manifests as widespread limb disease, with a two-year disease specific survival rate of 50%. cALCL can present as solitary, grouped, or multifocal skin nodules. Involvement of a draining lymph node alone is not associated with aggressive behavior. Histologically, a diffuse dermal infiltrate of large, pleomorphic, and CD30+ cells with prominent nucleoli and sometime horseshoe-shaped nuclei is seen (**Figures 6.56–6.58**). Background of inflammatory cells is frequently seen and exclusively subcutaneous presentation is rarely encountered. In order to be classified as ALCL, >75% of tumor cells should

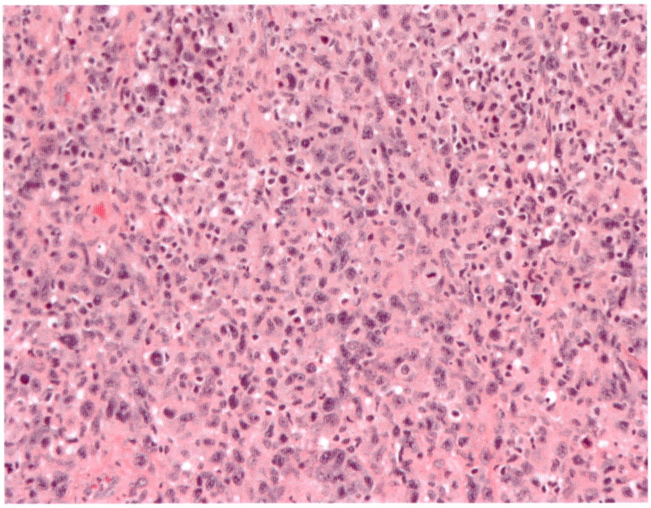

Figure 6.56 A diffuse infiltrate of large and pleomorphic cells is seen in the dermis in anaplastic large cell lymphoma (X200).

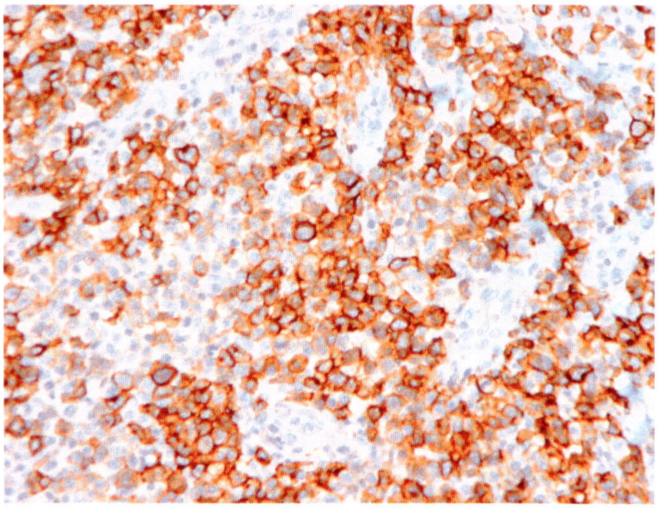

Figure 6.57 Anaplastic large cell lymphoma. The tumor cells are positive for CD30 (X200).

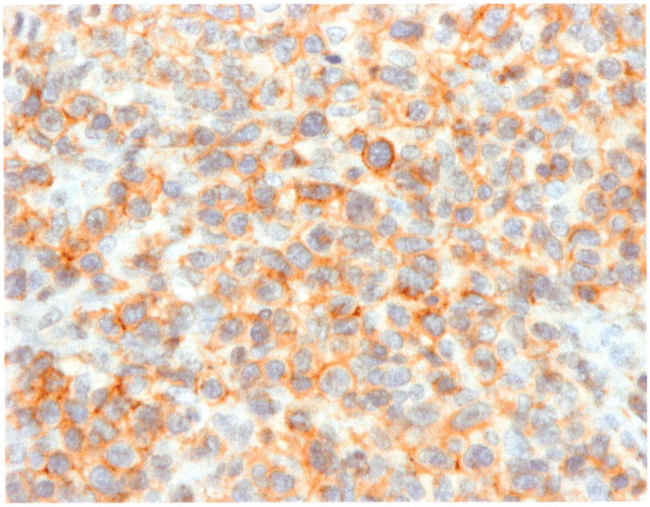

Figure 6.58 Anaplastic large cell lymphoma. They are also positive for CD4 (X200).

react with CD30 antibody on both the cell membrane and Golgi region. Although the tumor cells are often CD4+, a cytotoxic phenotype CD8+ as well as CD4+CD8+ and CD4-CD8- phenotypes can be seen.[108] CD3 may be negative or weakly expressed due to genetic alterations of the T-cell receptor (TCR). In many cases, there is also a loss of other T-cell antigens, such as CD7 and CD5. There have been reports of rare instances of cALCL with a null-cell phenotype and T-cell receptor (TCR) gamma delta. Patients who get treatment with the CD30-specific antibody drug conjugate, Brentuximab vedotin, may have a reduction or absence of CD30 antibody expression in their tissue.[109] ALCL can be stratified genetically based on rearrangements of the *ALK*, *TP63*, and or *DUSP22* genes; the last two rearrangements define two subgroups of ALK-ALCL.[100] The ALK immunohistochemistry is a highly effective method for identifying *ALK* rearrangement, while the p63 stain may reveal *TP63* rearrangement in approximately 75% of patients. Whereas cases of systemic ALCL possessing a t(2;5)(p23;q35) translocation between nucleophosmin (*NPM*) gene and anaplastic lymphoma kinase (*ALK*) are invariably ALK positive, cALCL and LyP are typically negative for ALK (**Table 6.5**).[110] Nuclear and cytoplasmic ALK staining has been reported in pediatric cALCL with *ALK* rearrangement.[111] Rearrangement of *DUSP22::IRF4* locus on 6p25.3 can be detected in 20–57% of cALCL; additionally it is also observed in approximately one quarter of patients with systemic ALCL and a small subset of patients with lymphomatoid papulosis and mycosis fungoides with large cell transformation.[112] Frequently 6p25.3 in cALCL adjoined the FRA7H fragile site on chromosome 7 displaying a distinct "biphasic morphologic pattern" (larger transformed lymphocytes diffusely infiltrating the dermis and smaller cells infiltrating the epidermis as in pagetoid reticulosis).[113] As observed in LyP with *DUSP22* rearrangement, cALCL with this rearrangement exhibits the presence of LEF1 and the absence of TIA-1 or STAT3.[100] The clinical outcome of cALCL is similar regardless of the presence or absence of *DUSP22* rearrangement. EMA is usually negative in cALCL in contrast to being positive in 60% of systemic ALCL.[114] Although intravascular spread can be commonly identified in cutaneous CD30+ lymphoproliferative disorders, an intravascular CD30+ large T-cell lymphoma is a rare entity that should be taken into account.[115,116] Distinguishing cALCL from LyP and various reactive processes would require clinicopathologic correlation. The presence of epidermotropic CD30+ cells and clinical history of patches and plaques of MF would support transformed MF over ALCL. Recent comparative transcriptional analysis had identified a diagnostic model incorporating BATF3 and TCF7 immunostains to separate ALCL from CD30+ transformed MF.[117] CD30+ transformed MF shows TCF7+ exhausted T-cells with B-cell infiltration and absence of BATF3 staining, whereas ALCL shows BATF3 expression inducing MYC activity leading to promote tumor growth and TCF7-. Systemic ALK- ALCL with *TP63* rearrangement is associated with aggressive behavior; however, its detection in cALCL is extremely rare. WHO discourages a diagnosis of cALCL in a patient with MF and suggests that CD30+ transformed MF is the most appropriate classification for these instances. An infectious etiology would

Table 6.5 Immunoprofile of cutaneous versus systemic anaplastic large cell lymphoma (ALCL)

	CD30	ALK	EMA	CD2/CD4/CD5	CD8
Cutaneous ALCL	+	-	-	+	-
Systemic ALCL with t(2;5)	+	+	+	+	-
Systemic ALCL without t(2;5)	+	-	-	+	-

be in the differential diagnosis of the neutrophilic-rich variant of ALCL. Monoclonal TCR gene rearrangements are present in the majority of cALCL.

Cutaneous anaplastic large cell lymphoma

- CD30+, ALK-, EMA-, LEF1+/-
- CD2+ CD4+ CD5+ CD43+ CD8-

Intravascular CD30-Positive Lymphoma

This is a rare form of intravascular lymphomas, as most cases are of B-cell linage. Cutaneous lesions range from erythematous patches, plaques and nodules. Approximately eleven cases have been reported in the literature, including six cases restricted to the skin.[118] These cases were characterized by a predominance of CD4 and CD30 positive lymphocytes; with only one case showing intravascular CD8 positive ALCL.[116] Expression of ALK-1 and EMA, commonly seen in sALCL, is uncommonly reported. Cytotoxic markers and EBER are negative. Pertinent staging workup is crucial to distinguish it from ALK-negative sALCL as it has unfavorable diagnosis.[118] Rare case of intravascular large B cell lymphoma has demonstrated CD30 expression.[119]

6.4 Cutaneous Peripheral T-Cell Lymphoma, Not Otherwise Specified

Cutaneous peripheral T-cell lymphoma, not otherwise defined (NOS), refers to a group of lymphomas that cannot be classified into the existing categories of CTCL and do not exhibit disease outside of the skin at the time of diagnosis. The optimal way to categorize this diverse collection of neoplasms is still up for debate.[120] This is an aggressive lymphoma with most of the patients dying within a few months from diagnosis.[121] Possibility of mycosis fungoides, cutaneous CD4+ small/medium T-cell lymphoproliferative disorder, cutaneous aggressive epidermotropic CD8+ cytotoxic T-cell lymphoma, cutaneous anaplastic large cell lymphoma, and cutaneous extranodal NK/T-cell lymphoma must be excluded.[122,123]

The most common clinical presentation is generalized plaques, papules, or tumors in adults in the sixth decade.[124] While multiple lesions present on trunk and extremities, solitary tumors are located on extremities and sometimes of the head and neck.[124]

The diagnosis is one of exclusion, therefore, there are no characteristic histopathologic features. Focal epidermotropism can be seen in a third of cases.[124] The tumor cells are CD2+ CD3+, and negative for cytotoxic markers.[124] A dense infiltrate of BetaF1+ CD4+/- CD8- lymphoid cells is typically noted in the dermis and often extends to the subcutaneous tissue.[122,123] CD4-CD8+ phenotype is seen in a third of cases and CD4+CD8+ is seen in 10% of cases.[124] They are CD30-ALK-, frequently CD5-CD7- while CD56+/- TIA1+ granzyme B+ perforin + and EBV- (**Figures 6.59–6.62**).[122,123]

Primary cutaneous peripheral T-cell lymphoma, not otherwise specified

- CD2+, CD3+, BetaF1+, CD4+/-, CD5+/-, CD56+/-, TIA1+, granzyme B+, perforin +
- CD8-, CD30-, ALK-

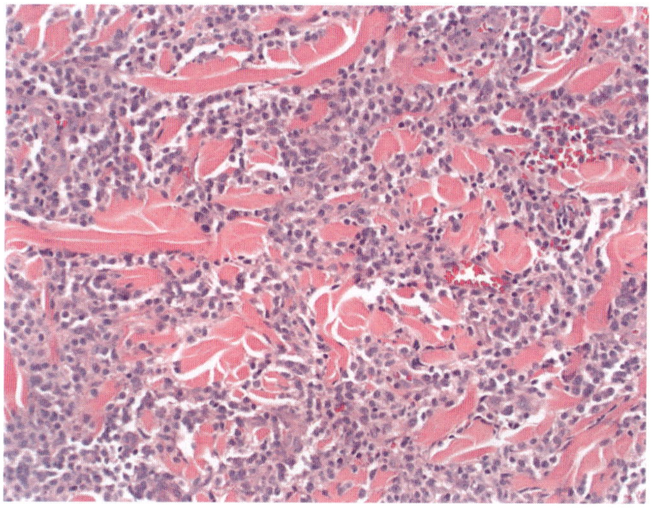

Figure 6.59 A diffuse infiltrate of pleomorphic cells is seen in the dermis in cutaneous peripheral T-cell lymphoma, not otherwise specified (X200).

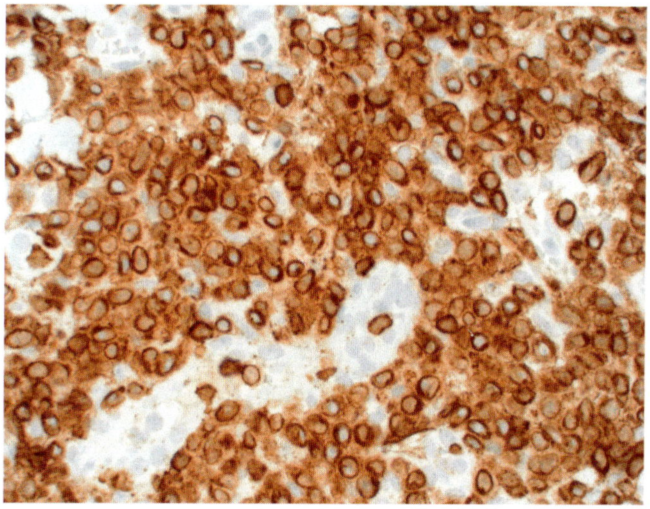

Figure 6.60 Cutaneous peripheral T-cell lymphoma, not otherwise specified. The tumor cells are positive for CD3 (X200).

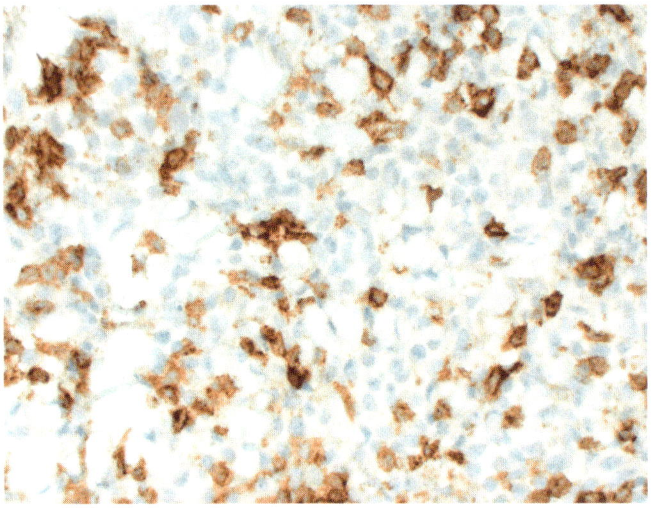

Figure 6.61 Cutaneous peripheral T-cell lymphoma, not otherwise specified. They are focally positive for CD4 (X200).

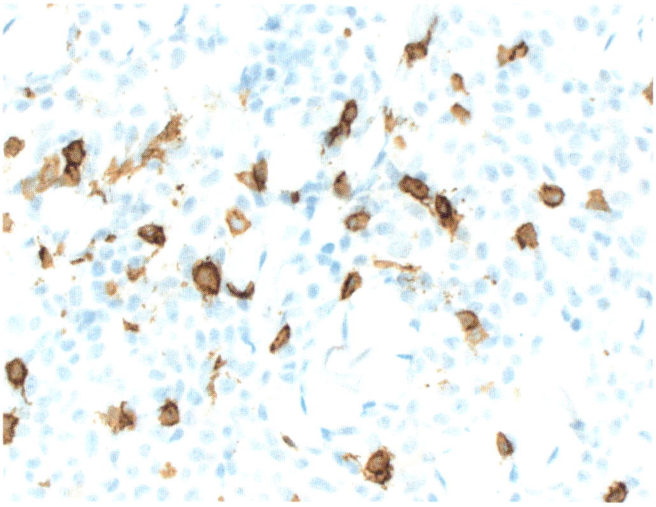

Figure 6.62 Cutaneous peripheral T-cell lymphoma, not otherwise specified. CD56 decorates occasional tumor cells (X200).

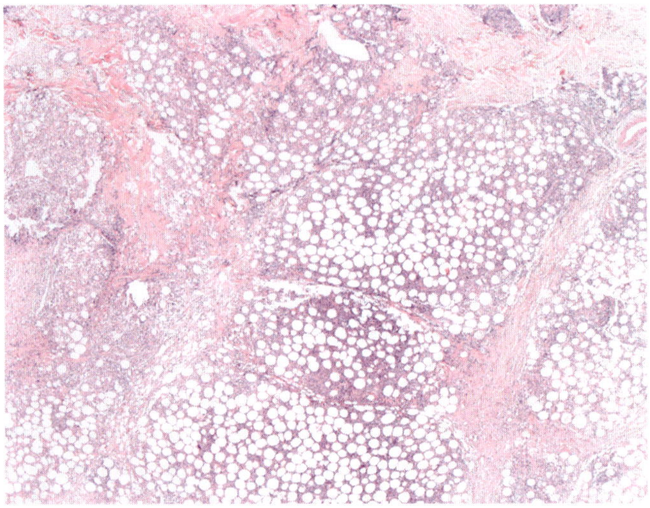

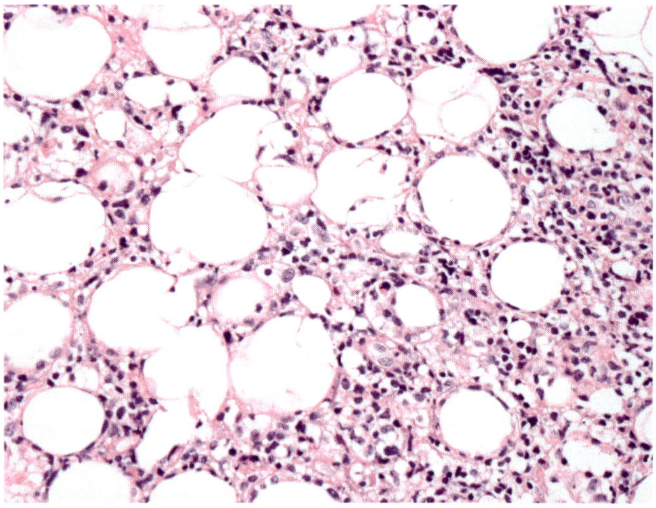

Figures 6.63 and 6.64 Atypical cells are seen infiltrating the subcutaneous tissue in subcutaneous panniculitis-like T-cell lymphoma (X40 and X400).

6.5 Subcutaneous Panniculitis-Like T-Cell Lymphoma

Subcutaneous panniculitis-like T-cell lymphoma (SPTCL) presents as tender non-ulcerated nodules involving the lower extremities, followed by upper extremities and trunk.[125] Constitutional symptoms are common and hemophagocytic lymphohistiocytosis can be seen in 20–30% of cases. [125] The disease is more common in Asia, affects women more frequently than men, with the median age of 35 years. Pediatric patients can be affected. This lymphoma is indolent with a five-year overall survival rate of over 80%.

The neoplastic cells of subcutaneous panniculitis-like T-cell lymphoma (SPTCL) are small to medium and pleomorphic lymphoid cells. They surround or rim the adipocytes of the subcutaneous tissue and are frequently accompanied by karryorhexis and fat necrosis imparting a lobular panniculitis appearance (**Figures 6.63–6.64**).[2,125] They exhibit an alpha-beta cytotoxic T-cell phenotype: CD3+, CD4-, CD8+, BetaF1+ (TCR beta), TIA-1+, Granzyme B+, and CD56- (**Figures 6.65–6.69**).[125] Although the CD8+ phenotype is the most common for SPTCL, there have been reported cases of CD4+CD8- SPTCL. CD2, CD5, and CD7 expression is variably reduced. TCR gene rearrangement analysis has demonstrated TCR-gamma clonality in approximately 75% of cases.[125] The differential diagnosis would include cutaneous gamma-delta T-cell lymphoma and lupus panniculitis (**see Chapter 5**). The distinction between SPTCL and lupus profundus is not always clear with some cases with overlap histologic and molecular findings; thus, some experts have proposed the existence of a continuum of subcutaneous T-cell dyscrasias ranging from lupus profundus to SPTCL.[126,127,128] The detection of hot spots defined as the coexpression of Ki-67 and CD8 antibodies by lymphocytes have been described as a helpful marker in the diagnosis of subcutaneous panniculitis like T cell lymphoma (**Figure 6.66**).[129] Germline mutations of the *HAVCR2* gene have been documented in younger patients (<30 years), with increased chance of developing hemophagocytic lymphohistiocytosis and shorter relapse-free survival. On the other hand, patients with *HVACR2* wild type show upregulation of genes linked with autoimmunity.[130]

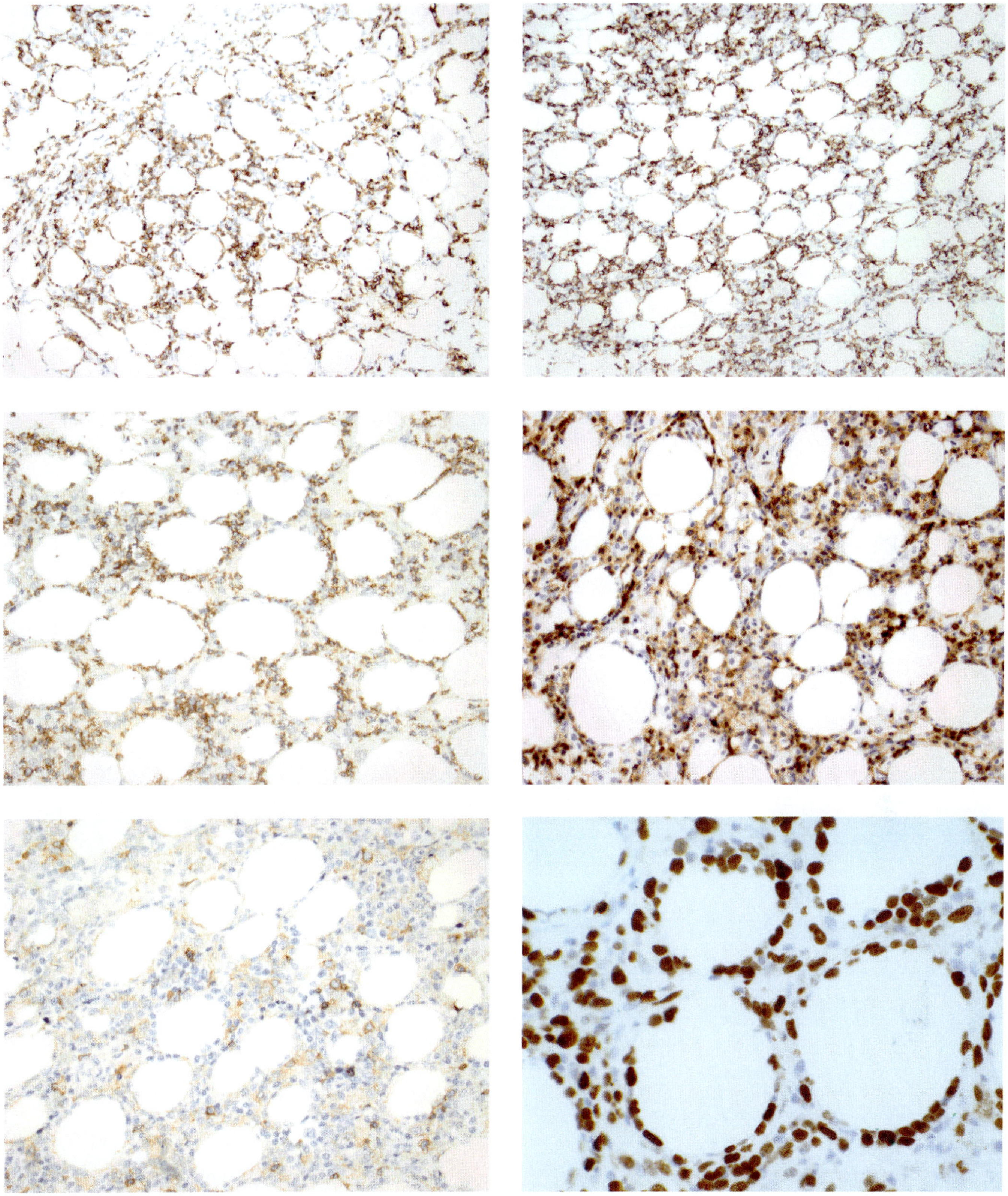

Figures 6.65–6.70 *Subcutaneous panniculitis-like T-cell lymphoma.* The tumor cells are positive for CD3 (6.65, X200), CD8 (6.66, X200), TIA1 (6.67, X400), and T-cell receptor beta (6.68, X400); and negative for CD4 (6.69, X400). Ki-67 highlights the rimming lymphocytes (6.70, X400).

Subcutaneous panniculitis-like T-cell lymphoma

- CD3+, CD8+, BetaF1+, TIA–1+, and Granzyme B+
- "Hot spots": Ki–67+, CD8+ lymphocytes riming the adipocytes.
- TCR gamma-, CD4-, CD56-

6.6 Cutaneous Gamma Delta T-Cell Lymphoma

Cutaneous γ/δ T-cell lymphoma (CGD-TCL) is a clonal proliferation of mature, activated γ/δ T-cells with a five-year survival rate of 11%.[2,125,131] Nevertheless, there have been documented cases with indolent behavior.[132] Commonly, there are generalized skin lesions that resemble panniculitis or MF, often accompanied by ulceration and spreading to mucosal and extranodal areas. At the time of initial presentation, the lower limbs are the most frequently affected area, followed by the upper extremities and trunk.

From a histological perspective, there are three distinct patterns of infiltration that can be identified: epidermotropic, dermal, and subcutaneous. The epidermotropic pattern might vary from a small number of malignant cells lining the basal layer to a significant lichenoid infiltrate accompanied by necrosis and ulceration (**Figures 6.71–6.74**). Pautrier microabscesses are

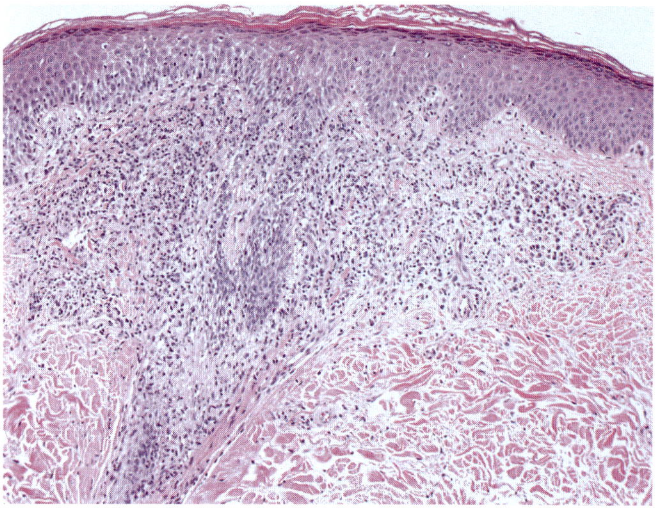

Figures 6.71 Cutaneous gamma delta T-cell lymphoma Epidermotropic and folliculotropic atypical lymphocytic infiltrate (X100).

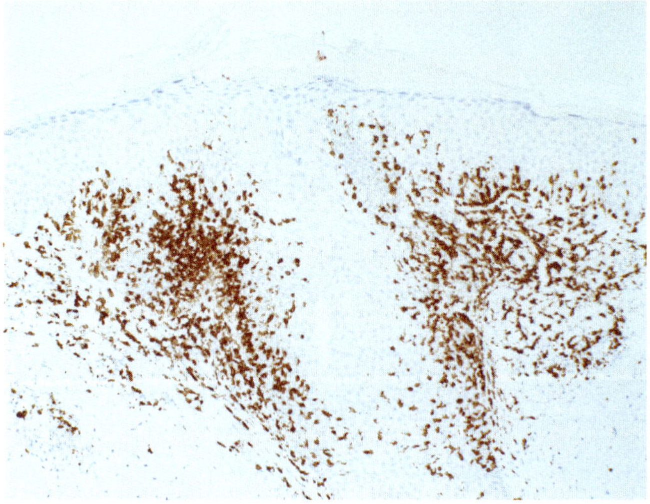

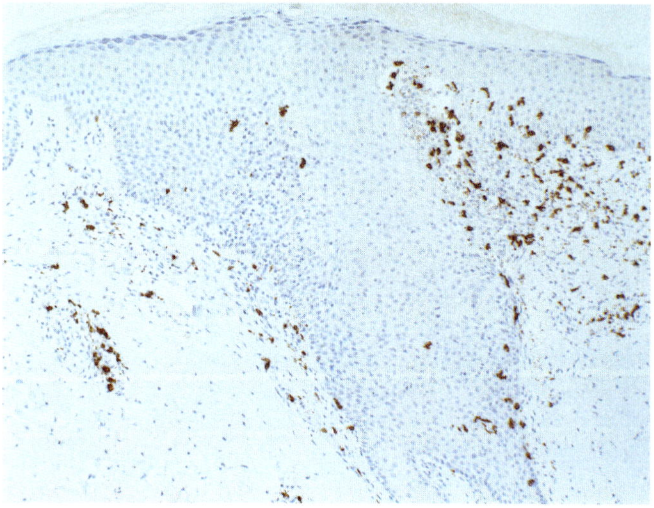

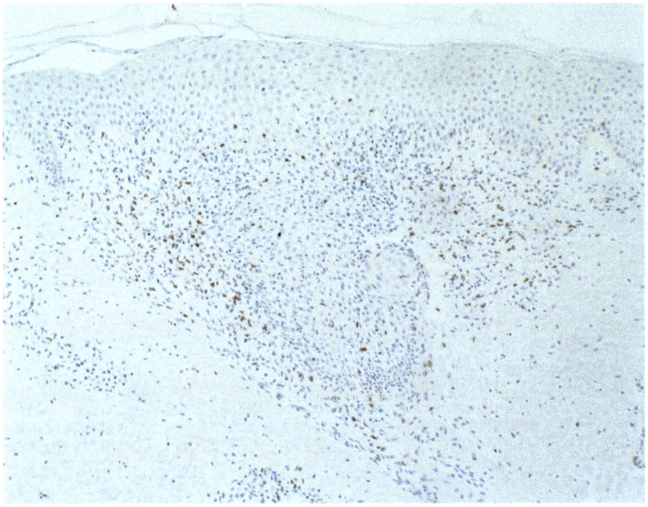

Figure 6.72–6.74 Cutaneous gamma delta T-cell lymphoma The lymphocytes were diffusely CD3 positive (Fig 6.72, X100) with scattered CD8 positive lymphocytes (Fig 6.73, X100) that are reactive with BF-1 (Fig 6.74, X100).

rarely observed. The clinical behavior of this variant is more indolent.[133] The subcutaneous variant can be associated with dermal or epidermal involvement and rimming of adipocytes by medium to large, atypical lymphocytes is not common as seen in SPTCL. Instead, it frequently manifests as a diffuse infiltration with areas of apoptosis and necrosis. Cytophagic histiocytes can be found in cases with clinical hemophagocytic syndrome, which is observed in 25% of patients. CGD-TCL expresses a mature γ/δ T-cell phenotype: CD3+, CD56+, TIA1+, Granzyme B+, TCR gamma+, CD4-, CD5-, CD7-, CD8-, and BetaF1- (**Figures 6.75–6.79**).[125,134,135] Demonstration of TCR γ and/or δ by the tumoral T-cells is an essential diagnostic criterion, the mere negative BF-1 is not sufficient.[124] There are three Vδ isoforms as part of the T cell receptor. Vδ 1 γ/δ T-cells are mainly found in mucosal sites, while Vδ 2 γ/δ cells constitute the majority of circulating γ/δ T lymphocytes. Recent studies have shown that the epidermotropic and or dermal subtypes derive from Vδ 1 γ/δ T-cells; while the subcutaneous subtype, with worst prognosis originates from Vδ 2 γ/δ T-cells. Furthermore, all the Vδ 2 lymphomas were accompanied by Vγ 3 chain, rarely seen in peripheral cells. Conversely, Vδ 1 lymphomas were paired with either the Vγ 3 or Vγ 5. The recognition of different populations of γ/δ T cells in the different subtypes lead to the hypothesis of common antigenic triggers for each tumor variant.[70] TCR gene rearrangement analysis has demonstrated TCR-gamma clonality in approximately 75% of cases.[124] Epstein Barr virus (EBV) testing is typically negative.[134] Other CTCL such as MF or LyP, may seldom exhibits γ/δ phenotype, but they still display their distinctive clinical features.[136] Hepatic γ/δ T-cell lymphoma does not involve the skin. In addition, they express TIA1 but not granzyme B and perforin. Extranodal NK/T-cell lymphoma would be EBV+ and TCR gamma-. Irrespectively of tumor subtypes, all displayed targetable mutations in the JAK/STAT, MAPK, MYC and chromatin modifications pathways.

Cutaneous gamma delta T-cell lymphoma

- CD3+, CD56+, TIA1+, Granzyme B+, TCR delta+
- CD4-, CD5-, CD7-, CD8-, BetaF1-, EBER-

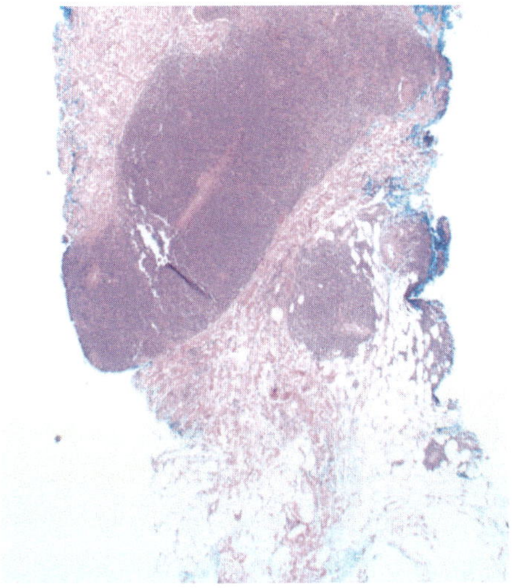

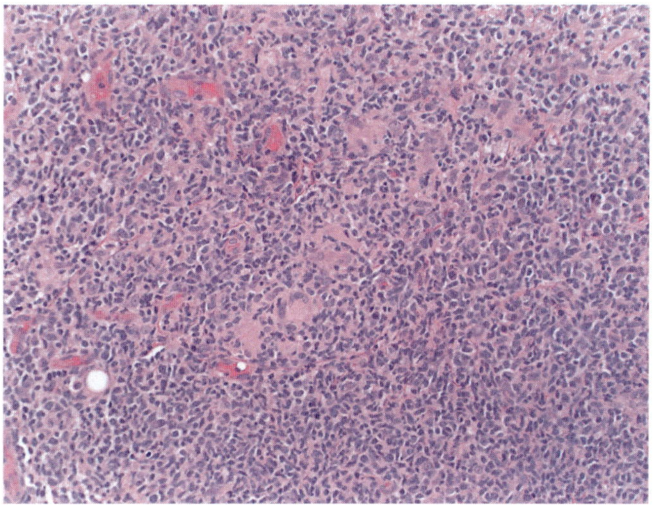

Figures 6.75–6.76 Florid nodular infiltrate in dermis with extension to the subcutaneous tissue is seen in cutaneous gamma delta T-cell lymphoma (X20, X200).

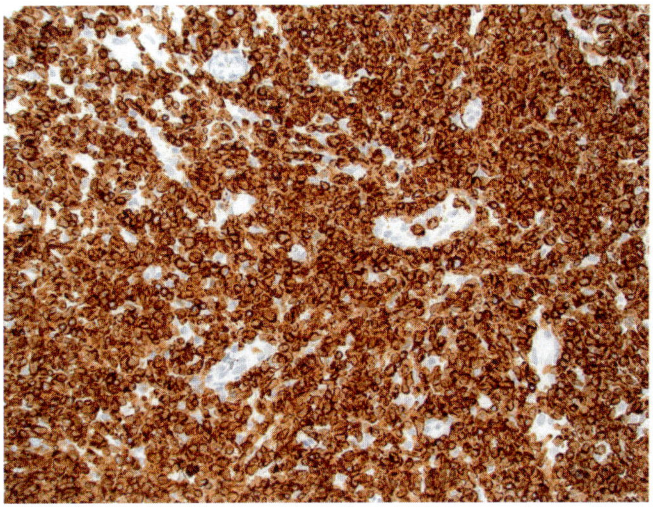

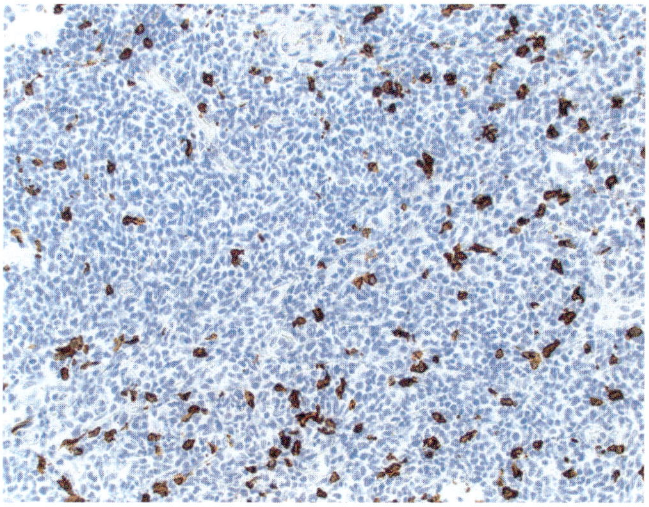

Figures 6.77–6.78 Cutaneous gamma delta T-cell lymphoma. The infiltrate is positive for CD3 with scattered CD8 positive cells (X200, X200).

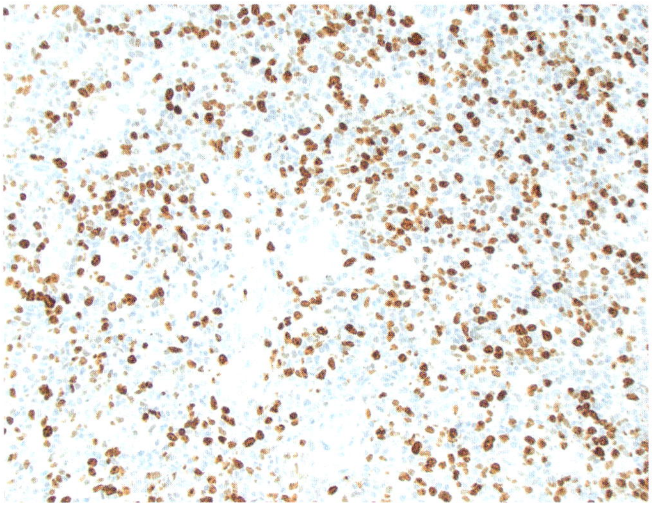

Figure 6.79 Cutaneous gamma delta T-cell lymphoma. High Ki-67 proliferation index is noted (X200).

6.7 Cutaneous CD8+ Aggressive Epidermotropic Cytotoxic T-Cell Lymphoma

Primary cutaneous CD8+ aggressive epidermotropic cytotoxic T-cell lymphoma presents clinically similar to cutaneous gamma delta T-cell lymphoma; eruptive ulcerated plaques and nodules which are associated with an aggressive clinical course and poor prognosis.[137,138] Involvement of mucosa is frequent as well as the spread to the central nervous system, genitalia, lung, and spleen; however, lymph node involvement is uncommon. The average lifespan of these patients is one year.[137] A lichenoid or nodular infiltrate of small, medium, or large atypical lymphoid cells is seen in the dermis with noticeable epidermotropism. (**Figures 6.76–6.77**). Angiocentricity and angioinvasion are frequently observed. Derived from the cytotoxic T-cells, the tumor cells are CD3+, CD7+, CD8+, BetaF1+, TIA-1+, granzyme B+, CD45RA+, CD45RO-, CD4-, CD30-, CD56-, TCR gamma-, and EBER- (**Figures 6.78–6.85**).[138] In contrast to other

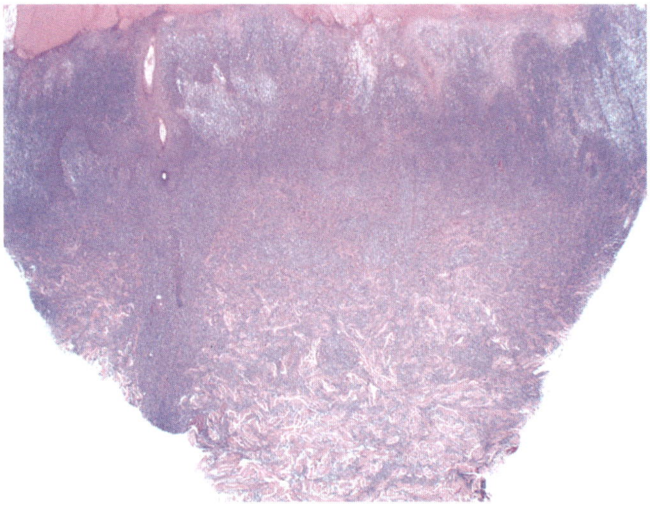

Figure 6.80 Cutaneous CD8+ aggressive epidermotropic cytotoxic T-cell lymphoma is characterized by a diffusely proliferation of atypical lymphoid infiltrate with associated ulceration (X40).

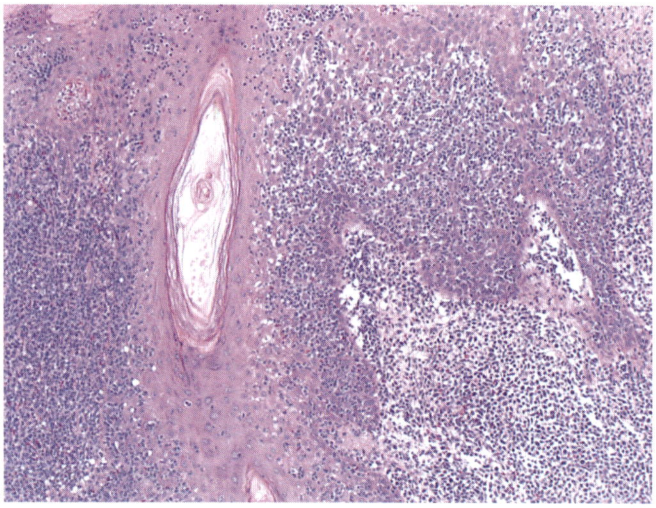

Figure 6.81 Cutaneous CD8+ aggressive epidermotropic cytotoxic T-cell lymphoma. Exuberant epidermotropism of atypical cells is seen (X100).

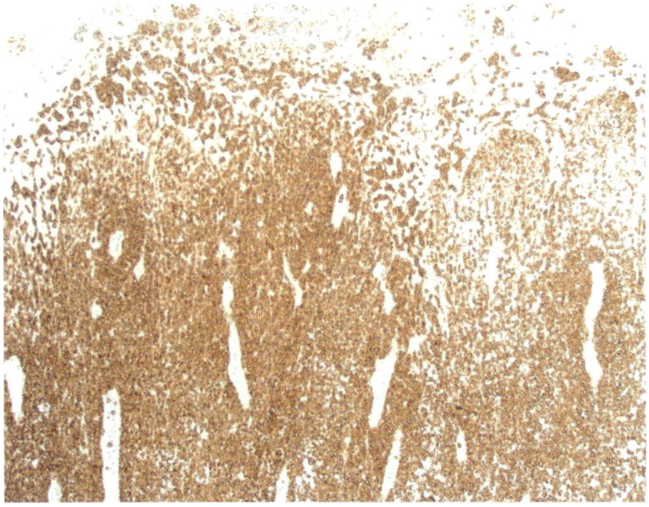

Figure 6.82 Cutaneous CD8+ aggressive epidermotropic cytotoxic T-cell lymphoma. The tumor cells are diffusely positive for CD8.

Figure 6.83 Cutaneous CD8+ aggressive epidermotropic cytotoxic T-cell lymphoma. Marked reduction of CD5 expression is noted (X100).

Table 6.6 Immunoprofiles of CD8+ lymphoid lesions[134,137]

	CD2	CD3	CD4	CD5	CD8	BF1	CD45RA	CD45RO	CD30	Cytotoxic markers
Cutaneous CD8+ aggressive epidermotropic cytotoxic T-cell lymphoma	-	+	-	-	+	+	+	-	-	+
Acral CD8+ T-cell lymphoproliferative disorder	+	+	-	+	+	+	ND	ND	-	+
CD8+ mycosis fungoides	+	+	-	+	+	+	-	+	-	-
Lymphomatoid papulosis type D	+	+	-	+/-	+	+	-	-	+	-

ND: not done

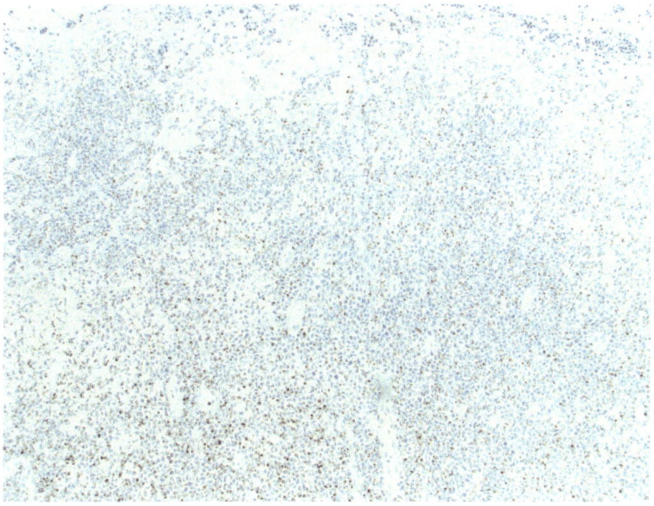

Figure 6.84 Cutaneous CD8+ aggressive epidermotropic cytotoxic T-cell lymphoma. TIA-1 is positive (X100).

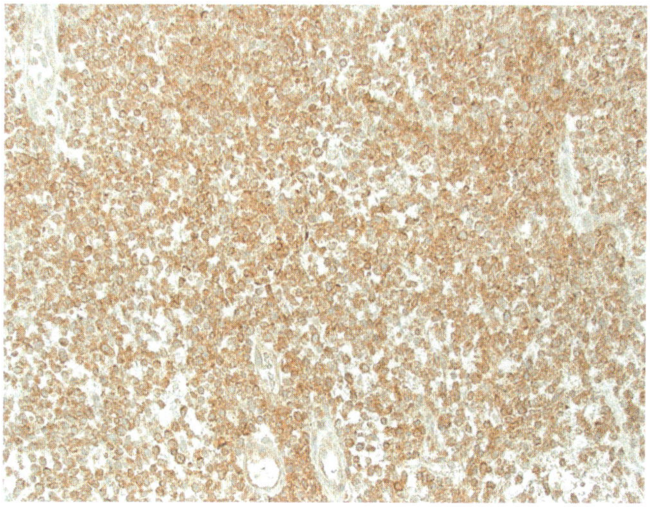

Figure 6.85 Cutaneous CD8+ aggressive epidermotropic cytotoxic T-cell lymphoma. BetaF1 decorates the majority of tumor cells (X100).

T-cell lymphomas, CD7 is usually preserved but CD3, CD2, and CD5 are not (**Figure 6.83**). The main histologic differential diagnosis would be CD8+ mycosis fungoides and lymphomatoid papulosis type D. CD8+ mycosis fungoides would typically express CD2 and CD45RO; and exhibit loss of CD7.[138] A high Ki-67 proliferation index, at least 50% translated into rapidly evolving ulcerated tumors, seen in CD8+ aggressive epidermotropic cytotoxic T-cell lymphoma is not a typical feature of CD8+ variant of mycosis fungoides which typically present with hypo and hyperpigmented non erosive patches and plaques.[138] Lymphomatoid papulosis type D would express CD30 (**Table 6.6**).[97] JAK2 and SH2B3 abnormalities are mutually exclusive and detected in three quarter of patients and sometime associated with co-activation of the NFkB pathway, this is not only of diagnostic relevance but also offers therapeutic potential.[139,140]

Cutaneous CD8+ aggressive epidermotropic cytotoxic T-cell lymphoma

- CD3+, CD7+, CD8+, CD45RA+, BetaF1+, TIA1+, granzyme B+, perforin+, TIA1+
- CD2-, CD4-, CD5-, CD30-, CD56-, CD45RO-, TCR gamma-, EBER-

6.8 Cutaneous Acral CD8+ T-Cell Lymphoproliferative Disorder

In 2007, Petrella and colleagues documented four cases of cutaneous lymphoid proliferation that preferentially involved the ear.[141] This disease was termed indolent CD8+ lymphoid proliferation of the ear (face). Additional cases involving the hands, feet, heel, and eyelids have been reported prompting a proposed new name "indolent CD8-positive proliferation of acral sites."[142–144] To emphasize the indolent clinical behavior with cutaneous relapses but exceptional extracutaneous dissemination, the 5th edition of the WHO classification (2022) and the 2022 International Consensus Classification (ICC) of mature lymphoid neoplasms proposed "primary cutaneous acral CD8+ T-cell lymphoproliferative disorder."[145,146]

In contrast to the clinical history of slow growing reddish-purple nodule/plaque, histology resembles a high-grade lymphoma.[141,142,147,148] A dense and diffuse infiltrate of small- to medium-sized lymphoid cells without epidermotropism and presence of a grenz zone is typically seen in the dermis (**Figure 6.86**).[141,142,147] Histiocytes, eosinophils and a polyclonal population of plasma cells can be seen; however, in a minor degree. Subcutaneous tissue can be involved but rimming of adipocytes by neoplastic cells is not seen.[147] The immunoprofile is CD8+, CD3+,

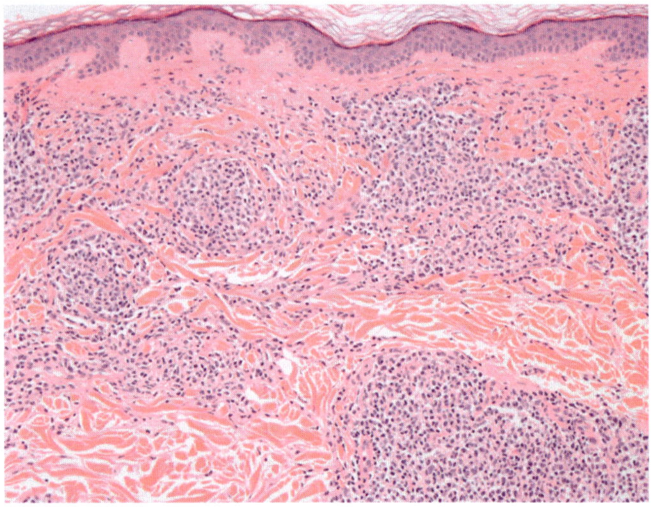

Figure 6.86 Cutaneous acral CD8+ T-cell lymphoproliferative disorder is characterized by infiltrate of small- to medium-sized lymphoid cells without epidermotropism (X200).

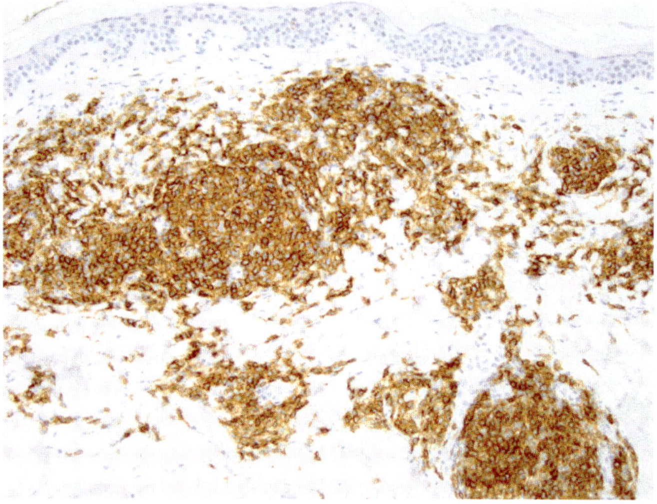

Figure 6.87 Cutaneous acral CD8+ T-cell lymphoproliferative disorder. The tumor cells are strongly positive for CD8 (X200).

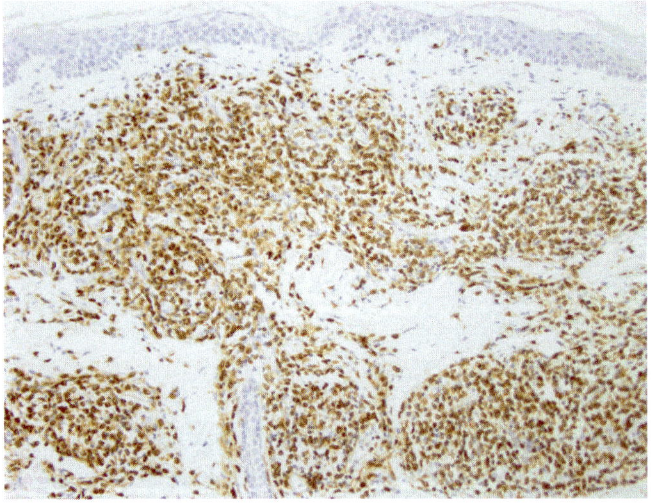

Figure 6.88 Cutaneous acral CD8+ T-cell lymphoproliferative disorder. They are positive for BetaF1 (X200).

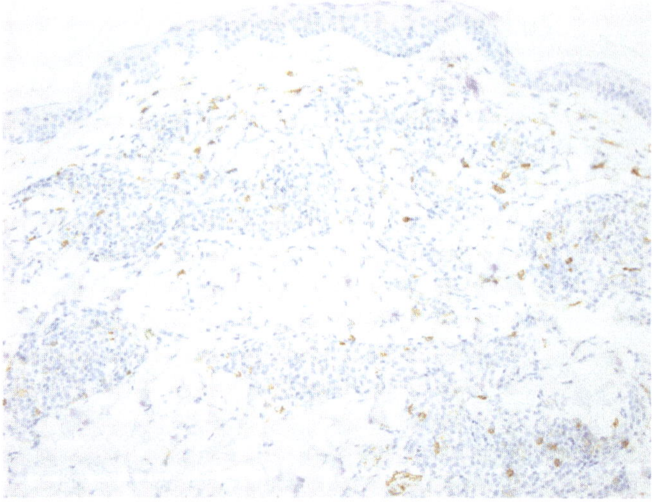

Figure 6.89 Cutaneous acral CD8+ T-cell lymphoproliferative disorder. The tumor cells are negative for CD56 (X200).

TIA1+, CD56-, and EBV-. Often, they lack one or more of CD2, CD5, and CD7 antigen. While positive for CD8 and TIA-1, they do not express CD56 in contrast to cutaneous CD8+ aggressive epidermotrophic cytotoxic T-cell lymphoma (**Figures 6.87–6.89**).[149] Loss of some of the T-cell antigens and Granzyme B expression can be observed; however other cytotoxic protein (e.g. granzyme B or perforin) are not present.[141,142,144,147,149] The Ki67 proliferation index is typically low, ranging up to 40%.[150] CD68 has a Golgi dot-like staining in tumor cells.[150] T-cell receptor gene rearrangement is clonal in the majority of studied cases.[141,147]

A number of cutaneous lymphoid neoplasms can express CD8 including gamma delta T-cell lymphoma, primary cutaneous aggressive cytotoxic CD8+ T-cell lymphoma, subcutaneous panniculitis-like T-cell lymphoma, CD8+ variant of prolymphocytic leukemia, pagetoid reticulosis, CD8+ mycosis fungoides, and CD8+CD30+ lymphoproliferative disease. CD8+ aggressive epidermotropic cytotoxic lymphoma is characterized by marked epidermotropism, aggressive biologic course, and CD56 expression (**Table 6.7**).[149] Subcutaneous panniculitis-like T-cell lymphoma would have a similar immunoprofile yet it would involve mainly the subcutaneous tissue. Cutaneous gamma delta T-cell lymphoma would be commonly CD8- and CD56+. CD8-positive T-cell type of nasal-type T/NK-cell lymphomas can be excluded by the negative Epstein-Barr virus expression. [141,142] While *Borrelia burgdorferi*-induced pseudolymphoma preferentially affects the ear, PCR analysis for *Borrelia burgdorferi* DNA was negative in one studied case.[147]

Cutaneous acral CD8+ T-cell lymphoproliferative disorder

- CD3+, CD4-, CD8+, TIA–1+, Granzyme B-, perforin-
- Golgi dot-like CD68 expression in the tumor cells
- The proliferation is typically negative for CD56 and granzyme B and with a low Ki–67 proliferation index in contrast to CD8+ aggressive epidermotropic T-cell lymphoma.

Table 6.7 Comparison of histologic and immunohistochemical features of cutaneous acral CD8+ lymphoproliferative disorder versus cutaneous CD8+ aggressive epidermotropic T-cell lymphoma.[141,142,144,147,149,150]

	Cutaneous acral CD8+ T-cell lymphoproliferative disorder	Cutaneous CD8+ aggressive epidermotropic T-cell lymphoma
Grenz zone	present	absent
Epidermotropism	absent	present
CD8	+	+
Granzyme B	-/+	+
TIA–1	+	+
CD56	-	-
CD68	Golgi dot-like staining	-
Ki67 proliferation	low	high
Clonality	clonal	clonal
Biologic course	indolent	aggressive

6.9 Cutaneous CD4+ Small- to Medium-Sized T-Cell Lymphoproliferative Disorder

This cutaneous indolent CD4+ small- to medium T-cell proliferation (PCSM-LPD) is considered as a lymphoproliferative disorder rather than a lymphoma and must be distinguished from mycosis fungoides.[145,146,151,152] Presently, it is recognized as one of the most frequent CTCL variants, approximately 6%. Typically, it affects individuals in their fifth decade of life, with no preference for gender. It presents as a solitary or localized nodule, papule or plaque involving head, neck, upper trunk or upper extremities.[153] Relevant is the absence of patches and plaques as seen in patient suffering for mycosis fungoides.

A dense, nodular, or diffuse lymphoid infiltrate typically fills the entire dermis and the superficial aspect of the subcutaneous tissue (**Figure 6.90**). Occasionally, it can present as a subepidermal band-like infiltrate. Beside the small to medium pleomorphic T-cells, a component of inflammatory cells in the form of small CD8+ lymphocytes, plasma cells, eosinophils and histiocytes is seen. Epidermotropism is limited to absence, when extensive a diagnosis of mycosis fungoides should be considered. The neoplastic cells exhibit a T-helper phenotype (CD4+), with loss of CD5 and/or CD7 expression in some cases.[151] CD30 is negative. They also express follicular T-cell markers including PD1, CXCL13, ICOS, and Bcl-6, representing 30% or less of the infiltrate and arranging as single cells or small clusters; the latter forming small pseudorosettes around large B-cells (**Figures 6.91–6.93**).[154] PD1+ cells make up the clonal T-cell population present at different locations or times in the same patient.[155] The Ki-67 proliferation index is <30%. PCSM-LPD may include a clonal B-cell population with light chain restricted plasma cells, raising the differential diagnosis of marginal zone B-cell lymphoma/ lymphoproliferative disorder.[156]

Cutaneous CD4+ small- to medium-sized T-cell lymphoproliferative disorder

- Predominance of CD4+ T-cells admixed with B-cells
- Follicular T-helper cell phenotype: PD1+, ICOS/CD278+/-, Bcl6+, CD10-
- CD8-, TIA1-, CD7-, CD10-, CD30-
- Clonal TCR and IgH gene rearrangements can be detected.
- Absence of lymphoid follicles

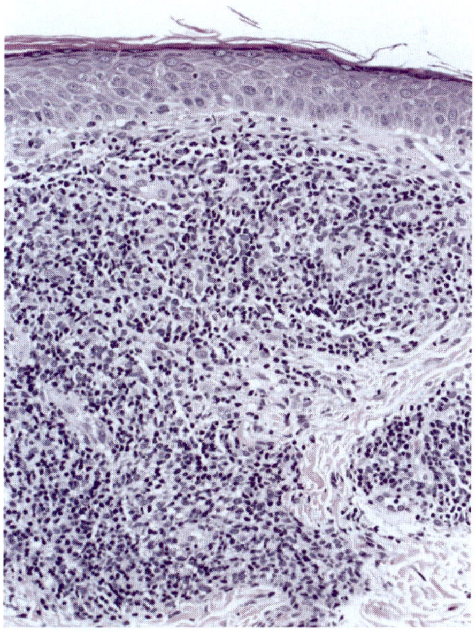

Figure 6.90 Cutaneous CD4+ small- to medium-sized T-cell lymphoproliferative disorder. Dermal based lymphocytic infiltrate of small to medium sized cells (x200).

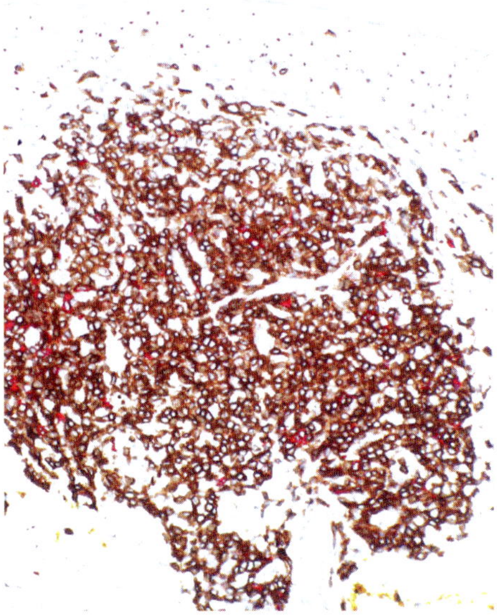

Figure 6.91 Cutaneous CD4+ small- to medium-sized T-cell lymphoproliferative disorder. CD3/CD20 double stains shows a predominantly T-cell infiltrate (CD3 with brown chromogen) with scattered CD20 positive lymphocytes (CD20 red chromogen) (x200).

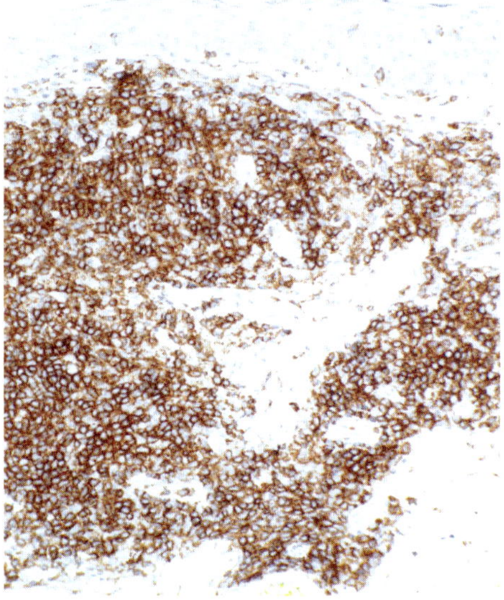

Figure 6.92 Cutaneous CD4+ small- to medium-sized T-cell lymphoproliferative disorder. CD4 reacts with the majority of the dermal infiltrate (x200).

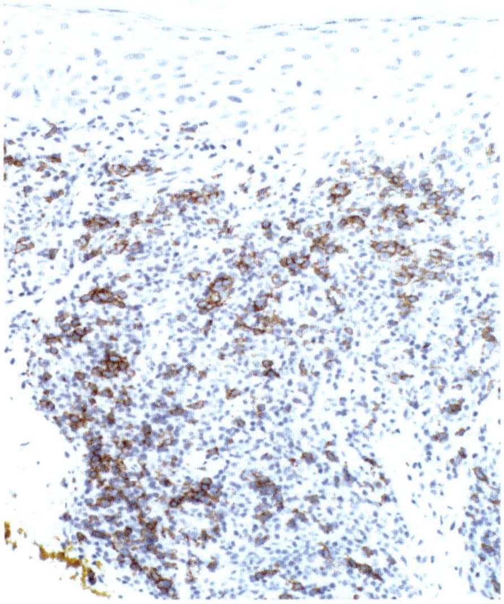

Figure 6.93 Cutaneous CD4+ small- to medium-sized T-cell lymphoproliferative disorder. PD-1 displays reactivity in single cells and clusters (x200).

Cutaneous Extranodal NK/T-Cell Lymphoma, Nasal Type

Extranodal NK/T-cell lymphoma is a cytotoxic lymphoma that commonly involves the aerodigestive tract with skin as the most common site of secondary involvement. Extranodal NK/T-cell lymphoma affects men of East Asia more commonly than other ethnic groups. There are two clinical subtypes, nasal and extra-nasal. In the nasal subtype, 80% of the cases, the lesions start in the nasal cavity then invade into the nasal floor, destroy the palate, and create the "lethal midline granuloma." In advanced disease, regional lymph nodes and distant organs including skin, gastrointestinal tract, testis, liver, spleen, and bone morrow, can be affected. In the extra-nasal subtype, 20% of the cases, skin, gastrointestinal tract, testis, and other sites can be the initial affected site.[157] Skin is the primary disease site in only 10% of cases.[158,159] The clinical presentation typically consists of ulcerative violaceous plaques or nodules affecting trunk and extremities.[160–162] The majority of patients dies within a few months following diagnosis.

A dense and nodular dermal and subcutaneous infiltrate of medium-sized atypical lymphoid cells is seen often with an angiocentric pattern (**Figure 6.94**). Ulceration and extensive necrosis are noted. Epidermotropism can be noted. The prominent background inflammatory cells can mimic an inflammatory process. The neoplastic cells can range from small to medium, large, and even anaplastic in size. Most cases of cutaneous extranodal NK/T-cell lymphoma, nasal type, exhibits an NK phenotype and association with EBV.[163] The neoplastic cells are positive for CD2, CD3ε, CD56, TIA1, granzyme B, and EBER (**Figures 6.95–6.97**); while they are negative for CD3, CD4, CD5, CD7, CD8, CD20, CD30, BetaF1, and TCR gamma.[164,165] Some T- and NK-cell associated antigens such as CD4, CD8, CD16, and CD57 are negative. Cytotoxic markers such as TIA1, granzyme B, and perforin are positive. CD30 expression can be seen in approximately half of the cases.[166]

Cutaneous extranodal NK/T-cell lymphoma, nasal type

- CD2+, CD56+, TIA1+, granzyme B+, and EBER+
- CD3-, CD4-, CD5-, CD7-, CD8-, CD20-, CD30-, BetaF1-, and TCR gamma-

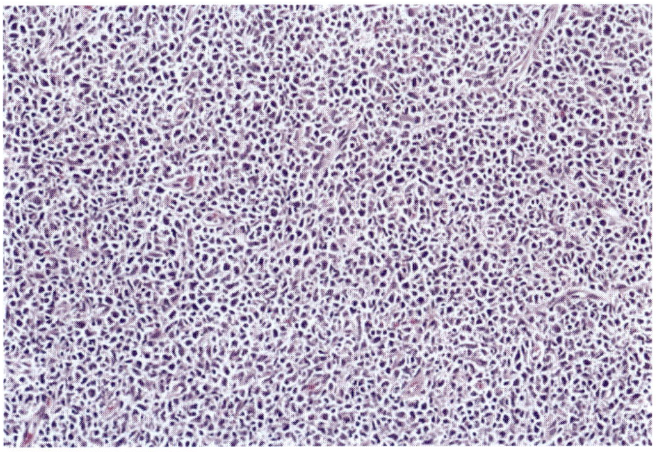

Figure 6.94 A dense infiltrate of atypical lymphoid cells in an angiocentric pattern in cutaneous extranodal NK/T lymphoma, nasal type (X100).

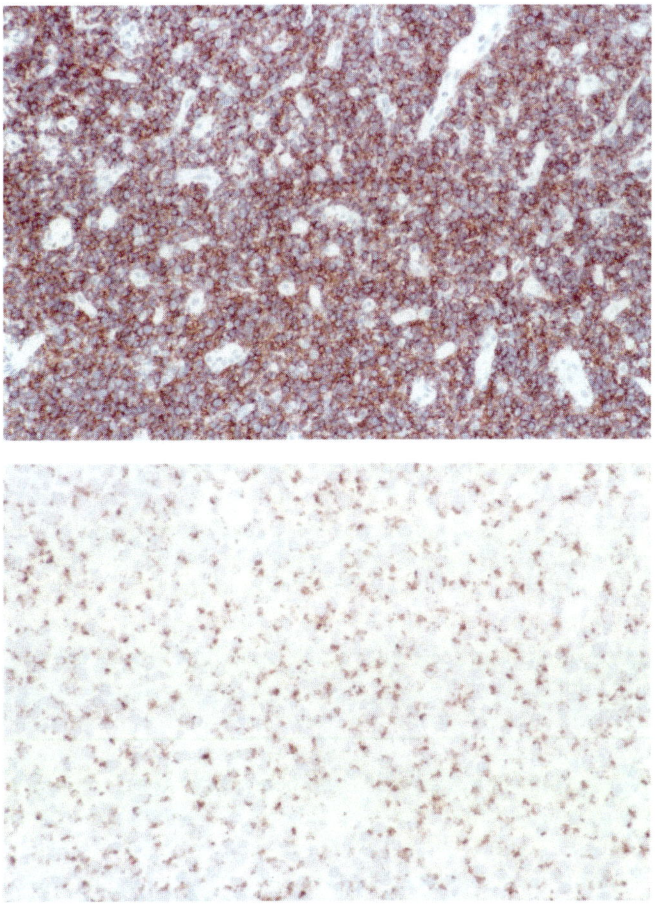

Figures 6.95 and 6.96 Cutaneous extranodal NK/T lymphoma, nasal type. The tumor cells are positive CD56 (X100) and TIA1 (X200).

Intravascular T/NK Lymphoma

Intravascular NK/T cell lymphoma (IVNKTL) is a rare and highly aggressive lymphoma typically affecting small to medium sized vessels. Since its initial description by Santucci and colleagues in 2003, there have been approximately 27 thoroughly documented cases published.[167] According to the latest WHO classification of lymphoid neoplasms, IVNKTL is now classified

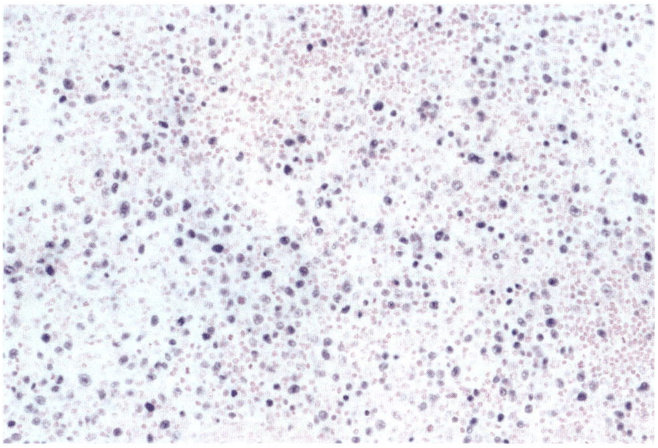

Figure 6.97 Cutaneous extranodal NK/T lymphoma, nasal type. EBER *in situ* hybridization is diffusely positive (X100).

as a subtype of aggressive NK-cell leukemia. In addition to skin lesions that vary from erythema to plaques and nodules, additional organs that are affected include the central nervous system (CNS), as well as the bone marrow, lungs, and kidneys. Skin biopsy is the most effective diagnostic tool, when cutaneous lesions are absent diagnoses can be reach by bone marrow or brain biopsy.[168] Histologically, proliferation of atypical lymphoid cells with elongated nuclei displaying single or multiple nucleoli and pale to eosinophilic cytoplasm can be seen in vessels. The neoplastic cells express CD2, CD3ε, CD56, and cytotoxic molecules such as TIA-1, perforin, and granzyme B. They typically fail to express surface CD4, CD5, CD8, betaF1, and TRC delta. EBV/EBER is positive in most of the cases. Genetic landscape studies on IVNKTL have shown mutations in regulator genes as well as suppressor and oncogenes like HRA, MDM2, and VEGFA.[169]

Intravascular NK/T-cell lymphoma

- Immunophenotype: CD3+, CD43+, CD56+, TIA1+, perforin+, granzyme B+, EBER+, CD30-/+, CD4-, CD5-, CD7-, CD8-, CD20-, CD79a-

6.10 Secondary Cutaneous Involvement of T-Cell and NK-Cell Lymphomas/Leukemias

Cutaneous HTLV-1 Adult T-Cell Leukemia/Lymphoma

Cutaneous adult T-cell leukemia/lymphoma has an association with the retrovirus human T-cell lymphotropic virus-1 (HTLV-1) and is endemic in southwestern Japan, the Caribbean islands, South America and Central Africa.[170,171] The prognosis of ATLL is in general poor, but indolent variants have been published. In the WHO classification there are four variants: acute leukemic, chronic leukemic, lymphomatous, and smoldering.[172]

The skin as well as peripheral blood, bone marrow, lymph node, spleen, liver, and other internal organs may be involved. In half the cases, the cutaneous lesions of ATLL resemble those of MF and Sezary syndrome clinically.[173] The lesions can be patches, plaques, papules, nodules, tumoral or erythrodermic, with nodulotumoral type associated with poor prognosis. [173]

On histologic sections an infiltrate of atypical cerebriform pleomorphic cells is seen commonly with epidermotropism and Pautrier microabscesses. Tumor nodule extending to the subcutaneous fat can be seen in some cases. Since the clinical presentation and histopathology are similar to MF, serologic testing for HTLV-1 antibodies is essential for diagnosis. In addition to possessing a T-helper phenotype (CD3+ CD4+ CD8-) with a CD4:CD8 ratio greater than or equal to 20:1, the neoplastic cells often express CD25, CD30 and PD1.[170,172] Loss of CD7 expression, CD4-CD8+, CD4+CD8+, and CD4-CD8- phenotypes can be seen. They have been reported to have a T-regulatory phenotype (CD4+ CD25+ FoxP3+). Decreased CD7 expression and increased CADM1 expression are more frequently seen in aggressive ATLL tumors.[174]

The differential diagnosis includes MF, Sezary syndrome, primary cutaneous anaplastic large cell lymphoma, and peripheral T-cell lymphoma not otherwise specified. The presence of HTLV-1 antibody or monoclonal integration of pro-viral HTLV-1 DNA helps to confirm the diagnosis.[175,176]

Cutaneous HTLV–1 adult T-cell leukemia/lymphoma

- CD3+, CD4+, CD5+, CD25+/-, CD30+/-
- CD8-, CD20-, CD79a-

Angioimmunoblastic T-Cell Lymphoma

Angioimmunoblastic T-cell lymphoma is an aggressive peripheral T-cell lymphoma of follicular helper T lymphocytes that accompanied by a proliferation of high endothelial venules (venules with prominent endothelial lining). It is primarily nodal with frequent hepatic and splenic involvement and associated hypergammaglobulinemia. The low number of published cases has resulted in limited information regarding prognosis of cases with mainly cutaneous involvement; however, it is generally considered an aggressive lymphoma with poor prognosis. Cutaneous manifestations, although not characteristic, can be the first manifestation of a systemic lymphoma.[177] Cutaneous manifestations range from maculopapular eruptions to purpura and even erythroderma. It affects elderly adults in the form of erythematous papules, plaques, or tumors, simulating other T-cell lymphomas.

Histologic sections show a nodular to diffuse infiltrate of small, medium or large pleomorphic lymphocytes admixed with inflammatory cells (plasma cells, eosinophils, and histiocytes). The histologic pattern typically shows hyperplasia of thick-walled venules associated with either sparse or dense dermal infiltrate comprised of large pleomorphic cells admixed with histiocytes, plasma cells, and eosinophils.[177]

The proliferative follicular helper T lymphocytes are CD3+, CD4+, CD5+, and CD8-. The neoplastic T-cells often express other T follicular helper markers with PD1 and ICOS being more sensitive than CD10 and CXCL13.[178] Aggregates of polyclonal B-cell lymphocytes can be seen. Around the high endothelial venules, a CD21 positive follicular dendritic cells may be also detected. Helpful histologic features include vascular hyperplasia, expansile CD21+ dendritic meshwork, co-expression of CD10, and germinal center T-helper cell markers (CXCL13, PD1, Bcl6) by the tumor cells. Expression of germinal-center T-helper-cell markers such as PD1 and CXCL13 has been reported to be helpful in distinguish angioimmunoblastic T-cell lymphoma from peripheral T-cell lymphoma, not otherwise specified.[179,180] Occasional cases can be positive for EBV.[180]

6.11 EBV-Positive Lymphoproliferative Diseases

Hydroa Vacciniforme Lymphoproliferative Disorder

This rare form of lymphoproliferative disorder affects predominantly children in Latin America and Asia with the clinical presentation resembling hydroa vacciniforme.[181] The median age is 16 years and there is a male predominance.[182] It has previously been classified as a lymphoma in the 2008 WHO classification. There are two subtypes, classic and systemic. Recurrent papulovesicular eruptions are seen on sun-exposed skin, especially the face with prominent swelling, which resolve as atrophic scars in the classic form.[181] Seasonal variation is noted with eruption more common in spring and summer. Classic form follows a relapsing course with complete resolution by adolescence or adulthood. In the systemic form, non-sun-exposed skin as well as liver, spleen, and lymph node are affected.[183] Onset age of greater than nine years and *BXLF1* expression, EBV-encoded immediate-early gene transcript are markers of poor survival.[184]

It has a prolonged course with an outcome between aggressive cutaneous cytotoxic NK/T cell lymphoma and more indolent types of cutaneous T-cell lymphomas.[183] Epidermal degeneration, vesiculation, and sometimes ulceration are seen. A dense infiltrate of atypical lymphoid cells is noted in the dermis and often the subcutaneous tissue. The neoplastic cells are CD2+, CD3+, CD4-, CD8+/-, CD56+/-, and CD30+/-. In many cases the CD8+ cytotoxic tumor cells express granzyme B, TIA1, and perforin. In a small subset, the tumor cells have an NK-cell phenotype (CD56- CD5- TCR -). *In situ* hybridization for EBV is invariably positive. [181] Clonal TCR rearrangement is detected in most cases.

Hydroa vacciniforme-like lymphoproliferative disorder

- Cytotoxic phenotype: CD8+, TIA1+, granzyme B+, perforin+
- NK-cell phenotype: CD56-, CD5-, TCR-
- All cases EBER+

Lymphomatoid Granulomatosis

Lymphomatoid granulomatosis is a rare, aggressive EBV-associated B-cell predominant LPD most commonly affecting the lungs, but also involving the skin in up to 50% of cases, with skin lesions preceding the development of lung lesions in 10–15% of cases.[185] Clinically, it often presents as widespread, multifocal erythematous papulonodular or plaque-like rash often associated with systemic symptoms.[185] Histologically, it is characterized by dermal- and subcutaneous-based angioinvasive lymphocytic inflammation with associated necrosis and admixed histiocytes, plasma cells, and rare granulocytes and eosinophils.[185] Granulomas are rarely encountered. The infiltrate is predominantly composed of small CD4+ T cells infiltrating the vasculature with a variable amount of atypical CD20+ B cells. EBER ISH highlights rare, scattered B cells, which are more conspicuous in biopsied nodular skin lesions. The absence of EBV positivity should not preclude the diagnosis in an otherwise classic presentation.[185] B-cell clonality has been demonstrated in pulmonary lesions of lymphomatoid granulomatosis with an absence of T-cell clonality, leading to the classification of a B-cell LPD with a prominent T-cell background component.[185]

Lymphomatoid granulomatosis

- Dermal to subcutaneous angioinvasive mixed inflammation should prompt a panel of T-cell (CD3, CD4, CD8) and B-cell markers (CD20) coupled with EBER to assist in the diagnosis, especially in the context of pulmonary involvement

6.12 Cutaneous Lymphoproliferative Disorders Associated with Immunodeficiency and Dysregulation

EBV-Positive Mucocutaneous Ulcer

EBV-positive mucocutaneous ulcer can affect the cutaneous as well as mucosal sites (oral, upper aerodigestive tract, and gastrointestinal tract). [186,187] It arises in association with autoimmunity, therapy-related immune suppression, post-organ transplantation, and HIV infection.[186,188] The typical presentation is a well-circumscribed and painful ulcer in cutaneous or mucosal sites without systemic symptoms in an elderly individual (>70 years).[186]

On histologic sections, a polymorphous infiltrate of small to large lymphoid cells, variable number of immunoblasts, admixed with plasma cells, histiocytes, and eosinophils is seen beneath an ulcer. Necrosis, vascular thrombosis, and angioinvasive can be seen.[188] The atypical large B-cells are CD20+EBV+, and sometimes CD30+ yet CD15-.[186,188]

The differential diagnosis includes EBV-positive diffuse large B-cell lymphoma, other methotrexate-induced cutaneous B-cell lymphoproliferative disorders that are not EBV-related.[187] Clonal TCR or IgH gene rearrangements can be detected in 30–50% of cases.[186]

EBV-positive mucocutaneous ulcer

- Well-circumscribed ulcer in cutaneous or mucosal sites
- Polymorphous infiltrate with CD20+CD30+/– large atypical cells
- EBV+

6.13 Case Studies

Case 6.1

Clinical history: A 78-year-old man presented with left upper arm nodule.

Description: Histologic sections showed a diffuse proliferation of atypical lymphoid cells with numerous mitotic figures (**Figures 6.98 and 6.99**). These small to medium atypical lymphoid cells were CD20+ CD5+ Cyclin

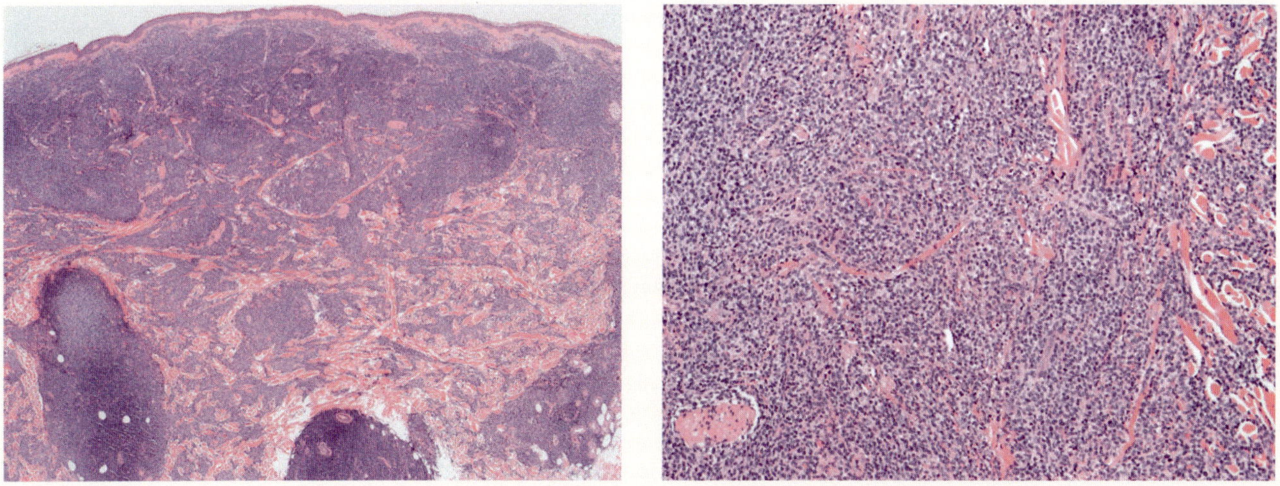

Figures 6.98 and 6.99 A diffuse proliferation of atypical lymphoid cells is seen replacing the dermis (X40 and X200).

D1+ SOX11+ Bcl2+ and CD3- Bcl6- (**Figures 6.100–6.103**). A year and three months ago he presented with an enlarged left inguinal lymph node. At that time the tumor cells were positive for CD20, CD5, cyclin D1, SOX11, CD43, and Bcl2. They were negative for Bcl6, CD23, and CD10. Flow cytometric analysis demonstrated a clonal CD20+ B-cell population that co-express CD5 and surface lambda light chain. Fluorescence *in situ* hybridization demonstrated fusion of *CDND1* (11q23) and *IGH* (14q32.3). These findings are supportive of mantle cell lymphoma and the immunoprofile is similar to that of skin lymphoma.

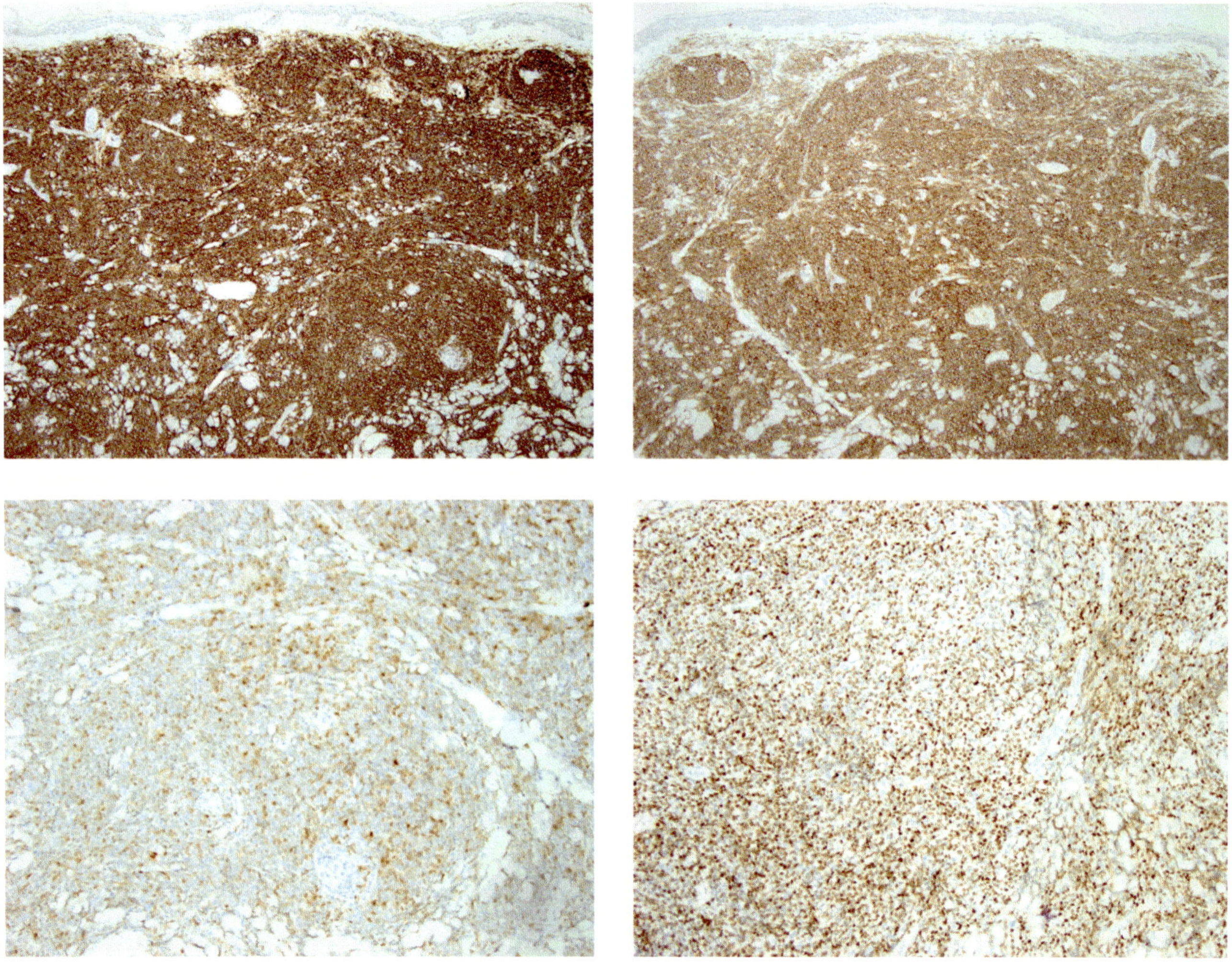

Figures 6.100–103 The tumor cells are strongly positive for CD20 (Fig 6.100, X100), CD5 (Fig 6.101, X100), cyclin D1 (Fig 6.102, X200) and Sox11 (Fig 6.103, X200).

Diagnosis: Cutaneous involvement by nodal mantle cell lymphoma.

Discussion: Deriving from the inner mantle zone of lymphoid follicles mantle cell lymphoma is rare and cutaneous manifestation can be the first presentation of the disease.[189] Mantle cell lymphoma is a B-cell lymphoma that expresses CD20, CD5, and not CD23. It harbors a characteristic translocation t(11;14)(q13;q32) that results in overexpression of cyclin D1 in greater than 95% of cases.[189] For cases that lack this translocation Sox11 immunostain has recently been shown to be a helpful diagnostic marker.[190] It is now understood that differential Sox11 expression is a result of development from a different pathway. Classical mantle cell lymphoma is composed of *IGHV*-unmutated B-cells that typically express Sox11.[191] A subset of mantle cell lymphoma arises from *IGHV*-mutated B-cells that do not express Sox11.[191]

Case 6.2

Clinical history: A 77-year-old man with a long history of mycosis fungoides presented with progressive nodules. On physical examination multiple erythematous scaly plaques were seen on his trunk and extremities (**Figure 6.104**). In addition, several ulcerated nodules were seen on his chest (**Figure 6.105**).

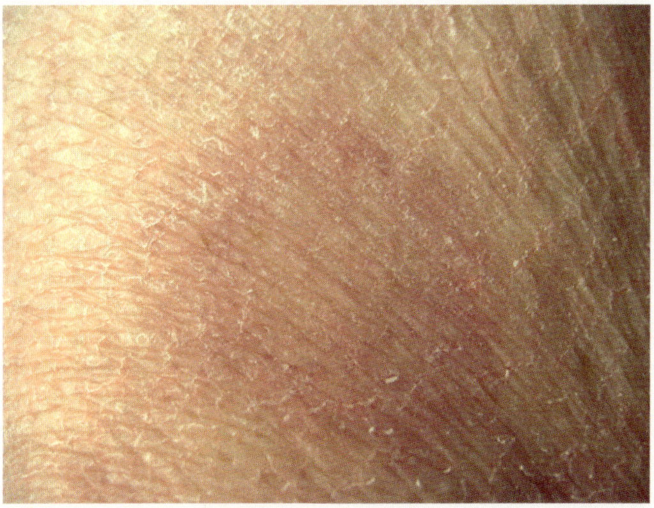

Figure 6.104 Erythematous scaly plaque on the patient's extremity (courtesy of Whitney A. High, MD, JD, Departments of Dermatology and Pathology, University of Colorado School of Medicine, Denver, Colorado, USA).

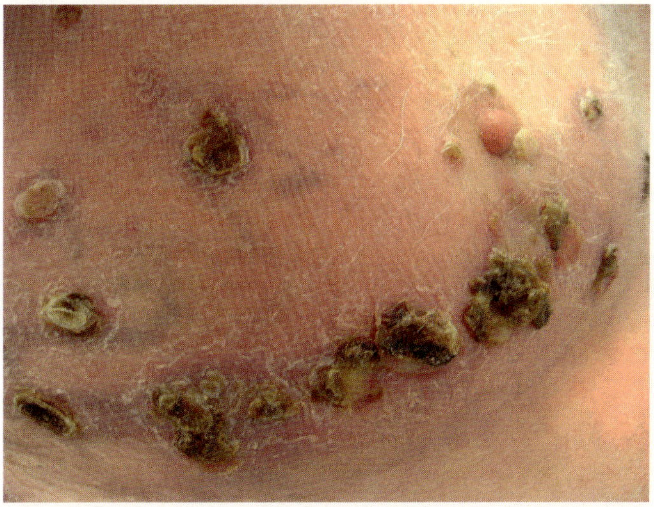

Figure 6.105 Ulcerated nodules on the patient's chest (Courtesy of Whitney A. High, MD, JD, Departments of Dermatology and Pathology, University of Colorado School of Medicine, Denver, Colorado, USA).

Description: The biopsy of the background erythematous and scaly plaques showed a patchy band-like infiltrate of atypical CD3+CD4+CD8- lymphoid cells in the superficial dermis and focal epidermotropism (**Figure 6.106**). The biopsy of the nodule showed a dense infiltrate of large pleomorphic cells admixed with lymphocytes and neutrophils below an ulcerated epidermis (**Figure 6.107**). This population of CD30+ tumor cells comprised of approximately 60% of the dermal infiltrate (**Figure 6.108**). They were also positive for CD3, CD4, and CD25 and negative for ALK1. T-cell receptor gamma gene rearrangement analysis revealed the same clonal population in the patch stage as well as the tumor nodule.

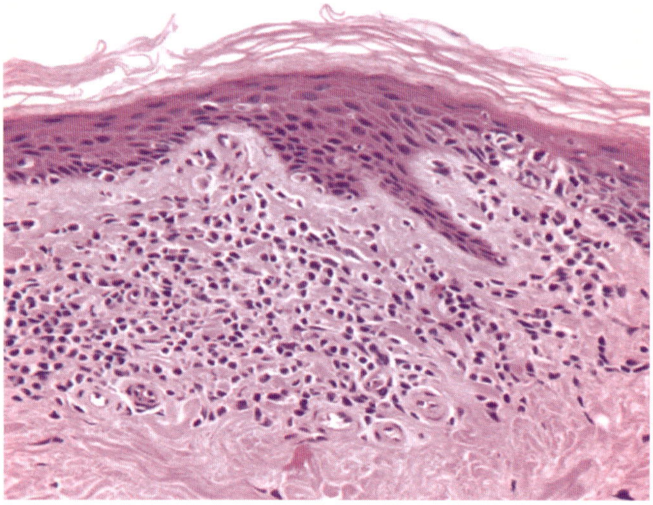

Figure 6.106 Patchy band-like infiltrate of atypical lymphoid cells with focal epidermotropism (X200).

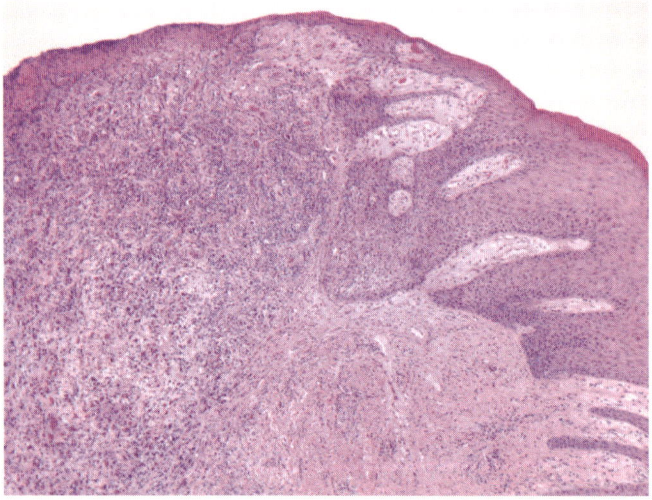

Figure 6.107 Dense infiltrate of large pleomorphic cells (X100).

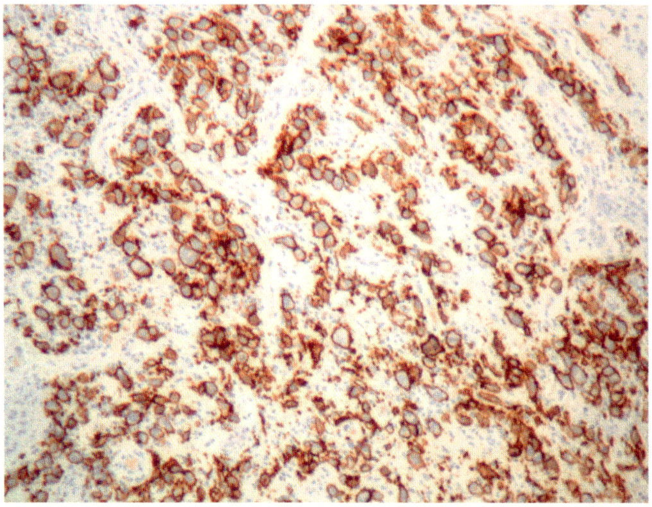

Figure 6.108 The tumor cells are strongly positive for CD30 (X200).

Diagnosis: Transformed mycosis fungoides.

Discussion: Large cell transformation of MF can be seen in advanced stage and is a marker of poor prognosis.[85] It is usually associated with multiple skin plaques or tumors. Large cell transformation is defined by a population of large cells, immunoblast or pleomorphic in appearance, CD30 positive or negative, in greater than 25% of the tumor cells.[85] A cell diameter of greater than 35um has been defined as large.[192] CD30 expression can be seen and its lack of expression has been reported to be associated with poor prognosis.[84] The presence of nodules together with patches and plaques typically seen in MF is supportive of large cell transformation of MF rather than CD30-positive anaplastic large cell lymphoma. CD68 would be helpful in highlighting the prominent histiocytes in histiocyte-rich or granulomatous MF. CD30 expression can be seen in other non-MF lymphomas such as cutaneous EBV+ diffuse large B-cell lymphoma of the elderly and hydroa vacciniforme-like lymphoproliferative disorder. Although CD30+ tumor cells would raise the possibility of anaplastic large cell lymphoma, the expression of CD30 has to be seen in 75% or greater of the tumor cells to support this diagnosis.

Case 6.3

Clinical history: A 61-year-old man presented with a 2.5 × 2.5 cm purpuric patch on his left chest.

Description: Histologic sections showed aggregates of plasma cells at the periphery of homogeneous dermal and perivascular materials in the dermis (**Figures 6.109 and 6.110**). Congo red stain demonstrates these dermal deposits to be amyloid (**Figure 6.111**). Kappa and lambda *in situ* hybridization demonstrated the plasma cell infiltrate to be monotypic for kappa light chain (**Figures 6.112 and 6.113**). Subsequent bone marrow biopsy was negative for significant plasma cell infiltrate.

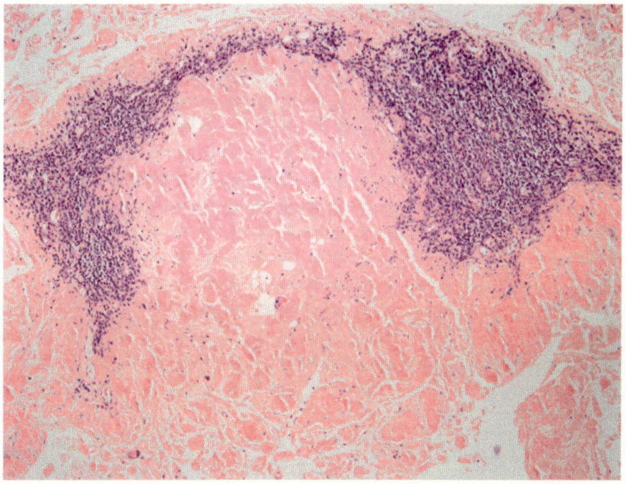

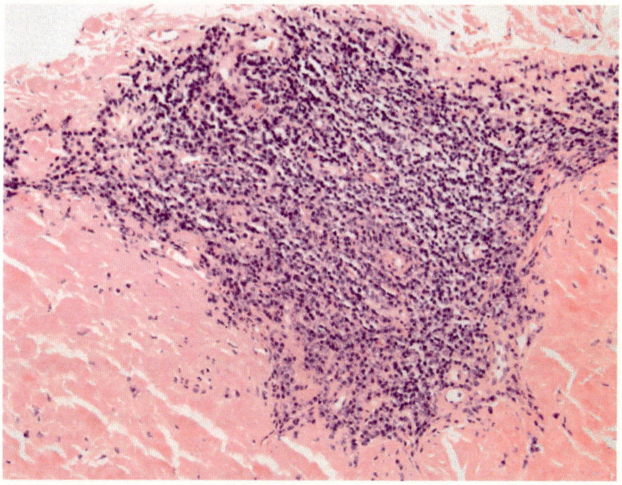

Figures 6.109 and 6.110 A prominent infiltrate of plasma cells is seen in association with amorphous and eosinophilic materials (X100 and X200).

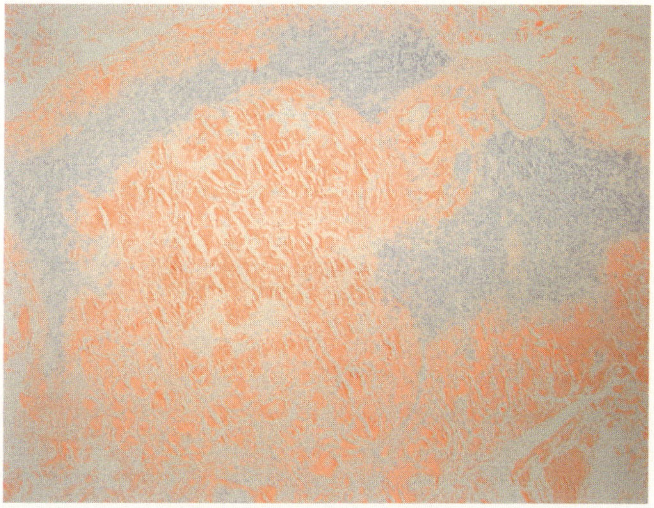

Figure 6.111 Congo red special stain highlights the amyloid deposit (X100).

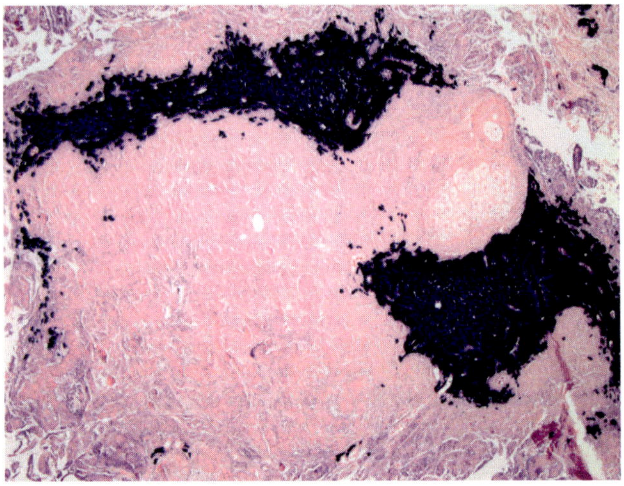

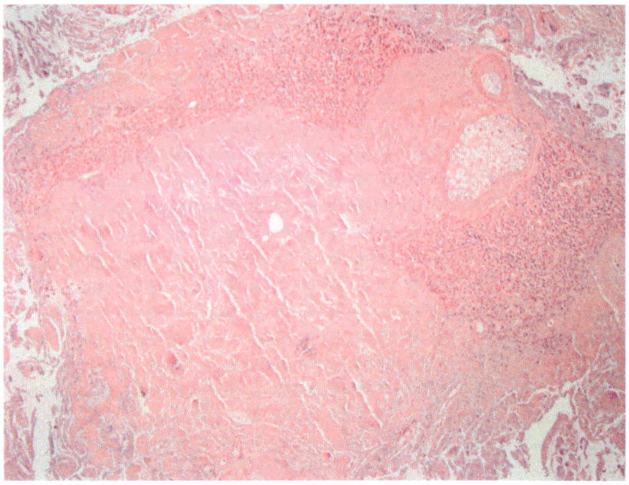

Figures 6.112 and 6.113 Kappa and lambda *in situ* hybridization demonstrates kappa light chain restriction (X100).

Diagnosis: Plasmacytoma with associated amyloidosis.

Discussion: Cutaneous plasmacytoma without bone marrow involvement is exceeding rare; thus, some have proposed that it is likely a marginal zone lymphoma with prominent plasma cell differentiation.[192] It is classified as a provisional entity in the EORTC classification and a peripheral B-cell lymphoma in the REAL and WHO classification.[1] It can present as a solitary cluster of plaques or nodules on the head and trunk of elderly males. A proliferation of mature and immature CD38+, CD138+, MUM1+, and CD79a+/- plasma cells is seen expanding the dermis.[193] Amyloid deposition is often seen in the setting of cutaneous involvement by multiple myeloma especially in vascular walls. Multiple myeloma is a plasma cell dyscrasia mainly involving the bone marrow; however, extramedullary such as cutaneous involvement is an indicator of poor prognosis.[194] Other conditions with prominent dermal infiltrate of plasma cells include IgG4-related skin disease, plasmablastic lymphoma, and cutaneous marginal zone B-cell lymphoma. IgG4-related skin disease is characterized by prominent IgG4+ plasma cells (IgG4:IgG ratio greater than 40%), storiform fibrosis, obliterative phlebitis, and elevated serum IgG4 level.[195]

Case 6.4

Clinical history: A ten-year-old girl with non-resolving hematoma on the left leg (**Figure 6.114**).

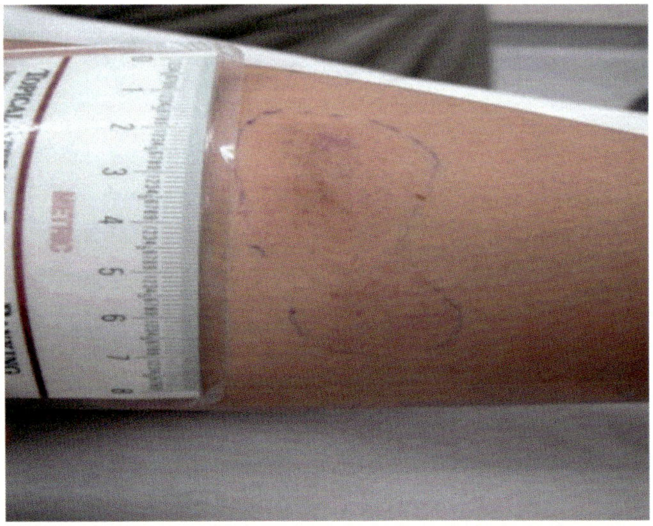

Figure 6.114 A non-resolving "hematoma" is seen on the patient's leg.

Description: The sections showed a predominantly perivascular dermal monomorphous infiltrate of medium sized neoplastic cells extending to the subcutaneous tissue (**Figure 6.115**). The epidermis was within normal limits. Intratumoral hemorrhage was noted. High power examination showed blastoid cells admixed with reactive lymphocytes (**Figure 6.116**). The neoplastic cells expressed CD4, CD56, and CD123. TdT reactivity demonstrated the origin from precursor cells. CD3, CD20, TIA-1 and myeloperoxidase were negative (**Figures 6.117–6.121**).

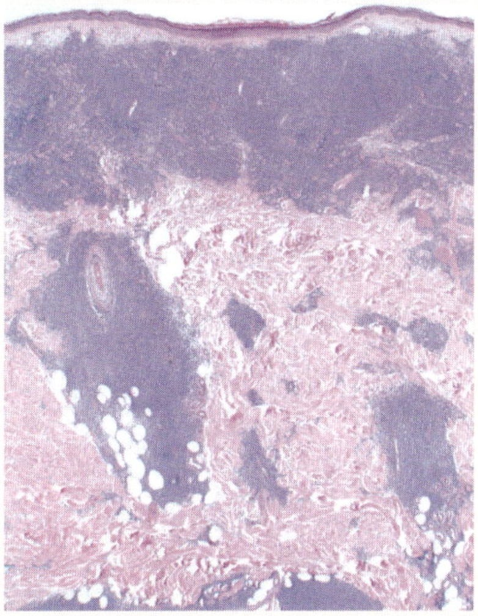

Figure 6.115 A dense lymphoid infiltrate is seen extending from the upper dermis to the subcutaneous tissue.

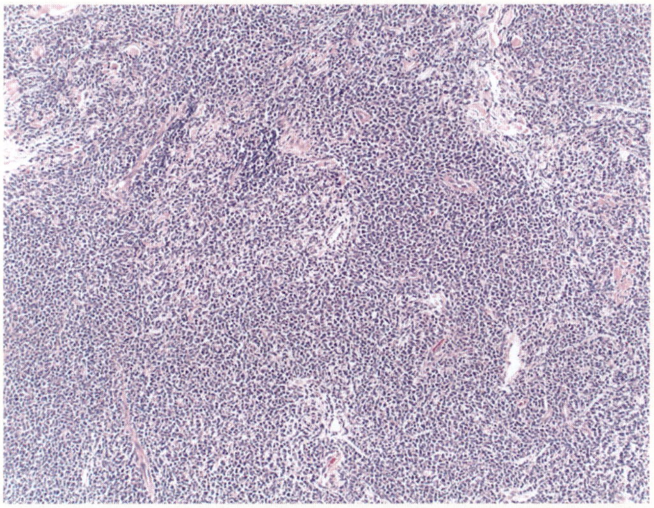

Figure 6.116 The cells are medium in size and blastoid in appearance (X100).

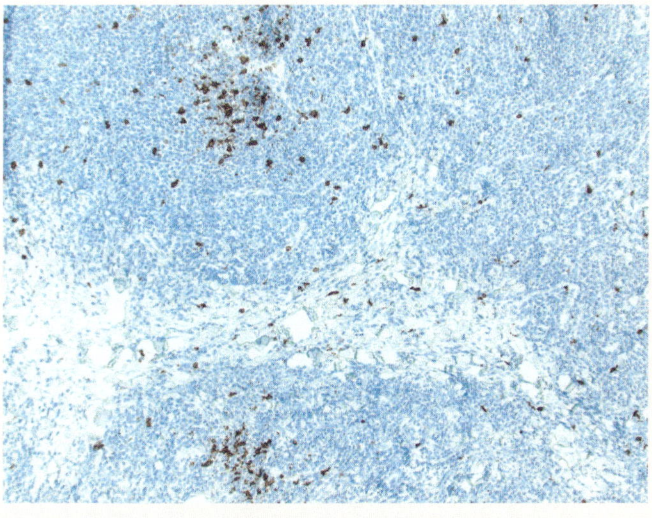

Figure 6.117 Isolated lymphocytes are CD3 positive (X100).

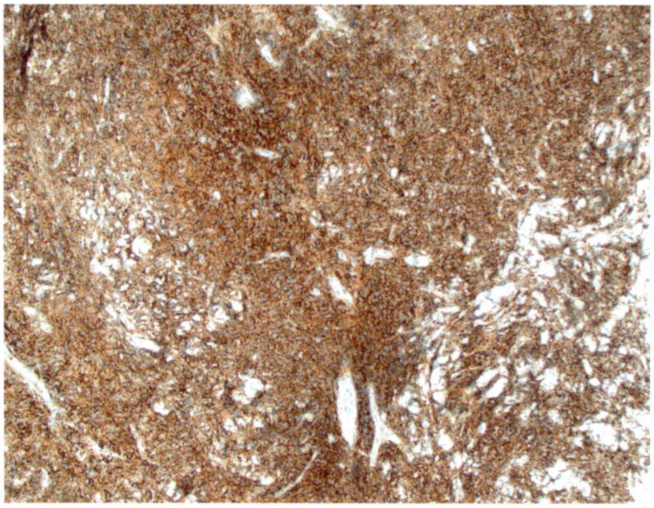

Figure 6.118 The majority of the lymphocytes are CD4 positive (X100).

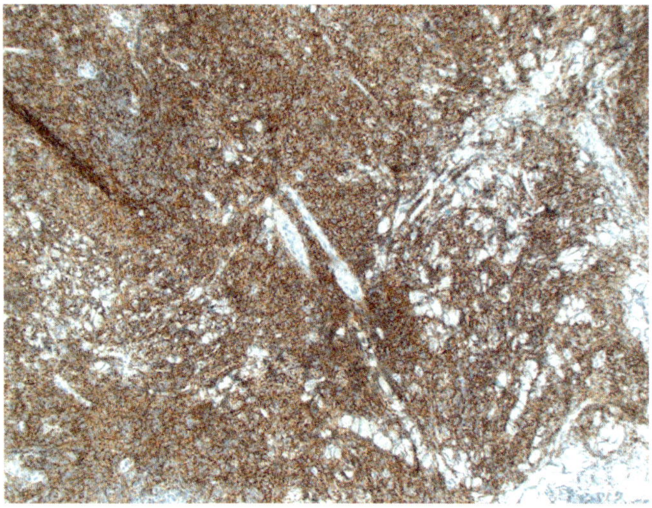

Figure 6.119 CD56 is seen in most of the lymphocytes (X100).

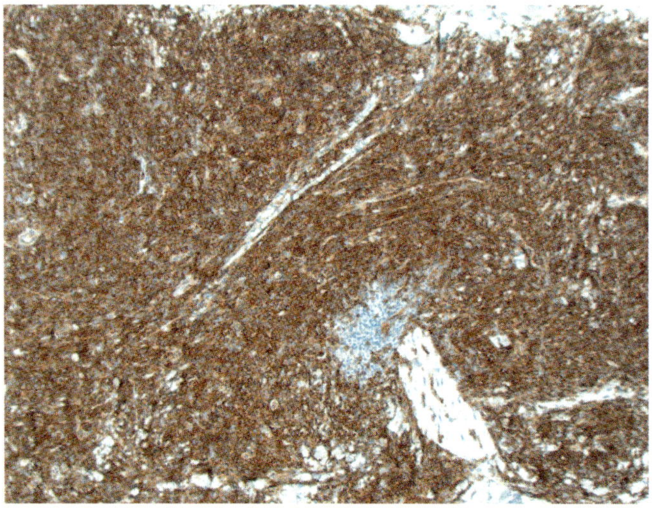

Figure 6.120 CD123 decorates the tumor cells (X100).

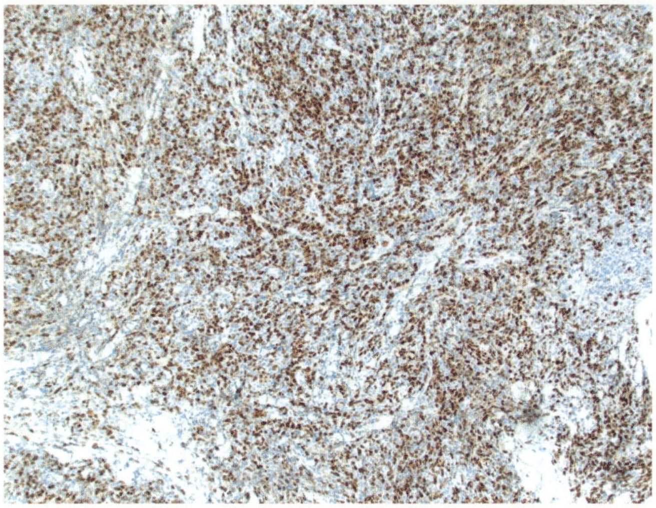

Figure 6.121 The lymphocytes are TdT positive (X100).

Diagnosis: Blastic plasmacytoid dendritic cell neoplasm.

Discussion: Blastic plasmacytoid dendritic cell neoplasm is a rare disease with very poor prognosis. Commonly, it affects adults and elderly patients; however, pediatric cases as represented by this case can also occur. Localized or generalized plaques and tumors with hemorrhagic or "bruise-like" appearance are characteristic clinical presentations.[196] Early cases present as perivascular infiltrate of blastoid medium-size cells that evolves to pandermal infiltrates with extension to the subcutis. Although the combination of CD4, CD56, and CD123 reactivity is the classic profile in this neoplasm, negative cases has been published.[197] Therefore these three markers need to be part of a panel in conjunction with markers for lymphoid and myeloid antigens. Of note, myeloid leukemia can be positive for CD4 and CD123. The three classical antigens should be used in conjunction with T-cell leukemia/lymphoma (TCL)-1 and blood dendritic cell antigen 2 (BDCA-2, CD303) positive in blastic plasmacytoid dendritic cell neoplasm and commonly negative in myelogenous leukemia. This overlap in immunohistochemical stains is not surprising in view of the relationship seen between these two diseases using whole exome sequencing analysis.

Case 6.5

Clinical history: A 35-year-old female presented with papulosquamous eruption follow by enlargement of a lymph node.

Description: The skin showed a pan-dermal perivascular aggregates of medium sized lymphocytes admixed with eosinophils (**Figures 6.122 and 6.123**). The lymph node demonstrated small to medium sized pleomorphic lymphocytes intermingled with plasma cells, histiocytes, immunoblasts, and eosinophils. High endothelial venules were seen. The neoplastic cells reacted with CD3, CD4, CD10 and CXCL13 (**Figures 6.124–6.127**). The same clonal rearrangement was seen in the lymph node and skin.

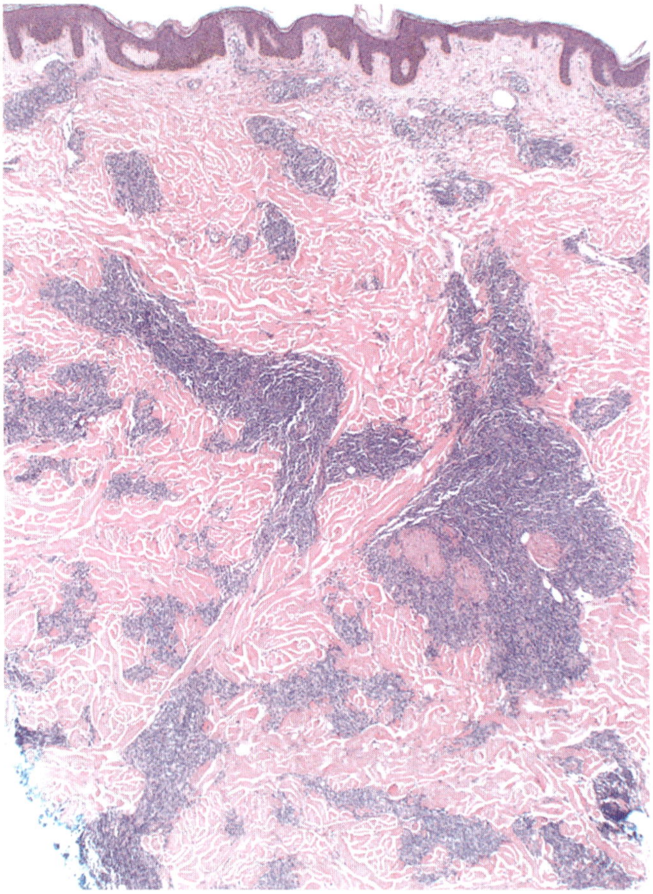

Figure 6.122 A dense nodular infiltrate affects the dermis (X40).

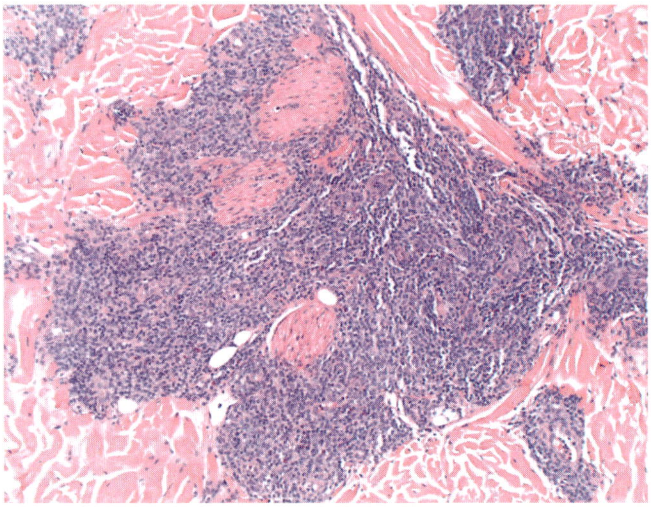

Figure 6.123 The cells are medium in size admixed with eosinophils (X100).

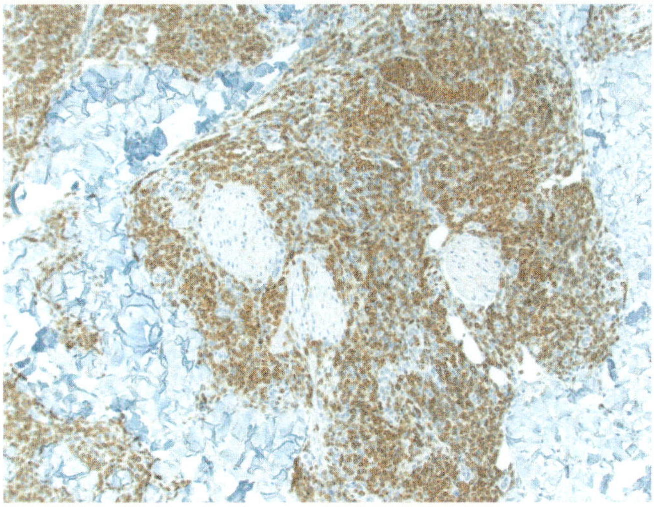

Figure 6.124 The majority of the lymphoid cells are CD3 positive (X100).

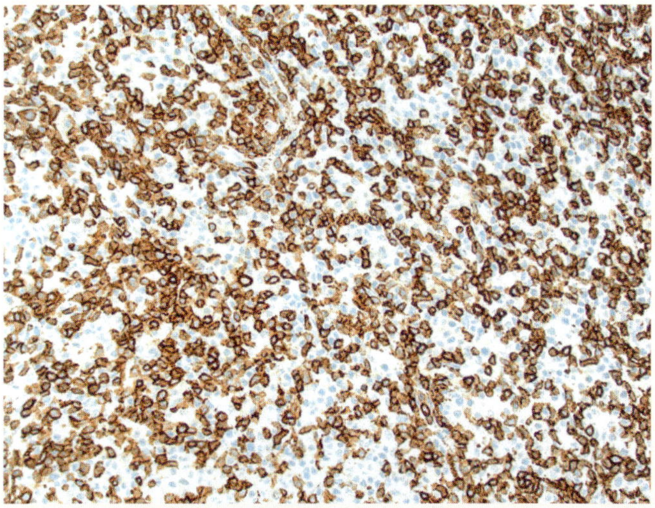

Figure 6.125 CD4 decorates the infiltrate (X200).

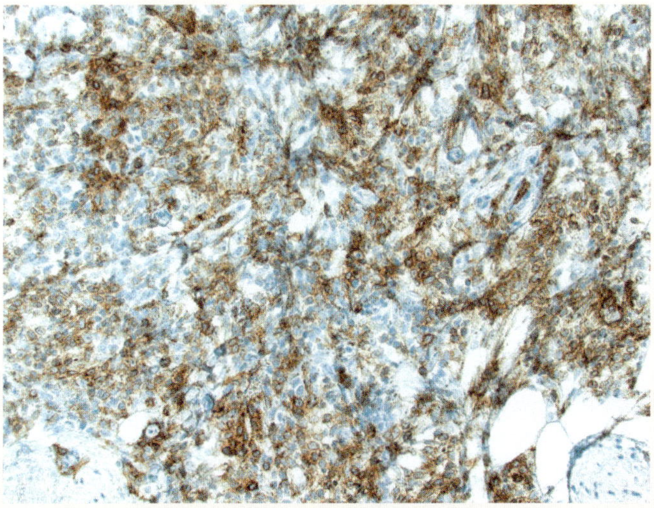

Figure 6.126 CD10 expression is seen in most of the lymphocytes (X200).

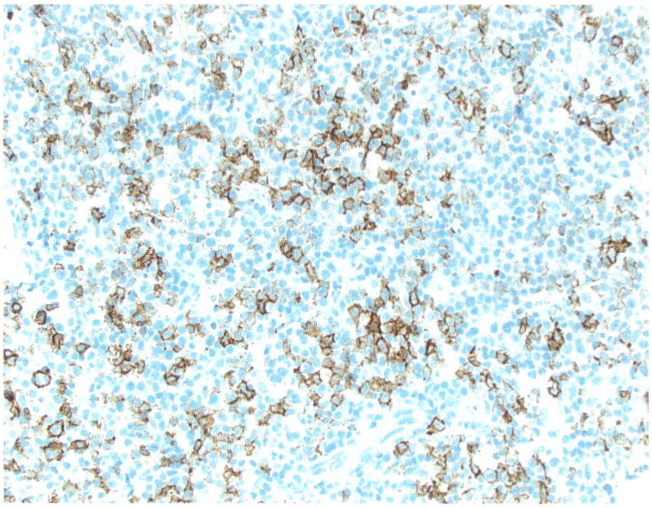

Figure 6.127 CXCL13 highlights some of the lesional cells (X200).

Diagnosis: Cutaneous involvement by angioimmunoblastic T-cell lymphoma.

Discussion: Angioimmunoblastic T-cell lymphoma is an aggressive peripheral T-cell lymphoma with poor prognosis. The tumor cells exhibit a follicular helper T lymphocyte phenotype characterized by expression of CD3, CD4, CD10, Bcl6, PD1 and chemokine ligand CXCL13. Expression of germinal-center T-helper-cell markers such as PD1 and CXCL13 has been reported to be helpful in distinguish angioimmunoblastic T-cell lymphoma from peripheral T-cell lymphoma, not otherwise specified.

Case 6.6

Clinical history: A 40-year-old man with a long history of an erythematous plaques that had evolved to a peduncular mass in the inguinal area (**Figure 6.128**). No lymphadenopathy was identified.

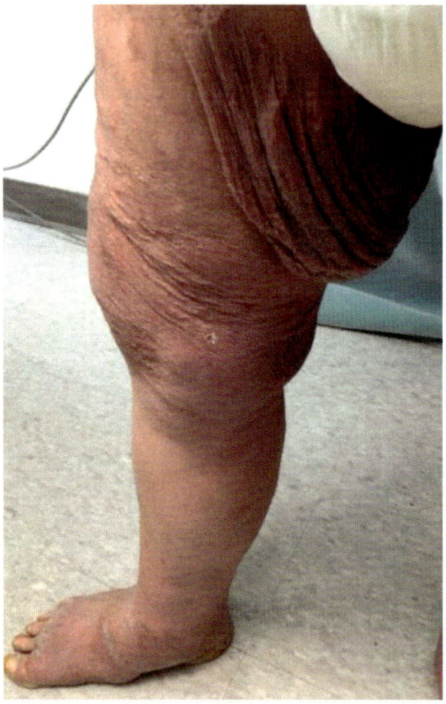

Figure 6.128 A pedunculated mass affects the inguinal area of a 40-year-old man.

Description: The biopsy of the pedunculated mass shows a dermal based infiltrate of multinucleated giant cells admixed with atypical lymphocytes (**Figure 6.129**). Only focal epidermotropism is noted. Decreased density of elastic fibers is seen (**Figure 6.130**). Immunohistochemical stains show that the lymphocytic infiltrate is CD3+CD4+CD8- (**Figures 6.131–6.133**). T-cell receptor gamma gene rearrangement analysis is clonal.

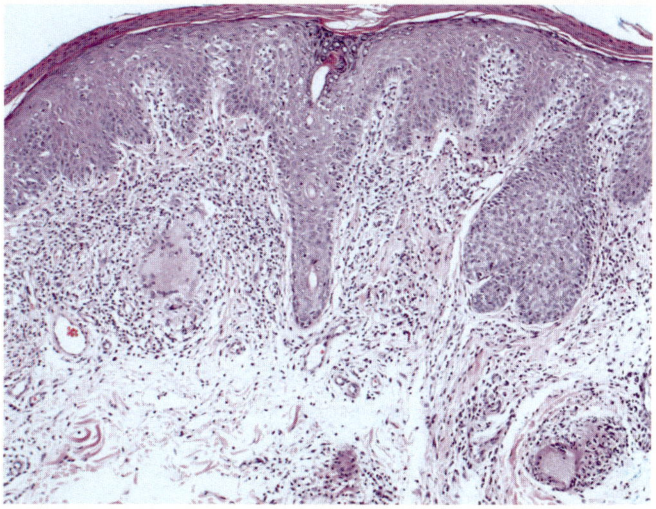

Figure 6.129 An infiltrate of atypical lymphocytes admixed with multinucleated giant cells is seen (X100).

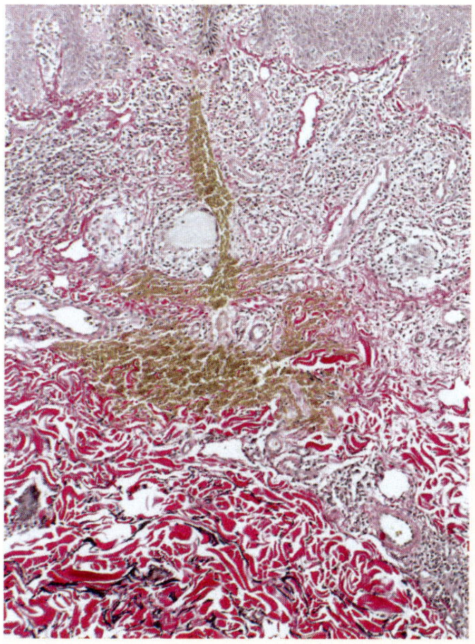

Figure 6.130 A reduction of dermal elastic fibers is noted (X100).

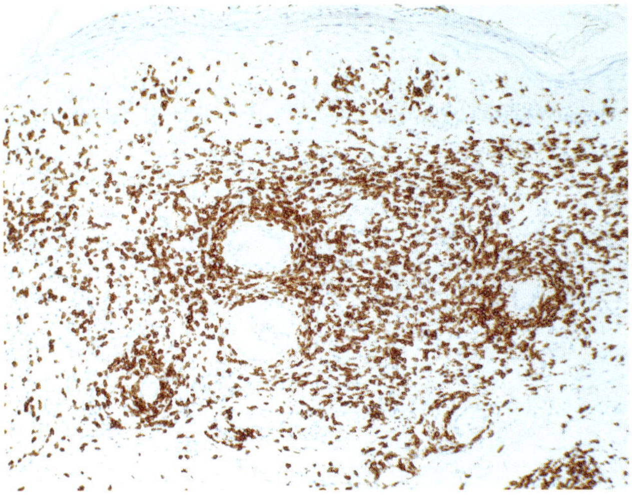

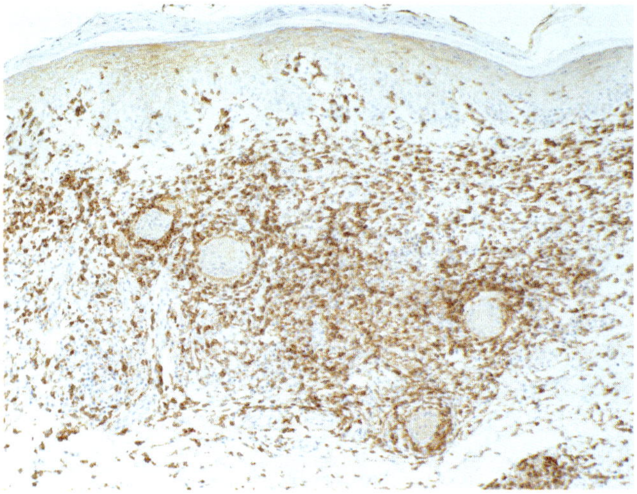

Figures 6.131 and 6.132 The atypical lymphoid cells are positive for CD3 and CD4 (X100, X100).

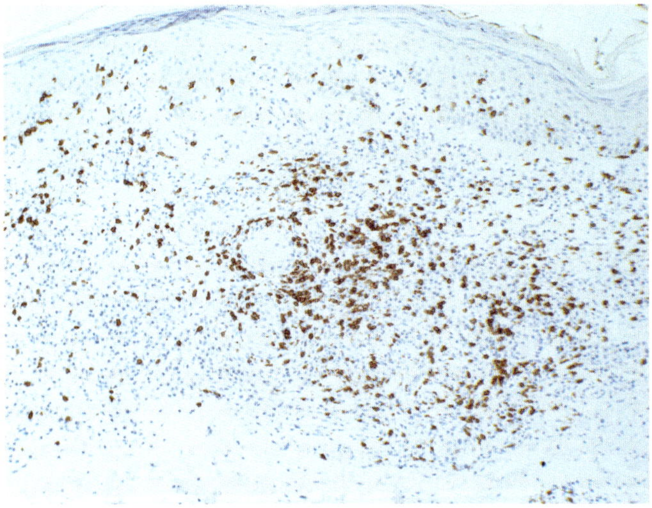

Figure 6.133 They are negative for CD8 (X100).

Diagnosis: Granulomatous slack skin.

Discussion: GSS is a rare variant of MF affecting predominantly young males. It manifests first with patches and plaques that evolve into the characteristic pendulous skin folds as in this patient.[81] The biopsy usually shows a prominent dermal infiltrate of multinucleated giant cells admixed with histiocytes showing elastophagocytosis. The dermal lymphocytic infiltrate may not demonstrate significant nuclear atypia, making these cases difficult to diagnose in the absence of clinical information.[82] The diagnostic difficulty increases as some of the biopsies may lack epidermotropism. The immunophenotype has a classic MF profile with CD3+, CD4+, CD8- and CD45RO+. Rare cases of CD8+ are seen. The loss of pan T-cell markers like CD5 and CD7 in conjunction with detection of clonality will support the diagnosis of GSS. The clinical presentation is of paramount importance to reach a final diagnosis. Although this is an indolent and slowly progressive lymphoma, it is often treatment-resistant.[83]

Case 6.7

Clinical history: A 65-year-old female present with multiple erythematous plaques with follicular prominence, papules and acneiform lesions in head and neck areas as well as upper trunk. No nodules or lymphadenopathy was identified.

Description: The biopsy of one of the erythematous plaques shows hair follicles distended by mucin with peri and intrafollicular atypical lymphocytic infiltrate (**Figures 6.134–6.135**). The infiltrate is mild and affects the superficial to mid dermis and is composed of small- to medium-sized lymphocytes. The infiltrate is positive for CD3 and CD4, while negative for CD7 (**Figures 6.136–6.137**). T-cell receptor gamma gene rearrangement analysis is positive.

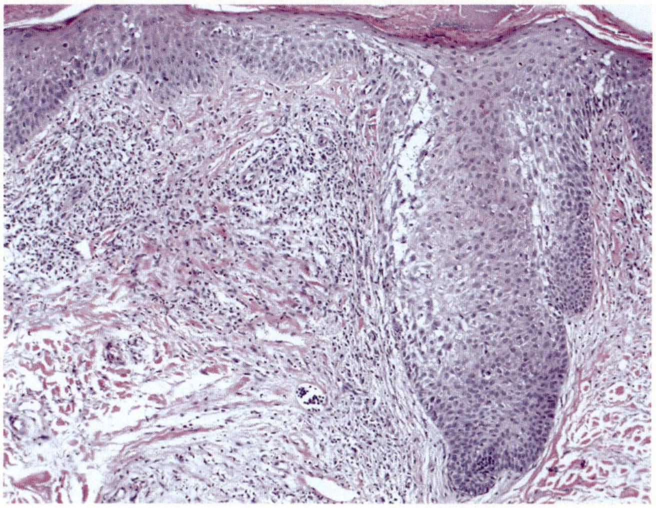

Figure 6.134 An atypical lymphoid infiltrate of small to medium sized lymphocytes is seen affecting the hair follicle (X100).

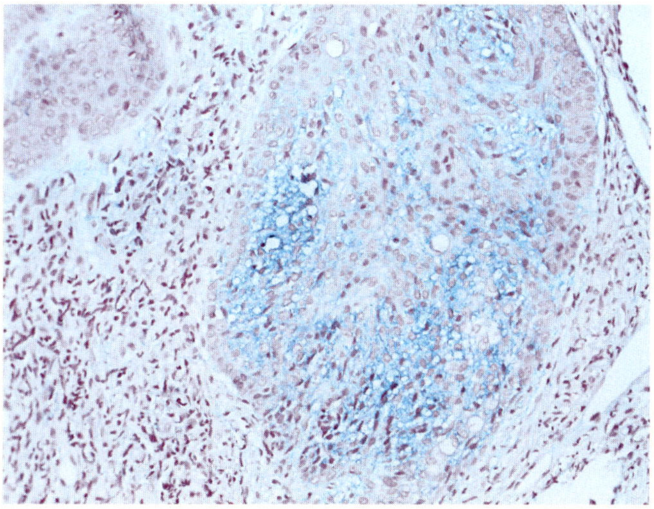

Figure 6.135 Colloidal iron highlights the mucin deposition within hair follicular epithelium (X200).

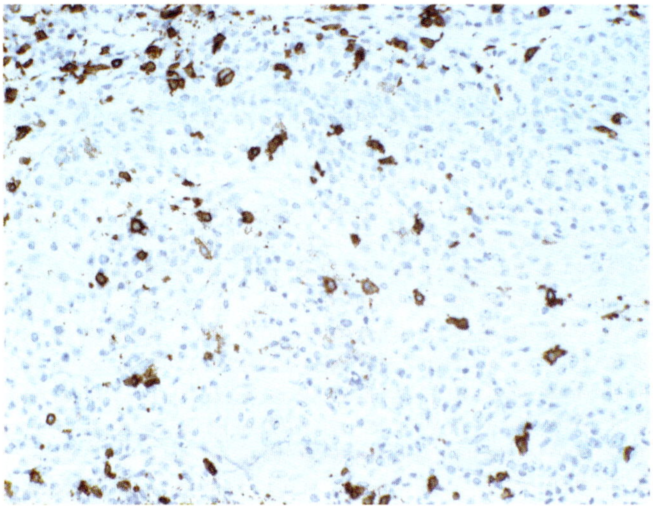

Figure 6.136 CD4 highlights the atypical lymphoid cells (X200).

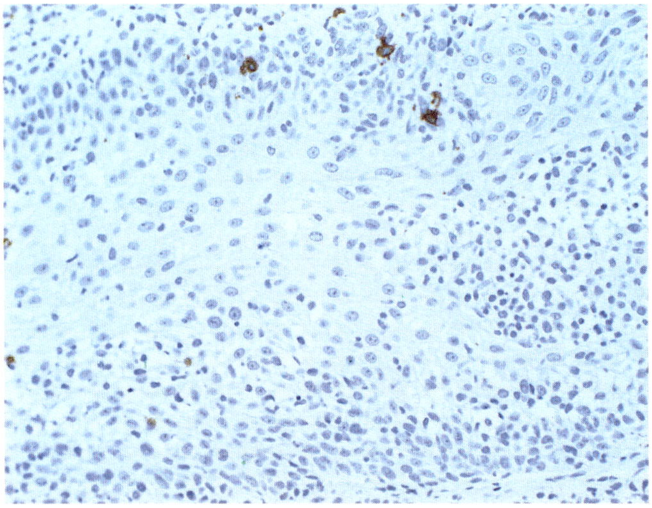

Figure 6.137 Loss of CD7 expression is noted (X200).

Diagnosis: Folliculotropic mycosis fungoides.

Discussion: Folliculotropic MF is the most common variant with a wide range of clinical presentations. Histologic sections are characterized by peri and intrafollicular atypical lymphoid infiltrate, sometime associated with follicular mucinosis, like in this case.[77] Biopsies may also show cysts, granulomatous inflammation, follicular hyperplasia, and eosinophilic folliculitis like changes. The immunoprofile is typically CD4+ alpha/beta TCR +. The presence of follicular mucinosis has been associated with reduced disease progression and therefore better prognosis. Recent studies have proposed to separate folliculotropic MF into early and late stages, as they differ in prognosis and treatment recommendations.[77] Patients with erythematous plaques, papules, keratosis pilaris like or acneiform like lesions are early stage and have favorable prognosis while plaques, nodules, tumors, erythroderma, or extracutaneous involvement have advanced stage disease. Clinically this patient belongs to the group of early stage. Plaque stage lesions have been separated into early stage with superficial to mid dermal intra or perifollicular few mainly small lymphoid cells associated with good prognosis whereas dense, confluent deep follicular infiltrates of medium to large lymphocytes are late stage.[77]

References

1. Swerdlow SH, Campo E, Harris NL, et al. WHO classification of tumors haematopoietic and lymphoid tissues. Lyon: IARC, 2008.
2. Willemze R, Cerroni L, Kempf W, et al. The 2018 update of the WHO-EORTC classification for primary cutaneous lymphomas. *Blood* 2019; **133**: 1703–14.
3. Swerdlow SH, Campo E, Pileri SA, et al. The 2016 revision of the World Health Organization classification of lymphoid neoplasms. *Blood* 2016; **127**: 2375–90.
4. Kempf W, Mitteldorf C, Cerroni L, et al. Classifications of cutaneous lymphomas and lymphoproliferative disorders: An update from the EORTC cutaneous lymphoma histopathology group. *J Eur Acad Dermatol Venereol* 2024; **38**: 1491–503.
5. Cerroni L, Signoretti S, Hofler G, et al. Primary cutaneous marginal B-cell lymphoma: a recently described entity of low-grade malignant cutaneous B-cell lymphoma. *Am J Surg Pathol* 1997; **21**: 1307–15.
6. Takino H, Li C, Hu S, et al. Primary cutaneous marginal zone B-cell lymphoma: a molecular and clinicopathological study of cases from Asia, Germany, and the United States. *Mod Pathol* 2008; **21**: 1517–26.
7. Edinger JT, Kant JA, Swerdlow SH. Cutaneous marginal zone lymphomas have distinctive features and include 2 subsets. *Am J Surg Pathol* 2010; **34**: 1830–41.
8. Carlsen ED, Swerdlow SH, Cook JR, Gibson SE. Class-switched primary cutaneous marginal zone lymphomas are frequently IgG4-positive and have features distinct from IgM-positive cases. *Am J Surg Pathol* 2019; **43**: 1403–12.
9. de Leval L, Harris NL, Longtine J, Ferry JA, Duncan LM. Cutaneous B-cell lymphomas of follicular and marginal zone types: Use of Bcl-6, CD10, Bcl-2, and CD21 in differential diagnosis and classification. *Am J Surg Pathol* 2001; **25**: 732–41.
10. Cerroni L, Arzberger E, Putz B, et al. Primary cutaneous follicular center cell lymphoma with follicular growth pattern. *Blood* 2000; **95**: 3922–8.
11. Brenner I, Roth S, Puppe B, Wobser M, Rosenwald A, Geissinger E. Primary cutaneous marginal zone lymphomas with plasmacytic differentiation show frequent IgG4 expression. *Mod Pathol* 2013; **26**: 1568–76.
12. Geyer JT, Ferry JA, Longine JA, Flotte TJ, Harris NL, Zukerberg LR. Characteristics of cutaneous marginal zone lymphomas with marked plasmacytic differentiation and a T cell-rich background. *Am J Clin Pathol* 2010; **133**: 59–69.
13. Kutzner H, Kerl H, Pfaltz MC, Kempf W. CD123-positive plasmacytoid dendritic cells in primary cutaneous marginal zone B-cell lymphoma: diagnostic and pathogenetic implications. *Am J Surg Pathol* 2009; **33**: 1307–13.
14. Falini B, Agostinelli C, Bigerna B, et al. IRTA1 is selectively expressed in nodal and extranodal marginal zone lymphomas. *Histopathology* 2012; **61**: 930–41.
15. Hoefnagel JJ, Vermeer MH, Janssen PM, Fleuren GJ, Miejer CJ, Willemze R. Bcl-2, Bcl-6 and CD10 expression in cutaneous B-cell lymphoma: further support for a follicle centre cell origin and differential diagnostic significance. *Br J Dermatol* 2003; **149**: 1183–91.
16. Zinzani PL, Quaglino P, Pimpinelli N, et al. Prognostic factors in primary cutaneous B-cell lymphoma: the Italian Study Group for Cutaneous Lymphomas. *J Clin Oncol* 2006; **24**: 1376–82.
17. Massone C, Fink-Puches R, Laimer M, Rütten A, Vale E, Cerroni L. Miliary and agminated-type primary cutaneous follicle center lymphoma: report of 18 cases. *J Am Acad Dermatol* 2011; **65**: 749–55.
18. Massone C, Fink-Puches R, Cerroni L. Atypical clinical presentation of primary and secondary cutaneous follicle center lymphoma (FCL) on the head characterized by macular lesions. *J Am Acad Dermatol* 2016; **75**: 1000–6.
19. Charli-Joseph Y, Cerroni L, LeBoit PE. Cutaneous spindle-cell B-cell lymphomas: most are neoplasms of follicular center cell origin. *Am J Surg Pathol* 2015; **39**: 737–43.
20. Lawnicki LC, Weisenburger DD, Aoun P, Chan WC, Wickert RS, Greiner TC. The t(14;18) and bcl-2 expression are present in a subset of primary cutaneous follicular lymphoma: association with lower grade. *Am J Clin Pathol* 2002; **118**: 765–72.
21. Szablewski V, Ingen-Housz-Oro S, Baia M, Delfau-Larue MH, Copie-Bergman C, Ortonne N. Primary cutaneous follicle center lymphomas expression Bcl2 protein frequently harbor Bcl2 gene break and may present 1p36 deletion: a study of 20 cases. *Am J Surg Pathol* 2016; **40**: 127–36.
22. Koens L, Vermeer MH, Willemze R, Jansen PM. IgM expression on paraffin sections distinguishes primary cutaneous large B-cell lymphoma, leg type from primary cutaneous follicle center lymphoma. *Am J Surg Pathol* 2010; **34**: 1043–8.
23. Robson A, Shukur Z, Ally M, et al. Immunocytochemical p63 expression discriminates between primary cutaneous follicle center cell and diffuse large B-cell lymphoma-leg type, and is of the TAp63 isoform. *Histopathology* 2016; **69**: 11–19.
24. Fink-Puches R, Wolf IH, Zalaudek I, Kerl H, Cerroni L. Treatment of primary cutaneous B-cell lymphoma with rituximab. *J Am Acad Dermatol* 2005; **52**: 847–53.
25. Kempf W, Kazakov DV, Rutten A, et al. Primary cutaneous follicle center lymphoma with diffuse CD30 expression: a report of 4 cases of a rare variant. *J Am Acad Dermatol* 2014; **71**: 548–54.
26. Grange F, Beylot-Barry M, Courville P, et al. Primary cutaneous diffuse large B-cell lymphoma, leg type: clinicopathologic features and prognositc analysis in 60 cases. *Arch Dermatol* 2007; **143**: 1144–50.
27. Senff NJ, Hoefnagel JJ, Jansen PM, et al. Reclassification of 300 primary cutaneous B-Cell lymphomas according to the new WHO-EORTC classification for cutaneous lymphomas: comparison with previous classifications and identification of prognostic markers. *J Clin Oncol* 2007; **25**: 1581–7.
28. Hoefnagel JJ, Dijkman R, Basso K, et al. Distinct types of primary cutaneous large B-cell lymphoma identified by gene expression profiling. *Blood* 2005; **105**: 3671–8.
29. Seçkin D, Barete S, Euvrard S, et al. Primary cutaneous posttransplant lymphoproliferative disorders in solid organ transplant recipients: a multicenter European case series. *Am J Transplant* 2013; **13**: 2146–53.
30. Mareschal S, Pham-Ledard A, Viailly PJ, et al. Identification of somatic mutations in primary cutaneous diffuse large B-cell lymphoma, leg type by massive parallel sequencing. *J Invest Dermatol* 2017; **137**: 1984–94.
31. Ferreri AJ, Dognini GP, Campo E, et al. Variations in clinical presentation, frequency of hemophagocytosis and clinical behavior of intravascular

lymphoma diagnosed in different geographical regions. *Haematologica* 2007; **92**: 486–92.

32. Ferreri AJM, Campo E, Seymour JF, et al. Intravascular lymphoma: clinical presentation, natural history, management and prognostic factors in a series of 38 cases, with special emphasis on the "cutaneous variant." *Br J Haematol* 2004; **127**: 173–83.
33. Qiu L, Wang SA, Vega F, et al. From the archives of MD Anderson Cancer Center: intravascular large B-cell lymphoma with numerous circulating lymphoma cells. *Ann Diagn Pathol* 2022; **58**: 151934.
34. Rajyaguru DJ, Bhaskar C, Borgert AJ, Smith A, Parsons B. Intravascular large B-cell lymphoma in the United States (US): a population-based study using Surveillance, Epidemiology, and End Results program and National Cancer Database. *Leukemia Lymphoma* 2017; **58**: 2080–8.
35. Han Y, Li Q, Wang D, Peng L, Huang T, Ou C, Yang K, Wang J. Case report: intravascular large B-cell lymphoma: a clinicopathologic study of four cases with review of additional 331 cases in the literature. *Front Oncol* 2022; **12**: 883141. doi: 10.3389/fonc.2022.883141.
36. Geer M, Roberts E, Shango M, et al. Multicentre retrospective study of intravascular large B-cell lymphoma treated at academic institutions within the United States. *Br J Haematol* 2019; **86**: 255–62.
37. Rozenbaum D, Tung J, Xue Y, Hoang MP, Kroshinsky D. Skin biopsy in the diagnosis of intravascular lymphoma: a retrospective diagnostic accuracy study. *J Am Acad Dermatol* 2021; **85**: 665–70.
38. Breakell T, Waibel H, Schliep S, et al. Intravascular large B-cell lymphoma: a review with a focus on the prognostic value of skin involvement. *Curr Oncol* 2022; **29**: 2909–19.
39. Tanaka M, Miyagaki T, Okano T, Takeuchi S, Kadono T. Predictive factors and scoring system for intravascular large B-cell lymphoma among suspected cases: a single-center retrospective analysis. *Int J Dermatol* 2024; **63**: 79–84.
40. Murase T, Yamaguchi M, Suzuki R, et al. Intravascular large B-cell lymphoma (IVLBCL): a clinicopahologic study of 96 cases with special reference to the immunophenotypic heterogeneity of CD5. *Blood* 2007; **109**: 895–902.
41. Ferry JA, Sohani AR, Longtine JA, Schwartz RA, Harris NL. HHV8-positive, EBV-positive Hodgkin lymphoma-like large B-cell lymphoma and HHV8-positive intravascular large B-cell lymphoma. *Mod Pathol* 2009; **22**: 618–26.
42. Sander CA, Kaudewitz P, Kutzner H, et al. T-cell-rich B-cell lymphoma presenting in skin: a clinicopathologic analysis of six cases. *J Cutan Pathol* 1996; **23**: 101–8.
43. Achten R, Verhoef G, Vanuytsel L, de Wolf-Peeters C. T-cell/histiocyte-rich large B-cell lymphoma: a distinct clinicopathologic entity. *J Clin Oncol* 2002; **20**: 1269–77.
44. Dunphy CH, Nahass GT. Primary cutaneous T-cell-rich B-cell lymphomas with flow cytometric immunophenotypic findings: report of 3 cases and review of the literature. *Arch Pathol Lab Med* 1999; **123**: 1236–40.
45. Hoeller S, Tzankov A, Pileri SA, Went P, Dirnhofer S. Epstein-Barr virus-positive diffuse large B-cell lymphoma in elderly patients is rare in Western populations. *Hum Pathol* 2010; **41**: 352–7.
46. Oyama T, Ichimura K, Suzuki R, et al. Senile EBV+ B-cell lymphoproliferative disorders: a clinicopathologic study of 22 patients. *Am J Surg Pathol* 2003; **27**: 16–26.
47. Uccini S, Al-Jadiry MF, Scarpino S, et al. Epstein-Barr virus-positive diffuse large B-cell lymphoma in children: a disease reminiscent of Epstein-Barr virus-positive diffuse large B-cell lymphoma of the elderly. *Hum Pathol* 2015; **46**: 716–24.
48. Gibson SE, Hsi ED. Epstein-Barr virus-positive B-cell lymphoma of the elderly at a United States tertiary medical center: an uncommon aggressive lymphoma with a nongerminal center B-cell phenotype. *Hum Pathol* 2009; **40**: 653–61.
49. Nicolae A, Pittaluga S, Abdullah S, et al. EBV-positive large B-cell lymphomas in young patients: a nodal lymphoma with evidence for a tolerogenic immune environment. *Blood* 2015; **126**: 863–72.
50. Batuello C, Mason EF. Diagnostic utility of CD200 immunohistochemistry in distinguishing EBV-positive large B-cell lymphoma from classic Hodgkin lymphoma. *Am J Clin Pathol* 2023; **160**: 284–91.
51. Morscio J, Dierickx D, Nijs J, et al. Clinicopathologic comparison of plasmablastic lymphoma in HIV-positive, immunocompetent, and posttransplant patients: single-center series of 25 cases and meta-analysis of 277 reported cases. *Am J Surg Pathol* 2014; **38**: 875–86.
52. Gilaberte M, Gallardo F, Bellosillo B, et al. Recurrent and self-healing cutaneous monoclonal plasmablastic infiltrates in a patient with AIDS and Kaposi sarcoma. *Br J Dermatol* 2005; **153**: 828–32.
53. Castillo JJ, Bibas M, Roberto N Miranda RN. The biology and treatment of plasmablastic lymphoma. *Blood* 2015; **125**: 2323–30.
54. Delecluse HJ, Anagnostopoulos I, Dallenbach F, et al. Plasmablastic lymphomas of the oral cavity: a new entity associated with the human immunodeficiency virus infection. *Blood* 1997; **89**: 1413–20.
55. Liu W, Lacouture ME, Jiang J, et al. KSHV/HHV8-associated primary cutaneous plasmablastic lymphoma in a patient with Castleman's disease and Kaposi's sarcoma. *J Cutan Pathol* 2006; **33**: 46–51.
56. Garcia-Reyero J, Magunacelaya NM, de Villambrosia SG, et al. Genetic lesions in MYC and STAT3 drive oncogenic transcription factor overexpression in plasmablastic lymphoma. *Haematologica* 2021; **106**: 1120–8.
57. Loghavi S, Alayed K, Aladily TN, et al. Stage, age, and EBV status impact outcomes of plasmablastic lymphoma patients: a clinicopathologic analysis of 61 patients. *J Hematol Oncol* 2015: **8**: 65.
58. Frontzek F, Staiger AM, Zapukhlyak M, et al. Molecular and functional profiling identifies therapeutically targetable vulnerabilities in plasmablastic lymphoma. *Nat Commun* 2021; **12**: 5183. doi: 10.1038/s41467-021-25405-w.
59. Sen F, Medeiros LJ, Lu D, Lai R, Katz R, Abruzzo LV. Mantle cell lymphoma involving skin: cutaneous lesions may be the first manifestation of disease and tumors often have blastoid cytologic features. *Am J Surg Pathol* 2002; **26**: 1312–18.
60. Sander B, Quintanilla-Martinez L, Ott G, et al. Mantle cell lymphoma: a spectrum from indolent to aggressive disease. *Virchows Arch* 2016; **468**: 245–57.

61. Fried LJ, Criscito MC, Stevenson ML, Pomeranz MK. Chronic lymphocytic leukemia and the skin: implications for the dermatologist. *Int J Dermatol* 2022; **61**: 519–31.

62. Menter T, Trivedi P, Ahmad R, et al. Diagnostic utility of lymphoid enhancer binding factor 1 immunohistochemistry in small B-cell lymphomas. *Am J Clin Pathol* 2017; **147**: 292–300.

63. Rodriguez-Pinilla SM, Ortiz-Romero PL, et al. TCR-gamma expression in primary cutaneous T-cell lymphomas. *Am J Surg Pathol* 2016; **37**: 375–84.

64. Falini B, Flenghi L, Pileri S, et al. Distribution of T cells bearing different forms of the T cell receptor gamma/delta in normal and pathological human tissues. *J Immunol* 1989; **143**: 2480–8.

65. Zackheim HS, Amin S, Kashani-Sabet M, McMillan A. Prognosis in cutaneous T-cell lymphoma by skin stage: long-term survival in 489 patients. *J Am Acad Dermatol* 1999; **40**: 418–25.

66. Quaglino P, Pimpinelli N, Berti E, et al; Gruppo Italiano Linfomi Cutanei. Time course, clinical pathways, and long-term hazards risk trends of disease progression in patients with classic mycosis fungoides: a multicenter, retrospective follow-up study from the Italian Group of Cutaneous Lymphomas. *Cancer* 2012; **118**: 5830–9.

67. Saleh JS, Subtil A, Hristov AC. Primary cutaneous T-cell lymphoma: a review of the most common entities with focus on recent updates. *Hum Pathol* 2023; **138**: 76–102.

68. Vonderheid EC, Pavlov I, Delgado JC, et al. Prognostic factors and risk stratification in early mycosis fungoides. *Leuk Lymphoma* 2014; **55**: 44–50.

69. Merrill ED, Agbay R, Miranda RN, et al. Primary cutaneous T-cell lymphomas showing gamma-delta (gamma delta) phenotype and predominantly epidermotropic pattern are clinicopathologically distinct from classic primary cutaneous gamma delta T-cell lymphomas. *Am J Surg Pathol* 2017; **41**: 204–15.

70. Daniels J, Doukas PG, Escala MEM, et al. Cellular origins and genetic landscape of cutaneous gamma delta T cell lymphomas. *Nat Commun* 2020; **11**: 1806. doi: 10.1038/s41467-020-15572-7.

71. Guitart J, Chung C, Torres-Cabala CA. The dilemma of primary gamma delta epidermotropic T-cell lymphoma: distinction from mycosis fungoides, signs of cytotoxicity, and need for more detailed analysis. *J Cutan Pathol* 2022; **49**: 419–20.

72. Lee SC, Berg KD, Racke FK, Griffin CA, Eshleman JR. Pseudo-spikes are common in histologically benign lymphoid tissues. *J Mol Diagn* 2000; **2**: 145–52.

73. Posnett DN, Sinha R, Kabak S, Russo C. Clonal populations of T cells in normal elderly humans: the T cell equivalent to "benign monoclonal gammapathy." *J Exp Med* 1994; **179**: 609–18.

74. Scarisbrick JJ, Hodak E, Bagot M, et al. Blood classification and blood response criteria in mycosis fungoides and Sézary syndrome using flow cytometry: recommendations from the EORTC cutaneous lymphoma task force. *Eur J Cancer* 2018: **93**: 47–56.

75. Cerroni L, Fink-Puches R, Back B, Kerl H. Follicular mucinosis: a critical reappraisal of clinicopathologic features and association with mycosis fungoides and Sezary syndrome. *Arch Dermatol* 2002; **138**: 182–9.

76. van Santen S, Jansen PM, Quint KD, Vermeer MH, Willemze R. Plaque stage folliculotropic mycosis fungoides: histopathologic features and prognostic factors in a series of 40 patients. *J Cutan Pathol* 2020; **47**: 241–50.

77. Charli-Joseph Y, Kashani-Sabet M, McCalmont TH, et al. Association of a proposed new staging system for folliculotropic mycosis fungoides with prognostic variables in a US cohort. *JAMA Dermatol* 2021; **157**: 157–65.

78. Pileri A, Facchetti F, Rutten A, et al. Syringotropic mycosis fungoides: a rare variant of the disease with peculiar clinicopathologic features. *Am J Surg Pathol* 2011; **35**: 100–9.

79. Haghighi B, Smoller BR, LeBoit PE, Warnke RA, Sander CA, Kohler S. Pagetoid reticulosis (Woringer-Kolopp disease): an immunophenotypic, molecular, and clinicopathologic study. *Mod Pathol* 2000; **13**: 502–10.

80. El Shabrawi-Caelen L, Cerroni L, Medeiros LJ, McCalmont TH. Hypopigmented mycosis fungoides: frequent expression of a CD8 T-cell phenotype. *Am J Surg Pathol* 2002; **26**: 450–7.

81. Shah A, Safaya A. Granulomatous slack skin disease: a review in comparison with mycosis fungoides. *J Eur Acad Dermatol Venereol* 2012; **26**: 1472–8.

82. Kempf W, Ostheeren-Michaelis S, Paulli M, et al. Granulomatous mycosis fungoides and granulomatous slack skin: a multicenter study of the cutaneous lymphoma histopathology task force group of the European organization for research and treatment of cancer (EORTC). *Arch Dermatol* 2008; **144**: 1609–17.

83. Battesti G, Ram-Wolff C, Dobos G, et al. Granulomatous slack skin: clinical retrospective study of 8 cases of the Cutaneous Lymphoma French Study Group. *Eur J Cancer* 2021; **156**: S35-6.

84. Benner MA, Jansen PM, Vermeer MH, et al. Prognostic factors in transformed mycosis fungoides: a retrospective analysis of 100 cases. *Blood* 2012; **119**: 1643–9.

85. Vergier B, De Muret A, Beylot-Barry M, et al. Transformation of mycosis fungoides: clinicopathologic and prognostic features of 45 cases. *Blood* 2009; **95**: 2212–18.

86. Jullié ML, Carlotti M, Vivot A Jr, et al. CD20 antigen may be expressed by reactive or lymphomatous cells of transformed mycosis fungoides: diagnostic and prognostic impact. *Am J Surg Pathol* 2013; **37**: 1845–54.

87. Klemke CD, Booken N, Weiss C, et al. Histopathological and immunophenotypical criteria for the diagnosis of Sezary syndrome in differentiation from other erythrodermic skin diseases: a European Organisation for Research and Treatment of Cancer (EORTC) Cutaneous Lymphoma Task Force Study of 97 cases. *Br J Dermatol* 2015; **173**: 93–105.

88. Cetinozman F, Jansen PM, Vermeer MH, et al. Differential expression of programmed death-1 (PD-1) in Sezary syndrome and mycosis fungoides. *Arch Dermatol* 2012; **148**: 1379–85.

89. Capriotti E, Vonderheid EC, Thoburn CJ, Wasik MA, Bahler DW, Hess AD. Expression of T-plastin, FoxP3 and other tumor-associated markers by leukemic T-cells of cutaneous T-cell lymphoma. *Leuk Lymphoma* 2008; **49**: 1190–201.

90. Gros A, Laharanne E, Vergier M, et al. TP53 alterations in primary and secondary Sezary syndrome: a diagnostic tool for the assessment of malignancy in patients with

erythroderma. *PLoS One* 2017; **12**: e0173171. doi: 10.1371/journal.pone.0173171.

91. Goodlad JR, Cerroni L, Swerdlow SH. Recent advances in cutaneous lymphoma-implications for current and future classifications. *Virchows Arch* 2023; **482**: 281–98.
92. Dobos G, de Masson A, Ram-Wolff C, et al. Epidemiological changes in cutaneous lymphomas: an analysis of 8593 patients from the French Cutaneous Lymphoma Registry. *Br J Dermatol* 2021; **184**: 1059–67.
93. Bekkenk MW, Geelen FA, van Voorst Vader PC, et al. Primary and secondary cutaneous CD30(+) lymphoproliferative disorders: a report from the Dutch Cutaneous Lymphoma Group on the long-term follow-up data of 219 patients and guidelines for diagnosis and treatment. *Blood* 2000; **95**: 3653–61.
94. Sciallis AP, Law ME, Inwards DJ, et al. Mucosal CD30-positive T-cell lymphoproliferations of the head and neck show a clinicopathologic spectrum similar to cutaneous CD30-positive T-cell lymphoproliferative disorders. *Mod Pathol* 2012; **25**: 983–92.
95. Melchers RC, Willemze R, Bekkenk MW, et al. Frequency and prognosis of associated malignancies in 504 patients with lymphomatoid papulosis. *J Eur Acad Dermatol Venereol* 2020; **34**: 260–6.
96. El Shabrawi-Caelen L, Kerl H, Cerroni L. Lymphomatoid papulosis: reappraisal of clinicopathologic presentation and classification into subtypes A, B, and C. *Arch Dermatol* 2004; **140**: 441–7.
97. Saggini A, Gulia A, Argenyi Z, et al. A variant of lymphomatoid papulosis simulating primary cutaneous aggressive epidermotropic CD8+ cytotoxic T-cell lymphoma. Description of 9 cases. *Am J Surg Pathol* 2010; **34**: 1168–75.
98. Sharaf MA, Romanelli P, Kirsner R, Miteva M. Angioinvasive lymphomatoid papulosis: another case of a newly described variant. *Am J Dermatopathol* 2014; **36**: e75–77.
99. Karai LJ, Kadin ME, Hsi ED, et al. Chromosomal rearrangements of 6p25.3 define a new subtype of lymphomatoid papulosis. *Am J Surg Pathol* 2013; **37**: 1173–81.
100. Feldman AL, Oishi N, Ketterling RP, Ansell SM, Shi M, Dasari S. Immunohistochemical approach to genetic subtyping of anaplastic large cell lymphoma. *Am J Surg Pathol* 2022; **46**: 1490–9.
101. Kempf W, Mitteldorf C, Karai LJ, Robson A. Lymphomatoid papulosis – making sense of the alphabet soup: a proposal to simplify terminology. *J Dtsch Dermatol Ges* 2017; **15**: 390–4.
102. Smoller BR, Longacre TA, Warnke RA. Ki-1 (CD30) expression in differentiation of lymphomatoid papulosis from arthropod bite reactions. *Mod Pathol* 1992; **5**: 492–6.
103. Werner B, Massone C, Kerl H, Cerroni L. Large CD30-positive cells in benign, atypical lymphoid infiltrates of the skin. *J Cutan Pathol* 2008; **35**: 1100–7.
104. Kempf W, Kazakov DV, Palmedo G, Fraitag S, Schaerer L, Kutzner H. Pityriasis lichenoides et varioliformis acuta with numerous CD30(+) cells: a variant mimicking lymphomatoid papulosis and other cutaneous lymphomas. A clinicopathologic, immunohistochemical, and molecular biological study of 13 cases. *Am J Surg Pathol* 2012; **36**: 1021–9.
105. Kempf W. CD30+ lymphoproliferative disorders: histopathology, differential diagnosis, new variants, and simulators. *J Cutan Pathol* 2006; **33**: 58–70.
106. Kempf W, Kutzner H, Cozzio A, et al. MUM1 expression in cutaneous CD30+ lymphoproliferative disorders: a valuable tool for the distinction between lymphomatoid papulosis and primary cutaneous anaplastic large-cell lymphoma. *Br J Dermatol* 2008; **158**: 1280–7.
107. Kempf W, Pfaltz K, Vermeer MH, et al. EORTC, ISCL, and USCLC consensus recommendations for the treatment of primary cutaneous CD30-positive lymphoproliferative disorders: lymphomatoid papulosis and primary cutaneous anaplastic large-cell lymphoma. *Blood* 2011; **118**: 4024–35.
108. Massone C, Cerroni L. Phenotypic variability in primary cutaneous anaplastic large T-cell lymphoma: a study on 35 patients. *Am J Dermatopathol* 2014; **36**: 153–7.
109. Kaimi Y, Takahashi Y, Taniguchi H, et al. Loss of or decrease in CD30 expression in four patients with anaplastic large cell lymphoma after brentuximab vedotin-containing therapy. *Virchows Arch* 2024; **484**: 465–73.
110. ten Berge RL, Oudejans JJ, Ossenkoppele GJ, et al. ALK expression in extranodal anaplastic large cell lymphoma favours systemic disease with (primary) nodal involvement and a good prognosis and occurs before dissemination. *J Clin Pathol* 2000; **53**: 445–50.
111. Oschlies I, Lisfeld J, Lamant L, et al. ALK-positive anaplastic large cell lymphoma limited to the skin: clinical, histopathological and molecular analysis of 6 pediatric cases: a report from the ALCL99 study. *Haematologica* 2013; **98**: 50–6.
112. Miyagaki T, Inoue N, Kamijo H, et al. Prognostic factors for primary cutaneous anaplastic large-cell lymphoma: a multicentre retrospective study from Japan. *Br J Dermatol* 2023; **189**: 612–20.
113. Díaz de la Pinta FJ, Rodríguez Moreno M, Salgado RN, et al. Anaplastic large cell lymphomas with the 6p25.3 rearrangement are a heterogeneous group of tumours with a diverse molecular background. *Hum Pathol* 2023; **137**: 71–8.
114. de Bruin PC, Beljaards RC van Heerde P, et al. Differences in clinical behaviour and immunophenotype between primary cutaneous and primary nodal anaplastic large cell lymphoma of T-cell or null cell phenotype. *Histopathology* 1993; **23**: 127–35.
115. Ferrara G, Ena L, Cota C, Cerroni L. Intralymphatic spread is a common finding in cutaneous CD30+ lymphoproliferative disorders. *Am J Surg Pathol* 2015; **39**: 1511–17.
116. Samols MA, Su A, Ra S, Cappel MA, et al. Intralymphatic cutaneous anaplastic large cell lymphoma/lymphomatoid papulosis: expanding the spectrum of CD30-positive lymphoproliferative disorders. *Am J Surg Pathol* 2014; **38**: 1203–11.
117. Lai P, Liu F, Liu X, Sun J, Wang Y. Differential molecular programs of cutaneous anaplastic large cell lymphoma and CD30-positive transformed mycosis fungoides. *Front Immunol* 2023; **14**: 1270365. doi: 10.3389/fimmu.2023.1270365.
118. Banafshay K, Maldonado D, Tarbox M. Cutaneous intravascular CD-30-positive anaplastic large cell lymphoma: a case report and literature review. *Cureus* 2023; **15**: e44450.
119. Provasi M, Bagnoli F, Fanoni D, et al. CD30 expression in a case of intravascular large B-cell lymphoma, cutaneous variant. *J Cutan Pathol* 2019; **46**: 447–51.

120. Kempf W, Mitteldorf C, Cerroni L, et al. Classifications of cutaneous lymphomas and lymphoproliferative disorders: An update from the EORTC cutaneous lymphoma histopathology group. *J Eur Acad Dermatol Venereol* 2024; **38**: 1491–503.
121. Bekkenk MW, Vermeer MH, Jansen PM, et al. Peripheral T-cell lymphomas unspecified presenting in the skin: analysis of prognostic factors in a group of 82 patients. *Blood* 2003; **102**: 2213–19.
122. Hagiwara M, Takata K, Shimoyama Y, et al. Primary cutaneous T-cell lymphoma of unspecified type with cytotoxic phenotype: clinicopathological analysis of 27 patients. *Cancer Sci* 2009; **100**: 33–41.
123. Savage KJ, Ferreri AJ, Zinzani PL, Pilari SA. Peripheral T-cell lymphoma- not otherwise specified. *Crit Rev Oncol Hematol* 2011; **79**: 321–9.
124. Kempf W, Mitteldorf C, Battistella M, et al. Primary cutaneous peripheral T-cell lymphoma, not otherwise specified: results of a multicentre European Organization for Research and Treatment of Cancer (EORTC) cutaneous lymphoma taskforce study on the clinico-pathological and prognostic features. *J Eur Acad Dermatol Venereol* 2021; **35**: 658–68.
125. Willemze R, Jansen PM, Cerroni L, et al. Subcutaneous panniculitis-like T-cell lymphoma: definition, classification, and prognostic factors: an EORTC Cutaneous Lymphoma Group Study of 83 cases. *Blood* 2008; **111**: 838–45.
126. Bosisio F, Boi S, Caputo V, et al. Lobular panniculitic infiltrates with overlapping histopathologic features of lupus panniculitis (lupus profundus) and subcutaneous T-cell lymphoma: a conceptual and practical dilemma. *Am J Surg Pathol* 2015; **39**: 206–11.
127. Magro CM, Schaefer JT, Morrison C, Porcu P. Atypical lymphocytic lobular panniculitis: a clonal subcutaneous T-cell dyscrasia. *J Cutan Pathol* 2008; **35**: 947–54.
128. Machan S, Rodriguez M, Alonso-Alonso R, et al. Subcutaneous panniculitis-like T-cell lymphoma, lupus erythematosus profundus, and overlapping cases: molecular characterization through the study of 208 genes. *Leuk Lymphoma* 2021; **62**: 2130–40.
129. LeBlanc RE, Tavallaee M, Kim YH, Kim J. Useful parameters for distinguishing subcutaneous panniculitis-like T-Cell lymphoma from lupus erythematosus panniculitis. *Am J Surg Pathol* 2016; **40**: 745–54.
130. Koh J, Jang I, Mun S, et al. Genetic profiles of subcutaneous panniculitis-like T-cell lymphoma and clinicopathological impact of HAVCR2 mutations. *Blood Adv* 2021; **5**: 3919–30.
131. Salhany KE, Macon WR, Choi JK, et al. Subcutaneous panniculitis-like T cell lymphoma: clinicopathologic, immunophenotypic, and genotypic analysis of alpha/beta and gamma/delta subtypes. *Am J Surg Pathol* 1998; **22**: 881–93.
132. Torres-Cabala CA, Huen A, Iyer SP, Miranda RN. Gamma/delta phenotype in primary cutaneous T-cell lymphomas and lymphoid proliferations: challenges for diagnosis and classification. *Surg Pathol Clin* 2021; **14**: 177–94.
133. Endly DC, Weenig RH, Peters MS, Viswanatha DS, Comfere NI. Indolent course of cutaneous gamma-delta T-cell lymphoma. *J Cutan Pathol* 2013; **40**: 896–902.
134. Guitart J, Weisenburger DD, Subtil A, et al. Cutaneous gamma/delta T-cell lymphomas. A spectrum of presentations with overlap with other cytotoxic lymphomas. *Am J Surg Pathol* 2012; **36**: 1656–65.
135. Toro JR, Beaty M, Sorbara L, et al. Gamma delta T-cell lymphoma of the skin: a clinical, microscopic, and molecular study. *Arch Dermatol* 2000; **136**: 1024–32.
136. Rodriguez-Pinilla SM, Ortiz-Romero PL, Monsalvez V, et al. TCR-gamma expression in primary cutaneous T-cell lymphomas. *Am J Surg Pathol* 2013; **37**: 375–84.
137. Berti E, Tomasini D, Vermeer MH, Meijer CJLM, Alessi E, Willemze R. Primary cutaneous CD8-positive epidermotropic cytotoxic T cell lymphomas: a distinct clinicopathological entity with an aggressive clinical behavior. *Am J Pathol* 1999; **155**: 483–92.
138. Robson A, Assaf C, Bagot M, et al. Aggressive epidermotropic cutaneous CD8+ lymphoma: a cutaneous lymphoma with distinct clinical and pathological features. Report of an EORTC Cutaneous Lymphoma Task Force Workshop. *Histopathology* 2015; **67**: 425–41.
139. Lee K, Evans MG, Yang L, et al. Primary cytotoxic T-cell lymphomas harbor recurrent targetable alterations in the JAK-STAT pathway. *Blood* 2021; **138**: 2435–40.
140. Bastidas Torres AN, Cats D, Out-Luiting JJ, et al Deregulation of JAK2 signaling underlies primary cutaneous CD8(+) aggressive epidermotropic cytotoxic T-cell lymphoma. *Haematologica* 2022; **107**: 702–14.
141. Petrella T, Maubec E, Cornillet-Lefebvre P, et al. Indolent CD8-positive lymphoid proliferation of the ear: a distinct primary cutaneous T-cell lymphoma? *Am J Surg Pathol* 2007; **31**: 1887–92.
142. Greenblatt D, Ally M, Child F, et al. Indolent CD8+ lymphoid proliferation of acral sites: a clinicopathologic study of six patients with some atypical features. *J Cutan Pathol* 2013; **40**: 248–58.
143. Wobser M, Petrella T, Kneitz H, et al. Extrafacial indolent CD8-positive cutaneous lymphoid proliferation with unusual symmetrical presentation involving both feet. *J Cutan Pathol* 2013; **40**: 955–61.
144. Hagen JW, Magro CM. Indolent CD8+ lymphoid proliferation of the face with eyelid involvement. *Am J Dermatopathol* 2014; **36**: 137–41.
145. Alaggio R, Amador C, Anagnostopoulos I, et al. The 5th edition of the World Health Organization classification of hematolymphoid tumors: lymphoid neoplasms. *Leukemia* 2022; **36**: 1720–48.
146. Campo E, Jaffe ES, Cook JR, et al. The International Consensus Classification of mature lymphoid neoplasms: a report from the Clinical Advisory Committee. *Blood* 2022; **140**: 1229–53.
147. Beltraminelli H, Mullegger R, Cerroni L. Indolent CD8+ lymphoid proliferation of the ear: a phenotypic variant of the small-medium pleomorphic cutaneous T-cell lymphoma? *J Cutan Pathol* 2010; **37**: 81–4.
148. Kempf W, Petrella T, Willemze R, et al. Clinical, histopathological and prognostic features of primary cutaneous acral CD8+T-cell lymphoma and other dermal CD8+cutaneous lymphoproliferations: results of an EORTC Cutaneous Lymphoma Group workshop. *Br J Dermatol* 2022; **186**: 887–97.
149. Li JY, Guitart J, Pulitzer MP, et al. Multicenter case series of indolent small/medium-sized CD8+ lymphoid proliferations with predilection for the

ear and face. *Am J Dermatopathol* 2014; **36**: 402–8.

150. Wobser M, Roth S, Reinartz T, Rosenwald A, Goebeler M, Geissinger E. CD68 expression is a discriminative feature of indolent cutaneous CD8-positive lymphoid proliferation and distinguishes this lymphoma subtype from other CD8-positive cutaneouslymphomas. *Br J Dermatol* 2015; **172**: 1573–80.
151. Beltraminelli H, Leinweber B, Kerl H, Cerroni L. Primary cutaneous CD4+ small/medium-sized pleomorphic T cell lymphoma: a cutaneous nodular proliferation of pleomorphic T lymphocytes of undetermined significance? A study of 136 cases. *Am J Dermatopathol* 2009; **31**: 317–22.
152. William VL, Torres-Cabala CA, Duvic M. Primary cutaneous small- to medium-sized CD4+ pleomorphic T-cell lymphoma: a retrospective case series and review of the provisional cutaneous lymphoma category. *Am J Clin Dermatol* 2011; **12**: 389–401.
153. Beltzung F, Ortonne N, Pelletier L, et al. Primary cutaneous CD4+small/medium T-cell lymphoproliferative disorders: a clinical, patho logic and molecular study of 60 cases presenting with a single lesion:a multicenter study of the French Cutaneous Lymphoma Study Group. *Am J Surg Pathol* 2020; **44**: 862–72.
154. Rodriguez-Pinilla SM, Roncador G, Rodriguez-Peralto IJ, et al. Primary cutaneous CD4+ small/medium-sized pleomorphic T-cell lymphoma expresses follicular T-cell markers. *Am J Surg Pathol* 2009; **33**: 81–90.
155. Oschlies I, Kock K, Wuseke T, et al. Cyclin D1 expression, cell proliferation, and clonal persistence characterize primary cutaneous CD4+ small or medium T-cell lymphoproliferative disorder. *Histopathology* 2023; **82**: 485–94.
156. Obiorah IE, Karrs J, Brown L, et al. Overlapping features of primary cutaneous marginal zone lymphoproliferative disorder and primary cutaneous CD4+ small/medium T-cell lymphoproliferative disorder: a diagnostic challenge examined by genomic analysis. Am J Surg Pathol 2022. *Am J Surg Pathol* 2023; **47**: 344–53.
157. Suzuki R, Suzumiya J, Yamaguchi M, et al. Prognostic factors for mature natural killer (NK) cell neoplasms: aggressive NK cell leukemia and extranodal NK cell lymphoma, nasal type. *Ann Oncol* 2010; **21**: 1032–40.
158. Takata K, Hong ME, Sitthinamsuwan P, et al. Primary cutaneous NK/T-cell lymphoma, nasal type and CD56-positive peripheral T-cell lymphoma: a cellular lineage and clinicopathologic study of 60 patients from Asia. *Am J Surg Pathol* 2015; **39**: 1–12.
159. Lee WJ, Jung JM, Won CH, et al. Cutaneous extranodal natural killer/T-cell lymphoma: a comparative clinicohistopathologic and survival outcome analysis of 45 cases according to the primary tumor site. *J Am Acad Dermatol* 2014; **70**: 1002–9.
160. Stoll JR, Willner J, Oh Y, et al. Primary cutaneous T-cell lymphomas other than mycosis fungoides and Sézary syndrome. Part I: clinical and histologic features and diagnosis. *J Am Acad Dermatol* 2021; **85**: 1073–90.
161. Ngamdamrongkiat P, Sukpanichnant S, Chairatchaneeboon M, Khuhapinant A, Sitthinamsuwan P. Cutaneous involvement of extranodal NK/T cell lymphoma, nasal type, a clinical and histopathological mimicker of various skin diseases. *Dermatopathology* 2022; **9**: 307–20.
162. Plaza JA, Gru AA, Sangueza OP, et al. An update on viral-induced cutaneous lymphoproliferative disorders. CME Part I. *J Am Acad Dermatol* 2023; **88**: 965–80.
163. Gualco G, Domeny-Duarte P, Chioato L, et al. Clinicopathologic and molecular features of 122 Brazilian cases of nodal and extranodal NK/T-cell lymphoma, nasal type, with EBV subtyping analysis. *Am J Surg Pathol* 2011; **35**: 1195–203.
164. Schwartz EJ, Molina-Kirsch H, Zhao S, et al. Immunohistochemical characterization of nasal-type extranodal NK/T-cell lymphoma using a tissue microarray: an analysis of 84 cases. *Am J Clin Pathol* 2008; **130**: 343–51.
165. Ohno T, Yamaguchi M, Oka K, Miwa H, Kita H, Shirakawa S. Frequent expression of CD3 epsilon in CD3 (Leu 4)-negative nasal T-cell lymphoma. *Leukemia* 1995; **9**: 44–52.
166. Kawamoto K, Miyoshi H, Suzuki T, et al. Frequent expression of CD30 in extranodal NK/T-cell lymphoma: Potential therapeutic target for anti-CD30 antibody-based therapy. *Hematol Oncol* 2018; **36**: 166–73.
167. Marshall EH, Brumbaugh B, Holt A, Chen ST, Hoang MP. Cutaneous intravascular hematolymphoid entities: a review. *Diagnostics* 2024; **14**: 679. doi: 10.3390/diagnostics14070679.
168. Na JM, Jung W, Kim M, et al. Intravascular NK/T-cell lymphoma: a case report and literature review. *J Pathol Transl Med* 2023; **57**: 332–6.
169. Fujikura K, Yoshida M, Uesaka K. Transcriptome complexity in intravascular NK/T-cell lymphoma. *J Clin Pathol* 2020; **73**: 671–5.
170. Marchetti MA, Pulitzer MP, Myskowski PL, et al. Cutaneous manifestations of human T-cell lymphotrophic virus type-1-associated adult T-cell leukemia/lymphoma: a single-center, retrospective study. *J Am Acad Dermatol* 2015; **72**: 293–301.
171. Malpica L, Enriquez DJ, Castro DA, et al. Real-world data on adult T-cell leukemia/lymphoma in Latin America: a study from the Grupo de Estudio Latinoamericano de Linfoproliferativos. *JCO Glob Oncol* 2021: 7: 1151–66.
172. Tokura Y, Sawada Y, Shimauchi T. Skin manifestations of adult T-cell leukemia/lymphoma: clinical, cytological and immunological features. *J Dermatol* 2014; **41**: 19–25.
173. Sawada Y, Hino R, Hama K, et al. Type of skin eruption is an independent prognostic indicator for adult T-cell leukemia/lymphoma. *Blood* 2011; **117**: 3961–7.
174. Kobayashi S, Nakano K, Watanabe E, et al. CADM1 expression and stepwise downregulation of CD7 are closely associated with clonal expansion of HTLV-I-infected cells in adult T-cell leukemia/lymphoma. *Clin Cancer Res* 2014; **20**: 2851–61.
175. Takatori M, Sakihama S, Miyara M, et al. A new diagnostic algorithm using biopsy specimens in adult T-cell leukemia/lymphoma: combination of RNA in situ hybridization and quantitative PCR for HTLV-1. *Mod Pathol* 2021; **34**: 51–8.
176. Yamada K, Miyoshi H, Yoshida N, et al. Human T-cell lymphotropic virus HBZ and tax mRNA expression are associated with specific clinicopathological features in adult T-cell leukemia/lymphoma. *Mod Pathol* 2021; **34**: 314–26.
177. Botros N, Cerroni L, Shawwa A, et al. Cutaneous manifestations of angioimmunoblastic T-cell lymphoma: clinical and pathological characteristics. *Am J Dermatopathol* 2015; **37**: 274–83.

178. Oishi N, Sartori-Valinotti JC, Bennani NN, et al. Cutaneous lesions of angioimmunoblastic T-cell lymphoma: Clinical, pathological, and immunophenotypic features. *J Cutan Pathol* 2019; **46**: 637–44.

179. Yu H, Shahsafaei A, Dorfman DM. Germinal-center T-helper-cell markers PD-1 and CXCL13 are both expressed by neoplastic cells in angioimmunoblastic T-cell lymphoma. *Am J Clin Pathol* 2009; **131**: 33–41.

180. Brown HA, Macon WR, Kurtin PJ, Gibson LE. Cutaneous involvement by angioimmunoblastic T-cell lymphoma with remarkable heterogeneous Epstein-Barr virus expression. *J Cutan Pathol* 2001; **28**: 432–8.

181. Magana M, Massone C, Magana P, Cerroni L. Clinicopathologic features of hydroa vacciniforme-like lymphoma: a series of 9 patients. *Am J Dermatopathol* 2016; **38**: 20–5.

182. Liu Y, Ma C, Wang G, Wang L. Hydroa vacciniforme-like lymphoproliferative disorder: Clinicopathologic study of 41 cases. *J Am Acad Dermatol* 2019; **81**: 534–40.

183. Quintanilla-Martinez L, Ridaura C, Nagl F, et al. Hydroa vacciniforme-like lymphoma: a chronic EBV+ lymphoproliferative disorder with risk to develop a systemic lymphoma. *Blood* 2013; **122**: 3101–10.

184. Miyake T, Yamamoto T, Hirai Y, et al. Survival rates and prognostic factors of Epstein-Barr virus-associated hydroa vacciniforme and hypersensitivity to mosquito bites. *Br J Dermatol* 2015; **172**: 56–63.

185. Rysgaard CD, Stone MS. Lymphomatoid granulomatosis presenting with cutaneous involvement: A case report and review of the literature. *J Cutan Pathol* 2015; **42**: 188–93.

186. Dojcinov SD, Venkataraman G, Raffeld M, Pittaluga S, Jaffe ES. EBV positive mucocutaneous ulcer–a study of 26 cases associated with various sources of immunosuppression. *Am J Surg Pathol* 2010; **34**: 405–17.

187. Satou A, Banno S, Kohno K, et al. Primary cutaneous methotrexate-associated B-cell lymphoproliferative disorders other than EBV-positive mucocutaneous ulcer: clinical, pathological, and immunophenotypic features. *Pathology* 2021; **53**: 595–601.

188. Ikeda T, Gion Y, Sakamoto M, et al. Clinicopathological analysis of 34 Japanese patients with EBV-positive mucocutaneous ulcer. *Mod Pathol* 2020; **33**: 2437–48.

189. Sen F, Medeiros LJ, Lu D, Lai R, Katz R, Abruzzo LV. Mantle cell lymphoma involving skin: cutaneous lesions may be the first manifestation of disease and tumors often have blastoid cytologic features. *Am J Surg Pathol* 2002; **26**: 1312–18.

190. Soldini D, Valera A, Sole C, et al. Assessment of Sox11 expression in routine lymphoma tissue sections: characterization of new monoclonal antibodies for diagnosis of mantle cell lymphoma. *Am J Surg Pathol* 2014; **38**: 86–93.

191. Jares P, Colomer D, Campo E. Molecular pathogenesis of mantle cell lymphoma. *J Clin Invest* 2012; **122**: 3416–23.

192. Salhany KE, Sousar JB, Greer JP, Casey TT, Fields JP, Collins RD. Transformation of cutaneous T cell lymphoma to large cell lymphoma. A clinicopathologic and immunologic study. *Am J Pathol* 1988; **132**: 265–77.

193. Hussong JW, Perkins SL, Schnitzer B, Hargreaves H, Frizzera G. Extramedullary plasmacytoma. A form of marginal zone cell lymphoma? *Am J Clin Pathol* 1999; **111**: 111–16.

194. Jurczyszyn A, Olszewska-Szopa M, Hundria V, et al. Cutaneous involvement in multiple myeloma: a multi-institutional retrospective study of 53 patients. *Leuk Lymphoma* 2016; **57**: 2071–6.

195. Deshpande V, Zen Y, Chan JK, et al. Consensus statement on the pathology of IgG4-related disease. *Mod Pathol* 2012; **25**: 1181–92.

196. Deconinck E, Petrella T, Ottou FG. Blastic plasmacytoid dendritic cell neoplasm: clinical presentation and diagnosis. *Hematol Oncol Clin North Am* 2020; **34**: 491–500.

197. Julia F, Dalle S, Duru G, et al. Blastic plasmacytoid dendritic cell neoplasms: clinico-immunohistochemical correlations in a series of 91 patients. *Am J Surg Pathol* 2014; **38**: 673–80.

Chapter 7

Melanocytic Neoplasms

Mai P. Hoang

7.1 Introduction

In recent years there have been several new immunohistochemical markers made available for the diagnosis of melanocytic lesions. Immunostains are helpful in the distinction of benign from atypical melanocytic proliferation and of melanocytic versus non-melanocytic lesions. The immunostains routinely used in diagnosing melanocytic lesions are outlined in **Table 7.1**. Currently S100 protein is the most sensitive melanocytic marker with polyclonal antibodies against S100B most commonly used in the majority of clinical laboratories.[1] Although with great sensitivity S100 protein has low specificity; thus, other melanocytic markers such as Sox10, Melan-A (melanoma antigen recognized by T cells), Mart-1, HMB-45, and microphthalmia transcription factor (MiTF) are included in the work-up panel (**Table 7.2**).[2–30] The sensitivity of Melan-A, Mart-1, MiTF and HMB-45 is lower for desmoplastic melanoma and metastatic melanoma in comparison to conventional epithelioid primary melanoma (**Table 7.2**). HMB-45 (anti-gp100) is a premelanosome marker since it reacts with the multivesicular stage I melanosomes and fibrillary matrix in stage II melanocytes.[31] Mart-1 and Melan-A antibodies label clear cell sarcomas and a subset of perivascular epithelioid cell tumors (PEComas) in addition to melanocytic proliferations.[14] Both MiTF (microphthalmia transcription factor) and Sox10, being nuclear stains, are superior to Melan-A/Mart-1 in quantitation of junctional melanocytes. Sox10, a nuclear transcription factor expressed in cells destined for glial, schwannian, and melanocytic differentiation has been shown to be more specific than S100 and with similar sensitivity in detecting melanocytic lesions.[32] One should be aware that malignant melanomas can exhibit aberrant expression of epithelial markers including cytokeratin and epithelial membrane antigen (EMA), and others such as desmin, smooth muscle actin, CD10, MUM1, Bcl-2, and CD68 (**Table 7.3**).[2–19,26,33,34]

Table 7.1 Commonly used melanocytic markers

Antibody	Commonly used clones	Staining pattern
HMB–45	HMB–45	cytoplasmic
Melan-A	A103	cytoplasmic
Mart–1	M2–7C10	cytoplasmic
MiTF	C5/D5, 34CA5	nuclear
S100	Polyclonal, 4C4.9	cytoplasmic
Sox10	N–20	nuclear
Tyrosinase	T311	cytoplasmic
p75/CD271/nerve growth factor receptor	EP1039Y	cytoplasmic
PRAME	EPR20330	nuclear
NKI/C3 or CD63	NKI/C3	cytoplasmic

A combination of stains can be performed on the same tissue section. Melanoma marker cocktails are comprised of a combination of two or more monoclonal antibodies. Although they have high sensitivity one must be aware of their low specificity due to reactivity to multiple antibodies. Dual staining for D2-40 and S100 protein or Mart-1/Melan-A has been reported to highlight lymphatic invasion in melanoma (**Figure 7.1**).[35] MIB-1 (anti-Ki-67) nuclear staining is seen in cells during the proliferative cell cycle (G1, M, G2, and S phases) but is absent in the

Table 7.2 Summary of melanocytic-associated markers [2–30]

Markers	Primary epithelioid melanoma	Desmoplastic or spindle melanoma	Metastatic melanoma	Normal structures	Tumors
S100	86–100%	90–95%	79–98%	Schwann cells Neural progenitor cells Chondrocytes Adipocytes Myoepithelial cells Langerhans cells Dendritic cells of both skin and lymph node	Granular cell tumor Myoepithelioma Parachordoma Dendritic cell sarcoma Histiocytic neoplasms
Melan-A/ Mart-1	85–97%	7–15%	63–88%	Dendritic cells of skin	Clear cell sarcoma PEComas Atypical fibroxanthoma
HMB-45	71–93%	0–5%	55–86%	NA	Clear cell sarcoma PEComas Melanocytic schwannoma
Tyrosinase	30–90%	0–30%	26–93%	NA	Clear cell sarcoma
MiTF	97–100%	0%	84–88%	Mast cells Histiocytes Fibroblasts Dendritic cells of lymph nodes Schwann cells Smooth muscle cells of uterus and bladder Renal tubular cells	Clear cell sarcoma Angiomyolipoma Lymphangiomyomas
Sox10	97–100%	97–100%	97–100%	Eccrine glands	Clear cell sarcomas MPNST Granular cell tumors Myoepithelioma
p75/ NGFR	ND	100%		Peripheral nerves	Type C or neurotized nevus cells
PNL2	78–100%	0–6%	75–100%	NA	Clear cell sarcoma PEComa Melanocytic schwannoma Renal angiomyolipoma
KBA.62	93%	82–100%	83–91%	NA	Clear cell sarcoma Well differentiated SCC Leiomyosarcoma Nodular fasciitis Neurofibromas Schwannoma MPNST
NKI/C3	90%	50%	90–93%	Peripheral nerves	PEComas
CD146 (Mel-CAM)	100%	82%	100%	Endothelial cells Smooth muscle cells Myoepithelial cells Schwann cells	Clear cell sarcoma Melanotic schwannoma Leiomyosarcomas Angiosarcomas

ND: not done, NA: not applicable, NFGR: nerve growth factor receptor, GFAP: glial fibrillary acidic protein, MPNST: malignant peripheral nerve sheath tumor, SCC: squamous cell carcinoma

Table 7.3 Expression of non-melanocytic markers in melanomas [2–19, 26, 33, 34]

	Primary epithelioid melanoma	Desmoplastic or spindle melanoma	Metastatic melanoma
Bcl2	61%	ND	77%
CD68	90%	83%	92%
CD99	27%	ND	10%
CD117	72%	ND	74%
CEA	8–42%	78%	37%

Table 7.3 (cont.)

	Primary epithelioid melanoma	Desmoplastic or spindle melanoma	Metastatic melanoma
Desmin	25%	20%	ND
EMA	7–19%	43%	24%
Factor XIIIa	ND	0–30%	ND
GFAP	9%	11%	ND
Keratin (AE1/AE3)	10–45%	0–27%	12%
MUM1	92–95%	33%	81–86%
Neurofilament	2–19%	0–10%	0%
SMA	1%	52%	ND
Synaptophysin	32%	25%	ND
TFF1	1%	ND	7%

ND: not documented

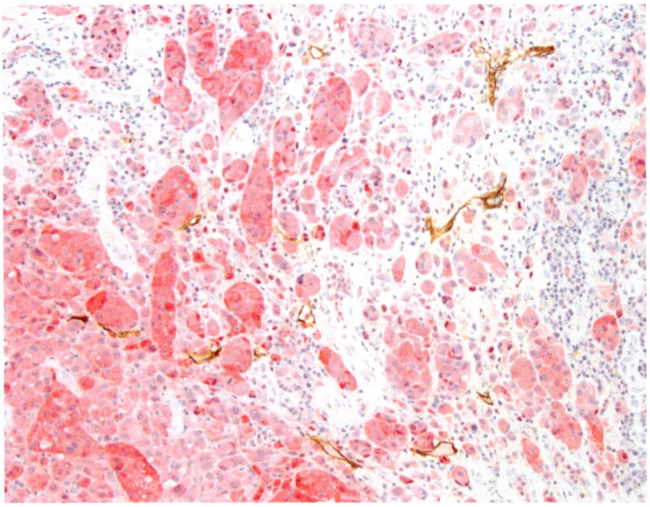

Figure 7.1 In a combined S100 and D2-40 stain, S100 highlights the atypical melanocytes while D2-40 highlights the lymphatic vessels (X200).

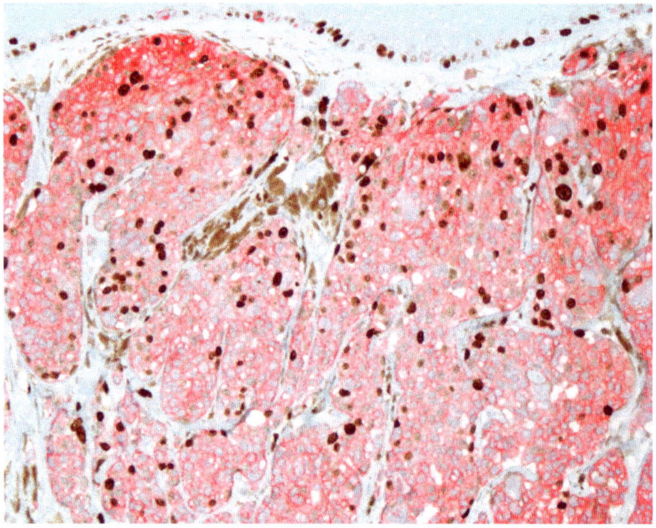

Figure 7.2 A combined Mart-1 and Ki-67 stain demonstrates an increased proliferation index within the dermal melanocytes (X200).

G0 resting phase.[36] Phosphohistone H3 (PHH3) is a marker of mitotic phase of the cell cycle.[37] Mart1/Ki67 and Mart1/PHH3 double stains have been shown to be helpful diagnostic adjuncts (**Figures 7.2**).[37]

Diagnostic utility of Sox10 immunostain

Nuclear Sox10 expression has similar sensitivity but with better specificity than S100 in the evaluation of melanocytic lesions (**Figures 7.3 and 7.4**).[21,30,32,38] Sox10 expression is seen in 90–100% of primary and metastatic melanomas, 100% spindle cell melanomas, 78–100% desmoplastic melanomas, and 57–100% clear cell sarcomas (**Table 7.4**).[21,30,32,39] In addition, Sox10 expression can be seen neural tumor and cutaneous adnexal neoplasms (**Figure 7.4**). In specimens from sun-damaged skin, Sox10 is better than Melan-A in detecting melanocytes.[38] Evaluation of excision margins with a nuclear stain such as Sox10 immunostain has been shown to be superior to cytoplasmic stain since one can quantify the melanocytes density as well as assessing the nuclear size of the melanocytes.[40] Of potential diagnostic pitfall, Sox10 expression

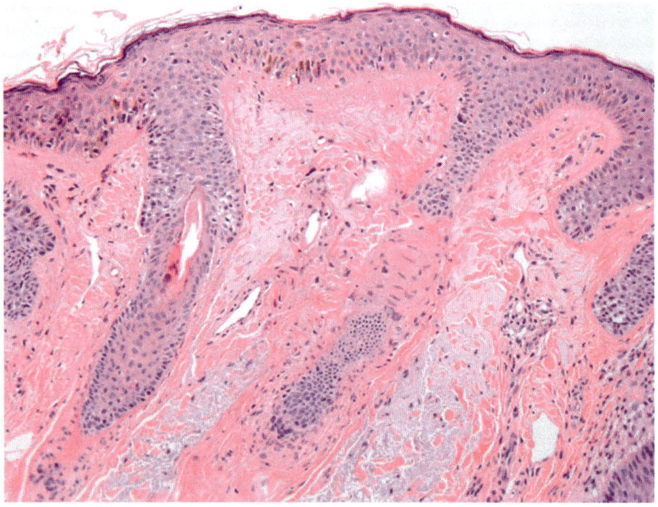

Figure 7.3 *Melanoma in situ, lentigo maligna type*. Severely atypical melanocytes are seen at the dermal epidermal junction within sun-damaged skin (X200).

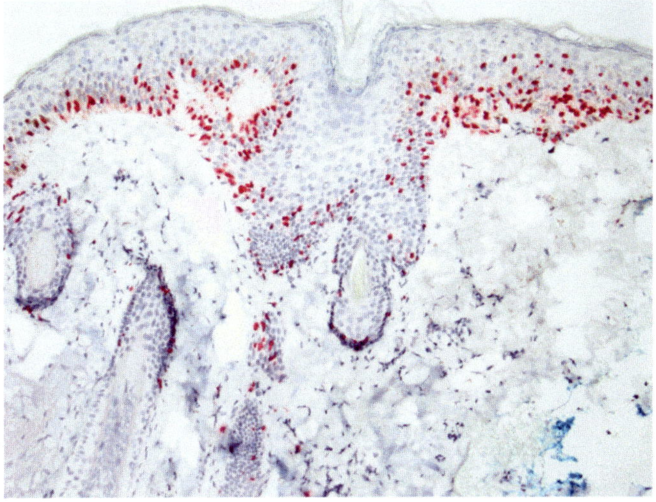

Figure 7.4 *Melanoma in situ, lentigo maligna type.* Increased density of melanocytes with enlarged nuclear size at the dermal epidermal junction is demonstrated by Sox10 immunostain (X200).

Table 7.4 Sox10 expression in neural and non-melanocytic neoplasms

Tumor type	Positivity	References
Granular cell tumor	100%	Shin 2012[21], Miettinen 2015[30]
Neurofibroma	98–100%	Shin 2012[21], Miettinen 2015[30]
Schwannoma	95–100%	Shin 2012[21], Miettinen 2015[30]
Malignant peripheral nerve sheath tumor	22–100%	Shin 2012[21], Miettinen 2015[30]
Chondroid syringoma	60–100%	Evangelista 2017[7], Lezcano 2017[8]
Cylindroma and spiradenoma	85–100%	Cassarino 2017[6], Evangelista 2017[7], Lezcano 2017[8]
Digital papillary adenocarcinoma	100%	Evangelista 2017[7]
Hidradenoma	9–40%	Cassarino 2017[6], Evangelista 2017[7], Lezcano 2017[8]
Hidradenoma papilliferum	75–100%	Cassarino 2017[6], Lezcano 2017[8]
Adenoid cystic carcinoma	96–100%	Hsieh 2016[9], Lee 2019[10], Ohtomo 2013[11]
Myoepithelioma	100%	Ohtomo 2013[11]

can be frequently seen in scar tissue, representing staining of fibrohistiocytes in scar.[41] In the differential diagnosis for spindle cell melanocytic lesions, except for neural tumors, Sox10 expression is typically negative in soft tissue tumors (**Table 7.4**).[30,32,39]

7.2 Diagnostic Utility of PRAME Immunostain

Stain evaluation

Many studies have defined positive PRAME expression to be >75% of the tumor cell nuclei stained positively regardless of staining intensity.[42,43] A meta-analysis by Kunc et al[44] suggests that 3+/50% cut-off would be better in practice than 4+/75% cut-off.

Primary melanoma

PRAME expression is seen in 59–100% of primary melanomas[42,43,45]; however, its expression is seen in 0–35% of desmoplastic melanomas[42,43], 56% spindle cell melanomas[46], 60–80% of Spitz melanomas[43, 47], blue nevus-like melanoma[48], deep penetrating nevus-like melanoma [48], sinonasal melanoma[49], oral melanoma [50], and conjunctival melanoma (**Table 7.5**). [51]

Metastatic melanoma

PRAME expression is seen in 87–100% of metastatic melanomas (**Figures 7.5 and 7.6**).[42,43,52]

Nevi

PRAME expression can be seen in 0–13.6% of melanocytic nevi.[42,43]

Ambiguous melanocytic lesions

In challenging melanocytic proliferation, PRAME expression does not correlate with morphologic features in majority of cases. These lesions include Spitz nevi, atypical Spitz nevi, acral melanoma *in situ* and superficially invasive melanomas.[42,43,53]

Non-melanocytic lesions

PRAME expression can be seen in a variety of soft tissue lesions including dermatofibrosarcoma protuberans (0–50%)[54–56], cellular neurothekeoma[57] atypical fibroxanthoma (4–70%)[46,54,55], pleomorphic dermal sarcoma (4%)[46], vascular tumors (13–67%)[46,55,56], leiomyosarcoma (0–13%)[53,54], rhabdomyosarcoma

Table 7.5 PRAME expression in melanocytic proliferation

		References
Primary melanoma	59–89.9%	Chen 2023[43], Lezcano AJSP 2018[42]
Superficial spreading melanoma	92.5–100%	Lezcano AJSP 2018[42], Chen 2023[43]
Nodular melanoma	90–91.4%	Lezcano AJSP 2018[42], Chen 2023[43]
Lentigo maligna melanoma	80–93.5%	Lezcano AJSP 2018[42], Chen 2023[43], Gradecki 2021
Acral lentiginous melanoma	87.8–100%	Lezcano AJSP 2018[42], Chen 2023[43], Rothrock 2022[45]
Desmoplastic melanoma	0–35%	Lezcano AJSP 2018[42], Chen 2023[43]
Spindle cell melanoma	56%	Hrycai 2022[46]
Subungual melanoma	73–100%	Rothrock 2022[45]
Spitz melanoma	60–82%	Chen 2023[43], Koh 2022[47]

Table 7.5 (cont.)

		References
Blue nevus-like melanoma	62.5%	Kline 2022[48]
Deep penetrating nevus-like melanoma	50%	Kine 2022[48]
Melanoma arising in congenital nevus	100%	Chen 2023[43]
Mucosal melanoma	96.2–99%	Chen 2023[43], Kaczorowski 2022[56]
Sinonasal melanoma	100%	Scheurleer 2023[49]
Oral melanoma	90%	Schmitt 2022[50]
Uveal melanoma	80%	Chen 2023[43]
Conjunctival melanoma	70%	Sekoranja 2021[51]
Primary dedifferentiated melanoma	100%	Hornick ASJP 2023[52]
Clear cell sarcoma of soft parts	0–10.5%	Cammareri 2023[54], Chen 2023[43], Kline 2022[48]
Perivascular epithelioid cell tumors/ PEComa	88.9%	Kline 2022[48]
Metastatic melanoma	87–100%	Lezcano AJSP 2018[42], Chen 2023[43], Kaczorowski 2022[56], Hornick 2023[52]
Nodal nevi	0–2%	Lezcano AJSP 2018[42], Chen 2023[43]
Dysplastic nevi	0–18%	Lezcano AJSP 2018[42], Chen 2023[43]
Conjunctival primary acquired melanosis with atypia	17.4–100%	Sekoranja 2021[51]
Conjunctival primary acquired melanosis without atypia	0–45%	Sekoranja 2021[51]
Melanocytic nevi	2–13.6%	Chen 2023[43], Lezcano AJSP 2018[42]
Common nevi	2–10%	Lezcano AJSP 2018[42], Chen 2023[43]
Blue nevi	0%	Lezcano AJSP 2018[42], Chen 2023[43]
Cellular blue nevi	0%	Kaczorowski 2022, Kline 2022[48]
Spitz nevi	0–20%	Lezcano AJSP 2018[42], Chen 2023[43], Koh 2022[47]
Atypical Spitz nevi	0%	Chen 2023[43], Koh 2022[47]
Deep penetrating nevi	0%	Lezcano AJSP 2018[42], Kline 2022[48]
Recurrent nevi	0–6.7%	Lezcano AJSP 2018[42], Chen 2023[43]
Congenital nevi	0%	Lezcano AJSP 2018[42], Kaczorowski 2022[56]
Acral nevi	0–7%	Chen 2023[43], Rothrock 2022[45]
Conjunctival nevi	0–30% focal	Sekoranja 2021[51]
Oral nevi	0%	Schmitt 2022[50]
Oral melanotic macule	0%	Schmitt 2022 [50]

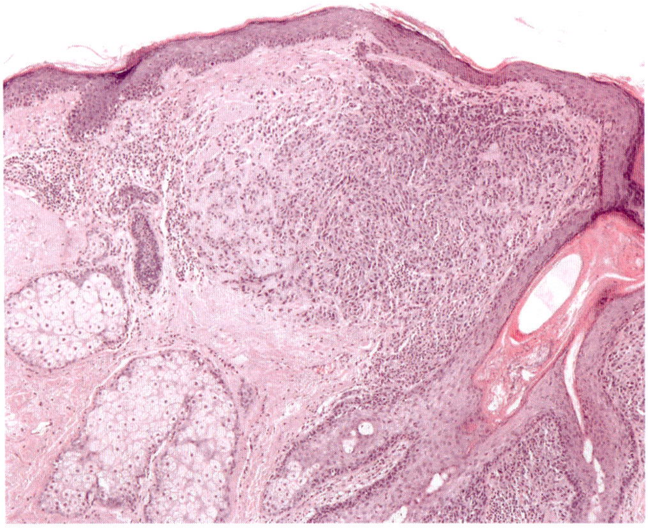

Figure 7.5 An invasive melanoma is seen in the dermis (X100).

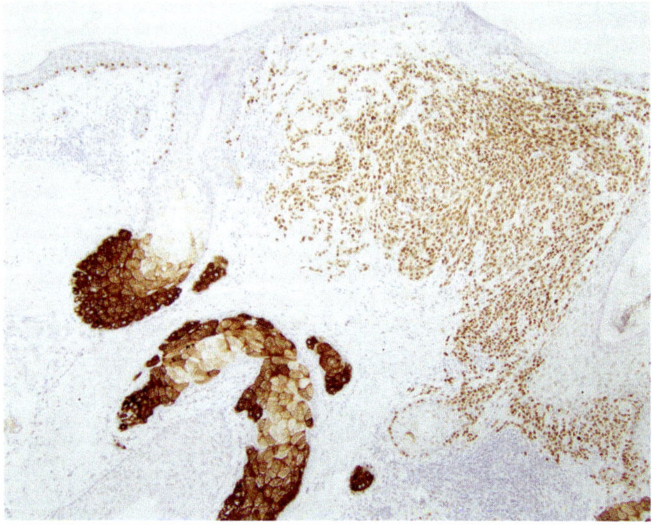

Figure 7.6 *Invasive melanoma.* PRAME highlights the invasive melanoma cells as well as the in-situ component. Note the strong staining of the sebaceous glands serving as internal positive control (X100).

Table 7.6 PRAME expression in non-melanocytic proliferation

	Percent positivity	References
Cellular neurothekeoma	27%	Cesinaro 2021[57]
Desmoid fibromatosis	0%	Kaczorowski 2022[56]
Dermatofibrosarcoma protuberans	0–50%	Cammareri 2023[54], Elsensohn 2021[55], Kaczorowski 2022[56]
Atypical fibroxanthoma	4–70%	Cammareri 2023[54], Elsensohn 2021[55], Hrycaj 2022[46]
Pleomorphic dermal sarcoma	4%	Hrycaj 2022[46]
Epithelioid sarcoma	0%	Kaczorowski 2022[56]
Kaposi sarcoma	20%	Cammareri 2023[54]
Angiosarcoma	13–67%	Cammareri 2023 [54], Kaczorowski 2022[56], Hrycaj 2022[46]
Leiomyosarcoma	0–13%	Cammareri 2023[54], Kaczorowski 2022[56], Elsensohn 2021[55]
Malignant peripheral nerve sheath tumor	18–75%	Cammareri 2023[54], Kaczorowski 2022[56], Hrycaj 2022[46]
Pleomorphic rhabdomyosarcoma	67%	Cammareri 2023[54]
Alveolar rhabdomyosarcoma	26–33%	Cammareri 2023[54], Kaczorowski 2022[56]
Embryonal rhabdomyosarcoma	32–100%	Cammareri 2023[54], Kaczorowski 2022[56]
Synovial sarcoma	70–100%	Cammareri 2023[54], Kaczorowski 2022[56]
Myxoid liposarcoma	100%	Cammareri 2023[54]
Low-grade fibromyxoid sarcoma	20%	Cammareri 2023[54]
Intimal sarcoma	100%	Cammareri 2023[54]
Biphenotypic sinonasal sarcoma	100%	Cammareri 2023[54]
Undifferentiated pleomorphic sarcoma	6–17%	Cammareri 2023[54], Kaczorowski 2022[56]
Ewing sarcoma	20%	Cammareri 2023[54]
CIC-rearranged sarcoma	100%	Cammareri 2023[54]
BCOR-sarcoma	40%	Cammareri 2023[54]
SMARCA4-deficient undifferentiated tumor	100%	Cammareri 2023[54]
NTRK-rearranged spindle cell neoplasm	50%	Cammareri 2023[54]
Basal cell carcinoma	62–86%	Elsensohn 2021[55], Kaczorowski 2022[56]
Squamous cell carcinoma	36%	Elsensohn 2021[55]
Basosquamous carcinoma	40%	Elsensohn 2021[55]
Merkel cell carcinoma	30–57%	Elsensohn 2021[55], Kaczorowski 2022[56]
Sebaceous carcinoma	25%	Elsensohn 2021[55]

(32–100%)[54,56], and malignant peripheral nerve sheath tumor (18–75%) (**Table 7.6**).[46,54,56]

Its expression can also be seen in various carcinoma such as basal cell carcinoma (62–86%)[55,56], basosquamous carcinoma (40%)[55], Merkel cell carcinoma (30–57%)[55,56], sebaceous carcinoma (25%)[55], squamous cell carcinoma (36%).[55]

PRAME immunostain

Diagnostic pearls

- PRAME is typically negative in clear cell sarcoma.

Limitations

- PRAME expression is not seen in all melanomas.
- PRAME expression can be seen in melanocytic nevi.
- In challenging melanocytic proliferation, PRAME expression does not correlate with morphologic features in many cases.
- PRAME expression can be seen a variety of non-melanocytic lesions including soft tissue lesions and carcinomas.

7.3 Evaluation of Atypical Junctional Melanocytic Proliferation

The distinction between pigmented actinic keratosis or solar lentigo and melanoma *in situ* (MIS) is of clinical importance since the diagnosis of MIS will result in wider excision. A high density of mildly to moderately atypical junctional melanocytes can be seen on chronically sun exposed skin without a clinically apparent melanocytic lesion.[58] Thus, pigmented actinic keratosis and solar lentigo can histologically mimic MIS. In addition, the pigmented epidermal keratinocytes on sun-damaged skin can be labeled by Melan-A resulting in over-diagnosing pigmented actinic keratosis or solar lentigo as malignant melanoma *in situ*.[59] Melan A can also highlight the melanin pigment within dermal macrophages.[60] In these settings, markers with nuclear staining such as MiTF, Sox10, and PRAME have been demonstrated to be superior by not only quantifying the junctional melanocytes but also outline their nuclear shape and size (**Figures 7.3–7.6**).[61] Nuclear PRAME expression has recently been reported to be helpful in diagnosing lentigo maligna and assessing surgical excision margins (**Figure 7.6**).[62] MiTF and Sox10 are most helpful in highlighting the density of the atypical melanocytes at the dermal-epidermal junction for margin evaluation, whereas in a pigmented actinic keratosis or lentigo Sox10 or MiTF with red chromogen highlights the non-confluent junctional melanocytic proliferation (**Figures 7.7 and 7.8**). PRAME can be helpful in distinguishing melanocytic pseudonests of lichenoid dermatitis.[63] In small biopsies, MiTF has been reported to exhibit better sensitivity than Sox10 in detecting junctional melanocytes.[61] In the setting of superficially invasive melanoma Sox10 has the advantage of labeling the spindle or desmoplastic melanoma cells in the dermis that would typically be negative for MiTF.[64]

Evaluation of atypical junctional melanocytic proliferation

- Sox10, MiTF, and PRAME being nuclear stains are superior to Melan-A in labeling melanocytes at the dermal epidermal junction.

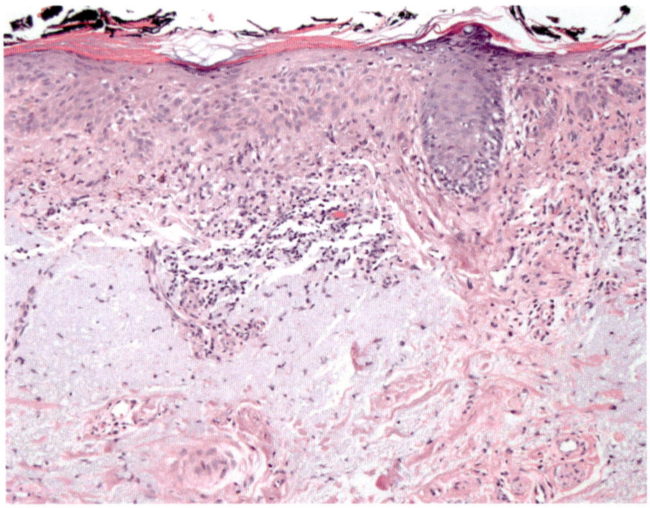

Figure 7.7 *Pigmented actinic keratosis.* Dysplastic keratinocytes with cytoplasmic melanin pigment are seen at the basal aspect of the epidermis (X200).

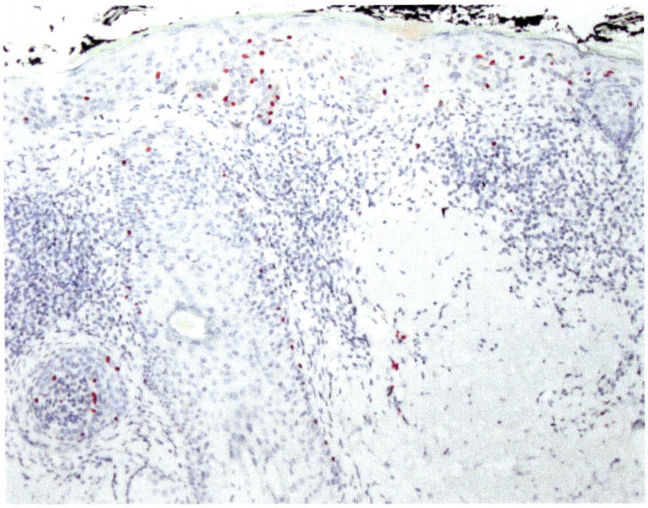

Figure 7.8 *Pigmented actinic keratosis.* Sox10 immunostain highlights only a mild increase in the number of junctional melanocytes (X200).

7.4 Nevoid Melanoma versus Melanocytic Nevus

Benign dermal melanocytic proliferation typically would exhibit "maturation," i.e. the cells or nests become smaller with progressive dermal depth. HMB-45 staining often mirrors this pattern with immunoreactivity seen in the intraepidermal and superficial dermal components in benign lesions and one can use this staining pattern in the diagnosis of melanocytic nevus versus melanoma. However, diffuse HMB-45 staining pattern is not specific for melanoma but can be seen in Spitz nevi, blue and deep penetrating nevi, and congenital nevi.[20,65,66] One setting is the diagnosis of nevoid melanoma which has minimal intraepidermal component and the dermal component appears to exhibit maturation. In contrast to a dermal nevus which exhibits progressive loss of HMB-45 staining, these cases usually have an irregular HMB-45 staining pattern.[67] In these settings, it is not the actual percentage of Ki-67-positive cells but the pattern of Ki-67 labeling would be diagnostically helpful. Similar numbers Ki-67-positive cells would be seen in the upper and lower dermal areas in melanoma cases.[67]

Because tumor thickness is the most important prognostic factor, it is important to accurately determine the extent of dermal involvement by melanoma cells. In this setting a panel of HMB-45 and Ki-67 can be of diagnostic help in the distinction of an invasive melanoma versus a severely atypical compound dysplastic nevus. In some cases it is difficult to distinguish whether the dermal component is all nevus or part of it represents invasive melanoma cells. While the dermal component of an atypical melanocytic nevus often exhibits diminishing gradient of HMB-45 staining, a reflection of maturation, the cells of an invasive melanoma often express HMB-45 (**Figures 7.9 and 7.10**). PRAME staining is positive in the invasive melanoma component while negative in the associated dermal nevus component.[42,43] Ki-67 proliferative index can be higher in the invasive melanoma component if these dermal nests are of sufficient size. In a lesion with marked host response, double labeling of Ki-67 and Melan-A or Mart-1 would be helpful in distinguishing

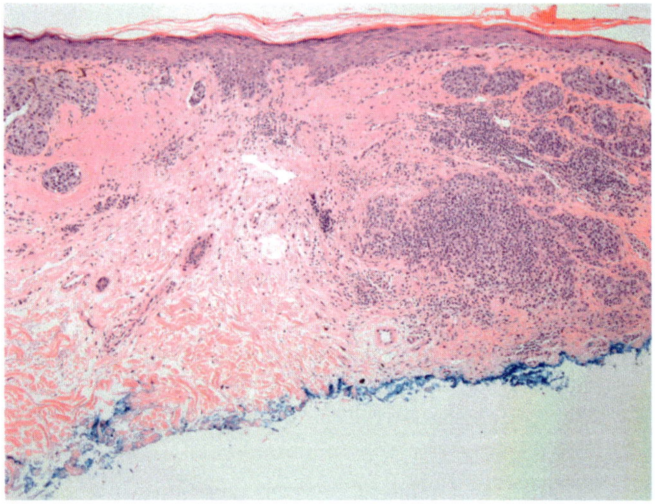

Figure 7.9 *Melanoma with associated dermal nevus.* In addition to a superficially invasive melanoma, an associated dermal proliferation of uniform melanocytes is seen below (X100).

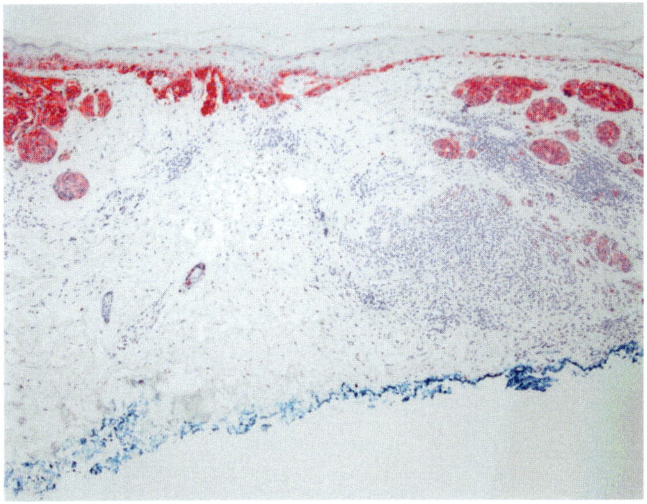

Figure 7.10 *Melanoma with associated dermal nevus.* Whereas the invasive melanoma component is strongly positive for HMB-45, only the superficial aspect of the dermal nevus component exhibits focal HMB-45 positivity (X100).

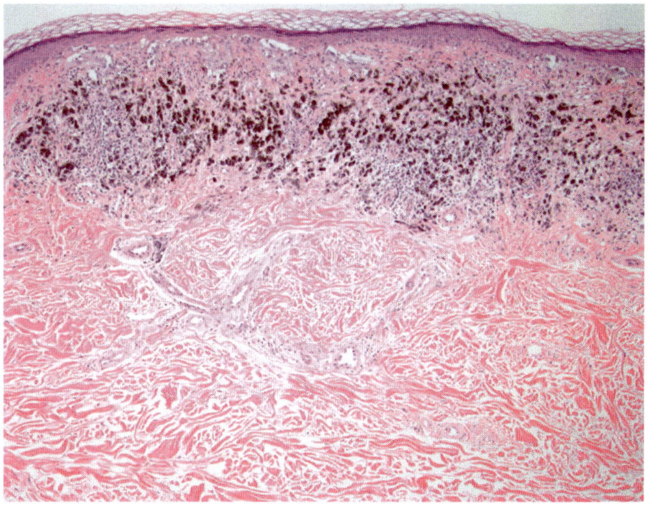

Figure 7.11 *Melanoma in situ with regression.* Below the junctional proliferation of severely atypical melanocytes, a dense and band-like infiltrate of lymphocytes, histiocytes and prominent melanophages is seen consistent with inflammatory regression (X100).

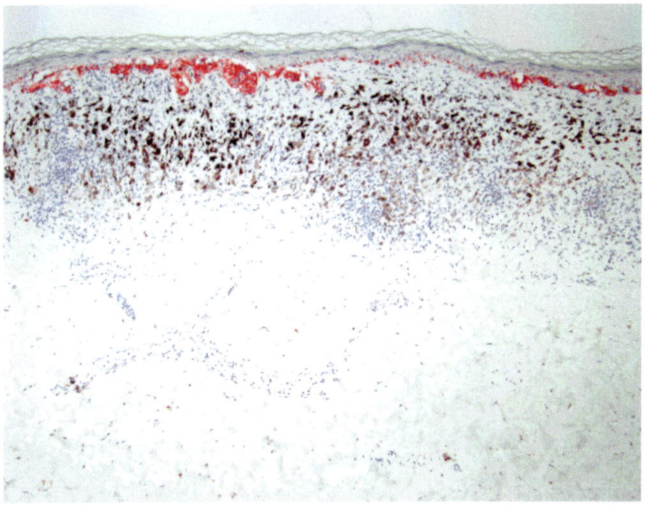

Figure 7.12 *Melanoma in situ with regression.* Melan A highlights only the atypical junctional melanocytes but none in the inflammatory dermal regression (X100).

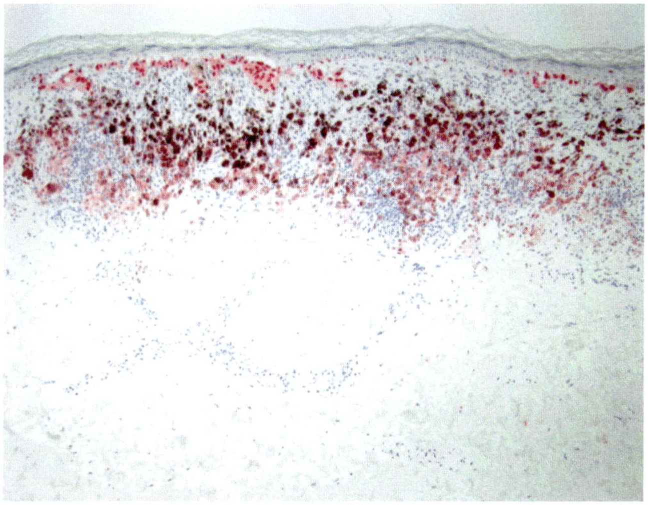

Figure 7.13 *Melanoma in situ with regression.* MiTF highlights the atypical junctional melanocytes as well as the dermal melanophages (X100).

proliferating melanocytes from lymphocytes In the setting of marked dermal regression, Melan-A, MiTF or Sox10 would aid in visualizing the residual invasive melanocytes although MiTF can label the dermal macrophages (**Figures 7.11, 7.12 and 7.13**).

Melanoma versus melanocytic nevus

- HMB–45 staining in both the superficial and deep aspect of melanoma, whereas only the superficial aspect of dermal nevus.
- HMB–45 and PRAME staining are often positive in the invasive melanoma component while typically negative in the dermal nevus component.
- Similar numbers Ki–67-positive cells would be seen in the upper and lower dermal areas in nevoid melanoma cases.

7.5 Melanocytoma/Dermal Melanocytic Proliferation

Deep Penetrating Nevus/WNT-activated Deep Penetrating/Plexiform Melanocytoma

Deep penetrating nevus (DPN), a rare subtype of melanocytic nevus, occurs in young adults as small, dome-shaped, and pigmented nodule. DPN affects mostly the head and neck area (33%) and the upper and lower extremity (31%).[68] It has been classified as a WNT-activated deep penetrating/plexiform melanocytoma (naevus) in the 5th edition WHO Classification of Skin Tumors (**Table 7.7**).[69,71–73]

Histopathologically, there are two subtypes including deep penetrating type and plexiform spindle cell subtype. The lesion is predominantly dermal with an inverted triangle shape

Table 7.7 Comparison of deep penetrating nevus, deep penetrating melanocytoma, and malignant deep penetrating nevus[69, 71–73]

	Deep penetrating nevus	Deep penetrating melanocytoma	Malignant deep penetrating nevus
Classification (WHO)	Low-grade intermediate/ melanocytoma	High-grade intermediate/ melanocytoma	Melanoma
Dermal mitoses	0–2 per mm2	> 2 per mm2	> 2 per mm2
Cytologic atypia	Mild to moderate	Mild to moderate, rarely severe	Often severe
Marked inflammation	Infrequent	Infrequent	Present
Ki67 proliferation index	< 5%	< 10%	>= 10%
p16 expression	Intact	Intact or partially lost	Absent or partially lost
PRAME expression [71]	Absent	Usually absent	Usually positive
Beta-catenin nuclear expression	Present	Present	Present/absent
TERT-promoter mutation	Absent	Usually absent	Usually present
Copy number variant [72,73]	0–1	1–2	>= 3

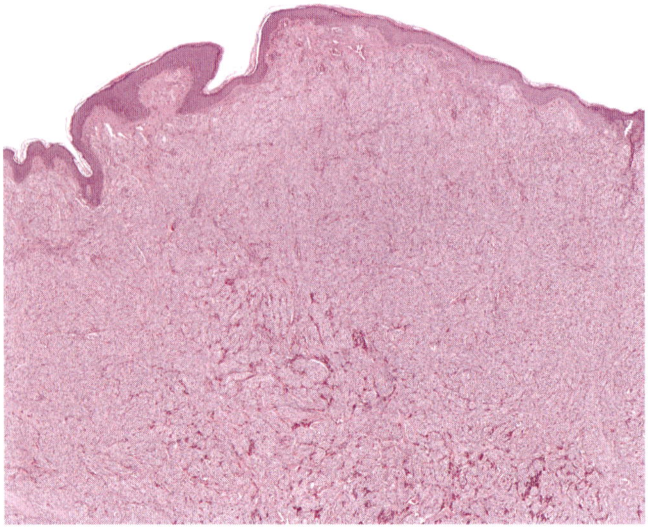

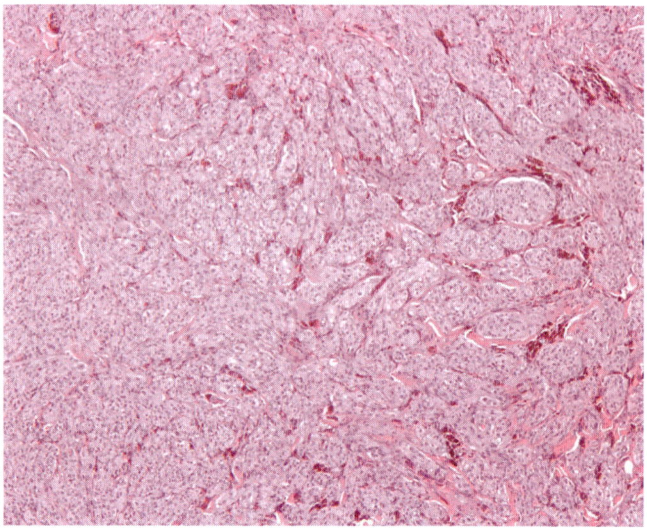

Figures 7.14 and 7.15 *Deep penetrating nevus.* An inverted triangular proliferation of spindled and epithelioid melanocytes is seen in the dermis (X100, X400).

extending to deep dermis or subcutaneous tissue in the deep penetrating subtype. Nests or small fascicles of large spindled or epithelioid melanocytes with pigmented cytoplasm and prominent nucleoli are seen associated with variable number of melanophages. In the plexiform spindle cell subtype the proliferation exhibits a fascicular architecture often extending along hair follicles, adnexal structure, nerves, or blood vessels. DPN is often seen as a component of a combined nevus. Features of an atypical DPN (high-grade deep penetrating melanocytoma) include large size, asymmetry, sheet-like growth, >2 mitoses per squared millimeter, and cytologic atypia (**Figures 7.14 and 7.15**).

Studies have shown that activation of both MAP kinase and WNT/beta-catenin pathways is the underlying molecular mechanism of DPN.[70] Mutations of the beta-catenin pathway result in a lesion with increased cytoplasm and pigmentation, and nuclear cyclin D1 expression.[70] Additional oncogenic mutations including *TERT* promoter mutations and *CDKN2A* inactivation were seen in melanoma arising in association with DPN.

When the WNT/beta-catenin pathway is activated, beta-catenin enters the nucleus and interacts with transcription factors including lymphoid enhancer-binding factor 1 (LEF1). LEF1 has been shown to be important in tumorigenesis and epithelial-mesenchymal transition.[71] Beta-catenin (**Figure 7.16**), LEF1, and cyclin D1 (**Figure 7.17**) immunostains have been reported to be helpful in the distinction of DPN versus mimics (**Table 7.8**). Diffuse HMB-45 expression is seen. Distinction of from malignant deep penetrating tumor would have treatment implication. Complete loss of p16, positive PRAME expression, presence of *APC* mutation or *TERT* promoter, are supportive of malignant deep penetrating tumor.[73]

Deep penetrating nevus

- Deep penetrating nevus is often seen as a component of combined nevus.
- Beta-catenin, LEF1, and cyclin D1 expression is seen in deep penetrating nevus in contrast to histologic mimics.

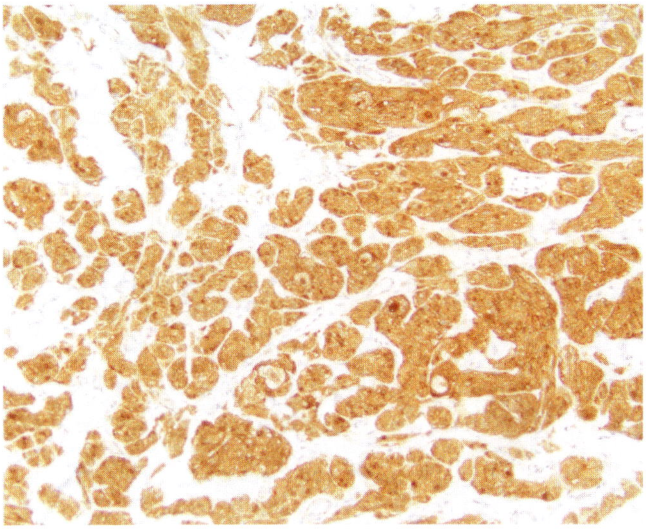

Figure 7.16 *Deep penetrating nevus.* Nuclear as well as cytoplasmic beta-catenin expression is seen (X200).

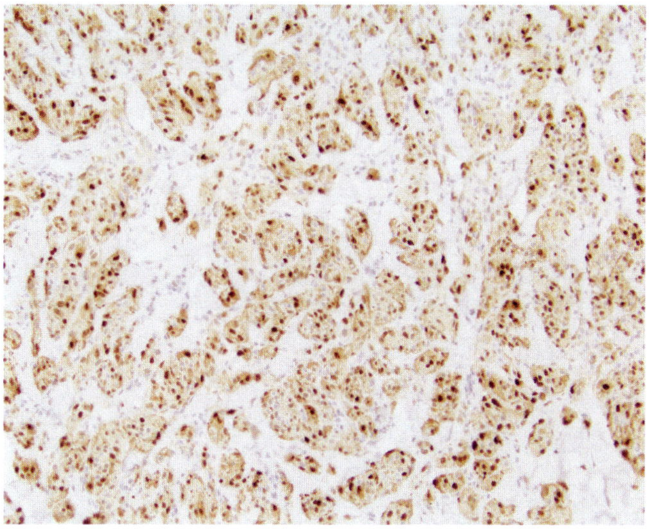

Figure 7.17 *Deep penetrating nevus.* Diffuse nuclear cyclinD1 expression is noted (X200).

Table 7.8 Expression of beta-catenin, LEF1, and cyclin D1 in deep penetrating nevus and histologic mimics.

	Beta-catenin	LEF1	Cyclin D1	reference
Deep penetrating nevi	14/14 (100%)	13/14 (92.8%)		Raghavan 2020[74]
	98/100 (98%)		82/82 (100%)	De la fouchardiere 2019[75]
		9/9 (100%)		Vanderbeck 2023[71]
Cellular blue nevi	0/19 (0%)	0/19 (0%)		Raghavan 2020[74]
Blue nevi	0/15 (0%)	0/15 (0%)		Raghavan 2020[74]
		6/16 (37.5%)		Vanderbeck 2023[71]
Congenital nevi	0/12 (0%)	0/12 (0%)		Raghavan 2020[74]
Spitz nevi and tumors				De la fouchardiere 2019[75]
Pigmented epithelioid melanocytoma	0/6 (0%)		1/1 (100%)	De la fouchardiere 2019[75]
Melanoma	1/12 (8.3%)	9/12 (75%)		Raghavan 2020[74]
	2/16 (12.5%)		8/8 (100%)	De la fouchardiere 2019[75]

Pigmented epithelioid melanocytoma

Pigmented epithelioid melanocytoma (PEM) was first reported in 2004 as an indolent tumor with frequent regional lymph node involvement but rarely with distant metastasis.[76] PEM has a predilection with young patients with a median age of 27 years. Although the extremities are the most involved site, back, trunk, scalp, genital sites, and oral mucosa have been reported.[76] Blue-black, >1cm, plaques or nodules are seen. PEM can recur locally, spread to regional lymph node, and rarely metastasize to distant sites.[76]

In the WHO Classification of Skin Tumors[69], there are two pigmented epithelioid melanocytoma (PEM) genetic models: (1) protein kinase cAMP-dependent type I regulatory subunit alpha (*PRKAR1A*) inactivation and (2) protein kinase C alpha (*PRKCA*) fusion, both located on 17q24.2.[77] PEM can be either "pure" or "combined" or in combination with a nevus which usually harboring a *BRAF*V600E mutation.[77] Recent study has shown that the associated nevus can be a common nevus, blue nevus, Spitz nevus, and even *PRKCA*-fused PEM, supporting the notion that *PRKAR1A* inactivation can occur as a secondary event in various melanocytic neoplasms.[78]

In pure PEM, a sheet-like proliferation of heavily pigmented epithelioid and spindled melanocytes is seen in the dermis (**Figures 7.18 and 7.19**). In combined PEM, the associated nevus is typically the common nevus, but it can be blue nevus, Spitz nevus, or congenital nevus. Extension into the subcutaneous fat is seen along hair follicles, pilar muscle, and adnexal structures. The proliferation is comprised of three types of cells: (1) dendritic cells, (2) pigmented polygonal cells, and (3) epithelioid cells with abundant cytoplasm and prominent vesicular nuclei. Mitotic activity is not prominent. The *PRKCA* fusion type usually present as solid nodule of monomorphic melanocytes in young patients.[77] *PRKAR1A*-mutated lesion often has an associated nevus component.[79]

PEM typically expresses Sox10, S100, Mart-1, and variably for HMB-45. Loss of PrkAr1a expression can detect 80% of *PRKAR1A* inactivation and is typically seen in all Carney complex associated PEMs, and 82% of sporadic PEMs (**Figure 7.20**).[80] PEMs with fusion do not show R1alpha loss of expression.

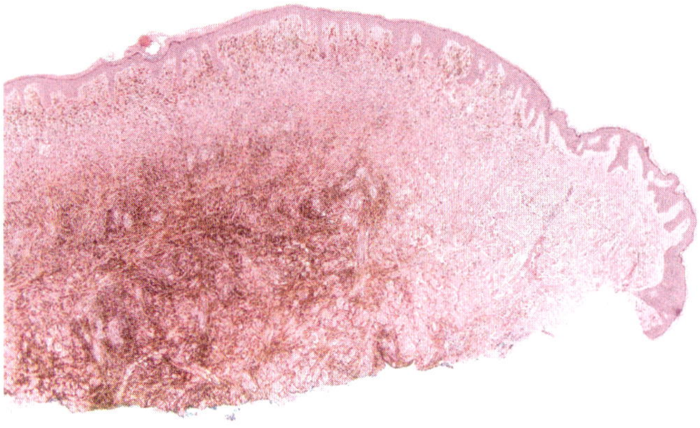

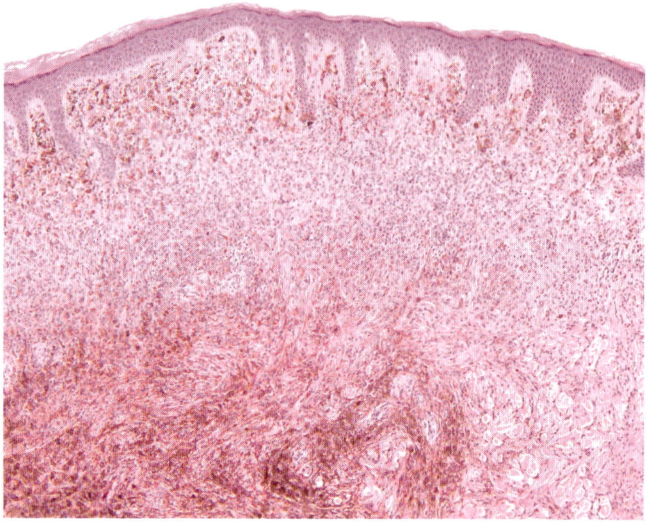

Figures 7.18 and 7.19 *Pigmented epithelioid melanocytoma.* A proliferation of heavily pigmented melanocytes is seen in the dermis (X40, X100).

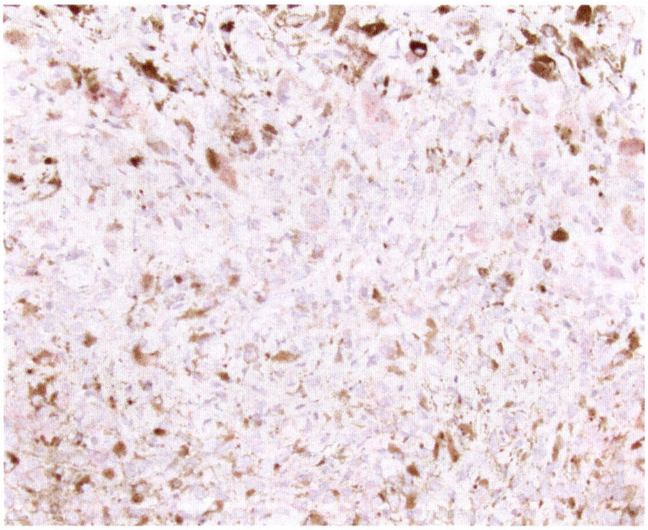

Figure 7.20 *Pigmented epithelioid melanocytoma.* Loss of PRKAR1A nuclear expression is seen (X400).

The histologic differential diagnosis of PEM includes cellular blue nevus, atypical cellular blue nevus, deep penetrating nevus (DPN), combined nevus, cutaneous neurocristic hamartoma, DPN-like melanoma, and PEM-like melanoma.

Fascicular proliferation of spindled but not epithelioid melanocytes is seen in *CYSLTR2*-mutant cutaneous melanocytic neoplasms (cellular blue nevi, atypical cellular blue nevi, blue nevus-like melanomas).[81] *PRKAR1A* or *PRKCA*, but not *GNAQ*, *GNA11*, *CYSLTR2*, and *PLCB4*, is associated with PEM. PEM-like melanoma is also in the differential diagnosis.[82] Although PEM-like morphology can be seen, genetic alteration involving *TERT* promoter, *CDKN2A*, or both is seen in majority of cases.[82] Frequently affected genes in PEM includes *BRAF*, *MAP2K1*, *GNAQ*, *CTNNB1*, *NRAS*, *NF1*, and *NTRK1*.

Pigmented epithelioid melanocytoma

- PEM can be either "pure" or "combined" or in combination with a nevus which usually harboring a *BRAF*V600E mutation.
- Combined PEMs are typically *PRKAR1A*-mutated, and the type associated with Carney complex.
- Loss of R1alpha expression is typically seen in 82% of sporadic PEMs and all Carney complex associated PEMs.
- Sentinel lymph node may be positive; however, risk of distant metastasis is low.

BAP1-inactivated melanocytic tumor

BAP1 (BRCA1-associated protein 1) located on 3p21 is a tumor suppressor gene whose germline mutations have resulted in an autosomal dominant cancer susceptibility syndrome. Individuals with *BAP1* germline mutations have increased incidence of uveal and cutaneous melanomas, renal cell carcinomas, mesotheliomas, lung cancer, and others.[83] *BAP1*-inactivated melanocytic tumor (BIMT) can be either sporadic or in association with *BAP1*-inactivating autosomal dominant cancer syndrome. BIMTs present as flesh-colored papule or nodule on the head and neck, trunk, and upper extremities without age or gender predilection.[83] Most follow an indolent biologic course; however, rare *BAP1*-inactivated melanomas have been reported.[83,84]

BIMT can display several morphologic patterns. Often these lesions are "combined" nevus with a proliferation of epithelioid melanocytes associated with a conventional dermal nevus. A well-demarcated dermal nodule of epithelioid melanocytes can be seen with a dermal nevus (**Figures 7.21 and 7.22**). In another pattern, nests of epithelioid melanocytes are seen in a background of dermal nevus with features of congenital onset.[85] A "pure" pattern comprising of only BAP1-negative epithelioid melanocytes can be seen.[86] Multinucleated

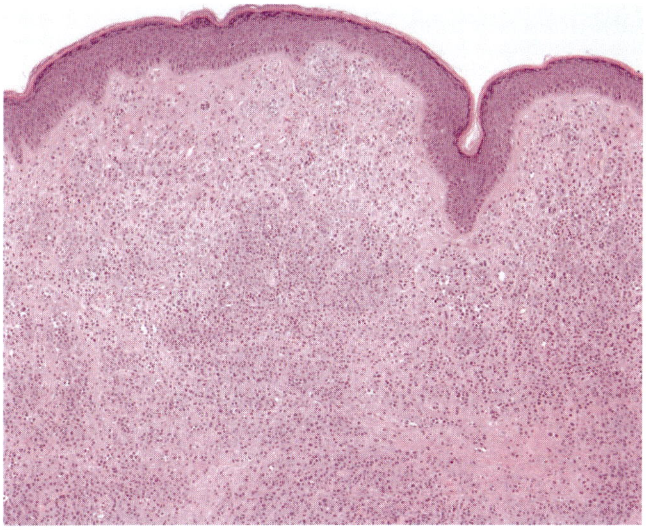
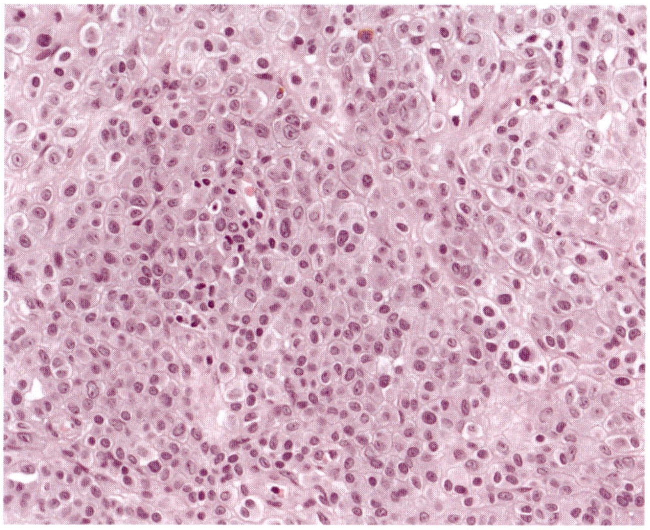

Figures 7.21 and 7.22 *BAP1-inactivated melanocytic tumor.* A proliferation of epithelioid melanocytes is seen in the dermis (X100, X400).

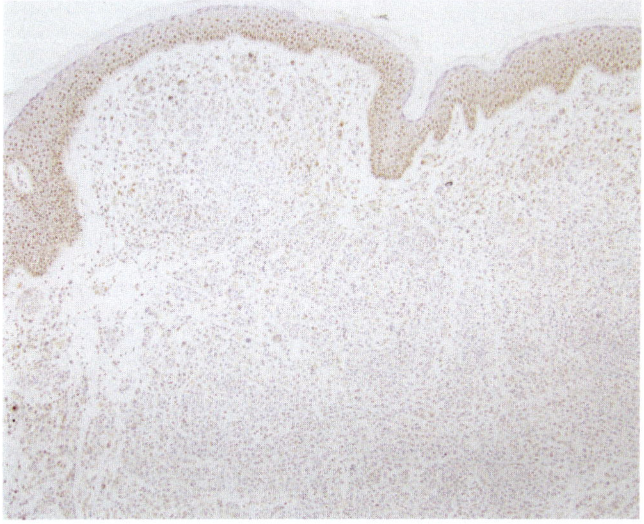

Figure 7.23 *BAP1-inactivated melanocytic tumor.* Loss of BAP1 nuclear expression by the lesional cells is seen (X100).

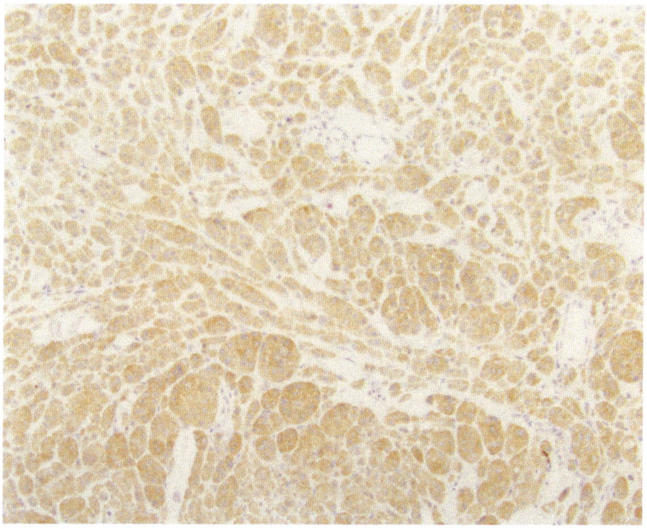

Figure 7.24 *BAP1-inactivated melanocytic tumor.* Diffuse BRAFV600E expression is noted (X200).

or giant cells, pseudonuclear inclusions, adipocytic metaplasia, and associated lymphohistiocytic response are often seen.[85] Mitotic activity is low.[85,86] A junctional component is more often seen in lesions of patients with germline *BAP1* mutation.[87]

BAP1 protein loss is accepted to be the result of biallelic inactivation of *BAP1*. The epithelioid neoplastic cells exhibit loss of BAP1 nuclear expression (**Figure 7.23**). A perinuclear BAP1 staining has been reported to be specific for BIMT.[88] The background nevus as well as the epithelioid proliferation often exhibit BRAFV600 expression (**Figure 7.24**).

BAP1-inactivated melanocytic tumor

- The epithelioid neoplastic cells exhibit loss of BAP1 nuclear expression.
- The background nevus as well as the epithelioid proliferation often exhibit BRAFV600 expression.

Clear cell tumor with melanocytic differentiation (*ACTIN::MITF*, *MITF::CREM*)

Clear cell tumor with melanocytic differentiation and *MITF::CREM* translocation is a recently reported entity in rare cases.[89] Clear cell tumor with melanocytic differentiation and *ACTIN::MITF* translocation is another closely related tumor.[89] Melanocytic differentiation in these dermal based tumors has been attributed to increased MITF function as a result of gene fusion. Both present as non-ulcerated and non-pigmented cutaneous nodule.[89]

Clear cell tumor with melanocytic differentiation and *MITF::CREM* translocation often affects the distal extremities. It is a poorly circumscribed dermal nodule is noted in the dermis and subcutaneous tissue comprised of a sheet-like proliferation of epithelioid to spindle tumor cells. Clear cell morphology can be prominent.[89] Perineural invasion and prominent mitotic figures can be seen.[89] Ulceration, lymphovascular invasion, and necrosis were not reported.[89] Diffuse and strong Sox10, S100, and MiTF expression is seen.[89] HMB-45 positivity is patchy.

Clear cell tumor with melanocytic differentiation and *ACTIN::MITF* translocation commonly affects the distal extremities and trunk. A dermal tumor with prominent clear cell change is noted. Mitosis is infrequent. Ulceration, perineural invasion, lymphovascular invasion, and necrosis are not typically seen.[89] S100, MiTF, HMB-45, and Melan-A expression are seen.[89]

The differential diagnosis includes clear cell sarcoma which typically harbors *EWSR1::ATF1*, *EWSR1::CREB1*, and *EWSR1::CREM*.[90] Another tumor in the differential diagnosis is cutaneous melanocytic tumor with *CRTC1::TRIM11* fusion.[91] PEComas would express MiTF or TFE3, but not S100.[92] Cellular blue nevi, Spitz tumors, and melanomas are also in the differential diagnosis.

Clear cell tumor with melanocytic differentiation and *MITF::CREM* or *ACTIN::MITF* translocation

- Diffuse and strong Sox10, S100, Melan-A, and MiTF expression

Cutaneous melanocytic tumor with *CRTC1::TRIM11* fusion

Cutaneous melanocytic tumor with *CRTC1::TRIM11* fusion, first reported in 2018, is an indolent tumor that rarely recurs or metastasizes.[91] Yang et al [93] reported a case of metastasizing tumor. There is a female predilection, and the median age is 44 years.[91] Children can be involved. It presents at a flesh-colored nodule on trunk or extremities with an average size of 8.4 mm.[91]

Histopathologically, a well-circumscribed nodular proliferation of spindle and epithelioid cell with pink cytoplasm is seen in the dermis (**Figure 7.25**). Epidermal involvement can be seen. The spindle tumor cells are arranged in nests or fascicles (**Figure 7.26**). There are less than 5 mitoses per 10 high power fields. Ulceration, perineural invasion and lymphovascular invasion are typically not seen.[91] The tumor cells exhibit strong and diffuse Sox10 expression, and inconsistently for S100, MiTF, HMB-45 and Melan-A (**Figures 7.27 and 7.28**). The histologic differential diagnoses include atypical Spitz tumor, cutaneous clear cell

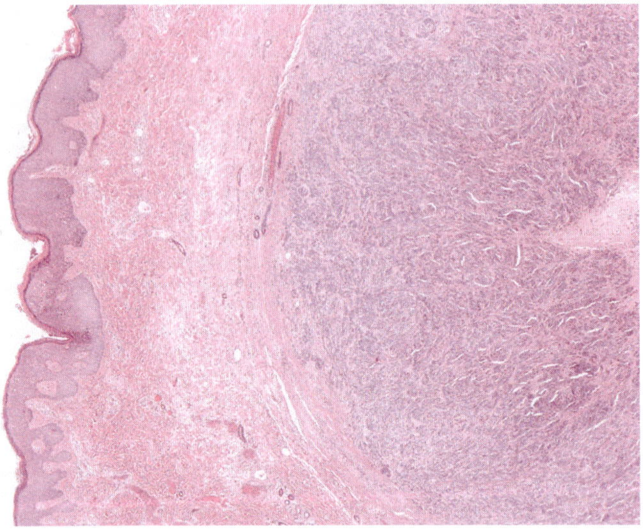

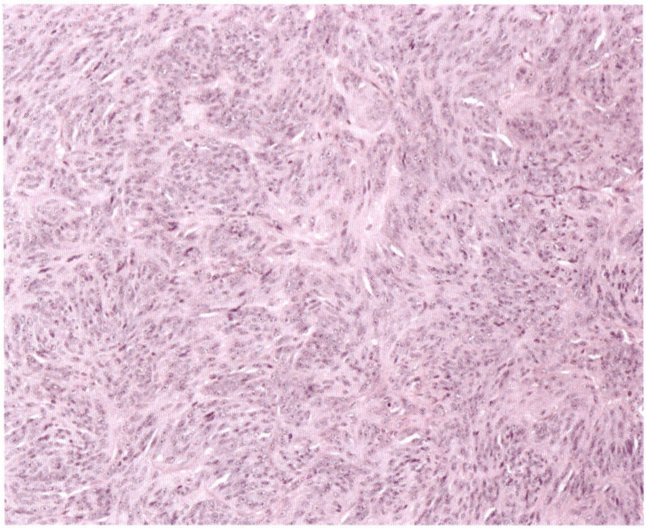

Figures 7.25 and 7.26 Cutaneous melanocytic tumor with *CRTC1::TRIM11* fusion. A well-demarcated nodule of spindled cells arranging in fascicles is seen in the dermis (X40, X200).

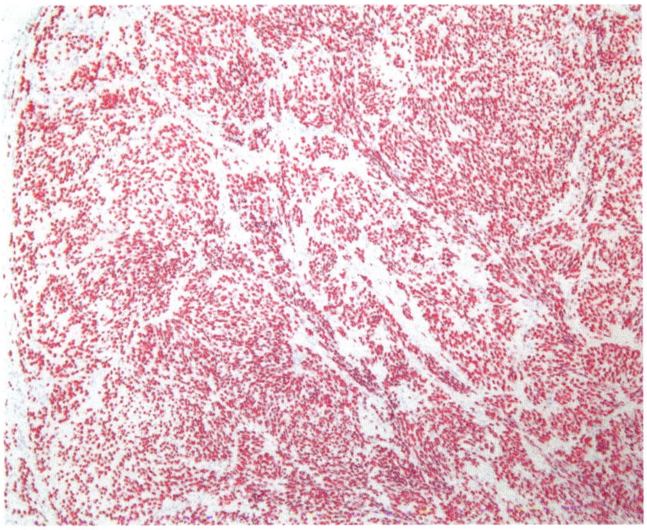

Figure 7.27 Cutaneous melanocytic tumor with *CRTC1::TRIM11* fusion. Diffuse Sox10 expression is seen (X200).

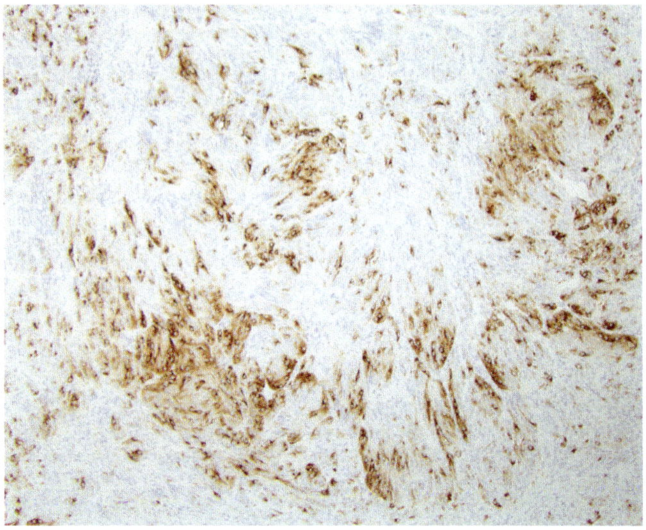

Figure 7.28 Cutaneous melanocytic tumor with *CRTC1::TRIM11* fusion. Patchy HMB-45 expression is noted (X100).

sarcoma, primary dermal and metastatic melanoma, myoepithelial tumor, and paraganglioma-like dermal melanocytic tumor.

Cutaneous melanocytic tumor with *CRTC1::TRIM11* fusion

- Strong and diffuse Sox10 expression is typically seen; however, S100, MiTF, HMB-45 and Melan-A expression is inconsistent.

7.6 Benign versus Atypical Proliferative Nodule Arising in a Congenital Nevus

Discrete dermal nodular proliferations or "proliferative nodules" can be seen in congenital nevi. These proliferations are usually self-limited and may occasionally regress spontaneously. Some proliferative nodules exhibit atypical histologic appearance which makes the histologic distinction from malignant melanoma a diagnostic challenge. Several studies have shown that the Ki-67 index is a helpful marker for distinguishing melanocytic nevi from malignant melanoma.[94] Histone H3 protein is maximally phosphorylated during the mitotic phase of the cell cycle, making the PHH3 a specific marker for mitosis.[95] The PHH3 marker has been studied in melanocytic lesions and has been found to be useful in rapid determination of mitotic index.[95] Congenital melanocytic nevus has been shown to express minimal reactivity for Ki-67.[96] Up to date there have been few series reporting immunohistochemical analyses of proliferative nodules.[96,97] The immunohistochemical analyses by Herron and colleagues[97] indicated that congenital melanocytic nevus and proliferative nodule share similar expression of Ki-67, p16, p21, p27, c-Myc, Bax, CD95, and Bcl-2. However, Phadke et al.[96] found in their series that atypical proliferative nodules have a significantly higher Ki-67% (7% vs. 1%) and PHH3 (5 vs. 1) expression than the benign proliferative nodule and the background congenital melanocytic nevus. The mean Ki-67% expression of atypical proliferative nodules is significantly different from previously reported invasive melanoma cases (7% vs. 37%) (**Figures 7.29 and 7.30**).[94] These immunohistochemical results suggest that atypical proliferative nodules represent a distinctive clonal population within congenital melanocytic nevus with biologic behavior possibly residing between benign nevus and malignant melanoma, and thus best be treated as a borderline lesion.

Proliferative nodule arising within a congenital nevus

- Atypical proliferative nodules have a significantly higher Ki-67% and PHH3 expression than the background congenital nevus

7.7 Spitz Tumors

A spectrum of tumors ranging from benign, indeterminate to melanomas can be seen in Spitz melanocytic tumors. Spitz tumors typically follow an indolent clinical course with only rare malignant cases reported in the literature.[98] Kinase fusions are frequently documented in most Spitz tumors including receptor tyrosine kinases *ALK*, *NTRK1*, *NTRK2*, *NTRK3*, *RET*, *MET*, *MERTK*, *FGFR1*, and *ROS1*; serine threonine kinases *BRAF*, *ERBB4*, *PRKDC* and *MAP3K8*.[99] Some fusions are associated with distinct histologic appearance. These findings suggest that gene fusions may play a role in tumorigenesis, histomorphologic patterns and may be site-specific. In Spitz tumors ALK, ROS1, and pan-TRK immunoreactivity is typically correlated with an associated gene fusion; however, a positive immunostaining does not equate to the presence of gene rearrangement. Quan et al.[99] have shown that Spitzoid neoplasms with either *BRAF* or *NRAS* mutation typically follow an aggressive biological course. Therefore, BRAFV600E immunoreactivity would not support the diagnosis of Spitz tumor. Desmoplastic Spitz nevus often harbor 11p gain involving *HRAS* gene.[100]

ALK

ALK (anaplastic lymphoma kinase, receptor tyrosine kinase) fusions have been detected in up to 13% of acral lentiginous melanomas. *ALK* fusions are detected in 8–11%, 5–16% and 1–3%

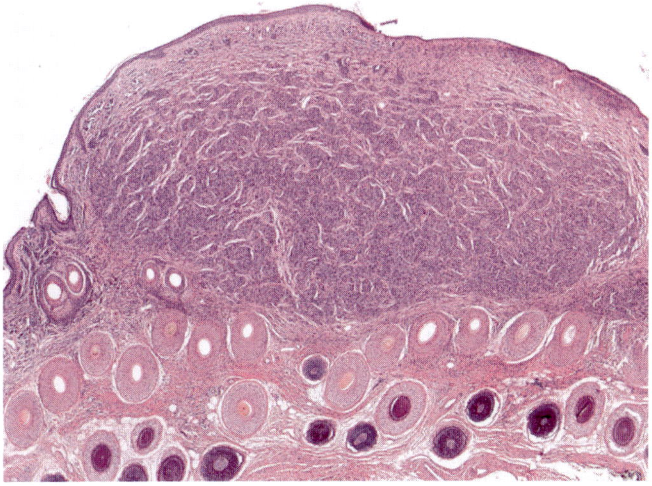

Figure 7.29 *Atypical proliferative nodule arising in a congenital nevus.* A well-demarcated and nodular proliferation of melanocytes is seen in the background of dermal congenital nevus (X40).

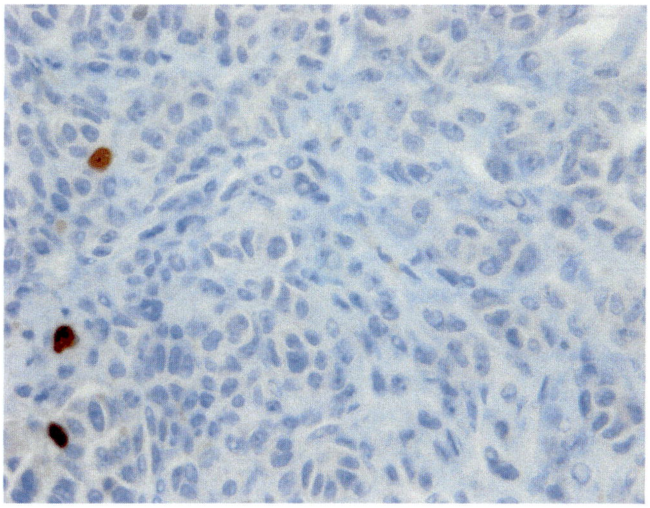

Figure 7.30 *Atypical proliferative nodule arising in a congenital nevus.* Ki-67 demonstrates a low Ki-67 proliferation index (X400).

of Spitz nevi, atypical Spitz tumors and 1–3% Spitz melanomas, respectively.[101]

Spitz tumors with ALK-overexpression are typically located on the lower extremity, exophytic, wedge-shaped. They have a plexiform architecture, infiltrative growth at the periphery of the lesion, spindle cell morphology, moderate cytologic atypia, and associated epidermal hyperplasia (**Figures 7.31 and 7.32**).[102] Immunohistochemistry with D5F3 and 5A4 monoclonal antibodies has been shown to be helpful in detecting *ALK* fusion (**Figures 7.33 and 7.34**).[103]

ROS1

ROS1 (ROS proto-oncogene 1, receptor tyrosine kinase) fusions can be detected in Spitz nevi, desmoplastic Spitz nevi, pigmented spindle cell nevi, and atypical Spitz tumors.[103] Spitz tumors with ROS1-overexpression often exhibit plaque-like or nodular pattern, pagetoid spread, transepidermal elimination of tumor nests, spindle, or mixed spindle/epithelioid morphology, small to intermediate in size, and low to moderate cytologic atypia (**Figure 7.35**).[104] Myxoid change can be seen. Majority of lesions with *ROS1* fusion exhibits ROS1 staining.[104] Immunostaining with D4D6 monoclonal antibody has 97.4% sensitivity in detecting *ROS1* fusion (**Figure 7.36**).[103]

NTRK

Spitz tumors with NTRK1 (neutrotrophic receptor tyrosine kinase 1) overexpression often exhibit exophytic/verrucous architecture,[102] lobulated nests, filigree-like and thin rete ridges, Kamino bodies, nevoid cells with scant cytoplasm, moderate cytologic atypia, and rosette-like structures (**Figures 7.37 and 7.38**).[105] Spitz tumors with *NTRK2* fusion have horizontally oriented junctional nests, lentiginous proliferation within follicular epithelium, hyaline globules, and polygonal melanocytes with prominent dendritic processes.[106] NTRK3 overexpressed tumors have Reed nevus-like features, pseudo-schwannoma pattern, and spindle morphology.[107] Pan-TRK immunostain, EPR17341 monoclonal antibody, has been shown to be reliable in the detection of *NTRK* fusions (**Figures 7.39 and 7.40**).[108]

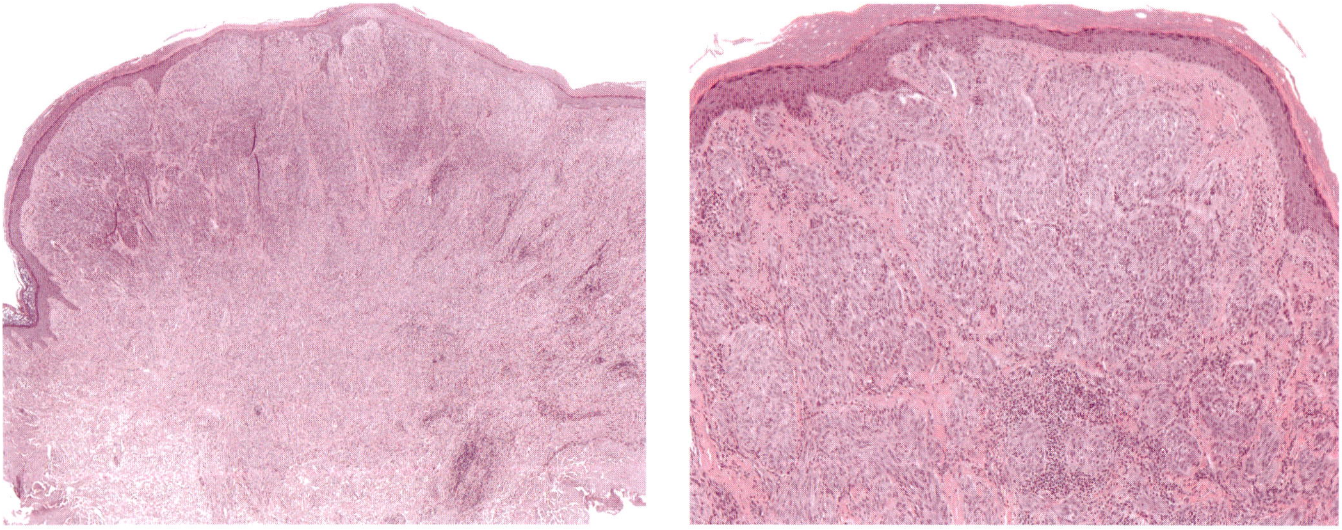

Figures 7.31 and 7.32 ALK-positive Spitz tumor. A plexiform proliferation of spindle and epithelioid melanocytes in the dermis (X40, X100).

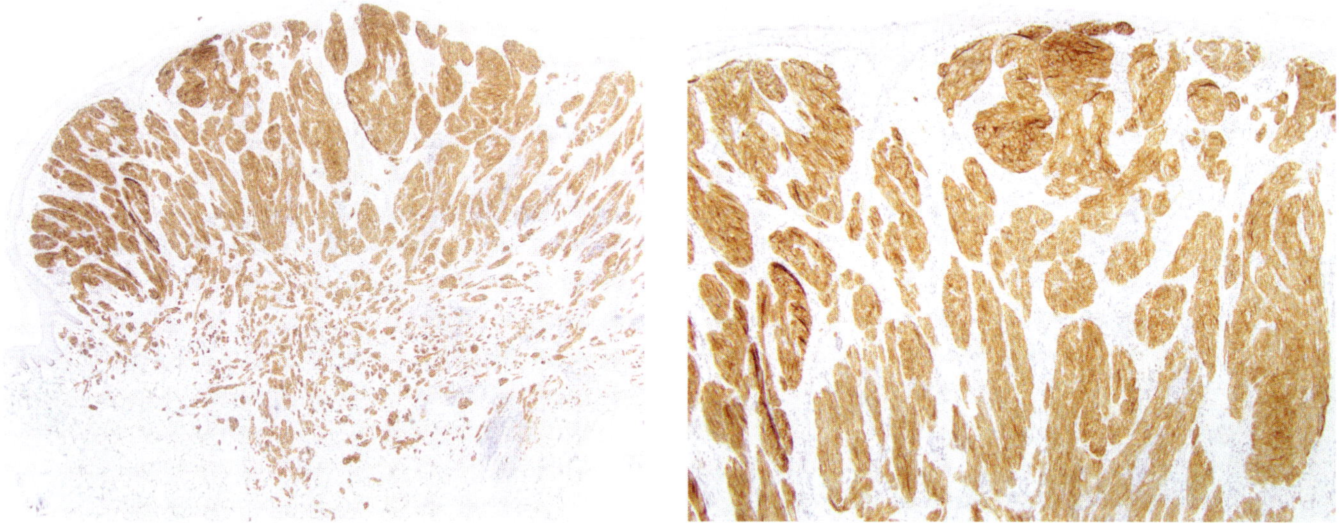

Figures 7.33 and 7.34 ALK-positive Spitz tumor. Diffuse and strong ALK expression is noted (X40).

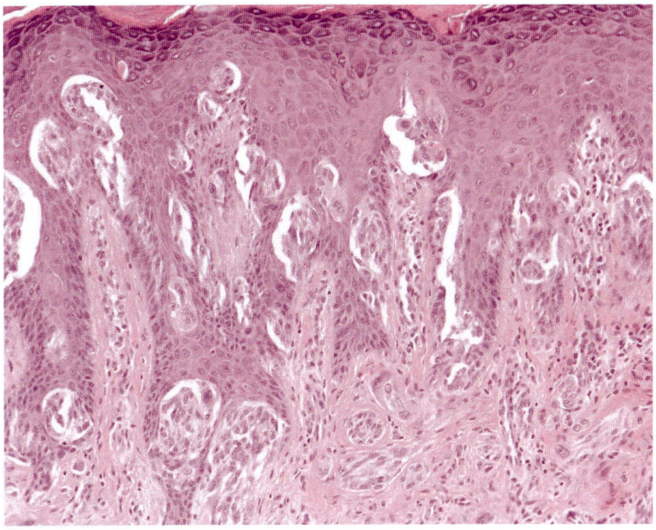

Figure 7.35 ROS1-positive Spitz tumor. A compound Spitzoid proliferation within the epidermis and in the dermis (X200).

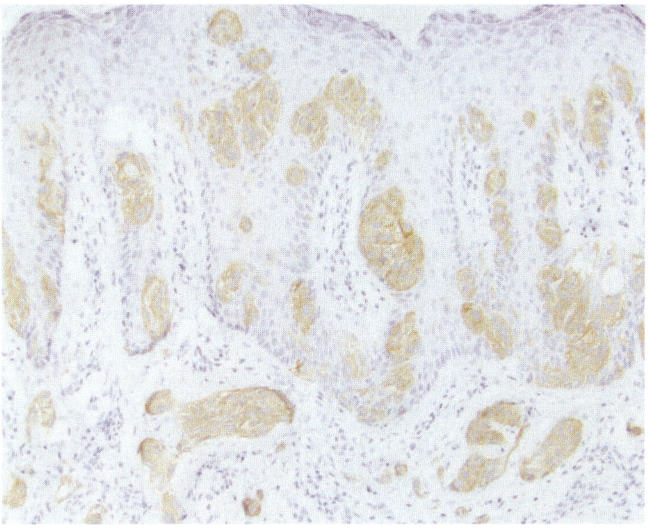

Figure 7.36 ROS1-positive Spitz tumor. ROS1 cytoplasmic expression by the tumor cells is seen (X200).

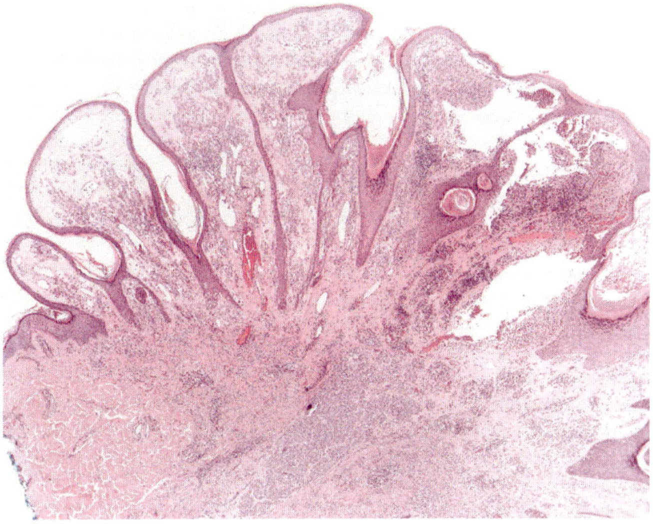

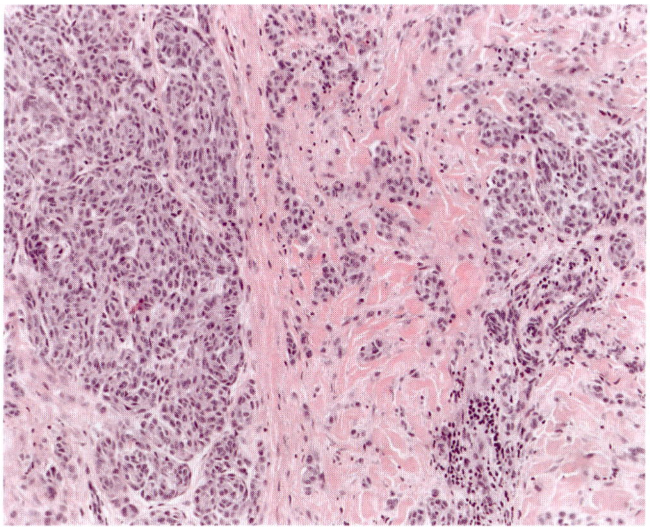

Figures 7.37 and 7.38 Pan-TRK-positive Spitz tumor. An exophytic and verrucous proliferation of spindle and epithelioid cells is seen (X40, X200).

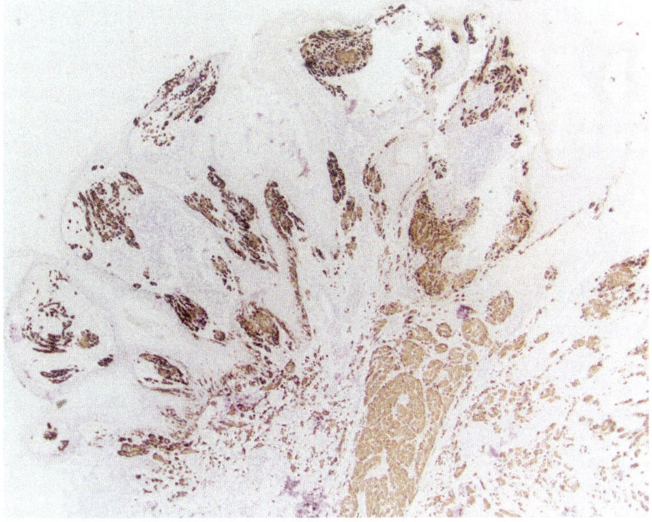

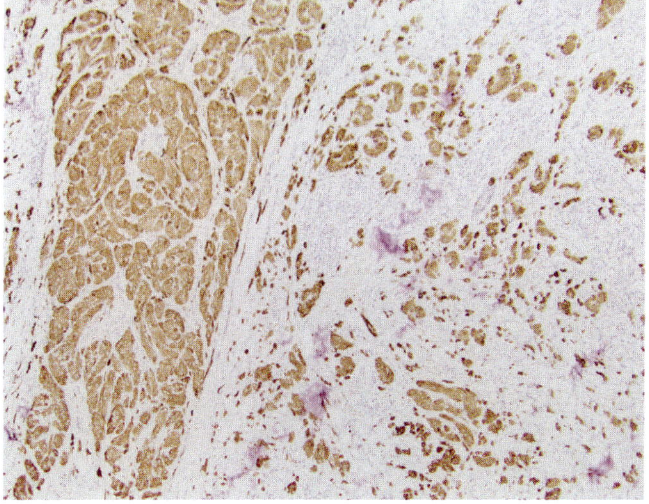

Figures 7.39 and 7.40 Pan-TRK-positive Spitz tumor. Strong cytoplasmic pan-TRK expression by the tumor cells is noted (X40, X100).

BRAF

BRAF (B-Raf proto-oncogene, serine/threonine kinase) fusions are common kinase translocations in tumors. Although estimated to occur in 2.6–6.7% of all melanomas, the frequency of *BRAF* fusions is higher in melanomas occurring in younger females and in Spitz neoplasms.[109] *BRAF*-rearranged Spitz tumors have sheet-like growth, plaque-like/nodular growth pattern, intermediate to large size, severe cytologic atypia, epithelioid morphology, and associated fibrosis.[102,109]

MAP3K8

Of the Spitz neoplasms with *MAP3K8* (Mitogen-activated protein kinase 8) fusions, 52% were Spitz melanomas, 40% AST, and 8% Spitz nevi.[103] On histologic sections, these tumors are nodular with a nested dermal pattern, ulcerated, epithelioid morphology, moderate to severe cytologic atypia [103] and multinucleate cells, and with p16 loss. [110]

MET

Spitz nevi with *MET* fusions are symmetric dome-shaped lesions with epidermal hyperplasia, large nests, and intermediate to large epithelioid melanocytes.[111]

RAF1

RAF1 fusions though uncommon have been reported in cutaneous melanomas including those with Spitzoid morphology.[112] In a genetic analysis of 7119 melanomas, 8 primary cutaneous melanomas with *RAF1* gene rearrangement were identified, 7 of which displayed an epithelioid morphology.[112] *RAF1* fusion has been reported in 2 Spitz nevi and one Spitz melanoma: *CTDSPL::RAF1* fusion and two novel *PPAP2B::RAF1* and *ATP2B4::RAF1* fusions.[113] Two of these three Spitz lesions with *RAF1* fusion were comprised of mainly dermal proliferation of epithelioid neoplastic cells.[113]

RET

2–3% of Spitz melanocytic tumors harbor *RET* fusion.[103] The histology of *RET* fused Spitz nevi is not specific. They are often well-circumscribed, symmetric, compound lesions comprised of large expansile nests of small to intermediate epithelioid tumor cells.[114]

MAP2K1

Most Spitz neoplasms with *MAP2K1* mutations are AST or Spitz melanoma.[103] In a series of six melanocytic neoplasms with *MAP2K1* in frame deletions, Spitzoid morphology and prominent pigmentation were noted in majority of cases.[115] Deep penetrating nevi-like architecture was noted in half of the cases.[115] Some can have features of both Spitz nevi and dysplastic nevi.

Spitz tumors

- ALK-overexpressed Spitz tumors often have a plexiform appearance characterized by intersecting fascicles of spindle melanocytes.
- NTRK1-overexpressed Spitz tumors have filigree-like epidermal rete ridges, pronounced dermal maturation, and occasional rosettes.
- *NTRK3* fusions are often detected in pigmented Spitz nevi. Pseudo-schwannoma appearance is often seen.
- *BRAF*-rearranged tumors have sheet-like growth, fibrotic stroma, and epithelioid neoplastic cells with severe cytologic atypia.

7.8 Atypical Spitz Tumor versus Spitz Melanoma

Despite frequent sentinel lymph node involvement, atypical Spitz tumor (AST) do not exhibit similarly poor prognosis as noted for conventional melanoma; thus, the distinction between AST and Spitzoid melanoma is important.[116] Histologic features that favor the diagnosis of atypical Spitz tumors include: asymmetry, expansile growth, Clark level IV or V, absence of maturation, nuclear pleomorphism, atypical and deep mitotic figures with more than six noted per squared millimeters (**Figures 7.41 and 7.42**).[117]

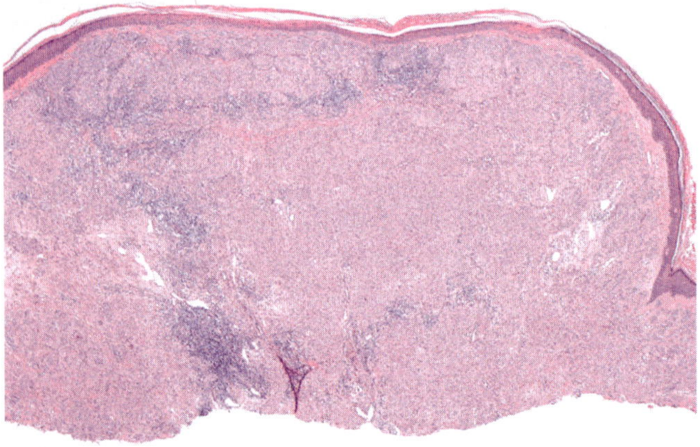

Figure 7.41 Atypical Spitz tumor. A nodular and expansile proliferation of spindle melanocytes is seen in the dermis (X40).

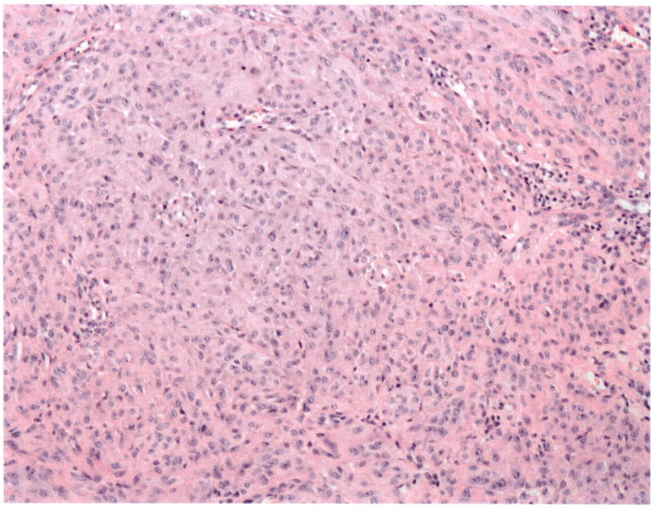

Figure 7.42 Atypical Spitz tumor. The cells are uniformly atypical with abundant eosinophilic cytoplasm (X200).

Immunostains including HMB-45, Ki-67, p16, p21, and PHH3 have been reported as helpful ancillary tests in the distinction between Spitz nevus versus Spitz tumor and Spitzoid melanoma. Intradermal Spitz nevi would exhibit a stratified HMB-45 staining pattern.[94] Ki-67 highlights only the superficial component of Spitz nevi similar to that observed in dermal nevi.[94] Vollmer et al.[118] found that a Ki-67 proliferation index of over 10% favors melanoma while a proliferation index below 2% favors a Spitz nevus. Kapur et al.[94] found significant difference in Ki-67% staining in Spitz nevi versus atypical Spitz nevi/tumors (5% versus 10%). p16 is typically strongly expressed in conventional nevi whereas loss of both nuclear and cytoplasmic p16 staining has been reported to be specific for melanoma.[119] p21 is overexpressed in Spitz nevi in comparison to melanoma.[94] In a recent study of 66 melanocytic lesions by Nasr et al.[95] PHH3 labeled only the superficial aspect of Spitz nevi yet all of melanoma. Kapur et al.[94] reported significant difference in fatty acid synthase expression between atypical Spitz nevi/tumors and malignant melanoma. In a study of Spitz tumors versus malignant melanoma, loss of both nuclear and cytoplasmic dermal reactivity of S100A6 is highly associated with melanoma.[119] PRAME expression can be seen in atypical Spitz tumors.[43,47]

Several chromosomal copy number changes can be seen in ASTs. Studies have shown that ASTs with 6p25 or 11q13 gains or homozygous 9p21 deletions would possess a worse prognosis in comparison to ASTs without these findings.[120] ASTs can have isolated 6q23 deletions but have not been shown to have higher risk for aggressive biologic course.[121,122] In a series by Shen et al.[122] with a median follow-up of 2 years, 6/11 ASTs with 6q23 had positive sentinel lymph node biopsy yet none developed in transit or distant metastasis. BAP1 and p16 immunostains can be used as screening tests for some of these chromosomal abnormalities. Loss of p16 staining is consistently seen in ASTs with homozygous 9p21 deletions while p16 expression is variably noted in up to 67% of ASTs with heterozygous 9p21 deletions (**Figure 7.43**). Thus, although loss of p16 expression is not synonymous with homozygous 9p21 deletions, diffuse p16 expression would exclude homozygous 9p21 deletions.[121] BRAFV600E immunostain might add additional diagnostic information since *BRAF* mutations can be detected in Spitzoid melanomas but absent in atypical Spitz nevi. Immunohistochemistry and molecular studies can aid in the distinction of Spitz melanoma versus Spitzoid melanoma with kinase fusions and *BRAF*V600 mutation is more frequently seen in Spitz melanoma and Spitzoid melanoma, respectively (**Table 7.9**).

Atypical Spitz tumors

- Atypical Spitz tumors likely exhibit higher Ki–67 proliferation index.
- Loss of p16 expression is not typically seen in Spitz nevi but can be in atypical Spitz tumor with homozygous 9p21 deletion.
- BRAFV600E immunostain might add additional diagnostic information since *BRAF* mutations can be detected in Spitzoid melanomas but absent in atypical Spitz nevi.

Table 7.9 Distinction between Spitz melanoma versus Spitzoid melanoma

	Spitz melanoma	Spitzoid melanoma
Histologic features	Spitzoid features	Spitzoid features
Immunohistochemical findings	BRAFV600E negative Can be positive for ALK, ROS1, or pan-TRK	Often BRAFV600E positive Can be NRASQ61 R positive Often PRAME positive
Molecular alterations	Kinase fusions such as *BRAF* or *MAP3K8* Low tumor mutational burden	Often *BRAF*, *NRAS*, *NF1* driver mutations Chromosomal copy number gain High tumor mutational burden Frequent *TERT* promoter mutations

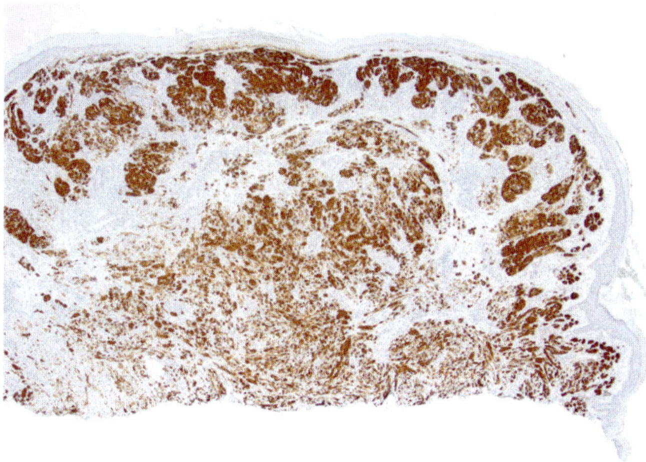

Figure 7.43 Atypical Spitz tumor. Strong and diffuse p16 expression is noted in the tumor cells (X40).

7.9 Nail Melanocytic Lesions

Increased pigment production within the nail matrix from lentigo, melanocytic nevus, atypical melanocytic hyperplasia, or melanoma will result in longitudinal melanonychia clinically. Of the single digit longitudinal melanonychia, melanoma accounts for 6% of the cases in adults whereas it is extremely rare in children.[123] Lentigo is diagnosed when there is increased melanin pigmentation or single melanocytes at the junction; nevus when there are prominent nests; and atypical junctional melanocytic hyperplasia when there is increased number of single melanocytes. The presence of lentiginous proliferation, increased number, dendritic morphology, pagetoid upward migration, and cytologic atypia is supportive of melanoma *in situ* of the matrix.[124]

A nuclear stain such as Sox10 is most helpful in demonstrating the density and size of junctional melanocytes. HMB45 and Melan-A have been reported to be more sensitive than S100 protein in highlighting the intraepithelial melanocytic proliferation of the nail.[125] Using a cutoff value of 10%, PRAME has been shown to be a good discriminator between subungual melanocytic proliferation and subungual melanoma *in situ*. However, in another study of 127 benign and malignant acral melanocytic lesions, PRAME expression did not correlate in a subset of lesions including Spitz nevi, *in situ* melanoma, and thin invasive melanoma.[53]

7.10 Nodal Nevus versus Metastatic Melanoma

In the setting of sentinel lymph node biopsy, the distinction between capsular nevus versus metastatic melanoma has important treatment and prognostic implication. Also known as nodal melanocytic nevus and capsular nevus rest, nevus cell aggregates were found in 3% of 100 consecutive dissections for melanomas in a 10-year retrospective examination of lymphadenectomy[126] and in 22% of 208 lymphadenectomy of melanoma patients in a subsequent study.[127] Nodal nevi are typically confined to the fibrous capsule whereas metastatic melanoma would be present in the subcapsular sinus; however, nodal nevi can be seen within the parenchyma (**Figures 7.44, 7.45, 7.46, and 7.47**).[128] Since nodal nevi are frequently observed in patients with melanoma-associated nevi, it has been postulated that nodal nevus arises due to mechanical transport of nevus cells.[129]

Nodal nevi are typically positive for S100, Sox10, and Mart-1/Melan-A, are usually negative for HMB-45, and exhibit minimal (less than 1%) Ki-67 proliferation index.[128,129,130] One caveat is that melanoma cells can be negative for HMB-45 and accurate determination of Ki-67 proliferation index can be difficult in small aggregates of melanocytes; thus the immunohistochemical findings must be correlated with the cells' morphology and location. Sox10 and S100 are best markers in the setting of desmoplastic melanoma since this subtype of melanoma is typically negative for Melan-A/Mart-1 and HMB-45. PRAME has been shown to be negative in nodal nevi while positive in nodal metastasis.[42,43] When the metastases have been treated, tumor necrosis, marked histiocytic infiltration and melanophages can be seen. In this setting an immunostain utilizing a red or alkaline phosphatase chromogen would be invaluable in assessing for residual tumor.

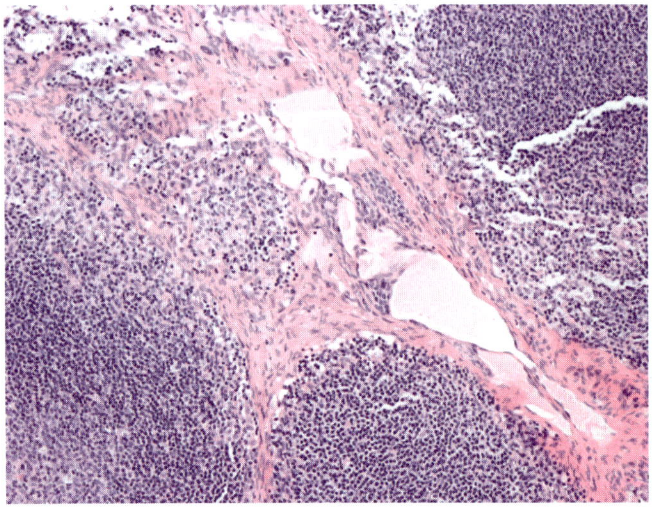

Figure 7.44 Capsular nevus. Aggregates of benign nevus cells are seen within the lymph node capsule and surrounding vascular structure (X200).

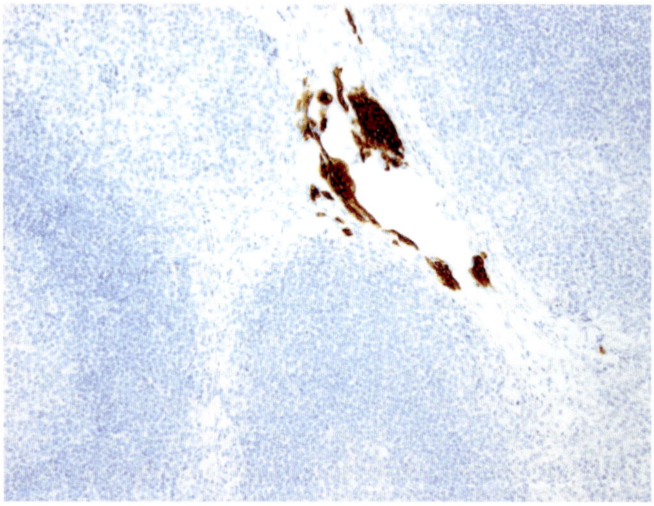

Figure 7.45 Capsular nevus. The nodal nevus cells are strongly positive for Mart-1 (X200).

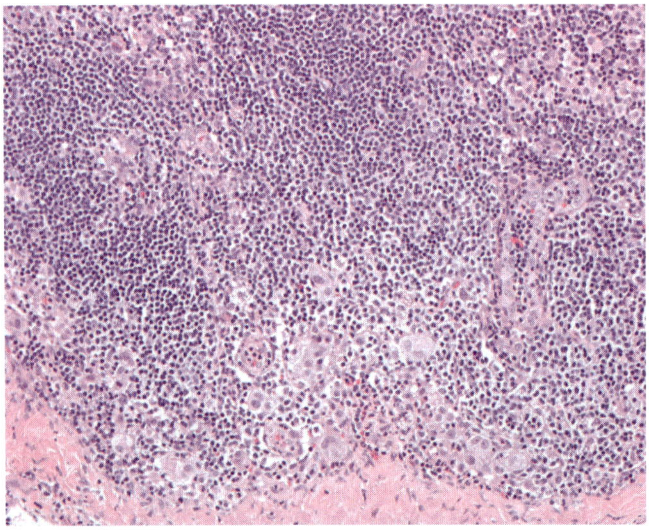

Figure 7.46 Capsular nevus. Microscopic foci of metastatic melanoma within a sentinel lymph node (X100).

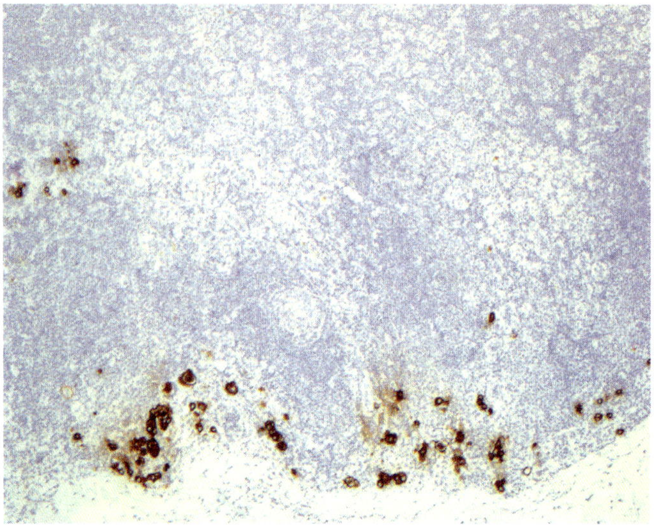

Figure 7.47 Capsular nevus. The tumor cells are strongly positive for HMB-45 (X100).

Investigations of the utility of a variety of markers including p16, NM23, IMP-3 (insulin-like growth factor-II messenger RNA-binding protein-3), Sox2, nestin, and 5-hydroxymethylcytosine in the distinction of metastases versus nodal nevi have been performed. Mihic-Probst et al.[130] reported nuclear and cytoplasmic p16 staining in all 18 nodal nevi while all 26 melanoma metastases were negative; however, cytoplasmic staining was seen in 25/26 metastases thus interpretation can be difficult. A study reported p16 to be a helpful marker with p16 expression noted in studied nodal nevi while absent in 5 melanoma metastases.[131] While none of the benign nodal nevi expressed IMP3, 70% (21/30) of metastatic melanoma in lymph node was positive for IMP3.[132] Complete loss of 5-hydroxymethylcytosine nuclear staining would be suggestive of metastatic melanoma.[133] Although these results are promising, these markers are not routinely used in clinical practice due to availability.

Capsular nevus

- Capsular nevi are negative for HMB–45 and PRAME, while metastatic melanoma often HMB–45 and PRAME positive.

7.11 Desmoplastic Melanoma versus Mimics

Sox 10 has shown to exhibit great sensitivity in detecting desmoplastic melanoma and distinguishing it from mimics. Almost all desmoplastic melanomas express S-100 protein strongly and diffusely in the dermis. In addition, the presence of rare tumor cells positive for HMB-45, MiTF, or Melan-A/Mart-1 can be helpful; however, HMB-45 is typically negative and Melan-A is positive only focally in 7% of desmoplastic melanoma cases.[134] Recently, p75 has been reported to be superior to S100 in diagnosing spindle cell and desmoplastic melanoma (**Figures 7.48 and 7.49**).[135] S-100 and p75 positive cells can be seen in scar tissue; therefore, Sox10 would be the better marker in the distinction between dermal scar versus desmoplastic melanoma.[136]

Desmoplastic melanoma

- Desmoplastic melanoma is invariably positive for S100, p75, and Sox10; while only focally positive or negative for MiTF, Melan-A/Mart–1, and HMB–45.

7.12 Clear Cell Sarcoma

Clear cell sarcoma is a rare soft tissue sarcoma of young adults that often arises in the distal extremities and involves the tendons and aponeuroses. Histologically it is characterized by nests of spindled neoplastic cells with eosinophilic cytoplasm and occasional multinucleated giant cells. The tumor cells are invariably positive for S-100, HMB-45, KBA62, and PN2; and often for Melan-A and MiTF (**Table 7.10**) (**Figures 7.50, 7.51, 7.52 and 7.53**).[137–141] They are negative for SMA, desmin, and keratins (**Table 7.10**).[137–141] Melanosomes can be demonstrated ultrastructurally in clear cell sarcoma. Often the distinction of clear cell sarcoma from metastatic melanoma can be difficult. In these setting, genetic studies for recurrent translocation involving the *EWSR1* gene located on chromosome 22q12 is helpful.[142] Although expressing melanocytic markers, clear cell sarcoma exhibits a distinctive cytogenetic abnormality, a fusion of *EWS* gene on 22q12 with the *ATF1* gene on 12q13 in the majority of cases and another fusion of *EWS* to *CREB1* gene on 2q13 in a minority of cases.[142] While *BRAF* and *NRAS* mutations can be detected in melanomas, these mutations are typically absent in clear cell sarcoma.[143] While clear cell sarcomas are diffusely positive for S100, HMB-45 and Melan-A; PEComas are typically negative for Sox10 and focally positive for HMB-45. In addition, clear cell sarcomas are negative for muscle markers. Clear cell sarcomas are typically negative for PRAME with expression seen in a small subset of tumors.[43,48,54]

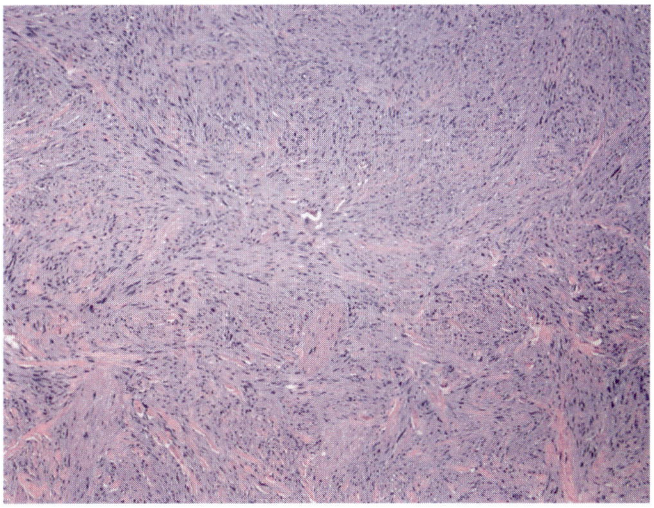

Figure 7.48 Desmoplastic melanoma. A diffuse proliferation of spindle melanocytes in the dermis (X100).

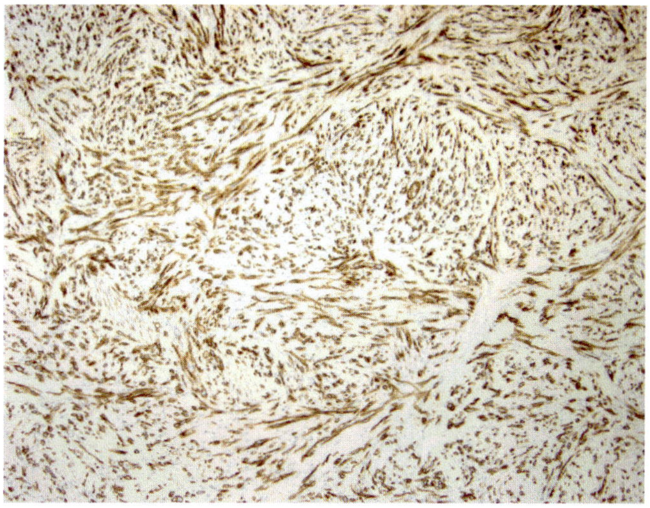

Figure 7.49 Desmoplastic melanoma. Diffuse and strong p75 expression by the tumor cells (X100).

Table 7.10 Immunoprofile of clear cell sarcoma and PEComa[48,139–148]

Immunostain	Clear cell sarcoma	PEComa
S100	99%	32%
HMB–45	96%	96%, focal
MiTF	77%	100%
Melan-A	81%	27%
Sox10	57%	0%
PRAME	negative	89%
NKI/C3	ND	100%
PNL2	100%	ND
KBA62	94%	ND
Keratin	2%	0%
SMA	0%	36%, focal
Desmin	0%	28%
Calponin	ND	16%
Caldesmon	ND	0%

ND: not documented, SMA: smooth muscle actin

Clear cell sarcoma

- Molecular analyses are essential for diagnosis since clear cell sarcoma has the same immunoprofile as metastatic melanoma.
- The presence of t(12;22)(q13;q13) (*EWS::ATF1*) gene fusion allows a definitive diagnosis of clear cell sarcoma.
- Clear cell sarcoma is typically negative for PRAME expression while melanoma is positive.

7.13 Perivascular Epithelioid Cell Tumors (PEComa)

Perivascular epithelioid cell tumors (PEComas) are rare mesenchymal neoplasms. Whereas PEComas also include angiomyolipoma, clear cell sugar tumor, and lymphangioleiomyoma in other organs, cutaneous PEComas refers to tumors with perivascular epithelioid or spindled neoplastic cells with clear or eosinophilic cytoplasm. Cutaneous PEComas have a female

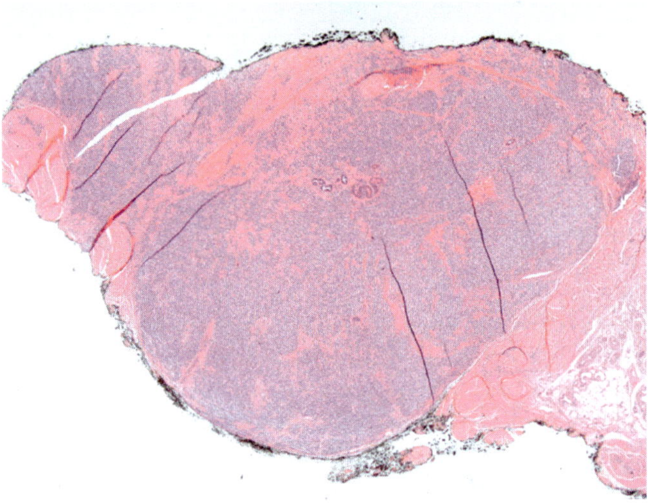

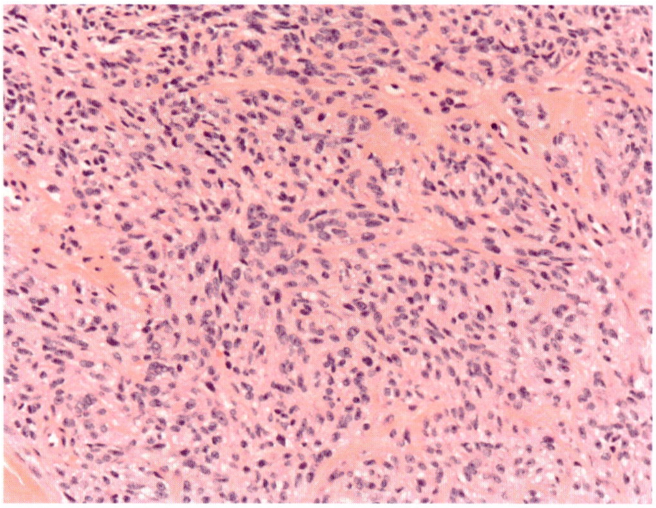

Figures 7.50 and 7.51 Clear cell sarcoma. A nodular proliferation of tumor cells, some with clear cytoplasm, is seen in the deep soft tissue (X20, X200).

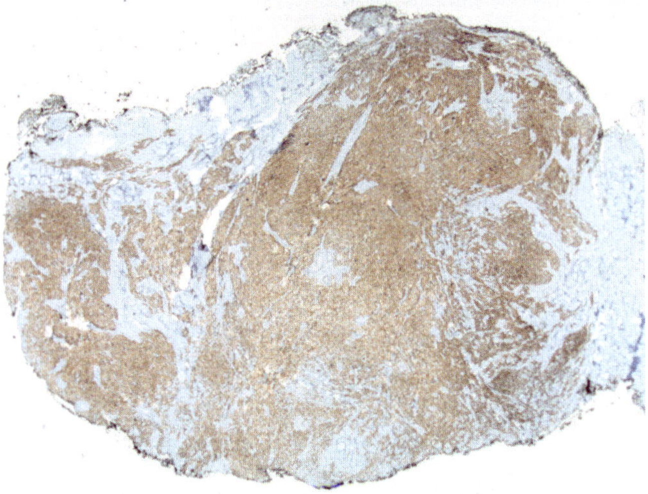

Figure 7.52 Clear cell sarcoma. Diffuse and strong HMB-45 expression by the tumor cells (X20).

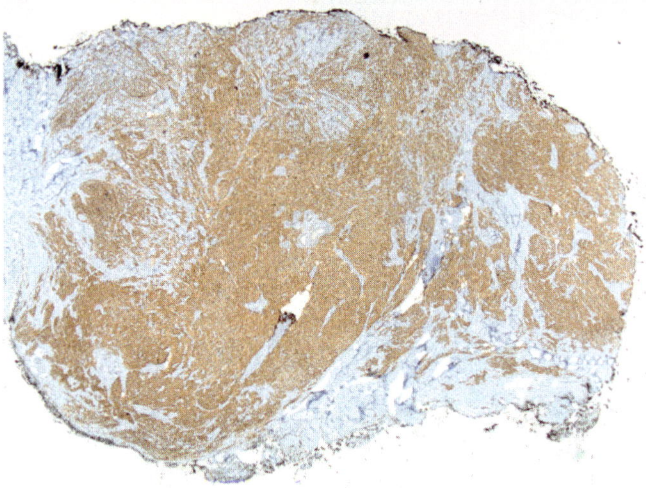

Figure 7.53 Clear cell sarcoma. Diffuse and strong Mart-1 expression by the tumor cells (X20).

predilection, occur commonly on the lower extremities, and less commonly the upper extremities and back.[144]

Histopathologically, PEComas are dermal tumors comprised of sheets, cords, and/or nests of epithelioid cells with clear to eosinophilic cytoplasm surrounded by vascular network. PEComas are positive for both melanocytic and smooth muscle markers with MiTF, HMB-45 and SMA being most sensitive (**Table 7.10**) (**Figures 7.54, 7.55, 7.56 and 7.57**).[144–146] Although they can express S100, MiTF, HMB-45, Melan-A, and NKIC3, PEComas are typically negative for Sox10.[144,145] In tumors with predominant spindle morphology strong SMA expression together with focal expression of melanocytic markers is noted. In tumors with epithelioid morphology, strong expression of MiTF and HMB45 is noted while SMA expression is only focally seen. Because of this unusual immunoprofile PEComas have been thought to derive from pluripotent stem cells that can express both a melanocytic as well as smooth muscle phenotype. A negative SMA expression does not exclude the diagnosis of PEComa. Most cutaneous PEComas behave in a benign fashion. In the few malignant cutaneous PEComas reported, the expression of HMB45, Melan-A, and SMA is still retained.[147,148] The dual expression of S100 and myogenic markers rules out a melanocytic neoplasm. The differential diagnosis also includes clear cell dermatofibroma, metastatic renal cell carcinoma, and alveolar soft part sarcoma. While alveolar soft part sarcoma can be positive for cathepsin K as noted in PEComa, they are invariably positive for TFE3.[149] PEComa expresses strong CD10 which can be mistaken for metastatic renal cell carcinoma.[150] The majority of PEComa express PRAME (89%).[48]

PEComa

- A rare mesenchyma neoplasm that has dual expression of melanocytic (S100, MiTF, HMB45, Melan-A) and myogenic (SMA, desmin) markers.
- It typically is negative for Sox10.

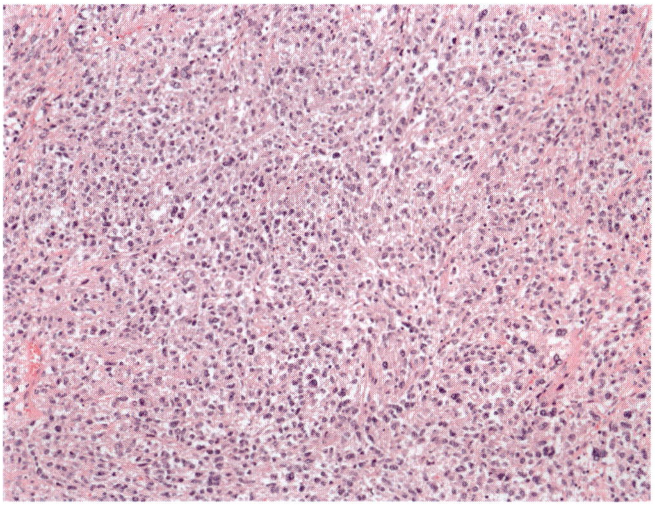

Figure 7.54 Perivascular epithelioid cell tumors (PEComa). Perivascular epithelioid neoplastic cells with eosinophilic cytoplasm are noted (X200).

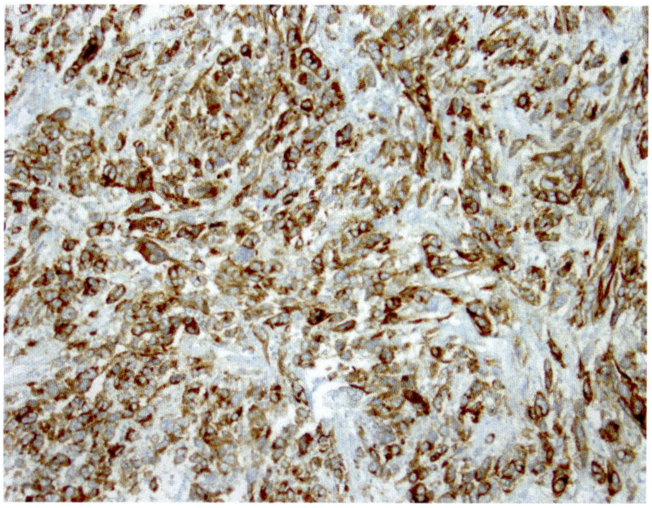

Figure 7.55 Perivascular epithelioid cell tumors (PEComa). Strong and diffuse HMB45 expression by the tumor cells (X200).

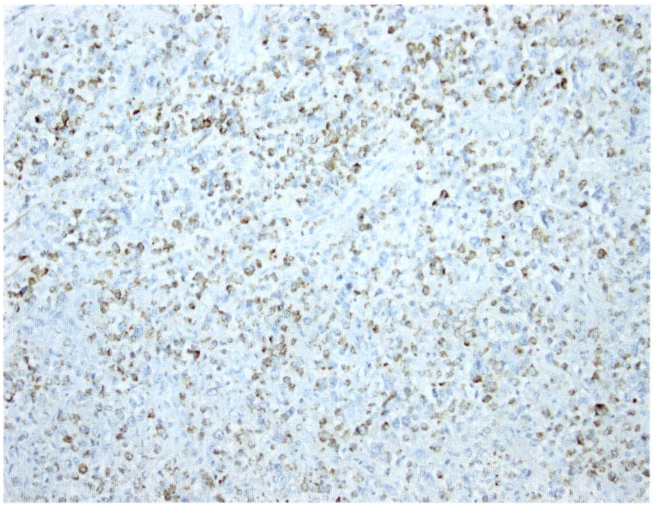

Figure 7.56 Perivascular epithelioid cell tumors (PEComa). The tumor cells are positive for desmin (X200).

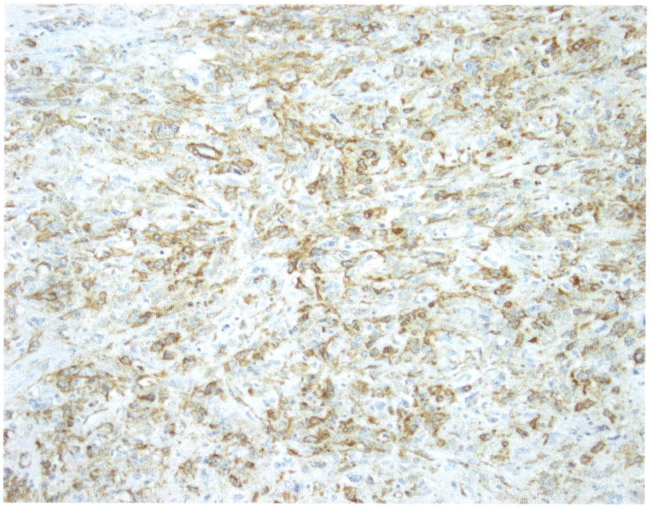

Figure 7.57 Perivascular epithelioid cell tumors (PEComa). Diffuse SMA expression (X200).

7.14 Melanoma versus Non-melanocytic Tumors

The differential diagnosis of a spindle cell melanoma and desmoplastic melanoma would include sarcomatoid carcinoma, atypical fibroxanthoma (AFX), and leiomyosarcoma. A helpful diagnostic immunohistochemical panel would include p40, keratin 903, keratin 5/6, Sox10, S100, and CD10 (**see Chapter 3**). p40, keratin 903 and keratin 5/6 would stain sarcomatoid carcinoma while Sox10 and S100 would stain a spindle cell melanoma. MiTF[151] and Melan-A[29] expression can be seen in AFX. Keratin AE1/AE3 and EMA expression have been reported in rare cases of AFX.[152] The differential diagnosis of melanoma would sometimes include Merkel cell carcinoma, lymphoproliferative disorders, myoepithelial neoplasms, epithelioid sarcoma and other sarcomas with round cell morphology such as those of the family of Ewing sarcoma/primitive neuroectodermal tumors (**see Chapter 9**). In the setting of a metastatic undifferentiated melanoma, often there is complete lack of expression of any melanocytic markers such as S100 and Sox10. Immunostains detecting specific mutations such as *BRAF*V600E and *NRAS*Q61 R have been reported to be potentially helpful since these mutations are commonly detected in melanomas and not non-melanocytic mimics.[153]

A number of soft tissue tumors can express melanocytic markers which include melanotic schwannoma.[154] Melanotic schwannomas exhibit diffuse Melan-A and HMB-45 expression, also Sox10 and S100. Epithelioid schwannomas are typically diffusely positive for Sox10 and S100, yet negative for Melan-A, MiTF, and HMB-45. Malignant peripheral nerve sheath tumor exhibits focal or patchy immunoreactivity for Sox10 or S100. Loss of H3K27me3 is highly specific for MPNST though not sensitive. Cutaneous syncytial myoepitheliomas are positive for S100.[154] Clear cell sarcoma of soft tissue expresses Sox10 and S100.

7.15 Case Studies

Case 7.1

Case history: 73-year-old man with a pigmented lesion on his right superior parietal scalp. A skin biopsy performed at the outside laboratory showed a malignant spindle cell tumor consistent with melanoma. A wide excision and sentinel lymph node biopsy were performed.

Description: A proliferation of atypical spindle cells is seen extending from the superficial dermis to the subcutaneous tissue (**Figures 7.58 and 7.59**). These spindle tumor cells exhibit strong nuclear Sox10 expression (**Figure 7.60**). These findings are consistent with a spindle cell melanoma. Similarly atypical spindle cells are seen within the capsular sinus of the sentinel lymph node (**Figure 7.61**). These cells are positive for S100 and Sox10 (**Figures 7.62 and 7.63**) and negative for Mart-1 (**Figure 7.64**), supportive of metastatic melanoma.

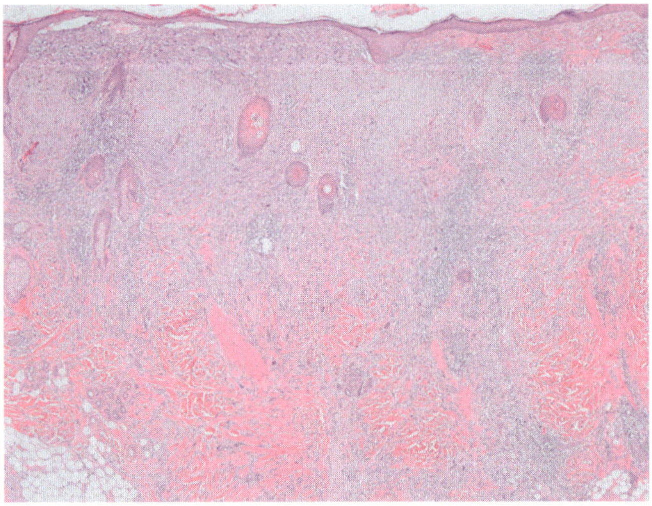

Figure 7.58 A proliferation of atypical spindle cells is seen extending from the superficial dermis to the subcutaneous tissue (X40).

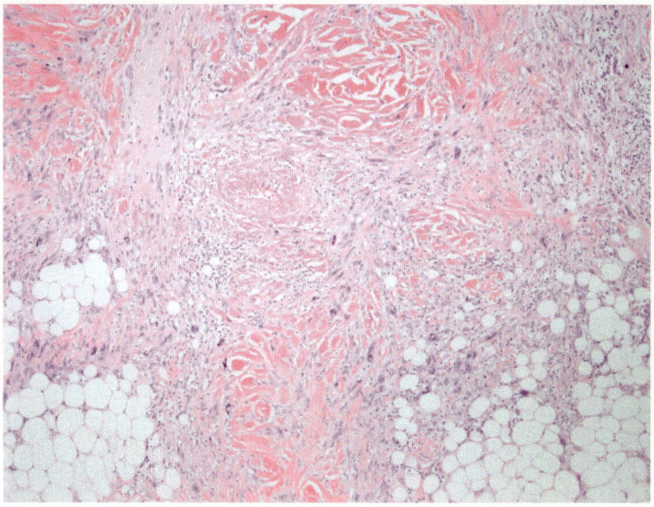

Figure 7.59 Some of the tumor cells are pleomorphic and hyperchromatic (X100).

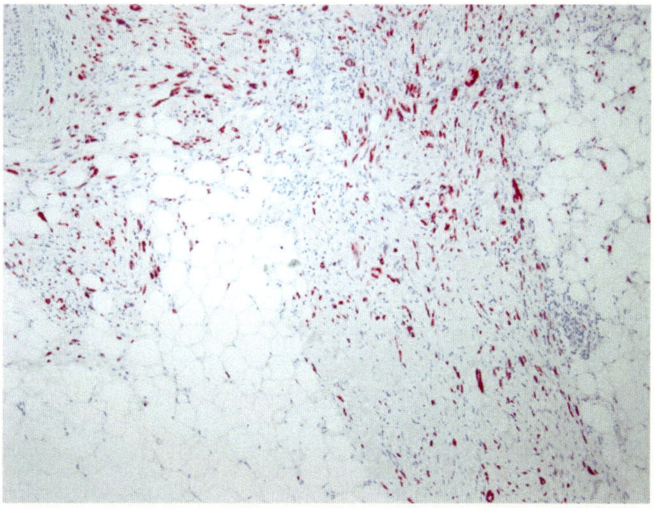

Figure 7.60 They exhibit strong nuclear Sox10 expression (X100).

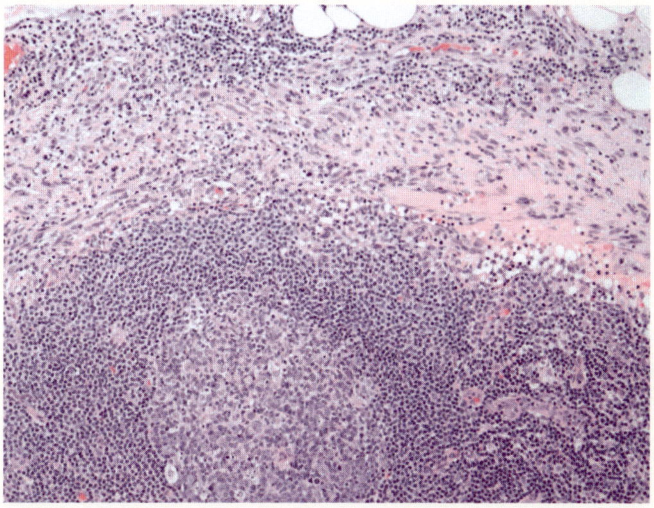

Figure 7.61 A similarly atypical and spindle proliferation is noted within the sinus of the sentinel lymph node (X200).

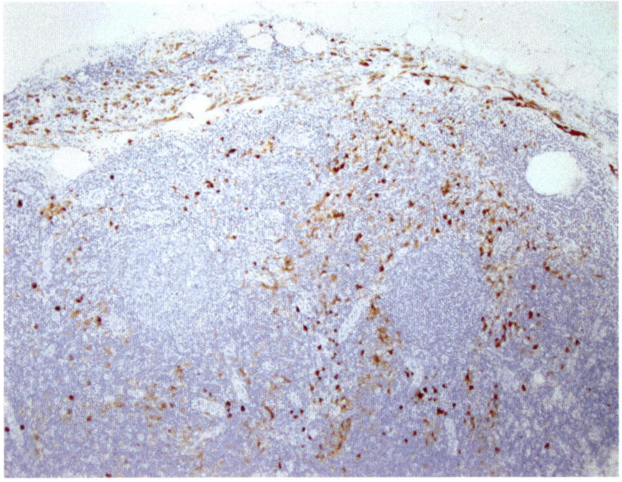

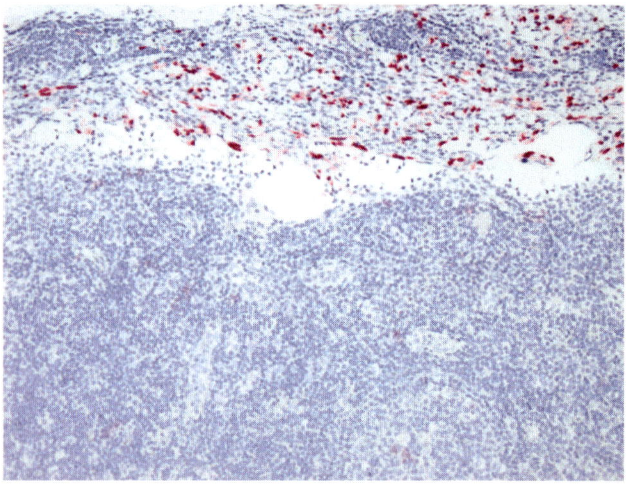

Figures 7.62 and 7.63 These tumor cells are strongly positive for S100 and Sox10 (X100, X200).

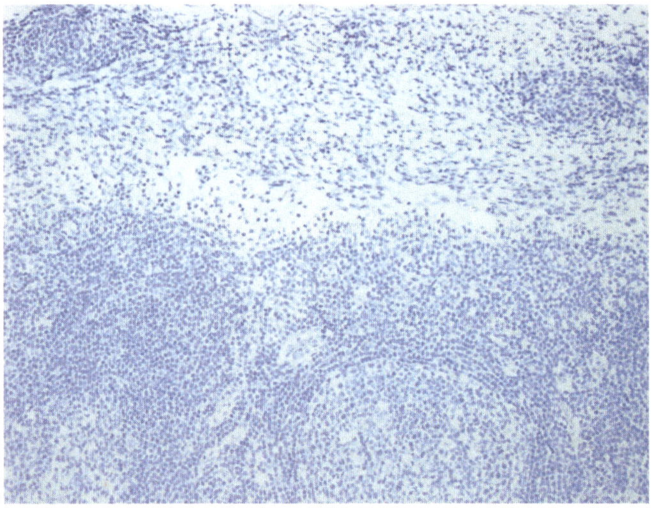

Figure 7.64 They are negative for Mart-1 (X200).

Diagnosis: Spindle cell melanoma with metastasis in sentinel lymph node.

Discussion: Sox10 and S100 are the best markers in the setting of spindle or desmoplastic melanoma since this subtype of melanoma is often negative for Melan-A, Mart-1, MiTF, and HMB-45. This case highlights the importance of including a sensitive although not specific melanocytic marker such as S100 in the sentinel lymph node protocol as well as in the initial work-up of any spindle cell neoplasm.

Case 7.2

Case history: A 77-year-old man presented with a nodule on his left temporoparietal scalp. The patient has immunosuppression following cardiac transplant.

Description: Histologic sections of an excisional biopsy show a diffuse proliferation of pleomorphic tumor cells in the dermis (**Figures 7.65 and 7.66**). The tumor exhibits focally cytoplasmic expression for high molecular weight keratin 903 (**Figure 7.67**) and diffuse nuclear positivity for p63 (**Figure 7.68**). The tumor cells are positive for CD10 and CD68. They are negative for S100, desmin, smooth muscle actin, cytokeratin cocktail, epithelial membrane antigen, and CD34.

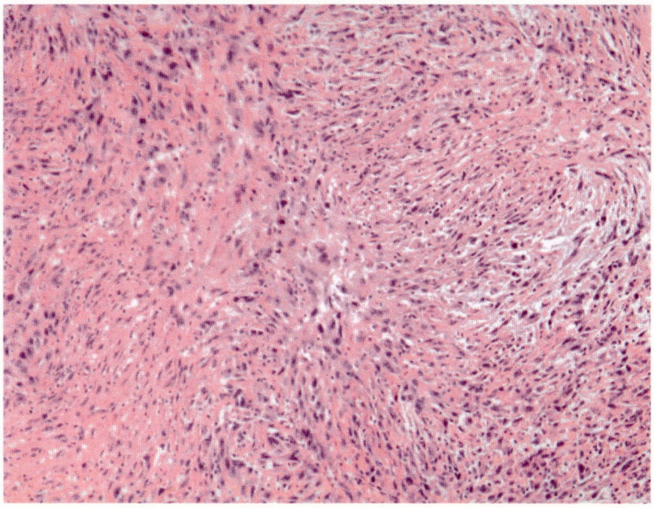

Figure 7.65 A diffuse proliferation of pleomorphic tumor cells (X100).

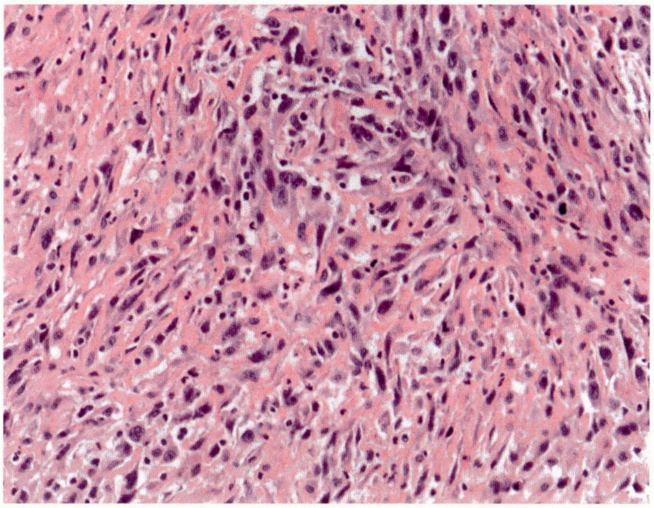

Figure 7.66 The nuclei are hyperchromatic and very irregular (X200).

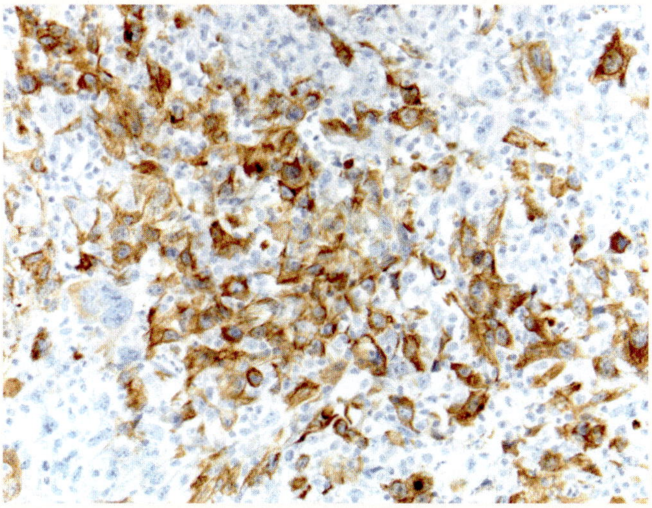

Figure 7.67 Expression of keratin 903 is focally seen (X200).

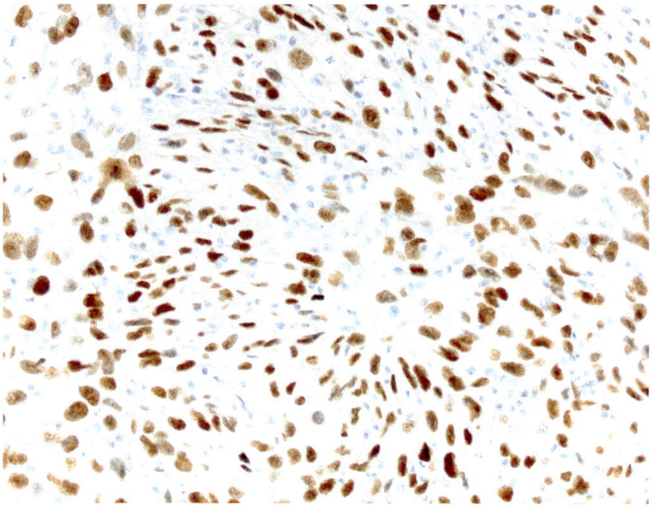

Figure 7.68 Diffuse p63 expression is noted (X200).

Diagnosis: Sarcomatoid carcinoma.

Discussion: The differential diagnosis of a dermal spindle cell neoplasm would include sarcomatoid carcinoma, spindle cell melanoma, leiomyosarcoma, and atypical fibroxanthoma. Recently p40 has been shown to be a helpful marker, in addition to p63, in labelling sarcomatoid squamous cell carcinoma;[155] since sarcomatoid SCC may show only focal positivity for high molecular weight cytokeratin. Sox10 and S100 would be sensitive markers for spindle cell melanoma. A smooth muscle tumor would express desmin in addition to smooth muscle actin. Only when epithelial, melanocytic, and myogenic markers are negative, AFX would be the diagnosis in the context of a positive CD10 expression. A helpful diagnostic immunohistochemical panel would include p40, keratin 903, keratin 5/6, Sox10, S100, and CD10.

Case 7.3

Case history: A 55-year-old man presented with a pigmented lesion on his left trunk.

Description: A proliferation of atypical epithelioid tumor cells is seen within the epidermis and in the dermis (**Figure 7.69**). At high magnification many of the tumor cells have clear cytoplasm (**Figures 7.70 and 7.71**). The tumor cells are positive for S100 supportive of the diagnosis of melanoma (**Figure 7.72**).

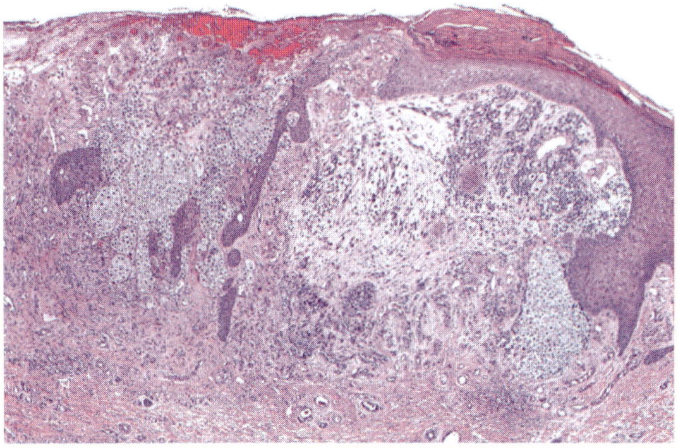

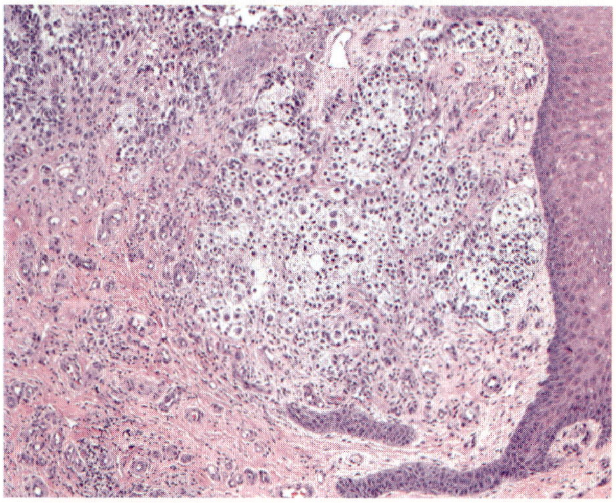

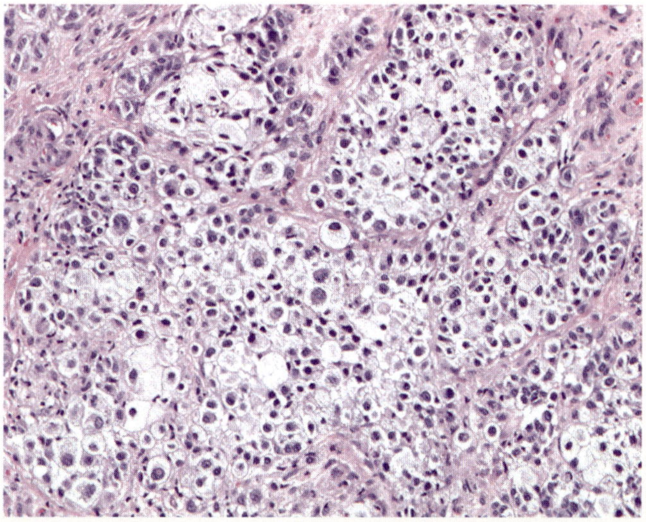

Figures 7.69, 7.70 and 7.71 A proliferation of tumor cells many with clear cytoplasm is seen within the epidermis and within the dermis (X40, X100, X200).

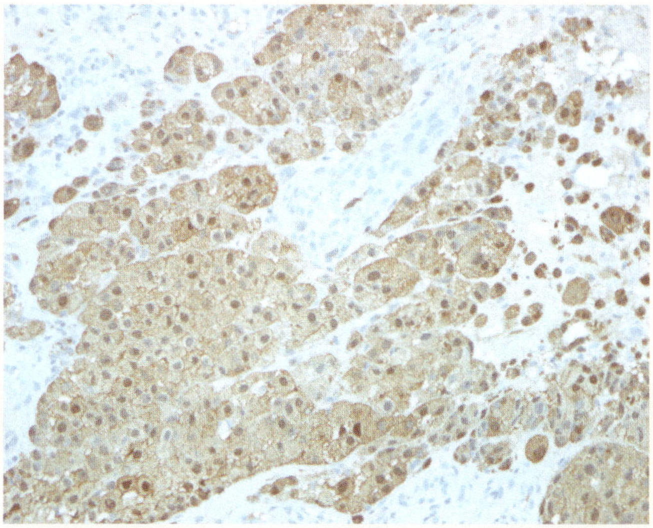

Figure 7.72 The tumor cells uniformly express S100 (X200).

Diagnosis: Balloon cell melanoma.

Discussion: Balloon cell melanoma is a rare variant of melanoma that presents as soft or firm skin nodule.[156] In order to render the diagnosis of primary balloon cell melanoma, one must identify the clear cell or balloon cell change in greater than 50% of the tumor cells.[157] Melanin pigment might not be prominent. Many cytoplasmic membrane-bound vacuoles with rare abnormal premelanosomes would be seen on ultrastructural examination.[156]

Case 7.4

Case history: A 71-year-old woman presented with a 3mm tan-brown macule on her left lower lip. The clinical differential diagnosis included lentigo versus nevus versus lentigo maligna.

Description: Histologic sections show a proliferation of atypical keratinocytes within the epidermis (**Figure 7.73**). Although more staining is noted on Melan-A immunostain (**Figure 7.74**), Sox10 immunostain shows only a mildly increased number of melanocytes at the dermal epidermal junction (**Figure 7.75**).

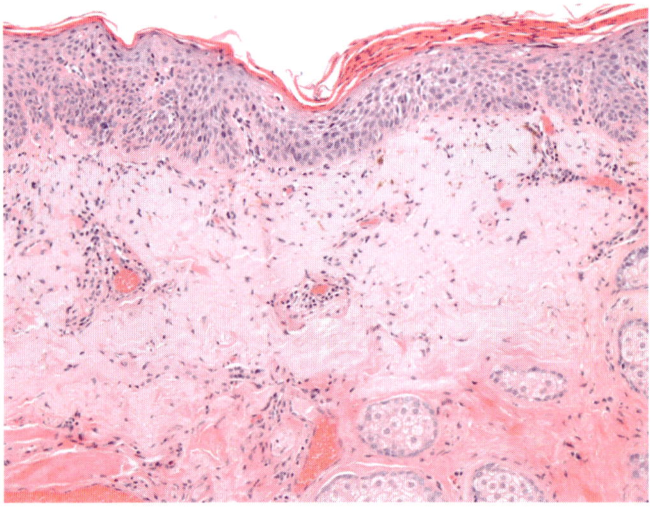

Figure 7.73 A proliferation of atypical keratinocytes is seen within the epidermis and there is marked underlying dermal solar elastosis (X200).

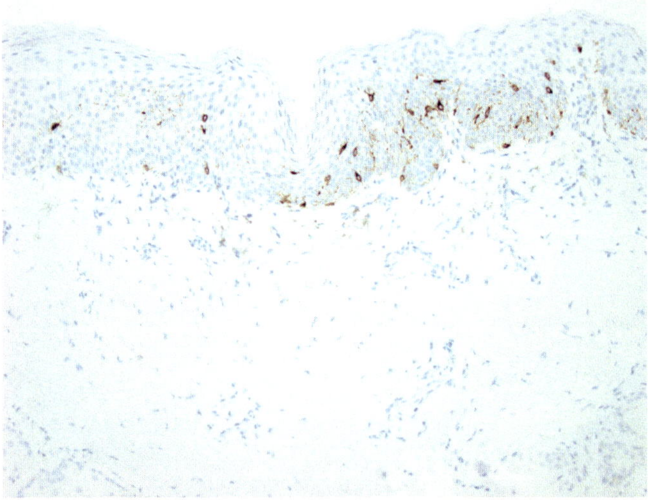

Figure 7.74 Melan A immunostain highlights a notable number of cells within the epidermis (X200).

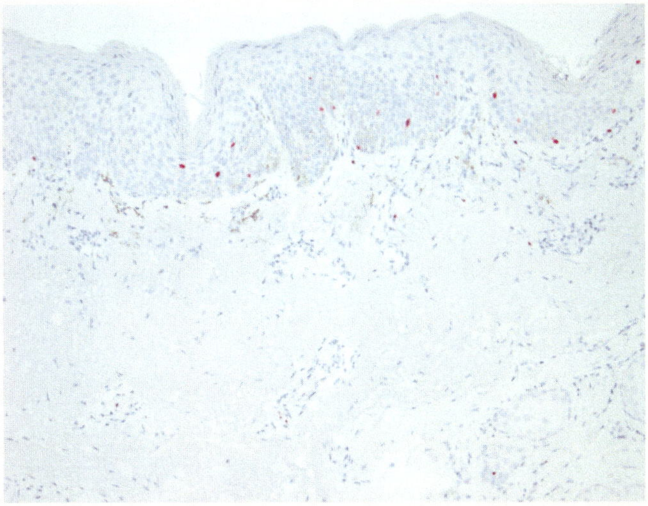

Figure 7.75 Sox10 immunostain demonstrates only mild junctional melanocytic hyperplasia (X200).

Diagnosis: Pigmented actinic keratosis.

Discussion: It has been reported that Melan-A and Mart-1 stains can label the pigmented keratinocytes in the setting of pigmented actinic keratosis or solar lentigo.[59] This can result in overdiagnosing the lesion as lentigo maligna or melanoma *in situ*. Therefore, in assessing the melanocytic proliferation at the dermal epidermal junction, especially in margin evaluation, immunostains with nuclear expression such as MiTF and Sox10 are superior to cytoplasmic stains in quantifying the density of melanocytes.

Case 7.5

Case history: A 49-year-old man presented with a right posterior shoulder lesion.

Description: A diffuse proliferation of atypical melanocytes without maturation is seen in the dermis (**Figure 7.76**). The tumor cells are deceptively uniform (**Figure 7.77**). Rare dermal mitotic figure is identified (**Figure 7.78**). Diffuse Melan-A, HMB-45 (**Figure 7.79**), and PRAME (**Figure 7.80**) staining are seen (**Figures 7.79 and 7.80**). Ki67 proliferation index is focally increased in the dermal component (**Figure 7.81**). BAP1 and p16 staining is retained.

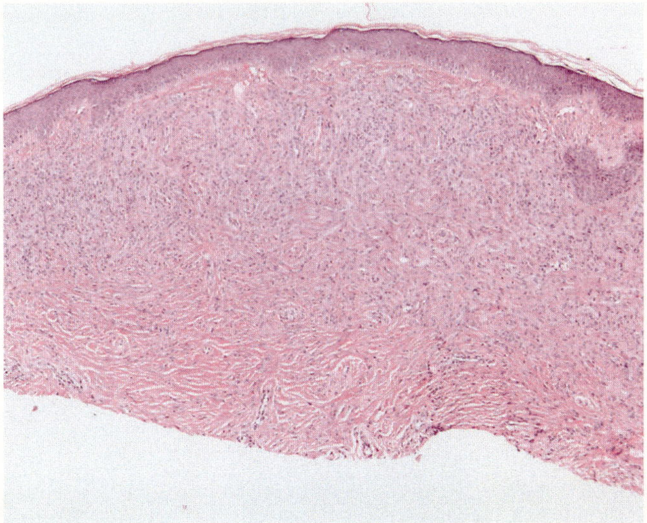

Figure 7.76 A diffuse proliferation of atypical melanocytes without maturation is seen in the dermis (X100).

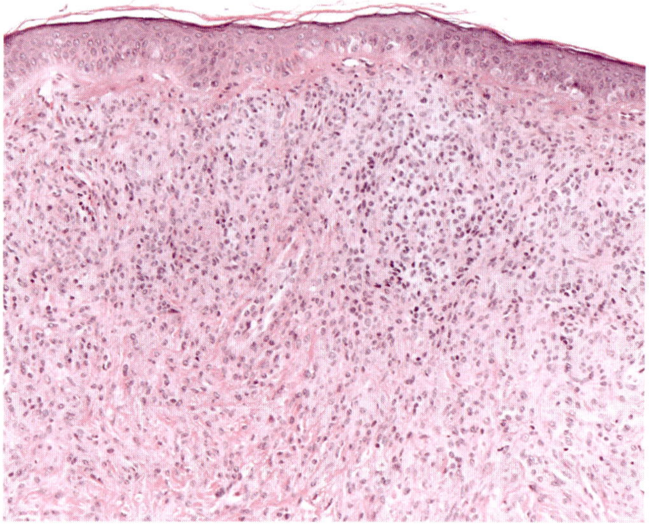

Figure 7.77 The tumor cells are deceptively uniform (X200).

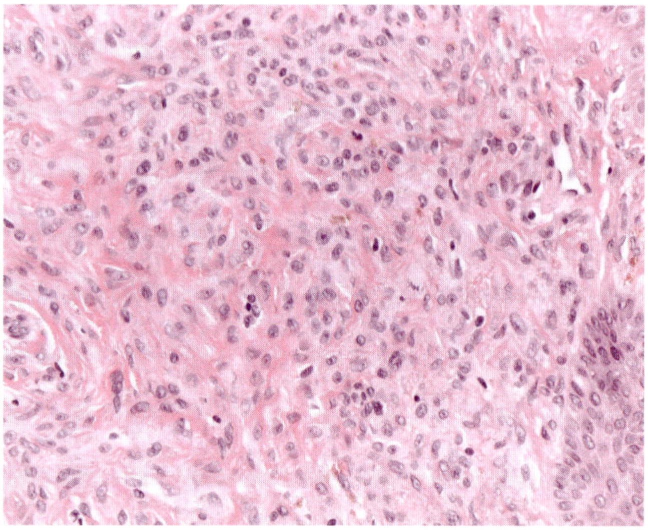

Figure 7.78 Dermal mitotic figure is noted (X400).

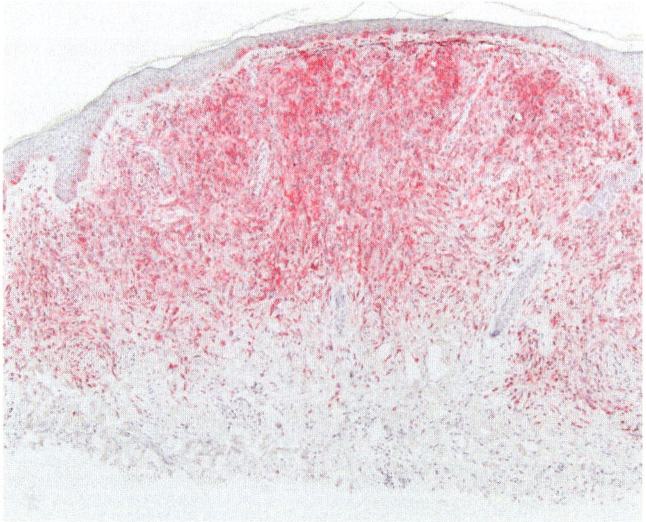

Figure 7.79 Diffuse HMB-45 staining is seen (X100).

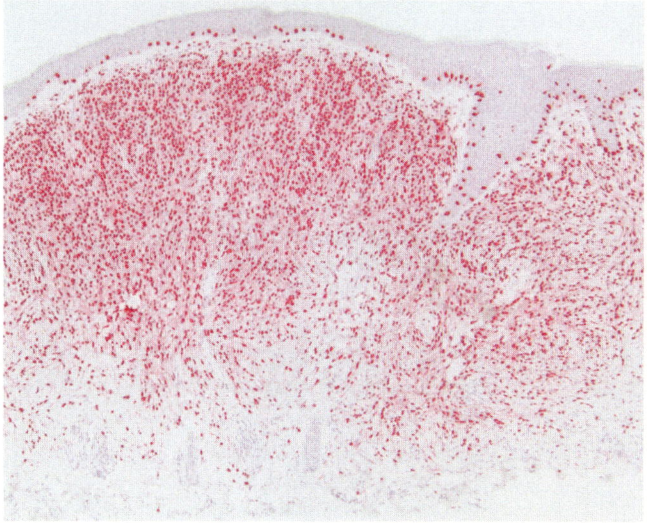

Figure 7.80 Diffuse PRAME staining (X100).

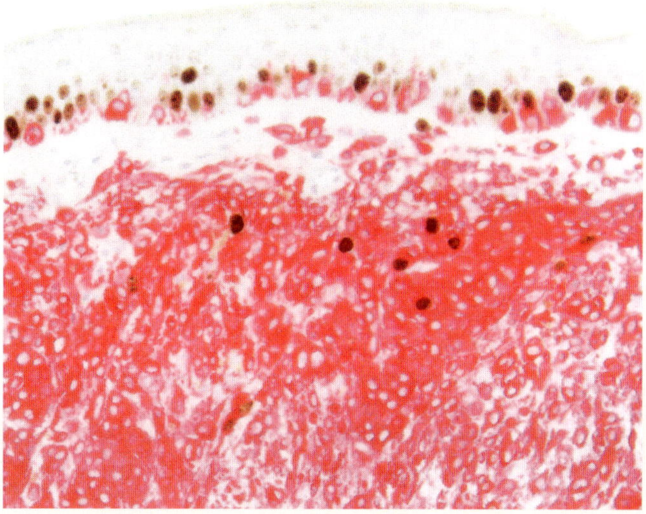

Figure 7.81 Focal increased KI67 proliferation index (X400).

Diagnosis: Nevoid melanoma.

Discussion: A proliferation of uniform melanocytes is a characteristic of nevoid melanoma. Mitoses are rare. Hyperchromatic and atypical melanocytes are seen at the advancing edge. Ancillary studies including diffuse HMB-45 expression and increased dermal Ki-67 proliferation index can be helpful diagnostic clues.

References

1. Timar J, Udvarhelyi N, Banfalvi T, Gilde K, Orosz Z. Accuracy of the determination of S100B protein expression in malignant melanoma using polyclonal or monoclonal antibodies. *Histopathology* 2004; **44**: 180–4.
2. Anstey A, Cerio R, Ramnarain N, Orchard G, Smith N, Jones EW. Desmoplastic malignant melanoma. an immunocytochemical study of 25 cases. *Am J Dermatopathol* 1994; **16**: 14–22.
3. Aung PP, Sarlomo-Rikala M, Lasota J, Lai JP, Wang ZF, Miettinen M. KBA62 and PNL2: 2 new melanoma markers-immunohistochemical analysis of 1563 tumors including metastatic, desmoplastic, and mucosal melanomas and their mimics. *Am J Surg Pathol* 2012; **36**: 265–72.
4. Busam KJ, Iversen K, Coplan KC, Jungbluth AA. Analysis of microphthalmia transcription factor expression in normal tissues and tumors, and comparison of its expression with S-100 protein, gp100, and tyrosinase in desmoplastic melanoma. *Am J Surg Pathol* 2001; **25**: 197–204.
5. Cohen-Knafo E, al Saati T, Aziza J, et al. Production and characterization of an antimelanoma monoclonal antibody KBA.62 using a new melanoma cell line reactive on paraffin wax embedded sections. *J Clin Pathol* 1995; **48**: 826–31.
6. Ferenczi K, Lastra RR, Farkas T, et al. MUM-1 expression differentiates tumors in the PEComa family from

clear cell sarcoma and melanoma. *Int J Surg Pathol* 2012; **20**: 29–36.

7. Koch MB, Shih IM, Weiss SW, Folpe AL. Microphthalmia transcription factor and melnoma cell adhesion molecule expression distinguish desmoplastic/spindle cell melanoma from morphologic mimics. *Am J Surg Pathol* 2001; **25**: 58–64.
8. Mangini J, Li N, Bhawan J. Immunohistochemical markers of melanocytic lesions: a review of their diagnostic usefulness. *Am J Dermatopathol* 2002; **24**: 270–81.
9. Miettinen M, Fernandez M, Franssila K, Gatalica Z, Lasota J, Sarlomo-Rikala M. Microphthalmia transcription factor in the immunohistochemical diagnosis of metastatic melanoma: comparison with four other melanoma markers. *Am J Surg Pathol* 2001; **25**: 205–11.
10. Nonaka D, Chiriboga L, Rubin BP. Differential expression of S100 protein subtypes in malignant melanoma, and benign and malignant peripheral nerve sheath tumors. *J Cutan Pathol* 2008; **35**: 1014–19.
11. Orchard GE. Comparison of immunohistochemical labelling of melanocyte differentiation antibodies melan-A, tyrosinase and HMB45 with NKIC3 and S100 protein in the evaluation of benign and malignant melanoma. *Histochem J* 2000; **32**: 475–81.
12. Pages C, Rochaix P, al Saati T, et al. KBA.62: a useful marker for primary and metastatic melanomas. *Hum Pathol* 2008; **39**: 1136–42.
13. Plaza JA, Suster D, Perez-Montiel D. Expression of immunohistochemical markers in primary and metastatic malignant melanoma: a comparative study in 70 patients using a tissue microarray technique. *Appl Immunohistochem Mol Morphol* 2007; **15**: 421–5.
14. Rochaix P, Lacroiz-Triki M, Lamant L, et al. PNL2, a new monoclonal antibody directed against a fixative-resistant melanocyte antigen. *Mod Pathol* 2003; **16**: 481–90.
15. Sundram U, Harvell JD, Rouse RV, Natkunam Y. Expression of the B-cell proliferation marker MUM1 by melanocytic lesions and comparison with S100, gp100 (HMB45), and MelanA. *Mod Pathol* 2003; **16**: 802–10.
16. Shih IM, Nesbit M, Herlyn M, Kurman RJ. A new Mel-CAM (CD146)-specific monoclonal antibody, MN-4, on paraffin-embedded tissue. *Mod Pathol* 1998; **11**: 1098–106.
17. Shin J, Vincent JG, Cuda JD, et al. Sox10 is expressed in primary melanocytic neoplasms of various histologies but not in fibrohistiocytic proliferations and histiocytoses. *J Am Acad Dermatol* 2012; **67**: 717–26.
18. Wick MR, Swanson PE, Rocamora A. Recognition of malignant melanoma by monoclonal antibody HMB-45: an immunohistochemical study of 200 paraffin-embedded cutaneous tumors. *J Cutan Pathol* 1988; **15**: 201–7.
19. Zubovits J, Buzney E, Yu L, Duncan LM. HMB-45, S-100, NK1/C3, and MART-1 in metastatic melanoma. *Hum Pathol* 2004; **35**: 217–23.
20. Skelton 3rd HG, Smith KJ, Barrett TL, Lupton GP, Graham JH. HMB-45 staining in benign and malignant melanocytic lesions: a reflection of cellular activation. *Am J Dermatopathol* 1991; **13**: 543–50.
21. Romano RC, Carter JM, Folpe AL. Aberrant intermediate filament and synaptophysin expression is a frequent event in malignant melanoma: an immunohistochemical study of 73 cases. *Mod Pathol* 2015; **28**: 1033–42.
22. Ben-Izhak O, Stark P, Levy R, et al. Epithelial markers in malignant melanoma: a study of primary lesions and their metastases. *Am J Dermatopathol* 1994; **16**: 241–6.
23. Sanders DS, Evans AT, Allen CA, et al. Classification of CEA-related positivity in primary and metastatic malignant melanoma. *J Pathol* 1994; **172**: 343–8.
24. Carlson JA, Dickersin GR, Sober AJ, Barnhill RL. Desmoplastic neurotrophic melanoma. *Cancer* 1995; **75**: 478–94.
25. Bishop PW, Menasce LP, Yates AJ, Win NA, Banerjee SS. An immunophenotypic survey of malignant melanomas. *Histopathology* 1993; **23**: 159–66.
26. Shah IA, Gani OS, Wheler L. Comparative immunoreactivity of CD68 and HMB-45 in malignant melanoma, neural tumors and nevi. *Pathol Res Pract* 1997; **193**: 497–502.
27. Donato R, Sorci G, Riuzzi F, et al. S100B's double life: intracellular regulator and extracellular signal. *Biochim Biophys Acta* 2009; **1793**: 1008–22.
28. Ohsie SJ, Sarantopoulos GP, Cochran AJ, et al. Immunohistochemical characteristics of melanoma. *J Cutan Pathol* 2008; **35**: 433–44.
29. Thum C, Hollowood K, Birch J, Goodlad JR, Brenn T. Aberrant Melan-A expression in atypical fibroxanthoma and undifferentiated pleomorphic sarcoma of the skin. *J Cutan Pathol* 2011; **38**: 954–60.
30. Miettinen M, McCue PA, Sariomo-Rikala M, et al. Sox-10 – a marker for not only schwannian and melanocytic neoplasms but also myoepithelial cell tumors of soft tissue: a systematic analysis of 5134 tumors. *Am J Surg Pathol* 2015; **39**: 826–35.
31. Lee ZH, Hou L, Moellmann G, et al. Characterization and subcellular localization of human Pmel 17/silver, a 110-kDa (pre)melanosomal membrane protein associated with 5,6-dihydroxyindole-2-carboxylic acid (DHICA) converting activity. *J Invest Dermatol* 1996; **106**: 605–10.
32. Nonaka D, Chiriboga L, Rubin BP. Sox10: a pan-schwannian and melanocytic marker. *Am J Surg Pathol* 2008; **32**: 1291–8.
33. Busam KJ, Kucukgol D, Sato E, Frosina D, Teruya-Feldstein J, Jungbluth AA. Immunohistochemical analysis of novel monoclonal antibody PNL2 and comparison with other melanocyte differentiation markers. *Am J Surg Pathol* 2005; **29**: 400–6.
34. Banerjee SS, Harris M. Morphological and immunophenotypic variations in malignant melanoma. *Histopathology* 2000; **36**: 387–402.
35. Petitt M, Allison A, Shimoni T, Uchida T, Raimer S, Kelly B. Lymphatic invasion detected by D2-40/S100 dual immunohistochemistry does not predict sentinel lymph node status in melanoma. *J Am Acad Dermatol* 2009; **61**: 819–28.
36. Gerdes J, Lemke H, Baisch H, Wacker HH, Schwab U, Stein H. Cell cycle analysis of a cell proliferation-associated human nuclear antigen defined by the monoclonal antibody Ki-67. *J Immunol* 1984; **133**: 1710–15.
37. Ikenberg K, Pfaltz M, Rakozy C, Kempf W. Immunohistochemical dual staining as an adjunct in assessment of mitotic activity in melanoma. *J Cutan Pathol* 2012; **39**: 324–30.
38. Saleem A, Narala S, Raghavan SS. Immunohistochemistry in melanocytic lesions: updates with a practical review for pathologists. *Semin Diagn Pathol* 2022; **39**: 239–247.
39. Karamchandani JR, Nielsen TO, van de Rijn M, West RB. Sox10 and S100 in the diagnosis of soft-tissue neoplasms. *Appl Immunohistochem Mol Morphol* 2012; **20**: 445–50.

40. Siarov J, Neittaanmäki N, Mölne J, Gillstedt M, Paoli J. Digital quantification of melanocytic density in resection margins of lentigo maligna using SOX10 versus hematoxylin-eosin staining. *Am J Dermatopathol* 2021; **43**: 273–7.
41. Behrens EL, Boothe W, D'Silva N, Walterscheid B, Watkins P, Tarbox M. SOX-10 staining in dermal scars. *J Cutan Pathol* 2019; **46**: 579–85.
42. Lezcano C, Jungbluth AA, Nehal KS, Hollmann TJ, Busam KJ. PRAME expression in melanocytic tumors. *Am J Surg Pathol* 2018; **42**: 1456–65.
43. Chen YP, Zhang WW, Qiu YT, Ke LF, Chen H, Chen G. PRAME is a useful marker for the differential diagnosis of melanocytic tumours and histological mimics. *Histopathology* 2023; **82**: 285–95.
44. Kunc M, Żemierowska N, Skowronek F, Biernat W. Diagnostic test accuracy meta-analysis of PRAME in distinguishing primary cutaneous melanomas from benign melanocytic lesions. *Histopathology* 2023; **83**: 3–14.
45. Rothrock AT, Torres-Cabala CA, Milton DR, et al. Diagnostic utility of PRAME expression by immunohistochemistry in subungual and non-subungual acral melanocytic lesions. *J Cutan Pathol* 2022; **49**: 859–67.
46. Hrycaj SM, Szczepanski JM, Zhao L, et al. PRAME expression in spindle cell melanoma, malignant peripheral nerve sheath tumour, and other cutaneous sarcomatoid neoplasms: a comparative analysis. *Histopathology* 2022; **81**: 818–25.
47. Koh SS, Lau SK, Scapa JV, Cassarino DS. PRAME immunohistochemistry of spitzoid neoplasms. *J Cutan Pathol* 2022; **49**: 709–16.
48. Kline N, Menge TD, Hrycaj SM, et al. PRAME expression in challenging dermal melanocytic neoplasms and soft tissue tumors with melanocytic differentiation. *Am J Dermatopathol* 2022; **44**: 404–10.
49. Scheurleer WFJ, Braunius WW, Tijink BM, et al. PRAME staining in sinonasal mucosal melanoma: a single-center experience. *Head Neck Pathol* 2023; **17**: 401–8.
50. Schmitt TA, Lee JC, Martinka M, Ko KYC. PRAME immunohistochemistry is useful in differentiating oral melanomas from nevi and melanotic macules. *J Cutan Pathol* 2023; **50**: 275–8.
51. Šekoranja D, Hawlina G, Pižem J. PRAME expression in melanocytic lesions of the conjunctiva. *Histopathology* 2021; **79**: 989–96.
52. Hornick JL, Plaza JA, Mentzel T, Gru AA, Brenn T. PRAME expression is a useful tool in the diagnosis of primary and metastatic dedifferentiated and undifferentiated melanoma. *Am J Surg Pathol* 2023; **47**: 1390–7.
53. Santandrea G, Valli R, Zanetti E, Ragazzi M, et al. Comparative analysis of PRAME expression in 127 acral and nail melanocytic lesions. *Am J Surg Pathol* 2022; **46**: 579–90.
54. Cammareri C, Beltzung F, Michal M, et al. PRAME immunohistochemistry in soft tissue tumors and mimics: a study of 350 cases highlighting its imperfect specificity but potentially useful diagnostic applications. *Virchows Arch* 2023; **483**: 145–56.
55. Elsensohn A, Hanson J, Ferringer T. Preferentially expressed antigen in melanoma expression in nonmelanoma skin cancers and melanocytes in surrounding skin. *J Cutan Pathol* 2021; **48**: 1150–5.
56. Kaczorowski M, Chłopek M, Kruczak A, Ryś J, Lasota J, Miettinen M. PRAME expression in cancer. A systematic immunohistochemical study of >5800 epithelial and nonepithelial tumors. *Am J Surg Pathol* 2022; **46**: 1467–76.
57. Cesinaro AM, Piana S, Paganelli A, Pedroni G, Santandrea G, Maiorana A. PRAME expression in cellular neurothekeoma: a study of 11 cases. *J Cutan Pathol* 2022; **49**: 338–42.
58. Hendi A, Wada DA, Jacobs MA, et al. Melanocytes in nonlesional sun-exposed skin: a multicenter comparative study. *J Am Acad Dermatol* 2011; **65**: 1186–93.
59. Beltraminelli H, Shabrawi-Caelen LE, Kerl H, Cerroni L. Melan-a-positive "pseudomelanocytic nests": a pitfall in the histopathologic and immunohistochemical diagnosis of pigmented lesions on sun-damages skin. *Am J Dermatopathol* 2009; **31**: 305–8.
60. Yan S, Brennick JB. False-positive rate of the immunoperoxidase stains for MART1/MelanA in lymph nodes. *Am J Surg Pathol* 2004; **28**: 596–600.
61. Buonaccorsi JN, Prieto VG, Torres-Cabala C, Suster S, Plaza JA. Diagnostic utility and comparative immunohistochemical analysis of MiTF and Sox10 to distinguish melanoma in situ and actinic keratosis: a clinicopathological and immunohistochemical study of 70 cases. *Am J Dermatopathol* 2014; **36**: 124–30.
62. Gradecki SE, Valdes-Rodriguez R, Wick MR, Gru AA. PRAME immunohistochemistry as an adjunct for diagnosis and histological margin assessment in lentigo maligna. *Histopathology* 2021; **78**: 1000–8.
63. Roy SF, Panse G, McNiff JM. PRAME immunohistochemistry can distinguish melanocytic pseudonests of lichenoid reactions from melanoma in situ. *J Cutan Pathol* 2023; **50**: 450–4.
64. Ramos-Herberth FI, Karamchandani J, Kim J, Dadras SS. Sox10 immunostaining distinguishes desmoplastic melanoma from excision scar. *J Cutan Pathol* 2010; **37**: 944–52.
65. Harvell JD, Bastian BC, LeBoit PE. Persistent (recurrent) Spitz nevi: a histopathologic, immunohistochemical, and molecular pathologic study of 22 cases. *Am J Surg Pathol* 2002; **26**: 654–61.
66. Wood WS, Tron VA. Analysis of HMB-45 immunoreactivity in common and cellular blue nevi. *J Cutan Pathol* 1991; **18**: 261–3.
67. Prieto VG, Shea CR. Use of immunohistochemistry in melanocytic lesions. *J Cutan Pathol* 2008; **35**: 1–10.
68. Cosgarea I, Griewank KG, Ungureanu L, Tamayo A, Siepmann T. Deep penetrating nevus and borderline-deep penetrating nevus: a literature review. *Front Oncol* 2020; **10**: 837. doi: 10.3389/fonc.2020.00837.
69. World Health Organization. Elder DE, Massi D, Scoyler RA, Williemze R, eds. WHO Classification of Skin Tumors. 4th ed. Lyon, France: IARC, 2018.
70. Yeh I, Lang UE, Durieux E, et al. Combined activation of MAP kinase pathway and β-catenin signaling cause deep penetrating nevi. *Nat Commun* 2017; **8**: 644. doi: 10.1038/s41467-017-00758-3.
71. Vanderbeck K, Rothrock AT, Cho WC, et al. PRAME and LEF1 in combined deep penetrating nevus and combined blue nevus: utility and pitfalls. *Am J Dermatopathol* 2023; **45**: 549–56.
72. Magro CM, Abraham RM, Guo R, et al. Deep penetrating nevus-like borderline tumors: a unique subset of ambiguous melanocytic tumors with malignant potential and normal cytogenetics. *Eur J Dermatol* 2014; **24**: 594–602.
73. Ebbelaar CF, Schrader AMR, van Dijk M, et al. MOLecular Evaluation of Melanocytic Ambiguous Tumors (MOLEMAT) investigators: towards diagnostic criteria for malignant deep penetrating melanocytic tumors using single nucleotide polymorphism array and next-generation sequencing. *Mod Pathol* 2022; **35**: 1110–20.

74. Raghavan SS, Saleem A, Wang JY, Rieger KE, Brown RA, Novoa RA. Diagnostic utility of LEF1 immunohistochemistry in differentiating deep penetrating nevi from histologic mimics. *Am J Surg Pathol* 2020; **44**: 1413–18.
75. de la Fouchardière A, Caillot C, Jacquemus J, et al. β-Catenin nuclear expression discriminates deep penetrating nevi from other cutaneous melanocytic tumors. *Virchows Arch* 2019; **474**: 539–50.
76. Zembowicz A, Carney JA, Mihm MC. Pigmented epithelioid melanocytoma: a low-grade melanocytic tumor with metastatic potential indistinguishable from animal-type melanoma and epithelioid blue nevus. *Am J Surg Pathol* 2004; **28**: 31–40.
77. Cohen JN, Joseph NM, North JP, Onodera C, Zembowicz A, LeBoit PE. Genomic analysis of pigmented epithelioid melanocytomas reveals recurrent alterations in PRKAR1A, and PRKCA genes. *Am J Surg Pathol* 2017; **41**: 1333–46.
78. de la Fouchardiere A, Tirode F, Castillo C, et al. Attempting to solve the pigmented epithelioid melanocytoma (PEM) conundrum: PRKAR1A inactivation can occur in different genetic backgrounds (common, blue, and Spitz subgroups) with variation in their clinicopathologic characteristics. *Am J Surg Pathol* 2022; **46**: 1106–15.
79. Isales MC, Mohan LS, Quan VL, et al. Distinct genomic patterns in pigmented epithelioid melanocytoma: a molecular and histologic analysis of 16 cases. *Am J Surg Pathol* 2019; **43**: 480–8.
80. Zembowicz A, Knoepp SM, Bei T, et al. Loss of expression of protein kinase a regulatory subunit 1alpha in pigmented epithelioid melanocytoma but not in melanoma or other melanocytic lesions. *Am J Surg Pathol* 2007; **31**: 1764–75.
81. Goto K, Pissaloux D, Paindavoine S, Tirode F, de la Fouchardière A. CYSLTR2-mutant cutaneous melanocytic neoplasms frequently simulate "pigmented epithelioid melanocytoma," expanding the morphologic spectrum of blue tumors: a clinicopathologic study of 7 cases. *Am J Surg Pathol* 2019; **43**: 1368–76.
82. Williams EA, Shah N, Danziger N, et al. Clinical, histopathologic, and molecular profiles of PRKAR1A-inactivated melanocytic neoplasms. *J Am Acad Dermatol* 2021; **84**: 1069–71.
83. Wiesner T, Obenauf AC, Murali R, et al. Germline mutations in BAP1 predispose to melanocytic tumors. *Nat Genet* 2011; **43**: 1018–21.
84. Aung PP, Nagarajan P, Tetzlaff MT, et al. Melanoma with loss of BAP1 expression in patients with no family history of BAP1-associated cancer susceptibility syndrome: a case series. *Am J Dermatopathol* 2019; **41**: 167–79.
85. Piris A, Mihm MC Jr, Hoang MP. BAP1 and BRAFV600E expression in benign and malignant melanocytic proliferations. *Hum Pathol* 2015; **46**: 239–45.
86. Donati M, Martinek P, Steiner P, et al. Novel insights into the BAP1-inactivated melanocytic tumor. *Mod Pathol* 2022; **35**: 664–75.
87. Garfield EM, Walton KE, Quan VL, et al. Histomorphologic spectrum of germline-related and sporadic BAP1-inactivated melanocytic tumors. *J Am Acad Dermatol* 2018; **79**: 525–34.
88. Gammon B, Traczyk TN, Gerami P. Clumped perinuclear BAP1 expression is a frequent finding in sporadic epithelioid Spitz tumors. *J Cutan Pathol* 2013; **40**: 538–42.
89. de la Fourchardière A, Pissaloux D, Tirode F, Hanna J. Clear cell tumor with melanocytic differentiation and MITF-CREM translocation: a novel entity similar to clear cell sarcoma. *Virchows Arch* 2021; **479**: 841–6.
90. Zucman J, Delattre O, Desmaze C, et al. EWS and ATF-1 gene fusion induced by t(12;22) translocation in malignant melanoma of soft parts. *Nat Genet* 1993; **4**: 341–5.
91. Hanna J, Ko JS, Billings SD, Boivin F, et al. Cutaneous melanocytic tumor with CRTC1::TRIM11 translocation: an emerging entity analyzed in a series of 41 Cases. *Am J Surg Pathol* 2022; **46**: 1457–66.
92. Argani P, Aulmann S, Illei PB, et al. A distinctive subset of PEComas harbors TFE3 gene fusions. *Am J Surg Pathol* 2010; **34**: 1395–406.
93. Yang L, Yin Z, Wei J, et al. Cutaneous melanocytic tumour with CRTC1::TRIM11 fusion in a case with recurrent local lymph node and distant pulmonary metastases at early stage: aggressive rather than indolent? *Histopathology* 2023; **82**: 368–71.
94. Kapur P, Selim MA, Roy LC, Yegappan M, Weinberg AG, Hoang MP. Spitz nevi and atypical Spitz nevi/tumors: a histologic and immunohistochemical analysis. *Mod Pathol* 2005; **18**: 197–204.
95. Nasr MR, El-Zammar O. Comparison of PHH3, Ki-67, and survivin immunoreactivity in benign and malignant melanocytic lesions. *Am J Dermatopathol* 2008; **30**: 117–22.
96. Phadke PA, Rakheja D, Le LP, et al. Proliferative nodules arising within congenital melanocytic nevi: a histologic, immunohistochemical, and molecular analyses of 43 cases. *Am J Surg Pathol* 2011; **35**: 656–69.
97. Herron MD, Vanderhooft SL, Smock K, Zhou H, Leachman SA, Coffin C. Proliferative nodules in congenital melanocytic nevi: a clinicopathologic and immunohistochemical analysis. *Am J Surg Pathol* 2004; **28**: 1017–25.
98. Hung T, Piris A, Lobo A, et al. Sentinel lymph node metastasis is not predictive of poor outcome in patients with problematic spitzoid melanocytic tumors. *Hum Pathol* 2013; **44**: 87–94.
99. Quan VL, Zhang B, Zhang Y, et al. Integrating next generation sequencing with morphology improves prognostic and biologic classification of Spitz neoplasms. *J Invest Dermatol* 2020; **140**: 1599–608.
100. Bastian BC, LeBoit PE, Pinkel D. Mutations and copy number increase of HRAS in Spitz nevi with distinctive histopathological features. *Am J Pathol* 2000; **157**: 967–72.
101. Wiesner T, Kutzner H, Cerroni L, Mihm Jr MC, Busam KJ, Murali R. Genomic aberrations in Spitzoid melanocytic tumors and their implications for diagnosis, prognosis and therapy. *Pathology* 2016; **48**: 113–31.
102. Amin SM, Haugh AM, Lee CY, et al. A comparison of morphologic and molecular features of BRAF, ALK, and NTRK1 fusion Spitzoid neoplasms. *Am J Surg Pathol* 2017; **41**: 491–8.
103. Hagstrom M, Fumero-Velázquez M, Dhillon S, Olivares S, Gerami P. An update on genomic aberrations in Spitz naevi and tumours. *Pathology* 2023; **55**: 196–205.
104. Gerami P, Kim D, Compres EV, et al. Clinical, morphologic, and genomic findings in ROS1 fusion Spitz neoplasms. *Mod Pathol* 2021; **34**: 348–57.
105. Yeh I, Busam KJ, McCalmont TH, et al. Filigree-like rete ridges, lobulated nests, rosette-like structures, and exaggerated maturation characterize Spitz tumors with NTRK1 fusion. *Am J Surg Pathol* 2019; **43**: 737–46.
106. Mansour B, Vanecek T, Kastnerova L, Nosek D, Kazakov DV, Donati M. Spitz

tumor With SQSTM1::NTRK2 fusion: a clinicopathological study of 5 cases. *Am J Dermatopathol* 2023; **45**: 306–10.

107. de la Fouchardière A, Tee MK, Peternel S, et al. Fusion partners of NTRK3 affect subcellular localization of the fusion kinase and cytomorphology of melanocytes. *Mod Pathol* 2021; **34**: 735–47.

108. Hechtman JF, Benayed R, Hyman DM, et al. Pan-Trk immunohistochemistry Is an efficient and reliable screen for the detection of NTRK fusions. *Am J Surg Pathol* 2017; **41**: 1547–51.

109. Roy SF, Milante R, Pissaloux D, et al. Spectrum of melanocytic tumors harboring BRAF gene fusions: 58 cases with histomorphologic and genetic correlations. *Mod Pathol* 2023; **36**: 100149. doi: 10.1016/j.modpat.2023.100149.

110. Houlier A, Pissaloux D, Masse I, et al. Melanocytic tumors with MAP3K8 fusions: report of 33 cases with morphological-genetic correlations. *Mod Pathol* 2020; **33**: 846–57.

111. Yeh I, Botton T, Talevich E, et al. Activating MET kinase rearrangements in melanoma and Spitz tumours. *Nat Commun* 2015; **6**: 7174. https://doi.org/10.1038/ncomms8174

112. Williams EA, Shah N, Montesion M, et al. Melanomas with activating RAF1 fusions: clinical, histopathologic, and molecular profiles. *Mod Pathol* 2020; **33**: 1466–74.

113. Donati M, Nosek D, Olivares S, et al. Spitz tumor with RAF1 fusion: A report of 3 cases. *Ann Diagn Pathol* 2023; **67**: 152215. doi: 10.1016/j.anndiagpath.2023.152215.

114. Kim D, Compres EV, Zhang B, et al. A series of RET fusion Spitz neoplasms with plaque-like silhouette and dyscohesive nesting of epithelioid melanocytes. *Am J Dermatopathol* 2021; **43**: 243–51.

115. Sunshine JC, Kim D, Zhang B, et al. Melanocytic neoplasms with MAP2K1 in frame deletions and Spitz morphology. *Am J Dermatopathol* 2020; **42**: 923–31.

116. Ludgate MW, Fullen DR, Lee J, et al. The atypical Spitz tumor of uncertain biologic potential: a series of 67 patients from a single institution. *Cancer* 2009; **115**: 631–41.

117. Massi D, Tomasini C, Senetta R, et al. Atypical Spitz tumors in patients younger than 18 years. *J Am Acad Dermatol* 2015; **72**: 37–46.

118. Vollmer RT. Use of Bayes rule and MIB-1 proliferation index to discriminate Spitz nevus from malignant melanoma. *Am J Clin Pathol* 2004; **122**: 499–505.

119. George E, Polissar NL, Wick M. Immunohistochemical evaluation of p16INK4A, E-cadherin, and cyclin D1 expression in melanoma and Spitz tumors. *Am J Clin Pathol* 2010; **133**: 370–9.

120. Gerami P, Scolyer RA, Xu X, et al. Risk assessment for atypical spitzoid melanocytic neoplasms using FISH to identify chromosomal copy number aberrations. *Am J Surg Pathol* 2013; **37**: 676–84.

121. Yazdan P, Cooper C, Sholl LM, et al. Comparative analysis of atypical Spitz tumors with heterozygous versus homozygous 9p21 deletions for clinical outcomes, histomorphology, BRAF mutation, and p16 expression. *Am J Surg Pathol* 2014; **38**: 638–45.

122. Shen L, Cooper C, Bajaj S, et al. Atypical spitz tumors with 6q23 deletions: a clinical, histological, and molecular study. *Am J Dermatopathol* 2013; **35**: 804–12.

123. Cooper C, Arva NC, Lee C, et al. A clinical, histopathologic, and outcome study of melanonychia striata in childhood. *J Am Acad Dermatol* 2015; **72**: 773–9.

124. Tan KB, Moncrieff M, Thompson JF, et al. Subungual melanoma: a study of 124 cases highlighting features of early lesions, potential pitfalls in diagnosis, and guidelines for histologic reporting. *Am J Surg Pathol* 2007; **31**: 1902–12.

125. Theunis A, Richert B, Sass U, Lateur N, Sales F, Andre J. Immunohistochemical study of 40 cases of longitudinal melanonychia. *Am J Dermatopathol* 2011; **33**: 27–34.

126. Ridolfi RL, Rosen PP, Thaler H. Nevus cell aggregates associated with lymph nodes: estimated frequency and clinical significance. *Cancer* 1977; **39**: 164–71.

127. Carson KF, Wen DR, Li PX, et al. Nodal nevi and cutaneous melanoma. *Am J Surg Pathol* 1996; **20**: 834–40.

128. Biddle DA, Evans HL, Kemp BL, et al. Intraparenchymal nevus cell aggregates in lymph nodes: a possible diagnostic pitfall with malignant melanoma and carcinoma. *Am J Surg Pathol* 2003; **27**: 673–81.

129. Holt JB, Sangueza OP, Levine EA, et al. Nodal melanocytic nevi in sentinel lymph nodes: correlation with melanoma-associated cutaneous nevi. *Am J Clin Pathol* 2004; **121**: 58–63.

130. Mihic-Probst D, Saremaslani P, Komminoth P, Heitz PU. Immunostaining for the tumour suppressor gene p16 product is a useful marker to differentiate melanoma metastasis from lymph-node nevus. *Virchows Arch* 2003; **443**: 745–51.

131. See SHC, Finkelman BS, Yeldandi AV. The diagnostic utility of PRAME and p16 in distinguishing nodal nevi from nodal metastatic melanoma. *Pathol Res Pract* 2020; **216**: 153105. doi: 10.1016/j.prp.2020.153105.

132. Mentrikoshi MJ, Ma L, Pryor JG, et al. Diagnostic utility of IMP3 in segregating metastatic melanoma from benign nevi in lymph nodes. *Mod Pathol* 2009; **22**: 1582–7.

133. Lee JJ, Granter SR, Laga AC, et al. 5-hydroxymethylcytosine expression in metastatic melanoma versus nodal nevus in sentinel lymph node biopsies. *Mod Pathol* 2015; **28**: 218–29.

134. Kucher C, Zhang PJ, Pasha T, et al. Expression of Melan-A and Ki-67 in desmoplastic melanoma and desmoplastic nevi. *Am J Dermatopathol* 2004; **26**: 452–7.

135. Lazova R, Tantcheva-Poor I, Sigal AC. P75 nerve growth factor receptor staining is superior to S100 in identifying spingle cell and desmoplastic melanoma. *J Am Acad Dermatol* 2010; **63**: 852–8.

136. Chorny JA, Barr RJ. S100-positive spindle cells in scars: a diagnostic pitfall in the re-excision of desmoplastic melanoma. *Am J Dermatopathol* 2002; **24**: 309–12.

137. Bianchi G, Charoenlap C, Cocchi S, et al. Clear cell sarcoma of soft tissue: a retrospective review and analysis of 31 cases treated at Istituto Ortopedico Rizzoli. *Eur J Surg Oncol* 2014; **40**: 505–10.

138. Hisaoka M, Ishida T, Kuo TT, et al. Clear cell sarcoma of soft tissue: a clinicopathologic, immunohistochemical, and molecular analysis of 33 cases. *Am J Surg Pathol* 2008; **32**: 452–60.

139. Granter SR, Weilbaecher KN, Quigley C, Fletcher CD, Fisher DE. Clear cell sarcoma shows immunoreactivity for microphthalmia transcription factor: further evidence for melanocytic differentiation. *Mod Pathol* 2001; **14**: 6–9.

140. Aung PP, Sarlomo-Rikala M, Lasota J, Lai JP, Wang ZF, Miettinen M. KBA62

and PNL2: 2 new melanoma markers-immunohistochemical analysis of 1563 tumors including metastatic, desmoplastic, and mucosal melanomas and their mimics. *Am J Surg Pathol* 2012; **36**: 265–72.

141. Karamchandani JR, Nielsen TO, van de Rijn M, West RB. Sox10 and S100 in the diagnosis of soft-tissue neoplasms. *Appl Immunohistochem Mol Morphol* 2012; **20**: 445–50.
142. Wang WL, Mayordomo E, Zhang W, et al. Detection and characterization of EWSR1/ATF1 and EWSR1/CREB1 chimeric transcripts in clear cell sarcoma (melanoma of soft parts). *Mod Pathol* 2009; **22**: 1201–9.
143. Yang L, Chen Y, Cui T, et al. Identification of biomarkers to distinguish clear cell sarcoma from malignant melanoma. *Hum Pathol* 2012; **43**: 1463–70.
144. Charli-Joseph Y, Saggini A, Vemula S, Weier J, Mirza S, LeBoit PE. Primary cutaneous perivascular epithelioid cell tumor: a clinicopathological and molecular reappraisal. *J Am Acad Dermatol* 2014; **71**: 1127–36.
145. Llamas-Velasco M, Mentzel T, Requena L, Palmedo G, Kasten R, Kutzner H. Cutaneous PEComa does not harbour TFE3 gene fusions: immunohistochemical and molecular study of 17 cases. *Histopathology* 2013; **63**: 122–9.
146. Mentzel T, Reisshauer S, Rutten A, Hantschke M, Soares de Almeida LM, Kutzner H. Cutaneous clear cell myomelanocytic tumour: a new member of the growing family of perivascular peithelioid cell tumours (PEComas). Clinicopathological and immunohistochemical analysis of seven cases. *Histopathology* 2005; **46**: 498–504.
147. Greveling K, Winnepennickx VJ, Nagtzaam IF, et al. Malignant perivascular epithelioid tumor: a case report of a cutaneous tumor on the cheek of a male patient. *J Am Acad Dermatol* 2013; **69**: e262-4.
148. Calder KB, Schlauder S, Morgan MB. Malignant perivascular epithelioid cell tumor ("PEComa"): a case report and literature review of cutaneous/subcutaneous presentations. *J Cutan Pathol* 2008; **35**: 499–503.
149. Martignoni G, Gobbo S, Camparo P, et al. Differential expression of cathepsin K in neoplasms harboring TFE3 gene fusions. *Mod Pathol* 2011; **24**: 1313–19.
150. Fernandez-Flores A, Nguyen CM, Cassarino DS. Cutaneous PEComas express CD10: implications for the classification of PEComas and the differential diagnosis with metastatic renal cell carcinoma. *Am J Dermatopathol* 2016; **38**: 645–52.
151. Tallon B, Beer TW. MiTF positivity in atypical fibroxanthoma: a diagnostic pitfall. *Am J Dermatopathol* 2014; **36**: 888–91.
152. Suarez-Vilela D, Izquierdo FM, Escobar-Stein J, Mendez-Alvarez JR. Atypical fibroxanthoma with T-cytotoxic inflammatory infiltrate and aberrant expression of cytokeratin. *J Cutan Pathol* 2011; **38**: 930–2.
153. Uquen A, Sassolas B, Mondine P, et al. NRASQ61 R and BRAFV600E mutation-specific immunohistochemistry is a helpful tool to diagnose metastatic undifferentiated/dedifferentiated melanomas. *Am J Surg Pathol* 2016; **40**: 1004–5.
154. Saleh JS, Whittington CP, Bresler SC, Patel RM. Mesenchymal tumours with melanocytic expression: a potential pitfall in the differential diagnosis of malignant melanoma. *Pathology* 2023; **55**: 258–68.
155. Henderson SA, Torres-Cabala CA, Curry JL, et al. p40 is more specific than p63 for the distinction of atypical fibroxanthoma from other cutaneous spindle cell malignancies. *Am J Surg Pathol* 2014; **38**: 1102–10.
156. Kao GF, Helwig EB, Graham JH. Balloon cell malignant melanoma of the skin. A clinicopathologic study of 34 cases with histochemical, immunohistochemical, and ultrastructural observations. *Cancer* 1992; **69**: 2942–52.
157. Plaza JA, Torres-Cabala C Evans H, Diwan HA, Suster S, Prieto VG. Cutaneous metastases of malignant melanoma: a clinicopathologic study of 192 cases with emphasis on the morphologic spectrum. *Am J Dermatopathol* 2010; **32**: 129–36.

Chapter 8

Soft Tissue Neoplasms

Jakob M. T. Moran, Joana Pardal, and Mai P. Hoang

Introduction

Pathologists often encounter soft tissue neoplasms while examining biopsies and excisions from the skin. Soft tissue neoplasms are classified along their line of differentiation and include fibroblastic, myofibroblastic and fibrohistiocytic tumors, smooth muscle tumors, skeletal muscle tumors, neural tumors, lipomatous tumors, vascular tumors, pericytic and perivascular tumors, and tumors of uncertain differentiation. These tumors can be categorized as benign, intermediate (locally recurrent/aggressive), intermediate (rarely metastasizing), and malignant (locally recurrent/aggressive with significant metastatic potential).

Accurate histologic diagnosis, grading, and staging is imperative for proper prognostication and treatment. A number of grading and staging systems exist; however, the Fédération Nationale des Centres de Lutte Contre Le Cancer (FNCLCC) grading system is referenced by the College of American Pathologists synoptic reports, the World Health Organization (WHO) classification of tumors and is incorporated into the American Joint Committee on Cancer (AJCC) staging manual. The FNCLCC grading system assigns a grade based on necrosis, mitotic activity, and degree of differentiation.[1] The 8th edition of the AJCC staging manual for soft tissue sarcomas incorporates grade, anatomic site, size, node status, and the presence of metastasis.[2]

The expanding array of molecular diagnostic techniques continues to identify numerous novel gene alterations, enabling recognition and classification of distinct tumor entities. For example, *ALK* translocations have been identified in epithelioid fibrous histiocytomas, allowing distinction from conventional fibrous histiocytomas (dermatofibromas) and its subtypes.[3] Other examples of diagnostic entities defined by novel gene alterations include *EWSR1::SMAD3* rearranged fibroblastic tumors which demonstrate strong Erg expression by immunohistochemistry[4] and *NTRK*-rearranged spindle cell neoplasms (lipofibromatosis-like neural tumor) which demonstrate co-expression of CD34 and S100.[5]

In this chapter we will review many (but not all) soft tissue neoplasms which can be encountered in the skin including recently categorized ones as well as established entities and highlight important immunohistochemical markers (**Table 8.1**).

Table 8.1 Summary of available soft tissue markers in clinical immunohistochemistry laboratory

Antibody	Commonly used clones	Staining pattern	Normal structures
ALK	5A4, 1A4, D5F3	cytoplasmic	NA
Beta-catenin	14, EP35	cytoplasmic, membranous, nuclear	fibroblasts, endothelial cells
CADM3	polyclonal	cytoplasmic	
Caldesmon	h-CD, EP19	cytoplasmic	smooth muscle cells
Calponin	CALP, EP798Y	cytoplasmic	smooth muscle cells
Calretinin	5A5, CAL6, 2E7	cytoplasmic	axons, ganglion cells
CD31	JC70A, 1A10	cytoplasmic	endothelial cells
CD34	QBEnd/10	cytoplasmic	endothelial cells

Table 8.1 (cont.)

Antibody	Commonly used clones	Staining pattern	Normal structures
CD57	NK–1, TB01	membranous	natural killer cells, cytotoxic lymphocytes
CD68	KP1, PG-M1, 514H12	cytoplasmic	histiocytes, monocytes
CD99	12E7, O13, EPR3097Y	membranous staining	basal squamous epithelial cells
CD163	10D6, MRQ–26	cytoplasmic	histiocytes, monocytes
CDK4	DCS–35, EP180	nuclear	NA
Claudin 1	polyclonal	membranous	keratinocytes, epithelial cells
Clusterin	41D	cytoplasmic	
C-MYC	9E10, Y69	nuclear	NA
CSF–1	21113	cytoplasmic	
DDIT3	OTI2D3	cytoplasmic	
Desmin	D33, DE-R–11	cytoplasmic	smooth muscle cells
D2–40	D2–40	cytoplasmic	lymphatic endothelial cells
Erg	EPR3864	nuclear	endothelial cells
Factor XIIIa	EP3372	nuclear	histiocytes, dermal dendrocytes
Fascin	55K2	cytoplasmic	dendritic cells
FH	polyclonal	cytoplasmic	
FLI1	G146–222, MRQ–1	nuclear	endothelial cells, lymphocytes
FOSB	5g4	cytoplasmic	
GFAP	EP13, GA5	cytoplasmic	neurons
GLUT1	Polyclonal, EP141	membranous	erythrocytes
H3K27me3	(lys27)(c36b11)	nuclear	
Inhibin alpha	R1	cytoplasmic	trophoblasts of placenta
INI1	25, MRQ–27	nuclear	endothelial cells, lymphocytes
MDM2	BSB–64	nuclear	endothelial cells, lymphocytes
MSA (muscle specific actin)	HHF35	cytoplasmic	smooth muscle cells
MUC4	8G7, EP256	cytoplasmic, membranous	colonic epithelium
MyoD1	EP212, 5.8A	nuclear	NA
Myogenin (Myf–4)	F5D, EP162, LO26	nuclear	NA
Myoglobin	polyclonal	cytoplasmic	skeletal muscle
Myosin, smooth muscle	SMMS–1, S131	cytoplasmic	follicular dendritic cells of tonsils or lymph node
Neurofilament	2F11	cytoplasmic	axons, ganglion cells
NKI/C3 (CD63)	NKI/C3	cytoplasmic	
Pan-TRK	EPR17341	cytoplasmic	
p16	E6h4	cytoplasmic	
PRKAR1A	OTI6C7	cytoplasmic	
PGP 9.5	BSB–46, polyclonal	cytoplasmic	peripheral nerves
PROX1	4G10	cytoplasmic	lymphatic endothelial cells
PRDM10	polyclonal	cytoplasmic	
PTEN	6H2.1	cytoplasmic	
RB	1F8	nuclear	
ROS1	D4d6	cytoplasmic	
S100	4C4.9, polyclonal	cytoplasmic, nuclear	peripheral nerves, dendritic cells, melanocytes
SMA	1A4	cytoplasmic	smooth muscle cells
SOX10	EP268, BC34, SP267, polyclonal	nuclear	melanocytes, peripheral nerves, eccrine glands
SSTR2 (somatostatin receptor type 2)	EP149	cytoplasmic, membranous	pancreatic islet cells

Table 8.1 (cont.)

Antibody	Commonly used clones	Staining pattern	Normal structures
STAT6	EP325, polyclonal	nuclear	NA
TFE3	MRQ–37, EP285	nuclear	germ cell of testis
TLE1	1F5, M101	nuclear	NA
Vimentin	V9, Vim 3B4	cytoplasmic	all B- and T-cells
WT–1	6FH2, WT49	nuclear	epithelial and smooth muscle cells of fallopian tubes

NA: not applicable

8.1 Fibroblastic, Myofibroblastic, and Fibrohistiocytic Neoplasms

Dermatofibroma (Fibrous Histiocytoma)

Dermatofibroma, also known as fibrous histiocytoma, is a common mesenchymal neoplasm of the skin that occurs over a broad age range with several histologic variants including clear cell, granular, lipidized, palisading, myxoid, atypical, aneurysmal, deep, and cellular.[6] The "conventional" or "common" dermatofibroma is characterized by a proliferation of spindle cells in the papillary/reticular dermis with admixed histiocytes, dendrocytes, and myofibroblasts with peripheral trapping of collagen and overlying epidermal hyperplasia with hyperpigmentation (**Figure 8.1**).[6] The atypical, aneurysmal, deep, and cellular variants of dermatofibroma deserve special attention as they have a high rate of local recurrence (~20%) and, very rarely, can metastasize.[6–9] The atypical variant of dermatofibroma features atypical/pleomorphic cells as the name suggests and can also demonstrate necrosis. The aneurysmal variant of dermatofibroma demonstrates spaces filled with blood and hemosiderin. The deep variant of dermatofibroma is typically well-circumscribed and centered in the deep dermis/subcutaneous tissue. The cellular variant of dermatofibroma is more cellular than the "conventional" or "common" dermatofibroma, may be mitotically active and can show focal entrapment of the subcutis.[6–9] Other subtypes of dermatofibroma rarely recur (reported rate of <2%).[6]

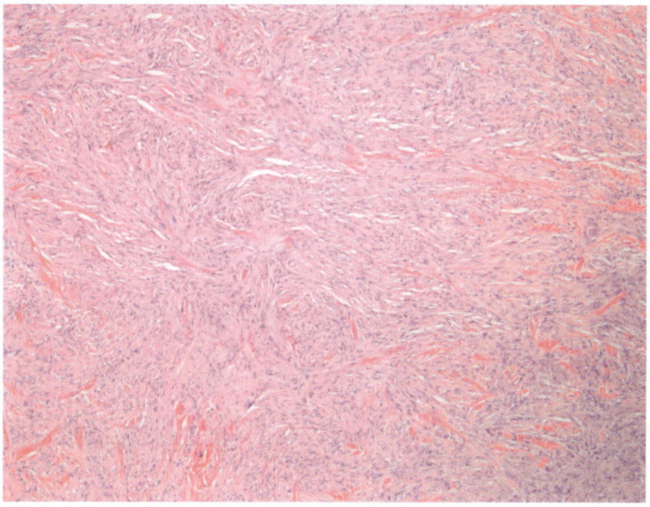

Figure 8.1 Dermatofibroma is characterized by a proliferation of bland spindle cells (X100).

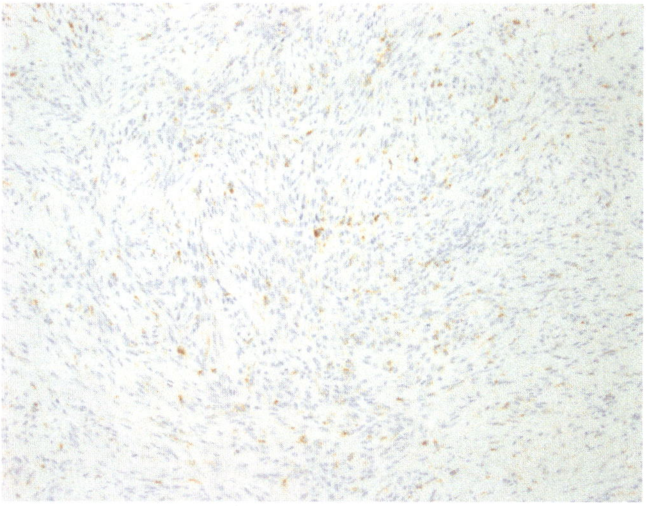

Figure 8.2 Dermatofibroma. The tumor cells are positive for CD68 (X200).

No single immunohistochemical marker is diagnostic for dermatofibroma but immunohistochemistry is helpful in highlighting components of the lesion including histiocytes (CD68+/CD163+) (**Figure 8.2**), dendrocytes (factor 13a+), and myofibroblasts (focal SMA expression).[10] Although sensitive, factor 13a is not a specific marker for dermatofibroma since its expression has been reported in angiofibroma, xanthogranuloma, angiomatoid fibrous histiocytoma, and some atypical fibroxanthoma. Immunohistochemistry is also helpful in excluding entities in the differential diagnosis including spindle cell carcinoma (keratin+, p40+, p63+), melanoma (Sox10+, S100+, HMB-45+, Melan-A+), smooth muscle neoplasms (SMA+, h-caldesmon+), and vascular lesions (Erg+, CD34+, CD31+).

Dermatofibrosarcoma protuberans (DFSP) is diffusely positive for CD34, infiltrates the subcutaneous tissue in a "honeycomb" fashion and often harbors a *COL1A1::PDGFB* gene rearrangement.[11] Dermatofibroma is typically negative or focally positive for CD34 (**Figure 8.3**), although variants such as cellular dermatofibroma and deep fibrous histiocytoma can demonstrate stronger and more diffuse CD34 expression.[12] Factor 13a+ dendrocytes are almost always identified in dermatofibroma and cellular dermatofibromas while they are typically absent or rare in DFSP. However, none of these markers is superior to CD34 in the distinction of dermatofibroma versus DFSP.

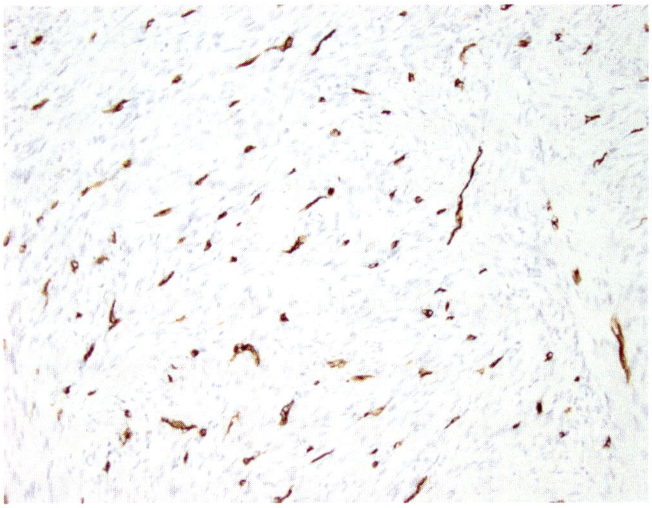

Figure 8.3 Dermatofibroma. They are negative for CD34 (X200).

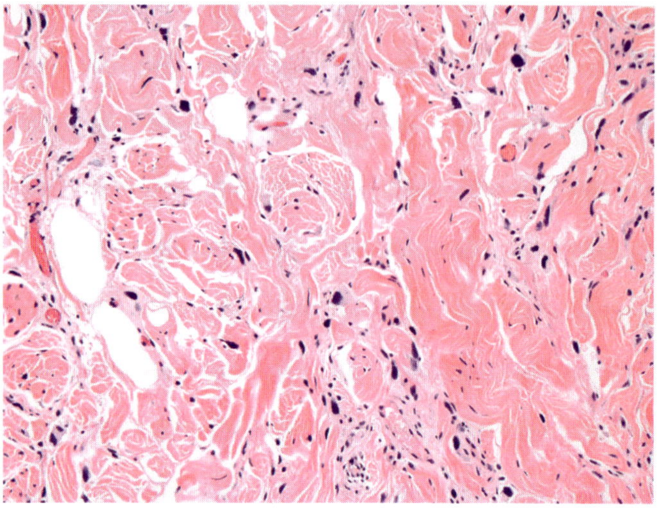

Figure 8.4 Occasional pleomorphic and multinucleated tumors cells are seen in a fibrotic background in pleomorphic fibroma (X200).

Atypical, aneurysmal, and cellular variants of dermatofibroma can be difficult to distinguish from intermediate and malignant cutaneous neoplasms such as atypical fibroxanthoma or pleomorphic dermal sarcoma, especially on small or superficial biopsies. Atypical fibroxanthoma and pleomorphic dermal sarcoma typically occur in older patients in sun-exposed areas while dermatofibromas typically occur in young to middle aged adults.[13] Of note, although CD10 positivity has been reported in atypical fibroxanthomas, dermatofibromas also stain for CD10.[14]

Dermatofibroma

CD68+/CD163+ (histiocytes), factor 13a+ (dendrocytes), CD34-

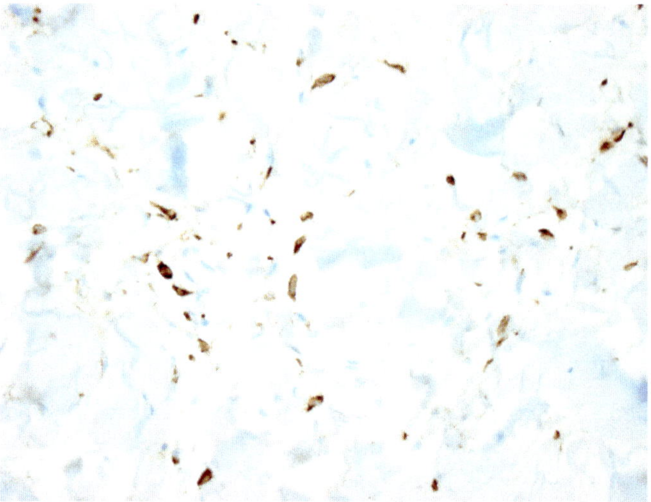

Figure 8.5 Pleomorphic fibroma. The pleomorphic tumor cells are positive for CD163 (X200).

Pleomorphic Fibroma

Pleomorphic fibroma is a benign fibroblastic tumor that exhibits an exophytic architecture. Although hypocellular at low magnification, large, pleomorphic, and sometimes multinucleated tumor cells are seen at high magnification (**Figure 8.4**).[15] Mitotic figures are rarely seen. Smooth muscle actin expression (SMA), which can be weak, has been observed as well as CD34 expression.[15] Pleomorphic fibromas can express CD163 (**Figure 8.5**) and are negative for CD68, S100, and desmin.[15] The differential diagnosis would include an atypical dermatofibroma, multinucleate cell angiohistiocytoma, and an atypical lipomatous tumor.[15,16] Dermatofibromas are cellular lesions with CD68+ histiocytes, factor 13a+ dendrocytes and are CD34- while pleomorphic fibroma is hypocellular and CD34+ and is without CD68+ histiocytes and factor 13a+ dendrocytes.[15] Multinucleate cell angiohistiocytoma has multinucleated giant cells but also has a vascular component with numerous small-medium sized vessels and the spindle and multinucleated tumor cells of multinucleate cell angiohistiocytoma are positive for CD68 and negative for CD34.[16] An atypical lipomatous tumor has hyperchromatic, pleomorphic cells but also has an adipocytic component that is readily identifiable as well as *MDM2/CDK4* gene amplification which can be detected by immunohistochemistry (IHC) or fluorescence *in-situ* hybridization (FISH).[17] Pleomorphic fibromas also have deletion of *RB1* which can be evident by Rb loss of expression.[18]

Pleomorphic fibroma

CD34+ CD163 + SMA+/- CD68- factor 13a- Rb- (loss of nuclear expression)

Sclerotic Fibroma

Sclerotic fibroma can be either sporadic or associated with Cowden syndrome.[19] Sclerotic fibromas are circumscribed, hypocellular dermal nodules with eosinophilic and sclerotic collagen bundles arranged in a storiform pattern and separated by prominent clefts (**Figure 8.6**). This histologic appearance can be seen focally in a variety of lesions including sclerotic lipomas, sclerotic neurofibroma, and fibroma of tendon sheath. In

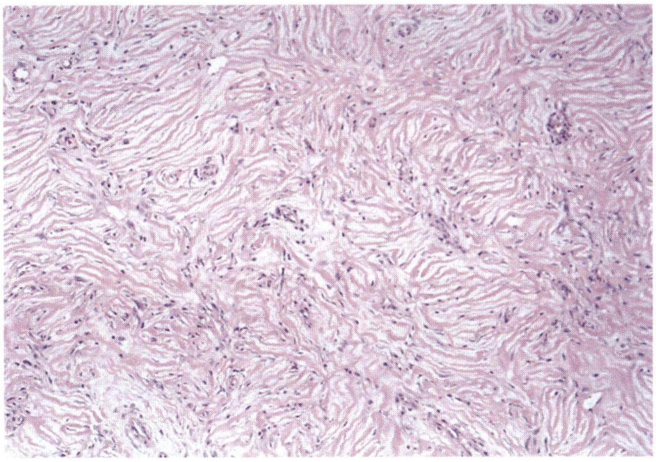

Figure 8.6 A hypocellular dermal proliferation of collagen arranged in a storiform pattern in sclerotic fibroma (X100).

sclerotic fibromas, rare factor 13a+ cells can be identified and the lesional cells stain variably for CD34 (**Figure 8.7**).[19] Sclerotic fibromas can be associated with Cowden syndrome and loss of PTEN by immunohistochemistry may identify syndromic individuals.[20] The differential diagnosis includes a sclerotic dermatofibroma and peripheral nerve sheath tumors such as perineurioma (Glut-1+, Claudin-1+, EMA+).

Sclerotic fibroma

Rare factor 13a+ CD34+/-

PTEN expression is frequently lost in syndrome cases.

Desmoplastic Fibroblastoma (Collagenous Fibroma)

Desmoplastic fibroblastoma (also known as collagenous fibroma) is a hypocellular, benign lesion composed of spindle cells in a fibrous/fibromyxoid background.[21] Variable staining for SMA (diffuse to focal) and S100 (faint) has been reported.[21] The tumor is negative for desmin, keratin, and CD34.[21] The differential diagnosis includes desmoid fibromatosis (β-catenin nuclear positivity), neurofibroma (S100+, Sox10+), fibroma of tendon sheath (associated with a tendon), and low-grade fibromyxoid sarcoma (MUC4+). Of note, recurrent translocations involving *FOSL* have been reported in desmoplastic fibroblastomas and FOSL immunostain may aid in diagnosis.[22]

Desmoplastic fibroblastoma

FOSL+ SMA +/- CD34- desmin- S100-

Medallion-Like Dermal Dendrocyte Hamartoma

Medallion-like dermal dendrocyte hamartoma also known as plaque-like CD34+ dermal fibroma is a very rare lesion that presents mainly on the trunk or proximal extremities.[23] A band-like proliferation in the superficial dermis is noted at low magnification. Concentric arrangement of monomorphous spindle cells is seen around dermal blood vessels. The tumor cells express CD34, factor 13a (variable) and fascin; and they are negative for S100, CD1a, and CD68 (**Figures 8.8** and **8.9**).[23] Since the lesion expresses CD34 a clinically important differential diagnosis

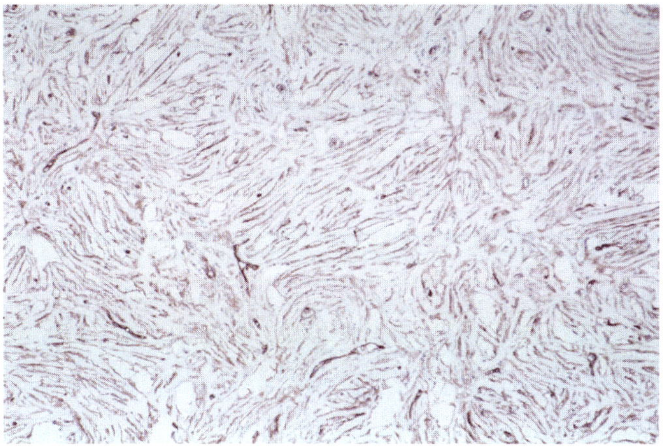

Figure 8.7 Sclerotic fibroma. The tumor cells are CD34 positive (X200).

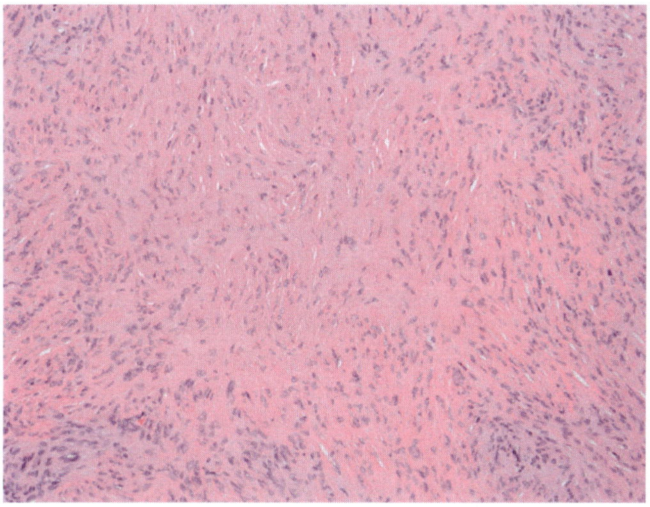

Figure 8.8 A proliferation of uniform spindle cells is seen in the dermis of medallion-like dermal dendrocyte hamartoma (X200).

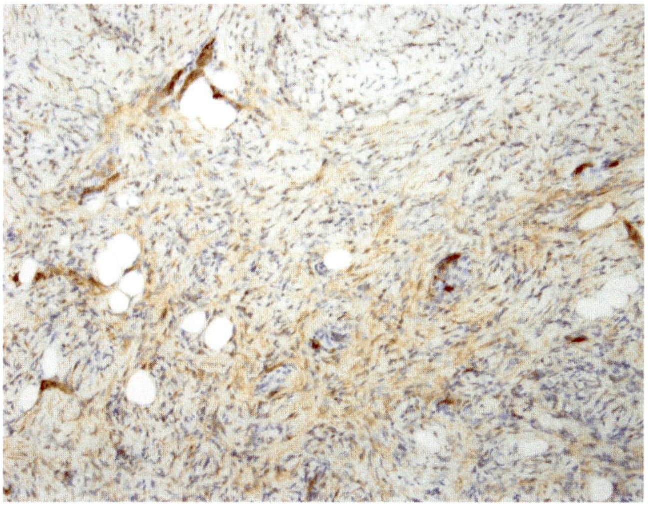

Figure 8.9 Medallion-like dermal dendrocyte hamartoma. The tumor cells exhibit fascin positivity (X200).

would be DFSP. Molecular analyses for a *COL1A1::PDGFB* gene rearrangement would be negative in medallion-like dermal dendrocyte hamartoma in contrast to the atrophic or superficial variant of DFSP.[23] The differential diagnosis also includes fibroblastic connective tissue nevus and dermatomyofibroma, both of which have been reported to express CD34 and SMA.[24]

Medalion-like dermal dendrocyte hamartoma

CD34+ fascin+ factor 13a+/-

Superficial CD34+ Fibroblastic Tumor

Superficial CD34+ fibroblastic tumor typically occurs in the superficial aspects of the lower extremities.[25] The tumor may be infiltrative or circumscribed and the tumor cells can demonstrate significant nuclear pleomorphism; however mitoses are infrequent, and necrosis is rare.[25] The tumor cells are positive for CD34 and are often positive for keratins.[25] The tumors cells are reportedly negative for desmin, SMA, ERG, and S100.[25] A subset of these tumors demonstrates *PRDM10* rearrangement and PRDM10 nuclear staining has been reported to be specific.[26] SynCAM3 (CADM3) has also been reported in superficial CD34+ fibroblastic tumors.[26] Because of the pleomorphism that can be seen in superficial CD34+ fibroblastic tumors, the differential diagnosis includes intermediate and malignant neoplasms including epithelioid sarcoma (keratin+, CD34+, INI1 loss), atypical fibroxanthoma/pleomorphic dermal sarcoma (CD34-), and DFSP (CD34+ but with diffuse infiltration of the subcutis). A rare case of lymph node metastasis has been reported.[25] Molecular analysis for *PRDM10* rearrangements may be of utility in challenging cases.

Superficial CD34+ fibroblastic tumor

CD34+, keratin +, PRDM10+

Fibroblastic Connective Tissue Nevus

Fibroblastic connective tissue nevus is a benign lesion that typically presents in the deep dermis and subcutis. The tumor demonstrates a proliferation of spindle cells that entraps the subcutis and adjacent cutaneous adnexal structures.[27] CD34 is often expressed and SMA expression is variable/focal.[27] The tumor cells are reportedly negative for desmin and S100.[27] The differential diagnosis includes medallion-like dermal dendrocyte hamartoma/plaque-like CD34+ dermal fibroma (CD34+ fascin+), scar (CD34-, SMA+/-, S100+/-),[28] dermatomyofibroma (CD34+ SMA+), leiomyoma (desmin+, SMA+, h-caldesmon+), and *NTRK*-rearranged spindle cell neoplasm (CD34+ S100+, pan-TRK+).

Fibroblastic connective tissue nevus

CD34+, SMA+/−

Solitary Fibrous Tumor

Solitary fibrous tumor (SFT) can affect many organs, including the skin, usually the head and neck region, and typically follows a benign biologic course.[29,30] Of note, assessment of metastatic risk is dependent on clinical and histologic features including the age of the patient, tumor size, necrosis, and mitotic count.[30] Histopathologically, a "patternless" pattern with a "staghorn" (hemangiopericytoma-like) vascular pattern is characteristically described, however a wide range of histologic appearances has been reported (**Figure 8.10**).[30] The tumor can have a biphasic appearance – highly cellular areas with hemangiopericytomatous pattern alternate with hypocellular areas. The tumor cells typically express CD34 (diffuse) and demonstrate STAT6 nuclear staining due to the *NAB2::STAT6* gene fusion product that is found in solitary fibrous tumors (**Figure 8.11**).[29,31] They are negative for S100, factor 13a, lysozyme, keratin, EMA, desmin, calretinin, and HBME1.[29] There is variable expression

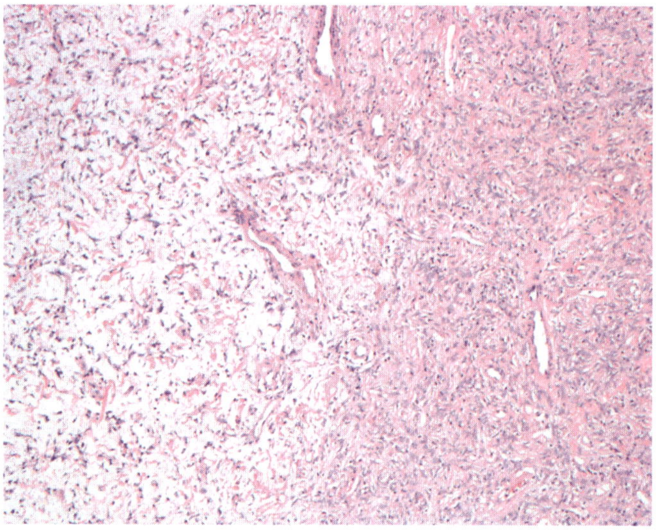

Figure 8.10 Solitary fibrous tumor is characterized by a biphasic appearance – cellular area with hemangiopericytomatous pattern alternate with hypocellular area (X100).

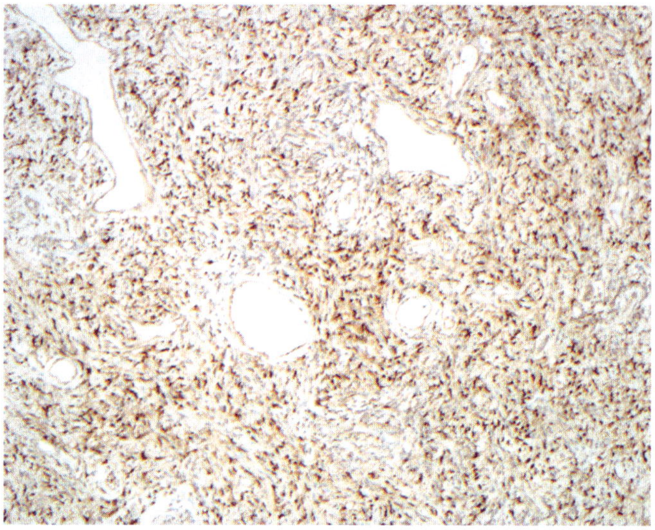

Figure 8.11 Solitary fibrous tumor. Diffuse nuclear Stat6 expression is seen (X100).

for CD99, Bcl-2, and SMA.[29] Although other entities such as DFSP may enter the differential diagnosis, STAT6 immunohistochemistry has been shown to be highly sensitive and specific for solitary fibrous tumor.[31]

Solitary fibrous tumor

CD34+ STAT6+

Multinucleate Cell Angiohistiocytoma

It is not clear whether multinucleate cell angiohistiocytoma is a vascular or fibrohistiocytic proliferation. Multinucleate cell angiohistiocytoma exhibits pleomorphic and multinucleated cells in a background of dilated dermal vasculature, dermal fibrosis and lymphohistiocytic infiltrate.[32] Due to its expression of estrogen receptor, some have speculated that it is a reactive process.[33] The vascular component stains with CD31 and CD34, while the multinucleated cells are variably positive for CD68 and factor 13a while negative for CD34 (see **Case Study 1**).[32]

Multinucleate cell angiohistiocytoma

CD68+/- factor 13a+/- CD34-

Fibrous Hamartoma of Infancy

Fibrous hamartoma of infancy is a benign fibrous proliferation that usually occurs in infancy.[34] It is characterized by three distinctive histologic components: (1) trabeculae of fibrous bands composed of spindled myofibroblastic cells that can be positive for SMA and CD34, (2) whorls of round immature cells within a myxoid matrix that can also be positive for CD34 and bcl2, and (3) mature adipose tissue (S100 +).[34] Presence of the three histologic components is diagnostic.

Fibrous hamartoma of infancy

Fibrous component: SMA+/- CD34+/-

Immature myxoid/mesenchymal component: SMA +/- CD34+/-

Adipocytic component: S100+

Calcifying Aponeurotic Fibroma

Calcifying aponeurotic fibroma is a rare soft tissue tumor that mainly presents in children and has a predilection for the hands and feet. On histologic sections the tumor is characterized by spindle and epithelioid fibroblasts surrounding foci of cartilaginous metaplasia and mineralization. The tumor cells are positive for CD99, S100, and CD68 and they variably express SMA, CD34, CD57, EMA, and progesterone receptor.[35] *FN1::EGF* gene fusions have also been identified in calcifying aponeurotic fibromas.[36] The histologic differential diagnosis includes lipofibromatosis (CD34+ with adipocytes and without cartilaginous metaplasia), *NTRK*-rearranged spindle cell neoplasm (S100+ CD34+), and palmar/plantar fibromatosis (absence of cartilaginous metaplasia).

Calcifying aponeurotic fibroma

SMA+ CD34+

Tenosynovial Giant Cell Tumor (Giant Cell Tumor of Tendon Sheath) and Giant Cell Tumor of Soft Tissue

Tenosynovial giant cell tumors (also referred to as giant cell tumor of tendon sheath) are lesions with synovial differentiation that occur in association with tendons and joints.[37] Two subtypes are recognized, localized and diffuse, with the latter associated with more aggressive behavior (destruction of joints, pain, decrease in quality of life).[38] Histologically, these tumors are composed of a mix of cells including large mononuclear cells, multinucleated giant cells and macrophages/histiocytes in a background of inflammation (**Figure 8.12**).[37] The large mononuclear cells are typically positive for clusterin, desmin, and D2-40, the multinucleated giant cells are positive for CD68 and CD45 (LCA) (**Figure 8.13**) and the macrophages/ histiocytes are positive for CD68, CD163, and CD45 (LCA).[39] *CSF1* rearrangements have been identified in tenosynovial giant cell tumors and immunohistochemistry for CSF1 may be of diagnostic utility.[37]

The histologic differential diagnosis includes giant cell tumor of soft tissue; however, radiologic correlation and immunohistochemistry (CSF1, clusterin) should be able to distinguish most cases. Giant cell tumor (GCT) of soft tissue is morphologically similar to GCT of bone but does not harbor *H3F3A* gene mutations which are seen in GCTs of bone.[40] Histologically, GCTs of soft tissue demonstrate a multilobulated growth pattern with mononuclear cells and giant cells in a fibrous, vascularized stroma (**Figure 8.12**).[40] Often, there is a peripheral rim of bone.[40] CD68 can be positive in the mononuclear and giant cells (**Figure 8.13**), however, histologic features and radiographic appearance are the key diagnostic criteria.[41]

Tenosynovial giant cell tumor/Giant cell tumor of tendon sheath

- Clusterin+ desmin +/- CSF1+

Giant cell tumor of soft tissue

- CD68+ H3F3A G34 W-

Desmoid Fibromatosis

Desmoid fibromatosis, distinct from palmar/plantar fibromatosis, is a locally aggressive neoplasm that commonly harbors mutations in the WNT/β-catenin pathway (either *CTNNB1* or *APC* mutations).[42] Histologically, long "sweeping" fascicles of banal-appearing spindled cells are described (**Figure 8.14**).[42]

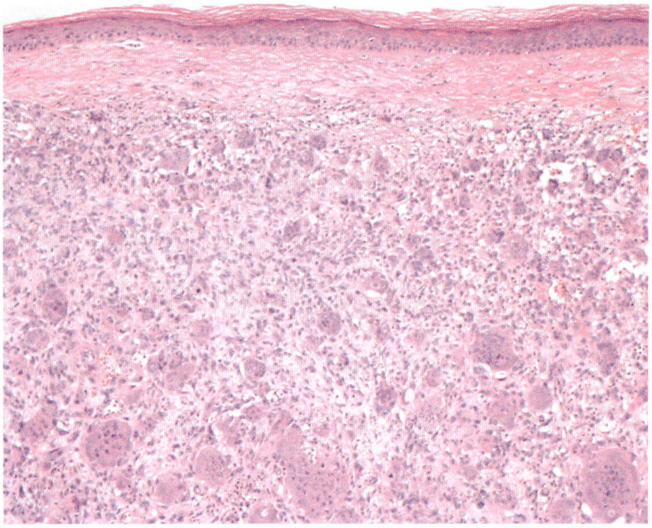

Figure 8.12 A proliferation mononuclear cells as well as multinucleated giant cells is seen in the dermis in giant cell tumor of soft tissue (X100).

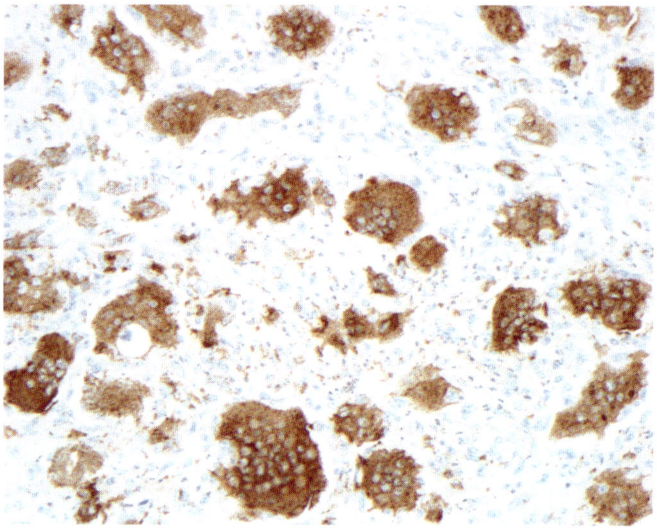

Figure 8.13 Giant cell tumor of soft tissue. The multinucleated giant cells are positive for CD68 (X200).

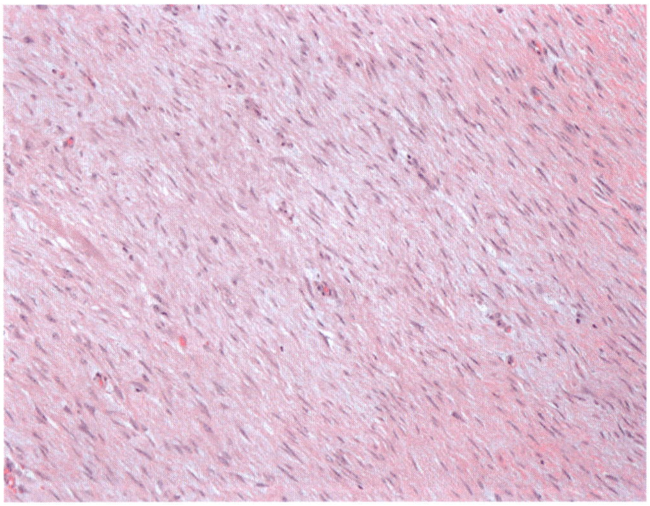

Figure 8.14 Slender spindle cells are seen among keloidal collagen bundles in fibromatosis (X200).

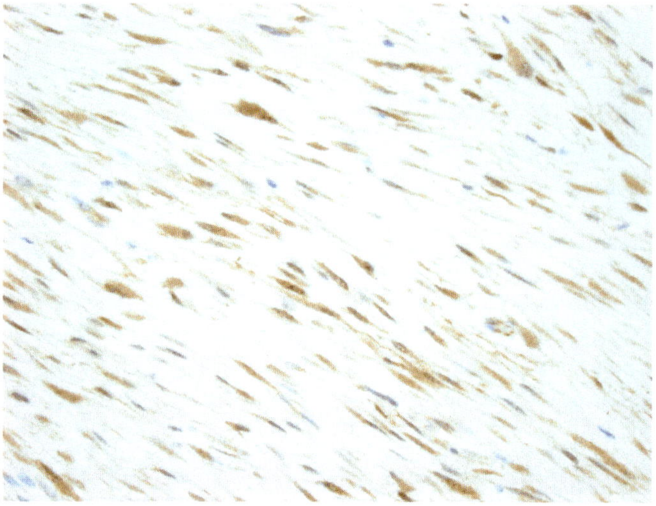

Figure 8.15 Fibromatosis. Nuclear β-catenin expression is seen (X400).

Nuclear positivity for β-catenin is frequently identified **(Figure 8.15)** and the cells can be positive for SMA.[43] Of note, β-catenin nuclear staining can be seen in 30% of low-grade myofibroblastic sarcoma, and 22% of solitary fibrous tumor.[42] The differential diagnosis includes solitary fibrous tumor (CD34+ STAT6+), hypertrophic scar (β-catenin-), nodular fasciitis (*USP6* rearrangements with different histologic appearance), and smooth muscle tumors (desmin+ SMA+) among others. Only cytoplasmic β-catenin expression is seen in some of the histologic mimics including scar, nodular fasciitis, myofibroma, and leiomyosarcoma.[44] Molecular profiling for alterations in the WNT/β-catenin pathway coupled with histology may be needed in difficult cases.

Palmar/plantar fibromatosis is distinct in clinical behavior from desmoid fibromatosis and typically occurs on the palms and plantar surface.[45] Palmar/plantar fibromatosis can show nuclear positivity for β-catenin, however, mutations in *CTNNB1* and *APC* are not identified (in contrast with desmoid fibromatosis).[45]

Desmoid fibromatosis

- β-catenin nuclear staining, SMA +/-

Inclusion Body Fibromatosis (Infantile Digital Fibromatosis)

Infantile digital fibroma/fibromatosis is a myofibroblastic proliferation that typically involves the digits of infants and young children and can persist or recur in up to 74% of cases. The most characteristic histologic finding is the presence of round, eosinophilic inclusion bodies within the cytoplasm that stain purple/red on Masson trichrome stain. The tumor cells express vimentin, SMA, and calponin; variably desmin; variably β-catenin, h-caldesmon, CD10, and CD34.[46] The differential diagnosis includes palmar/plantar fibromatosis (absence of inclusion bodies).

Inclusion body fibromatosis (infantile digital fibromatosis)

- SMA+, calponin+, desmin+/-

Nodular Fasciitis

Nodular fasciitis is a reactive or pseudosarcomatous proliferation of fibroblasts and myofibroblasts, often associated with an antecedent trauma. Rarely nodular fasciitis can present as a dermal lesion.[47] Histopathologically it demonstrates a "tissue culture" pattern with extravasated red blood cells in a collagenous to myxoid background (**Figure 8.16**). The tumor cells are typically positive for SMA (**Figure 8.17**); and desmin and h-caldesmon are usually negative.[47] *USP6* rearrangements (particularly *MYH9::USP6*) are frequently identified.[47] The histologic differential diagnosis includes desmoid fibromatosis (β-catenin+), peripheral nerve sheath tumors such as neurofibroma (S100+, Sox-10+), proliferative fasciitis/myositis (SMA+ but with ganglion-like cells), inflammatory myofibroblastic tumor (ALK+/-, SMA +/- keratin +/-), and reactive processes. Of note, nodular fasciitis is not infrequently confused with a sarcoma.[48] In challenging cases, molecular analysis for *USP6* rearrangements may be helpful.

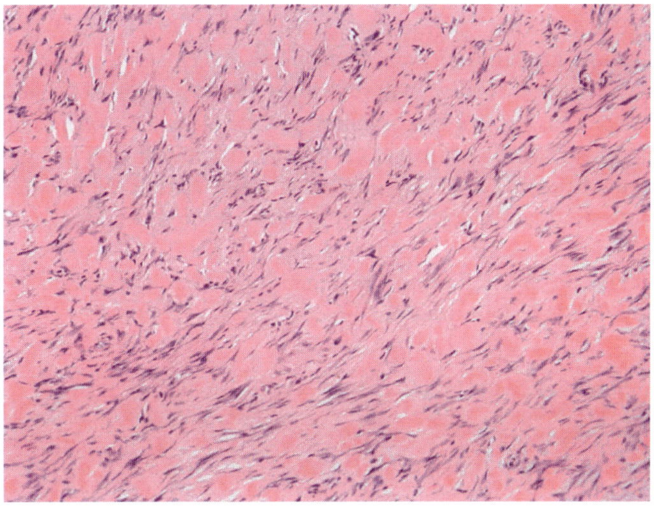

Figure 8.16 A proliferation of spindle fibroblasts and myofibroblasts in nodular fasciitis (X200).

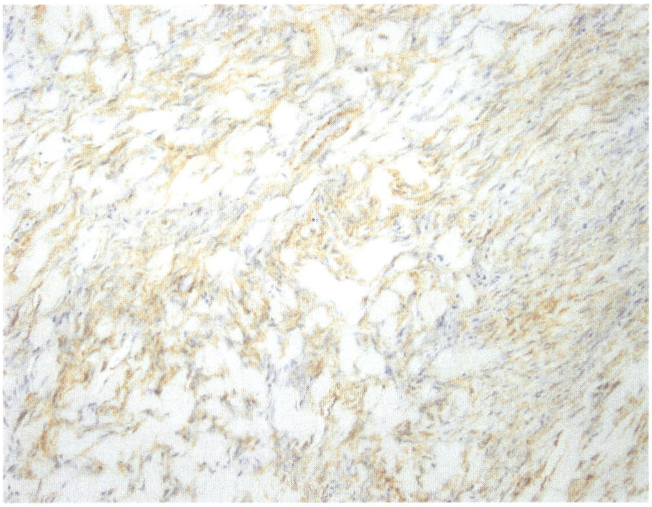

Figure 8.17 Nodular fasciitis. Cytoplasmic smooth muscle actin expression is seen (X200).

Nodular fasciitis

- SMA+

Proliferative Fasciitis and Proliferative Myositis

Proliferative fasciitis (if occurring in subcutis/fascia) and proliferative myositis (if occurring in muscle) demonstrate a proliferation of spindle cells with admixed ganglion-like cells (multinucleated cells with prominent nucleoli) in a collagenous to myxoid background.[49] The proliferation of spindle cells infiltrates surrounding tissue.[49] The lesional cells are typically positive for SMA and can be positive for desmin.[50] Relatively recent, recurrent *FOS* rearrangements have been identified in proliferative fasciitis/myositis and FOS immunohistochemistry may be of diagnostic utility.[51] Of note, proliferative fasciitis/myositis can be confused with sarcoma.[49]

Proliferative fasciitis/myositis

- SMA+ desmin -/+

Inflammatory Myofibroblastic Tumor

Inflammatory myofibroblastic tumors can show a spectrum of histologic appearances.[52] They typically demonstrate a multinodular yet well-demarcated proliferation of myofibroblastic cells in a myxoid to fibrous/collagenous background with abundant admixed inflammation (**Figure 8.18**).[52] There is variable expression of SMA, desmin, and cytokeratin. In the majority of lesions, *ALK* gene is fused with various genes including *TPM3*, *TPM4*, *CLTC*, *ATIC*, *RANBP2*, and *EML4*; this typically results in ALK expression by immunohistochemistry.[52] Recently *TFG::ROS1* and *ETV6::NTRK3* fusions have also been reported in a subset of cases.[53] By immunohistochemistry approximately 61% and 6% of inflammatory myofibroblastic tumors express ALK and ROS1, respectively (**Figure 8.19**).[53] The plasma cells are polyclonal and can express IgG4 in variable proportion. The histologic differential diagnosis includes reactive entities such as IgG4 related diseases (increase in IgG4 plasma cells with obliterative phlebitis and storiform fibrosis),[54] nodular fasciitis (*USP6* rearrangements), and sarcomas (such as low-grade myofibroblastic sarcoma). Molecular analysis for *ALK* rearrangements can be employed in challenging cases.

Inflammatory myofibroblastic tumor

- SMA+ desmin+/- keratins+/-
- Can be ALK+ or ROS1+

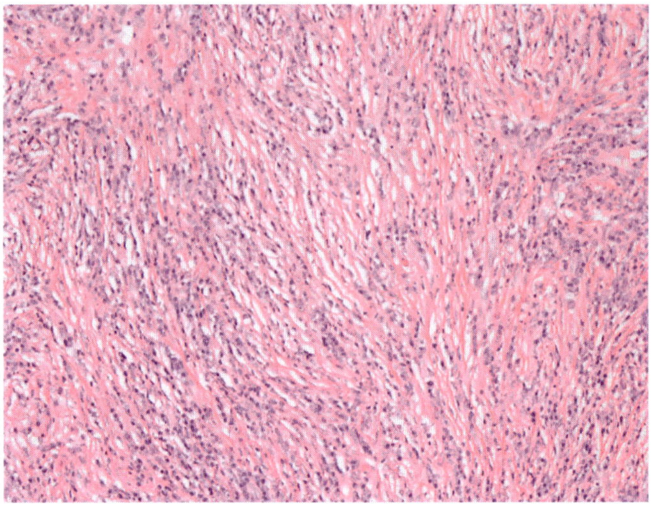

Figure 8.18 Inflammatory myofibroblastic tumor is characterized by a proliferation of spindle cells associated with abundant lymphoplasmacytic infiltrate (X200).

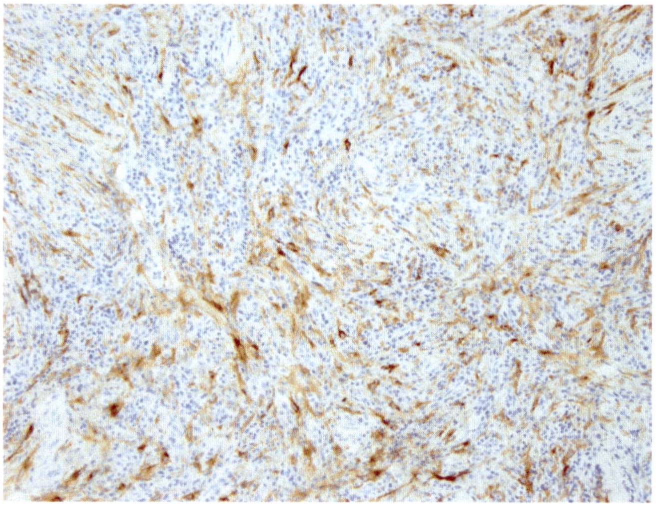

Figure 8.19 Inflammatory myofibroblastic tumor. ALK expression is noted in this case harboring *ALK* fusion (X200).

Myxoinflammatory Fibroblastic Sarcoma

Myxoinflammatory fibroblastic sarcoma (MIFS) is a locally destructive tumor that commonly occurs on acral areas.[55] Multiple cellular nodules of tumor are seen in the subcutaneous tissue. There is a spindled to epithelioid proliferation in a background of myxoid stroma and inflammation with scattered pleomorphic cells reminiscent of Reed-Sternberg cells, ganglion cells or virally infected cells (**Figure 8.20**).[55] There is variable expression for D2-40, CD68, CD163, factor 13a, CD34, cytokeratin, EMA, SMA, calponin, EGFR, clusterin, and CD117 (**Figures 8.21 and 8.22**).[56,57] The tumor is negative for CD15, CD30, CD45, Melan A, HMB45, desmin, CAM5.2, and glial fibrillary acidic protein.[56,57] Because of the variable expression, immunohistochemical studies are of limited utility but may be useful in excluding other entities such as vascular lesions (Erg+, CD34+, CD31+), epithelioid sarcoma (CD34+/- keratin+ INI-), and inflammatory myofibroblastic tumor (SMA+/-, ALK+/-).

Myxoinflammatory fibroblastic sarcoma

- Variable expression of CD34, CD68, SMA, D2–40, CD117, EMA

Superficial Acral Fibromyxoma

Superficial acral fibromyxoma exhibits a predilection for the digits and rarely occurs on the palms and soles (**Figure 8.23**).[58] A fascicular proliferation of spindle or stellate cells is seen within a hyalinized and myxoid stroma. The tumor cells express CD34 (**Figure 8.24**), and can be focally positive for EMA, SMA, and desmin.[58] They are negative for pan keratin, keratins AE1/AE3, CAM5.2, S100, MUC4, GFAP, claudin, and neurofilament.[58] Expression of CD10 and nestin in some cases have been recently reported. Of note, loss of *RB1* nuclear staining can be diagnostically helpful.[59] The histologic differential diagnosis includes cellular digital fibroma, cutaneous myxoma/superficial angiomyxoma (CD34- PRKAR1A loss),[58] perineurioma (claudin-1+, EMA+, GLUT-1+), and low-grade fibromyxoid sarcoma (MUC4+).[60]

Although cellular digital fibroma also expresses CD34 and factor 13a, it is less myxoid than superficial acral fibromyxoma and negative for EMA and CD99. Cellular myxoma of soft tissue is positive for CD34; however, it would harbor the *GNAS1*-activating mutation.[58] Sclerosing perineurioma would express claudin, EMA and GLUT1, and negative for CD34. Superficial acral fibromyxoma would be negative for MUC4, a marker for low-grade fibromyxoid sarcoma.[60]

Superficial acral fibromyxoma

- CD34+ Rb1 loss

Low Grade Fibromyxoid Sarcoma

Low grade fibromyxoid sarcoma (LGFMS) is a rare fibroblastic neoplasm with a predilection for young male adults and the deep soft tissues of extremities or trunk. It is comprised of monomorphic spindle cells within an alternating collagenous and myxoid stroma (**Figure 8.25**). Although it has bland histologic appearance which can be confused with a benign neoplasm, LGFMS can recur in 10% or metastasize in 5% of the cases, even when widely excised.[60] A recurrent and balanced translocation t(7;16) (q32-34;p11) involving *FUS* and *CREB3L2* or *CREB3L1* genes has been shown to be pathognomonic for LGFMS.[61] The mucin 4 (*MUC4*) gene, located on the long arm of chromosome 3 (3q29), has recently been shown to be upregulated in LGFMS and there was corresponding overexpression of MUC4 at the protein level.[61] Mucin 4 is a transmembrane glycoprotein expressed on many normal epithelia and is overexpressed or aberrantly expressed in many carcinomas. *MUC4* promotes cell proliferation and survival by interacting with the ErbB/HER2 family of growth factor receptors. The high

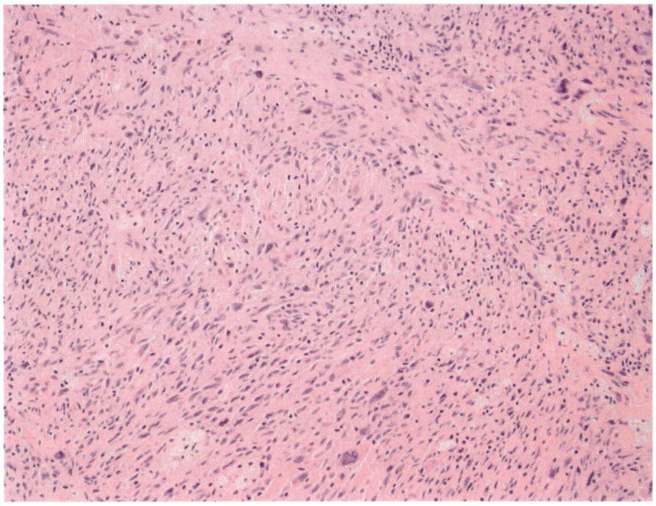

Figure 8.20 Myxoinflammatory fibroblastic sarcoma is characterized by markedly atypical cells and cellular spindle cells (X200).

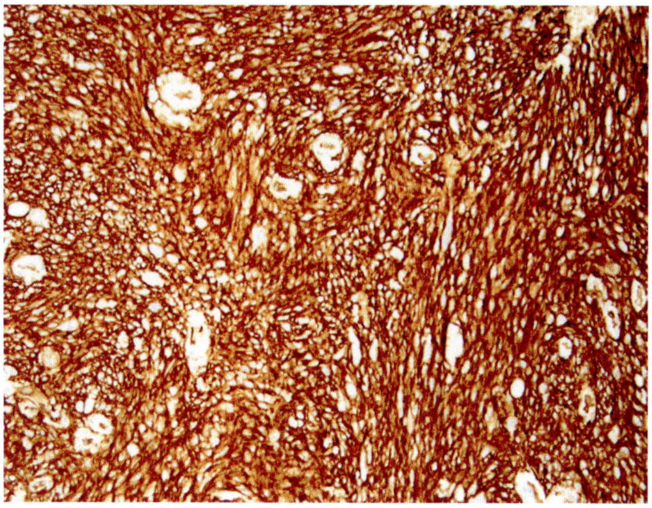

Figure 8.21 Myxoinflammatory fibroblastic sarcoma. Diffuse and strong CD34 expression (X200).

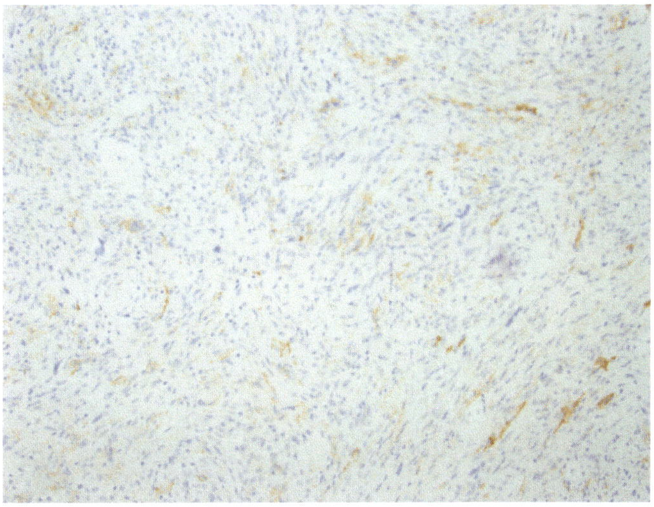

Figure 8.22 Myxoinflammatory fibroblastic sarcoma. Focal EMA positivity (X200).

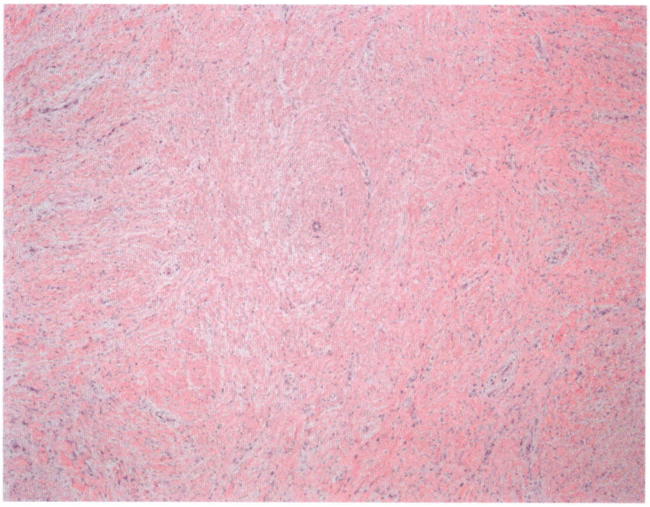

Figure 8.23 A proliferation of spindle or stellate cells in a collagenous and myxoid stroma in superficial acral fibromyxoma (X100).

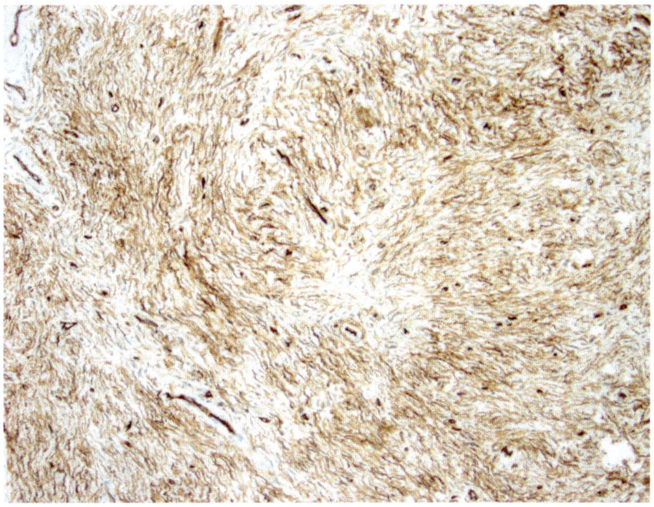

Figure 8.24 Superficial acral fibromyxoma. The tumor cells are positive for CD34 (X200).

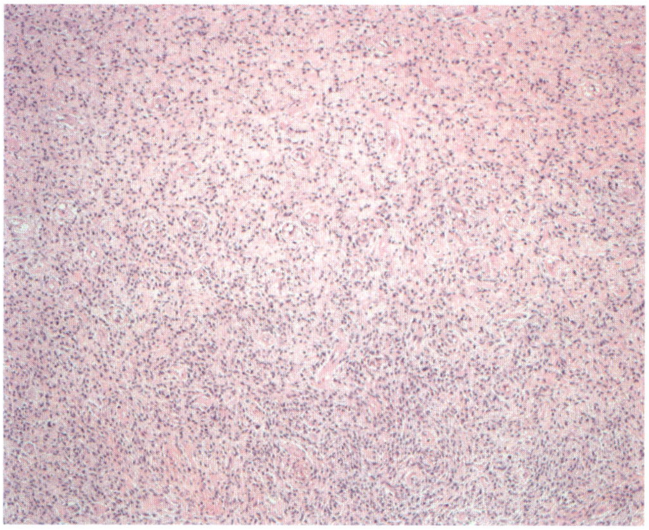

Figure 8.25 Bland and uniform spindle cells within a myxoid stroma in low grade fibromyxoid sarcoma (X100).

Table 8.2 MUC4 expression in low-grade fibromyxoid sarcoma

References	N	Sensitivity	Specificity
Moller 2011[69]	48	100%	100%
Doyle 2011[68]	309	100%	99%

specificity and sensitivity of MUC4 immunostain as a diagnostic marker for LGFMS has been confirmed in large series of LGFMS (**Figure 8.26**) (**Table 8.2**).[60]

Low grade fibromyxoid sarcoma

- MUC4+

Dermatofibrosarcoma Protuberans

Dermatofibrosarcoma protuberans (DFSP) is a tumor that often recurs locally and uncommonly metastasizes.[11] DFSP is composed of spindled cells that occupy the dermis and infiltrate into the subcutaneous tissue in a "honeycomb" pattern (**Figure 8.27**).[11] They are typically diffusely positive for CD34 (in contrast with dermatofibroma) (**Figure 8.28**) and are frequently without intermingled CD68/CD163+ histiocytes (**Figure 8.29**). A characteristic *COL1A1::PDGFB* gene rearrangement is identified.[11] Several variants of DFSP exist including myxoid, pigmented, atrophic and sclerosing.[62] Fibrosarcomatous transformation can be seen in 10–20% of DFSP and shows an abrupt transition from areas of conventional DFSP to more cellular, mitotically active areas with a "herringbone" pattern (**Figure 8.30**).[62] Fibrosarcomatous transformation portends a worse prognosis with an associated significant risk of metastasis.[62] Of note, CD34 expression can be lost in areas of fibrosarcomatous transformation (**Figure 8.31**).[62] The histologic differential diagnosis in the skin includes dermatofibroma (CD34- with numerous intermingled factor 13a dendrocytes). In challenging cases or in small biopsies, molecular studies to identify a *COL1A1::PDGFB* gene rearrangement can be of utility. Of interest, the sarcomatous

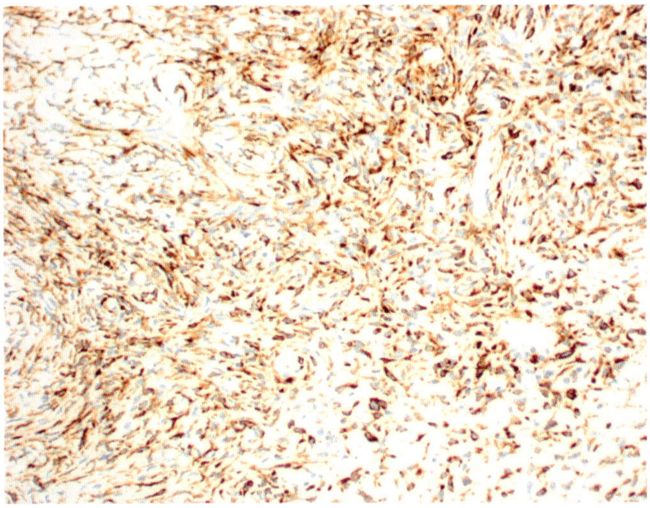

Figure 8.26 Low grade fibromyxoid sarcoma. Diffuse MUC4 expression is noted (X200).

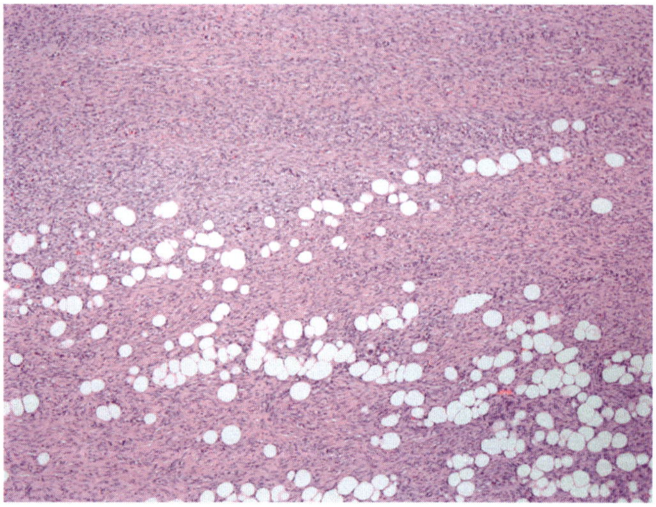

Figure 8.27 Storiform proliferation of spindle cells extending into the subcutaneous tissue in dermatofibrosarcoma protuberans (X100).

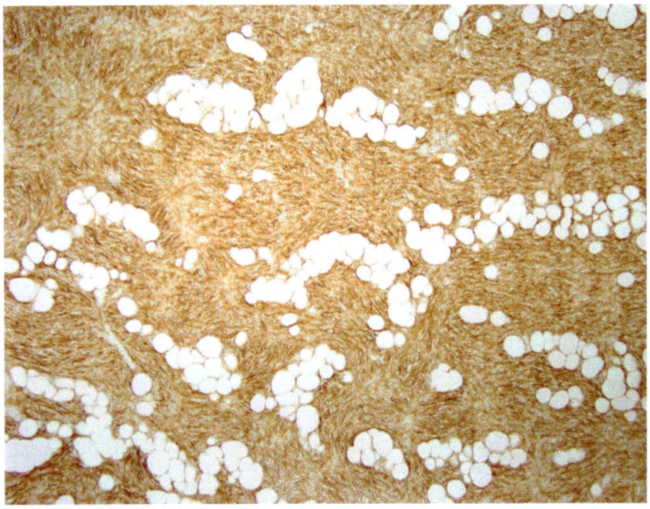

Figure 8.28 Dermatofibrosarcoma protuberans. Diffuse and strong CD34 expression by the tumor cells (X200).

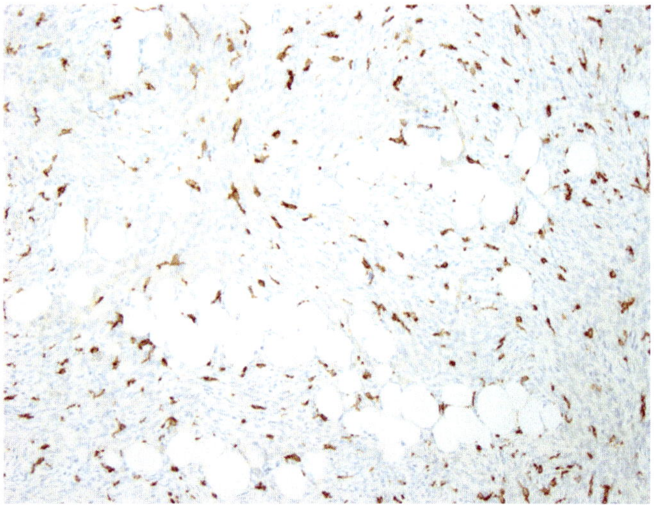

Figure 8.29 Dermatofibrosarcoma protuberans. They are negative for CD163 (X200).

areas harbor more frequently the *COL1A1::PFGFB* fusion gene than the conventional DFSP areas.[63]

Dermatofibrosarcoma protuberans

- CD34+
- Loss of CD34 expression in the fibrosarcomatous area

Giant Cell Fibroblastoma

Giant cell fibroblastoma is related to DFSP and "hybrid" lesions have been identified.[64] Giant cell fibroblastoma, like DFSP, also frequently harbors a *COL1A1::PDGFB* gene rearrangement.[64] Giant cell fibroblastoma commonly occurs in children but can occur in adults as well.[64] Histologically they are variably cellular lesions that infiltrate the dermis and subcutis.[64] Pseudovascular spaces lined by giant cells can be identified.[64] Like DFSP, the lesional cells are positive for CD34. The histologic differential diagnosis can include an atypical lipomatous tumor (MDM2+ CDK4+) and a vascular lesion (Erg+, CD31+).

Giant cell fibroblastoma

- CD34+

Plexiform Fibrohistiocytic Tumor

Plexiform fibrohistiocytic tumor is a tumor of dermis and subcutaneous tissue that occurs in children and young adults.[65] The tumor can recur and metastasize to regional lymph nodes but rarely metastasizes widely.[65] On histologic sections plexiform fibrohistiocytic tumor often has two components: (1) fascicles of spindle cells arranged in a plexiform pattern and (2) nodules of round histiocytic cells with osteoclast-like giant cells. While the spindle cells are positive for SMA, the mononuclear and multinucleated cells are positive for CD68 (**Figures 8.32 and 8.33**). Both cell types are negative for S100, HMB-45, lysozyme,

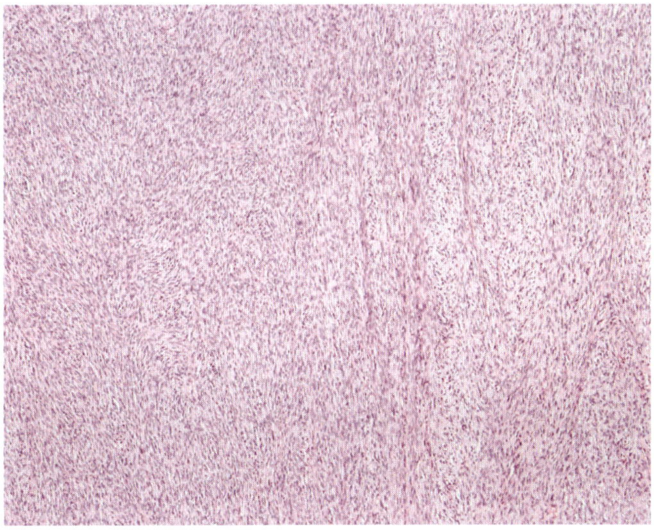

Figure 8.30 Dermatofibrosarcoma protuberans. Fibrosarcomatous transformation is characterized by cellular area with "herringbone" pattern (X100).

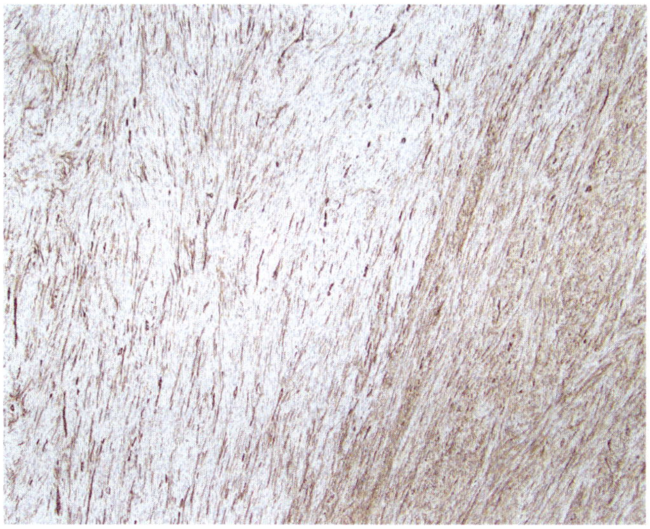

Figure 8.31 Loss of CD34 expression is noted in area of fibrosarcomatous transformation (X200).

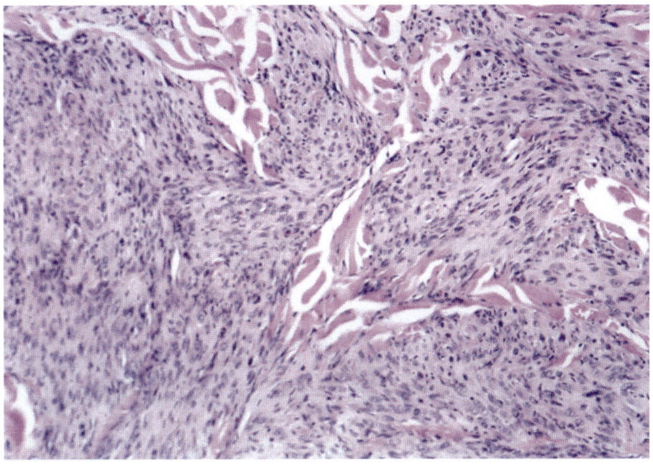

Figure 8.32 A dermal and plexiform proliferation of fibrohistiocytic cells seen in plexiform fibrohistiocytic tumor (X100).

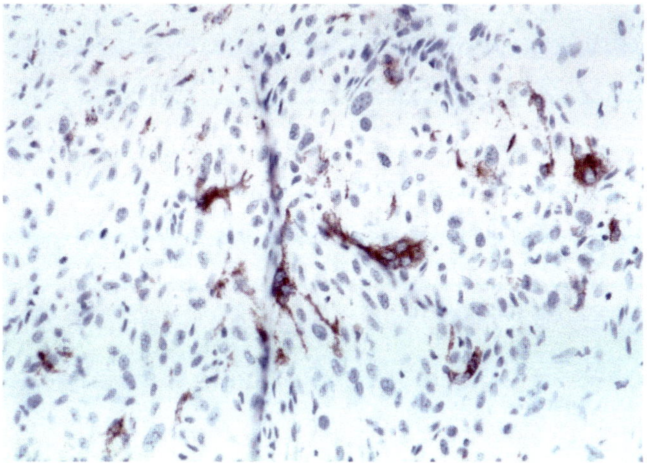

Figure 8.33 Plexiform fibrohistiocytic tumor. CD68 highlights the multinucleated giant cells (X200).

cytokeratins, desmin, factor 13a, factor VIII, and CD34. The differential diagnosis includes a melanocytic lesion (Sox10+, S100+, Melan-A+, HMB-45+) and a cellular neurothekeoma (MiTF+, CD63/NKI/C3+, and PGP9.5+).[65]

Plexiform fibrohistiocytic tumor

- Spindle cells: SMA+
- Mononuclear and multinucleated cells: CD68+

EWSR1::SMAD3 Rearranged Fibroblastic Tumor

These tumors tend to occur in the subcutaneous tissues of the distal extremities (hands/feet).[4] Histologically they are composed of cellular areas with spindled cells and hypocellular, hyalinized areas.[4] Characteristically, there is strong, diffuse expression of Erg in the lesional cells without staining for Sox10, S100, SMA, desmin, and keratins.[4] These unique immunohistochemical profile coupled with the histologic findings excludes many entities in the differential diagnosis. Additional molecular studies to identify a *EWSR1::SMAD3* gene rearrangement can be pursued in challenging cases.

***EWSR1::SMAD3* rearranged fibroblastic tumor**

- Erg+ SMA- CD34- S100- keratin-

Lipofibromatosis

Lipofibromatosis frequently occurs in in the distal extremities (hands/feet) of infants and children.[66] The lesion is composed of infiltrating bundles of fibroblastic spindled cells and adipose tissue.[66] The spindled cells are typically positive for CD34 and SMA and negative for desmin and keratins.[66] Of note, the spindled cells can exhibit focal, variable staining for S100.[66] The histologic differential diagnosis includes fibrous hamartoma of infancy (presence of primitive myxoid mesenchyme), lipofibromatosis-like neural tumor (CD34+ S100+, panTRK+/-), palmar/plantar fibromatosis (absence of adipocytic component), and inclusion body fibromatosis (presence of prominent cytoplasmic inclusions).

Lipofibromatosis

- CD34+ SMA+

NTRK-Rearranged Spindle Cell Neoplasm/ Lipofibromatosis-Like Neural Tumor

NTRK-rearranged spindle cell neoplasms (also known as lipofibromatosis-like neural tumor) occur in patients of a wide age range.[5] Histologically lipofibromatosis-like neural tumors resemble lipofibromatosis, however, lipofibromatosis-like neural tumors can demonstrate more cytologic atypia and mitotic activity (≤2/10hpf) (**Figure 8.34**).[5] Additionally, lipofibromatosis-like neural tumors have been reported to demonstrate CD34 and S100 reactivity (**Figure 8.35**) in the spindle cells and gene rearrangements involving *NTRK* have been reported (with corresponding panTRK immunohistochemical expression) (**Figure 8.36**).[5] Variable/multifocal staining for SMA has been reported.[5] The histologic differential diagnosis includes DFSP (CD34+ S100-), schwannoma/neurofibroma (Sox10+), malignant peripheral nerve sheath tumor (H3K27me3 loss and S100 variable), and lipofibromatosis (CD34+ S100 -/variable). In challenging cases, molecular analysis for an *NTRK* gene rearrangement can be helpful.

***NTRK*-rearranged spindle cell neoplasm/lipofibromatosis-like neural tumor**

- panTRK/NTRK+ CD34+ S100+ SMA+/-

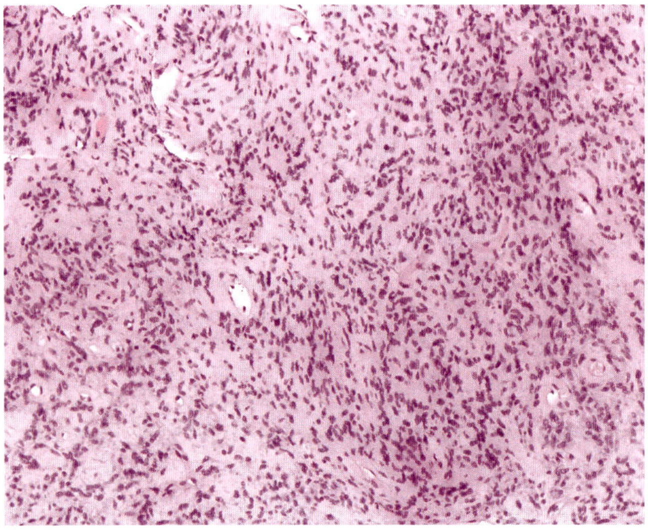

Figure 8.34 A low-grade spindle cell neoplasm with *EML4::NTRK3* fusion (X200).

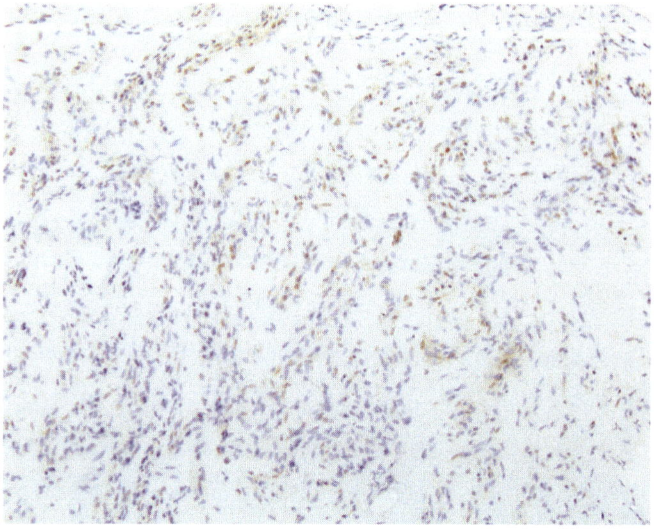

Figure 8.35 *NTRK*-rearranged spindle cell neoplasm. Focal S100 expression (X200).

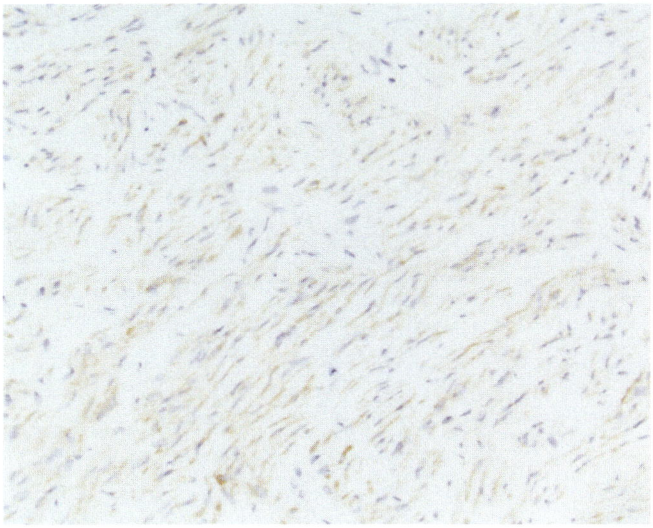

Figure 8.36 *NTRK*-rearranged spindle cell neoplasm. Diffuse pan-TRK expression (X200).

Dermatomyofibroma

Dermatomyofibromas are typically found as solitary lesions in children and young adults.[67] Dermatomyofibromas have a plaque-like outline and are composed of banal-appearing spindled cells, typically parallel to the epidermis.[67] Positive staining for calponin and variable staining for CD34 and SMA has been reported while desmin is negative.[67] The histologic differential diagnosis includes dermatofibroma (admixed factor 13a+ dendrocytes, CD68+ histiocytes with peripheral collagen trapping) and DFSP (diffuse CD34+ with infiltration of the subcutis).

Dermatomyofibroma

- Calponin+, CD34+/-, SMA+/-

Angiofibroma of Soft Tissue

Angiofibroma of soft tissue typically occurs in the lower extremities of adults.[68] Histologically they demonstrate a proliferation of spindled cells in a myxoid, collagenous or myxoid and collagenous background with prominent vessels.[68] Focal EMA expression is not infrequently seen while CD34, SMA, and desmin are frequently negative in the spindled cells (but can be focally positive).[68] A recurrent gene rearrangement involving *AHRR* and *NCOA2* has been consistently identified.[69] The differential diagnosis includes low-grade fibromyxoid sarcoma (MUC4+), myxoid liposarcoma (DDIT3+ with lipoblasts), myxofibrosarcoma (infiltrative growth pattern), and solitary fibrous tumor (STAT6+).

Angiofibroma of soft tissue

- EMA+/- CD34-/+ SMA-/+

Cellular Angiofibroma

Cellular angiofibroma typically occurs in the inguinal/genital region of men and women.[70] There are overlapping histologic and immunohistochemical features among cellular angiofibroma, spindle cell lipoma, and mammary type myofibroblastoma. A monoallelic loss of *RB1* and *FOXO1*, located on 13q14, has been documented in these tumors, suggesting that they are tumors within the same spectrum.[70]

Cellular angiofibroma is well-circumscribed with evenly distributed, small to medium-sized vessels with hyalinized walls. The tumor cells are spindled and bland and arranged in short intersecting fascicles **(Figure 8.37)**. Cytologic atypia and even sarcomatous change have been reported in a series of 13 cases from the vulva; however, follow-up of 7 cases with a median of 14 months did not show evidence of recurrence or metastases.[71] The sarcomatous component can resemble atypical lipomatous tumor, pleomorphic liposarcoma, and undifferentiated pleomorphic sarcoma. The lesional cells can express CD34, SMA and rarely, desmin **(Figures 8.38 and 8.39)**.[72] They may also express ER and PR and can show loss of Rb expression.[70,73] The differential diagnosis includes deep (aggressive) angiomyxoma (desmin+ with hypocellular and myxoid areas) and angiomyofibroblastoma (desmin+ with tumor cells surrounding vessels).

Cellular angiofibroma

- CD34+/-, SMA+/-, desmin-, Rb loss

Angiomyofibroblastoma

Angiomyofibroblastoma typically presents on the vulva of women during reproductive years. On histologic sections, they are well-demarcated masses with alternating hypercellular and hypocellular areas with multinucleated cells and epithelioid/ plasmacytoid cells that tend to aggregate around blood

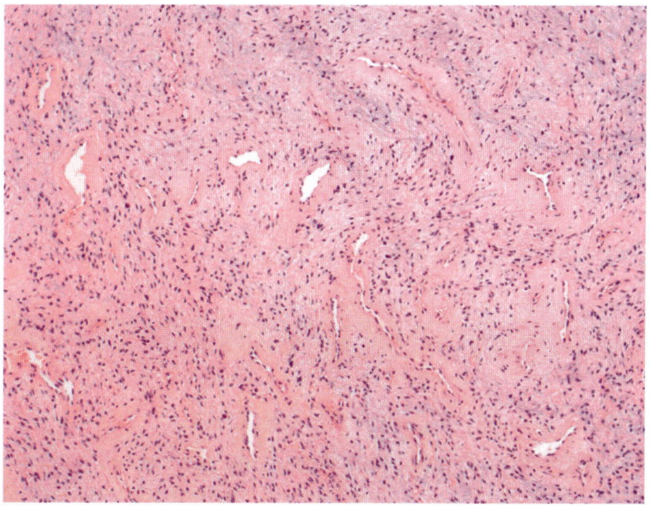

Figure 8.37 In cellular angiomyoma spindled and bland tumor cells are seen surrounding small to medium-sized vessels with hyalinized wall (X100).

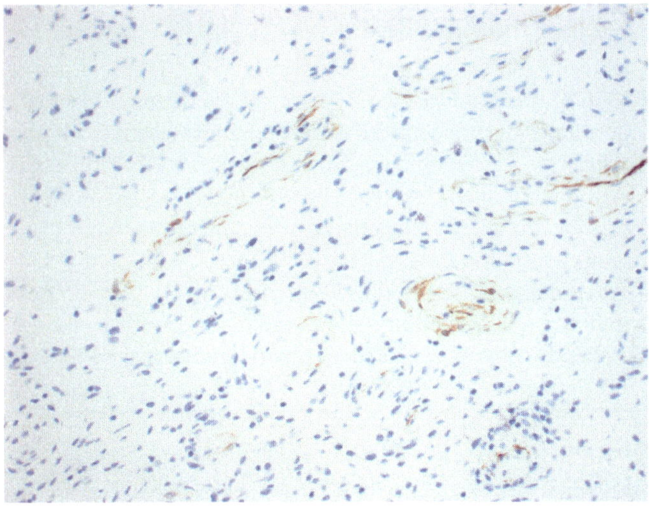

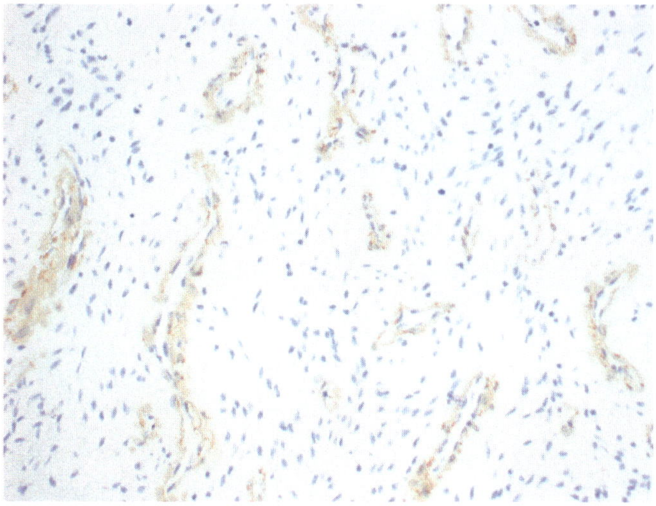

Figures 8.38 and 8.39 Cellular angiomyoma. The tumor cells are negative for desmin (X200) and smooth muscle actin (X200).

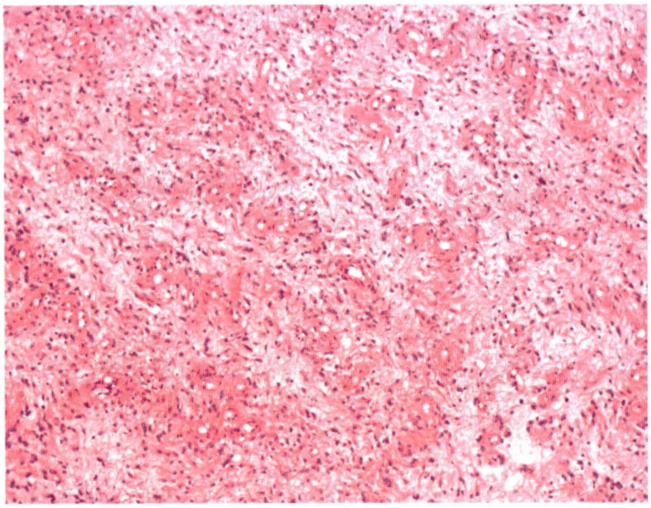

Figure 8.40 Alternating hypercellular and hypocellular areas are seen in angiomyofibroblastoma (X100).

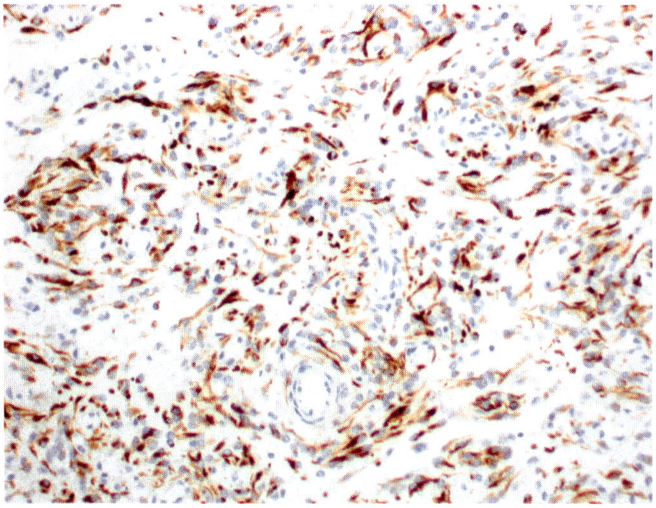

Figure 8.41 Angiomyofibroblastoma. The tumor cells are positive for desmin (X200).

vessels (**Figure 8.40**). The tumor cells are positive for desmin, and variably so for SMA, ER, and PR (**Figures 8.41 and 8.42**). They are typically negative for S100, CD34, EMA, and cytokeratin.[74,75] The differential diagnosis includes cellular angiofibroma (desmin- RB1 loss) and aggressive angiomyxoma (hypocellular and myxoid).

Angiomyofibroblastoma

- Desmin+, SMA+/-, CD34-

Low-Grade Myofibroblastic Sarcoma

Myofibroblastic sarcoma is a low-grade spindle cell sarcoma with myofibroblastic differentiation. Histologic examination shows a diffuse and infiltrative proliferation of atypical spindle tumor cells arranged in fascicles.[76] The tumor cells are typically

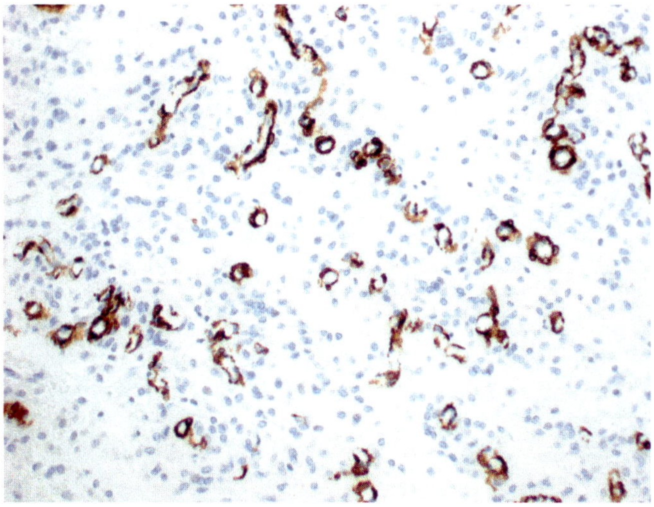

Figure 8.42 Angiomyofibroblastoma. They are negative for smooth muscle actin (X200).

positive for SMA, and calponin and can express desmin.[76] They are negative for h-caldesmon, S100, cytokeratin, and CD34.[76] They can show nuclear positivity for β-catenin.[77] The histologic differential diagnosis includes desmoid fibromatosis (β-catenin with WNT/β-catenin pathway mutations), leiomyosarcoma (desmin+, caldesmon+, SMA+), nodular fasciitis (*USP6* rearrangements), and reactive processes.

Myofibroblastic sarcoma

- SMA+, calponin+, desmin+/-

Myxofibrosarcoma

Myoxfibrosarcoma commonly arises in the extremities of older patients and can be low, intermediate, or high-grade.[78] Histologic examination shows a multinodular architecture with a proliferation of spindled to epithelioid, pleomorphic cells in a myxoid background.[78] The tumor cells can be positive for CD34 and SMA.[78,79] Myxofibrosarcoma frequently locally recurs and metastasizes.[78] The histologic differential diagnosis includes undifferentiated pleomorphic sarcoma (lack of myxoid background), low-grade fibromyxoid sarcoma (MUC4+), malignant peripheral nerve sheath tumor (Sox10/S100 patchy staining with H3K27me3 loss), and myxoid liposarcoma (DDIT3+ with lipoblasts and adipocytes).

Myxofibrosarcoma

- CD34+/- SMA+/-

8.2 Smooth Muscle Neoplasms

Smooth muscle neoplasms are typically positive for alpha-smooth muscle actin (SMA), desmin, and h-caldesmon.[80] Smooth muscle myosin can also be of utility in identifying smooth muscle differentiation.[80] Of note, expression of SMA and desmin can be seen in other tumors besides smooth muscle neoplasms.[80] Variable or loss of staining for immunohistochemical markers for smooth muscle differentiation can also be seen in moderately to poorly differentiated smooth muscle tumors.[80]

Leiomyoma

Cutaneous leiomyomas are well-differentiated, benign smooth muscle tumors that are thought to arise from normal structures such as arrector pilar smooth muscle (piloleiomyomas), dartoic/vulvar smooth muscle (genital leiomyomas), or areolar smooth muscle (nipple/mammary leiomyomas).[81] Histologically, the lesional cells are described with eosinophilic cytoplasm and "cigar"-shaped nuclei arranged in fascicles.[81] Although lesions can be poorly delineated (e.g. piloleiomyomas), significant mitotic activity or nuclear pleomorphism should be absent.[81] Leiomyomas should stain positively for SMA, desmin, and h-caldesmon. Leiomyomas of the vulva and areola express estrogen receptor and progesterone receptor.[82] The histologic differential includes dermatomyofibroma (SMA+/- and desmin-) and an atypical intradermal smooth muscle neoplasm/leiomyosarcoma (more significant mitotic activity and nuclear pleomorphism). Of note, the presence of multiple cutaneous leiomyomas should raise suspicion for hereditary leiomyomatosis, and renal cell carcinoma syndrome and cutaneous leiomyomas can show loss of fumarate hydratase (FH) by immunohistochemistry as well as increased expression of 2-succinocysteine (2SC).[83]

Leiomyoma

- SMA+ desmin+ h-caldesmon+

Atypical Intradermal Smooth Muscle Neoplasm/ Leiomyosarcoma

Cutaneous, well-differentiated smooth muscle tumors that are confined to the dermis and demonstrate more significant mitotic activity and nuclear pleomorphism than cutaneous leiomyomas can be classified as atypical intradermal smooth muscle neoplasms (**Figures 8.43 and 8.44**).[84] Atypical

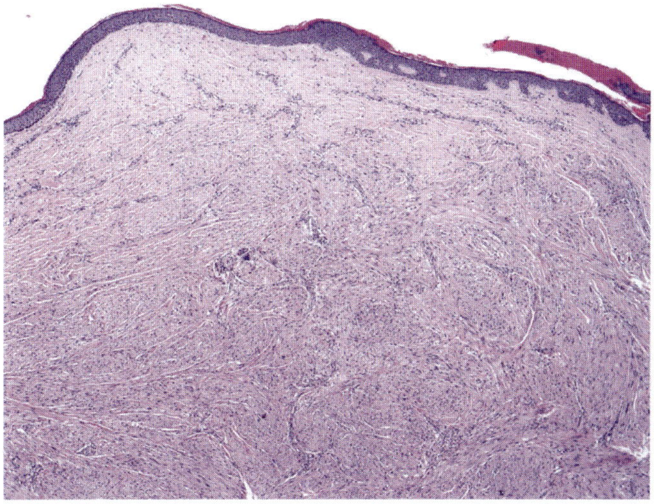

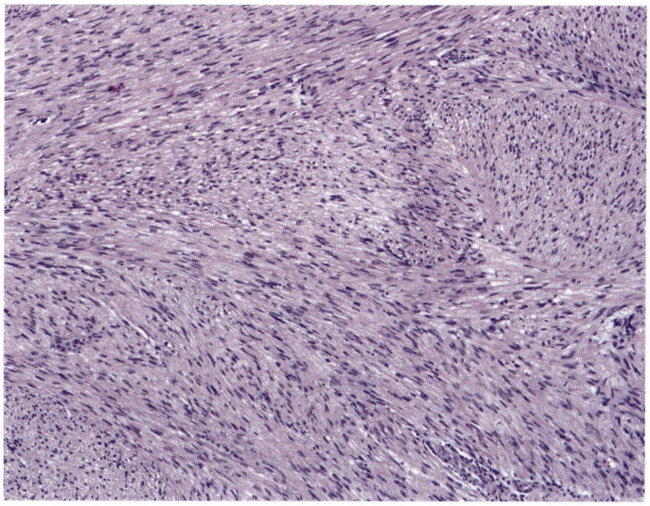

Figures 8.43 and 8.44 Proliferation of dermal fascicles of spindle cells in an atypical intradermal smooth muscle neoplasm (X40, X100).

intradermal smooth muscle neoplasms tend to recur locally and rarely metastasize which is why some have advocated pathologists avoid the term leiomyosarcoma to describe atypical smooth muscle tumors confined to the dermis.[84] Atypical smooth muscle tumors that extensively involve the subcutaneous tissue or that seem to arise in the subcutis may behave distinctly, with a possibly significant risk of metastasis.[84] Such subcutaneous lesions may justifiably be classified as leiomyosarcomas. Atypical intradermal smooth muscle tumors almost always express SMA, desmin, and caldesmon and can be focally positive for keratins (**Figure 8.45**).[84] The histologic differential diagnosis includes a cutaneous leiomyoma (less mitotic activity and nuclear pleomorphism).

EBV-Associated Smooth Muscle Tumor

Epstein-Barr virus (EBV)-associated smooth muscle tumors occur in immunosuppressed patients and present as circumscribed tumors with smooth muscle differentiation (**Figure 8.46**).[85] Admixed lymphocytes are commonly identified and background myxoid change can be seen.[85] These tumors express SMA (**Figure 8.47**), desmin and h-caldesmon and are positive for EBV by *in-situ* hybridization (**Figure 8.48**). Histologic findings including increased necrosis, mitotic activity, and nuclear pleomorphism can be seen although it is unclear if these findings impact prognosis and metastatic potential.[85] The differential diagnosis includes other smooth muscle tumors (SMA+, desmin+, h-caldesmon+ but EBV-).

Atypical intradermal smooth muscle neoplasm

- SMA+, desmin+, h-caldesmon+

EBV-associated smooth muscle tumor

- SMA+, desmin+, h-caldesmon+, EBV+ (in-situ hybridization)

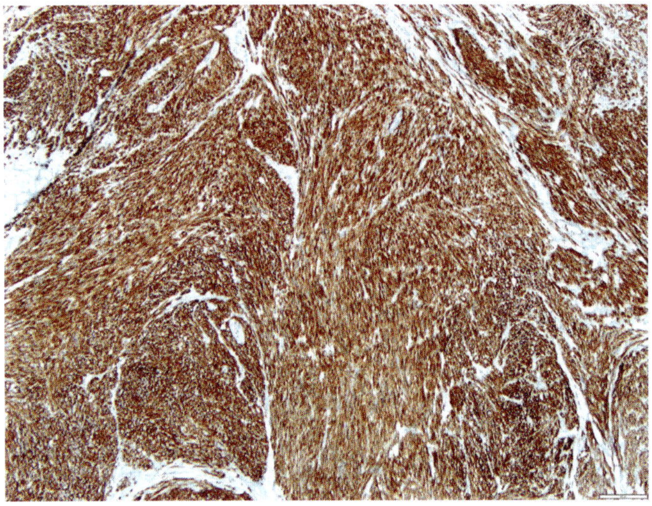

Figure 8.45 Atypical intradermal smooth muscle neoplasm. Diffuse and strong desmin expression (X100).

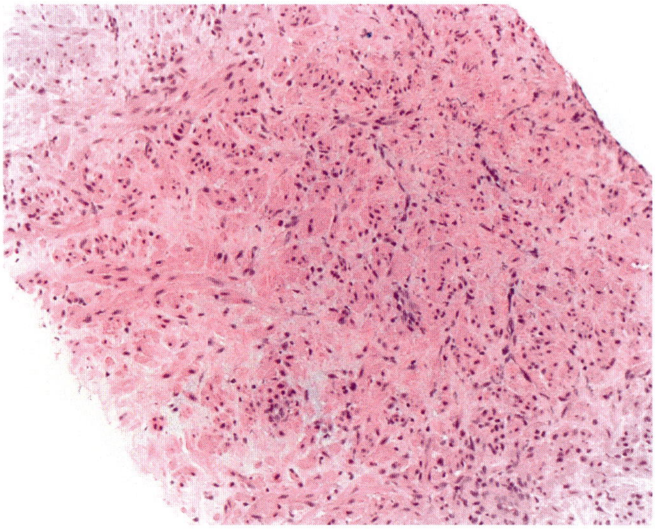

Figure 8.46 Atypical intradermal smooth muscle neoplasm. Bundles of smooth muscles with cigar-shaped nuclei and eosinophilic cytoplasm (X200).

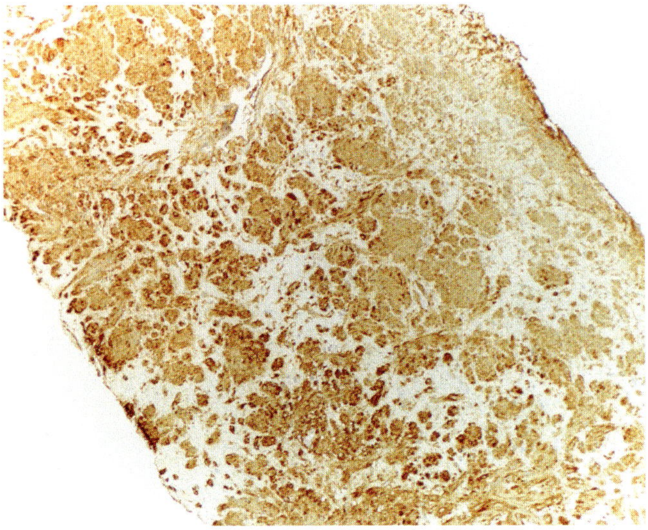

Figure 8.47 Atypical intradermal smooth muscle neoplasm. Strong, diffuse smooth muscle actin expression (X200).

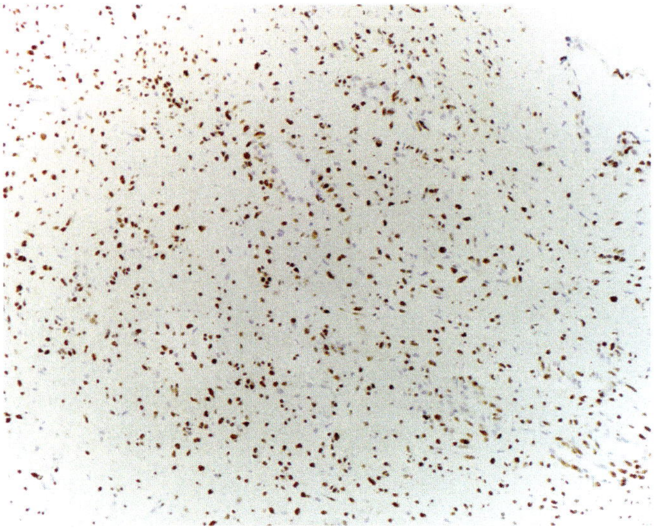

Figure 8.48 Ebstein-Barr virus (EBV) *in-situ* hybridization for is positive (nuclear expression) (X200).

8.3 Skeletal Muscle Neoplasms

Skeletal muscle tumors such as rhabdomyosarcoma are typically positive for desmin and myogenic-specific immunohistochemical markers include MyoD1 and myogenin.[80] Of note, rhabdomyosarcomatous differentiation can be seen in other tumors including liposarcoma, malignant peripheral nerve sheath tumor (Triton tumor), and melanoma.[80]

Rhabdomyoma

Rhabdomyomas are benign tumors with skeletal muscle differentiation and can be separated into adult-type, fetal-type, and genital-type. Adult-type rhabdomyomas are circumscribed with polygonal cells which can demonstrate cross-striations, rod-like structure, or vacuoles ("spider" cells).[86] Fetal type rhabdomyomas are also circumscribed and contain spindled/immature cells with skeletal muscle differentiation in a fibrous/myxoid background (**Figure 8.49**).[87] Slightly increased mitotic activity and some nuclear atypia can be identified in fetal type rhabdomyomas, but infiltrative growth should be absent.[87] Genital-type rhabdomyomas can occur in the female genital tract and male genital tract.[88] Genital-type rhabdomyomas occurring the female genital tract are typically polypoid and show rhabdomyoblasts with cross striations in a fibrous background.[88] Rhabdomyomas stain positively for desmin, myogenin, and MyoD1 (**Figure 8.50**). Rhabdomyomas are not infiltrative and typically do not show significantly elevated mitotic activity, hypercellularity, or severe nuclear pleomorphism, allowing separation from rhabdomyosarcoma.[87]

Rhabdomyoma

- Desmin+, myogenin+, MyoD1+

Rhabdomyosarcoma

Rhabdomyosarcomas are malignant soft tissue tumors that commonly occur in young individuals but also occurs in adults.[89] They have a number of subtypes including embryonal, alveolar, pleomorphic, and spindle cell/sclerosing (**Figure 8.51**). They are typically positive for desmin, myoD1, and myogenin (**Figures 8.52 and 8.53**).[80] Aberrant expression of S100, cytokeratin, synaptophysin, and NSE has been reported in rhabdomyosarcoma.[90]

Embryonal Rhabdomyosarcoma

Embryonal rhabdomyosarcoma commonly occurs in the head and neck area of young individuals.[89] Histologically, tumors show a mix of rhabdomyoblasts in various stages of differentiation in a myxoid background.[89] Botryoid embryonal rhabdomyosarcomas present as "grape-like" tumors and demonstrate condensation of tumor cells around epithelial structures (cambium layer).[89] The tumors stain positively for desmin, myogenin, and myoD1. The differential diagnosis includes other subtypes of rhabdomyosarcoma and may require molecular analysis to detect gene rearrangements.

Embryonal rhabdomyosarcoma

- Desmin+, myogenin+, myoD1+

Alveolar Rhabdomyosarcoma

Alveolar rhabdomyosarcoma also commonly occurs in young individuals and histological examination shows dyscohesive tumor cells in a background of fibrous septae, reminiscent of pulmonary alveolar spaces.[89] Gene rearrangements including *PAX3::FOXO1* and *PAX7::FOXO1* are commonly identified with the former portending a poorer prognosis.[89] By immunohistochemistry, diffuse, strong myogenin expression is characteristic with variable staining for desmin and myoD1.[89]

Alveolar rhabdomyosarcoma

- Myogenin+, desmin variable, myoD1 variable

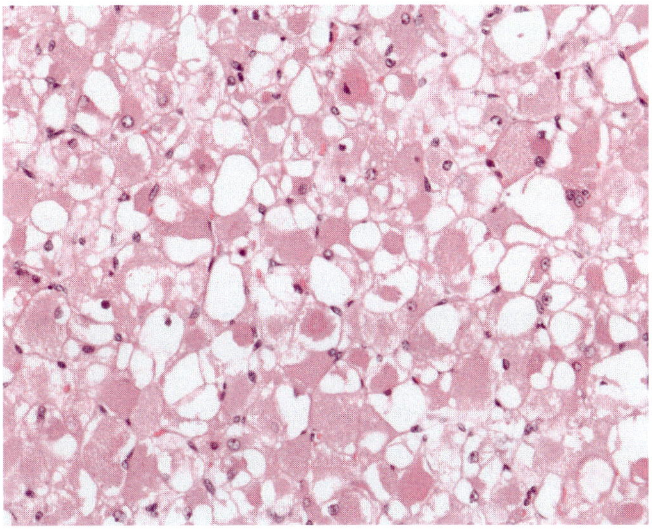

Figure 8.49 Rhabdomyoma. Eosinophilic and polygonal cells with skeletal muscle differentiation (X400).

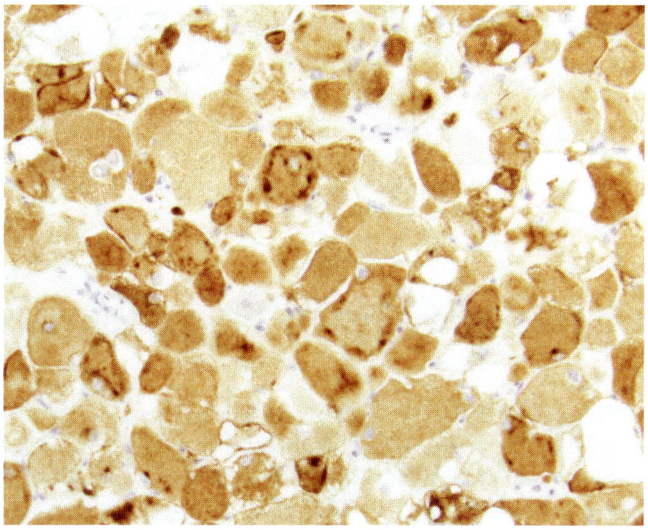

Figure 8.50 Rhabdomyoma. Strong desmin expression is noted (X400).

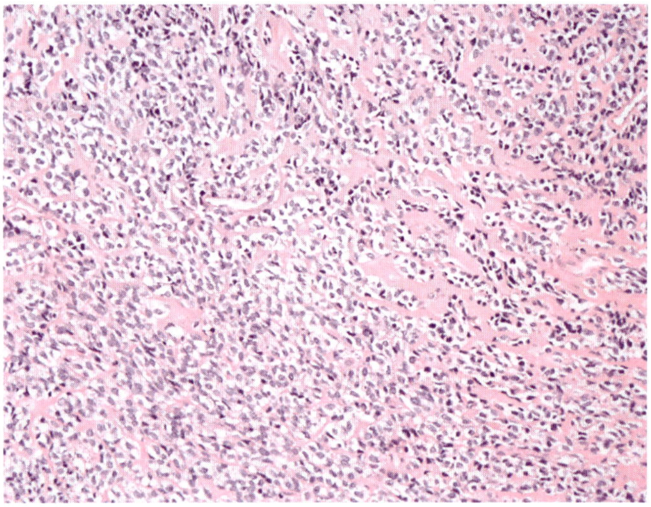

Figure 8.51 Round and hyperchromatic cells arranged in cellular nests are seen in rhabdomyosarcoma (X200).

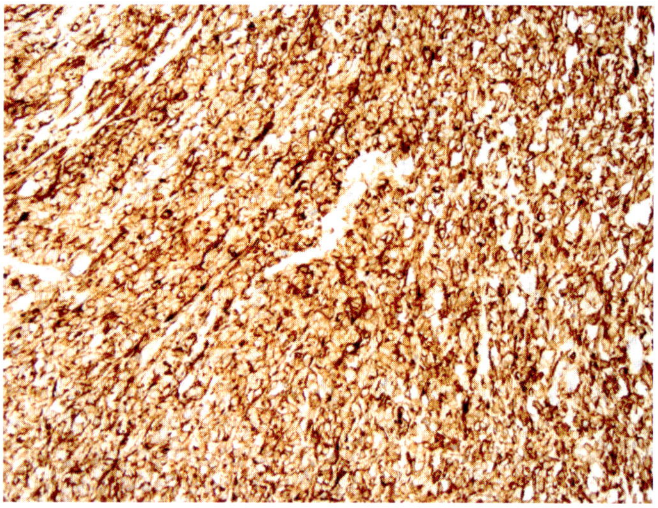

Figure 8.52 Rhabdomyosarcoma. Diffuse and strong desmin expression (X200).

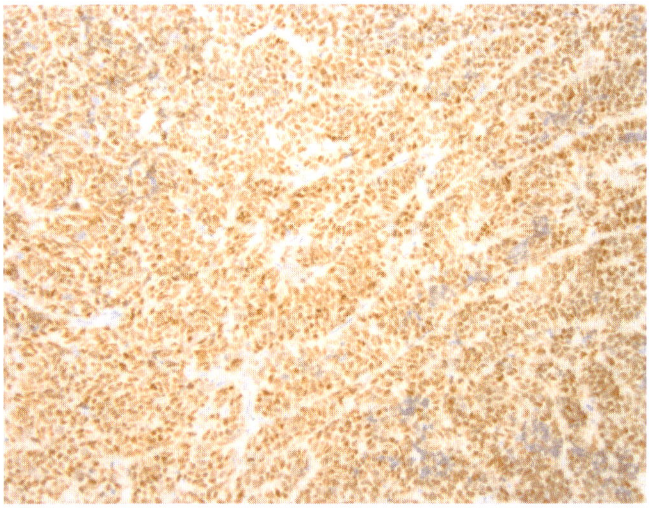

Figure 8.53 Rhabdomyosarcoma. Diffuse nuclear MyoD1 positivity (X200).

Pleomorphic Rhabdomyosarcoma

Pleomorphic rhabdomyosarcoma usually occurs in older adults and tumors show pleomorphic rhabdomyoblasts. Tumors are typically positive for desmin but staining for myogenin and myoD1 can be focal/limited. Recurrent molecular alterations have not been identified in pleomorphic rhabdomyosarcoma.[89] Clinical, histologic, and molecular data enable separation of pleomorphic rhabdomyosarcoma from other subtypes.

Pleomorphic rhabdomyosarcoma

- Desmin+, myogenin +/focal, myoD1 +/focal

Spindle Cell/Sclerosing Rhabdomyosarcoma

Spindle cell/sclerosing rhabdomyosarcoma can occur in the head and neck region of young individuals and adults.[91] Histologically they are characterized by fascicular proliferations of spindled rhabdomyoblasts which can occur in a background of hyalinization/sclerosis.[91] Undifferentiated areas of primitive cells can also be seen.[91] Molecularly, three separate groups are defined including those with *VGLL2* and *NCOA2* gene rearrangements, those with *MYOD1* L122 R mutations and those without any recurrent alterations.[91,92] By immunohistochemistry, tumors are positive for desmin and diffusely positive for myoD1 with variable/focal expression of myogenin.[91]

Spindle cell/sclerosing rhabdomyosarcoma

- Desmin+, myoD1 +, myogenin +/-

8.4 Neural Tumors

Neural tumors or tumors with nerve sheath differentiation are a heterogeneous group of tumors with both benign and malignant entities. Benign nerve sheath tumors like schwannoma and neurofibroma express S100 and Sox10 while entities like perineuriomas are S100 and Sox10 negative but express GLUT-1, claudin-1, and EMA.[80] Malignant nerve sheath tumors such as malignant peripheral nerve sheath tumor can lose expression of S100 and Sox10 and show loss of H3K27me3.[93]

Dermal Nerve Sheath Myxoma

Dermal nerve sheath myxoma is a peripheral nerve sheath tumor, predominantly developing on the extremities, particularly the fingers and knee. Histologic examination reveals a nodular to multinodular architecture pattern with abundant Schwann cells in a myxoid background (**Figure 8.54**).[94] Complete local excision with a margin of normal tissue is considered curative; a high local recurrence rate is seen when the lesion is incompletely excised.[94] By immunohistochemistry, lesional cells express S100, glial fibrillary acidic protein (GFAP), and Sox10 (**Figure 8.55**).[94,95] There is EMA reactivity in perineurial cells and CD34 expression in fibroblasts in the fibrous connective tissue bordering the myxoid nodules.[94] The histologic differential diagnosis includes neurofibroma (CD34+ fibroblasts and mast cells), superficial acral fibromyxoma (CD34+,

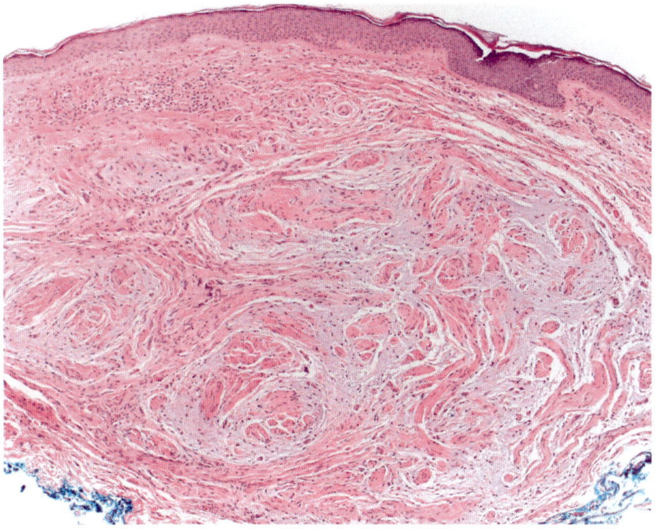

Figure 8.54 Dermal nerve sheath myxoma. Histologic sections show a multilobular proliferation of Schwann cells in a myxoid background (X100).

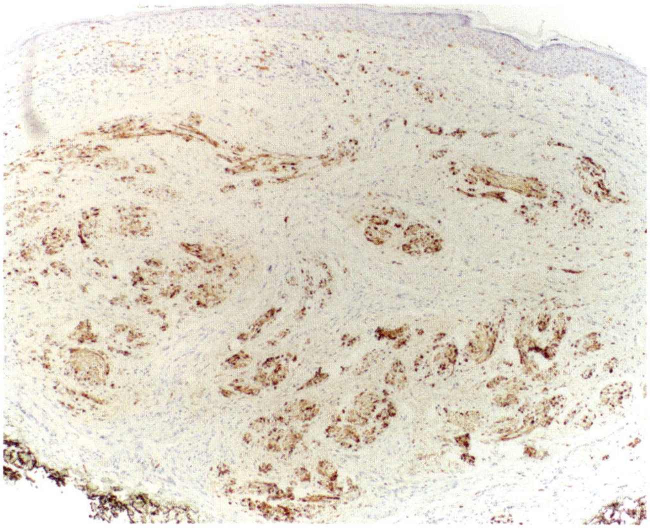

Figure 8.55 Dermal nerve sheath myxoma. S100 is positive in the Schwann cells (X100).

Rb loss, Sox10-, S100-), and cutaneous myxoma/superficial angiomyxoma (SMA+, CD34-, S100-, PRKAR1A loss).

Dermal nerve sheath myxoma

- S100+, Sox10+, GFAP+

Solitary Circumscribed Neuroma (Palisaded Encapsulated Neuroma)

Solitary circumscribed neuromas typically occur in the dermis of the skin and show a proliferation of Schwann cells that may be partially or completely encapsulated.[96] The Schwann cells are positive for S100 and Sox10 and entrapped neurofilaments can be highlighted with neurofilament protein.[96] The periphery of the lesion composed of perineural cells is positive for GLUT-1, EMA, and claudin-1. The histologic differential diagnosis includes neurofibroma (CD34+ intratumoral fibroblasts and mast cells) and schwannoma (prominent alternating hypocellular/hypercellular areas).

Solitary circumscribed neuroma

- S100+, Sox10+

Neurofibroma

Neurofibroma is a common benign nerve sheath tumor that is composed of an admixture of Schwann cells, axons, endoneurial fibroblasts, and perineurial-like cells. It can occur sporadically as a solitary polypoid or nodular soft lesion. It can present in the context of Neurofibromatosis 1 (NF1) or *von Recklinghausen* disease and is typically associated with a hyperpigmented epidermal macule, the "café-au-lait" spot.[97]

Neurofibromas can be localized, diffuse, or plexiform. The localized variant, the most common form of neurofibroma, is usually sporadic and does not have the risk to undergo malignant transformation. The diffuse and plexiform variants are often associated with neurofibromatosis. Importantly, the plexiform neurofibroma has a stronger association with neurofibromatosis and is more prone to malignant transformation than the other variants.[97] Other histologic variants include myxoid and pigmented neurofibroma.

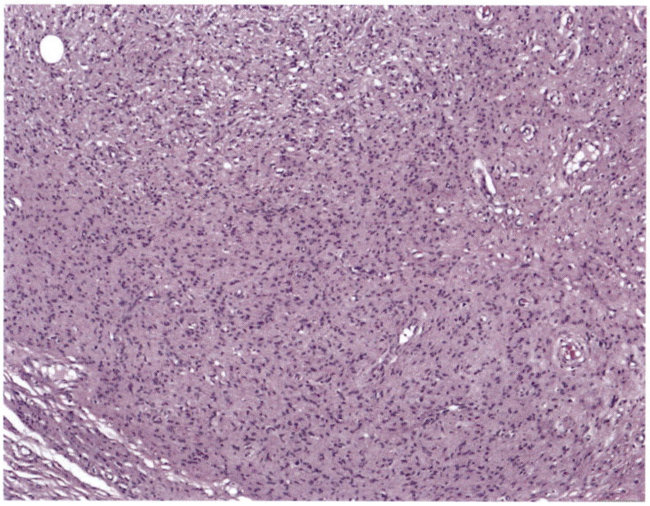

Figure 8.56 A proliferation of dermal bland spindle cells within a myxoid matrix in neurofibroma (X100).

Microscopically, neurofibromas are well-defined but non-encapsulated dermal or subcutaneous lesions that contain numerous small nerve fibers (**Figure 8.56**). Neurofibromas consist of bland spindle cells with wavy, tapered nuclei set in a fibrillary, collagenous, and sometimes myxoid stroma with scattered inflammatory cells (particularly mast cells). Mitotic figures are absent or rare. Of note, neurofibromas that demonstrate cytologic atypia, hypercellular areas, increased mitotic activity and loss of typical neurofibromatous architecture in the context of neurofibromatosis can be classified as atypical neurofibromas or atypical neurofibromatous neoplasm of uncertain biologic potential.[97]

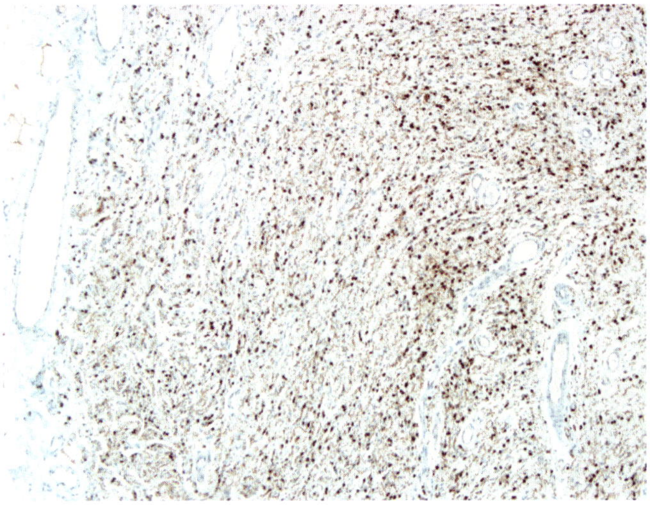

Figure 8.57 Neurofibroma. Strong S100 expression by the tumor cells (X200).

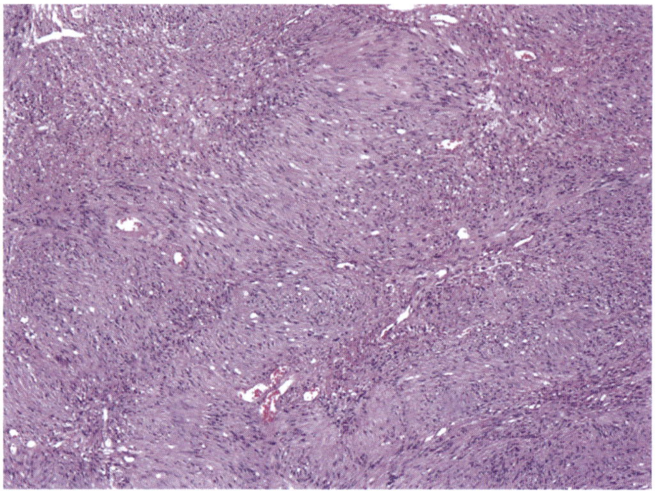

Figure 8.58 Schwannoma is characterized by cellular areas of nuclear palisade alternating with myxoid areas (X100).

The axons within neurofibromas stain with neurofilament, while the Schwann cells express S100, Sox10, CD57, and myelin basic protein (**Figure 8.57**).[95,98] Neurofibromas typically demonstrate a significant subpopulation of CD34-positive stromal cells, unlike most schwannomas.[99] In addition, the location of the expression of neurofilament has been reported to be useful in distinguishing neurofibroma from schwannoma, since the later displaces the nerve of origin and thus resulting in neurofilament expression at the periphery of the lesion. CD56 and calretinin are negative (or weakly focal) in neurofibroma and usually positive in schwannoma.[100] The histologic differential diagnosis includes schwannoma (diffuse S100+ and Sox10+ without entrapped neurofilament+ axons) and dermal nerve sheath myxoma (diffuse S100+ and Sox10+ without admixed fibroblasts and mast cells).

Neurofibroma

- S100+ Sox10+, CD34+ (fibroblasts/perineural cells), neurofilament+ (entrapped axons)

Schwannoma

Schwannoma is a benign peripheral nerve sheath tumor composed of Schwann cells, thought to arise eccentrically from the surface of peripheral nerves or nerve roots. It usually occurs sporadically but may also develop in association with neurofibromatosis type 2 (NF-2), with mutations in NF-2 and consequent loss of its protein product merlin. The presence of multiple cutaneous schwannomas has been termed schwannomatosis, in which germline aberrations in *INI1/SMARCB1* (22q11) may be involved.[101] Schwannomas usually occurs in the head and neck region and the flexor surfaces of the extremities, in the form of a solitary, slow-growing, painless subcutaneous mass. They affect patients of all ages with peaks between 20 and 50 without predilection to gender.

Grossly, schwannomas often present as a solitary encapsulated nodule. Histologically, schwannomas exhibit a biphasic appearance with cellular/Antoni A areas and hypocellular/Antoni B areas. Nuclear palisading (Verocay bodies), hyalinized vessels, and a fibrous capsule containing the parent nerve are classically seen (**Figure 8.58**). Neoplastic Schwann cells typically show bland spindle shaped nuclei, although degenerative changes, such as marked nuclear pleomorphism can be seen in longstanding lesions (so-called ancient schwannoma). Histologic variants include cellular schwannomas, melanotic schwannomas, plexiform schwannoma, and epithelioid schwannoma.

The tumor cells of schwannoma stain with S100, Sox10, myelin basic protein, and calretinin.[100] S100 is strongly and diffusely expressed by most cells in schwannoma (**Figures 8.59 and 8.60**). The perineural cells in the capsule stain with EMA.[102] The histologic differential diagnosis includes neurofibroma (less diffuse positivity for Sox10 and S100), perineurioma (Sox10-, S100-, claudin-1+, GLUT-1+, EMA+) and malignant peripheral nerve sheath tumor (Sox10/S100 variable, H3K27me3 loss).

Schwannoma

- S100+ Sox10+

Perineurioma

Perineurioma is a benign peripheral nerve sheath tumor composed of perineurial cells, which lie at the interface between epineurial and endoneurial tissues that surround both myelinated and unmyelinated axon-Schwann cell complexes of peripheral nerve. It is not associated with neurofibromatosis. Perineuriomas are divided into two groups: intraneural perineurioma and soft tissue perineurioma. Soft tissue perineurioma often involves the lower extremities and trunk as a painless, solitary nodule or mass.[103]

Histologically, soft tissue perineuriomas are sharply demarcated, non-encapsulated neoplasms, located within the subcutis or deep soft tissue, with rare tumors arising primarily in the

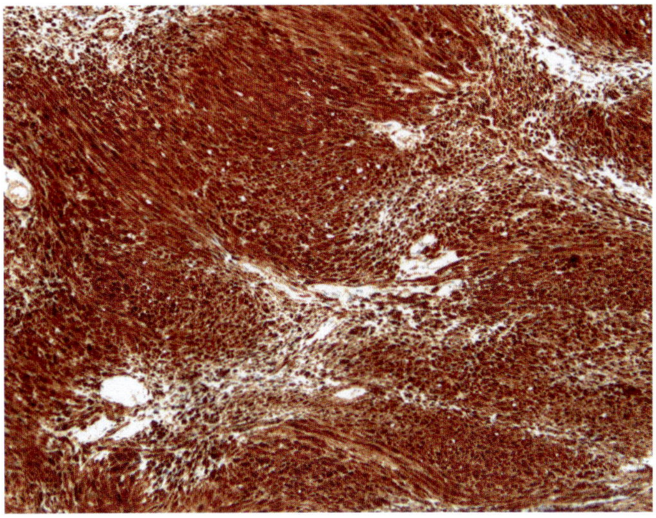

Figure 8.59 Schwannoma. S100 is diffusely and strongly positive (X100).

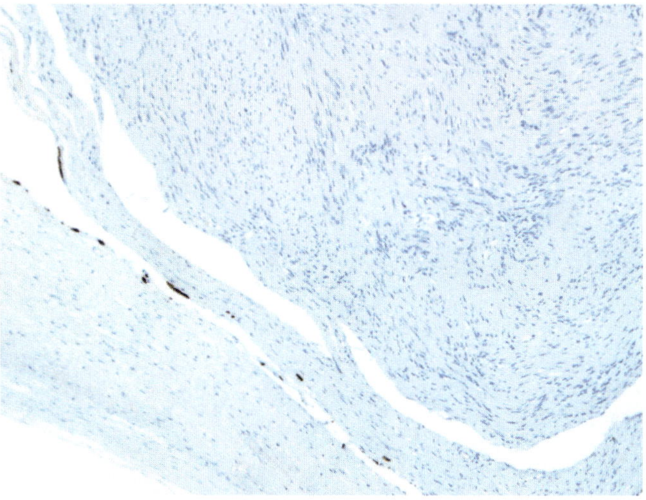

Figure 8.60 Schwannoma. Neurofilament highlights the displaced nerve of origin at the periphery of the tumor (X100).

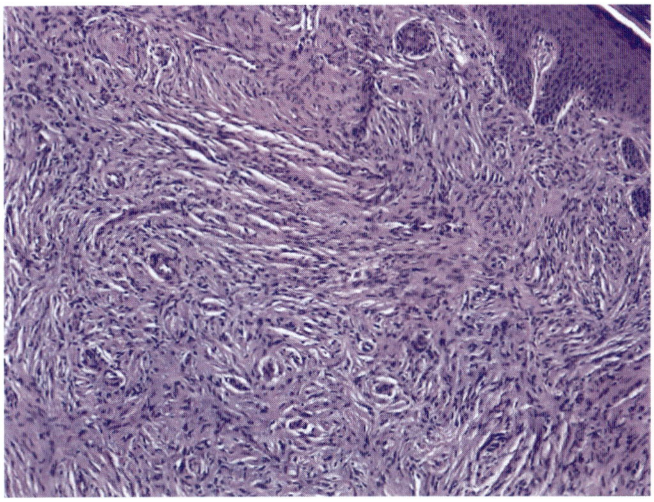

Figure 8.61 A proliferation of spindle cells arranged in storiform pattern in perineurioma (100X).

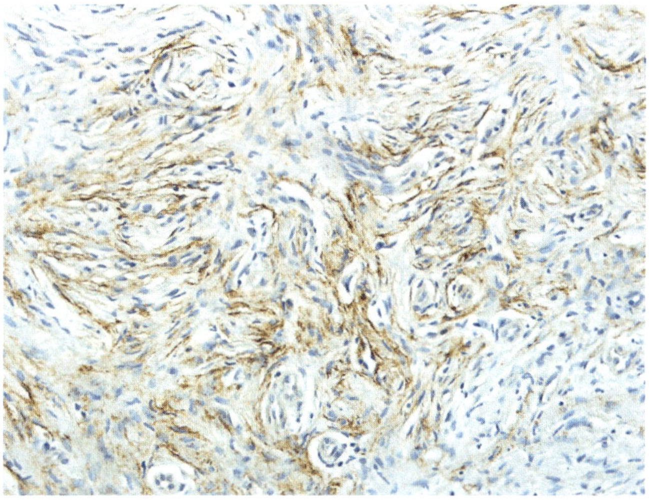

Figure 8.62 Perineurioma. The spindle cells are positive for EMA (200X).

dermis. They demonstrate a proliferation of spindle cells with wavy-shaped nuclei arranged in short fascicles, often with a lamellar, whorled or storiform architecture (**Figure 8.61**). The stroma varies from collagenous to myxoid and calcification can be seen. Mitoses are usually absent. In the intraneural subtype, the spindle cells form concentric layers around axons, forming characteristic pseudo-onion bulbs.[103]

All perineuriomas are EMA and type IV collagen positive and S100 and CD34 negative mirroring the immunoprofile of normal perineurial cells.[104] The expression of EMA can be strong, diffuse and membranous, reflecting the cell of origin (**Figure 8.62**). It is important to note that EMA expression in some perineuriomas may be difficult to evaluate at routinely used antibody concentrations. Axons at the center of pseudo-onion bulbs in intraneural perineurioma stain for neurofilament and S100 is expressed in residual Schwann cells. Perineuriomas lack S100 expression, a useful marker when distinguishing perineurioma from other benign peripheral nerve sheath tumors, namely schwannoma or neurofibroma.[103]

Perineurial cells differ from almost all other mesenchymal cell types by virtue of their formation of tight junctions. The expression of claudin-1, an integral structural component of tight junctions, has been described in normal perineurial cells and in a significant number of perineuriomas, even in rare cases that do not express EMA. In addition, Claudin-1 is negative in tumors that enter in the differential diagnosis, namely low-grade fibromyxoid sarcoma (MUC4+) and dermatofibrosarcoma protuberans (CD34+). In neurofibromas and schwannomas, it is only expressed in the few perineurial cells within or at the periphery of the lesion.[104] The expression of GLUT-1, a transmembrane protein that mediates facilitative transport of glucose, has been shown to be expressed in perineurial cells. GLUT-1 expression in perineurioma is useful in the setting of weak or absent EMA expression (**Figure 8.63**).[105]

Perineurioma

- EMA+ claudin–1 + Glut–1+ S100- Sox10-

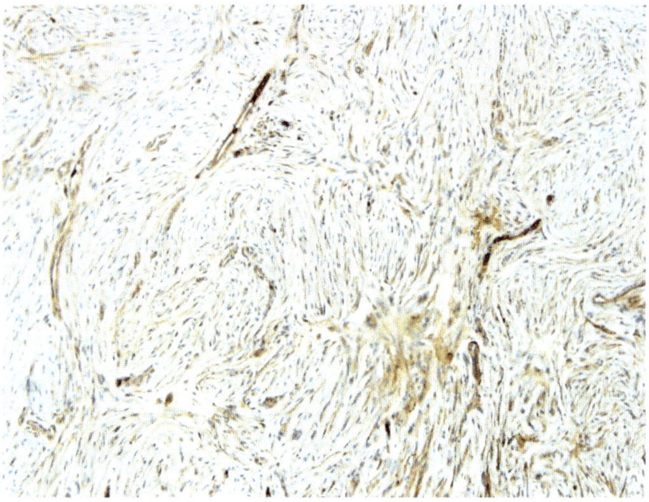

Figure 8.63 Perineurioma. They are focally positive for GLUT-1 (100X).

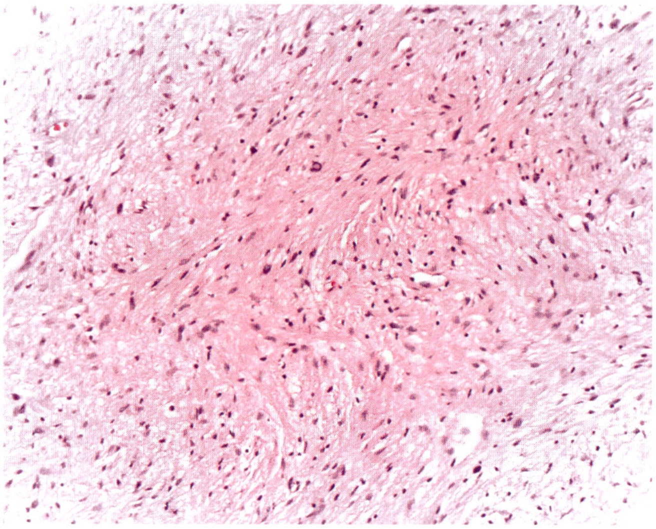

Figure 8.64 Hybrid nerve sheath tumor. Benign nerve sheath proliferation with two components, a Schwannian component with plump epithelioid cells and a perineural component with spindled cells (X200).

Hybrid Nerve Sheath Tumors

Hybrid nerve sheath tumors can be found in the dermis and subcutis in a variety of anatomic sites.[106] As the name implies, hybrid nerve sheath tumors feature combinations of benign nerve sheath tumors (neurofibroma, schwannoma, and perineurioma) and include schwannoma/perineurioma, neurofibroma/schwannoma and neurofibroma/perineurioma (**Figure 8.64**). Hybrid schwannoma/perineuriomas usually occur sporadically and harbor recurrent *VGLL3* rearrangements.[106] Hybrid neurofibroma/ schwannomas are associated with schwannomatosis and neurofibromatosis.[107] Hybrid neurofibroma/ perineuriomas are associated with neurofibromatosis type 1.[108]

Immunohistochemistry highlights the hybrid components of tumors with hybrid schwannoma/perineuriomas showing Sox10/S100+ Schwann cells intermingled with GLUT-1+, EMA+ perineurial cells. Hybrid neurofibroma/schwannomas show nodules of Sox10/S100+ Schwann cells in a background of neurofibroma (CD34+ fibroblasts and mast cells with entrapped NFP+ axons) (**Figure 8.65**). Claudin 1 highlights the perineural component while the Schwannian component is negative (**Figure 8.66**). Hybrid neurofibroma/perineuriomas resemble plexiform neurofibromas with neurofibromatous areas with entrapped perineural cells.[108] The histologic differential diagnosis includes non-hybrid nerve sheath tumors such as neurofibroma and schwannoma. Immunohistochemistry is needed to highlight the hybrid components.

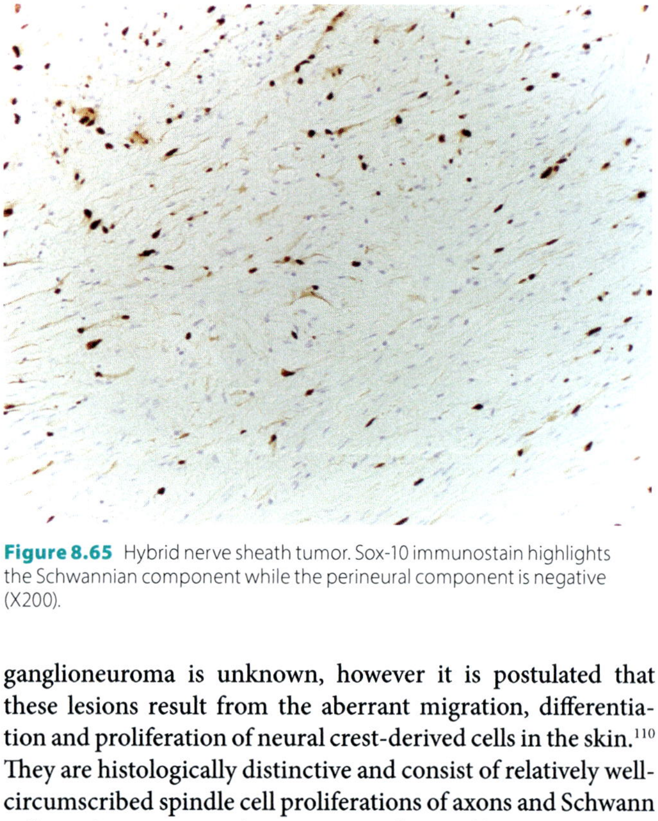

Figure 8.65 Hybrid nerve sheath tumor. Sox-10 immunostain highlights the Schwannian component while the perineural component is negative (X200).

Hybrid Nerve Sheath Tumors

- Sox10/ S100+ Schwann cells intermingled with Glut−1+, EMA+ perineurial cells

Cutaneous Ganglioneuroma

Primary cutaneous ganglioneuroma is an exceedingly rare benign neoplasms of the skin that can either be congenital or acquired later in life.[109] The pathogenesis of primary cutaneous ganglioneuroma is unknown, however it is postulated that these lesions result from the aberrant migration, differentiation and proliferation of neural crest-derived cells in the skin.[110] They are histologically distinctive and consist of relatively well-circumscribed spindle cell proliferations of axons and Schwann cells with interspersed mature ganglion cells. However, the ganglion cells can be found separate from the neuromatous component or represent the only proliferative component of the tumor, so-called ganglion cell choristoma.

The histologic differential diagnoses include ganglion cells entrapped by a plexiform neurofibroma in patients with neurofibromatosis, well-differentiated cutaneous neuroblastoma metastases, and ganglioneuromatous differentiation within a melanocytic lesion. These diagnoses can be differentiated from primary cutaneous ganglioneuroma, based on clinical and histological features.

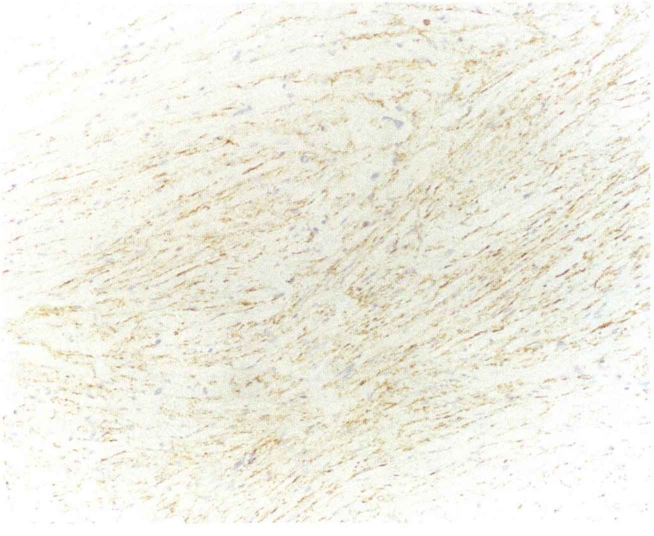

Figure 8.66 Hybrid nerve sheath tumor. Claudin-1 immunostain highlights the perineural component while the Schwannian component is negative (X200).

The fusiform or Schwann cells are strongly positive for S100, and the ganglion cells express CD56, NSE, CD117, synaptophysin, GFAP, neurofilament protein, PGP9.5, calretinin, and NeuN. One report described S100 expression in the ganglion cells and the spindle cells.[109]

Cutaneous ganglioneuroma

- S100+ Sox10+ Schwann cells
- CD56+ NSE+ calretinin+ ganglion cells

Cutaneous Meningioma

Cutaneous meningioma is a rare tumor indistinguishable from dural meningioma, which occurs in the skin and subcutaneous tissue. It is a benign lesion and usually do not recur. Cutaneous meningiomas can be derived from 1) ectopic arachnoid cells (type I), 2) arachnoid cells surrounding nerve bundles (type II), and 3) direct extension from a dural-based meningioma (type III). Type I is congenital and occupies an intermediate position in the spectrum between meningocele and extracranial meningioma (frequently called meningeal hamartomas), presents on the scalp and paravertebral regions of children. Type II consists of ectopic soft tissue meningiomas that extend to the skin by contiguity and usually occur on adults, around sensory organs of the head (eyes, ears, nose, and mouth). Type III is comprised of tumors that have extended into the dermis or subcutis from a primary intracranial meningioma.[111]

Cutaneous meningiomas are characterized by whorls of spindled to epithelioid cells on histologic sections. Histologically, type II and type III cutaneous meningiomas show similar histologic features as primary dural meningiomas. They are composed of lobules and sheets of uniform ovoid, epithelioid, or spindle cells in a whorled architecture, usually with an infiltrative growth pattern through the dermis and subcutaneous tissue. Type I lesions are usually confined to the deep dermis and subcutis and are composed of irregular, elongated, anastomosing, and dilated spaces resembling vascular channels dissecting between thickened collagen bundles.[111]

Like conventional meningioma, the lesional cells in cutaneous meningioma express EMA and p63 but are negative for keratin 5/6, S100, CD34, CD31, CD68, and the muscle markers SMA and desmin.[112]

One of the main differential diagnoses is the soft tissue perineurioma, not only because it shares some architectural features with cutaneous meningioma (mainly type II and type III) but also because it also expresses EMA. However, CD34 is expressed in the former (in the so-called endoneurial fibroblasts) and is usually absent in the latter. The expression of somatostatin receptor subtype 2 (SSTR2) and progesterone receptor would be supportive of meningioma over perineurioma.[113] Type I cutaneous meningioma can resemble an angiosarcoma, due to the pseudovascular appearance. However, angiosarcoma arises in older patients and usually expresses endothelial markers (CD31, CD34, FLI-1, Erg) and is not immunoreactive for EMA.

Cutaneous meningioma

- EMA+ SSTR2+

Granular Cell Tumor

Granular cell tumors are relatively common benign neoplasms postulated to be of Schwann cell origin. They most commonly arise in the skin, subcutaneous tissue, or tongue, are usually small, and are grossly firm with an ill-defined border, which may give a misleading impression of malignancy. The tumors occur most frequently in adults, and there is a female predilection. Many granular cell tumors are benign, and recurrences are uncommon, even following incomplete excision.[114]

Microscopically, conventional granular cell tumors present as poorly circumscribed and infiltrative neoplasms, centered in the dermis but frequently extending into deeper tissues. They are composed of sheets or nests of large polygonal epithelioid cells with indistinct cell borders with distinct granular and eosinophilic cytoplasm. Mitotic figures, pleomorphic cells and perineural growth can lead to an erroneous diagnosis of malignancy. The overlying epithelium often shows prominent pseudoepitheliomatous hyperplasia.[115]

The tumor cells are generally reactive for S100, reflecting schwannian differentiation.[115] In addition, tumor cells express NKI/C3, NSE, and CD68, nonspecific markers also present in other tumors with numerous lysosomes and granular cell change.[116] Granular cell tumors are consistently negative for GFAP, neurofilament, chromogranin, synaptophysin, cytokeratins, EMA, myoglobin, desmin, smooth muscle actin, HMB-45, and Melan-A. The tumor cells are positive for S100, neuron specific enolase, PGP9.5, NKI/C3, CD68, MiTF, Sox10, and inhibin alpha (**Figures 8.67 and 8.68**).[116]

The main differential diagnostic consideration is with other benign or malignant neoplasm that can show granular cell change, including dermatofibroma (SMA+, factor 13a+ dendrocytes,

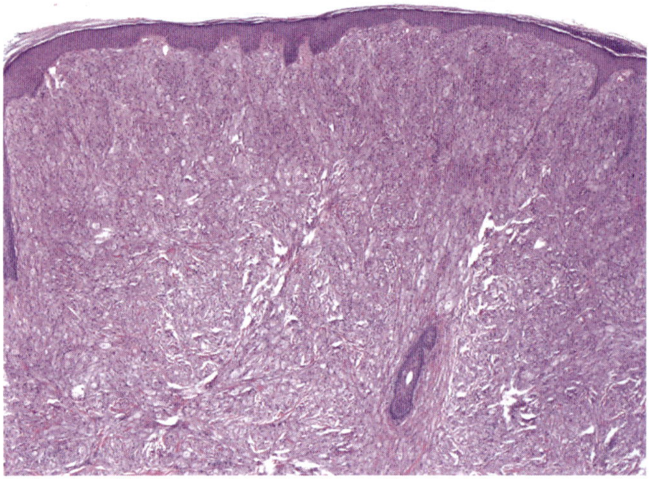

Figure 8.67 Epithelioid neoplastic cells with granular cytoplasm are characteristic of granular cell tumor (X20).

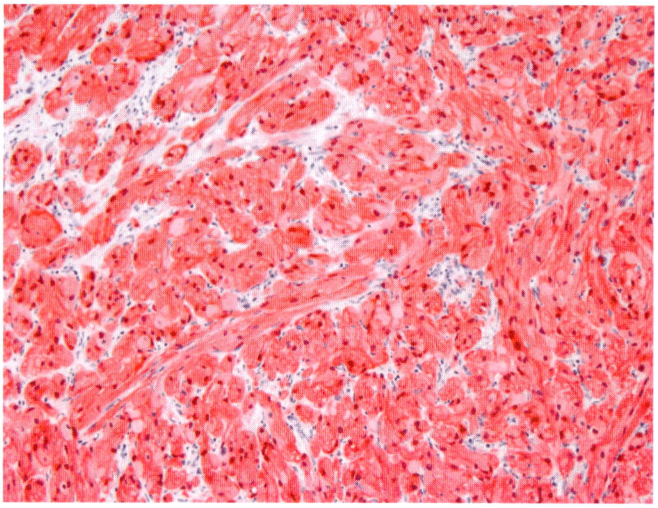

Figure 8.68 Granular cell tumor. Diffuse S100 positivity in the tumor cells (X200)

CD68+ histiocytes), cellular neurothekeoma (S100-), leiomyoma (SMA+, desmin+), and melanoma (Melan-A+, HMB-45+).

Granular cell tumor

- S100+ Sox10+ MiTF+ calretinin+ inhibin+

Malignant Granular Cell Tumor

Most cutaneous granular cell tumors are benign but rarely malignant cases have been reported. Malignant granular cell tumor is a distinct, extremely rare entity, classified as a high-grade sarcoma, with high rate of metastasis and local recurrence, with poor prognosis and short survival.[115]

The diagnosis of malignant granular tumor should be restricted to neoplasms that are histologically similar to benign granular cell tumors but that have three or more a histologic features of malignancy including necrosis, spindling, vesicular nuclei with prominent nucleoli, increased mitotic activity (greater than 2 mitoses/10 HPF), high nucleocytoplasmic ratio, and pleomorphism.[115] Tumors with some features of malignancy but with fewer than three are called *atypical granular cell tumor* and have good prognosis, with no metastases.[115]

The malignant granular cell tumors are positive for S100, NSE, CD56, CD57, p75, calretinin, NKI/C3, and CD68; and negative for SMA, desmin, EMA, cytokeratins, chromogranin, and HMB-45.[115] They express higher Ki-67 proliferation index and phosphohistone H3 than the benign or atypical counterpart.[115,117] The more problematic differential diagnoses include melanoma (Melan-A+ and HMB-45+) and MPNST with granular cell features (Sox10/S100 variable with loss of H3K27me3).

Malignant Peripheral Nerve Sheath Tumor

Malignant peripheral nerve sheath tumor (MPNST) has two subtypes, conventional and epithelioid. They usually arise from peripheral nerves and frequently metastasize and have an overall poor prognosis (five-year survival of 35–50%). Accounting for 5–10% of soft tissue sarcomas, conventional MPNSTs occur in association with neurofibromatosis 1 in 25–50% of cases.[118] MPNST often presents as an enlarging mass with pain more commonly noted in individuals with neurofibromatosis. They demonstrate cellular intersecting fascicles of atypical, spindled cells with alternating hypercellular and hypocellular areas that can impart a "marbled" appearance (**Figure 8.69**).

S100 staining is focal and identified in 50–90% of conventional MPNST, whereas epithelioid MPNSTs express strong and diffuse S100 staining in 87% of cases (**Figure 8.70**).[118] Sox10 expression is similarly focal in conventional MPNST and is less frequent (18%) while expression is usually strong and diffuse in epithelioid MPNST.[119] MPNSTs are negative for melanocytic markers such as MART-1/Melan-A, HMB-45, and MiTF.[118] There is variable staining for GFAP and EMA.[118] Complete loss of Sox10, neurofibromin or p16 expression, or the presence of EGFR immunoreactivity was reported to be specific for MPNST in comparison to cellular schwannoma.[119] Conventional MPNSTs show loss of H3K27me3 by immunohistochemistry (**Figure 8.71**) and epithelioid MPNSTs show loss of INI1 by immunohistochemistry.[120,121] The histologic differential diagnosis includes melanoma (Melan-A+, HMB-45+, Sox10+, S100+), cellular schwannoma (retention of H3K27me3 and diffuse Sox10+, S100+), synovial sarcoma (SSX+, SS18+), and other sarcomas. Clinical history and loss of H3K27me3 or INI1 is particularly helpful.

Malignant peripheral nerve sheath tumor

- Conventional: Focal S100+, focal Sox10+ and H3K27me3 loss of nuclear expression
- Epithelioid: Diffuse S100+, diffuse Sox10+ and loss of INI1

Malignant Melanotic Nerve Sheath Tumor

Malignant melanotic nerve sheath tumors (MMNST) typically occur in young adults and involve the spinal nerves.[122] Histologically they are composed of Schwann cells with

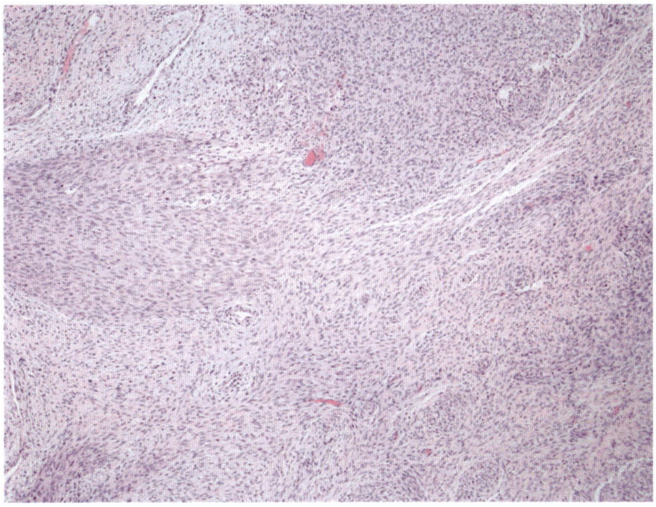

Figure 8.69 Malignant peripheral nerve sheath tumor is characterized by intersecting fascicles of spindled tumor cells (X100).

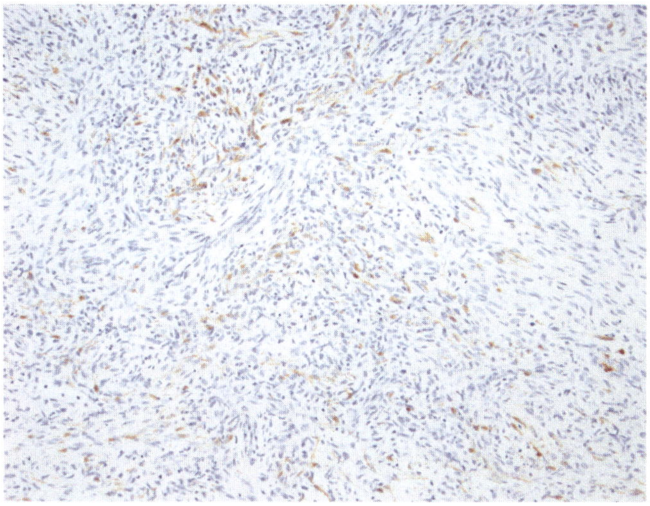

Figure 8.70 Malignant peripheral nerve sheath tumor. Focal S100 expression (X200).

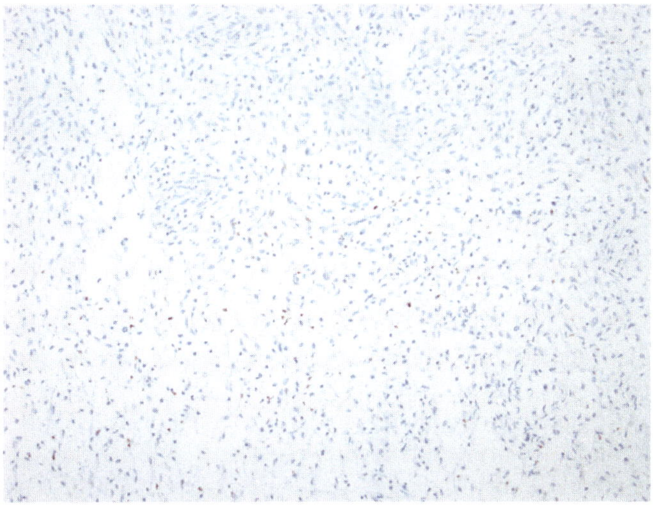

Figure 8.71 Malignant peripheral nerve sheath tumor. Marked loss of H3K27me3 expression (X200).

melanocytic differentiation and melanin production.[122,123] Psammomatous calcification can be seen.[123] By immunohistochemistry, tumors usually express melanocytic markers (Sox10, S100, Melan-A, HMB-45). An association with Carney complex has been identified and loss of PRKAR1A by immunohistochemistry can be found.[122] The histologic differential is melanoma and loss of PRKAR1A can be helpful but clinical correlation and molecular profiling may be needed in difficult cases.

Malignant melanotic nerve sheath tumor

- S100+, Sox10+, Melan-A+, HMB–45+, PRKAR1A loss

8.5 Lipomatous Tumors

Lipomatous tumors are neoplasms which contain adipocytes in varying stages of differentiation. Admixed elements such as myxoid areas, fibroblastic areas, and cartilage/bone can be seen. Adipocytes can be highlighted with S100 immunostain.[80]

Lipoma

Lipomas are benign tumors composed of well-differentiated adipocytes. They can occur in a variety of anatomic sites (e.g. trunk, extremities) and can be both superficial and deep (e.g. intramuscular).[124] The adipocytes can be highlighted with S100 and HMGA2 allows for distinction from non-neoplastic adipose tissue.[125] A number of subtypes with other admixed elements exist such as myolipoma, chondrolipoma and osteolipoma. The main differential diagnosis is with atypical lipomatous tumor/well-differentiated liposarcoma (ALT/WDLS) which are usually larger, deep-seated lesions with *MDM2* amplification. Of note, histiocytes in areas of fat necrosis in lipomas can be positive for MDM2 immunohistochemistry.[126] Cytogenetic/FISH analysis for *MDM2* amplification can be of utility.

Spindle Cell Lipoma/Pleomorphic Lipoma

Spindle cell or pleomorphic lipoma is a painless and slow-growing subcutaneous tissue tumor commonly occurring in men in the fifth to seventh decades, occurring primarily on shoulders, upper back, and back of the neck. It presents generally as a single lesion, with relatively small size, most often less than 5 cm in diameter. Less frequently, it can present as multiple lesions and can also occur as a familial disease. Uncommonly, spindle cell lipoma can be observed in a purely dermal location.[127]

Cytogenetically, spindle cell lipoma is characterized by monosomy or partial loss of chromosomes 13 and 16, including the *RB1* gene. These are the most common alterations and the same chromosomal alterations are also present in cellular angiofibroma and in mammary-type myofibroblastoma, strongly suggesting that these lesions form a family of histologically and cytogenetically related neoplasms.[128] Given their benign clinical behavior, conservative local excision is considered curative. Recurrence is exceptional, even after incomplete resection.[127]

Although spindle cell lipoma can grossly resemble lipomas, histologically, spindle cell lipomas are composed of lobules of mature fat interposed with areas of bland spindle cells arranged haphazardly and demonstrate areas of myxoid stroma. The stroma can contain coarse collagen fibers ("ropelike") (**Figure 8.72**). Scattered pleomorphic cells can be identified and mast cells are usually present throughout the stroma. Multiple variants including pseudoangiomatous, plexiform, vascular, and fibrous, have been described, which may broaden the potential differential diagnosis.[127]

The spindled cells are positive for CD34 (**Figure 8.73**) and negative for SMA, desmin, and S100.[129] Chen et al.[130] reported that the *RB1* deletion in spindle cell lipomas, pleomorphic lipomas, cellular angiofibromas, and mammary-type myofibroblastomas are associated with loss of Rb immunohistochemical expression. This can be useful since RB1 expression is maintained in histologic mimics.

Spindle cell lipoma

- CD34+ Rb1-

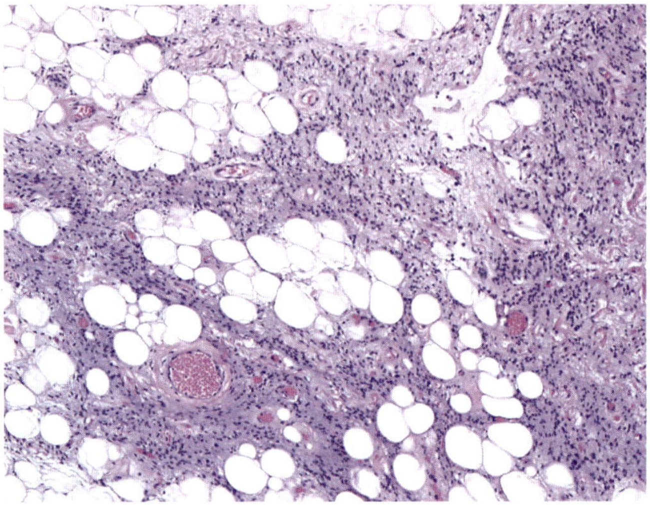

Figure 8.72 Spindle cells arranged in short bundles in spindle cell lipoma (X100).

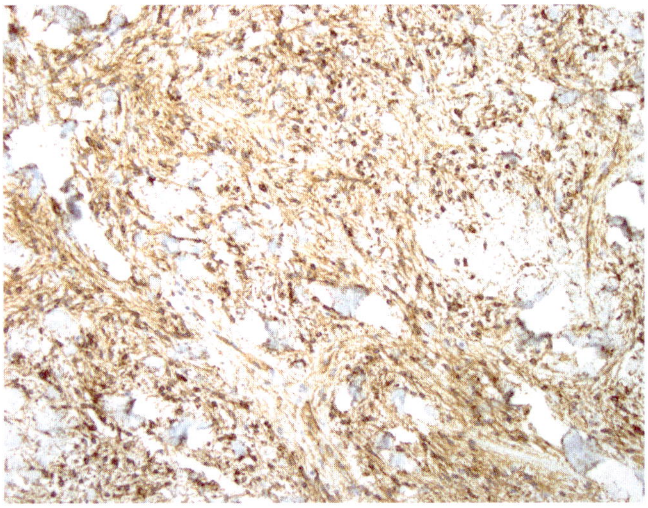

Figure 8.73 Spindle cell lipoma. Diffuse CD34 expression (X100).

Atypical Lipomatous Tumor/Well-Differentiated Liposarcoma

Atypical lipomatous tumor/well-differentiated liposarcoma (ALT/WDLS) is a tumor of intermediate malignant potential (commonly locally recurs) composed of adipocytes. Atypical lipomatous tumor should be used when referring to tumors in superficial locations (e.g. extremities) while well-differentiated liposarcoma should be used to refer to tumors in deep locations (e.g. retroperitoneum). Subcutaneous well-differentiated liposarcomas have a good prognosis with a tendency for local recurrence due to the frequent incomplete excision but they do not usually metastasize. Histologically, ALT/WLDS show adipocytes, fibrous septae and scattered, atypical, hyperchromatic nuclei.[131] By immunohistochemistry, the tumor cells express MDM2 and CDK4 strongly and amplification of *MDM2* and *CDK4* can be detected by cytogenics/FISH.[131] The histologic differential diagnosis includes lipoma (MDM2-, CDK4-) and spindle cell/pleomorphic lipoma (myxoid areas with CD34+ spindle cells).

Atypical lipomatous tumor/well-differentiated liposarcoma

- MDM2+ CDK4+

Dedifferentiated Liposarcoma

Dedifferentiated liposarcoma (DDLPS) arises from ALT/WDLPS and characteristically feature a sharp transition from areas of adipocytic differentiation to high-grade areas without adipocytic differentiation (**Figure 8.74**).[132] Identification of a dedifferentiated component is important as it confers a significant risk of metastasis and mortality.[132] Dedifferentiation is more commonly seen in deep-seated masses (LPS) but can rarely be seen in more superficial tumors of the extremities (ALT). Like ALT/WDLPS, DDLPS is positive for MDM2 and

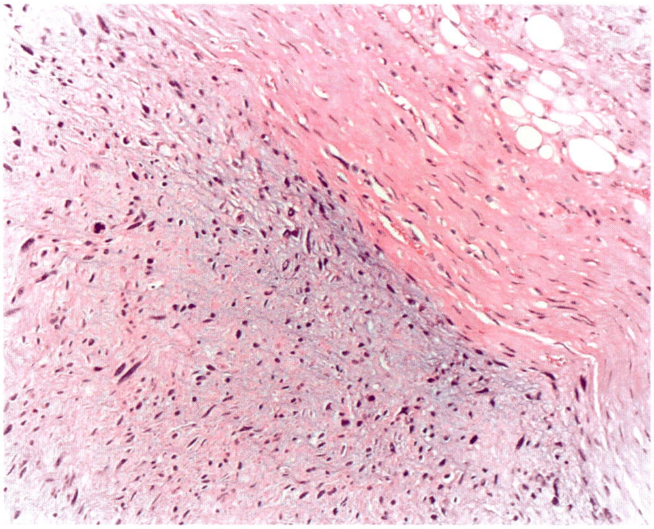

Figure 8.74 Non-lipogenic, high-grade tumor cells in a myxoid background (left-hand side) adjacent to lipogenic, well-differentiated liposarcoma (right-hand side), characteristic of dedifferentiated liposarcoma (X200).

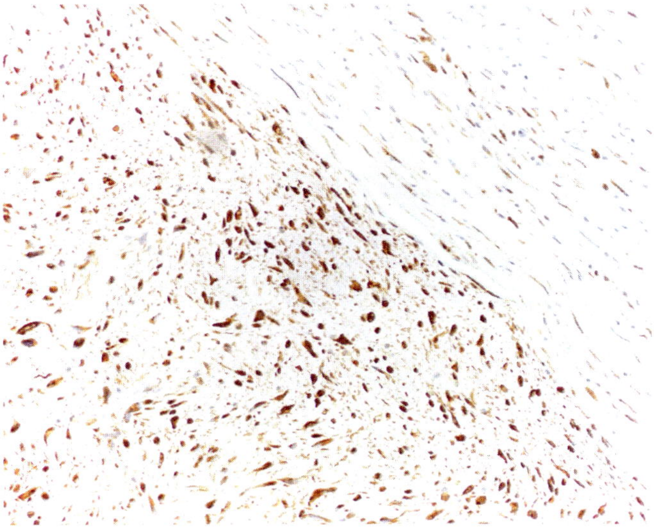

Figure 8.75 Strong expression of CDK4 can be seen in both well-differentiated liposarcoma (right-hand side) and dedifferentiated liposarcoma (left-hand side) (X200).

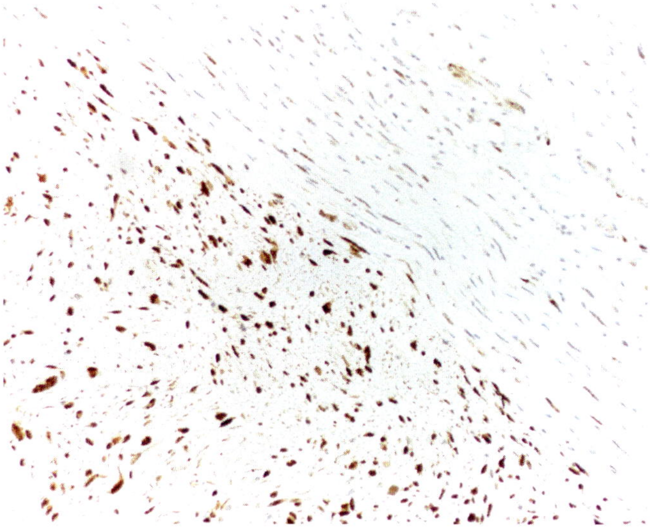

Figure 8.76 Strong expression of MDM2 is characteristic of both well-differentiated liposarcoma (right-hand side) and dedifferentiated liposarcoma (left-hand side) (X200).

CDK4 by immunohistochemistry (**Figures 8.75 and 8.76**) and has amplification of *MDM2/CDK4* due to supernumerary ring chromosomes.[133]

Dedifferentiated liposarcoma

- MDM2+ CDK4+

Myxoid Liposarcoma

Myxoid liposarcoma (MLPS) commonly occurs in the thigh.[134] Histologically they features ovoid cells in a myxoid background with small, delicate "chicken-wire" vasculature (**Figure 8.77**).[134] Pools of mucin and small lipoblasts can be seen.[134] High-grade myxoid liposarcoma (previously round cell liposarcoma) shows >5% areas with hypercellularity, significant mitotic activity and a less prominent myxoid background.[134] High-grade myxoid liposarcoma is associated with a poorer prognosis.[134] Myxoid liposarcomas harbor recurrent gene rearrangements involving *DDIT3* (with partners of *EWSR1* and *FUS*).[135] DDIT3 immunostain is a useful diagnostic marker (**Figure 8.78**).[135]

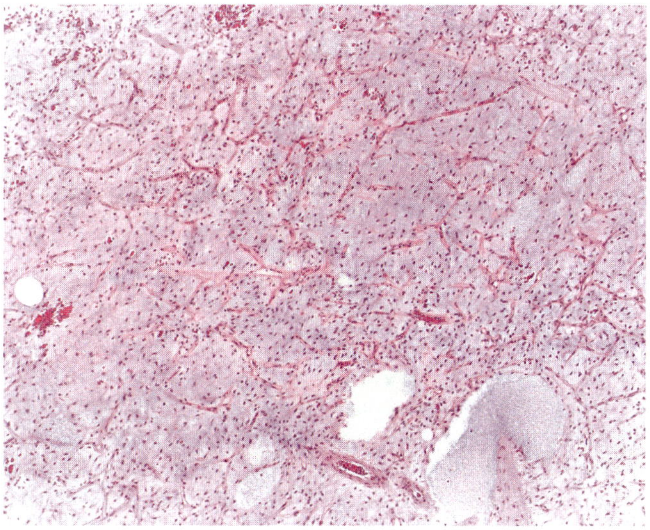

Figure 8.77 Small, epithelioid cells in a myxoid background with "chicken-wire" vasculature are commonly seen in myxoid liposarcoma (X100).

Myxoid liposarcoma

- DDIT3+

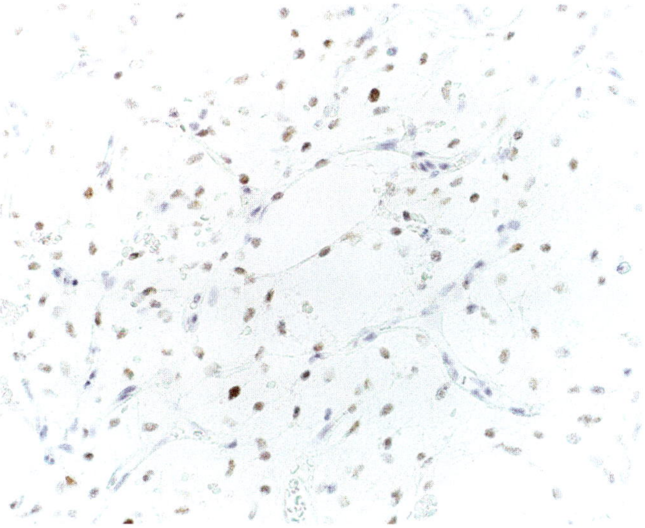

Figure 8.78 Myxoid liposarcoma. The neoplastic cells express DDIT3 (X400).

Pleomorphic Liposarcoma

Pleomorphic liposarcoma commonly occurs in the extremities and demonstrates pleormophic lipoblasts (**Figure 8.79**).[136] Unlike atypical lipomatous tumor, well-differentiated liposarcoma and dedifferentated liposarcoma, pleomorphic liposarcomas do not show amplification of *MDM2* and *CDK4*, allowing distinction between the entities (**Figure 8.80**).[137] By immunohistochemistry, the tumor cells can express SMA, S100, keratins, and desmin.[136]

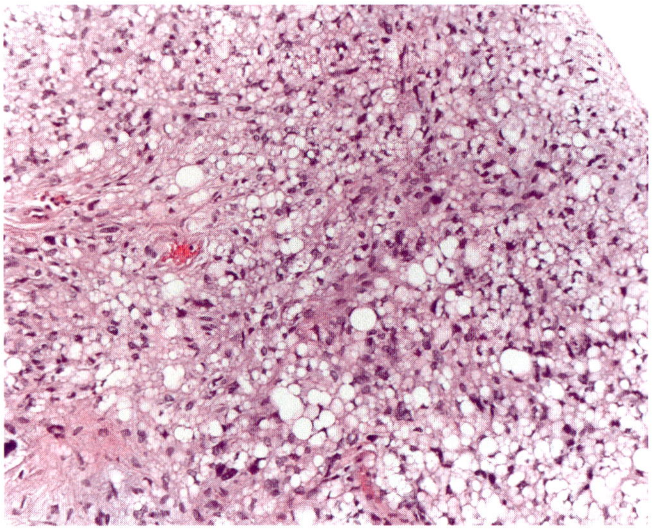

Figure 8.79 Pleomorphic liposarcoma is characterized by numerous pleomorphic lipoblasts (X200).

Figure 8.80 Pleomorphic liposarcoma. MDM2 immunostain is negative (X400).

Pleomorphic liposarcoma

- SMA+/-, S100+/-, MDM2-, CDK4-

8.6 Vascular Tumors

Acquired Progressive Lymphangioma

Acquired progressive lymphangioma or benign lymphangioendothelioma is a rare benign vascular lesion of the skin lesion with lymphatic differentiation that occurs mainly in adult patients.[138] It typically presents as a slow-growing, solitary, well-defined erythematous macule or plaque.[138] Recurrence is exceptional and the prognosis is generally excellent.

Histopathologically, anastomosing and tortuous vascular channels are seen dissecting the dermis and these histologic features can be mistaken for well-differentiated angiosarcoma or patch-stage Kaposi sarcoma (**Figure 8.81**). Mitotic figures are absent and stromal inflammation is not a feature. Some vascular spaces may have a layer of smooth muscle. Irregular and thin-walled vascular spaces are lined by flattened endothelial cells that are positive for D2-40, LYVE-1, and Prox-1; variably for CD31, CD34, and WT1 (**Figure 8.82**). They are negative for HHV-8.

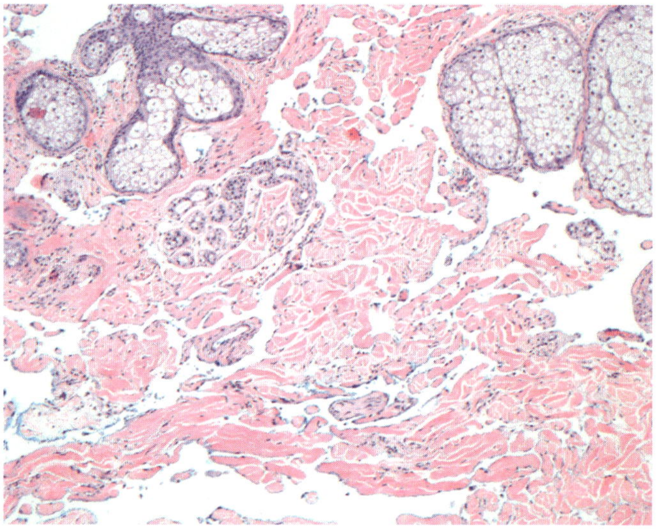

Figure 8.81 Irregular and anastomosing vascular channels dissect the dermis in acquired progressive lymphangioma (X100).

Acquired progressive lymphangioma/ benign lymphangioendothelioma

- D2–40+

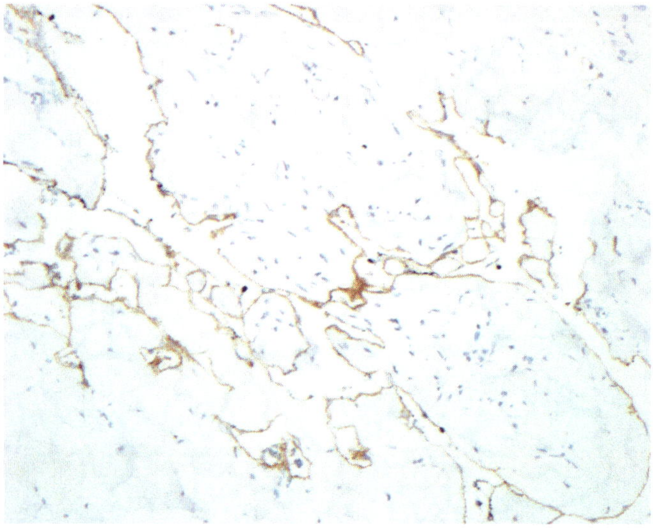

Figure 8.82 Acquired progressive lymphangioma. These vascular spaces are D2-40 positive (X200).

Lymphatic Malformation

Cutaneous lymphatic malformations can be divided into superficial and deep forms. Superficial lymphatic malformations are the most common variant of cutaneous lymphatic malformation. They are usually present at birth or arise in infancy or early childhood, with predilection for the proximal parts of the limbs and in the limb girdle regions.[139] Despite being a benign lesion, lymphatic malformation can cause significant morbidity because of the large size. They do not regress spontaneously, and surgery is the only effective treatment. Recurrence after excision is quite common.

Clinically, the lesion consists of numerous small vesicles or wart-like nodules grouped in a plaque. Histologically, it consists of dilated lymph vessels, lined by flat endothelial cells in a discontinuous layer, situated in the superficial dermis and frequently extending to the reticular dermis. They commonly appear to extend into the overlying epidermis. Scattered lymphoid aggregates are seen in the dermis.[139]

In most cases the diagnosis of lymphatic malformation can be made easily based only on histologic sections. The main differential diagnoses are cavernous hemangioma and venous malformation. Immunohistochemistry for lymphatic lineage markers such as D2-40 and Prox1 is ultimately the most reliable method to make this distinction (**Table 8.3**).[140,141]

Lymphatic malformation

- D2–40+ Prox1+

Table 8.3 Immunostains for lymphatics and blood vessels

Immunostain	Lymphatics	Blood vessels
CD31	+	++
CD34	-	++
Erg	-	++
Podoplanin (D2–40)	+	-
Prox–1	++	-

Lymphangioma and Lymphangiomatosis

Lymphangioma is comprised of dilated thin-walled lymphatic spaces, superficially as lymphangioma circumscriptum and deep as cavernous lymphangioma. While lymphangioma is localized, lymphangiomatosis can involve multiple tissue planes. Recurrence is higher for deep lesions. The lymphatic endothelium expresses D2-40, Prox1, CD31, and variably CD34.[141,142]

Arteriovenous Malformations

Arteriovenous malformation is a vascular congenital malformation characterized by an admixture of thin and thick-walled blood vessels. It can involve the skin, subcutaneous tissue, or bone and presents clinically in adults during the fifth and sixth decade of life as a solitary small, reddish our bluish papule of less than 1cm in diameter, most often on the head and neck (especially the lip) or extremities. The majority of the lesions are sporadic but inherited cases are associated with germline mutation.[143]

Histologically it is a well-circumscribed, nonencapsulated proliferation of thick-walled vessels resembling arteries and thin-walled vessels, involving the dermis or submucosa. Intraluminal microthrombi, dystrophic calcification, and lymphocytic infiltrate is occasionally seen. Frequently it is difficult to identify the arterial component and serial sectioning and stains for elastic fibers may be necessary. The endothelial cells express vascular markers like CD31, CD34, and Erg. Arteriovenous malformation can mimic infantile hemangioma, but the former is Glut1 negative.[144]

Arteriovenous malformations

- CD31+ CD34+ Erg+
- Glut1 -

Capillary Hemangioma

Capillary hemangiomas of the skin are often congenital lesions, with the exception of the acquired adult form (e.g. cherry angiomas), and are located in the skin or subcutaneous tissue. Most cutaneous hemangiomas may be classified by the sizes of their constituent vascular channels. Included in this category are a variety of entities with different clinical features, including pyogenic granuloma and its variants, acquired tufted angioma, glomeruloid hemangioma, infantile hemangioma, and cherry angioma. Lobular capillary hemangioma or pyogenic granuloma often presents as a solitary, pedunculated, or sessile growth.[145] Pyogenic granuloma has been thought to represent a reactive vascular proliferation in response to trauma, inflammatory dermatoses, viral infection, arthropod bite, and underlying neoplasm.[145] Pyogenic granuloma is characterized as a proliferation of vessels of different sizes and shapes, lined by prominent endothelium embedded in an edematous stroma. The endothelial cells invariably express general endothelial markers including CD31, CD34, and Erg (**Figures 8.83 and 8.84**).

Capillary hemangioma/ pyogenic granuloma

- CD31+ CD34+ Erg+

Targetoid Hemosiderotic Hemangioma

Targetoid hemosiderotic hemangioma, a benign non-recurring cutaneous hemangioma also known as hobnail hemangioma, is thought to be of lymphatic origin or lymphatic vascular malformation. Targetoid hemosiderotic hemangioma commonly occurs on extremities and trunk of male adults.[146]

Histopathology shows a biphasic appearance with dilated vascular channels seen superficially and narrower and elongated vascular structures in the deep aspect of the lesion (**Figure 8.85**). Hemosiderin deposition, fibrosis of dermal collagen, and associated lymphocytic infiltrate are often seen. The neoplastic endothelial cells express CD31 and D2-40 and variably for CD34 (**Figure 8.86**). The WT1 expression together with a low Ki67 proliferation index is supportive of a vascular malformation rather than a neoplastic lesion since WT1 expression is seen vascular tumors and typically negative in vascular malformation.[147] The differential diagnosis includes a low-grade

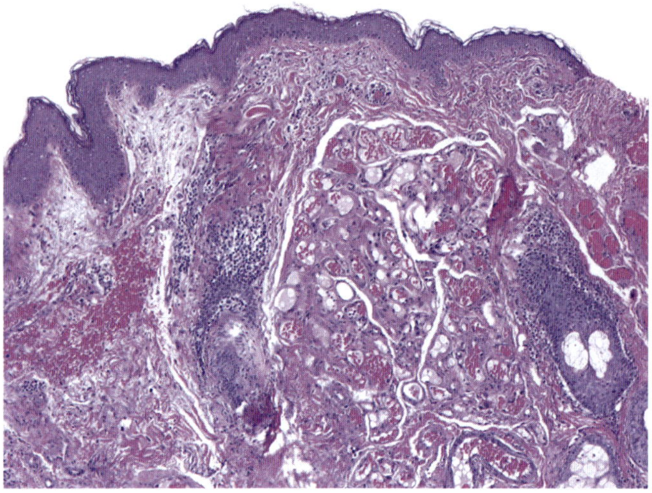

Figure 8.83 Capillary hemangioma is characterized by a lobular proliferation of well-formed vessels (X100).

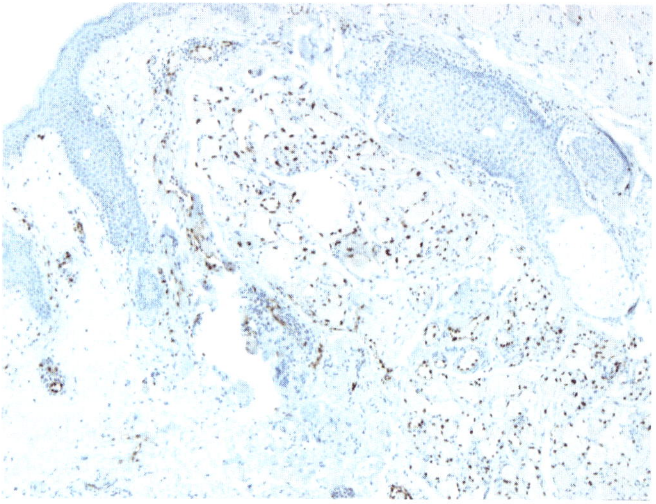

Figure 8.84 Capillary hemangioma. Erg highlights these dermal blood vessels (X100).

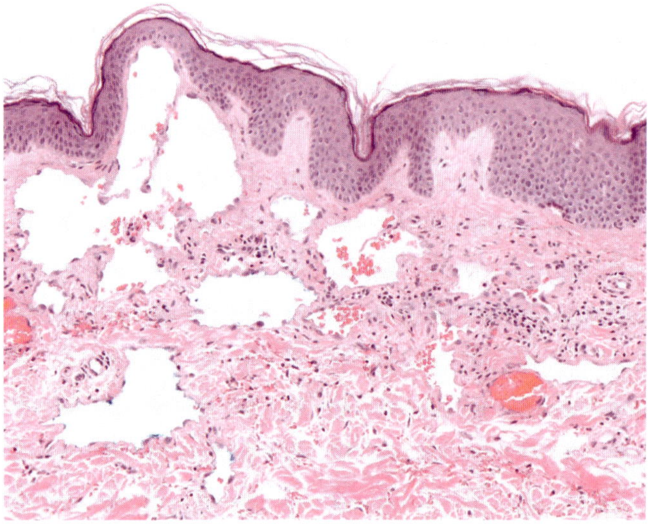

Figure 8.85 Targetoid hemosiderotic hemangioma is comprised of dilated vascular channels dissecting the dermis (X200).

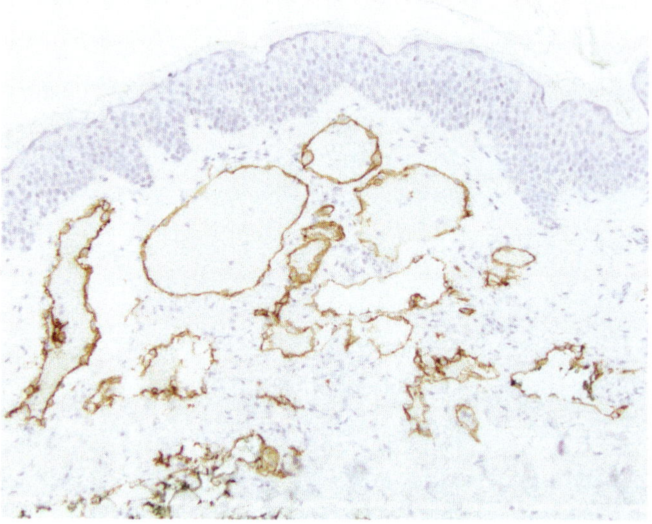

Figure 8.86 Targetoid hemosiderotic hemangioma. The endothelial cells express D2-40 (X200).

angiosarcoma, malignant endovascular papillary angioendothelioma or Dabska's tumor, and Kaposi sarcoma.

Targetoid hemosiderotic hemangioma

- CD31+ D2−40+ CD34-/+

Epithelioid Hemangioma

Epithelioid hemangioma, also known as histiocytoid hemangioma and angiolymphoid hyperplasia with eosinophilia, is an uncommon vascular neoplasm. Up to half of epithelioid hemangiomas harbor *FOS* and *FOSB* fusions.[148] The gene partners for *FOS* include *LMNA*, *MBNL1*, *VIM*, and lincRNA,[148] whereas *FOSB* is often fused to *ZFP36* or very rarely to *WWTR1* or *ACTB*.[149] Epithelioid hemangioma is characterized by a proliferation of thick-walled vessels lined by plump endothelial cells and associated with lymphohistiocytic infiltrate and prominent eosinophils. The endothelial cells are positive for CD31, FLI1, and Erg (**Figures 8.87 and 8.88**). Many cases also express keratin and EMA.

Epithelioid hemangioma

- Erg+

Infantile Hemangioma

Infantile hemangiomas are benign tumors of the vascular endothelium characterized by proliferative and involution phases. Starting in the first weeks of life, the lesions enlarge and reach maximum size by three to six months. A brief plateau period ensues and follows by total or partial involution by five to seven years of age, even without treatment.[150]

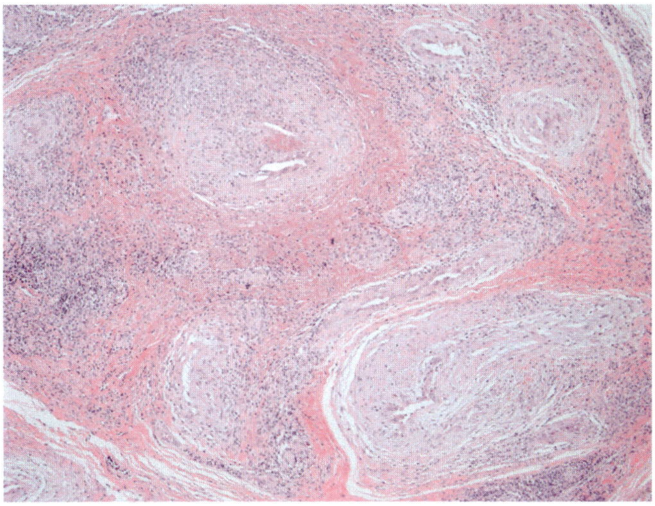

Figure 8.87 Thick-walled vessels lined by prominent endothelial cells are characteristic of epithelioid hemangioma (X100).

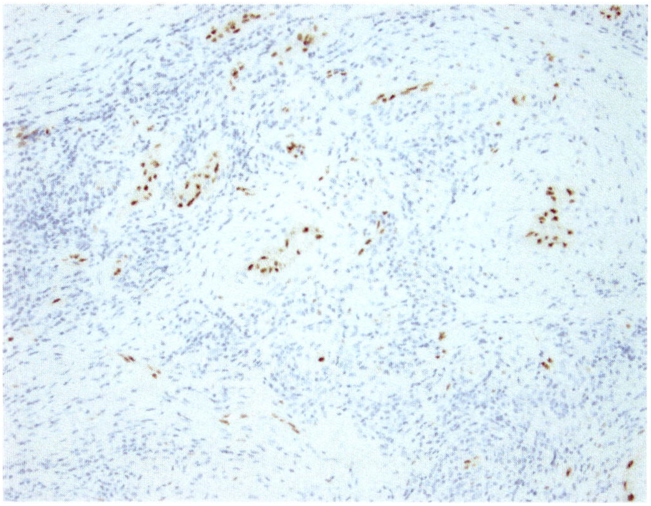

Figure 8.88 Epithelioid hemangioma. Erg highlights the endothelial cells (X200).

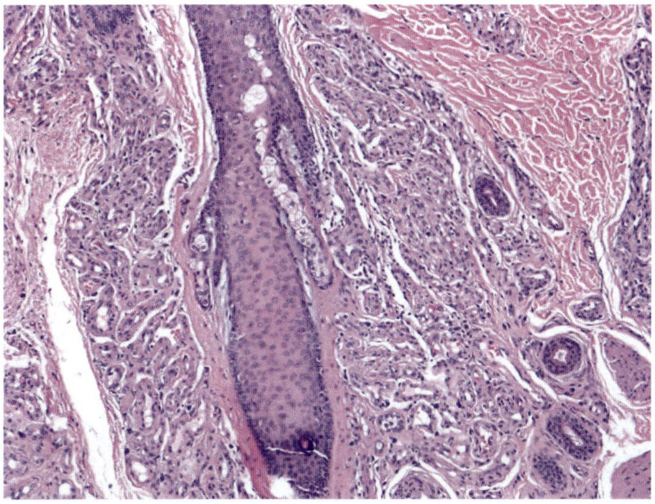

Figure 8.89 Plump endothelial cells are seen lining the vascular spaces in infantile hemangioma (X40).

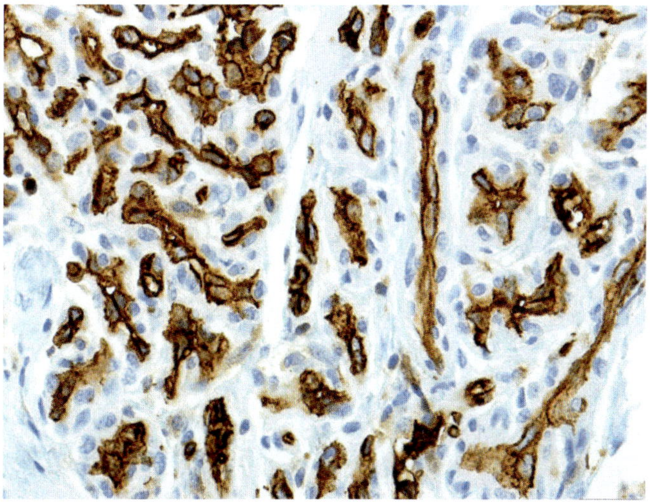

Figure 8.90 Infantile hemangioma. The vessels exhibit Glut1 positivity (X400).

The histopathologic composition of infantile hemangiomas varies with the age of the lesion. Early hemangiomas are highly cellular and are characterized by plump endothelial cells lining vascular spaces with small inconspicuous lumina (**Figure 8.89**). As the lesions mature, the lumina of the vessels enlarge and can assume a "cavernous" appearance that can be misinterpreted as a venous malformation. Regression is characterized as progressive interstitial fibrosis and adipose metaplasia.[151]

The immunophenotypic profile also depends on the clinical phase. Vascular markers (CD31, CD34, Factor VIII, Fli-1, and Erg) and smooth muscle actin are expressed during the proliferative and involution phases but not in involuted ones.[151] Glut1, a glucose transporter protein, is present in endothelial cells of placenta, retina, and blood-brain barrier, has been shown to be a specific marker for infantile hemangiomas.[151] The differential diagnosis of infantile hemangioma includes vascular malformations and congenital hemangiomas. Glut1 is not expressed in the vasculature of normal skin nor in other tumors or vascular malformations, non-involuting congenital hemangioma (NICH), and rapidly involuting congenital hemangioma (RICH) making it a diagnostically useful marker (**Figure 8.90**).[151]

Infantile hemangioma

- Glut1+

Kaposiform Hemangioendothelioma and Tufted Angioma

Kaposiform hemangioendothelioma and tufted angioma are now considered to be within the same spectrum of vascular neoplasms with cases exhibiting combined histologic appearance. It is a rare tumor affecting primarily children, frequently associated with Kasabach-Merritt phenomenon, a condition characterized by profound thrombocytopenia and life-threatening hemorrhage.[152] It presents most commonly as a soft tissue tumor but it frequently affects the dermis and subcutis most often on the extremities.[152] It is classified as a vascular tumor of intermediate malignancy. The outcome is strongly dependent on the site, clinical extent, and the development of consumption coagulopathy. Death occurs in about 10% of patients either from the local effects of disease or from complications of Kasabach-Merritt phenomenon.[152]

On the skin, it presents as an ill-defined violaceous plaque and histologically it has features common to both capillary hemangioma and Kaposi sarcoma. It is composed of spindled zones of fusiform endothelial cells with slight atypia, merging with glomeruloid nests of rounded or epithelioid endothelial cells and slit like vascular channels or rounded capillary-type vessels. Mitotic activity is variable but generally low. At the periphery it has a lymphatic component.[153] Kaposiform hemangioendothelioma is characterized by ill-defined lobules of spindle cells and interspersing thin-walled vessels within the deep dermis and subcutaneous tissue. Tufted angioma is comprised characteristically of multiple cellular capillary lobules ("cannon balls") in the dermis (**Figure 8.91**).

The tumors have both lymphatic and vascular components. The endothelial cells of kaposiform hemangioendotheliomas and tufted angioma are positive for lymphatic markers D2-40, LYVE-1, and Prox-1; and vascular markers Erg, CD31, and CD34 (**Figure 8.92**).[154] D2-40 and other lymphatic-specific endothelial markers, such as VEGFR-3 and LYVE-1 are expressed in the Kaposi-like component of kaposiform hemangioendothelioma, but not in the endothelial cells that form the nodules. They are negative for Glut-1 and HHV8, highlighting the importance of these two antibodies in differentiating kaposiform hemangioendothelioma from infantile hemangioma and Kaposi sarcoma (**Table 8.4**).[152,154]

Kaposiform hemangioendothelioma and tufted angioma

- D2–40+/- GLUT1-

Table 8.4 Summary of D2-40 and GLUT-1 immunoreactivity in vascular tumors

	D2–40	GLUT–1
Infantile hemangioma	–	+
Congenital hemangioma	–/+	–
Tufted angioma	+/–	–
Kaposiform hemangioendothelioma	+	–
Lobular capillary hemangioma (pyogenic granuloma)	–	–

Kaposi Sarcoma

There are four types of Kaposi sarcoma with different clinical and epidemiologic features and biologic behavior: the classical/endemic type of Kaposi sarcoma which affects mainly elderly patients; the African-endemic variant; Kaposi sarcoma associated with immunosuppressive drugs (iatrogenic) and AIDS-associated Kaposi sarcoma. Human herpes virus 8 (HHV8) is the etiologic agent of all subtypes.[155] The clinical presentation of the cutaneous lesions is similar in all the subtypes. They present as reddish-blue macules or plaques, which are often multiple and gradually enlarge, sometimes forming nodules.

The microscopic appearances of Kaposi sarcoma go through three phases. The patch stage of Kaposi sarcoma shows an increased number of irregular, jagged, vascular spaces lined by thin endothelial cells in the superficial dermis. The neoplastic vessels tend to dissect around pre-existing normal adnexae and blood vessels producing the so-called "promontory sign." Plaque lesions of Kaposi sarcoma show an increased number of spindle cells arranged in short fascicles between collagen bundles centered on proliferating vascular channels. In nodular stage, the spindle cells are arranged in interwoven fascicles with extravasated erythrocytes.

HHV8 immunostain detects the latent nuclear antigen (LANA-1) of HHV8 in the nuclei of neoplastic cells and exhibits 100% sensitivity and 100% specificity for Kaposi sarcoma.[156]

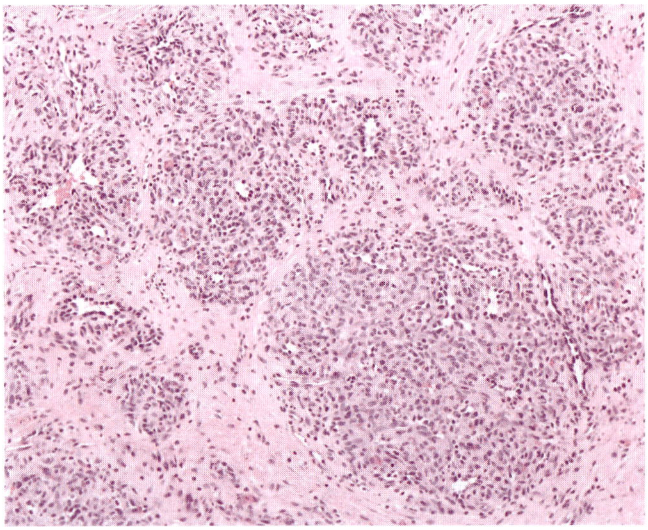

Figure 8.91 Tufted angioma is characterized by multiple cellular capillary lobules in the dermis (X200).

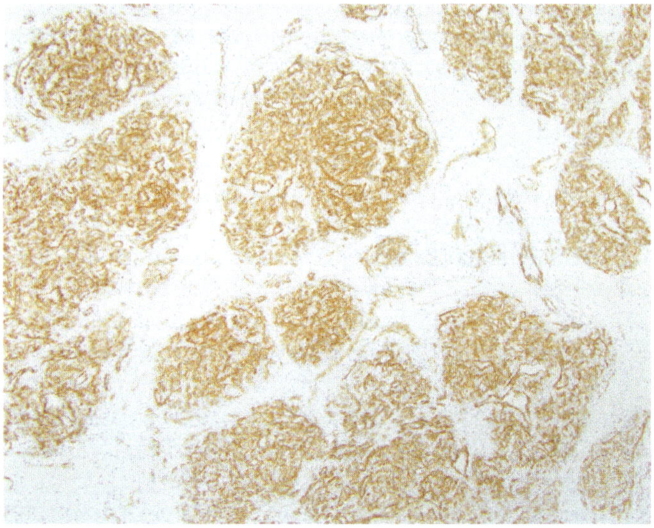

Figure 8.92 Tufted angioma. The endothelial cells express CD34 (X100).

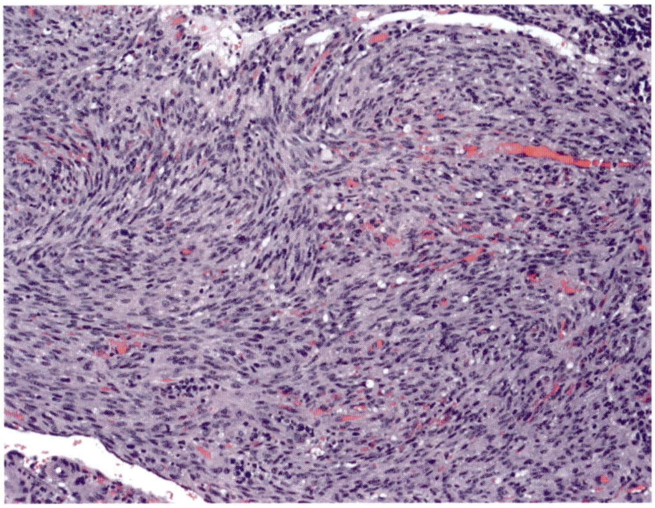

Figure 8.93 Intersecting fascicles of spindle neoplastic cells with associated extravasated erythrocytes characteristic of Kaposi sarcoma (X200).

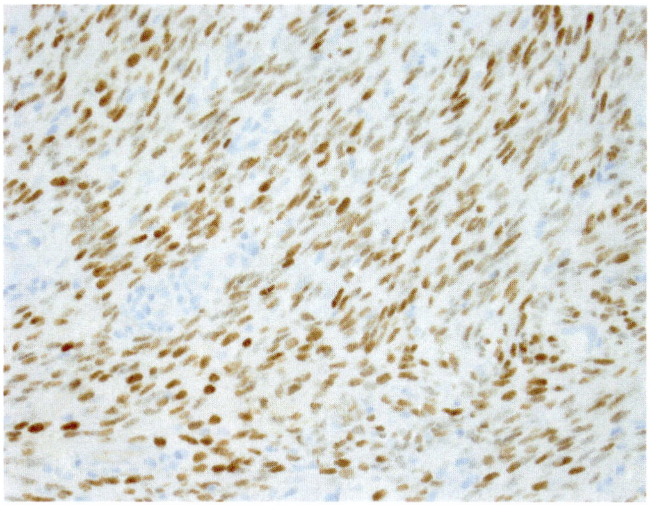

Figure 8.94 Kaposi sarcoma. Nuclear positivity with human herpesvirus 8 immunostain (X400).

The tumor cells express lymphatic markers including LYVE-1, D2-40 and Prox-1 as well as endothelial markers (CD31, CD34, and Erg) (**Figures 8.93 and 8.94**).[157]

The histologic differential diagnosis would include targetoid hemosiderotic hemangioma for patch-stage Kaposi sarcoma; tufted angioma, microvenular hemangioma, and acroangiodermatitis for plaque-stage; and bacillary angiomatosis, spindle cell hemangioma, kaposiform hemangioendothelioma, angiomatoid fibrous histiocytoma for nodular Kaposi sarcoma. The expression of HHV8 immunostain is helpful in distinguishing Kaposi sarcoma from various histologic mimics;[156] however, HHV8 expression has been reported in some angiosarcomas, hemangiomas, and dermatofibromas.[158]

Kaposi sarcoma

- HHV8+, D2–40+, CD31+, CD34+, Erg+

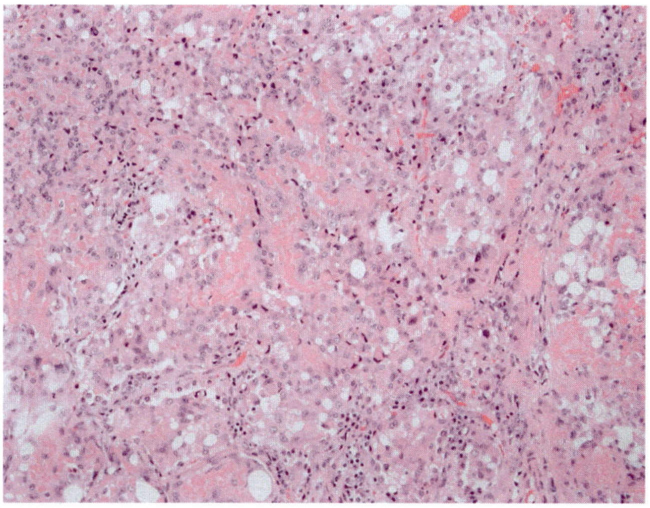

Figure 8.95 Epithelioid hemangioendothelioma. Epithelioid tumor cells contain vacuoles in their cytoplasm indicative of primitive vascular differentiation (X200).

Epithelioid Hemangioendothelioma

Epithelioid hemangioendothelioma is mainly a soft tissue tumor, but can occur in the skin, usually associated with an underlying bone or soft tissue tumor. Rare cases with exclusive cutaneous involvement have been described.[159] Presenting as circumscribed dermal or subcutaneous nodules epithelioid hemangioendothelioma often has a propensity for angiocentric growth, expanding the vessel wall and obliterating the lumen as they extend from the vascular lumen to the adjacent soft tissue. Many of the plump, epithelioid tumor cells contain vacuoles in their cytoplasm as a sign of primitive vascular differentiation (**Figure 8.95**).

The tumor cells express vascular endothelial markers such as CD31, CD34, Factor VIII, Fli-1, and Erg (v-ets erythroblastosis virus E26 homolog).[159,160] Epithelioid hemangioendothelioma expresses cytokeratin (CK) 18, CK7, and CK8 in 100%, 50%, and 10% of cases, respectively.[160] They are negative for CK14 and CK19.[160] The expression of cytokeratin is common and must be interpreted with caution when making the differential diagnosis with carcinoma.[160]

The differential diagnosis includes metastatic carcinoma, melanoma, epithelioid angiosarcoma and epithelioid sarcoma. A panel of immunohistochemical stains including broad spectrum keratins, S100, and Melan-A in addition to CD31 and CD34, would help either excluding or ruling in carcinoma and melanoma. Since epithelioid hemangioendothelioma also express keratin marker, using a broad panel of immunohistochemical markers is important. Epithelioid angiosarcoma would be comprised of a solid proliferation of atypical and mitotically active epithelioid endothelial cells. Epithelioid sarcoma would express CD34 and subsets of keratins; however, it would be negative for CD31.

Epithelioid hemangioendothelioma is characterized by recurrent translocations involving chromosomal regions 1p36.3 and 3q25, resulting in the formation of a *WWTR1::CAMTA1*

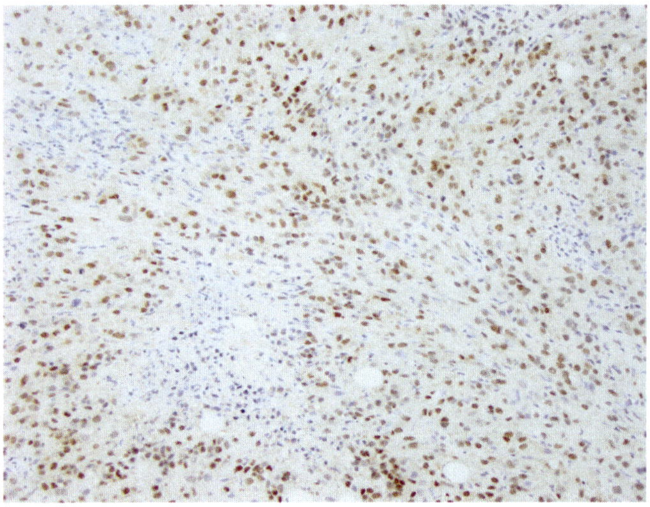

Figure 8.96 Epithelioid hemangioendothelioma. Nuclear CAMTA1 expression is seen (X200).

fusion gene in approximately 90% of cases and a small subset by a *YAP1::TFE3* fusion gene.[161,162] Epithelioid hemangioendothelioma with *YAP1::TFE3* fusion shows distinctive histology: solid growth pattern, neoplastic cells with eosinophilic cytoplasm, and forming vascular spaces.[162] The *WWTR1::CAMTA1* fusion, a feature of epithelioid hemangioendothelioma, has not been detected in epithelioid hemangioma, pseudomyogenic hemangioendothelioma (epithelioid sarcoma-like hemangioendothelioma), or epithelioid angiosarcoma; thus, it can be an ancillary molecular test in difficult cases.[161] Since most cases of epithelioid hemangioendothelioma harbor the *WWTR1::CAMTA1* fusion, there has been effort searching for a useful antibody to detect the protein product of this fusion. In fact, Doyle et al.[163] described the nuclear expression of a polyclonal anti-CAMTA1 antibody up to 86% of epithelioid hemangioendothelioma cases, and lack of expression in other epithelioid endothelial neoplasms in the differential diagnosis (**Figure 8.96**). The results of these studies suggested the potential role of CAMTA1 in confirming a diagnosis of epithelioid hemangioendothelioma, with high sensitivity and specificity.[163] Some cases of epithelioid hemangioendothelioma lack the *WWTR1::CAMTA1* fusion gene but instead have *TFE3*-rearrangements. Antonescu et al.[162] reported strong and diffuse nuclear TFE3 expression in cases with *TFE3*-rearrangements suggesting that this can be applied as a useful marker to diagnose tumors that harbor *TFE3*-rearrangements.

Epithelioid hemangioendothelioma

- CD31+, CD34+, Erg+, keratin 18+, keratin 7+/-
- CAMTA1+ in tumors with *CAMTA1* fusion

Hobnail Hemangioendotheliomas

Hobnail hemangioendotheliomas are locally aggressive, rarely metastasizing vascular neoplasms characterized by arborizing vascular channels lined by endothelial cells with a hobnail morphology. They include retiform hemangioendothelioma (RHE) and papillary intralymphatic angioendothelioma (PILA).

RHE occurs predominantly in young to middle-aged adults as asymptomatic single plaque-like lesion usually on limbs with higher incidence in lower limbs. They recur in up to 50% of cases but lymph node metastasis is rare. Histologically they present as poorly delineated dermal proliferation of interconnecting blood vessels lining by a single layer of bland hobnail endothelial cells.

PILA most often presents as an ill-defined violaceous or bluish papule or nodule with gradual enlargement, on distal extremities most frequently thigh but any anatomical site can be affected. Histologically PILA is characterized by dilated lymphatic channels resembling a cavernous lymphangioma in the dermis and subcutaneous tissue lined by a single layer of hobnail endothelial cells. Papillary projections into the vascular lumina are frequent.

Subsets of RHE demonstrate Yes-associated protein 1 (YAP1) rearrangements, most often *YAP1::MAML2* fusions.[164]

The endothelial cells of both PILA and RHE express endothelial markers (CD31, CD34, Erg, and FLI1) and lymphatic markers (D2-40, VEGFR3, and PROX1). Loss of expression of YAP1-cytoplasmic terminus may also be useful in the diagnosis of RHE and CHE.[165] Synaptophysin expression is described in hemangioendothelioma cases with hobnail morphology, a finding which in combination with shared *YAP1::MAML2* fusions supports a relationship with composite hemangioendothelioma.[166]

Hobnail hemangioendotheliomas

- Endothelial markers: CD31+ CD34+ Erg+ Fli–1+
- Lymphatic markers: D2–40+ VEGFR3+ Prox1+
- Synaptophysin +/-

Pseudomyogenic Hemangioendothelioma

Pseudomyogenic or cutaneous epithelioid sarcoma-like hemangioendothelioma is a rarely metastasizing vascular neoplasm of intermediate malignancy.[167] It tends to arise as painful or painless nodule in the lower limbs of young adults and children with a remarkable male predominance. Pseudomyogeneic hemangioendothelioma (PHE) can harbor *SERPINE1::FOSB* or *ACTB::FOSB* fusions, resulting in upregulation of *FOSB*.[168]

Histologically, PHE shows fascicular proliferation of plump spindle cells with eosinophilic cytoplasm arranged in short intersecting fascicles, sometimes mimicking rhabdomyoblasts, showing generally mild nuclear atypia and little mitotic activity (**Figure 8.97**). In addition to vascular markers Fli1, Erg, and CD31; expression of epithelial markers (keratin AE1/AE3, CAM5.2), smooth muscle actin focally, and INI1 is seen.[167] They are negative for EMA, D2-40, HHV8, S100, desmin, myogenin, MyoD1, CD99, and CD10 (**see Case Study 4**). Most tumors exhibit nuclear staining for FOSB (**Figure 8.98**).[169]

The histologic differential diagnosis of pseudomyogenic hemangioendothelioma includes epithelioid sarcoma, epithelioid hemangioendothelioma, and epithelioid angiosarcoma.

Table 8.5 Immunoprofile of epithelioid vascular neoplasms

	AE1/AE3	EMA	CD31	CD34	Fli1	Erg	FOSB	INI1	translocation
Pseudomyogenic hemangioendothelioma	+	-	+	-	+	+	+	+	t(7;19)(q22;q13)
Epithelioid sarcoma	+	+	-	+/-	+	-	-	-	not known
Epithelioid hemangioendothelioma	focal +	-	+	+	+	+	-	+	t(1;3)(p36.3;q25)
Epithelioid angiosarcoma	focal +	-	+	+	+	+	-	+	not known

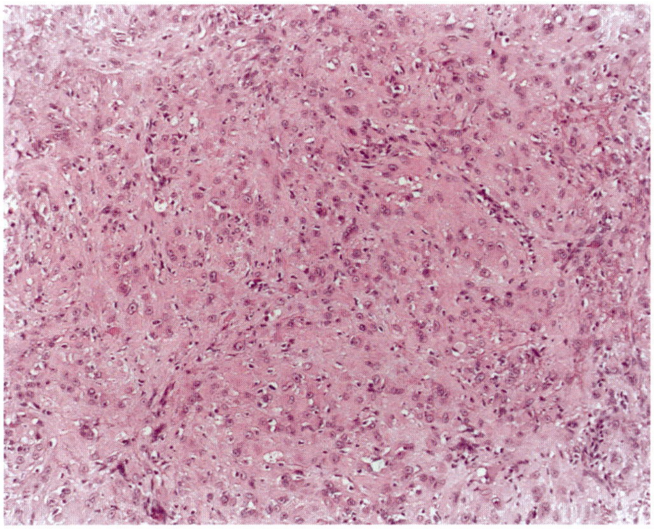

Figure 8.97 Pseudomyogenic hemangioendothelioma is characterized by a fascicular proliferation of epithelioid cells with abundant eosinophilic cytoplasm (X200).

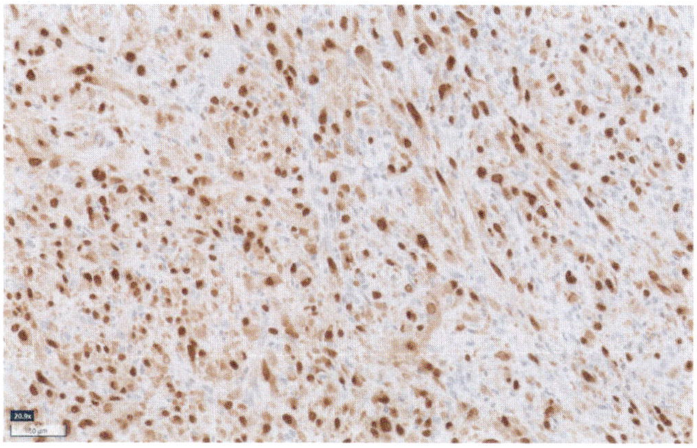

Figure 8.98 Pseudomyogenic hemangioendothelioma. The epithelioid cells are positive for FOSB (X200).

Epithelioid sarcoma would typically exhibit loss of INI1 expression, expresses EMA and CD34, and is negative for endothelial markers. Epithelioid hemangioendothelioma would express CD34 in 50% of cases and harbor *WWTR1::CAMTA1* fusion gene, whereas pseudomyogenic hemangioendothelioma is negative for CD34 and harbors *FOSB* translocation.[167] Although both epithelioid hemangioendothelioma and angiosarcoma can express keratins, the expression is typically focal (**Table 8.5**). [167]

Pseudomyogenic hemangioendothelioma

- FOSB+
- CD31+ Erg+ Fli1+ keratin AE1/AE3+ IN1+
- EMA- CD34-

Composite Hemangioendothelioma

Composite hemangioendothelioma is a locally aggressive rarely metastasizing malignant vascular tumor composed histologically of an admixture of benign, low-grade malignant and high-grade malignant vascular components. In a subset of cases neuroendocrine expression is present – so-called neuroendocrine composite hemangioendothelioma.

It most often occurs in distal extremities (hands and feet), or head and neck of adults in the fourth to fifth decade of life. The clinical presentation is usually as a slowly progressive solitary nodule but can be multiple. A subset of tumors harbors *YAP1::MAML2* gene fusions.[164] *PTBP1::MAML2* and *EPC1::PCH2* gene fusions have been identified in 3 cases and 1 case of neuroendocrine composite hemangioendothelioma, respectively.[165,170]

Histologically it is composed of a variable admixture of histological patterns, including retiform hemangioendothelioma, spindle cell hemangioma, epithelioid hemangioendothelioma, lymphangioma, hemangioma, and even well-differentiated angiosarcoma-like components. The tumor cells express endothelial markers (CD31, CD34, Erg, and FLI-1) and they are negative for CAMTA1. The neuroendocrine subtype composite hemangioendothelioma (a distinct subtype with aggressive clinical behavior) expresses synaptophysin but is usually negative for chromogranin.[170] Composite hemangioendothelioma with *YAP1::MAML2* fusions show loss of expression of YAP1 cytoplasmic-terminus.[164]

Composite hemangioendothelioma

- CD31+ CD34+ Erg+ FLI–1+
- Synaptophysin+ chromogranin – (in neuroendocrine subtype)

Cutaneous Angiosarcoma

Angiosarcomas are highly aggressive neoplasms that can be idiopathic or induced by sun exposure, radiation, and chronic lymphedema. Greater than 50% of cases are on cutaneous sites.

Clinically, the lesions appear as ill-defined bruise-like areas that simulate a hematoma. More advanced lesions present as indurate plaques with raised, nodular, and occasionally ulceration accompanied by smaller satellite lesions in the same vicinity.

Well-differentiated angiosarcomas appear as irregular, dilated vascular channels lined by flattened endothelial cells dissecting the dermis. These channels tend to communicate with each other, forming an anastomosing network. Poorly differentiated angiosarcomas demonstrate solid proliferations of polygonal or spindle-shaped pleomorphic endothelial cells, with prominent mitotic activity and poorly formed vascular spaces, which sometimes makes it difficult to distinguish them from carcinoma, melanoma, or a high-grade fibrosarcoma.

Most angiosarcomas express CD34 and variably for CD31, WT1, and Erg.[160] A diagnostic vascular panel includes CD31, Erg, and D2-40. Epithelioid angiosarcomas express CK8 and CK18 in approximately 50% of cases, EMA in 25%, and only rarely for CK7 and CK19, which can result in misdiagnosis as carcinoma.[171]

Cutaneous angiosarcoma

- CD34+, CD31+, WT1+, Erg+
- Epithelioid variant: CK8+/-, CK18+/-

Post-Radiation Vascular Lesions

Post-radiation angiosarcomas can develop after radiotherapy for benign or malignant conditions. Radiation-associated angiosarcoma usually start as violaceous infiltrating plaques or nodules. Because of similar physical findings, these lesions should be distinguished from hemangiomas or "simple bruises."

Several criteria must be present in order to associate radiotherapy with neoplastic development: (1) site of tumor must be within field of radiotherapy, (2) there must be at least three to five years' interval, and (3) the induced tumor has a different histology than the primary cancer. The latency period between radiation therapy and the onset of vascular lesions ranged from months to years.[172] Irregular, branched, and anastomosing vascular channels are seen in the dermis. The tumor is poorly defined and infiltrates the dermis. In some cases, it can present as a solid, undifferentiated, or spindled cell tumor and the vascular origin can be difficult to recognize. In these cases, immunohistochemistry using a panel of endothelial markers, including factors VIII, CD31, CD34, FLi-1, and Erg, may help in the diagnosis.

MYC amplification has been identified in 50% to 100% of post-radiation and lymphedema-associated angiosarcomas. Immunohistochemical stainings for MYC correlates with the presence or absence of *MYC* amplification and confirmation *MYC* amplification by FISH is diagnostically helpful.[173] MYC nuclear expression is typically seen in post-radiation angiosarcoma whereas this marker is negative in atypical vascular lesions status post radiation therapy (**Figures 8.99 and 8.100**). MYC expression has been reported in a subset of primary cutaneous angiosarcomas.[173] Post-radiation angiosarcoma would typically be MYC+Ki67 high while atypical post-radiation vascular lesions would be MYC-Ki67 low.

Post-radiation vascular lesions

- Post-radiation angiosarcomas: MYC+
- Post-radiation atypical vascular lesions: MYC-

Microvenular Hemangioma

Microvenular hemangioma is characterized by a poorly circumscribed proliferation of small blood vessels with inconspicuous lumina. The vascular channels are positive for factor VIII, CD34, and CD31.[174] While they are positive for WT1, they are negative for Glut1 and D2-40.[174]

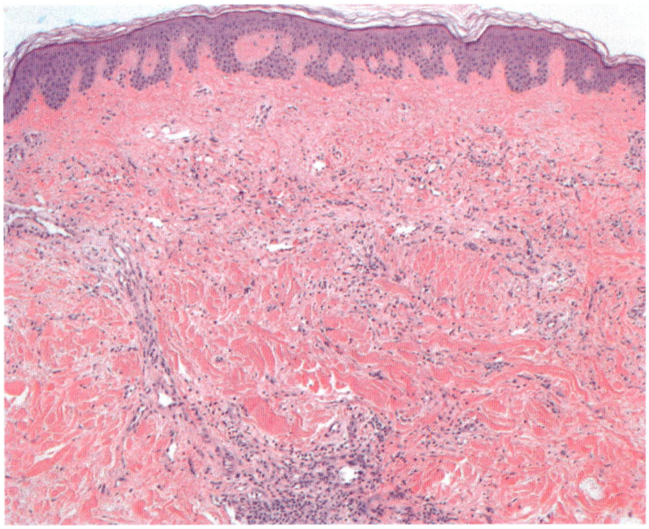

Figure 8.99 Post-radiation angiosarcoma. A proliferation of irregular vascular channels lined by plump endothelial cells is seen dissecting the dermis (X100).

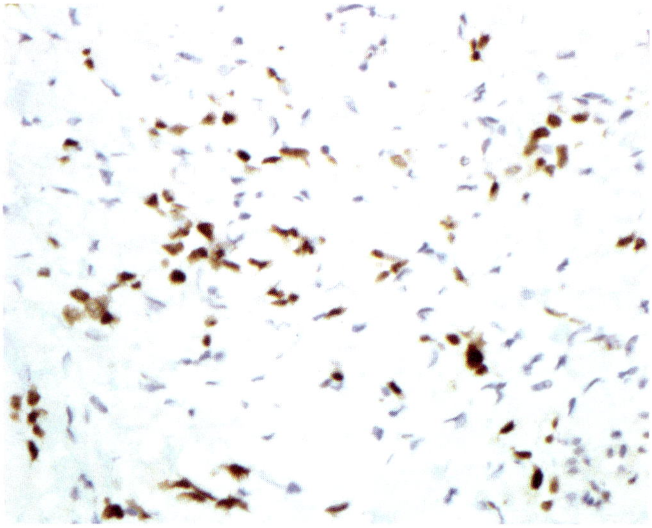

Figure 8.100 Post-radiation angiosarcoma. The endothelial cells are positive for c-MYC (X400).

Microvenular hemangioma

- CD34+ CD31+

Pseudolymphomatous Angiokeratoma

Pseudolymphomatous angiokeratoma, also known as acral pseudolymphomatous angiokeratoma of children is a benign cutaneous condition. It is clinically characterized by angiomatous papules with predilection for the hands and feet, particularly the digits of children. It also occurs in adults.[175] The etiology is unknown but the lesion is thought to develop after trauma.

Histologically, a nodular inflammatory cell infiltrate comprising B- and T-lymphocytes, plasma cells, and histiocytes in the papillary dermis and a proliferation of thick-walled blood vessels, sometimes with mitotic figures, is characteristic. Immunohistochemistry reveals a predominant T-cell population with a smaller component of B-cells. The T-cells are composed of equal numbers of CD4+ and CD8+ lymphocytes. PCR analyses for immunoglobulin heavy chain genes or T-cell receptor gamma genes re-arrangement show that these infiltrates are polyclonal.[175]

The clinical differential diagnosis includes other acquired angiomatous lesions that occur after trauma. However, the characteristic morphologic features of pseudolymphomatous angiokeratoma are usually sufficient to make the diagnosis.

Kimura Disease

Kimura disease is a rare benign chronic inflammatory disease that usually involves the deep subcutaneous tissue of the head and neck region with frequent regional lymphadenopathy or salivary gland enlargement. The etiology of this condition is unknown, but it may be an immune reaction to an unknown stimulus. It is classified as a benign reactive process, but it may recur locally.[176] It affects predominantly middle-aged Asian men.[189] It presents clinically as single or multiple red-violaceous nodules and, often associated with elevations of serum IgE levels and eosinophilia of the peripheral blood.[189]

Microscopically it is characterized by a prominent lymphoid component organized in follicles with germinal centers, admixed with reactive eosinophils sometimes with microabscesses and infiltration of germinal centers by eosinophils. The vascular component is seen between the follicles consisting of elongated capillary-sized vessels containing plump, cytologically bland endothelial cells.[176] Importantly the endothelial cells are not epithelioid, a feature that helps to distinguish from angiolymphoid hyperplasia with eosinophilia, a frequent differential diagnosis. During the late stages of the disease, a dense hyaline fibrosis supervenes.

Over the years, there has been considerable confusion between Kimura disease and angiolymphoid hyperplasia with eosinophilia, with a number of reports considering the two entities synonymously. However, it is now known that they are two entirely unrelated lesions clinically and histologically quite different.[176]

8.7 Pericytic and Perivascular Neoplasms

Pericytes are cells that surround blood vessels and control vascular permeability and stability. Pericytes and perivascular neoplasms usually stain positively for SMA and do not stain for desmin. Of note, perivascular epithelioid tumors (PEComas), which have a myomelanocytic phenotype (SMA+, Melan-A+) will not be reviewed in this section.

Myofibroma and Myofibromatosis

Myofibromas are benign lesions that most commonly occur in the pediatric population, although lesions can be seen in adults.[177] Histologically, they show a biphasic appearance with cellular areas with hemangiopericytoma-like vascular patterns and hypocellular myoid nodules (**Figure 8.101**). By immunohistochemistry they are positive for SMA (**Figure 8.102**) and are typically negative for desmin.[177] Caldesmon is usually negative and calponin expression can be focal (**Figure 8.103**). Of note, areas of increased mitotic activity, hypercellularity, infiltration, perineural entrapment and intravascular growth can be seen but do not indicate malignant transformation. Myofibromas

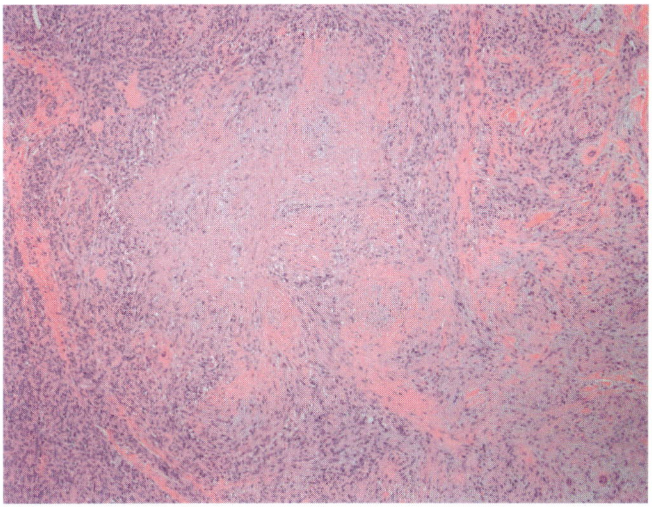

Figure 8.101 A proliferation of spindle cells with extensive hyalinization seen in myofibroma (X100).

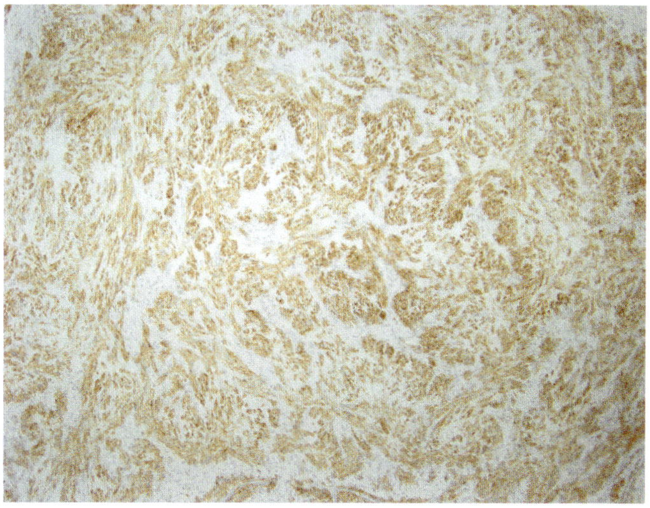

Figure 8.102 Myofibroma. Diffuse smooth muscle actin expression (X100).

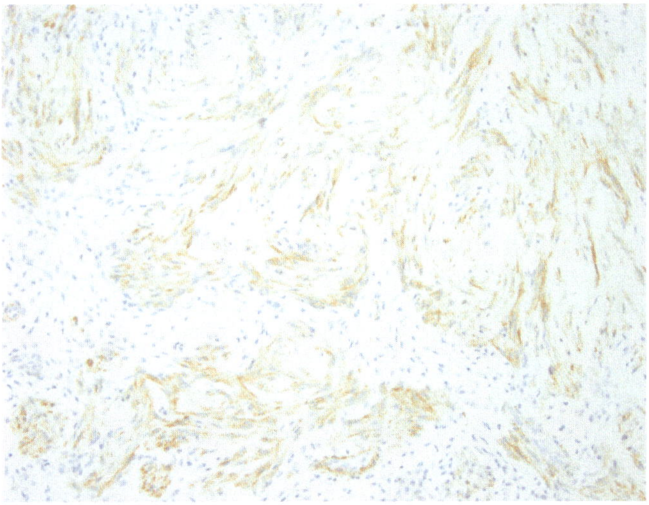

Figure 8.103 Myofibroma. Patchy calponin expression (X200).

harbor alterations in *PGDFRB* in the NOTCH pathway and immunohistochemistry for NOTCH3 can be used to identify myofibromas.[178] The histologic differential diagnosis includes myopericytoma (absence of myoid nodules), solitary fibrous tumor (STAT6+) and other myofibroblastic tumors.

Myofibroma and myofibromatosis

- SMA+, calponin+/-, h-caldesmon-, desmin-, S100-

Glomus Tumor

Glomus tumors are benign neoplasms that are derived from modified smooth muscle cells present in physiologic arteriovenous shunts, Sucquet-Hoyer canals, or from undifferentiated perivascular cells that can transform into glomus cells. They present as small, painful dermal neoplasms, particularly in the nail bed of the fingers, and other parts of the distal extremities, although they have been reported in every part of the body. Glomus tumors are comprised of glomus cells with round or polygonal shapes, eosinophilic cytoplasm and can be associated with vascular structures. Variants/subtypes include solid glomus tumor (with poor vasculature and scant smooth muscle component), glomangioma (with prominent vascular component), glomangiomatosis (resembling angiomatosis with abundant glomus cells), symplastic glomus tumor (striking nuclear atypia without other malignant features) or glomangiomyoma (with prominent vascular and smooth muscle components).[179]

The immunohistochemical phenotype of glomus tumor support a pericytic/perivascular phenotype: glomus cells express vimentin, smooth muscle actin, muscle-specific actin and h-caldesmon in virtually all glomus tumors (**Figures 8.104 and 8.105**). Desmin and CD34 are typically not expressed.

Malignant glomus tumors have atypical features including at least one of the following: deep-seated location with a size >2 cm, atypical mitotic figures, moderate to severe nuclear atypia and increased mitotic activity (>5/50 hpf).[179] The histologic differential diagnosis of glomus tumors includes cutaneous adnexal neoplasms (keratin+) and melanocytic nevi (Sox10+, S100+).

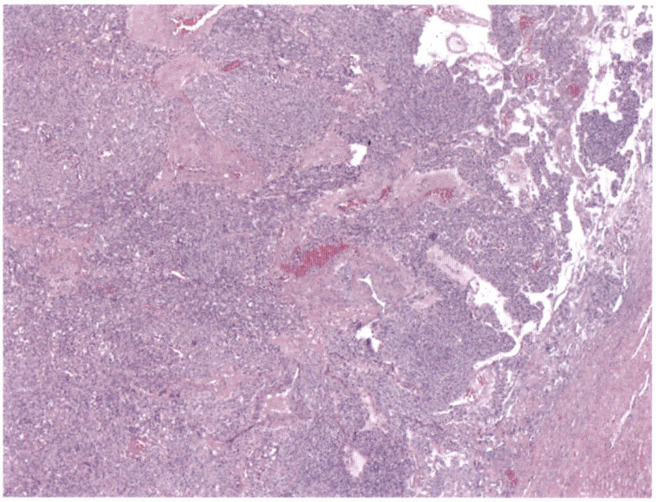

Figure 8.104 Uniformly shaped tumor cells are seen in glomus tumor (X100).

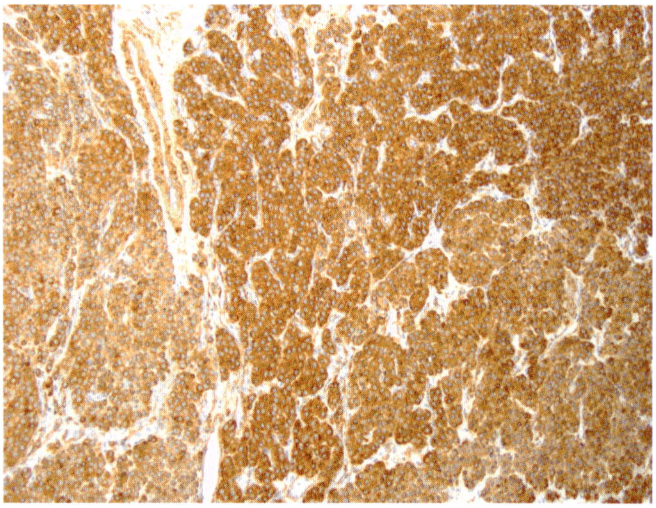

Figure 8.105 Glomus tumor. Diffuse smooth muscle actin expression (X200).

Glomus tumor

- SMA+, caldesmon+, desmin-

Myopericytoma

Myopericytomas are benign entities that commonly occur in the extremities and are typically found in the dermis and subcutis.[180] On histologic examination they are circumscribed and show perivascular, concentric growth around vessels (**Figure 8.106**).[180] By immunohistochemistry, myopericytomas are invariably positive for SMA, usually positive for h-caldesmon (**Figure 8.107**) and negative for desmin.[180] Very rare cases of malignant myopericytomas have been reported (high mitotic activity and metastatic disease). The histologic differential

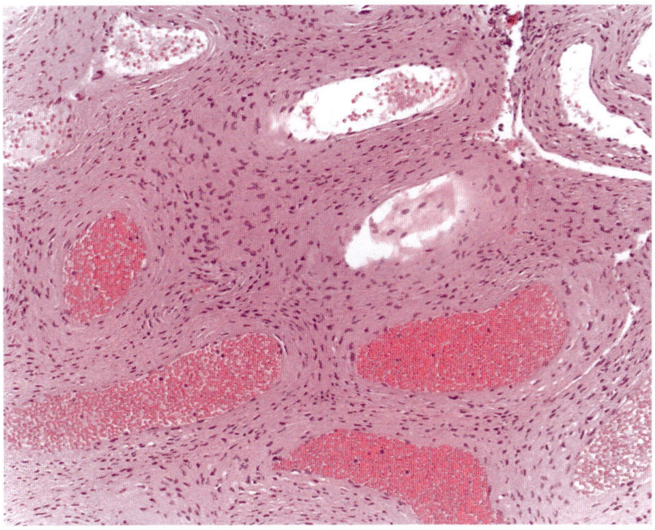

Figure 8.106 Myopericytomas characteristically show a proliferation of cells around vessels (X200).

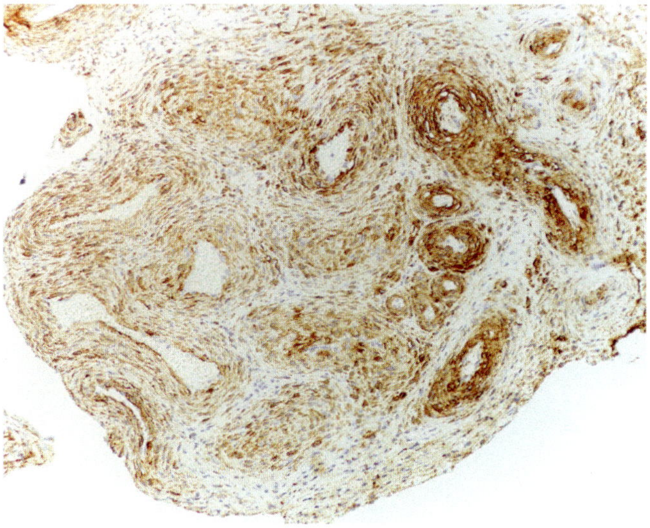

Figure 8.107 Myopericytoma. Caldesmon can be positive (X100).

diagnosis of myopericytoma includes myofibroma (presence of myoid nodules) and solitary fibrous tumor (STAT6+).

Myopericytoma

- SMA+, caldesmon+, desmin-

Angioleiomyoma

Angioleiomyomas can present as painful masses on the lower extremities. Three histologic subtypes have been identified including solid (proliferation of spindled smooth muscle cells compressing vessels), venous (proliferation of spindled smooth muscle cells with large, gaping vessels), and cavernous (dilated vessels with intermixed spindled smooth muscle cells).[181] By immunohistochemistry, angioleiomyomas are positive for SMA, h-caldesmon, and calponin with variable expression of desmin (dependent on subtype).[181] The histologic differential diagnosis includes PEComas (Melan-A+, HMB-45+) and myopericytoma (desmin-).

Angioleiomyoma

- SMA+, caldesmon+, calponin+, desmin+/-

8.8 Tumors of Uncertain Differentiation

Atypical Fibroxanthoma

Atypical fibroxanthoma (AFX) is a lesion that commonly occurs in older men at sun-exposed sites.[13] Histologic examination reveals a circumscribed proliferation of atypical pleomorphic cells centered in the dermis (**Figure 8.108**). A number of histologic variants exist including spindled, clear cell and myxoid; osteoclast-like giant cells can also be found.[13] Histologic features such as invasion into the subcutis, necrosis or lymphovascular/perineural invasion should prompt consideration of the diagnosis of pleomorphic dermal sarcoma (PDS).[13] Lesions without histologic features concerning for PDS can locally recur but rarely metastasize. AFX is a diagnosis of exclusion and other entities such as spindle cell squamous cell carcinoma (keratin+, p40+, p63+ with overlying in-situ component), melanoma (Sox10+, S100+, Melan-A+, HMB-45+), angiosarcoma (ERG+, CD31+), cutaneous metastases and leiomyosarcoma (SMA+, h-caldesmon+, desmin+) should be excluded. AFXs often stain positively for CD10, CD68 and CD163 (**see Case Study 5**).[182] In some cases there is focal aberrant expression of CD31, keratin AE1/AE3, EMA, MiTF (**Figure 8.109**), Melan-A and p63. p40 has been shown to be a more specific marker than p63 in highlighting sarcomatoid carcinoma, a lesion in the differential diagnosis of AFX.[183] SMA expression can be seen in AFX, however, other immunostains such as desmin and h-caldesmon should be employed to distinguish AFX from leiomyosarcoma.

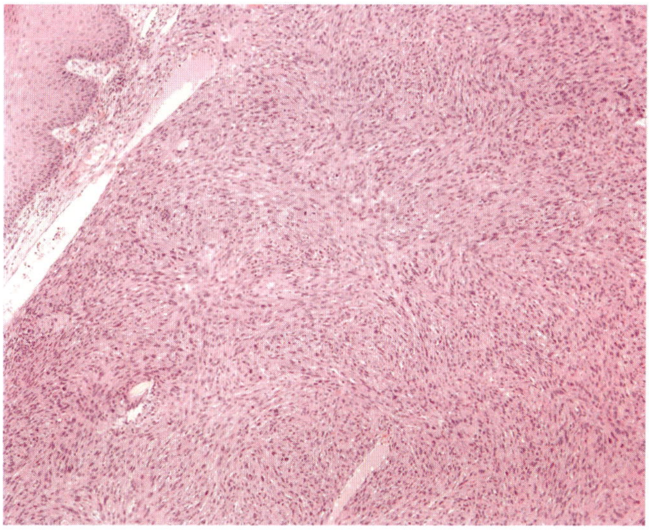

Figure 8.108 Atypical fibroxanthoma. An atypical proliferation of spindle tumor cells is seen in the dermis (X100).

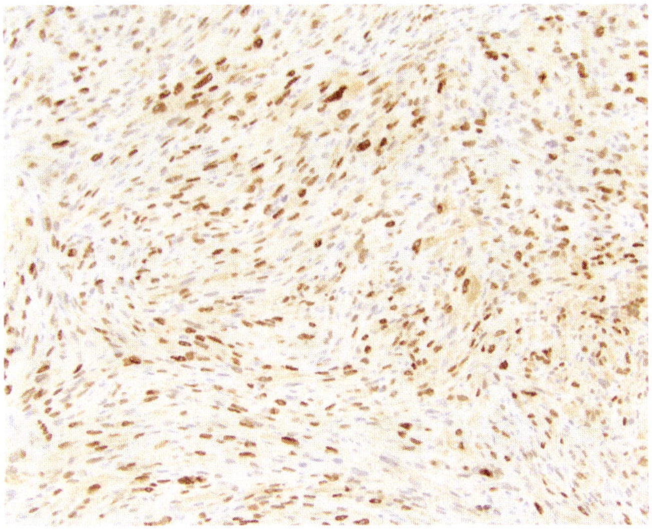

Figure 8.109 Atypical fibroxanthoma. Aberrant expression of MiTF can be seen in AFX (X200).

Atypical fibroxanthoma

- CD68+, CD10+, Sox10-, p40-

Pleomorphic Dermal Sarcoma

Pleomorphic dermal sarcoma, like atypical fibroxanthoma, occurs commonly in older males in sun-exposed areas.[13] On histologic examination pleomorphic dermal sarcoma show a proliferation of atypical, pleomorphic cells and shows features worrisome for more aggressive behavior including invasion into the subcutis, necrosis, or lymphovascular/perineural invasion.[13] These more aggressive histologic features confer a significant risk of local recurrence and metastasis.[13] Like AFX, pleomorphic dermal sarcoma is a diagnosis of exclusion and other entities such as spindle cell squamous cell carcinoma (keratin+, p40+, p63+ with overlying in-situ component), melanoma (Sox10+, S100+, Melan-A+, HMB-45+), angiosarcoma (ERG+, CD31+), cutaneous metastases and leiomyosarcoma (SMA+, h-caldesmon+, desmin+) should be excluded. Pleomorphic dermal sarcoma typically express CD10 and can express SMA but are almost always negative for keratins, S100, and desmin.[13]

Pleomorphic dermal sarcoma

- CD68+, CD10+, Sox10-, p40-

Angiomatoid Fibrous Histiocytoma

Angiomatoid fibrous histiocytoma is a rare tumor that primarily occurs in children and young adults. Although previously reported as angiomatoid malignant fibrous histiocytoma, it has been renamed since it has a low metastatic potential and an excellent biologic course. It typically presents as a slow growing and painless mass on the extremities. On histology, a multinodular and circumscribed lesion is comprised of sheets of round to spindle neoplastic cells and associated large cystic spaces filled with hemorrhage. It is surrounded by a dense fibrous pseudocapsule and often dense inflammatory infiltrate. Since it lacks a specific immunoprofile, immunohistochemistry can only be supportive but not diagnostic. There is variable expression of CD68, smooth muscle actin, h-caldesmon, calponin, desmin, EMA, and CD99. S100 protein, cytokeratins, CD31, and CD34 are typically negative.[184] ALK expression can be seen and can lead to confusion with inflammatory myofibroblastic tumor.[185] Three characteristic gene fusions, *EWSR1::CREB1*, *EWSR1::ATF1*, and rarely *FUS::ATF1*, have been reported in angiomatoid fibrous histiocytoma.[184] The differential diagnosis can include nodular fasciitis (*USP6* rearrangements without pseudocapsule), vascular lesions (ERG+, CD31), and rhabdomyosarcoma (myogenin+, myoD1+). Molecular analysis may be needed to confirm the diagnosis.

Angiomatoid fibrous histiocytoma

- Desmin +/- ALK +/- EMA+/-

Cutaneous Myxoma (Superficial Angiomyxoma)

Cutaneous myxoma or superficial angiomyxoma can be solitary/sporadic or multiple/associated with Carney complex. Cutaneous myxoma commonly affects the head and neck, trunk, and extremities of middle-aged adult males. Myxomas can recur if incompletely excised. On histologic sections a multinodular proliferation of spindle to stellate cells are seen within an abundant myxoid matrix (**Figure 8.110**). The spindle cells are thought to be myofibroblastic since they express smooth muscle actin. They are negative for S100 (**Figure 8.111**), CD34, CD68, and factor 13a.[186] Both sporadic cases and cases associated with Carney complex can show loss of PRKAR1A by immunohistochemistry.[187] The differential diagnosis includes a variety of myxoid lesions such as aggressive angiomyxoma (deep, site-specific location), focal cutaneous mucinosis (less cellular), dermal nerve sheath myxoma (Sox10+, S100+), superficial acral fibromyxoma (acral site and CD34+ with RB1 loss), and myxoid neurofibroma (Sox10+, S100+).

Cutaneous myxoma

- SMA+ PRKAR1A loss

Deep (Aggressive) Angiomyxoma

Deep (aggressive) angiomyxoma is a non-metastasizing tumor which can locally recur in 9–50% of cases decades after the initial excision.[188] Clinically, it often presents as a labial cyst in women in the fourth decade. The lesion has a gelatinous or myxoid appearance but can be fibrous in the setting of recurrence. Aggressive angiomyxoma is a poorly circumscribed and paucicellular neoplasm composed of bland spindle cells within a myxoid stroma. The border is irregular and infiltrative. The

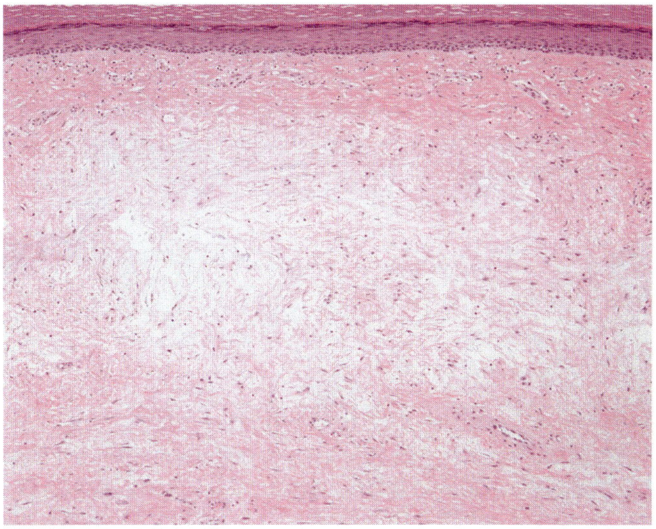

Figure 8.110 Cutaneous myxoma is characterized by a proliferation of stellate cells within a myxoid matrix (X100).

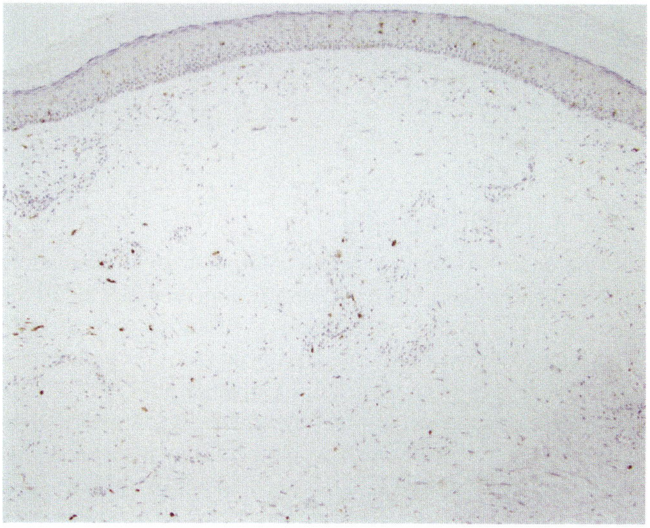

Figure 8.111 Cutaneous myxoma. S100 is negative (X100).

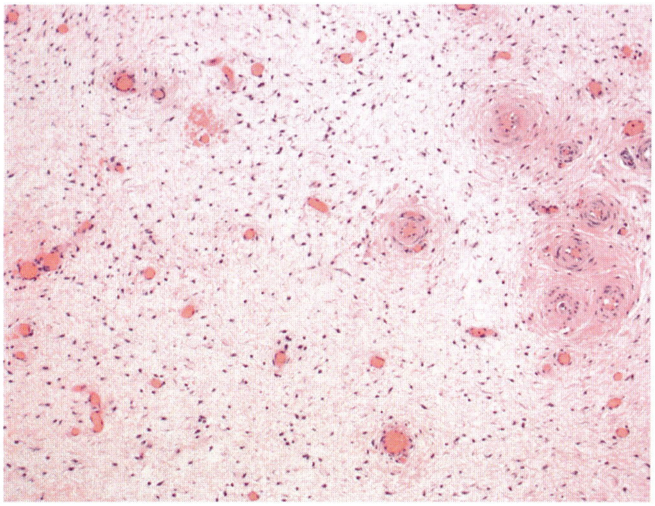

Figure 8.112 Paucicellular proliferation of bland spindle cells within a myxoid stroma in aggressive angiomyxoma (X100).

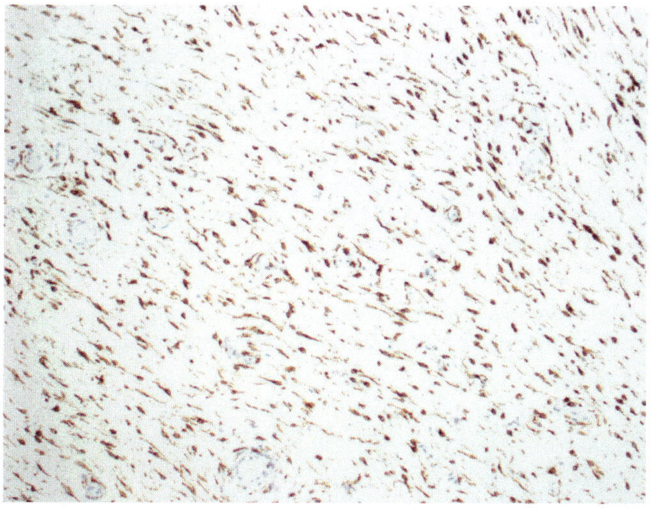

Figure 8.113 Aggressive angiomyxoma. Diffuse desmin expression (X100).

vessels are medium-sized, thick-walled and often hyalinized. Delicate bundles of smooth muscle are seen in loose clusters adjacent to these blood vessels.[188]

A number of genes including *HMGA2* on chromosome 12, especially region 12q13-15, have been implicated in the histogenesis of aggressive angiomyxoma.[189] Rearrangement of *HMGA2* and increased protein expression have been reported in 38–90% of aggressive angiomyxoma; thus, the marker has been suggested to be helpful in assessing margins.[189] The stromal cells often express desmin and smooth muscle actin (**Figures 8.112, 8.113, and 8.114**). They are negative for myosin, CD34, factor VIII, S100, NSE, and chromogranin.[188] Expression of estrogen and progesterone receptors is a frequent finding.[189] The histologic differential diagnosis includes superficial angiomyxoma (superficial and can show PRKAR1A loss), cellular angiofibroma (more cellular and can demonstrate Rb loss) and angiomyofibroblastoma (more cellular with perivascular growth of epithelioid cells).

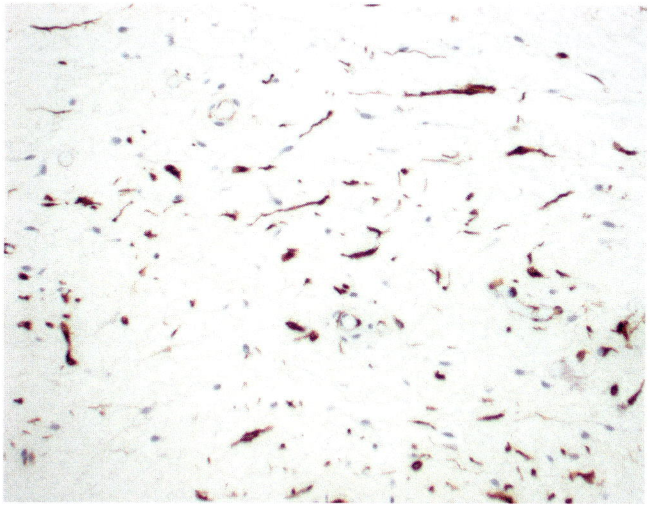

Figure 8.114 Aggressive angiomyxoma. Smooth muscle actin positivity (X200).

Aggressive angiomyxoma

- Desmin+, SMA+, HMGA2+, estrogen receptor+, progesterone receptor+

Cellular Neurothekeoma

Cellular neurothekeoma is a benign neoplasm of uncertain histogenesis, although some evidence suggests that they fall in the spectrum of fibrohistiocytic tumors.[190] Although once thought to be related to dermal nerve sheath myxomas, cellular neurothekeoma is now recognized as a distinct entity.[190] Cellular neurothekeomas usually occur in patients in the second decade, twice more common in women than in men and most commonly involve the head and neck, upper extremities, and shoulder region.[190] Clinically they presents as an asymptomatic, solitary, slow-growing, dome-shaped papule or nodule that is usually dermal-based but can involve superficial subcutis.

Histologically, the tumor has a multinodular, lobular, or plexiform pattern and is composed of nests of epithelioid or slightly spindle cells surrounded by densely hyaline collagen and a variably myxoid stroma (**Figure 8.115**). The tumor cells have abundant granular eosinophilic cytoplasm. The tumors can have an infiltrative appearance with some tumors entrapping fat, and occasional tumors (primarily from facial locations) infiltrating superficial skeletal muscle. Mitotic activity is usually less than 5/10 HPF, although a significant number show higher mitotic activity with no difference in the prognosis. A significant number of cases show cytologically atypical and pleomorphic cells, although this feature has not been proven to have prognostic significance.

The majority of cellular neurothekeoma express NKIC3, MiTF, and CD10; and they are invariably negative for S100, Melan A, and GFAP.[190] Hornick and Fletcher[190] found that all cellular neurothekeomas in their series were reactive for NKIC3 (**Figure 8.116**), 89% expressed NSE, and 57% demonstrated focal staining for SMA. Cellular neurothekeomas do not express S100 or GFAP, highlighting their lack of relationship with true nerve sheath tumors, including dermal nerve sheath myxoma.[190] The histologic differential diagnosis includes dermal nerve sheath myxoma (Sox10+, S100+), plexiform fibrohistiocytic tumor (presence of osteoclast-like giant cells and MiTF-) and melanocytic neoplasms such as Spitz lesions (Sox10+, S100+, Melan-A+, HMB-45+).

Cellular neurothekeoma

- NKIC3+ MiTF+ PRAME+ S100- Sox10-

Epithelioid Fibrous Histiocytoma

Epithelioid fibrous histiocytoma is a benign tumor distinct from other subtypes of fibrous histiocytomas.[3] They commonly occur on young/middle-aged individuals as a solitary nodule.[3] Histologically, they are composed of proliferation of epithelioid cells in the dermis often with an epidermal collarette (**Figure 8.117**).[3] Other variants including spindle-cell predominant and "chondroblastoma-like" have been reported. By immunohistochemistry they can be positive for EMA and CD30.[3] ALK immunostain is most helpful as it is expressed in most cases and corresponds with the *ALK* gene rearrangements found in these tumors (**Figure 8.118**).[3] The histologic differential diagnosis includes a melanocytic lesion (S100+, Sox10+, Melan-A+), epithelioid sarcoma (keratin+, INI1 loss), and a vascular lesion (Erg+, CD31+).

Epithelioid fibrous histiocytoma

- ALK+ EMA+/- CD30+/-

Non-Neural Granular Cell Tumor

Non-neural granular cell tumor (primitive polypoid granular cell tumor) is an intermediate grade lesion that can occur in young and adult individuals in a variety of anatomic locations.[191] On histologic examination the lesions can be polypoid and are

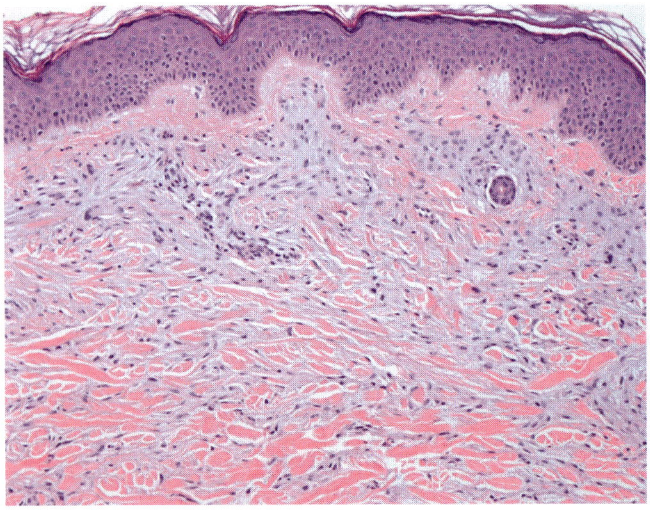

Figure 8.115 Cords of spindled and epithelioid tumor cells infiltrate the dermis in cellular neurothekeoma (X200).

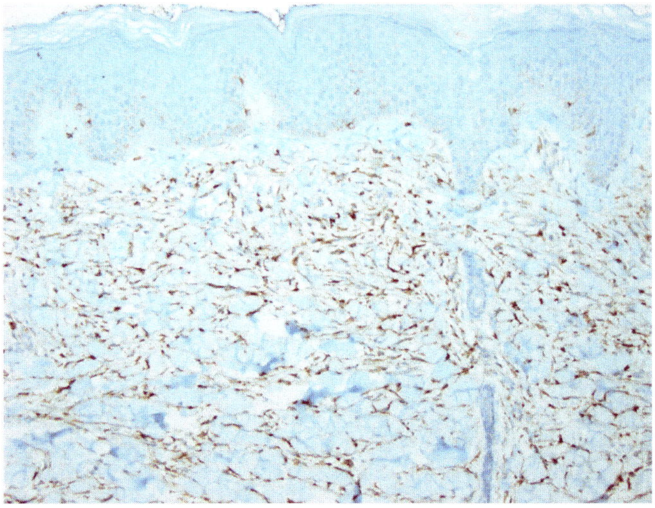

Figure 8.116 Cellular neurothekeoma. The tumor cells are positive for NKIC3 (X200).

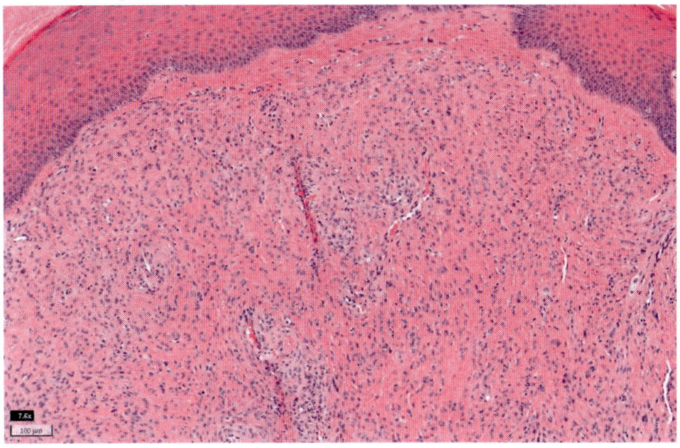

Figure 8.117 Epithelioid fibrous histiocytoma. Epithelioid cells with eosinophilic cytoplasm in a fibrous background are seen (X100).

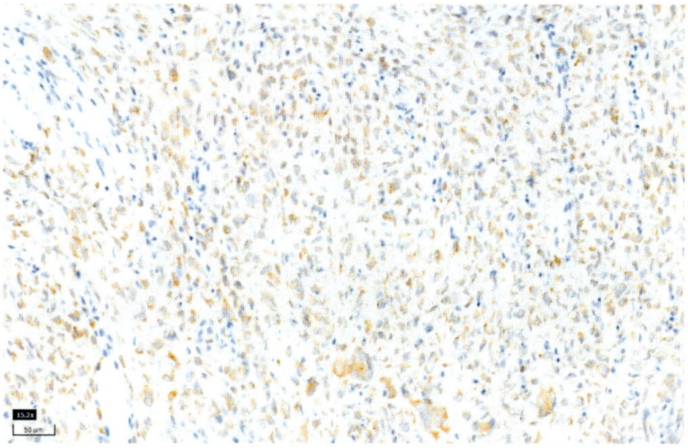

Figure 8.118 Epithelioid fibrous histiocytoma. The tumor cells are positive for ALK (X100).

composed of a proliferation of epithelioid to spindled cells with cytoplasmic granularity.[191] Mitotic activity can be elevated, and nuclear atypia can be present. [191] Unlike granular cell tumors, non-neural granular cell tumors do not express Sox10 or S100.[191] They are typically positive for NKIC3 and can express CD68 and NSE, although these markers are not specific to non-neural granular cell tumor.[191] Non-neural granular cell tumors do not express keratins, EMA, CD45, or SMA. A small series reported recurrent *ALK* gene fusions and ALK immunohistochemistry may be of utility.[192] The histologic differential diagnosis includes melanocytic lesions (Sox10+, S100+, Melan-A+, HMB-45+), granular cell tumor (Sox10+, S100+), and metastatic carcinomas (keratin+ and/or site-specific markers).

Non-neural granular cell tumor

- NKIC3+, CD68+, ALK+/-

8.9 Case Studies

Case 8.1

Case history: A 59-year-old woman presented with a 6-month to one-year history of four pink papules in a sporotrichoid pattern on her right index finger (**Figure 8.119**). They are painless, stable in size and occasionally pruritic. The clinical differential diagnosis includes atypical mycobacteria infection and lichen simplex chronicus.

Description: The biopsy shows a proliferation of ectatic dermal vessels with intervening occasional multinucleated cells (**Figures 8.120 and 8.121**). Factor 13a highlights the occasional multinucleated cells in the dermis (**Figure 8.122**). CD34 highlights the vascular proliferation.

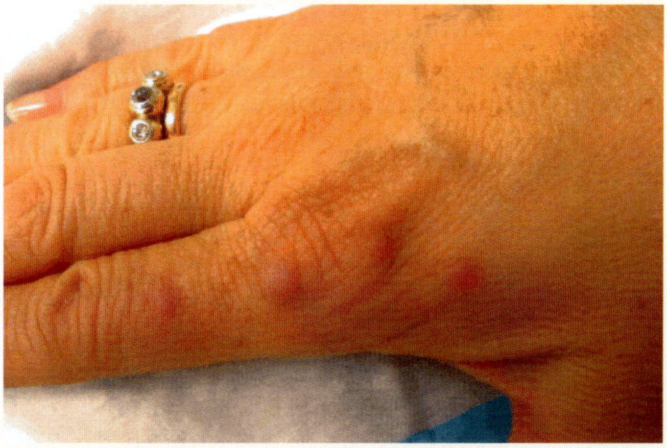

Figure 8.119 Four pink papules are seen on the lateral aspect of the patient's index finger in a linear or sporotrichoid pattern (courtesy of David M. Miller, M.D. Ph.D., Department of Dermatology, Massachusetts General Hospital, Boston, Massachusetts, USA).

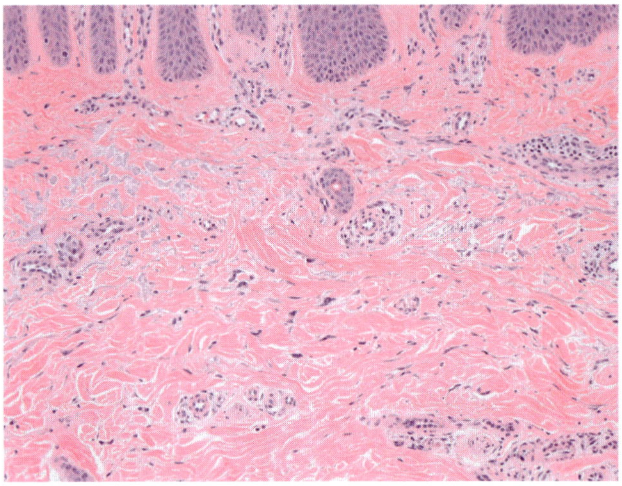
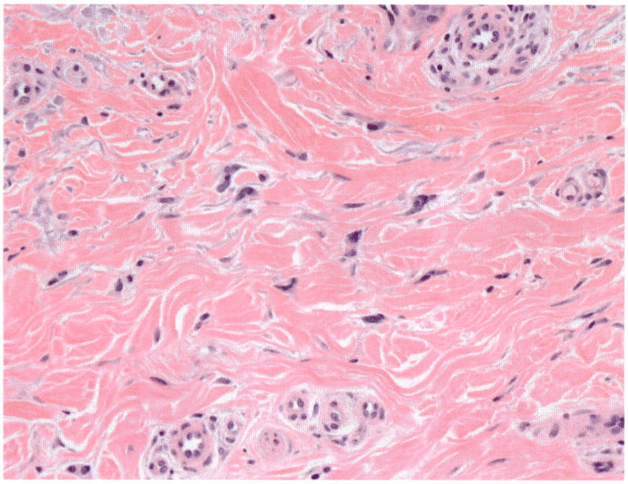

Figures 8.120 and 8.121 Multinucleated cells are seen in a background of dermal fibrosis and vascular proliferation (X200, X400).

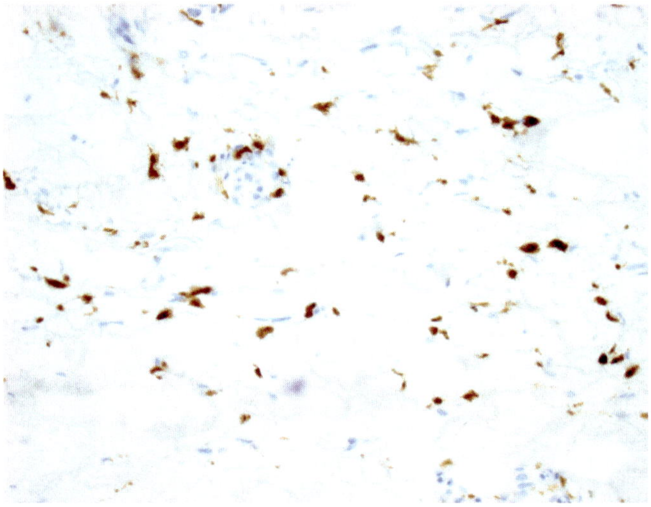

Figure 8.122 The multinucleated cells are positive for factor XIIIa (X200).

Diagnosis: Multinucleate cell angiohistiocytoma.

Discussion: It is not certain that multinucleate cell angiohistiocytoma is a vascular or fibrohistiocytic proliferation. Multinucleate cell angiohistiocytoma exhibits pleomorphic and multinucleated cells in a background of dilated dermal vasculature, dermal fibrosis and lymphohistiocytic infiltrate.[32] Due to its expression of estrogen receptor, some has speculated that it is a reactive process.[33]

Case 8.2

Case history: A 94-year-old man presented with a skin lesion on his left knee.

Description: Ectatic and interconnecting vascular channels are noted in the dermis (**Figure 8.123**). The dissecting vascular channels resemble a lymphatic proliferation (**Figure 8.124**). The neoplastic endothelial cells are positive for HHV8 (**Figure 8.125**), D2-40, and Erg.

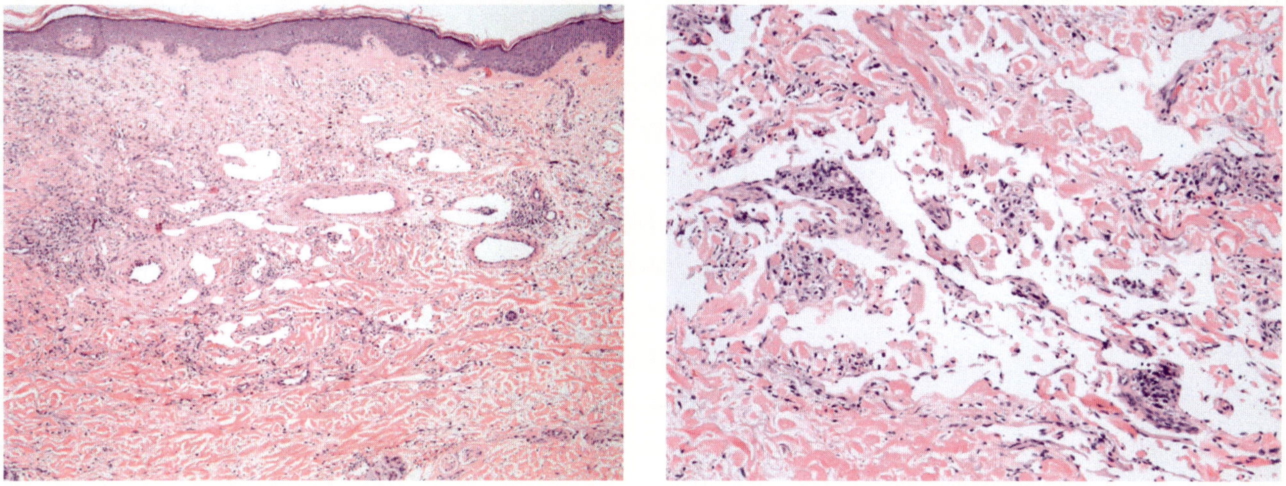

Figures 8.123 and 8.124 Interconnecting vascular channels are seen dissecting the dermis (X100, X200).

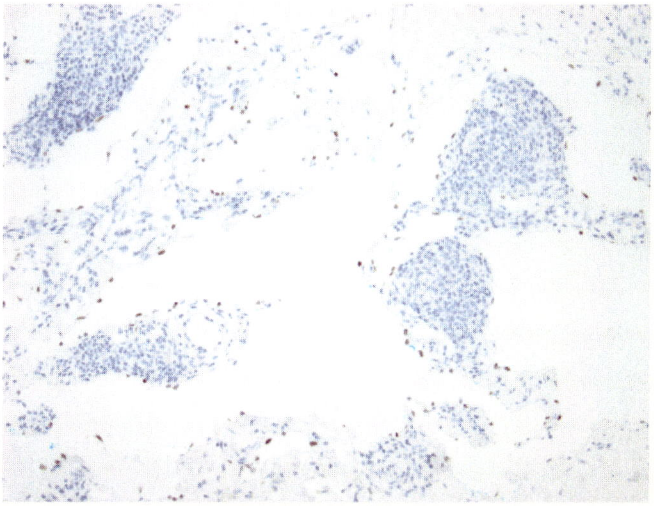

Figure 8.125 Nuclear staining with HHV8 immunostain of the neoplastic endothelial cells is seen (X200).

Diagnosis: Lymphangioma-like Kaposi sarcoma.

Discussion: A proliferation of well-formed capillaries arranged in lobules and absence of aggregates spindle cells is seen in the pyogenic granuloma-like and angiomatous variants of Kaposi sarcoma. These variants can mimic a benign vascular proliferation and HHV8 immunostain plays an important role in correctly diagnosing these lesions. Kaposi sarcoma can be subdivided into four epidemiologic groups: classic, African, acquired immunodeficiency syndrome (AIDS) associated, and iatrogenic. Classic Kaposi sarcoma occurs in elderly of Mediterranean or Ashkenazi Jewish descent and often presents with cutaneous lesions on distal extremities. This subgroup is associated with good prognosis. The age of our patient and the location of tumor are supportive of this case being a classic Kaposi sarcoma.

Case 8.3

Case history: A 34-year-old man, previously healthy, presents with multiple papules and plaques on the left lower leg (**Figure 8.126**). A computed tomography scan was performed showing invasion of muscle and bone. An incisional biopsy was performed.

Description: At low-power magnification we can see a predominantly subcutaneous proliferation that extended to the dermis (**Figure 8.127**). The tumor has a sheet-like architecture and is composed of plump spindle cells with vesicular nuclei, variably prominent nucleoli, and abundant brightly eosinophilic cytoplasm with a strikingly rhabdomyoblast-like appearance (**Figures 8.128 and 8.129**). The cells have mild nuclear atypia and there

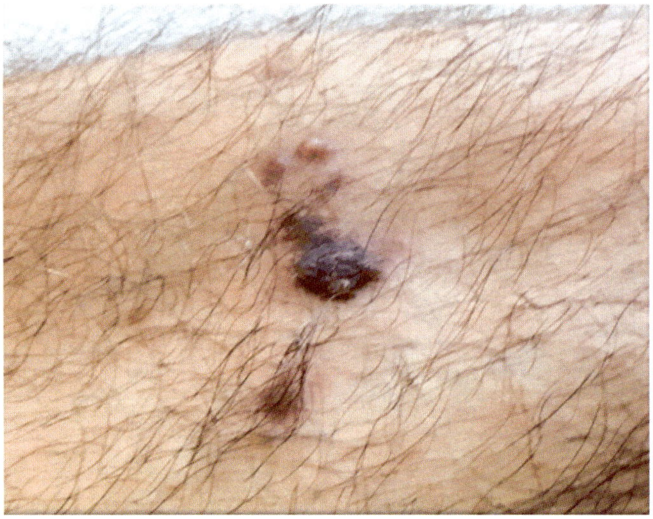

Figure 8.126 Multiple papules and plaques on the left lower leg (courtesy from Joana Gomes M.D., Assistant in Dermatology, Hospital de Braga, Braga, Portugal).

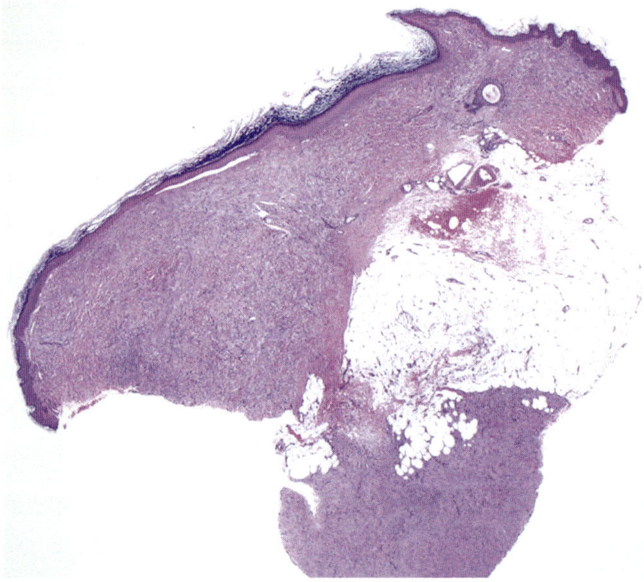

Figure 8.127 The tumor diffusely infiltrates the dermis and subcutaneous tissue (X200).

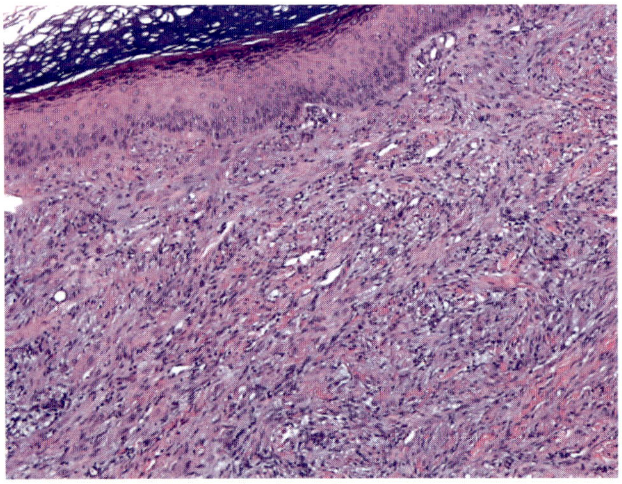

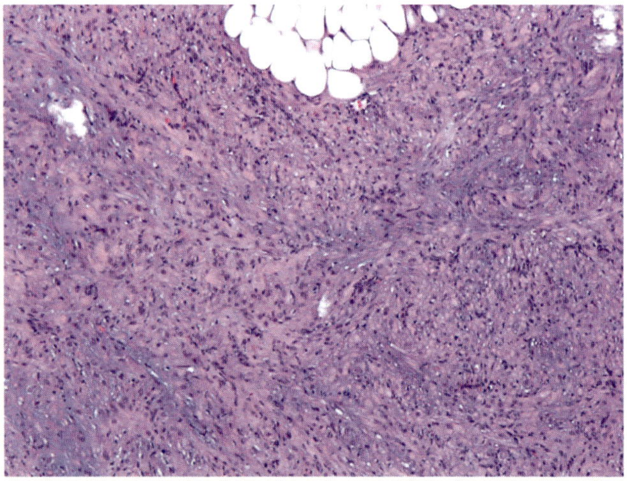

Figures 8.128 and 8.129 The tumor is composed of plump spindle cells with eosinophilic cytoplasm and epithelioid cells (X100, X100).

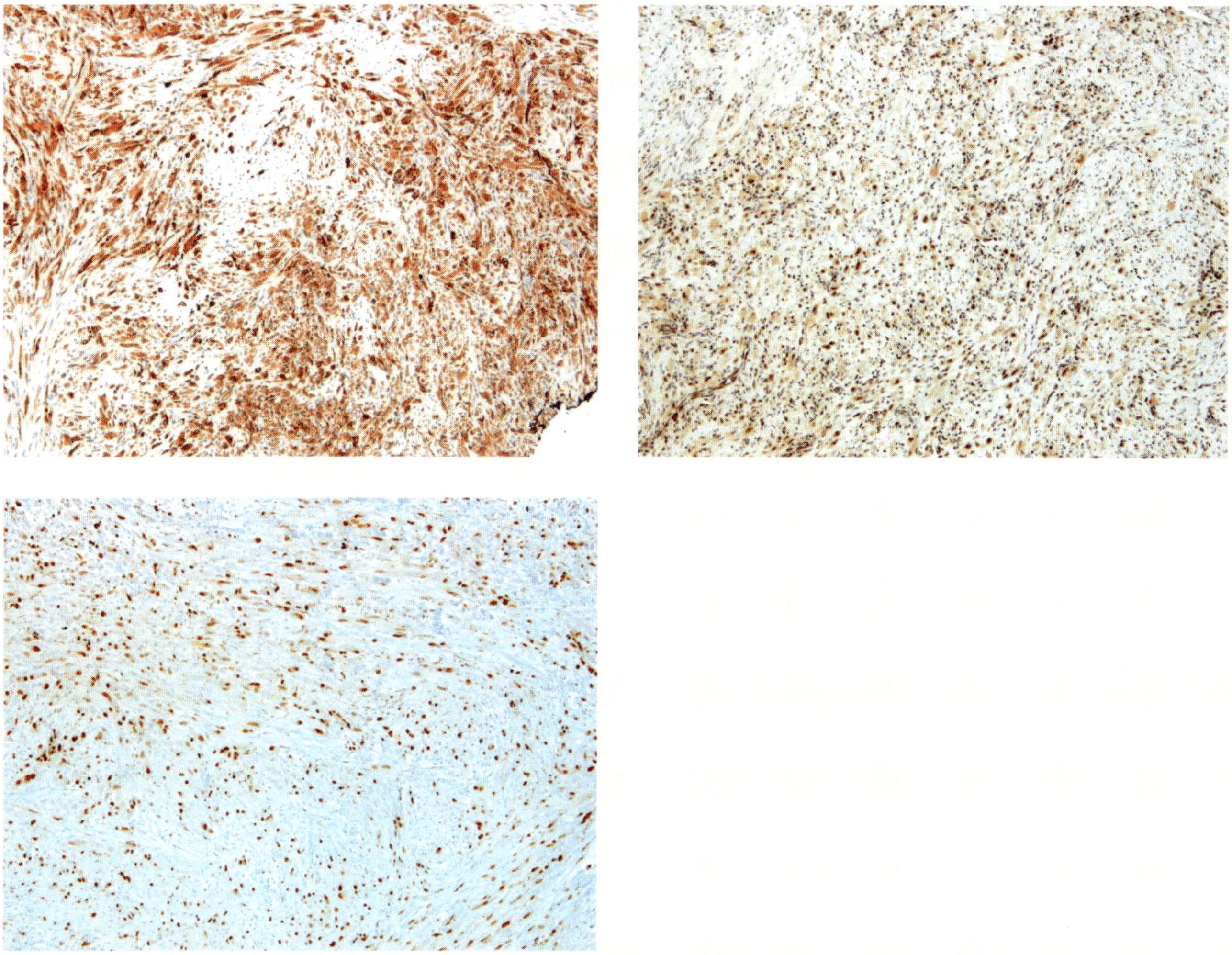

Figures 8.130–8.132 The tumor showed diffuse immunoreactivity for keratin AE1/AE3 (Figure 8.130), FLI1 (Figure 8.131) and ERG (Figure 8.132).

are no mitotic figures. An inflammatory infiltrate was also present. Both the spindle and the epithelioid cells were diffusely positive for AE1/AE3 (**Figure 8.130**), FLI1 (**Figure 8.131**), ERG (**Figure 8.132**), and FOSB. All markers of muscular differentiation (desmin, myogenin, MyoD1, and smooth-muscle actin), melanocytic markers (S100, HMB-45, and MelanA) were negative. CD31, CD34 were also negative, as well as CAMTA-1, EMA, and keratins MNF116 and CAM5.2. The expression of INI1 was preserved.

Diagnosis: Pseudomyogenic hemangioendothelioma.

Discussion: Pseudomyogenic hemangioendothelioma has also been termed epithelioid sarcoma-like hemangioendothelioma according to its morphological similarity to epithelioid sarcoma. In fact pseudomyogenic hemangioendothelioma shares some clinical and morphologic features with epithelioid sarcoma. However, the myoid-appearing plump spindle cell morphology is quite distinctive of pseudomyogenic hemangioendothelioma. Besides, the immunoprofiles of epithelioid sarcoma and pseudomyogenic hemandioendothelioma are different. Although both tumors express broad-spectrum keratins, epithelioid sarcoma shows loss of INI1 expression in more than 90% of cases, while pseudomyogenic hemandioendothelioma retains it. Epithelioid sarcoma is positive for EMA and often for CD34 and negative for other vascular tumors including FLI1, whereas pseudomyogenic hemangioendothelioma is positive for FLI1 and usually for CD31, but negative for EMA and CD34.[167] The differential diagnosis also includes epithelioid hemangioendothelioma, a tumor with very different clinical behavior and malignant potential. Nuclear expression of CAMTA-1, a recently described antibody, is a useful marker to confirm a diagnosis of epithelioid hemangioendothelioma, with high sensitivity and specificity.[163,169]

Case 8.4

Case history: A 68-year-old woman with a history of invasive mammary ductal carcinoma status post lumpectomy, subsequent chemotherapy, and radiotherapy. Four years later she presented with multiple violaceous papules and plaques on the left breast (**Figures 8.133 and 8.134**). An incisional biopsy was performed followed by a mastectomy.

Description: A densely cellular tumor involving the dermis and subcutaneous tissue seen at low magnification (**Figures 8.135 and 8.136**). The tumor is composed of spindle cells arranged predominantly in a fascicular pattern and vascular structures (**Figure 8.137**). There is significant nuclear atypia and pleomorphism. Mitotic figures are numerous. At the periphery there is a proliferation of thin-walled vascular structures with mild nuclear atypia and hyperchromasia (**Figure 8.138**). The neoplastic cells were strongly positive for ERG, FLI1, and CD31 (**Figure 8.139**).

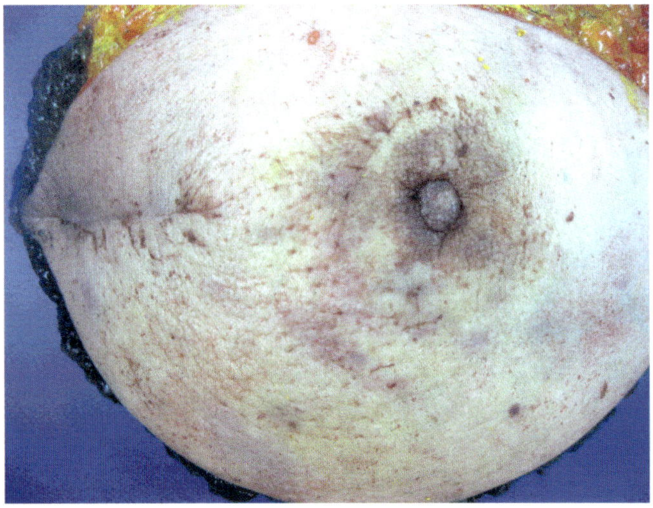

Figure 8.133 Violaceous plaques and nodules are seen on the skin after breast-conserving surgery and irradiation for carcinoma.

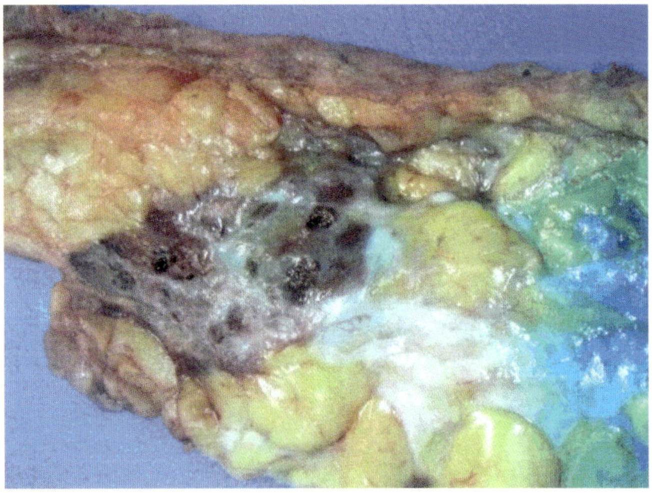

Figure 8.134 On cut section, the tumor has a microcystic appearance as a result of the presence of blood-filled spaces.

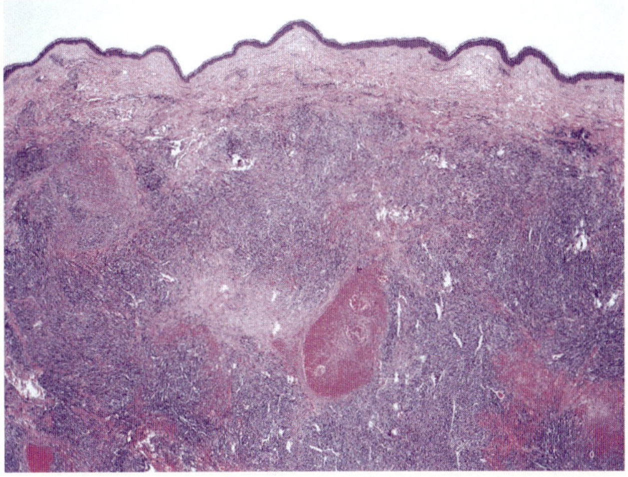

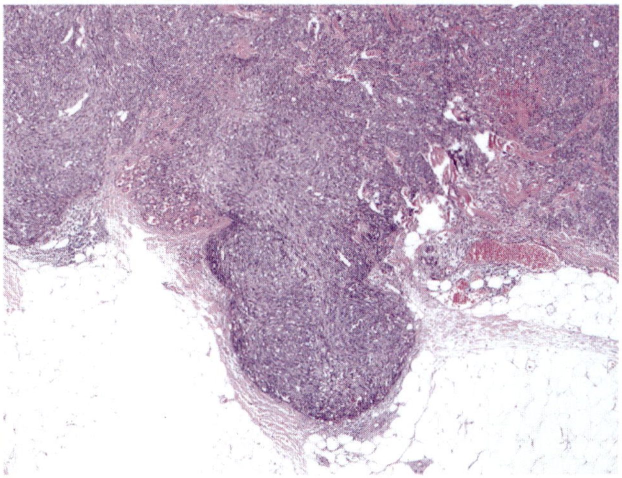

Figures 8.135 and 8.136 The tumor shows extensive infiltration of the dermis (X20) and subcutaneous tissue (X40).

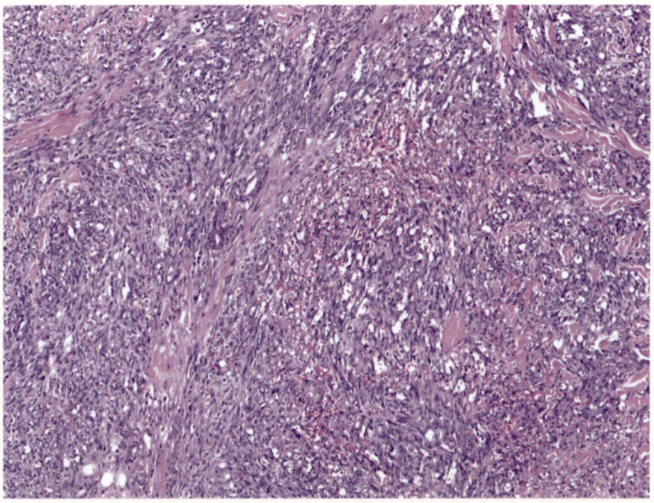

Figure 8.137 Spindle cells arranged in a fascicular pattern (X100).

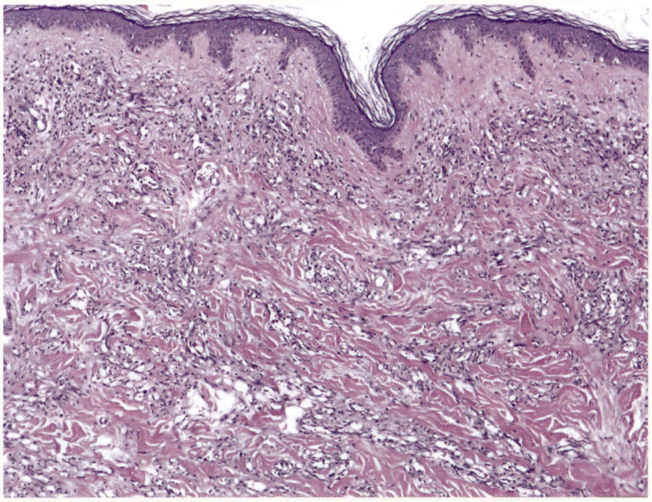

Figure 8.138 Atypical spindle cells dissect the dermis at the periphery of the lesion (X100).

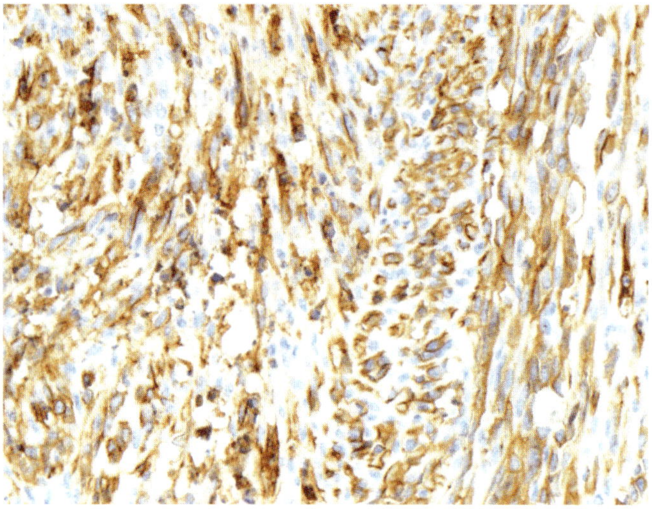

Figure 8.139 The tumor cells are strongly positive for CD31 (X200).

Diagnosis: Post-irradiation angiosarcoma.

Discussion: Post-irradiation angiosarcomas and atypical vascular proliferations can develop after radiotherapy for benign or malignant conditions, mainly for breast cancer, with a reported risk varying from 0.09% to 0.3%.[172] It typically begins as violaceous infiltrating plaques or nodules and histological it is like other cutaneous angiosarcomas arising outside the context of irradiation. The prognosis is poor with approximately 50% of patients experiencing recurrences and 40% metastases, most commonly to the lung, contralateral breast, and bone.

Case 8.5

Case history: A 50-year-old man presented with a scalp nodule.

Description: The skin biopsy shows a spindle cell neoplasm in the dermis (**Figure 8.140**). The tumor cells are positive for CD10 and focally for p63 (**Figures 8.141 and 8.142**). They are negative for S100, p40 (**Figure 8.143**), keratin 903, and keratin 5/6.

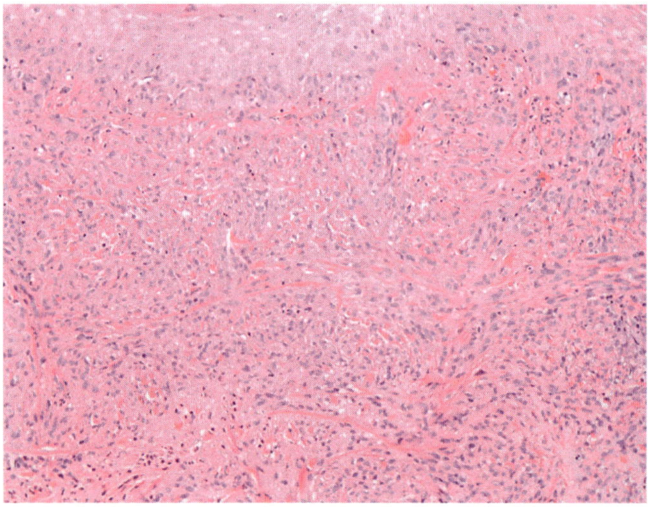

Figure 8.140 Pleomorphic spindle cells are noted in the dermis (X200).

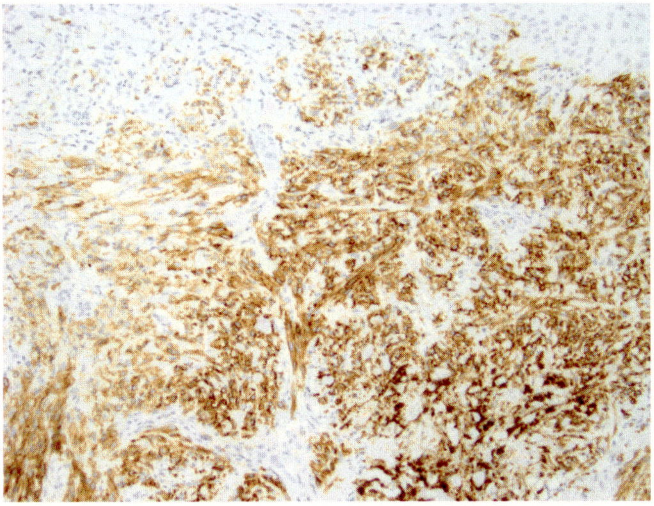

Figure 8.141 Diffuse cytoplasmic CD10 expression (X200).

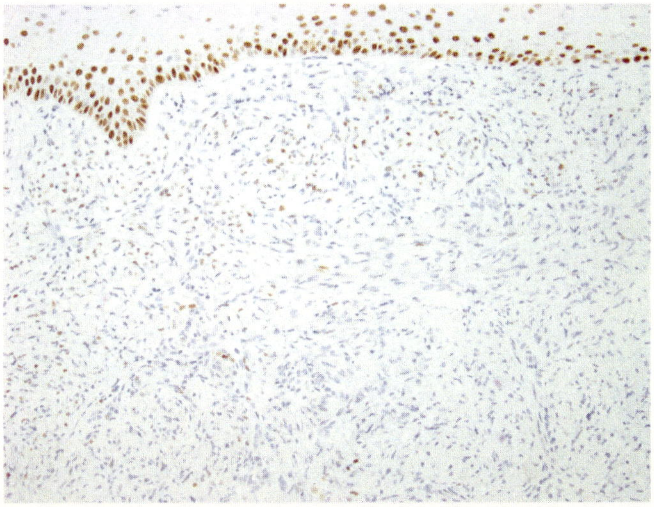

Figure 8.142 p63 highlights occasional tumor cells (X200).

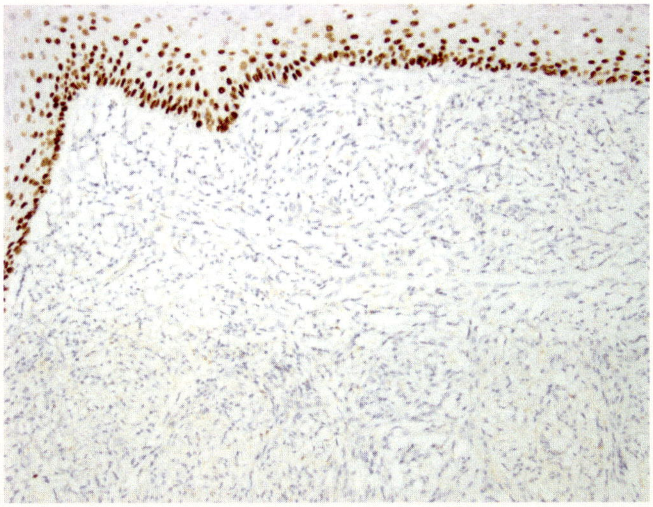

Figure 8.143 While the epidermal keratinocytes exhibit nuclear p40 staining, the tumor cells are negative (X200).

Diagnosis: Atypical fibroxanthoma.

Discussion: The focal p63 expression in this case highlights a potential diagnostic pitfall. The differential diagnosis of a dermal spindle cell lesion includes spindle cell melanoma, sarcomatoid carcinoma and atypical fibroxanthoma. Recently p40 has been shown to be a more specific marker than p63 in highlighting sarcomatoid carcinoma since p63 expression in atypical fibroxanthoma has been reported.[183]

Case 8.6

Case history: A 52-year-old woman presented with multiple papules on the trunk and extremities. She has previously undergone simple hysterectomy for leiomyomas.

Description: The skin biopsy shows proliferation of spindle cells in the dermis, without cytologic atypia, mitotic figures or necrosis (**Figures 8.144 and 8.145**). The tumor cells expressed desmin (**Figure 8.146**) confirming the muscular nature of the neoplasm. Since the patient had multiple skin lesions and a previous history of uterine leiomyomas, fumarate-hydratase immunostain was performed and the tumor cells exhibited loss of expression (**Figure 8.147**).[193] Genetic testing was performed and a heterozygous deletion in the exon 1 of FH gene was found.

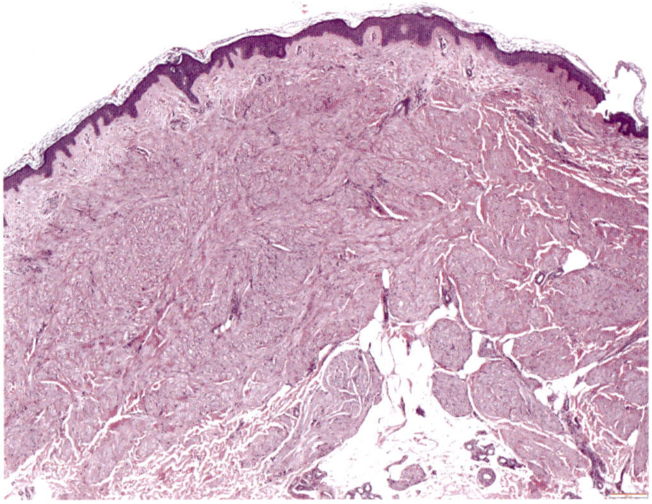

Figure 8.144 A spindle cell proliferation is seen in the dermis (X40).

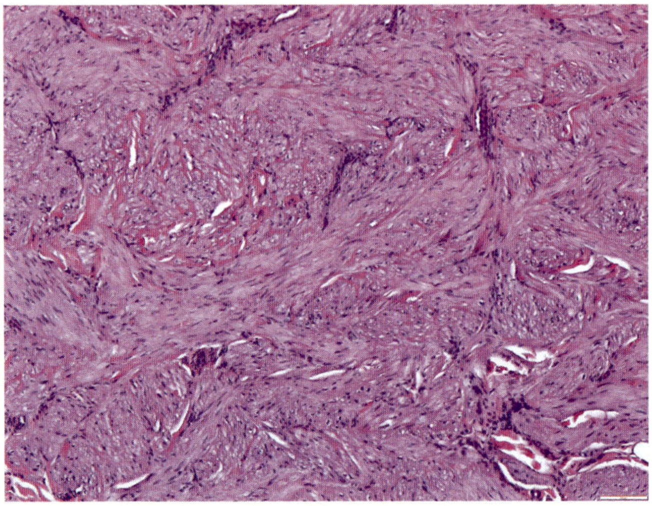

Figure 8.145 Intersecting fascicles of spindle cells are seen (X100).

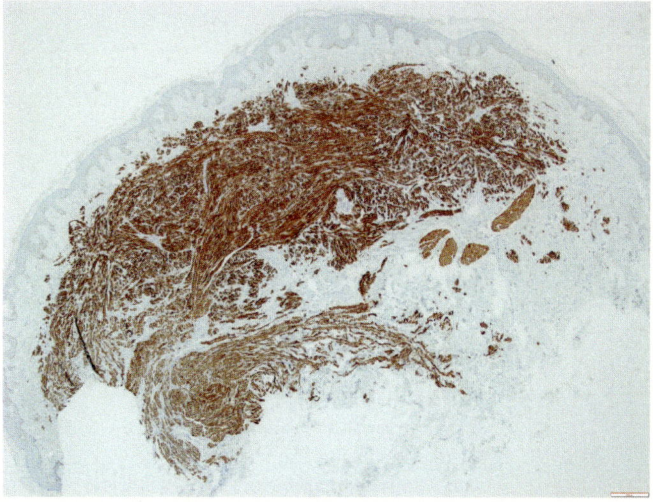

Figure 8.146 The tumor cells strongly express desmin (X40).

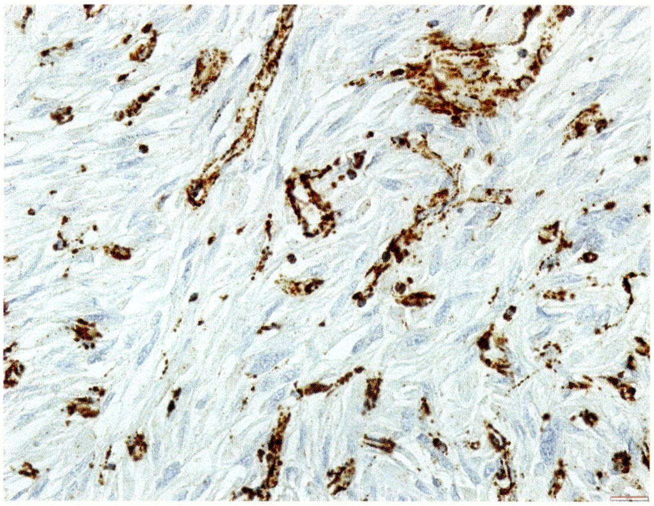

Figure 8.147 FH immunostain highlights only the intratumoral blood vessels but not the tumor cells (X400).

Diagnosis: Cutaneous leiomyoma with fumarate-hydratase loss in the setting of Hereditary Leiomyomatosis and Renal Cell Carcinoma Syndrome.

Discussion: In the setting of multiple cutaneous leiomyomas and specially when combined with uterine leiomyomas in women, fumarate-hydratase should be performed as a screening test for Hereditary Leiomyomatosis and Renal Cell Carcinoma syndrome, an autosomal dominant syndrome characterized by a germline or (in a subset) somatic mutations in the FH gene (chromosome 1q43). These molecular alterations confer an increased risk of cutaneous and uterine leiomyomas as well as highly aggressive subtype of renal cancer. A relatively high rate of FH germline mutation was reported in FH-negative uterine leiomyomas in young women.[194]

References

1. Guillou L, Coindre JM, Bonichon F, et al. Comparative study of the National Cancer Institute and French Federation of Cancer Centers Sarcoma Group grading systems in a population of 410 adult patients with soft tissue sarcoma. *J Clin Oncol* 1997; **15**: 350–62.
2. Amin MB, Edge SB, Greene FL, et al., eds. AJCC Cancer Staging Manual. 8th ed. New York: Springer; 2017.
3. Doyle LA, Mariño-Enriquez A, Fletcher CD, Hornick JL. ALK rearrangement and overexpression in epithelioid fibrous histiocytoma. *Mod Pathol* 2015; **28**: 904–12.
4. Michal M, Berry RS, Rubin BP, et al. EWSR1-SMAD3-rearranged fibroblastic tumor: an emerging entity in an increasingly more complex group of fibroblastic/myofibroblastic neoplasms. *Am J Surg Pathol* 2018; **42**: 1325–33.
5. Agaram NP, Zhang L, Sung YS, et al. Recurrent NTRK1 gene fusions define a novel subset of locally aggressive lipofibromatosis-like neural tumors. *Am J Surg Pathol* 2016; **40**: 1407–16.
6. Calonje E, Mentzel T, Fletcher CD. Cellular benign fibrous histiocytoma. Clinicopathologic analysis of 74 cases of a distinctive variant of cutaneous fibrous histiocytoma with frequent recurrence. *Am J Surg Pathol* 1994; **18**: 668–76.
7. Gleason BC, Fletcher CD. Deep "benign" fibrous histiocytoma: clinicopathologic analysis of 69 cases of a rare tumor indicating occasional metastatic potential. *Am J Surg Pathol* 2008; **32**: 354–62.
8. Calonje E, Fletcher CD. Aneurysmal benign fibrous histiocytoma: clinicopathological analysis of 40 cases of a tumour frequently misdiagnosed as a vascular neoplasm. *Histopathology* 1995; **26**: 323–31.
9. Kaddu S, McMenamin ME, Fletcher CD. Atypical fibrous histiocytoma of the skin: clinicopathologic analysis of 59 cases with evidence of infrequent metastasis. *Am J Surg Pathol* 2002; **26**: 35–46.
10. Sachdev R, Sundram U. Expression of CD163 in dermatofibroma, cellular fibrous histiocytoma, and dermatofibrosarcoma protuberans: comparison with CD68, CD34 and factor 13a. *J Cutan Pathol* 2006; **33**: 353–60.
11. Thway K, Noujaim J, Jones RL, Fisher C. Dermatofibrosarcoma protuberans: pathology, genetics, and potential therapeutic strategies. *Ann Diagn Pathol* 2016; **25**: 64–71.
12. Volpicelli ER, Fletcher CD. Desmin and CD34 positivity in cellular fibrous histiocytoma: an immunohistochemical analysis of 100 cases. *J Cutan Pathol* 2012; **39**: 747–52.
13. Miller K, Goodlad JR, Brenn T. Pleomorphic dermal sarcoma: adverse histologic features predict aggressive behavior and allow distinction from atypical fibroxanthoma. *Am J Surg Pathol* 2012; 36: 1317–26.
14. de Feraudy S, Mar N, McCalmont TH. Evaluation of CD10 and procollagen 1 expression in atypical fibroxanthoma and dermatofibroma. *Am J Surg Pathol* 2008; **32**: 1111–22.
15. Rudolph P, Schubert C, Zelger BG, et al. Different expression of CD34 and Ki-M1p in pleomorphic fibroma and dermatofibroma with monster cells. *Am J Dermatopathol* 1999; **21**: 414–19.
16. Puig L, Fernandez Figueras MT, Bielsa I, et al. Multinucleate cell angiohistiocytoma: a fibrohistiocytic proliferation with increased mast cell numbers and vascular hyperplasia. *J Cutan Pathol* 2002; **29**: 232–7.
17. Choi KY, Mack L, Caragea M, et al. MDM2 analysis in the management of benign lipomas versus atypical lipomatous tumors/well-differentiated liposarcomas: a useful prognostication tool? *Am J Surg* 2022; **224**: 747–50.
18. Hinds B, Agulló Pérez AD, LeBoit PE, McCalmont TH, North JP. Loss of retinoblastoma in pleomorphic fibroma: an immunohistochemical and genomic analysis. *J Cutan Pathol* 2017; **44**: 665–71.
19. Hanft VN, Shea CR, McNutt NS, et al. Expression of CD34 in sclerotic ("plywood') fibromas. *Am J Dermatopathol* 2000; **22**: 17–21.
20. Hartsough E, DeSimone MS, Lorenzo ME, et al. Utilizing PTEN immunohistochemistry as a screening test for Cowden syndrome. *Am J Clin Pathol* 2024; Jan 11:aqad177. doi: 10.1093/ajcp/aqad177.
21. Nielsen GP, O'Connell JX, Dickersin GR, Rosenberg AE. Collagenous fibroma (desmoplastic fibroblastoma): a report of seven cases. *Mod Pathol* 1996; **9**: 781–5.
22. Kato I, Yoshida A, Ikegami M, et al. FOSL1 immunohistochemistry clarifies the distinction between desmoplastic fibroblastoma and fibroma of tendon sheath. *Histopathology* 2016; **69**: 1012–20.
23. Kutzner H, Mentzel T, Palmedo G, et al. Plaque-like CD34-positive dermal fibroma ("medalion-like dermal dendrocyte hamartoma"): clinicopathologic, immunohistochemical, and molecular analysis of 5 cases emphasizing its distinction from superficial, plaque-like dermatofibrosarcoma protuberans. *Am J Surg Pathol* 2010; **34**: 190–201.
24. De Feraudy S, Fletcher CDM. Fibroblastic connective tissue nevus: a rare cutaneous lesion analyzed in a series of 25 cases. *Am J Surg Pathol* 2012; **36**: 1509–15.
25. Carter JM, Weiss SW, Linos K, DiCaudo DJ, Folpe AL. Superficial CD34-positive fibroblastic tumor: report of 18 cases of a distinctive low-grade mesenchymal neoplasm of intermediate (borderline) malignancy. *Mod Pathol* 2014; **27**: 294–302.
26. Perret R, Michal M, Carr RA, et al. Superficial CD34-positive fibroblastic tumor and PRDM10-rearranged soft tissue tumor are overlapping entities: a comprehensive study of 20 cases. *Histopathology* 2021; **79**: 810–25.
27. De Feraudy S, Fletcher CDM. Fibroblastic connective tissue nevus: a rare cutaneous lesion analyzed in a series of 25 cases. *Am J Surg Pathol* 2012; **36**: 1509–15.
28. Kamath NV, Ormsby A, Bergfeld WF, House NS. A light microscopic and immunohistochemical evaluation of scars. *J Cutan Pathol* 2002; **29**: 27–32.
29. Erdag G, Qureshi HS, Patterson JW, Wick MR. Solitary fibrous tumors of the skin: a clinicopathologic study of 10 cases and review of the literature. *J Cutan Pathol* 2007; **34**: 844–50.
30. Tariq MU, Din NU, Abdul-Ghafar J, Park YK. The many faces of solitary fibrous tumor; diversity of histological features, differential diagnosis and role of molecular studies and surrogate markers in avoiding misdiagnosis and predicting the behavior. *Diagn Pathol* 2021; **16**: 32. doi: 10.1186/s13000-021-01095-2.
31. Doyle LA, Vivero M, Fletcher CD, et al. Nuclear expression of STAT6 distinguishes solitary fibrous tumor from histologic mimics. *Mod Pathol* 2014; **27**: 290–5.
32. Frew JW. Multinucleate cell angiohistiocytoma: clinicopathological correlation of 142 cases with insights into etiology and pathogenesis. *Am J Dermatopathol* 2015; **37**: 222–8.

33. Cesinaro AM, Roncati L, Maiorana A. Estrogen receptor alpha overexpression in multinucleate cell angiohistiocytoma: new insights into the pathogenesis of a reactive process. *Am J Dermatopathol* 2010; **32**: 655–9.
34. Saab ST, McClain CM, Coffin CM. Fibrous hamartoma of infancy: a clinicopathologic analysis of 60 cases. *Am J Surg Pathol* 2014; **38**: 394–401.
35. Fetsch JF, Miettinen M. Calcifying aponeurotic fibroma: a clinicopathologic study of 22 cases arising in uncommon sites. *Hum Pathol* 1998; **29**: 1504–10.
36. Puls F, Hofvander J, Magnusson L, et al. FN1-EGF gene fusions are recurrent in calcifying aponeurotic fibroma. *J Pathol* 2016; **238**: 502–7.
37. Sugita S, Takenami T, Kido T, et al. Diagnostic utility of CSF1 immunohistochemistry in tenosynovial giant cell tumor for differentiating from giant cell-rich tumors and tumor-like lesions of bone and soft tissue. *Diagn Pathol* 2022; **17**: 88. doi: 10.1186/s13000-022-01266-9.
38. Stacchiotti S, Dürr HR, Schaefer IM, et al. Best clinical management of tenosynovial giant cell tumour (TGCT): a consensus paper from the community of experts. *Cancer Treat Rev* 2023; **112**: 102491. doi: 10.1016/j.ctrv.2022.102491.
39. Monaghan H, Salter DM, Al-Nafussi A. Giant cell tumour of tendon sheath (localised nodular tenosynovitis): clinicopathological features of 71 cases. *J Clin Pathol* 2001; **54**: 404–7.
40. Lee JC, Liang CW, Fletcher CD. Giant cell tumor of soft tissue is genetically distinct from its bone counterpart. *Mod Pathol* 2017; **30**: 728–33.
41. Hoang MP, Rogers BB, Albores Saavedra J. Giant cell tumor of the skin: a morphologic and immunohistochemical study of five cases. *Ann Diagn Pathol* 2002; **6**: 288–93.
42. Amary MF, Pauwels P, Meulemans E, et al. Detection of beta-catenin mutations in paraffin-embedded sporadic desmoid-type fibromatosis by mutation-specific restriction enzyme digestion (MSRED): an ancillary diagnostic tool. *Am J Surg Pathol* 2007; **31**: 1299–309.
43. An J, Woo HY, Lee Y, et al. Clinicopathological features of 70 desmoid-type fibromatoses confirmed by β-catenin immunohistochemical staining and CTNNB1 mutation analysis. *PLoS One* 2021; **16**: e0250619. doi: 10.1371/journal.pone.0250619.
44. Bhattacharya B, Dilworth HP, Iacobuzio-Donahue C, et al. Nuclear beta-catenin expression distinguishes deep fibromatosis from other benign and malignant fibroblastic and myofibroblastic lesions. *Am J Surg Pathol* 2005; **29**: 653–9.
45. Montgomery E, Lee JH, Abraham SC, Wu TT. Superficial fibromatoses are genetically distinct from deep fibromatoses. *Mod Pathol* 2001; **14**: 695–701.
46. Laskin WB, Miettinen M, Fetsch JF. Infantile digital fibroma/fibromatosis: a clinicopathological and immunohistochemical study of 69 tumors from 57 patients with long-term follow-up. *Am J Surg Pathol* 2009; **33**: 1–3.
47. Erickson-Johnson MR, Chou MM, Evers BR, et al. Nodular fasciitis: a novel model of transient neoplasia induced by MYH9-USP6 gene fusion. *Lab Invest* 2011; **91**: 1427–33.
48. Arbiser ZK, Folpe AL, Weiss SW. Consultative (expert) second opinions in soft tissue pathology. Analysis of problem-prone diagnostic situations. *Am J Clin Pathol* 2001; **116**: 473–6.
49. Wong NL, Di F. Pseudosarcomatous fasciitis and myositis: diagnosis by fine-needle aspiration cytology. *Am J Clin Pathol* 2009; **132**: 857–65.
50. el-Jabbour JN, Bennett MH, Burke MM, et al. Proliferative myositis: an immunohistochemical and ultrastructural study. *Am J Surg Pathol* 1991; **15**: 654–9.
51. Makise N, Mori T, Motoi T, et al. Recurrent *FOS* rearrangement in proliferative fasciitis/proliferative myositis. *Mod Pathol* 2021; **34**, 942–50.
52. Antonescu CR, Suurmeijer AJ, Zhang L, et al. Molecular characterization of inflammatory myofibroblastic tumors with frequent ALK and ROS1 gene fusions and rare novel RET rearrangement. *Am J Surg Pathol* 2015; **39**: 957–67.
53. Yamamoto H, Yoshida A, Taguchi K, et al. ALK, ROS1 and NTRK3 gene rearrangements in inflammatory myofibroblastic tumors. *Histopathology* 2016; **69**: 72–83.
54. Deshpande V, Zen Y, Chan J, *et al.* Consensus statement on the pathology of IgG4-related disease. *Mod Pathol* 2012; **25**: 1181–92.
55. Suster D, Michal M, Huang H, et al. Myxoinflammatory fibroblastic sarcoma: an immunohistochemical and molecular genetic study of 73 cases. *Mod Pathol* 2020; **33**: 2520–33.
56. Laskin WB, Fetsch JF, Miettinen M. Myxoinflammatory fibroblastic sarcoma: a clinicopathologic analysis of 104 cases, with emphasis on predictors of outcome. *Am J Surg Pathol* 2014; **38**: 1–12.
57. Kovarik CL, Barrett T, Auerbach A, Cassarino DS. Acral myxoinflammatory sarcoma: case series and immunohistochemical analysis. *J Cutan Pathol* 2008; **35**: 192–6.
58. Hollmann TJ, Bovee JVMG, Fletcher CDM. Digital fibromyxoma (superficial acral fibromyxoma): a detailed characterization of 124 cases. *Am J Surg Pathol* 2012; **36**: 789–98.
59. Agaimy A, Michal M, Giedl J, et al. Superficial acral fibromyxoma: clinicopathological, immunohistochemical, and molecular study of 11 cases highlighting frequent Rb1 loss/deletions. *Hum Pathol* 2017; **60**: 192–8.
60. Doyle LA, Moller E, Dal Cin P, et al. MUC4 is a highly sensitive and specific marker for low-grade fibromyxoid sarcoma. *Am J Surg Pathol* 2011; **35**: 733–41.
61. Möller E, Hornick JL, Magnusson L, et al. *FUS-CREB3L2/L1*-Positive sarcomas show a specific gene expression profile with upregulation of *CD24* and *FOXL1*. *Clin Cancer Res* 2011; **17**: 2646–56.
62. Trinidad CM, Wangsiricharoen S, Prieto VG, Aung PP. Rare variants of dermatofibrosarcoma protuberans: clinical, histologic, and molecular features and diagnostic pitfalls. *Dermatopathology* 2023; **10**: 54–62.
63. Segura S, Salgado R, Toll A, et al. Identification of t(17;22)(q22q13)(COL1A1/PDGFB) in dermatofibrosarcoma protuberans by fluorescence in situ hybridization in paraffin-embedded tissue microarrays. *Hum Pathol* 2011; **42**: 176–84.
64. Jha P, Moosavi C, Fanburg-Smith JC. Giant cell fibroblastoma: an update and addition of 86 new cases from the Armed Forces Institute of Pathology, in honor of Dr. Franz M. Enzinger. *Ann Diagn Pathol* 2007; **11**: 81–8.
65. Moosavi C, Jha P, Fanburg-Smith JC. An update on plexiform fibrohistiocytic tumor and addition of 66 new cases from the Armed Forces Institute of Pathology, in honor of

Frank M. Enzinger, MD. *Ann Diagn Pathol* 2007; **11**: 313–19.

66. Fetsch JF, Miettinen M, Laskin WB, et al. A clinicopathologic study of 45 pediatric soft tissue tumors with an admixture of adipose tissue and fibroblastic elements, and a proposal for classification as lipofibromatosis. *Am J Surg Pathol* 2000; **24**: 1491–500.
67. Mentzel T, Heinz K. Dermatomyofibroma: clinicopathologic and immunohistochemical analysis of 56 cases and reappraisal of a rare and distinct cutaneous neoplasm. *Am J Dermatopathol* 2009; **31**: 44–9.
68. Mariño-Enríquez A, Fletcher CD. Angiofibroma of soft tissue: clinicopathologic characterization of a distinctive benign fibrovascular neoplasm in a series of 37 cases. *Am J Surg Pathol* 2012; **36**: 500–8.
69. Jin Y, Möller E, Nord KH, Mandahl N, et al. Fusion of the AHRR and NCOA2 genes through a recurrent translocation t(5;8)(p15;q13) in soft tissue angiofibroma results in upregulation of aryl hydrocarbon receptor target genes. *Genes Chromosomes Cancer* 2012; **51**: 510–20.
70. Flucke U, van Krieken JH, Mentzel T. Cellular angiofibroma: analysis of 25 cases emphasizing its relationship to spindle cell lipoma and mammary type myofibroblastoma. *Mod Pathol* 2011; **24**: 82–9.
71. Chen E, Fletcher CD. Cellular angiofibroma with atypical or sarcomatous transformation: clinicopathologic analysis of 13 cases. *Am J Surg Pathol* 2010; **34**: 707–14.
72. Iwasa Y, Fletcher CD. Cellular angiofibroma: clinicopathologic and immunohistochemical analysis of 51 cases. *Am J Surg Pathol* 2004; **28**: 1426–35.
73. Laskin WB, Fetsch JF, Mostofi FK. Angiomyofibroblastomalike tumor of the male genital tract: analysis of 11 cases with comparison to female angiomyofibroblastoma and spindle cell lipoma. *Am J Surg Pathol* 1998; **22**: 6–16.
74. Laskin WB, Fetsch JF, Tavassoli FA. Angiofibroblastoma of the female genital tract: analysis of 17 cases including a lipomatous variant. *Hum Pathol* 1997; **28**: 1046–55.
75. Nielsen GP, Rosenberg AF, Young RH, et al. Angiomyofibroblastoma of the vulva and vagina. *Mod Pathol* 1996; **9**: 284–91.
76. Qiu X, Montgomery E, Sun B. Inflammatory myofibroblastic tumor and low-grade myofibroblastic sarcoma: a comparative study of clinicopathologic features and further observations on the immunohistochemical profile of myofibroblasts. *Hum Pathol* 2008; **39**: 846–56.
77. Carlson JW, Fletcher CD. Immunohistochemistry for beta-catenin in the differential diagnosis of spindle cell lesions: analysis of a series and review of the literature. *Histopathology* 2007; **51**: 509–14.
78. Mentzel T, Calonje E, Wadden C, et al. Myxofibrosarcoma: clinicopathologic analysis of 75 cases with emphasis on the low-grade variant. *Am J Surg Pathol* 1996; **20**: 391–405.
79. Smith SC, Poznanski AA, Fullen DR, et al. CD34-positive superficial myxofibrosarcoma: a potential diagnostic pitfall. *J Cutan Pathol* 2013; **40**: 639–45.
80. Miettinen M. Immunohistochemistry of soft tissue tumours: review with emphasis on 10 markers. *Histopathology* 2014; **64**: 101–18.
81. Malik K, Patel P, Chen J, Khachemoune A. Leiomyoma cutis: a focused review on presentation, management, and association with malignancy. *Am J Clin Dermatol* 2015; **16**: 35–46.
82. Chaudhary KS, Shousha S. Leiomyoma of the nipple, and normal subareola muscle fibers, are oestrogen and progesterone receptor positive. *Histopathology* 2004; **44**: 626–8.
83. Buelow B, Cohen J, Nagymanyoki Z, et al. Immunohistochemistry for 2-Succinocysteine (2SC) and Fumarate Hydratase (FH) in cutaneous leiomyomas may aid in identification of patients with HLRCC (Hereditary Leiomyomatosis and Renal Cell Carcinoma Syndrome). *Am J Surg Pathol* 2016; **40**: 982–8.
84. Kraft S, Fletcher CD. Atypical intradermal smooth muscle neoplasms: clinicopathologic analysis of 84 cases and a reappraisal of cutaneous "leiomyosarcoma." *Am J Surg Pathol* 2011; **35**: 599–607.
85. Pitjadi TM, Grayson W. Epstein-Barr virus-associated smooth muscle tumour: a case series with a significant proportion of tumours showing proclivity for cutaneous soft tissues. *Dermatopathology* 2019; **6**: 133–46. doi: 10.1159/000497075.
86. Yadav SK, Sood N. Multinodular adult rhabdomyoma in female: a rare case report. *J Oral Maxillofac Pathol* 2019; **23**: 54–7.
87. Kapadia SB, Meis JM, Frisman DM, Ellis GL, Heffner DK. Fetal rhabdomyoma of the head and neck: a clinicopathologic and immunophenotypic study of 24 cases. *Hum Pathol* 1993; **24**: 754–65.
88. Schoolmeester JK, Xing D, Keeney GL, Sukov WR. Genital rhabdomyoma of the lower female genital tract: a study of 12 cases with molecular cytogenetic findings. *Int J Gynecol Pathol* 2018; **37**: 349–55.
89. Skapek SX, Ferrari A, Gupta AA, et al. Rhabdomyosarcoma. *Nat Rev Dis Primers* 2019; **5**: 1. doi: 10.1038/s41572-018-0051-2.
90. Tsokos M, Linnoila RI, Chandra RS, Triche TJ. Neuron specific enolase in the diagnosis of neuroblastoma and other small round cell tumors in children. *Hum Pathol* 1984; **15**: 575–84.
91. Agaram NP, LaQuaglia MP, Alaggio R, et al. MYOD1-mutant spindle cell and sclerosing rhabdomyosarcoma: an aggressive subtype irrespective of age. A reappraisal for molecular classification and risk stratification. *Mod Pathol* 2019; **32**: 27–36.
92. Alaggio R, Zhang L, Sung YS, et al. A molecular study of pediatric spindle and sclerosing rhabdomyosarcoma: identification of novel and recurrent VGLL2-related fusions in infantile cases. *Am J Surg Pathol* 2016; **40**: 224–35.
93. Prieto-Granada CN, Wiesner T, Messina JL, et al. Loss of H3K27me3 expression is a highly sensitive marker for sporadic and radiation-induced MPNST. *Am J Surg Pathol* 2016; **40**: 479–89.
94. Fetsch JF, Laskin WB, Miettinen M. Nerve sheath myxoma: a clinicopathologic and immunohistochemical analysis of 57 morphologically distinctive, S100 protein- and GFAP-positive, myxoid peripheral nerve sheath tumors with a predilection for the extremities and a high local recurrence rate. *Am J Surg Pathol* 2005; **29**: 1615–24.
95. Miettinen M, McCue PA, Sarlomo-Rikala M, et al. Sox10–a marker for not only Schwannian and melanocytic neoplasms but also myoepithelial cell tumors of soft tissue: a systematic analysis of 5134 tumors. *Am J Surg Pathol* 2015; **39**: 826–35.

96. Koutlas IG, Scheithauer BW. Palisaded encapsulated ("solitary circumscribed") neuroma of the oral cavity: a review of 55 cases. *Head Neck Pathol* 2010; **4**: 15–26.

97. Higham CS, Dombi E, Rogiers A, et al. The characteristics of 76 atypical neurofibromas as precursors to neurofibromatosis 1 associated malignant peripheral nerve sheath tumors. *Neuro Oncol* 2018; **20**: 818–25.

98. Johnson MD, Glick AD, Davis BW. Immunohistochemical evaluation of Leu-7, myelin basic protein, S-100 protein, glial-fibrillary acidic-protein, and LN3 immunoreactivity in nerve sheath tumors and sarcomas. *Arch Pathol Lab Med* 1988; **112**: 155–60.

99. Hirose T, Tani T, Shimada T, et al. Immunohistochemical demonstration of EMA/Glut-1-positive perineurial cells and CD34 positive fibroblastic cells in peripheral nerve sheath tumors. *Mod Pathol* 2003; **16**: 293–8.

100. Fine SW, McClain SA, Li M. Immunohistochemical staining for calretinin is useful for differentiating schwannomas from neurofibromas. *Am J Clin Pathol* 2004; **122**: 552–9.

101. Boyd C, Smith MJ, Kluwe L, et al. Alterations in the SMARCB1 (INI1) tumor suppressor gene in familial Schwannomatosis. *Clin Genet* 2008; **74**: 358–66.

102. Theaker JM, Gatter KC, Puddle J. Epithelial membrane antigen expression by the perineurium of peripheral nerve and in peripheral nerve tumours. *Histopathology* 1998; **13**: 171–9.

103. Hornick JL, Fletcher CD. Soft tissue perineurioma: clinicopathologic analysis of 81 cases including those with atypical histologic features. *Am J Surg Pathol* 2005; **29**: 845–58.

104. Folpe AF, Billings SD, McKenney JF, et al. Expression of claudin-1, a recently described tight junction perineurioma from potential mimics. *Am J Surg Pathol* 2002; **26**: 1620–6.

105. Yamaguchi LI, Hasegawa T, Hirose T, et al. Sclerosing perineurioma: a clinicopathologic study of five cases and diagnostic utility of immunohistochemical staining for GLUT1. *Virchows Arch* 2003; **443**: 159–63.

106. Dickson BC, Antonescu CR, Demicco EG, et al. Hybrid schwannoma-perineurioma frequently harbors VGLL3 rearrangement. *Mod Pathol* 2021; **34**: 1116–24.

107. Harder A, Wesemann M, Hagel C, et al. Hybrid neurofibroma/schwannoma is overrepresented among schwannomatosis and neurofibromatosis patients. *Am J Surg Pathol* 2012; **36**: 702–9.

108. Kacerovska D, Michal M, Kuroda N, et al. Hybrid peripheral nerve sheath tumors, including a malignant variant in type 1 neurofibromatosis. *Am J Dermatopathol* 2013; **35**: 641–9.

109. Wallace CA, Hallman JR, Sangueza OP. Primary cutaneous ganglioneuroma: a report of two cases and literature review. *Am J Dermatopathol* 2003; **25**: 239–42.

110. Reed RJ. Neuromesenchyme: the concept of a neurocristic effector cell for dermal mesenchyme. *Am J Dermatopathol* 1983; **5**: 385–95.

111. López DA, Silvers DN, Helwig EB. Cutaneous meningiomas: a clinicopathologic study. *Cancer* 1974; **34**: 728–44.

112. Fox MD, Billings SD, Gleason BC, et al. Cutaneous meningioma: a potential diagnostic pitfall in p63 positive cutaneous neoplasms. *J Cutan Pathol* 2013; **40**: 891–5.

113. Agaimy A, Buslei R, Coras R, et al. Comparative study of soft tissue perineurioma and meningioma using a five-marker immunohistochemical panel. *Histopathology* 2014; **65**: 60–70.

114. Lack EE, Worsham GF, Callihan MD, et al. Granular cell tumor: a clinicopathologic study of 110 patients. *J Surg Oncol* 1980; **13**: 301–16.

115. Fanburg-Smith JC, Meis-Kindblom JM, Fante R, et al. Malignant granular cell tumor of soft tissue: diagnostic criteria and clinicopathologic correlation. *Am J Surg Pathol* 1998; **22**: 779–94.

116. Le BH, Boyer PJ, Lewis JE, et al. Granular cell tumors: immunohistochemical assessment of inhibin-alpha, protein gene product 9.5, S100 protein, CD68, and Ki-67 proliferation index with clinical correlation. *Arch Pathol Lab Med* 2004; **128**: 771–5.

117. Kapur P, Rakheja D, Balani JP, et al. Phosphorylated histone 3, Ki-67, p21, fatty acid synthase, and cleaved caspase-3 expression in benign and atypical granular cell tumors. *Arch Pathol Lab Med* 2007; **131**: 57–64.

118. Jo VY, Fletcher CD. Epithelioid malignant peripheral nerve sheath tumor: clinicopathologic analysis of 63 cases. *Am J Surg Pathol* 2015; **39**: 673–82.

119. Pekmezci M, Reuss DE, Hirbe AC, et al. Morphologic and immunohistochemical features of malignant peripheral nerve sheath tumors and cellular schwannomas. *Mod Pathol* 2015; **28**: 187–200.

120. Schaefer IM, Fletcher CD, Hornick JL. Loss of H3K27 trimethylation distinguishes malignant peripheral nerve sheath tumors from histologic mimics. *Mod Pathol* 2016; **29**: 4–13.

121. Schaefer IM, Dong F, Garcia EP, et al. Recurrent SMARCB1 inactivation in epithelioid malignant peripheral nerve sheath tumors. *Am J Surg Pathol* 2019; **43**: 835–43.

122. Torres-Mora J, Dry S, Li X, et al. Malignant melanotic Schwannian tumor: a clinicopathologic, immunohistochemical, and gene expression profiling study of 40 cases, with a proposal for the reclassification of "melanotic Schwannoma." *Am J Surg Pathol* 2014; **38**: 94–105.

123. Carney JA. Psammomatous melanotic schwannoma: a distinctive, heritable tumor with special associations, including cardiac myxoma and the Cushing syndrome. *Am J Surg Pathol* 1990; **14**: 206–22.

124. Kim KH, Kwon SH, Sim WY, Lew BL. The study of relationship between anatomical sites and depth of the lipoma. *Ann Dermatol* 2021; **33**: 562–7.

125. Dreux N, Marty M, Chibon F, et al. Value and limitation of immunohistochemical expression of HMGA2 in mesenchymal tumors: about a series of 1052 cases. *Mod Pathol* 2010; **23**: 1657–66.

126. Stojanov IJ, Mariño-Enriquez A, Bahri N, et al. Lipomas of the oral cavity: utility of MDM2 and CDK4 in avoiding overdiagnosis as atypical lipomatous tumor. *Head Neck Pathol* 2019; **13**: 169–76.

127. Fletcher CDM, Martin-Bates E. Spindle-cell lipoma: a clinicopathological study with some original observations. *Histopathology* 1987; **11**: 803–17.

128. Maggiani F, Debiec-Rychter M, Vanbockrijck M, et al. Cellular angiofibroma: another mesenchymal tumor with 13q14 involvement, suggesting a link with spindle cell lipoma and (extra)-mammary myofibroblastoma. *Histopathology* 2007; **51**: 410–12.

129. Suster S, Fisher C. Immunoreactivity for the human hematopoietic progenitor cell antigen (CD34) in lipomatous tumors. *Am J Surg Pathol* 1997; **21**: 195–200.

130. Chen BJ, Marino-Enriquez A, Fletcher CD, Hornick JL. Loss of retinoblastoma protein expression in spindle cell/pleomorphic lipomas and cytogenetically related tumors: an immunohistochemical study with diagnostic implications. *Am J Surg Pathol* 2012; **36**: 1119–28.

131. Sirvent N, Coindre JM, Maire G, et al. Detection of MDM2-CDK4 amplification by fluorescence in situ hybridization in 200 paraffin-embedded tumor samples: utility in diagnosing adipocytic lesions and comparison with immunohistochemistry and real-time PCR. *Am J Surg Pathol* 2007; **31**: 1476–89.

132. Henricks WH, Chu YC, Goldblum JR, Weiss SW. Dedifferentiated liposarcoma: a clinicopathological analysis of 155 cases with a proposal for an expanded definition of dedifferentiation. *Am J Surg Pathol* 1997; **21**: 271–81.

133. Chai H, Xu F, DiAdamo A, Grommisch B, Mao H, Li P. Cytogenomic characterization of giant ring or rod marker chromosome in four cases of well-differentiated and dedifferentiated liposarcoma. *Case Rep Genet* 2022; **2022**: 6341207. doi: 10.1155/2022/6341207.

134. Kilpatrick SE, Doyon J, Choong PF, et al. The clinicopathologic spectrum of myxoid and round cell liposarcoma: a study of 95 cases. *Cancer* 1996; **77**: 1450–8.

135. Scapa JV, Cloutier JM, Raghavan SS, et al. DDIT3 immunohistochemistry is a useful tool for the diagnosis of myxoid liposarcoma. *Am J Surg Pathol* 2021; **45**: 230–9.

136. Hornick JL, Bosenberg MW, Mentzel T, et al. Pleomorphic liposarcoma: clinicopathologic analysis of 57 cases. *Am J Surg Pathol* 2004; **28**: 1257–67.

137. Mariño-Enríquez A, Hornick JL, Dal Cin P, et al. Dedifferentiated liposarcoma and pleomorphic liposarcoma: a comparative study of cytomorphology and MDM2/CDK4 expression on fine-needle aspiration. *Cancer Cytopathol* 2014; **122**: 128–37.

138. Guillou L, Fletcher CD. Benign lymphangioendothelioma (acquired progressive lymphangioma): a lesion not to be confused with well-differentiated angiosarcoma and patch stage Kaposi's sarcoma: clinicopathologic analysis of a series. *Am J Surg Pathol* 2000; **24**: 1047–57.

139. Requena L, Sangueza OP, Cutaneous vascular anomalies. Part I. Hamartomas, malformations, and dilatation of preexisting vessels. *J Am Acad Dermatol* 1997; **37**: 523–49.

140. Fukunaga M : Expression of D2-40 in lymphatic endothelium of normal tissues and in vascular tumours. *Histopathology* 2005; **46**: 396–402.

141. Miettinen M, Wang ZF, Prox1 transcription factor as a marker for vascular tumors – evaluation of 314 vascular endothelial and 1086 nonvascular tumors. *Am J Surg Pathol* 2012; **36**: 351–9.

142. Hornick JL, Fletcher CD. Intraabdominal cystic lymphangiomas obscured by marked superimposed reactive changes: clinicopathological analysis of a series. *Hum Pathol* 2005; **36**: 426–32.

143. Thiex JB, Mulliken N, Revencu LM, et al. A novel association between RASA1 mutations and spinal arteriovenous anomalies. *Am J Neuroradiol* 2010; **31**: 775–9.

144. Vugt LJ, van der Vleuten CJM, Flucke U, Blokx WAM. The utility of GLUT1 as a diagnostic marker in cutaneous vascular anomalies: A review of literature and recommendations for daily practice. *Pathology Res Practice* 2017; **213**: 591–7.

145. Patrice SJ, Wiss K, Mulliken JB. Pyogenic granuloma (lobular capillary hemangioma): a clinicopathologic study of 178 cases. *Pediatr Dermatol* 1991; **8**: 267–76.

146. Mentzel T, Partanen TA, Kutzner H. Hobnail hemangioma ("targetoid hemosiderotic hemangioma"): clinicopathologic and immunohistochemical analysis of 62 cases. *J Cutan Pathol* 1999; **26**: 279–86.

147. Al Dhaybi R, Powell J, McCuaig C, Kokta V. Differentiation of vascular tumors from vascular malformations by expression of Wilms tumor 1 gene: evaluation of 126 cases. *J Am Acad Dermatol* 2010; **63**: 1052–7.

148. Huang SC, Zhang L, Sung YS, et al. Frequent FOS gene rearrangements in epithelioid hemangioma: a molecular study of 58 cases with morphologic reappraisal. *Am J Surg Pathol* 2015; **39**: 1313–21.

149. Agaram NP, Zhang L, Cotzia P, et al. Expanding the spectrum of genetic alterations in pseudomyogenic hemangioendothelioma with recurrent novel ACTB-FOSB gene fusions. *Am J Surg Pathol* 2018; **42**: 1653–61.

150. Frieden IJ, Haggstrom AN, Drolet BA, et al. Infantile hemangiomas: current knowledge, future directions. Proceedings of a research workshop on infantile hemangiomas, April 7–9, 2005, Bethesda, Maryland. *Pediatr Dermatol* 2005; **22**: 383–406.

151. North PE, Waner M, Mizeracki A, Mihm MC Jr. GLUT1: a newly discovered immunohistochemical marker for juvenile hemangiomas. *Hum Pathol* 2000; **31**: 11–22.

152. Lyon LL, North PE, Mac-Moune Lai F, et al. Kaposiform hemangioendothelioma: a study of 33 cases emphasizing its pathologic, immunophenotypic, and biologic uniqueness from juvenile hemangioma. *Am J Surg Pathol* 2004; **28**: 559–68.

153. Zukerberg LR, Nickoloff BJ, Weiss SW. Kaposiform hemangioendothelioma of infancy and childhood: an aggressive neoplasm associated with Kasabach–Merritt syndrome and lymphangiomatosis. *Am J Surg Pathol* 1993; **17**: 321–8.

154. Le Huu AR, Jokinen CH, Ruben BP, et al. Expression of prox1, lymphatic endothelial nuclear transcription factor, in kaposiform hemangioendothelioma and tufted angioma. *Am J Surg Pathol* 2010; **34**: 1563–73.

155. Chang Y, Cesarman E, Pessin MS, et al. Identification of herpesvirus-like DNA sequences in AIDS-associated Kaposi's sarcoma. *Science* 1994; **266**: 1865–9.

156. Cheuk W, Wong KO, Wong CS, Dinkel JE, Ben-Dor D, Chan JK. Immunostaining for human herpesvirus 8 latent nuclear antigen-1 helps distinguish Kaposi sarcoma from its mimickers. *Am J Clin Pathol* 2004; **121**: 335–42.

157. Reis RM, Reis-Filho JS, Longatto Filho A, et al. Differential Prox-1 and CD31 expression in mucosae, cutaneous and soft tissue vascular lesions and tumors. *Pathol Res Pract* 2005; **201**: 771–6.

158. Pantanowitz L, Pinkus GS, Dezube BJ, Tahan SR. HHV8 is not limited to Kaposi's sarcoma. *Mod Pathol* 2005; **18**: 1148–50.

159. Mentzel T, Beham A, Calonje E, et al. Epithelioid hemangioendothelioma of

skin and soft tissue: clinicopathologic and immunohistochemical study of 30 cases. *Am J Surg Pathol* 1997; **21**: 363–74.

160. Miettinen M, Fetsch JF. Distribution of keratins in normal endothelial cells and a spectrum of vascular tumors: implications in tumor diagnosis. *Hum Pathol* 2000; **31**: 1062–7.

161. Errani C, Zhang L, Sung YS, et al. A novel WWTR1-CAMTA1 gene fusion is a consistent abnormality in epithelioid hemangioendothelioma of different anatomic sites. *Genes Chromosomes Cancer* 2011; **50**: 644–53.

162. Antonescu CR, Le Loarer F, Mosquera JM, et al. Novel YAP1- TFE3 fusion defines a distinct subset of epithelioid hemangioendothelioma. *Genes Chromosomes Cancer* 2013; **52**: 775–84.

163. Doyle LA, Fletcher CDM, Hornick JL. Nuclear expression of CAMTA1 distinguishes epithelioid hemangioendothelioma from histologic mimics. *Am J Surg Pathol* 2016; **40**: 94–102.

164. Antonescu CR, Dickson BC, Sung YS, et al. Recurrent YAP1 and MAML2 gene rearrangements in retiform and composite hemangioendothelioma. *Am J Surg Pathol* 2020; **44**: 1677–84.

165. Anderson WJ, Fletcher CDM, Hornick JL. Loss of expression of YAP1 C-terminus as an ancillary marker for epithelioid hemangioendothelioma variant with YAP1-TFE3 fusion and other YAP1-related vascular neoplasms. *Mod Pathol* 2021; **34**: 2036–42.

166. Perry KD, Al-Lbraheemi A, Rubin BP, et al. Composite hemangioendothelioma with neuroendocrine marker expression: an aggressive variant. *Mod Pathol* 2017; **30**: 1589–602.

167. Hornick JL, Fletcher CD. Pseudomyogenic hemangioendothelioma: a distinctive often multicentric tumor with indolent behavior. *Am J Surg Pathol* 2011; **35**: 190–201.

168. Agaram NP, Zhang L, Cotzia P, et al. Expanding the spectrum of genetic alterations in pseudomyogenic hemangioendothelioma with recurrent novel ACTB-FOSB gene fusions. *Am J Surg Pathol* 2018; **42**: 1653–61.

169. Sugita S, Hirano H, Kikuchi N, et al. Diagnostic utility of FOSB immunohistochemistry in pseudomyogenic hemangioendothelioma and its histological mimics. *Diagn Pathol* 2016; **11**: 75. doi: 10.1186/s13000-016-0530-2.

170. Dermawan JK, Westra WH, Antonescu CR. Recurrent PTBP1::MAML2 fusions in composite hemangioendothelioma with neuroendocrine differentiation: a report of two cases involving neck lymph nodes. *Genes Chromosomes Cancer* 2022; **61**: 187–93.

171. Miettinen M, Wang ZF, Paetau A, et al. ERG transcription factor as an immunohistochemical marker for vascular endothelial tumors and prostatic carcinoma. *Am J Surg Pathol* 2011; **35**: 432–41.

172. Brenn T, Fletcher CD. Radiation-associated cutaneous atypical vascular lesions and angiosarcoma: clinicopathologic analysis of 42 cases. *Am J Surg Pathol* 2005; **29**: 983–9.

173. Shon W, Sukov WR, Jenkins SM, Folpe AL. MYC amplification and overexpression in primary cutaneous angiosarcoma: a fluorescence in-situ hybridization and immunohistochemical study. *Mod Pathol* 2014; **27**: 509–15.

174. Trindade F, Kutzner H, Requena L, Tellechea O, Colmenero I. Microvenular hemangioma: an immunohistochemical study of 9 cases. *Am J Dermatopathol* 2012; **34**: 810–12.

175. Hagari Y, Hagari S, Kambe N, et al. Acral pseudolymphomatous angiokeratoma of children: immunohistochemical and clonal analyses of the infiltrating cells. *J Cutan Pathol* 2002; **29**: 313–18.

176. Chen H, Thompson LD, Aguilera NS, Abbondanzo SL. Kimura's disease: a clinicopathologic study of 21 cases. *Am J Surg Pathol* 2004; **28**: 505–13.

177. Oudijk L, den Bakker MA, Hop WC, et al. Solitary, multifocal and generalized myofibromas: clinicopathological and immunohistochemical features of 114 cases. *Histopathology* 2012; **60**: E1–11.

178. Koo SC, Janeway KA, Harris MH, et al. A distinctive genomic and immunohistochemical profile for NOTCH3 and PDGFRB in myofibroma with diagnostic and therapeutic implications. *Int J Surg Pathol* 2020; **28**: 128–37.

179. Folpe AL, Fanburg-Smith JC, Miettinen M, Weiss SW. Atypical and malignant glomus tumors: analysis of 52 cases, with a proposal for the reclassification of glomus tumors. *Am J Surg Pathol* 2001; **25**: 1–12.

180. Mentzel T, Dei Tos AP, Sapi Z, Kutzner H. Myopericytoma of skin and soft tissues: clinicopathologic and immunohistochemical study of 54 cases. *Am J Surg Pathol* 2006; **30**: 104–13.

181. Matsuyama A, Hisaoka M, Hashimoto H. Angioleiomyoma: a clinicopathologic and immunohistochemical reappraisal with special reference to the correlation with myopericytoma. *Hum Pathol* 2007; **38**: 645–51.

182. Ørholt M, Abebe K, Aaberg F, et al. Immunohistochemical characteristics of atypical fibroxanthoma and pleomorphic dermal sarcoma: a systematic review and meta-analysis. *Am J Dermatopathol* 2022; **44**: 913–20.

183. Henderson SA, Torres-Cabala CA, Curry JL, et al. p40 is more specific than p63 for the distinction of atypical fibroxanthoma from other cutaneous spindle cell malignancies. *Am J Surg Pathol* 2014; **38**: 1102–10.

184. Thway K, Fisher C. Angiomatoid fibrous histiocytoma: the current status of pathology and genetics. *Arch Pathol Lab Med* 2015; **139**: 674–82.

185. Cheah AL, Zou Y, Lanigan C, et al. ALK expression in angiomatoid fibrous histiocytoma: a potential diagnostic pitfall. *Am J Surg Pathol* **43**: 93–101.

186. Calonje E, Guerin D, McCormick D, Fletcher CD. Superficial angiomyxoma: clinicopathologic analysis of a series of distinctive but poorly recognized cutaneous tumors with tendency for recurrence. *Am J Surg Pathol* 1999; **23**: 910–17.

187. Hafeez F, Krakowski AC, Lian CG, et al. Sporadic superficial angiomyxomas demonstrate loss of PRKAR1A expression. *Histopathology* 2022; **80**: 1001–3.

188. van Roggen JF, van Unnik JA, Briaire-de Bruijn IH, Hogendoorn PC. Aggressive angiomyxoma: a clinicopathological and immunohistochemical study of 11 cases with long-term follow-up. *Virchows Arch* 2005; **446**: 157–63.

189. Bigby SM, Symmans PJ, Miller MV, et al. Aggressive angiomyxoma of the female genital tract and pelvis: clinicopathologic features with immunohistochemical analysis. *Int J Gynecol Pathol* 2011; **30**: 505–13.

190. Hornick JL, Fletcher CD. Cellular neurothekeoma: detailed

characterization in a series of 133 cases. *Am J Surg Pathol* 2007; **31**: 329–40.

191. Chaudhry IH, Calonje E. Dermal non-neural granular cell tumour (so-called primitive polypoid granular cell tumour): a distinctive entity further delineated in a clinicopathological study of 11 cases. *Histopathology* 2005; **47**: 179–85.

192. Cohen JN, Yeh I, Jordan RC, et al. Cutaneous non-neural granular cell tumors harbor recurrent ALK gene fusions. *Am J Surg Pathol* 2018; **42**: 1133–42.

193. Llamas-Velasco M, Requena L, Kutzner H, et al. Fumarate hydratase immunohistochemical staining may help to identify patients with multiple cutaneous and uterine leiomyomatosis (MCUL) and hereditary leiomyomatosis and renal cell cancer (HLRCC) syndrome. *J Cutan Pathol* 2014; **41**: 859–65.

194. Liu C, Dillon J, Beavis AL, et al. Prevalence of somatic and germline mutations of Fumarate hydratase in uterine leiomyomas from young patients. *Histopathology* 2020; **76**: 354–65.

Chapter 9 Miscellaneous Tumors

Soma Jobbagy and Mai P. Hoang

Introduction

The histogenesis of a variety of tumors such as epithelioid sarcoma, alveolar soft part sarcoma, and synovial sarcoma remains unknown. Tumors of histiocytic origin include Erdheim-Chester disease and histiocytic sarcoma and dendritic cell tumors include Langerhans cell histiocytosis (LCH), follicular dendritic cell sarcoma, and interdigitating dendritic cell sarcoma. Despite their similar histopathologic appearance, tumors of histiocytic and dendritic cell origin have different immunoprofile and immunohistochemistry is essential in classifying these tumors. Leukemia cutis or granulocytic or myeloid sarcoma is comprised of immature myeloid precursor cells. Lymphoblastic lymphomas are derived from precursor B- or T-cell lymphocytes. Cutaneous involvement can be the sole manifestation of these diseases, during or after development of bone marrow leukemia. In this chapter these miscellaneous entities as well as Merkel cell carcinoma, myoepithelioma, myoepithelial carcinoma, Ewing sarcoma, and mast cell infiltrate are discussed.

9.1 Merkel Cell Carcinoma

Merkel cell carcinoma (MCC) or primary cutaneous neuroendocrine carcinoma is an uncommon and highly lethal tumor with ultraviolet radiation, immunosuppression, and Merkel cell polyomavirus (MCPyV) infection as risk factors.[1] Most present with localized cutaneous lesions; however, some present with regional lymph node or distant metastasis.[2] MCPyV-positive and MCPyV negative MCCs are now thought to represent distinct subtypes with divergent genetic origins.[2] These subtypes should be distinguished when rendering a diagnosis of MCC as MCPyV-negative MCCs have a worse prognosis than their MCPyV-positive counterparts.[3] MCPyV-positive MCCs are characterized by clonal integration of the MCPyV into epidermal cells with resultant expression of the small- and large T antigens, which are tumorigenic.[1] The majority of MCC from non-sun exposed areas harbor the Merkel cell polyomavirus, and MCPyV positivity is inversely correlated with sun damage.[3]

By contrast, MCPyV-negative MCCs have been described to harbor a UV-mutational signature with C>T transitions within pyrimidine runs, as well as *TP53* and *RB1* gene mutations. While MCC is typically considered a *de novo* neoplasm without a dysplastic precursor, some cutaneous neuroendocrine carcinomas (termed "combined" neuroendocrine carcinoma) have been described as arising from squamous dysplastic or neoplastic precursors.[4]

Histopathologically, epidermotropism can be seen in up to 30% of cases of MCC and can be suggestive of Pautrier microabscesses of mycosis fungoides.[5] Squamous, adnexal, and sarcomatous differentiation have been observed in MCC. Merkel cells can be found in the lower epidermis and the outer root sheath of hair follicles. Currently thought to originate from a totipotent stem cell, MCC can exhibit epithelial as well as neuroendocrine differentiation.

It often expresses low molecular weight keratins including keratins AE1/AE3, keratin 8/18 (CAM5.2), keratin 19, keratin 20, keratin MNF116, and epithelial membrane antigen (EMA) (**Figures 9.1, 9.2, and 9.3**) (**Table 9.1**).[6–27] Focal keratin 20 positivity can be seen up to 33% of pulmonary small cell carcinoma[28] and up to 23% of MCC can express keratin 7; however, MCC is invariably negative for thyroid transcription factor-1 (TTF1). Therefore, a panel including keratin 7, keratin 20, and TTF1 would be helpful in distinguishing MCC from pulmonary small cell carcinoma (**Table 9.2**). Recently POU4F3 has been reported to be a sensitive marker for Merkel cell carcinoma, helpful in the distinction from small cell lung carcinoma (**Figure 9.4**).[29] Neuroendocrine markers such as INSM1, chromogranin A

Table 9.1 Immunohistochemical profile of Merkel cell carcinoma[6–27, 29]

	Frequently positive	Can be positive
Epithelial markers	Keratin 20 (76–100%) Keratin CAM5.2 (100%) Keratin AE1/AE3 (100%) Keratin MNF116 (100%) Keratin 19 (100%) Pankeratin (83%) EMA (78%)	Keratin 7 (5–23%) Keratin 5/6 (0%) Keratin 17 (0%)
Neuroendocrine markers	NSE (100%) CD56 (94–100%) Synaptophysin (87–100%) Chromogranin A (73–100%) Neurofilament (22–50%)	
Infection marker	MCPyV (18–94%)	
Other markers	POU4F3 (98%) Bcl2 (100%) PAX8 (97%) Fli–1 (90%) Glypican 3 (77%) PAX5 (70.6–93.5%) TdT (53–78%) CD117 (53–95%) CD99 (13–100%) ALK (12.5–94%)	p63 (33%) NeuroD1 (20%) CD10 (7%) TTF1 (0–12%) ASCL1 (0%)

TTF1: thyroid transcription factor 1, NSE: neuron specific enolase, MCPyV: Merkel cell polyomavirus

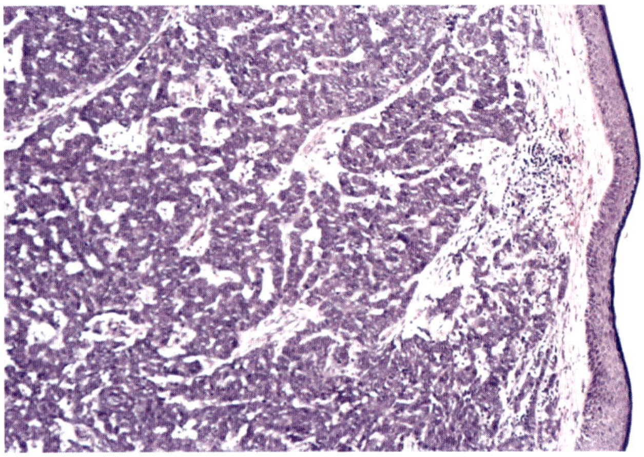

Figure 9.1 Cords of hyperchromatic neoplastic cells with high nuclear cytoplasmic ratio and neuroendocrine nuclear morphology are seen in this example of Merkel cell carcinoma (X100).

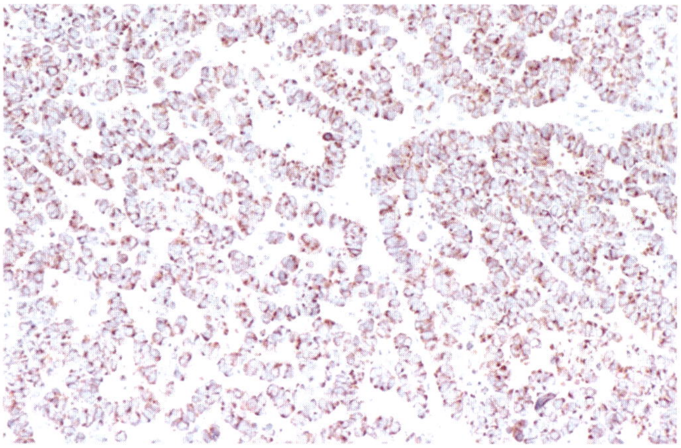

Figure 9.2 Dot-like cytoplasmic reactivity is noted with keratin AE1/AE3 (X200).

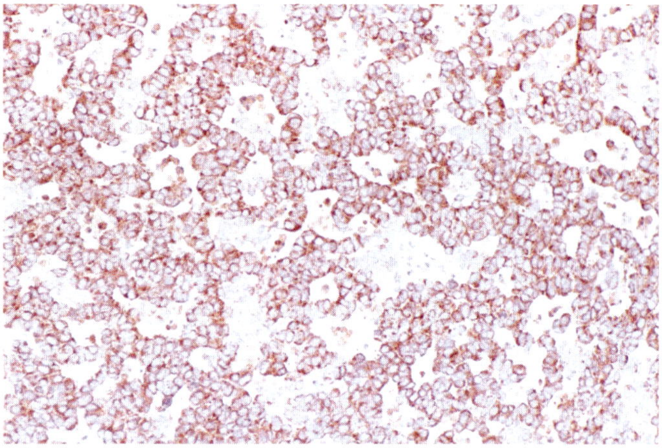

Figure 9.3 Similar dot-like cytoplasmic reactivity seen with keratin 20 (X200).

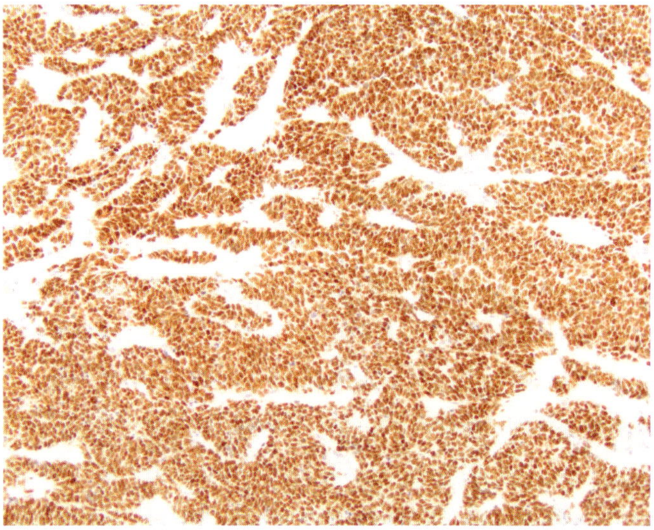

Figure 9.4 Strong nuclear POU4F3 expression (X200).

(**Figure 9.5**), synaptophysin, neuron-specific enolase, and CD56 are invariably positive. Neurofilament exhibits paranuclear dot-like positivity. Immunoreactivity for vasoactive intestinal peptide, calcitonin, and somatostatin can be seen. A series of 7 cases of MCC with keratin 7 expression yet negative for keratin 20 was reported by Caldder et al.[30] In addition, a rare case of keratin 20 negative and TTF1 positive MCC has also been reported.[31]

An immunostain against the MCPyV large T-antigen (antibody clones CM2B4, CM5E1 or Ab3) can demonstrate virus-association of the tumor **(Figure 9.6)**.[20] Although one report has indicated that Ab3 may be the most sensitive and specific, we have found clone CM2B4 to be most reliable.[20] While MCPyV DNA can be detected by PCR, the detection rate may be compromised by mutations and polymorphisms within the MCPyV DNA or by nucleic acid degradation during fixation and processing.[1] Molecular genetic techniques are not currently considered part of routine clinical evaluation for viral positivity.

Table 9.2 Differential diagnosis of Merkel cell carcinoma

	POU4F3	ASCL1	CK7	CK20	NF	BerEP4	S100	TTF1	CD45	Synaptophysin	CD56
Merkel cell carcinoma	+	-	-/+	+	+	-	-	-	-	+	+
Lung small cell carcinoma	-	+/-	+	-	-	-	-	+	-	+	+
Lymphoma	nd	nd	-	-	-	-	-	-	+	-	-/+
Melanoma	-	nd	-	-	-	-	+	-	-	-/+	-/+
Sweat gland carcinoma	nd	nd	+	-	-	-	-	-	-	-	-
Basal cell carcinoma	-	nd	-/+	-	-	+	-	-	-	-	-
Squamous cell carcinoma	nd	nd	-/+	-	-	-	-	-	-	-	-

NF: neurofilament, TTF1: thyroid transcription factor 1, nd: not documented

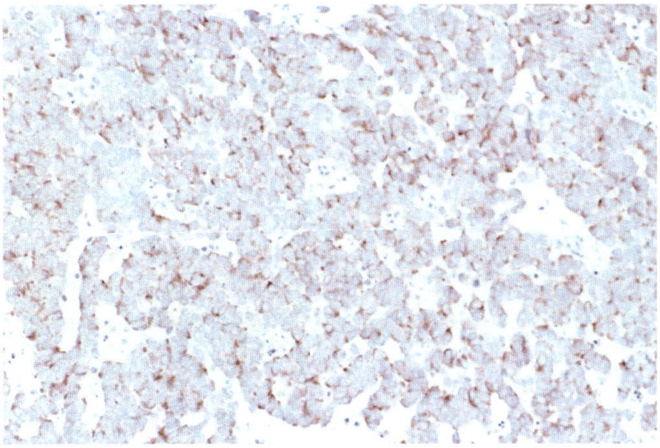

Figure 9.5 The tumor cells are positive for chromogranin (X200).

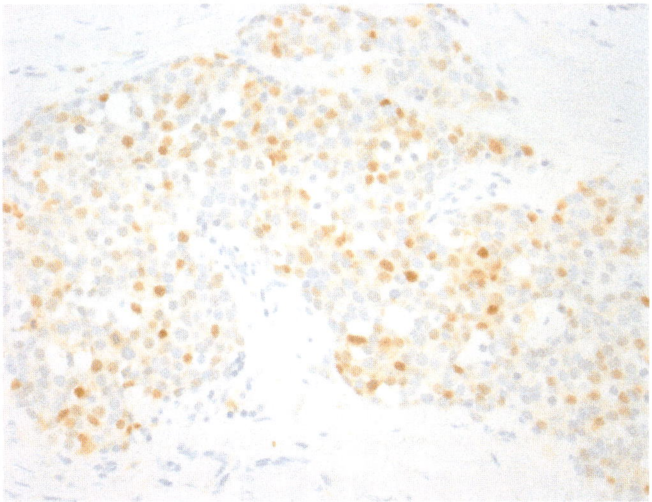

Figure 9.7 Aberrant TdT expression in Merkel cell carcinoma (X200).

Overlapping positive markers with hematolymphoid malignancies including terminal deoxynucleotidyl transferase (TdT) (**Figure 9.7**), PAX5, Bcl2, CD56, and anaplastic lymphoma kinase have been reported in MCC (**Table 9.1**).[6–27,29] A limited panel of CD45, CD20, PAX5, and TdT performed on a Merkel cell carcinoma could be misinterpreted as a lymphoblastic lymphoma. Merkel cell carcinoma is invariably negative for CD45 (LCA), CD20, and CD3.[32]

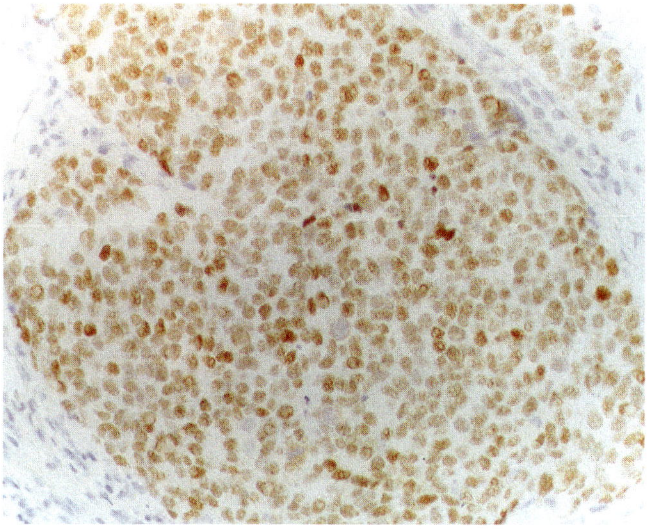

Figure 9.6 Immunohistochemistry for MCPyV large T-antigen (antibody clone CM2B4) in Merkel cell carcinoma shows strong positive nuclear staining indicative of viral positivity (X400).

Cutaneous NK/T cell lymphoma or blastic plasmacytoid dendritic cell neoplasm would be in the differential diagnosis due to CD56 expression; however, the expression of CD2, CD7, and cytoplasmic CD3 would help ruling in a NK/T cell lymphoma. Expression of Fli-1 and CD99 can raise the possibility of Ewing sarcoma/peripheral neuroectodermal tumor.

Merkel cell carcinoma

- MCPyV large T-antigen immunostaining positivity (virus positive) or UV-related signature, *TP53* and/or *RB1* mutation (virus negative)
- Positive with POU4F3, low molecular weight keratins including keratin AE1/AE3, keratin 8/18 (CAM5.2), keratin 19, keratin 20, keratin MNF116, and epithelial membrane antigen
- Neuroendocrine markers: chromogranin A+, synaptophysin+, neurofilament+, and CD56+
- Keratin 20 and neurofilament have characteristic perinuclear dot-like staining
- Invariably negative for thyroid transcription factor 1

9.2 Myoepitheliomas and Myoepithelial Carcinomas

Myoepitheliomas and myoepithelial carcinomas of the skin and soft tissue are uncommon.[33] They often present as painless soft tissue mass in an adult and without gender predilection.[34] They lack folliculosebaceous or apocrine differentiation or chondroid differentiation as seen in mixed tumor. While some of myoepitheliomas exhibit minimal cytologic atypia, others have malignant histopathologic features and are classified as malignant myoepitheliomas or myoepithelial carcinoma.[34] In the malignant tumors high grade cytologic atypia, multinodular and infiltrative architecture, and chondromyxoid or hyalinized stroma are seen (**Figures 9.8 and 9.9**). The tumor cells co-express Sox10, S100 (72–100%) (**Figure 9.10**), and epithelial markers including keratins (93–100%) (AE1/AE3, pan keratin, CAM5.2, keratin 14), and EMA (19–66%).[34,35] Most cases are positive for calponin (86–100%) while staining for smooth muscle actin (SMA) (36–64%), desmin (0–22%), and p63 (7–45%) (**Figure 9.11**) is seen only in a small subset of cases.[34] GFAP staining is variable (27–54%).[35] Loss of INI1 nuclear expression is seen in 9–22% of myoepitheliomas and myoepithelial carcinomas.[36] However, in INI1-deficient vulvar myoepithelial carcinomas EMA and SMA are the only markers consistently positive, while there is a limited expression of keratins, CD34, desmin, and S100 protein.[37]

EWSR1 gene rearrangements have been described in myoepithelial tumors of skin and soft tissue, including both benign myoepitheliomas and those with malignant potential. *EWSR1::PBX3* mutations are seen in up to 80% of cutaneous syncytial myoepitheliomas (**Figure 9.12**).[38] The most prevalent rearrangements in soft tissue myoepithelial tumors include t(6;22)(p21;q12) resulting in *EWSR1::POU5F1* and t(1;22)(q23;q12) resulting in *EWSR1::PBX1*. Each of these is observed in 16% of cases in the largest reported series of myoepithelial tumors.[39]

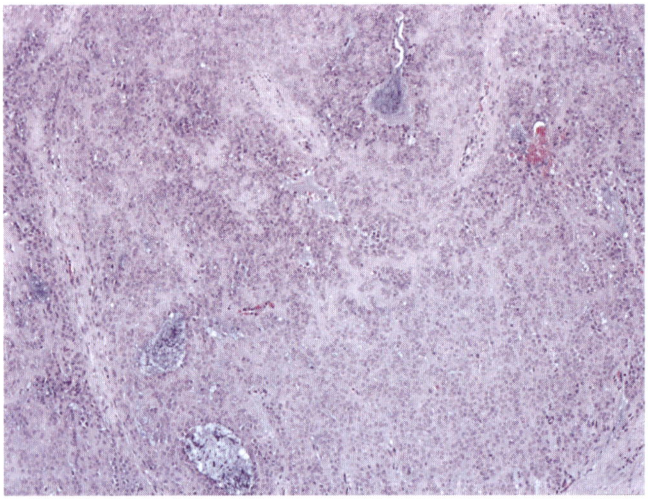

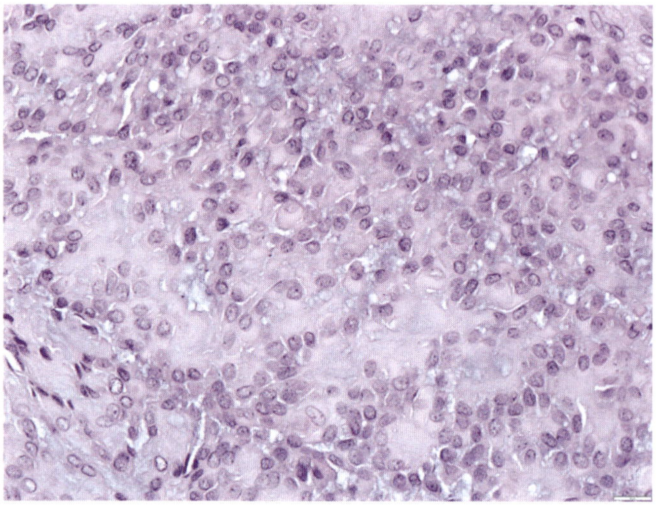

Figures 9.8 and 9.9 Myoepithelioma is characterized by a multinodular proliferation of plasmacytoid cells within a chondromyxoid stroma (courtesy of Joana Pardal M.D., Department of Pathology, Hospital S. João and Medical Faculty of Porto University, Porto, Portugal) (X100, X400).

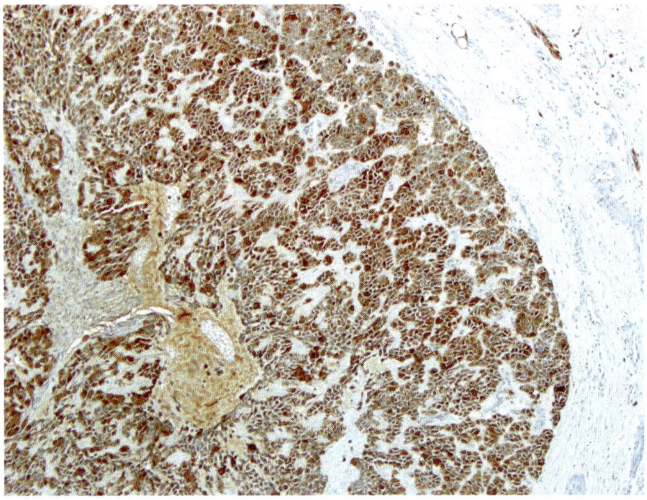

Figure 9.10 Diffuse S100 expression (X100) (courtesy of Joana Pardal M.D., Department of Pathology, Hospital S. João and Medical Faculty of Porto University, Porto, Portugal).

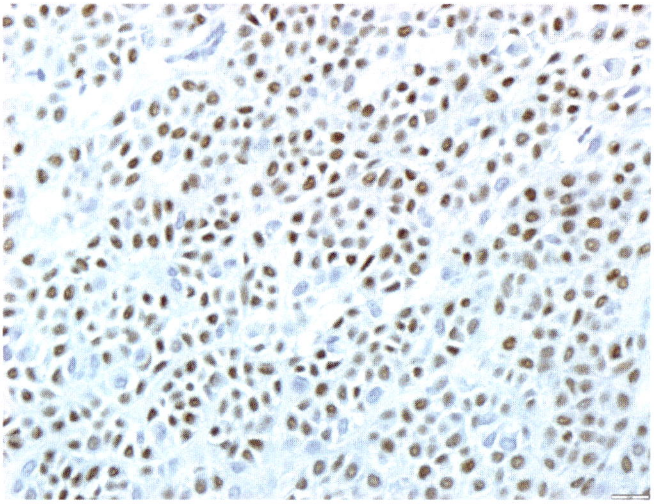

Figure 9.11 Strong nuclear p63 expression (X400) (courtesy of Joana Pardal M.D., Department of Pathology, Hospital S. João and Medical Faculty of Porto University, Porto, Portugal).

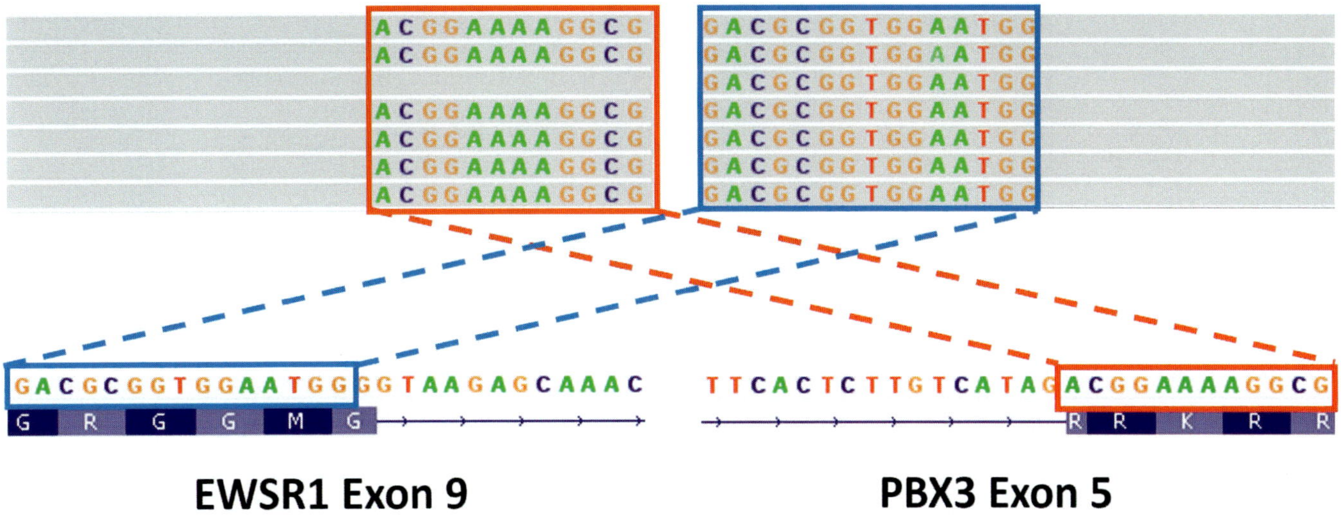

Figure 9.12 RNA-based next-generation sequencing demonstrates *EWSR1::PBX3* fusion involving *EWSR1* exon 9 and *PBX3* exon 5 (Integrated Genome Viewer).

Identification of the specific gene fusion may have prognostic significance. *EWSR1::POU5F1* tumors more frequently occur in children and young adults and are associated with malignancy. By contrast, tumors with *EWSR1/FUS::PBX1/3* fusions are typically benign.[40]

While salivary gland myoepithelial tumors, including pleomorphic adenoma and carcinoma *ex* pleomorphic adenoma, exhibit *PLAG1* or *HMGA2* rearrangements, these genetic alterations are typically absent in soft tissue myoepithelial tumors.[39] However, *PLAG1* rearrangements can be seen in a subset of cutaneous mixed tumors with prominent tubuloductal differentiation.[41]

EWSR1 rearrangement may be identified by *EWSR1* break-apart FISH with probes flanking the *EWSR1* break point. Dual-fusion FISH has also been used to identify specific fusion partners of *EWSR1*. Sequencing techniques, such as RT-PCR or anchored multiplexed sequencing can be used to identify or confirm fusion transcripts.

The differential diagnosis of a malignant myoepithelioma or myoepithelial carcinoma would include melanoma, metastatic carcinoma, and epithelioid sarcoma. While melanomas express S100 and Sox10, they are typically negative for keratins, GFAP, or myogenic markers. Expression of S100, GFAP, and calponin would exclude the possibility of metastatic carcinoma. While epithelioid sarcomas express keratin and EMA, they do not express Sox10, S100, GFAP, or myogenic markers. Unlike mixed tumor which expresses PLAG1 due to *PLAG1* rearrangement, up to 45% of myoepitheliomas and myoepithelial carcinomas harbor *EWSR1* gene rearrangement.[39]

Myoepitheliomas and myoepithelial carcinomas

- *EWSR1* rearrangement
- Keratin+, Sox10+, S100+, calponin+, EMA+/-, and GFAP+/-
- p63-/+ and INI1+

9.3 Epithelioid Sarcoma

Epithelioid sarcoma is a malignant soft tissue tumor of adolescents and young adults that has two histologic types: classic/distal-type and proximal-type. The classic or distal type is characterized by tumor nodules with central necrosis surrounded by epithelioid neoplastic cells (**Figure 9.13**). The proximal type exhibits a more aggressive biologic behavior and is comprised of markedly atypical epithelioid cells with cytoplasmic hyaline inclusion. The tumor cells express vimentin, CD34, EMA, keratin 8, keratin 19, and CA125.[42] Expression of beta-catenin by proximal-type allows differentiation from malignant rhabdoid tumor.[43]

SWI/SNF-related matrix-associated actin-dependent regulator of chromatin subfamily B member 1(SMARCB1), is also known as INI1, hSNF5, and BAP47. Mutation or loss of *SMARCB1* gene locus on chromosome 22q11.2 is characteristic of malignant rhabdoid tumor and the central nervous system counterpart, atypical teratoid/rhabdoid tumor.[44] SMARCB1/INI1 expression is seen in the nuclei of all normal cells and loss of its nuclear expression has been shown to be helpful in diagnosing pediatric atypical teratoid/rhabdoid tumors, malignant rhabdoid tumors of the kidney and extrarenal tissues, renal medullary carcinoma, both types of epithelioid sarcoma, epithelioid malignant peripheral nerve sheath tumors, and some myoepithelial soft tissue neoplasms.[44] Loss of SMARCB1/INI1 nuclear expression has been reported to be a diagnostic feature of both variants of epithelioid sarcoma (**Figure 9.14**).[44] While ERG is expressed in up to 54% of epithelioid sarcoma, SALL4 expression is seen in 71% of malignant rhabdoid tumors; thus a combination of ERG and SALL4 may be helpful in distinguishing epithelioid sarcoma from malignant rhabdoid tumor (**Table 9.3**).[45–47]

Due to the availability of SMARCB1/INI1 immunohistochemistry, molecular approaches are not usually needed to diagnose epithelioid sarcoma. Loss of protein expression is almost universal in epithelioid sarcoma, while inactivating mutations in the *SMARCB1* gene may only be seen in approximately half of tumors.[48]

Table 9.3 Tumors commonly with loss of INI1 expression[46,47]

Tumor type	Loss of INI1 expression
Malignant rhabdoid tumor and atypical teratoid/rhabdoid tumor	98%
Medullary carcinoma of the kidney	100%
Epithelioid sarcoma	80–93%
Synovial sarcoma	66%

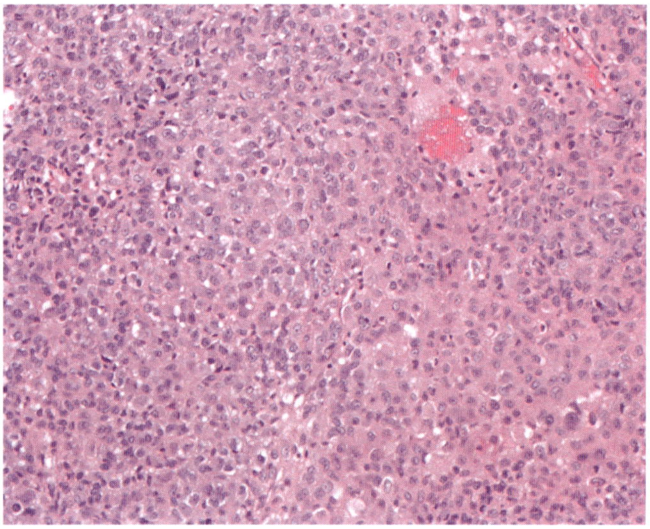

Figure 9.13 Epithelioid sarcoma is characterized by diffuse proliferation of epithelioid tumor cells (X200).

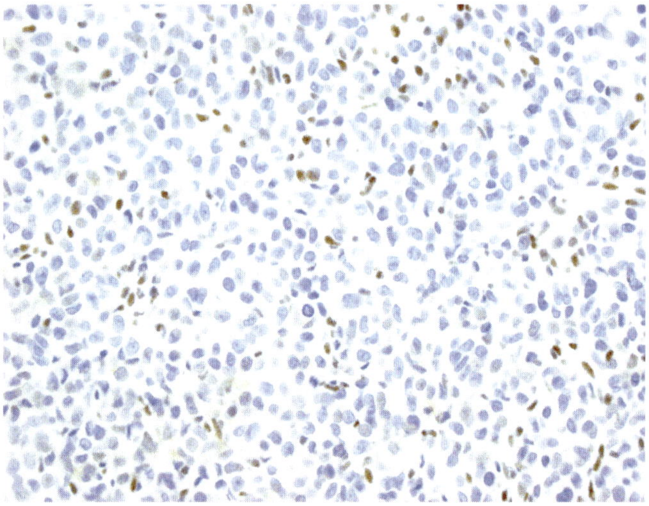

Figure 9.14 Loss of INI1 nuclear expression is observed in the tumor cells (X400).

Nonetheless, molecular techniques may be helpful in cases where SMARCB1/INI1 is retained by IHC but epithelioid sarcoma remains on the differential. Interphase FISH for *SMARCB1* can be performed on formalin-fixed, paraffin-embedded tissues. By FISH, biallelic deletion of *SMARCB1* is the most common pattern observed in epithelioid sarcoma although monoallelic deletions have also been described.[49] Multiplex ligation dependent probe amplification, a PCR-based technique, has been described as a reliable method of detecting *SMARCB1* copy number variation in formalin-fixed paraffin embedded tissues.[49] Sequencing-based techniques may be used to evaluate for *SMARCB1* polymorphism or as an unbiased method for detection of loss or mutation of other SWI/SNF family genes in rare cases SMARCB1-retained epithelioid sarcoma.[50]

Epithelioid sarcoma

- CD34+, EMA+, keratin 19+, and loss of INI1 nuclear expression

9.4 Ewing Sarcoma

Ewing sarcoma/peripheral neuroectodermal tumors (PNET) belongs to the group known as "small blue round cell tumors" (SBRCT). These mesenchymal neoplasms featuring round cell morphology include neuroblastoma, rhabdomyosarcoma, lymphoblastic lymphoma, esthesioneuroblastoma, desmoplastic round cell tumor, and Wilms' tumor; however, there is a considerable overlap in the immunoprofiles of these various tumors.[51,52] Ewing sarcoma/PNET are molecularly defined by chromosomal rearrangements resulting in in-frame fusions, particularly involving the amino-terminus of *FET* (*FUS*, *EWSR1*, *TAF15*) gene family members and the carboxyl terminus, including the DNA-binding domain, of *ETS* (Erythroblast Transformation Specific) gene family members (*FLI1*, *ERG*, *ETV1*, *ETV4*, *FEV*). The prototypical and most common fusion is t(11;22)(q24;q12), with resultant *EWSR1::FLI1*, which is observed in 90% of cases. *EWSR1::ERG* fusions account for a minority of Ewing sarcoma/PNET (5–10%).[53]

While cytogenetic and molecular techniques remain the "gold standard" for interrogation of *FET*/*ETS* gene family fusions, Ewing sarcoma/PNET have a characteristic immunophenotype which may be useful for initial diagnostic workup.

CD99 shows strong, diffuse membranous expression in 90–95% of cases of Ewing sarcoma/PNET. NKX2.2 is positive with staining in 93% of cases.[54] Immunostains specific for FLI1 or ERG may be positive depending on the specific fusion involved. FLI1 nuclear staining is present in 90% of tumors with *EWSR1::FLI1* fusion [52,55] while ERG nuclear staining has been reported in 88% of tumors harboring *EWSR1::ERG* fusion.[56]

The sensitivity and specificity of Fli-1 immunostain for Ewing sarcoma/PNET are 60–100% and 47–100%, respectively (**Figures 9.15 and 9.16**) (**Table 9.4**).[51–53,55,57] Importantly, Fli-1 positivity has

Table 9.4 FLI-1 expression in Ewing sarcoma/peripheral neuroectodermal tumor

References	N	Sensitivity	Specificity
Folpe 2000 [52]	132	71%	91%
Lombart-Bosch 2001 [55]	48	84%	69%
Rossi 2004 [51]	140	100%	47%*
Mhawech-Fauceglia 2006 [57]	58	98%	60%
Tomlins 2013 [53]	57	60%	100%

* Specificity increases to 62% if only 2–4+ is considered positive staining.

Table 9.5 The differential diagnosis of a small blue cell tumor

	CD99	Fli1	NKX2.2	Erg	WT1	desmin	MyoD1/ myogenin	TdT	keratin	S100
Ewing/PNET	+	+	+	-/+	-	-	-	-	+/-	-
Lymphoblastic lymphoma	+	+/-	-	-	-	-	-	+	-	-
Rhabdomyosarcoma	+/-	-	-	-	-	+	+	-	-	-
Desmoplastic small round cell tumor	+/-	+/-	-/+	-	+	+	-	-	+	
Melanoma	-	-	-	-	-	-	-	-	-	+

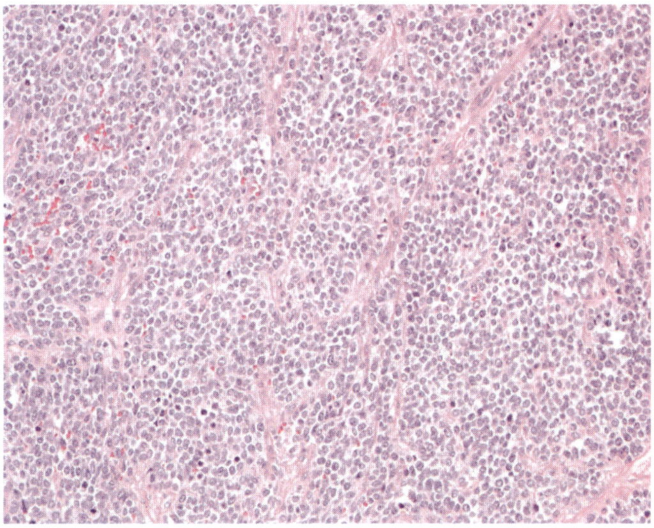

Figure 9.15 A proliferation of tumor cells with high nuclear cytoplasmic ratio seen in Ewing sarcoma/peripheral neuroectodermal tumor (X200).

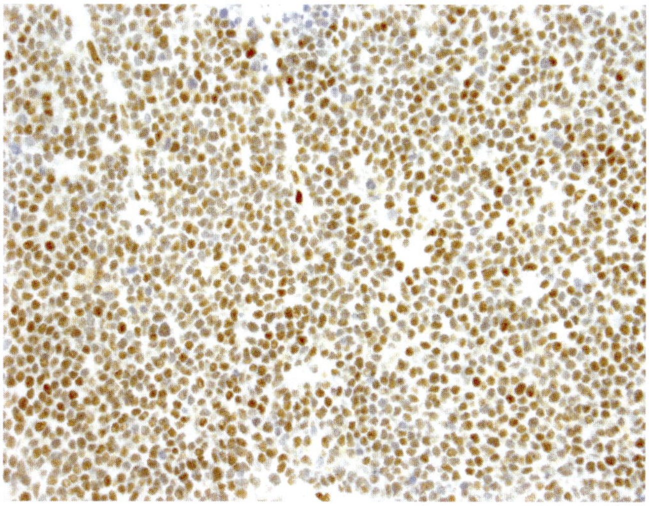

Figure 9.16 The tumor cells express diffuse and strong nuclear Fli-1 (X400).

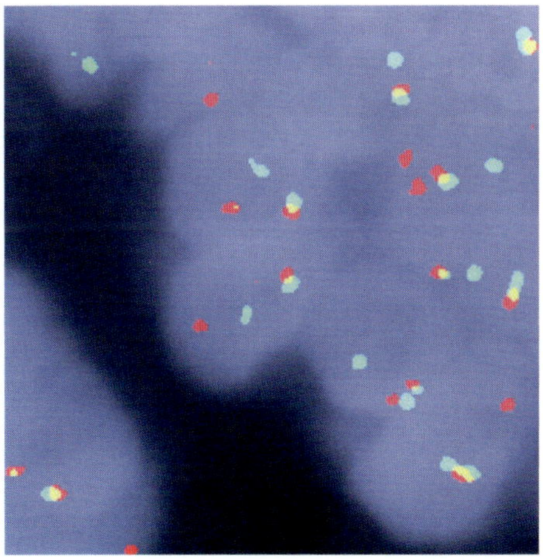

Figure 9.17 Ewing sarcoma with interphase fluorescence *in situ* hybridization (FISH) testing using break-apart probes for *EWSR1* shows separation of the red 5′ and green 3′ signals, indicative of *EWSR1* gene rearrangement.

been observed both in tumors with *EWSR1::FLI1* and *EWSR1::ERG* fusions, and cannot be considered mutation-specific due to significant cross-reactivity of the antibody between homologous C-terminal epitopes of Fli-1 and ERG (**Figure 9.17**).[56]

The low specificity of Fli-1 is due to the strong immunoreactivity detected in all endothelial neoplasms, including angiosarcoma, epithelioid hemangioendothelioma, and Kaposi sarcoma; however, this confirms the important role of Fli-1 immunostain as a very reliable nuclear marker of endothelial differentiation.[51] ERG immunostain has been reported to exhibit 88–96% sensitivity and 88–99% specificity in detecting *ERG* rearrangement.[56] The differential diagnosis of a small blue cell tumor would include Ewing sarcoma/PNET, melanoma, lymphoblastic lymphoma, desmoplastic small round cell tumor, and rhabdomyosarcoma (**Table 9.5**).

To definitively identify specific fusion events in Ewing sarcoma, interphase FISH with break-apart probes for *EWSR1*, PCR, and unbiased sequencing approaches (such as anchored multiplex PCR based sequencing, next generation sequencing may be pursued.

Ewing sarcoma

- CD99+, NKX2.2+, Fli1+

9.5 Alveolar Soft Part Sarcoma

Alveolar soft part sarcoma is a rare neoplasm of deep soft tissues with a characteristic histologic appearance and defining *ASPSCR1::TFE3* fusion. Nests of eosinophilic and polygonal neoplastic cells are demarcated by thin-walled vessels (**Figure 9.18**). Expression of S100 protein, neuron specific enolase, SMA, and desmin can be seen.[58] The tumor is negative for keratins, EMA, and MyoD1. The tumor cells contain Periodic acid-Schiff (PAS)-positive intracytoplasmic crystals and granules (**Figure 9.19**).

Table 9.6 TFE3 expression in alveolar soft part sarcoma and renal cell carcinoma with related translocation

References	N	ASPS	RCC*	Other tumors	Sensitivity	Specificity
Argani 2002 [62]	11	nd	11/11	nd	100%	nd
Argani 2003 [59]	1516	19/19	20/21	6/1476	97.5%	99.6%
Pang 2008 [63]	53	16/16	nd	1/37	100%	97%
Williams 2011 [61]	43	18/18	nd	5/25	100%	80%
Tsuji 2012 [64]	47	22/24	nd	2/23	92%	91%
Rekhi 2012 [60]	43	20/22	nd	6/21	91%	71%

* Renal cell carcinoma with *PRCC::TFE3*, *ASPL::TFE3*, and *PSF::TFE3* fusion transcripts nd: not documented

Table 9.7 Differential diagnosis of alveolar soft part sarcoma

	S100	Sox10	HMB45	MelanA	synaptophysin	TFE3
Alveolar soft part sarcoma	-	-	-	-	-	+
Granular cell tumor	+	+	-	-	-	-/+
Adrenocortical carcinoma	-	-	-	+	-	-/+
Paraganglioma	-*	-	-	-	+	-/+
Clear cell sarcoma/melanoma of soft tissue	+	+/-	+	+	-	-/+
PEComa	-/+	-	+	-/+	-	-/+

* sustentacular cells positive for S100

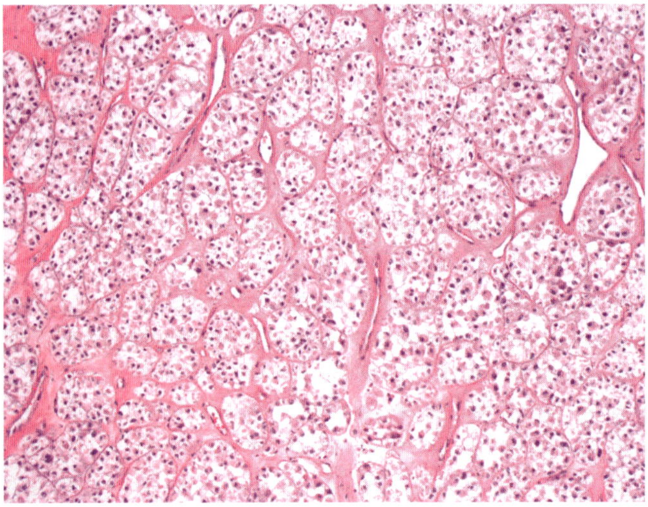

Figure 9.18 Nests of eosinophilic and polygonal neoplastic cells are demarcated by thin-walled vessels in alveolar soft part sarcoma (X100).

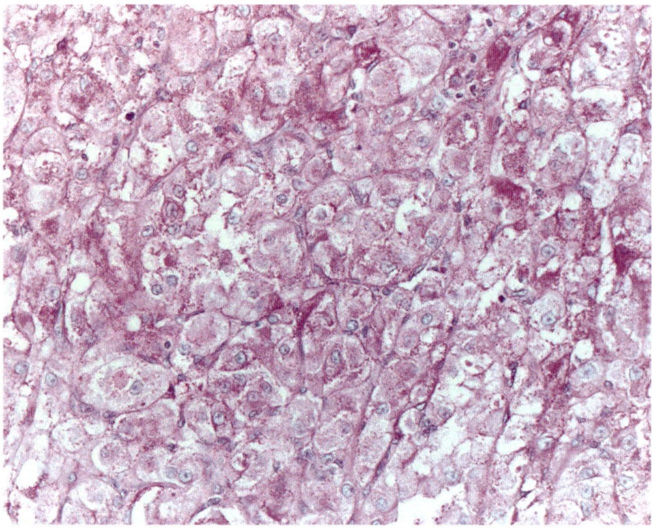

Figure 9.19 Periodic acid-Schiff stain highlights intracytoplasmic granules in alveolar soft part sarcoma (X400).

A structural rearrangement der(17)t(X;17)(p11.2;q25) gives rise to the fusion transcript *ASPSCR1::TFE3* (*ASPL* gene on 17q25 and *TFE3* gene on Xp11.1) and is specific for alveolar soft part sarcoma.[59] An antibody against TFE3 protein, a member of the basic helix-loop-helix family of transcription factors, has been shown to be a sensitive marker for alveolar soft part sarcoma (**Figure 9.20**).[59] Although sensitive (91–100%) TFE3 is not a specific marker for alveolar soft part sarcoma since other tumors in the histologic differential diagnosis can exhibit TFE3 nuclear expression. They include paraganglioma (75%), adrenocortical carcinoma (33–100%), and granular cell tumor (33–100%) (**Tables 9.6 and 9.7**).[60–64] However, these entities can easily be excluded by using S100 for sustentacular cells in paraganglioma, Melan A for adrenocortical carcinoma, and S100 and Sox10 for granular cell tumor.

Break-apart FISH probes for interrogation of *TFE3* gene rearrangements are available but are agnostic of the *TFE3* fusion partner. PCR and unbiased sequencing-based assays such as anchored multiplex PCR can also be used to document specific *TFE3* fusions. In very rare cases, non-*ASPSCR1* fusion partners of *TFE3* have been described.[65]

Alveolar soft part sarcoma

- TFE3+
- *TFE3* rearrangement (FISH) and/or *ASPSCR1::TFE3* fusion

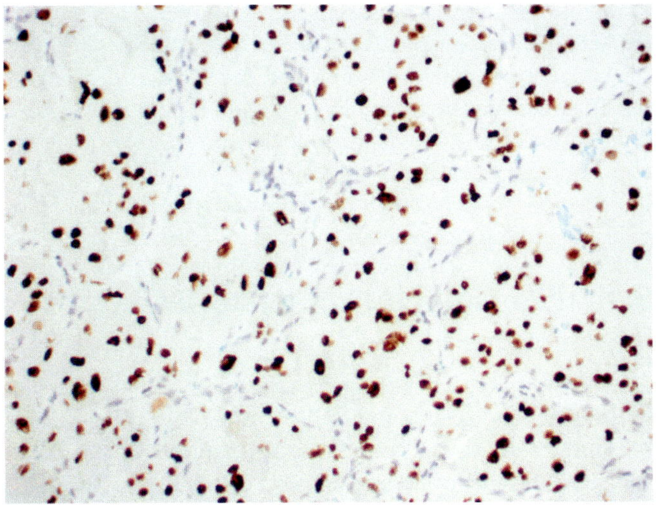

Figure 9.20 Strong nuclear TFE3 expression by the tumor cells (X200).

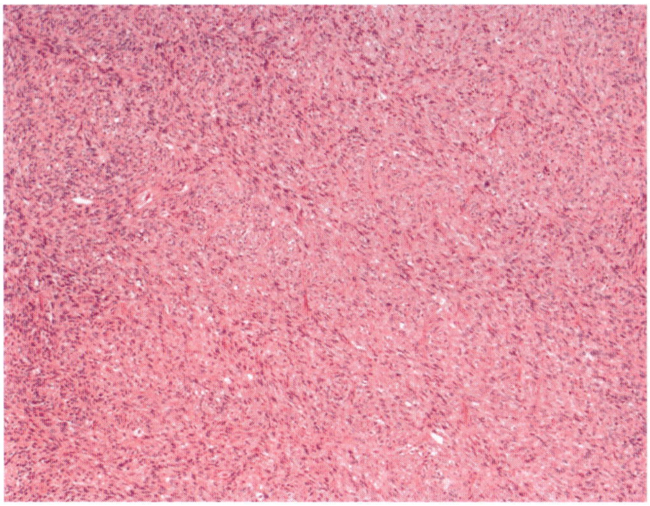

Figure 9.21 Intersecting fascicles of spindle tumor cells in synovial sarcoma (X100).

9.6 Synovial Sarcoma

Synovial sarcoma is an aggressive spindle cell neoplasm with a pathognomonic t(X;18)(p11;q11) translocation resulting in *SS18::SSX* fusion. Two types of neoplastic cells can be seen in synovial sarcoma: (1) epithelial cells resembling a carcinoma and (2) spindle cells resembling a fibrosarcoma. Depending on the proportion of these two types of cells, synovial sarcoma can be monophasic or biphasic (**Figure 9.21**). In the epithelial component expression of various keratins including keratin 7, 8, 14, 18, 19, and 20 can be seen.[66] Expression of EMA is frequently seen in the poorly differentiated form. Other markers that can be seen include S100 protein, CD99, Bcl2, and calponin.

Although the translocation t(X;18), between *SSX1* or *SSX2* gene on chromosome X to *SYT* gene on chromosome 18, is characteristic for synovial sarcoma; this translocation is not specific for synovial sarcoma and can be detected in malignant peripheral nerve sheath tumor (MPNST).[67] Historically, FISH, RT-PCR, or cytogenetics was the gold standard for detecting the t(X;18) fusion, these tests entail cost and time.

Recently, two rabbit monoclonal antibodies were developed which target either the *SS18::SSX* fusion site (clone E9X9V) or the conserved C-terminus of SSX proteins (clone E5A2C). The breakpoint specific E9X9V antibody is reported to be 95% sensitive and 100% specific for synovial sarcoma, while the SSX C-terminus specific E5A2C antibody demonstrates 100% sensitivity and 96% specificity.[68] When positive, these stains show nuclear staining.[68]

Gene microarray expression profiling studies have identified *TLE1* (Transducin-Like Enhancer of split 1) to be a discriminator for synovial sarcoma from histologic mimics.[69] Several studies have shown that TLE1 to be a sensitive marker for synovial sarcoma (82–100%) (**Figure 9.22**).[69,70] However, its specificity is lower in published studies.[69,70] Other soft tissue tumors that can exhibit TLE1 expression include schwannoma (27–100%), neurofibroma (100%), desmoplastic small round cell tumor (100%), low-grade fibromyxoid sarcoma (33%), Ewing sarcoma (8–40%), and MPNST (2–60%).[70] Given the availability of SS18::SSX and SSX-specific antibodies (**Figure 9.23**), TLE1 immunohistochemistry may play a secondary role.

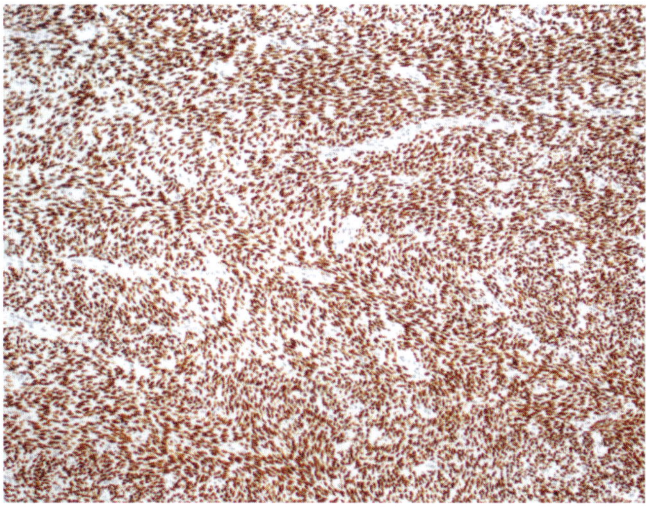

Figure 9.22 Diffuse and strong nuclear TLE1 expression (X200).

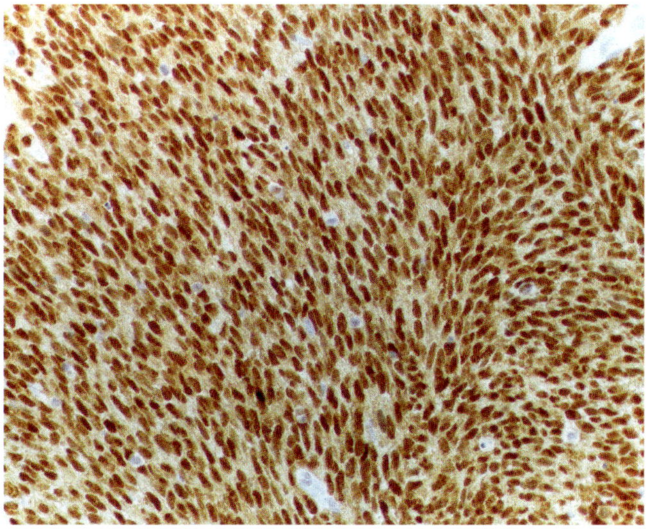

Figure 9.23 Immunohistochemistry for SSX (E5A2C) in synovial sarcoma shows strong positive nuclear staining.

The expression of keratins, especially 7 and 19, distinguishes synovial sarcoma from MPNST which would express neural markers (S100, Sox10) and leiomyosarcoma which would express muscle markers (desmin, SMA).

Synovial sarcoma

- SS18::SSX+ and/or SSX+
- *SS18::SSX*(1/2/4) fusion
- Keratin+ (especially keratins 7 and 19), EMA+, TLE1+

9.7 *NTRK*-Rearranged Spindle Cell Neoplasm

NTRK (neurotrophic tyrosine receptor kinase)-rearranged spindle cell neoplasms are an emerging classification of cutaneous spindle cell neoplasms, unified by the presence of *NTRK* fusions or other activating receptor tyrosine kinase mutations. These tumors are provisionally classified in the 2020 WHO classification of tumors as an emerging entity.[71]

Histologically, *NTRK*-rearranged spindle cell neoplasms exhibit a spectrum of morphologies. The most common appearance, which was historically termed lipofibromatosis-like neural tumor, is comprised of haphazardly oriented spindle cells with infiltrative growth into fat. Other features, such as stromal bands of hyalinized collagen, thin walled "staghorn" vessels, and perivascular hyalinization, can be seen but are not specific.[72,73]

The spindle cells show a variably CD34+ S100+ immunophenotype, with CD34 immunoreactivity reported in 89–92% of cases and S100 immunoreactivity reported in 64–100% of cases.[72,73] However, these are not required for the diagnosis. Demonstration of activating receptor tyrosine kinase fusion is considered an essential diagnostic criterium and can also guide therapy in cases where tyrosine kinase inhibitors are available. Molecular genetic testing is required for definitive diagnosis.[73] Immunostaining for Pan-TRK has been demonstrated to be a highly sensitive and specific adjunct test for molecular identification of *NTRK* rearrangements.[74] However, as IHC is not 100% sensitive or specific, confirmation with molecular genetic methods may be necessary.

The differential diagnosis for *NTRK*-rearranged spindle cell includes infantile fibrosarcoma, lipofibromatosis, and other spindle cell neoplasms without *NTRK* rearrangements or tyrosine kinase activation. Infantile fibrosarcoma is typically seen in the first year of life and has a characteristic *NTRK* fusion (*ETV6::NTRK3*). Recently, it has been proposed that classic infantile fibrosarcoma with *ETV6::NTRK3* fusion and other pediatric *NTRK*-rearranged neoplasms represent a spectrum of disease.[75]

9.8 Hemosiderotic Fibrolipomatous Tumor

Hemosiderotic fibrolipomatous tumor is a locally aggressive, non-metastasizing neoplasm of adipose tissue, spindled cells, and background chronic inflammation and hemosiderin. Hemosiderotic fibrolipomatous tumor has a strong predisposition to the distal lower extremity and is most commonly seen in females.[76] CD34 and calponin expression is typically seen in the spindle cell component.

While not essential for diagnosis, t(1;10)(p22;q24), *MGEA5*, or *TGFBR3* rearrangements can be seen in many cases of hemosiderotic fibrolipomatous tumor and can support the diagnosis. This rearrangement involves *TGFBR3* (1p22) and *MGEA5* (10q24) and has been documented in up to 86% of cases.[77] However, this rearrangement is uniquely not thought to result in a fusion transcript but leads to transcriptional upregulation of nearby proto-oncogenes.[77]

9.9 Pleomorphic Hyalinizing Angiectatic Tumor

Like hemosiderotic fibrolipomatous tumor, pleomorphic hyalinizing angiectatic tumor is a rare, locally aggressive, non-metastasizing neoplasm. It is also typically found in the subcutaneous tissue of the distal lower extremities, with affinity for the ankle and dorsal foot. On histology, pleomorphic hyalinizing angiectatic tumors consist of ectatic, thin-walled vessels with a fibrin-like hyaline lining and surrounding paucicellular stroma with embedded spindle cells. Pleomorphic hyalinizing angiectatic tumor and hemosiderotic fibrolipomatous tumor are classified separately in the 2020 WHO, however, tumors with areas of hemosiderotic fibrolipomatous tumor and pleomorphic hyalinizing angiectatic tumor comingling are frequently seen.

The same t(1;10)(p22;q24) involving *MGEA5* and *TGFBR3* which are described in hemosiderotic fibrolipomatous tumor are seen in pleomorphic hyalinizing angiectatic tumor. The clinical, histologic, and molecular overlap suggests that hemosiderotic fibrolipomatous tumor and pleomorphic hyalinizing angiectatic tumor are a spectrum of the same entity.[78,79]

Histiocytic and Dendritic Cell Neoplasms

The entities covered in this category are diverse clonal hematopoietics disorders derived from the monocytes, macrophages, and dendritic cells. They are termed "histiocytosis" and classified into five groups (**Table 9.8**).[80] In the 2022 World Health Organization classification of hematolymphoid neoplasms, tumors of histiocytic origin include Erdheim-Chester disease (ECD), Rosai-Dorfman disease (RDD) and histiocytic sarcoma and dendritic

Table 9.8 Histiocytic and dendritic cell neoplasms in the 2022 World Health Organization classification

L (Langerhans) group	Langerhans cell histiocytosis Indeterminate cell histiocytosis Erdheim-Chester disease Mixed Langerhans cell histiocytosis/ Erdheim Chester disease
C (Cutaneous and mucocutaneous) group	Cutaneous non-LCH Juvenile xanthogranuloma Benign cepthalic histiocytosis Cutaneous non-LCH with a systemic component
R (Rosai Dorfman disease) group	Rosai Dorfman disease
M group	Malignant histiocytoses
H group	Hemophagocytic lymphohistiocytosis Primary Secondary Malignancy associated

cell tumors include Langerhans cell histiocytosis (LCH), follicular dendritic cell sarcoma, and interdigitating dendritic cell sarcoma (**Table 9.8**).[81] LCH, histiocytic sarcoma and interdigitating dendritic cell sarcoma are thought to derive from bone marrow precursors; while follicular dendritic cell sarcoma and indeterminate dendritic cell sarcoma are thought to derive from stromal mesenchymal cells.[81] Despite their similar histopathologic appearance, tumors of histiocytic and dendritic cell origin have different immunoprofile (**Table 9.9**) and biologic behavior.

These histiocytic neoplasms can co-exist with one another. These mixed histiocytic neoplasms can be ECD/LCH, ECD/RDD, RDD/LCH, and ECD/RDD/LCH.[82] The underlying molecular alterations of these disorders involve the mitogen activated protein kinase (MAPK) signaling pathway. The association of LCH and ECD is linked to BRAFV600E mutation.[83] These common molecular alterations might account for the existence of mixed histiocytic neoplasms.

9.10 Langerhans Cell Neoplasms

Langerhans Cell Histiocytosis and Congenital Self-Healing Reticulohistiocytosis

Langerhans cell histiocytosis (LCH) is a clonal proliferation of Langerin (CD207)-positive Langerhans cells, antigen presenting cells located within the epidermis and dermis.[81] Although with similar histopathological appearance, the LCH lesions range from solitary to multiple and from spontaneous regression to aggressive biological course requiring chemotherapy.[81] The disease can be either single-system or multisystem. Multisystem LCH typically affects neonates and infants and involves bone, liver, spleen, and other organs in addition to skin. The solitary and self-limiting form of LCH is known as congenital self-healing reticulohistiocytosis (**see Case study 1**).[84]

The histology is characterized by oval cells with reniform nuclei (with nuclear groove) admixed with a variable number of eosinophils (**Figure 9.24**). The tumor cells are positive for CD1a and Langerin (CD207) (**Figure 9.25**), specific markers for Langerhans cells.[81] S100, CD31, CD45, and CD68 can be positive.[81] Birbeck granule seen on electron microscopy is a diagnostic ultrastructural feature (**Figure 9.26**). *BRAF*V600E mutation has been identified in 50–65% of LCH cases.[85] The main histologic differential diagnosis is the inflammatory CD1a+ dendritic cells with branching histologic appearance.

LCH is likely derived from a bone-marrow-derived myeloid dendritic cell and not from an epidermal Langerhans cell. MAPK pathway is central in LCH pathogenesis and greater than 85% of cases harbor MAPK pathway gene mutations.[86] *BRAF* p.V600E mutation is the most common, followed by *MAPT2K1*. *ARAF* mutation is infrequent. Tumors of adult patients can harbor *ERBB3*, *NRAS*, and *KRAS* mutations.

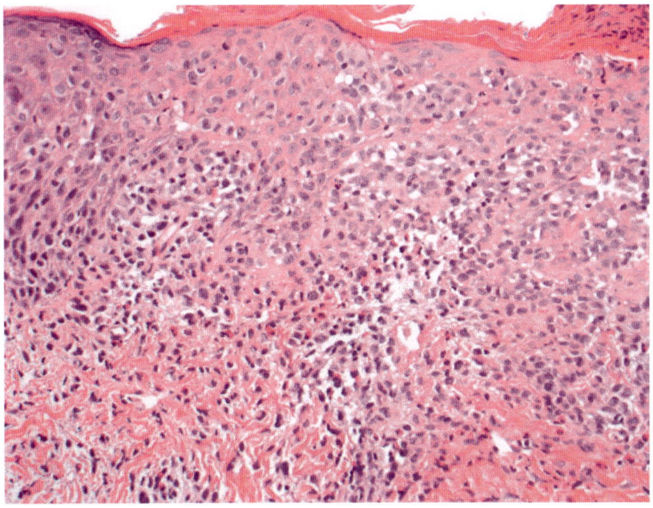

Figure 9.24 Neoplastic cells with abundant cytoplasm and reniform nuclei admixed with a variable number of eosinophils in Langerhans cell histiocytosis (X200).

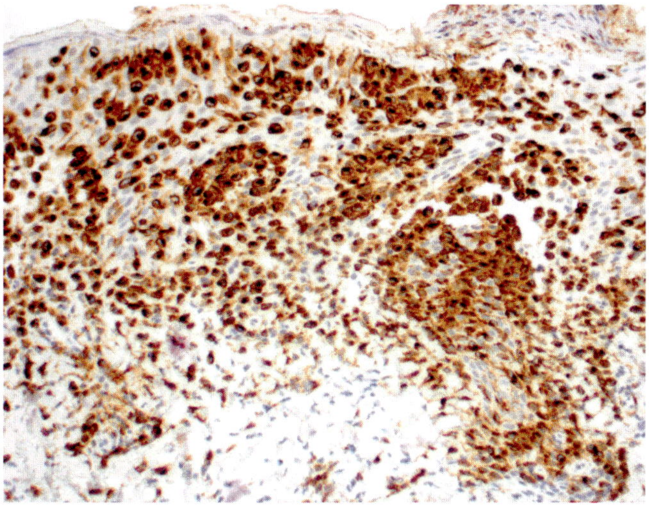

Figure 9.25 Langerin expression by the tumor cells (X200).

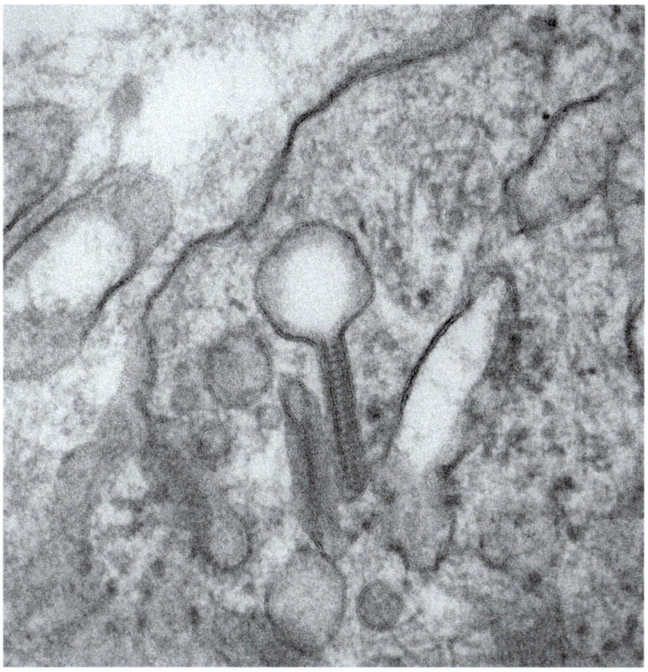

Figure 9.26 A Birbeck granule is seen ultrastructurally (X89,000) (Courtesy of Martin Selig, Electron Microscopy Laboratory, Massachusetts General Hospital, Boston, USA).

Table 9.9 The immunoprofile of tumors of histiocytic and dendritic cell origin

	CD1a	CD4	Braf v600e	CD21	CD23	CD35	CD31	CD43	CD45	CD68	CD163	lysozyme	langerin	S100	fascin	F13a
Langerhans cell histiocytosis	+	+	+	-	-	-	+	+	-/+	+/-	+/-	+/-	+	+	+	-
Langerhans cell sarcoma	+		-/+										+	+		
Erdheim Chester disease	-		+/-							+	+		-	-/+		
Follicular dendritic cell sarcoma	-	+		+	+	+	nd	nd	-	+/-	-	-	-	-/+	+	-
Interdigitating dendritic cell sarcoma	-	+		-	-	-	nd	nd	+/-	+/-	+	+/-	-	+	+	-
Indeterminate dendritic cell tumor	+	+	-	-	-	-	nd	nd	-	-/+	-	-/+	-	+	+	-
Histiocytic sarcoma	-	+/-		-	-	-	nd	+	+	+	+	+	-	+/-	nd	-
Rosai Dorfman disease	-									+	+		-	+		
Benign cephalic histiocytosis	-	nd		nd	nd	nd	nd	nd	nd	+	nd	nd	nd	-	nd	+
Progressive mucinous histiocytosis	-	nd		nd	nd	nd	+	nd	nd	+	nd	nd	nd	-	nd	-
Xanthogranuloma	nd	nd		nd	nd	nd	nd	nd	+	+	nd	nd	nd	-/+	nd	-
Reticulohistiocytoma	nd	nd		nd	nd	nd	nd	-	+	+	+	nd	nd	-/+	nd	-
Intralymphatic histiocytosis	nd	nd		nd	nd	nd	nd	nd	nd	+	nd	nd	nd	nd	nd	-

nd: not documented, F13: factor 13a

Langerhans cell histiocytosis

- CD1a+, langerin+, BRAFV600e+
- S100+, CD68+, CD31+, CD45+

Langerhans Cell Sarcoma

Langerhans cell sarcoma (LCS) is a malignant neoplasm of Langerhans cell origin, affecting mainly adults and slightly more male than female. It may originate *de novo* (primary LCS) or via progression of a low-grade LCH precursor (secondary LCS). Secondary LCS may also develop as trans-differentiation of other hematolymphoid neoplasms including chronic lymphocytic leukemia[87] and follicular lymphoma.[88] Most cases affect skin, lung, bone, and soft tissue.[81]

LCS is characterized by large, atypical cells with a Langerhans cell immunophenotype (CD1a+, S100+, Langerin+). Expression of CD68, cyclin D1, HLA-DR, and vimentin can be seen. The non-specific histology renders immunophenotypic confirmation essential when distinguishing LCS from malignant histiocytic neoplasms such as histiocytic sarcoma. Ultrastructural examination via electron microscopy can demonstrate Birbeck granules, which are rod-shaped inclusions associated with expression of Langerin and specific to Langerhans cells (**Figure 9.26**).[89]

MAPK pathway mutations, including mutations in *KRAS*, have been described in 90% of LCS. By contrast, the *BRAF*V600E mutation commonly observed in LCH has been reported only in a small subset (10%) of LCS.[90]

Langerhans cell sarcoma

- CD1a+, langerin+, S100+, CD68+, BRAFV600E-/+

9.11 Histiocytic Neoplasms

Histiocytic Sarcoma

Histiocytic sarcoma is a rare and aggressive non-Langerhans histiocytic disorder that commonly presents as solitary lesions in the skin, soft tissue, gastrointestinal tract, and central nervous system. Multifocal or systemic disease can also be seen.[91] Some histiocytic sarcoma can co-occur or precede lymphoid neoplasms including chronic lymphocytic leukemia/small lymphocytic lymphoma, B- and T-lymphoblastic leukemia/lymphoma, and follicular lymphoma.[92]

On histologic sections histiocytic sarcoma is a diffuse proliferation of large, atypical cells with pleomorphic nuclei and abundant eosinophilic cytoplasm. Due to morphologic overlap with other histiocytic or large cell neoplasms, immunohistochemistry is essential for diagnosing histiocytic sarcoma. The cells are positive for CD163, CD68, CD43, lysozyme, and PU.1.[87,93] Negative staining for CD1a and Langerin distinguishes histiocytic sarcoma from LCS, while negative staining for CD21 and CD35 distinguishes histiocytic sarcoma from follicular dendritic cell sarcoma.[91] There is variable expression with CD45, CD4 and S100.[93] ALK staining is negative in histiocytic sarcoma.

Mutations in the MAPK signaling pathway are frequent including *KRAS*, *NRAS*, *BRAF*, *MAP2K1*, *PTPN11*, *NF1*, and *CBL*. Mutations of *CDKN2A* and *TP53*, tumor suppressor genes, are also common.

Histiocytic sarcoma

- CD68+, CD163+, CD43+, lysozyme+, PU.1+
- CD1a-, langerin-, ALK-, CD21-, CD35-

Erdheim-Chester Disease

First described by William Chester in 1930, Erdheim-Chester disease is a rare, clonal non-Langerhans cells histiocytosis that most frequently involves bone (~95% of cases), followed by extra-skeletal (50–60%)[94] and cutaneous (25%) sites.[95–96] Somatic *BRAF* mutations have recently been identified in 54% of cases. Common features include bone sclerosis, orbital infiltration with proptosis, diabetes insipidus, cardiac involvement, and pulmonary infiltration.[81] Cutaneous manifestations, commonly xanthelasma (periorbital fatty deposits) and xanthomas (fatty deposits elsewhere in the body), can be seen in 30% of the patients. These lesions are indistinguishable from juvenile xanthogranuloma clinically and histopathologically.

Erdheim-Chester disease is characterized by tissue infiltrates of foamy histiocytes with varying amounts of intermixed Touton-type giant cells, plasma cells, and neutrophils (**Figure 9.27**) which can be indistinguishable from xanthogranuloma. Erdheim-Chester disease expresses histiocytic markers CD163, CD68 (**Figure 9.28**), CD4, and CD14; and is negative for CD1a and langerin.[94] Focal S100 positivity can be observed.

Erdheim-Chester disease

- CD68+, CD163+, CD4+, BRAFV600E +/-, S100-/+
- CD1a- and langerin-

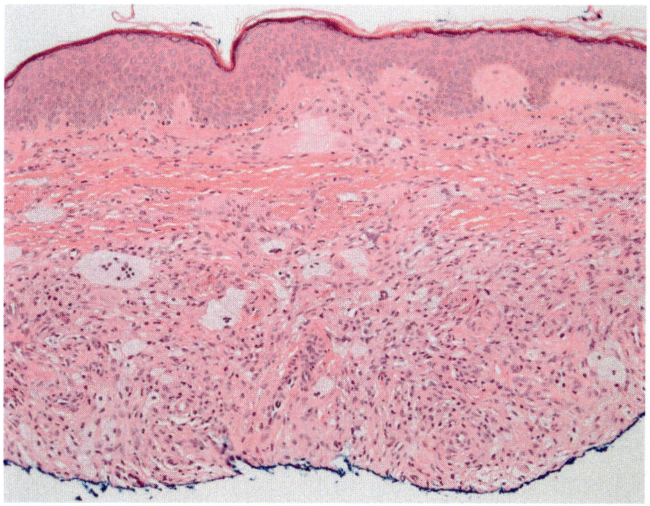

Figure 9.27 A dermal infiltrate of histiocytes with foamy cytoplasm is seen (X200).

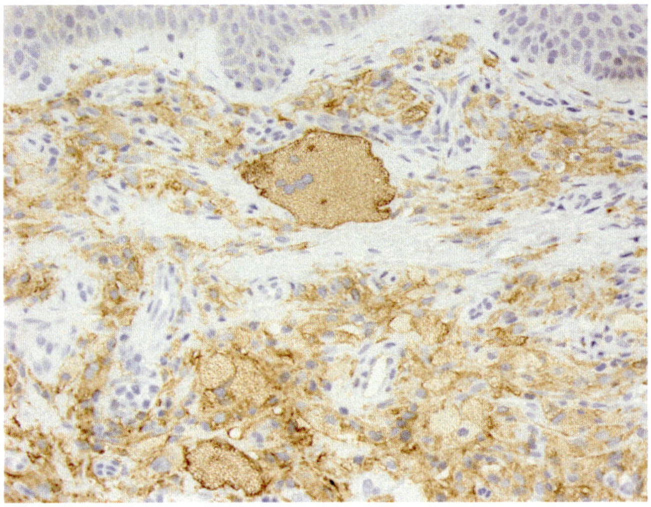

Figure 9.28 CD163 highlights the tumor cells (X400).

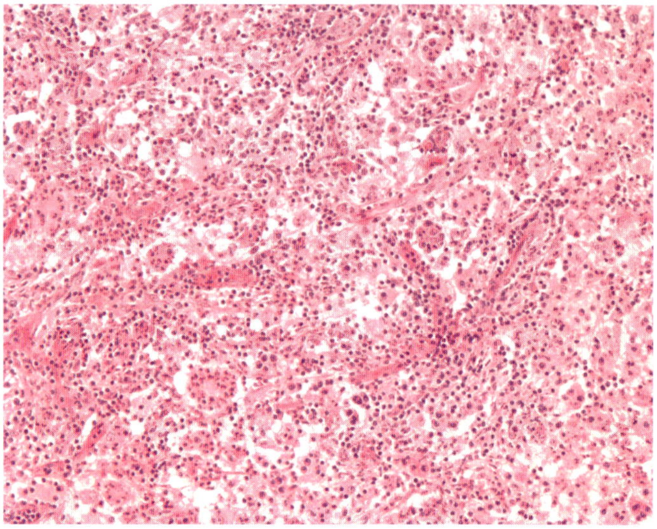

Figure 9.29 Rosai-Dorfman disease is characterized by large histiocytes exhibiting emperipolesis (X200).

Rosai-Dorfman Disease

First reported in 1969 by Rosai and Dorfman, sinus histiocytosis with massive lymphadenopathy is a rare benign lymphoproliferative process affecting mainly children and young adults. Bilateral neck lymphadenopathy together with fever and weight loss are the typical clinical presenting symptoms. It is usually a nodal disease but extranodal sites can be involved (~43%) including the skin, soft tissue, eyes, upper respiratory tract, eyes, brain, and bone.[97] The disease can be localized as one or multiple lesions, disseminated, and with or without systemic involvement.[97] Cutaneous Rosai-Dorfman disease most frequently presented as erythematous nodules on the face (38%).[98] Associated diseases include familial, neoplasia-associated, immune-related, and IgG4 related. Associated hematological malignancies can be seen in 7% of cases. [98]

Infection has been implicated in the etiology of Rosai-Dorfman disease including human herpes virus 6,[99] parvovirus B19,[100] and polyomavirus antigen,[101] cytomegalovirus (CMV), Epstein-Barr virus (EBV), and human immunodeficiency virus (HIV).[102]

It is characterized by S100+, CD68+, CD163+, CD1a-, and Langerin- histiocytes.[103] The large histiocytes exhibiting emperipolesis has been shown to be S100+ CD31+ (**Figures 9.29 and 9.30**).[104] Oct2 expression has been documented in 97% of cases.[105]

Although *BRAF* p.V600E mutation is rare, genetic alterations affecting *MAP2K1*, *KRAS*, *NRAS*, and *ARAF* can be seen in 10–30% of Rosai-Dorfman disease cases.[106] The *KRAS* and *MAP2K1* mutations in Rosai-Dorfman disease are mutually exclusive.[107]

Rosai-Dorfman disease

- S100+, CD68+, CD163+, Oct2+
- CD1a- and langerin-

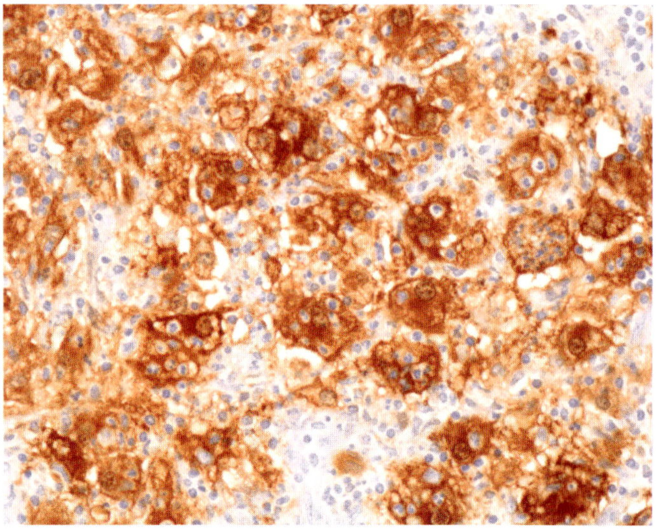

Figure 9.30 S100 highlights the histiocytes while the intracytoplasmic inflammatory cells are negative (X200).

ALK-Positive Histiocytosis

ALK-positive histiocytosis is a histiocytic neoplasm of unknown cellular origin, which clinically and histologically resembles other neoplasms in the juvenile xanthogranuloma (JXG) family. The tumors may be localized or multifocal and can be seen across a broad age range. Systemic presentation can rarely be seen.[108] Histologically, the lesions consist of histiocytes, lymphocytes, and occasional plasma cells (**Figure 9.31**). Scattered Touton giant cells may be present. Foamy changes can be seen within histiocytes, especially with chronicity.[108] By definition the lesional histiocytes are positive for ALK by immunohistochemistry (**Figure 9.32**).[108–110] *ALK* rearrangements can also be detected by FISH or by sequencing techniques. *KIF5B*::*ALK* fusion is most frequently observed, and isolated cases with *CLTC*::*ALK*, *TPM3*::*ALK*, *TFG*::*ALK*, *EML4*::*ALK*, *DCTN1*::*ALK*, and *TRIM33*::*ALK* fusions.[108,110] The tumor responses to ALK inhibition.[110] However, but molecular

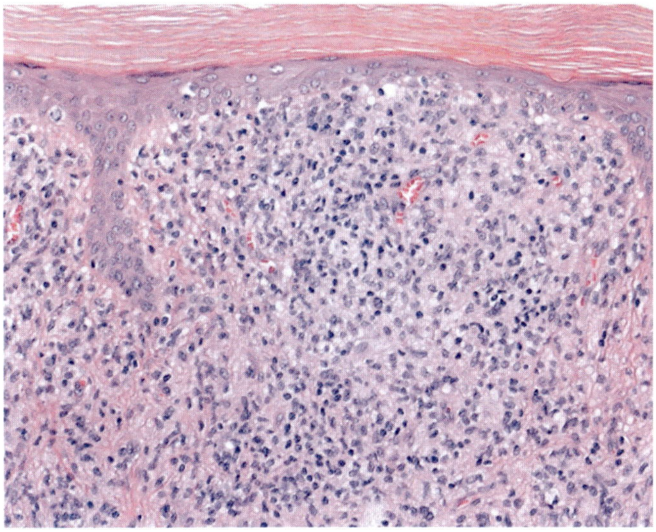

Figure 9.31 ALK-positive histiocytosis is characterized by a dense dermal proliferation of epithelioid to ovoid histiocytes with foamy and vacuolated cytoplasm (X200).

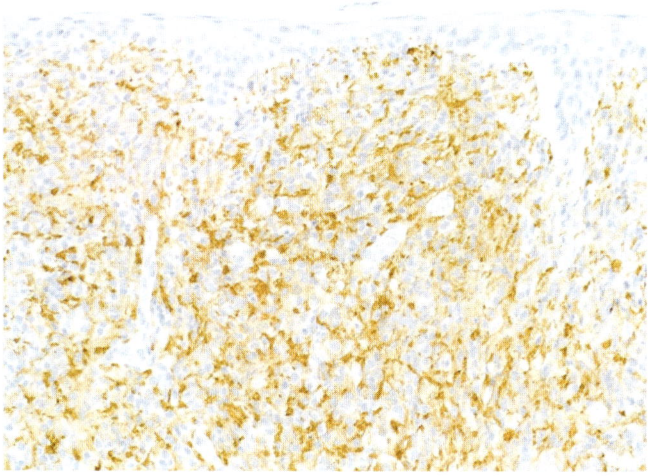

Figure 9.32 ALK immunohistochemistry (ALK1 clone, C-terminal epitope) shows positive staining (X200).

demonstration of a translocation is not an essential diagnostic feature. Histiocytic markers CD68 and CD163 are positive. Negative staining for Langerin (CD207), CD1a, and BRAF V600E are useful in excluding LCH. Of interest, a case of malakoplakia was reported to express ALK aberrantly.[111]

ALK-positive histiocytosis

- ALK+, CD68+, CD163+
- BRAFV600E-, S100-, CD1a-, and langerin-
- Associated with recurrent *KIF5B::ALK* fusion

Benign Cephalic Histiocytosis

Benign cephalic histiocytosis is a rare non-Langerhans cell histiocytosis that typically present as multiple small, yellow to brown, asymptomatic papules on the head and neck region of children. Proximal extremities and trunk can be involved.[112] It is limited to cutaneous sites and self-resolving.[112] On histologic section one would see a well-demarcated infiltrate of histiocytic cells admixed with eosinophils in the superficial to mid dermis (**Figure 9.33**). These histiocytes are positive for CD68 (**Figure 9.34**), Factor 13a, and fascin; and negative for CD1a, langerin and S100.[113]

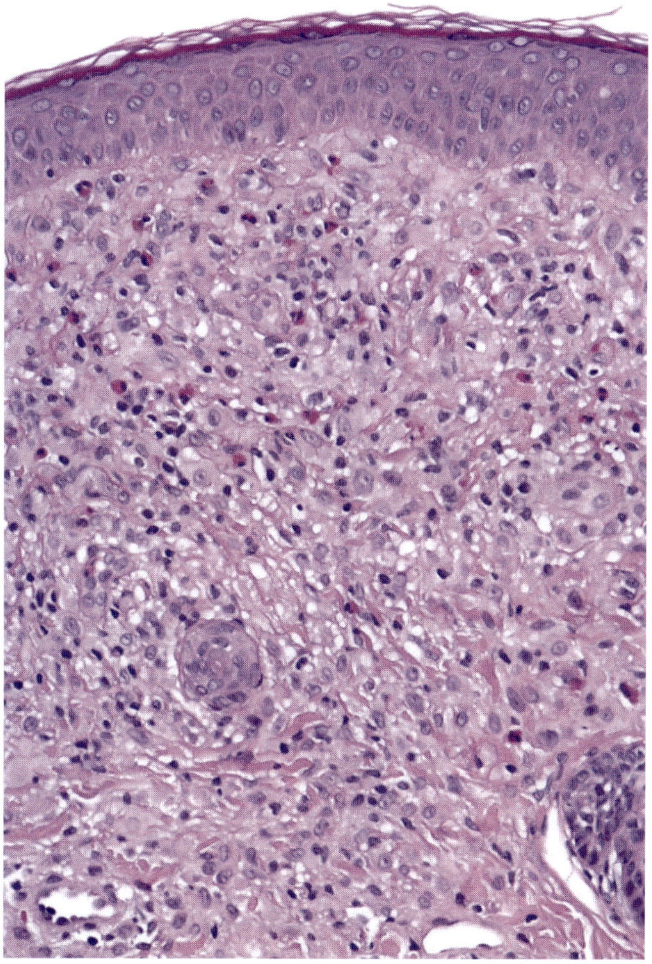

Figure 9.33 Benign cephalic histiocytosis is characterized by an infiltrate of histiocytic cells admixed with eosinophils in the superficial to mid dermis (X200).

Progressive Mucinous Histiocytosis

First reported by Bork and Hoede in 1988, there have been approximately 18 hereditary cases and 5 sporadic cases of progressive mucinous histiocytosis described in the literature.[114] The disease appears to affect mainly women and is inherited in an autosomal dominant fashion.[115] Red brown to skin colored papules are seen on the head and neck and extremities. A well demarcated infiltrate of histiocytes is seen in the dermis and associated with abundant dermal mucin (**Figure 9.35**). The tumor cells are positive for CD68 (**Figure 9.36**) and lysozyme; and negative for S100, CD1a, CD34, and Factor 13a.[114,115] Due to the presence of prominent dermal mucin deposition, the differential diagnosis would include papular mucinosis, scleromyxedema, granuloma annulare, and eruptive dermatofibroma. Clinical pathologic correlation is necessary to arrive at the correct diagnosis.

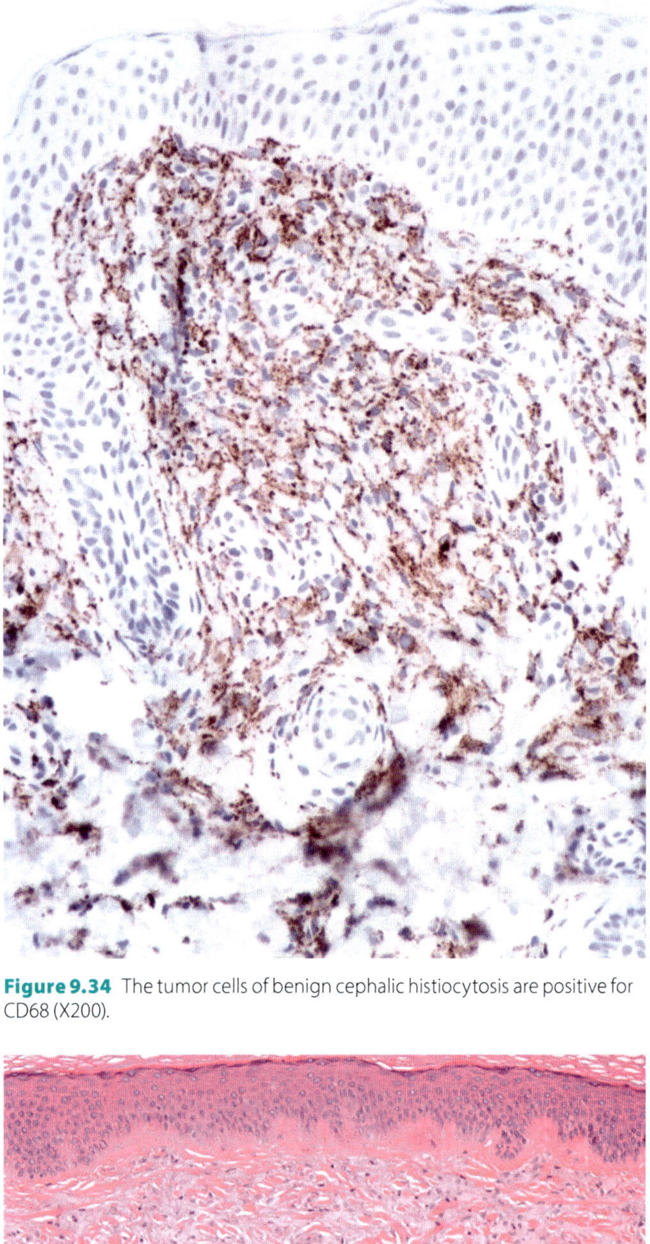

Figure 9.34 The tumor cells of benign cephalic histiocytosis are positive for CD68 (X200).

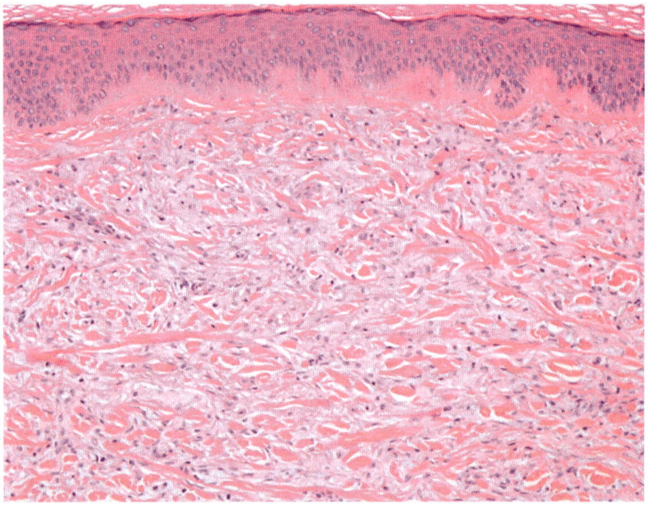

Figure 9.35 Progressive mucinous histiocytosis. An infiltrate of histiocytes with associated abundant mucin is seen in the dermis (X200).

Xanthogranuloma

In a series of 547 juvenile xanthogranuloma (JXG) lesions in 525 patients by Salari and Dehner,[116] the median age of the patients was 4.5 years, and head and neck region were affected in 41% of

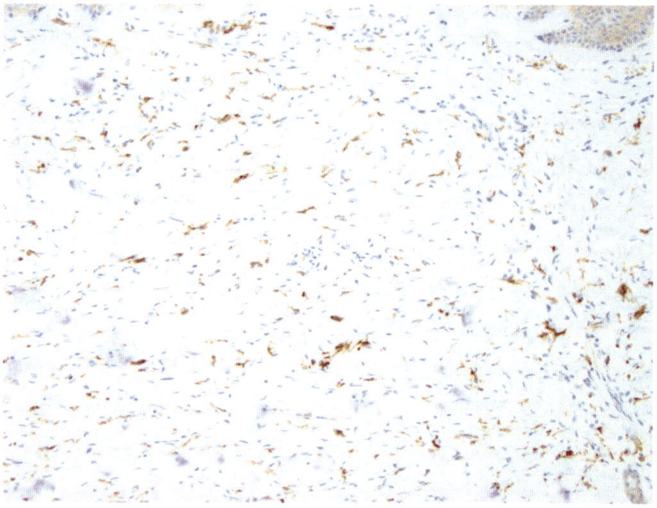

Figure 9.36 The tumor cells are positive for CD68 (X200).

cases. Cutaneous lesions were seen in 77% of cases. Cutaneous congenital JXG are often larger than 3cm.[117] They present as exophytic tumors, infiltrative plaques, agminated plaques, and subcutaneous tumors. They may spontaneously regress, and their clinical course is similar to that of JXG of infancy or childhood.[117] Systemic involvement can occur in 2–3% of cases with 35% presented at birth and 71% diagnosed within the first year of life.[118,119] In a meta-analysis of 159 patients with systemic JXG, the central nervous system, liver, lung, and eye are the commonly involved sites in descending order.[120]

The lesional cells of xanthogranuloma or JXG express factor 13a (94%), CD4 (97.6%), CD68 (99.5%), CD163 (100%), CD1a (0.9%), S100 (31.6%), and CD31 (71.4%) **(Figures 9.37 and 9.38)**.[116] They are negative for smooth muscle actin, CD1a, CD3, and CD34.[121] NTRK expression can be seen in xanthogranuloma, but S100 expression is usually negative in comparison to *NTRK*-rearranged spindle cell neoplasm.[121] PU.1 nuclear staining has been reported to be helpful in labeling histiocytosis in contrast to histiocyte-rich tumors.[123]

Xanthogranuloma

- Factor 13a+, CD4+, CD68+, CD163+, CD31+/-
- CD1a-, S100-

Reticulohistiocytoma

Reticulohistiocytoma can be either solitary or multicentric. The rare multicentric form is characterized by a generalized eruption of papulonodular lesions together with destructive arthropathy which can precede, develop concurrently, or follow the cutaneous eruption.[124] There is a predilection for female and Caucasian. Multicentric reticulohistiocytosis can be associated with underlying malignancy, systemic vasculitis, tuberculosis, diabetes mellitus, Sjogren syndrome, hypothyroidism, Wegener granulomatosis, lupus erythematosus and others.[124] Mucocutaneous nodules with predominant hand involvement were noted for the multicentric form.[124] Currently there are no diagnostic laboratory tests and treatment guidelines.

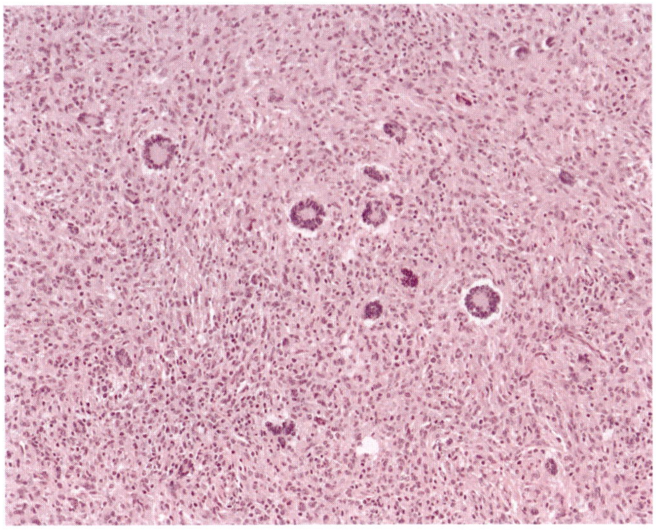

Figure 9.37 A nodular infiltrate of polygonal histiocytes, some with foamy cytoplasm (Touton giant cells), is seen in juvenile xanthogranuloma (X200).

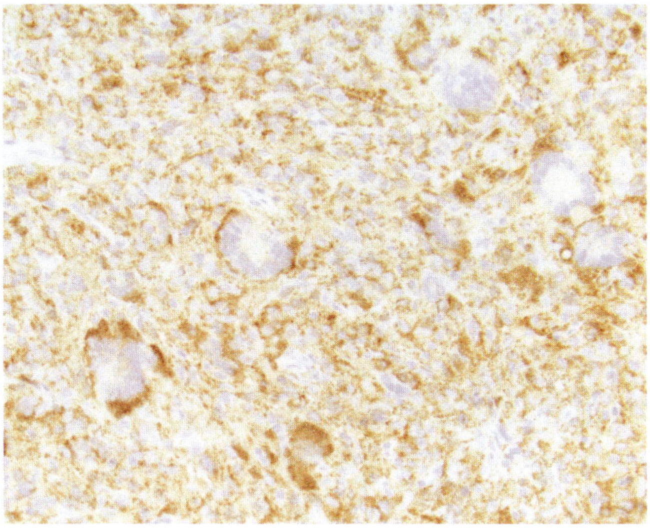

Figure 9.38 Strong CD163 expression by the tumor cells (X400).

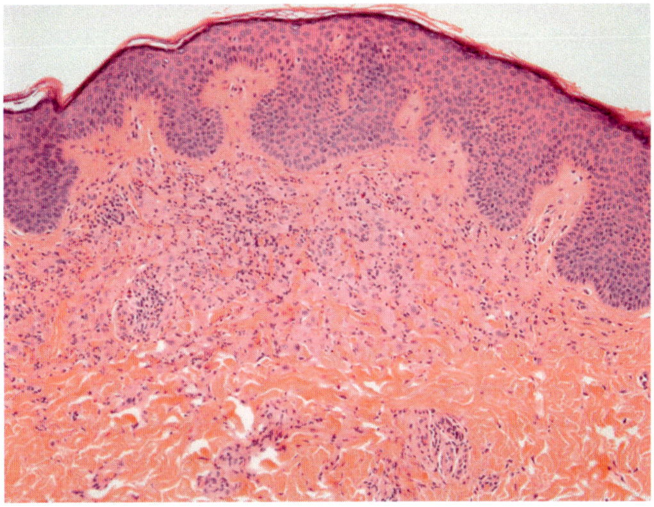

Figure 9.39 A proliferation of oncocytic histiocytes with "ground-glass" appearance is seen in the dermis in reticulohistiocytoma (X100).

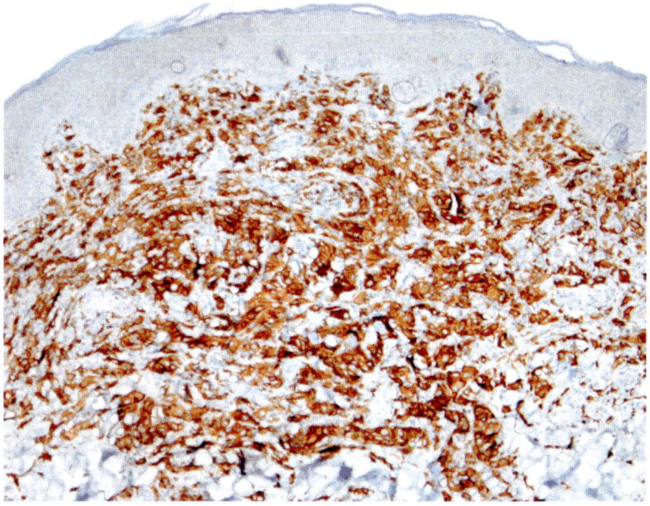

Figure 9.40 The tumor cells are strongly positive for CD163 (X100).

The histology of both forms shows a well-demarcated dermal nodule of large histiocytes with eosinophilic ground-glass cytoplasm (**Figure 9.39**). These histiocytes are positive for CD68, CD163 (**Figure 9.40**) factor 13a, lysozyme, alpha-1-antitrypsin, CD11b, CD14, and CD45; and they are negative for CD1a, CD34, and smooth muscle actin.[125] Although S100 expression as well as CD10 have been reported in some cases, it is typically negative in reticulohistiocytoma.[126]

Reticulohistiocytoma

- CD68+, CD163+, factor 13a+, lysozyme+, S100-/+
- CD1a-, CD34-

Kikuchi-Fujimoto Disease

Kikuchi-Fujimoto disease or histiocytic necrotizing lymphadenitis, first reported in 1972 by two Japanese pathologists Kikuchi and Fujimoto, often present with fever and lymphadenopathy.[127] In a meta-analyses of 244 cases reported in Pubmed over a 14-year period, about half of the cases were from East Asia.[127] Infectious etiologies, autoimmune diseases such as systemic lupus erythematosus, and Still disease have been implicated. DNA viruses including herpes simplex virus type 1 and 1, varicella-zoster virus, cytomegalovirus, Epstein-Barr virus, human herpes viruses 6 and 7, human papillomavirus, and hepatitis B virus have been documented.[128] RNA viruses include dengue virus, rubella virus, paramyxovirus, parainfluenza virus, HIV, and human T-lymphotropic virus type 1.[128] Next generation sequencing (NGS) assay, performed on formalin-fixed paraffin-embedded tissues of 64 patients, revealed detectable infectious agents in 9 cases: 6 bacterial and 3 viral.[128]

The most common extranodal site of involvement is the skin. The histologic sections of the cutaneous lesions often show a lymphohistiocytic infiltrate with karyorrhectic debris in the dermis and sometimes the subcutaneous tissue (**Figure 9.41**). The infiltrate contains CD68+ (**Figure 9.42**), CD163+ and

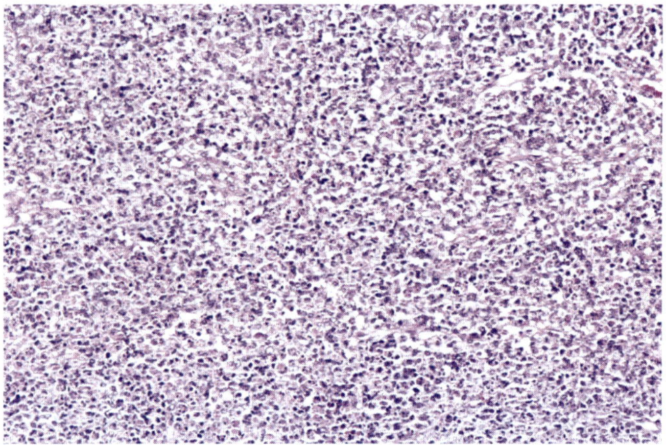

Figure 9.41 A lymphohistiocytic infiltrate with karyorrhectic debris is noted in the dermis in Kikuchi-Fujimoto disease (X100).

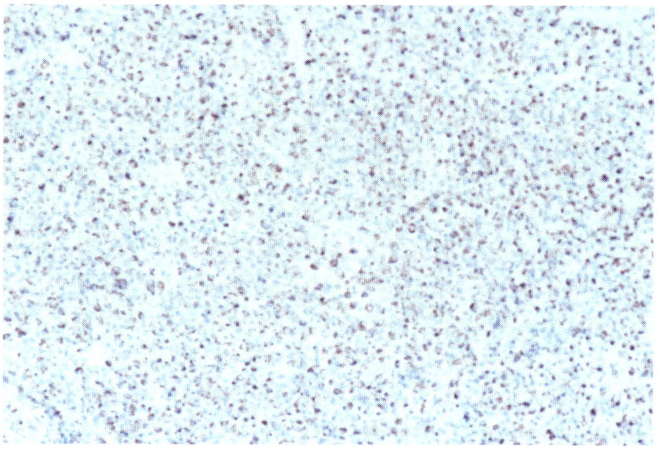

Figure 9.42 CD68 is positive (X200).

myeloperoxidase+ histiocytes, CD123+ plasmacytoid monocytes, and more CD8+ than CD4+ T-cells.[128]

Kikuchi-Fujimoto disease

- CD68+ CD163+

Intralymphatic Histiocytosis

Intralymphatic histiocytosis is a rare and reactive process that can present with or without a disease association. Also reported as "intravascular histiocytosis," "rheumatoid intravascular or intralymphatic histiocytosis of the skin," and "rheumatoid arthritis-associated intravascular histiocytopathy," this condition often occurs in females and with an association with rheumatoid arthritis but can be seen in association with osteoarthritis, joint replacements, metal implants, breast implants, Crohn disease, cellulitis, and various types of malignancies including Merkel cell carcinoma and melanoma.[129] It is characterized histopathologically by aggregates of histiocytes within the lumens of dilated blood vessels mostly lymphatics (**see Case Study 5**). While the vascular channels are positive for CD31, CD34, D2-40, LYVE-1, and Prox-1 confirming their lymphatic nature; the intravascular histiocytic cells are positive for CD68.[130] The main differential diagnosis would include intravascular B-cell lymphoma, intravascular T/NK-cell lymphoma and reactive intravascular CD30+ proliferation (**see Chapter 6**).

9.12 Dendritic Cell Neoplasms

Indeterminate Dendritic Cell Tumor

Indeterminate dendritic cell tumor (IDCT) or indeterminate cell histiocytosis was thought to represent a tumor of "indeterminate dendritic cells." It is a rare cutaneous histiocytic neoplasm which presents as solitary to generalized papules or nodules, on the trunk, extremities, and head and neck region. The clinical presentation is most often localized to skin, most often the scalp and upper extremities, but systemic presentation can be seen in 10% of cases.[131] Bone, spleen, lung, thyroid, parotid, and lymph node can be affected. Approximately 20% of cases are associated with non-Hodgkin lymphomas and acute/chronic myeloid neoplasms.[87]

Histologically, the lesions resemble xanthogranulomas, with a non-destructive dermal infiltrate of mononuclear cells of varying morphologies observed.[131] The cells of IDCT have features of both mononuclear-macrophage differentiation and dendritic cell differentiation, and a relationship has been proposed between the indeterminate cell and Langerhans cell.[132] Immunophenotypically, IDCT express the dendritic cell markers S100+ CD1a+ and the macrophage marker CD68+. Langerin (CD207) is negative, and no Birbeck granules are seen on electron microscopy, differentiating IDCT from LCH/LCS. BRAF V600E is not typically seen in IDCT but rare cases have been reported.[133]

IDCT is thought to arise from an immature Langerhans cell which expresses CD1a but not CD207/Langerin. Molecular analyses revealed a recurrent *ETV3::NCOA2* rearrangement, and *KRAS*, *NRAS*, *MAP2K1*, and *BRAF* mutation in isolated cases.[131]

Indeterminate dendritic cell tumor

- S100+, CD1a+, CD68+
- Langerin-, BRAFV600E-

Interdigitating Dendritic Cell Sarcoma

Follicular dendritic cells present antigens to B-cells while interdigitating dendritic cells present antigens to T-cells.[134] Cutaneous involvement by dendritic cell sarcomas, both follicular and interdigitating, are exceedingly rare. Cutaneous interdigitating dendritic cell sarcomas can be either solitary or diffuse nodules in adults, male more frequently than female.[135] Other sites such as liver, gastrointestinal tract, lung, spleen, parotid gland, bone marrow, soft tissue, and pleura can be involved. Approximately 13% has an association with chronic lymphocytic leukemia/small lymphocytic lymphoma.[87]

Interdigitating dendritic cell sarcomas are comprised of oval to spindle eosinophilic tumor cells forming whorls. They are S100+, fascin+, lysozyme+, beta-catenin+, p75+, CD45+, CD43+, and CD68+/-.[134] They are negative for follicular dendritic cell markers (CD21 and CD35) and Langerhans cell markers (CD1a and langerin). The extremely rare indeterminate dendritic cell sarcoma is CD1a+, CD68+, S100+, CD21-, CD35-, langerin-, CD30-, T- and B-cell markers-. Therefore, langerin is a helpful marker to distinguish interdigitating dendritic cell sarcoma from Langerhans cell histiocytosis. BRAFV600E immunostain can be positive in follicular dendritic cell sarcoma, as well as Langerhans cell histiocytosis, histiocytic sarcoma, disseminated juvenile xanthogranuloma, and Erdheim-Chester disease.

Mutations (*TET2*, *FBXW7*), gene rearrangement (*CBL::USP2*), and mutations of MAPK pathway genes (*BRAF* p.V600E, *KRAS*, *MAP2K1*, and *NRAS*) have been reported.[90]

Interdigitating dendritic cell sarcoma

- S100+ and one or more hematolymphoid (CD4, CD43, CD45) markers
- Negative for Langerhans cells (CD1a, langerin) and follicular dendritic cell (CD21, CD35) markers

9.13 Mast Cell Infiltrate

Mastocytosis is characterized by a clonal expansion of mast cells. In the WHO classification mastocytosis is classified as a myeloproliferative neoplasm and there are two variants, cutaneous and systemic mastocytosis.[81] Cutaneous mastocytosis is typically seen in children and subdivided into urticarial pigmentosa, diffuse cutaneous mastocytosis, and mastocytoma. The mast cell infiltrate is subtle in the adult form of cutaneous mastocytosis, telangiectasia macularis eruptive perstans. The frequency of systemic involvement is higher in adults than in children. On histologic sections the infiltrate ranges from aggregates of spindle shaped mast cells around dermal blood vessels to nodular infiltrate in mastocytoma (**Figure 9.43**). Systemic mastocytosis is characterized by extracutaneous involvement mainly the bone marrow.[81] The major diagnostic criterion for systemic mastocytosis is the presence of aggregate of at least 15 mast cells in extracutaneous tissues. The minor criteria include spindle shaped cells in >25% of the infiltrate and aberrant expression of CD25/CD2.[81]

Both benign and neoplastic mast cells express CD33, CD43, CD68, CD117 (**Figure 9.44**), and tryptase. They are negative for CD14, CD15, and myeloperoxidase. Tryptase is the most specific stain for mast cells while CD117 is most sensitive but not specific due to its expression in myeloblasts/early promyelocytes, erythroid progenitor cells, and melanocytes.[136] Neoplastic mast cells often express CD25 which is thought to be predictive of systemic disease and sometimes CD2 and CD4.[137,138] Strong CD30 expression has been reported in aggressive subtypes of systemic mastocytosis.[139]

Mast cell infiltrate

- Tryptase+, CD117+, CD2+, CD25+, CD3-, CD5-, CD7-
- A panel of tryptase, CD117, CD2, and CD25 for workup of systemic mastocytosis
- Both cutaneous and systemic mastocytosis may express CD4

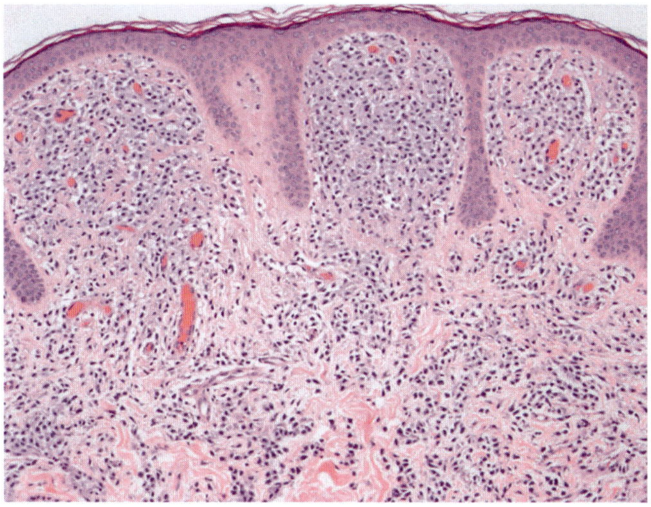

Figure 9.43 Mastocytosis. A dense infiltrate of mast cells is seen within the superficial dermis (X200).

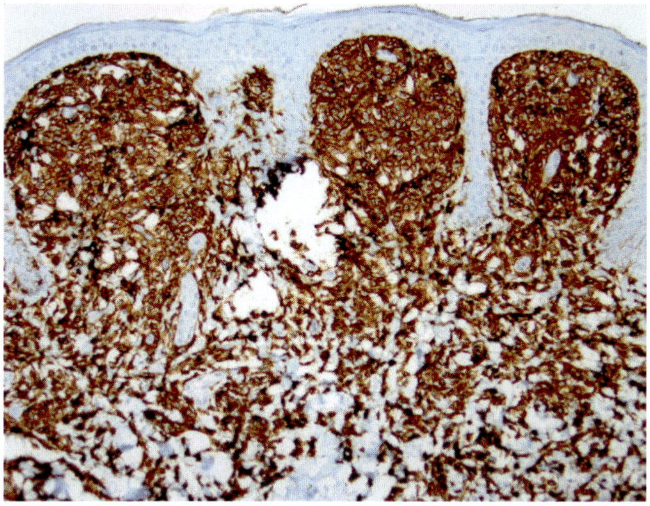

Figure 9.44 Mastocytosis. The neoplastic mast cells are strongly positive for CD117 (X200).

9.14 Cutaneous Involvement by Myeloid Neoplasm or Myeloid Sarcoma

The skin may be involved by mature or immature myeloid neoplasms, which may be infiltrative or tumor-forming in nature. Cutaneous involvement by a leukemic infiltrate is also termed leukemia cutis.[140] Myeloid neoplasms with maturation and without tumor formation include cutaneous involvement by chronic myelogenous leukemia (CMML), myelodysplastic syndrome (MDS), and myelodysplastic/myeloproliferative neoplasm (MDS/MPN). Infiltrative myeloid neoplasms without maturation (or >20% blasts) are best classified as cutaneous involvement by acute myelogenous leukemia (AML). Tumor forming myeloid neoplasms which destroy surrounding tissue architecture are best classified as myeloid sarcomas (**Table 9.10**).

Myeloid sarcoma is seen in up to 9% of patients with AML and can present before, during or after development of bone marrow leukemia.[141,142] Typically, myeloid sarcoma represents an aggressive presentation of AML.[143] However, myeloid sarcoma can also arise from patients with other myeloid neoplasms including

Table 9.10 Cutaneous involvement by myeloid sarcoma

Immunophenotype | Architecture	Infiltrative	Tumor-forming
Mature	Cutaneous involvement by myelodysplastic syndrome, myeloproliferative neoplasm, myelodysplastic/myeloproliferative neoplasm	Myeloid sarcoma
Immature/>20% Blasts	Cutaneous involvement by acute myelogenous leukemia	Myeloid sarcoma

Table 9.11 Summary of various hematolymphoid markers[144,145,147–150]

Line of differentiation	Supportive markers
Broad myeloid expression	CD13, CD33, CD43, CD68, myeloperoxidase
Immature granulocytic	CD34, CD117
Immature monocytic/monoblastic	CD11b, CD11c, CD15, CD64, CD117, lysozyme
Mature monocytic	CD14, CD68, CD163
Megakaryocytic	CD61
Erythroid	CD71, glycophorin A

MDS, MPN, or MDS/MPN including CMML. Occasionally, the cutaneous presentation is the first sign of the disease known as "aleukemic leukemia cutis." Clinically, cutaneous myeloid neoplasms present as papules or nodules. For myeloid sarcomas, gross pathological examination reveals a "fish-flesh" cut surface.

In myeloid neoplasms without architectural effacement of the skin, an interstitial infiltrate of atypical hematolymphoid cells is seen in the dermis and sometimes the subcutaneous tissue (**Figure 9.45**). The infiltrate consists of a variable combination of blasts admixed with hematolymphoid cells with myelomonocytic or monocytic differentiation.[151]

The immunophenotype of infiltrative or tumor-forming cutaneous myeloid neoplasms is dependent on the specific lineage and degree of differentiation. If fresh tissue is available, flow cytometry may be especially helpful due to the combination of many available antibodies, high sensitivity, and single-cell resolution.[144] Myeloid markers typically expressed across the myeloid neoplasms include CD13, CD33, CD43, and CD68.[145] Myeloid neoplasms with monocytic differentiation typically express CD4, CD11b, CD11c, and may express CD14, CD56, CD64, CD163, and lysozyme. Myeloid neoplasms with granulocytic differentiation typically express MPO, CD34, and CD117. Approximately 20–30% of myeloid sarcomas show aberrant cytoplasmic staining for NPM1, which is a surrogate marker for *NPM1* mutation.[146]

Because myeloid sarcoma is equivalent to a diagnosis of AML and AMLs are molecularly defined, complete cytogenetic and molecular genetic analyses is considered necessary for accurate classification, risk stratification, and treatment.[144,147]

Given their overlapping clinical and morphologic features, immunophenotyping is necessary to differentiate blastic plasmacytoid dendritic cell neoplasm (BPDCN) from myeloid sarcoma. Myeloid sarcomas would be expected to stain with lysozyme and/or myeloperoxidase. By contrast BPDCNs show immunoreactivity for MxA, TCL1, TCF4, TdT, and membranous staining for CD56 and CD123, and no staining for lysozyme or MPO.[148,150]

While MPO and CD33 highlight the myeloid or monocytic precursor cells, CD68 and lysozyme stain the mature histiomonocytic cells (**Figures 9.46 and 9.47**) (**Tables 9.11 and 9.12**).[112–117]

Myeloperoxidase can be seen in cells with monocytic differentiation; whereas CD68 and lysozyme would invariably be positive. In addition, expression of myeloperoxidase and CD34 were seen in 56% and 19%, respectively, in a series of 83 cases of cutaneous myeloid sarcoma.[143] Cutaneous infiltrate in patients

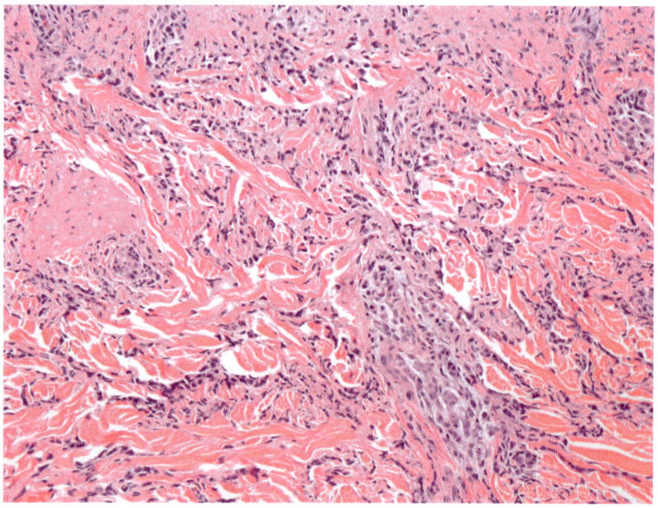

Figure 9.45 An interstitial infiltrate of atypical hematolymphoid cells is seen in the dermis of leukemia cutis (X200).

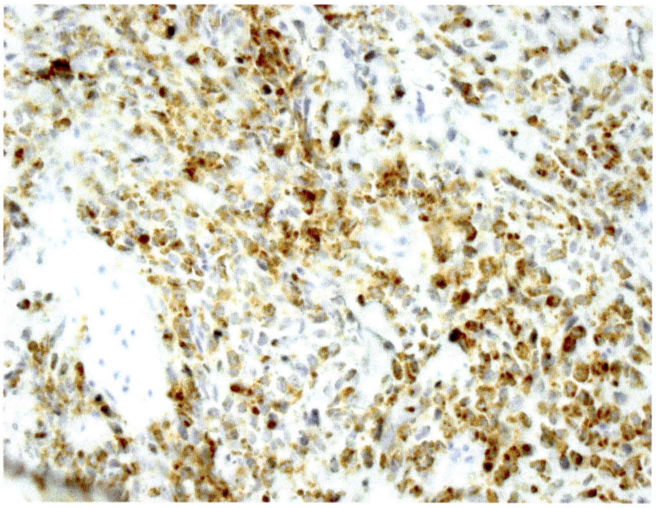

Figure 9.46 Leukemia cutis. The atypical hematolymphoid cells are positive for CD68 (X400).

with myelodysplastic syndrome or myeloproliferative disorders would express CD43, lysozyme, and myeloperoxidase. CD56 expression can frequently be seen and should not be mistaken as a natural-killer cell proliferation.[144,151] While the blasts would be CD34+ or CD117+ in the bone marrow, these markers are often negative in the cutaneous lesions.[151] Correlation with bone marrow findings is helpful in diagnosing leukemia cutis.

Table 9.12 Summary of marker expression in cutaneous leukemic/lymphomatous infiltrate[143, 145, 151–154, 162]

Marker	Myeloid sarcoma or leukemic infiltrate	B-cell lymphoblastic lymphoma	T-cell lymphoblastic lymphoma
CD1a	0%	0%	20–30%
CD3 cytoplasmic	0%	-	100%
CD4	1%	-/+	25–40%
CD8	nd	nd	30%
CD10	3%	92%	40%
CD14	35–60%	+/-	-
CD20	0%	+/-	-
CD33	60–93%	5–8%	15%
CD34	6–43%	70%	37–50%
CD43	97%	69%	97%
CD56	13–47%	-	+/-
CD68	94–100%	-	-
CD79a	10%	91%	8%
CD99	54%	+/-	+/-
CD117	10–80%	+/-	+/-
CD123	0%	31–61%	0%
CD163	25–58%	-	-
Lysozyme	91–100%	-	-
Myeloperoxidase	42–84%	-	-
Pax5	5%	99%	0%
TdT	31%	99%	95%

nd: not documented

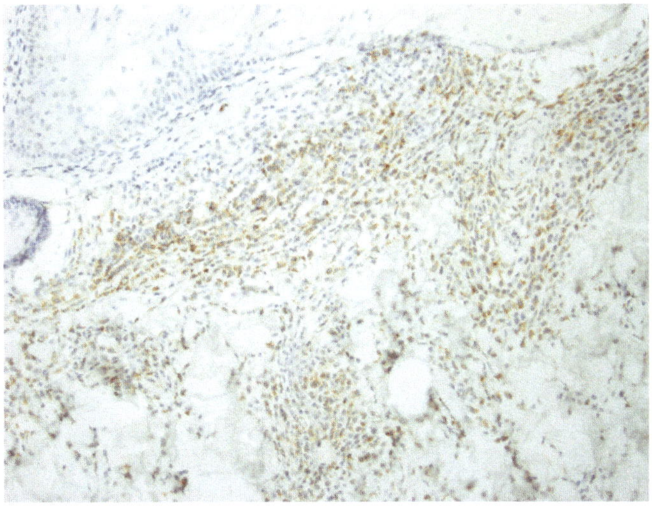

Figure 9.47 Leukemia cutis. They are also positive for myeloperoxidase supportive of myelomonocytic differentiation (X400).

Cutaneous involvement by myeloid neoplasm or myeloid sarcoma

- Immature granulocytic: CD34, CD117
- Immature monocytic/monoblastic: CD11b, CD11c, CD15, CD64, CD117, lysozyme
- Mature monocytic: CD14, CD68, CD163

9.15 Cutaneous Involvement by Lymphoblastic Lymphoma

Lymphoblastic lymphomas are derived from precursor B- or T-cell lymphocytes and possess an aggressive biologic behavior.[152,153] Up to one-third of B-lymphoblastic lymphomas have cutaneous involvement, and cutaneous involvement can be the sole manifestation of the disease especially with the B-cell variant accounting for 3.5–7% of lymphoma cases with cutaneous involvement.[154,155]

Ancillary techniques including flow cytometry and immunohistochemistry are considered essential for diagnosis of cutaneous lymphoblastic lymphoma.[156] The present classification relies on morphology and immunophenotype for broad classification as lymphoblastic lymphoma while specific molecular genetic alterations define subtypes with prognostic and/or therapeutic implications.[156]

On routine histology, a dense infiltrate of monomorphous and medium-sized neoplastic cells is seen in the dermis and subcutaneous tissue. Immunohistochemistry is specific for the lineage of origin and is also dependent on the degree of differentiation of the tumor cells. The tumor cells of B-cell lymphoblastic lymphoma are positive for precursor markers such as TdT, CD10 (common acute lymphoblastic leukemia/lymphoma antigen or CALLA), CD34, and CD99; and B-cell markers such as CD19, CD79a, and PAX5.[118,121] CD20 is typically negative.[157]

The differential diagnosis of B-cell lymphoblastic lymphoma would include mantle cell lymphoma, myelogenous leukemic infiltrate, blastic plasmacytoid dendritic cell neoplasm, Merkel cell carcinoma and metastatic neuroendocrine carcinoma, Ewing sarcoma/PNET, and rhabdomyosarcoma. While positive for B-cell marker, mantle cell lymphoma would express CD5 and cyclin D1 and would be negative for CD10 and TdT. Blastic plasmacytoid dendritic cell neoplasm would express CD4, CD56 and CD123. Neuroendocrine markers such as synaptophysin and chromogranin would be seen in Merkel cell carcinoma and metastatic neuroendocrine carcinoma. B-cell lymphoblastic lymphoma may express CD99 and lack expression of CD20, and this immunophenotypic overlap may result in misdiagnosis as Ewing sarcoma/PNET. In these cases, demonstration of clonal immunoglobulin heavy chain (IgH) rearrangement by PCR can support B-cell origin.[158] Evaluation for expression of myogenic markers such as MyoD1, myogenin, and desmin can be of help in cases where rhabdomyosarcoma is on the differential.

T-cell lymphoblastic lymphoma often present in the mediastinum and lymph nodes, and can have cutaneous involvement in approximately 4.3% of cases.[152,159,160] Rare cases of primary cutaneous cases of T-cell lymphoblastic lymphoma have been reported in children. The histologic pattern can be diffuse or infiltrative in a "single file" pattern of medium-sized neoplastic cells with scant cytoplasm. Lymphoblasts express T cell lineage markers CD3 (surface more commonly than cytosolic), CD5, and CD7.[161] They are invariably positive for TdT, CD1a, and CD117. CD2, CD34, and CD99 can be positive.[152,162] They can express CD79a and CD33 which can pose a diagnostic challenge. T-cell receptor (TCR) beta and TCR gamma gene rearrangements are seen in the majority of T-lymphoblastic leukemias, while a minority of cases may harbor TCR rearrangements together with immunoglobulin heavy chain (IgH) gene rearrangements.[163,164]

Cutaneous involvement by lymphoblastic lymphoma

- B-cell lymphoblastic lymphoma: TdT+, CD79a+, PAX5+, CD20+/-, CD10+, CD34+/-, CD99+/-; Absent surface immunoglobulin light chain expression; subtyping based on specific recurrent genetic abnormalities.
- T-cell lymphoblastic lymphoma: TdT+, CD3+, CD4+, CD8+/-, CD1a+/-, CD34+/-, CD99+/-; TCR gene rearrangement by PCR +/- IgH gene rearrangement by PCR (rare).

9.16 Case Studies

Case 9.1

Clinical history: A female infant was born with a 3mm firm red-brown nodule below her right knee (**Figure 9.48**). There is no evidence of systemic disease.

Description: The skin biopsy shows a dense infiltrate of mononuclear cells in the superficial and mid dermis (**Figure 9.49**). These histiocytic cells have abundant eosinophilic cytoplasm and reniform nuclei. They are strongly positive for S100 (**Figure 9.50**) and CD1a (**Figure 9.51**).

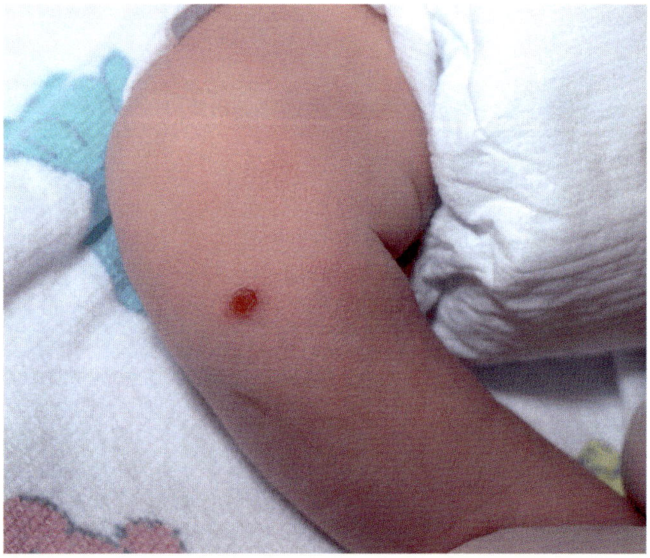

Figure 9.48 A red-brown nodule is noted on the infant's knee.

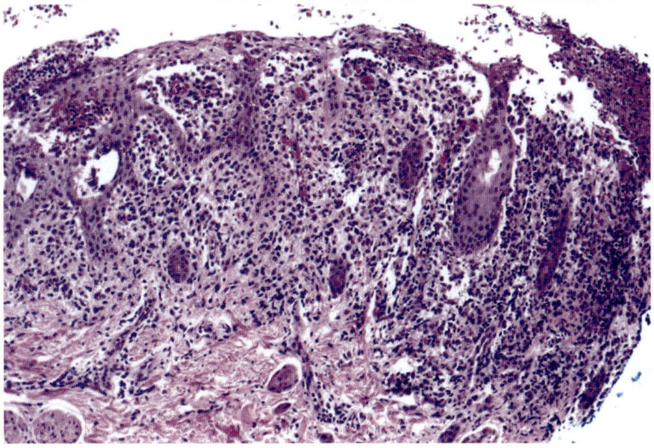

Figure 9.49 A band-like infiltrate of mononuclear cells is seen in the superficial dermis and infiltrate into the overlying epidermis (X100).

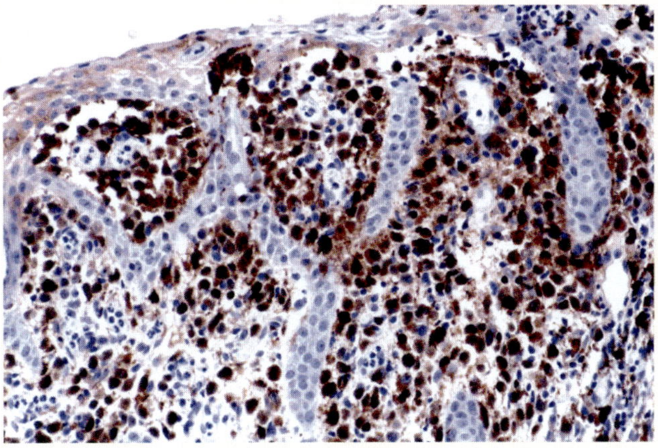

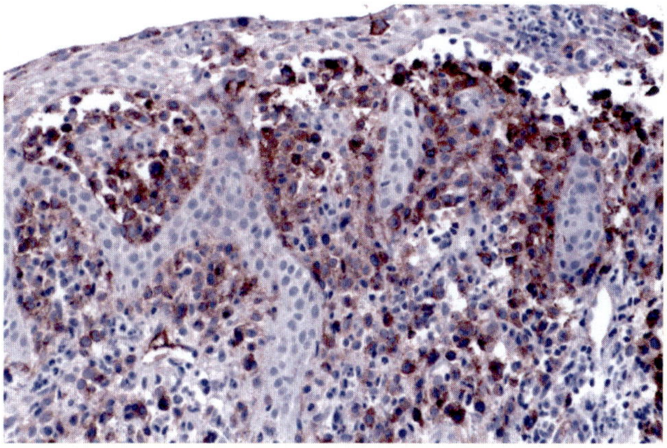

Figures 9.50 and 9.51 The tumor cells are strongly positive for S100 (X200) and CD1a (X200).

Diagnosis: Congenital self-healing reticulohistiocytosis.

Discussion: Congenital self-healing reticulohistiocytosis (CSHR) typically present as a solitary or widespread eruption of cutaneous red-brown nodules at birth or in the initial first weeks of life.[82] CSHR generally follow a benign clinical course with spontaneous regression of lesions without systemic involvement. Currently it is thought that CSHR and LCH represent different ends of a spectrum of the same condition. Long-term follow-up is essential since it is difficult to predict systemic involvement based on clinical and histologic findings. At the ultrastructural level, there appears to be a difference between LCH and CSRH. Although all the tumor cells express CD1a, only 5–25% of the tumor cells of CSRH contain Birbeck granules.[165] Concentrically laminated dense core bodies are seen in the same cells with Birbeck granules.[166] The differential diagnosis would include Langerhans and non-Langerhans histiocytosis. The CD1a expression would exclude the non-Langerhans histiocytoses such as juvenile xanthogranuloma.

Case 9.2

Clinical history: A 64-year-old woman with a history of chronic lymphocytic leukemia/small lymphocytic leukemia presented with a 2-year history of irritated plaques on her face and ears (**Figure 9.52**).

Description: A skin biopsy from her a plaque near her right eyebrow was performed. A dense and nodular infiltrate of small and medium lymphoid cells is noted in the dermis and extends to the subcutaneous tissue (**Figure 9.53**). The tumor cells strongly express CD20 (**Figure 9.54**), CD5 (**Figure 9.55**), LEF1, Bcl2, and focally CD23 (**Figure 9.56**). Ki-67 demonstrates a proliferation index of approximately 15%. CD3 highlights only scattered reactive T-lymphocytes. The tumors cells are negative for CD10, Bcl6, and cyclin D1.

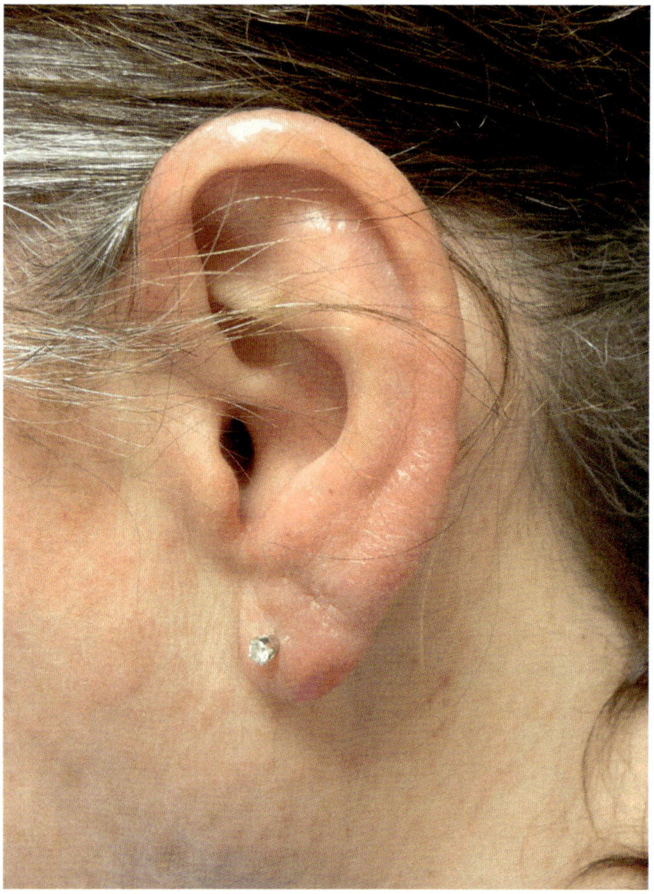

Figure 9.52 Erythematous plaques are seen on the patient's cheek and ear (Courtesy of Steven T. Chen M.D., Department of Dermatology, Massachusetts General Hospital, Boston, Massachusetts, USA).

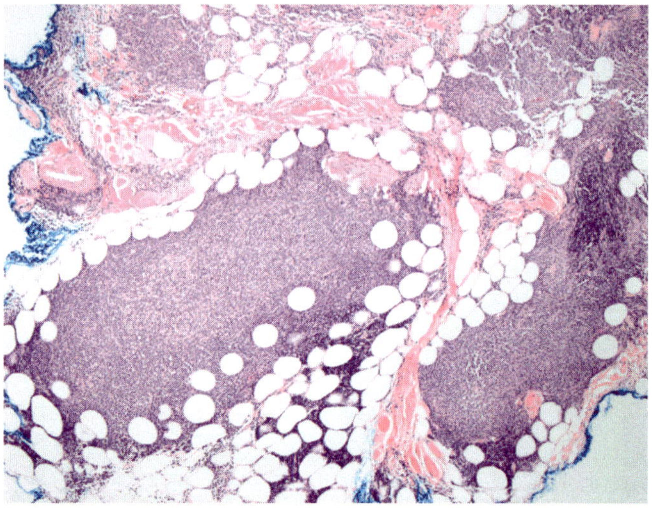

Figure 9.53 Nodules of atypical lymphoid cells are noted in the subcutaneous tissue (X100).

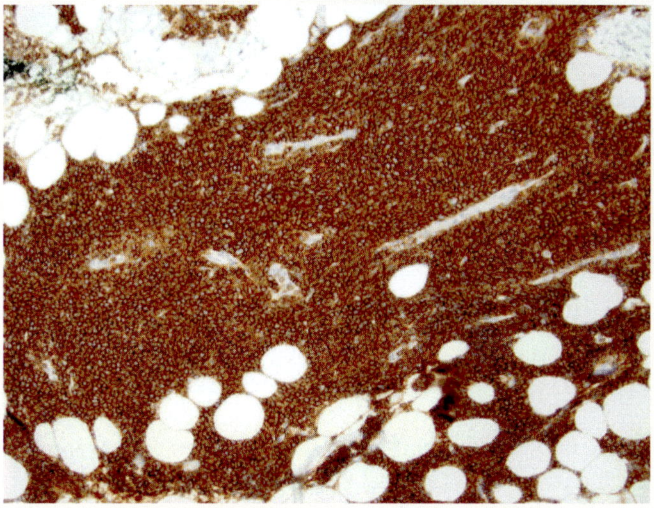

Figure 9.54 The tumor cells are strongly positive for CD20 (X200).

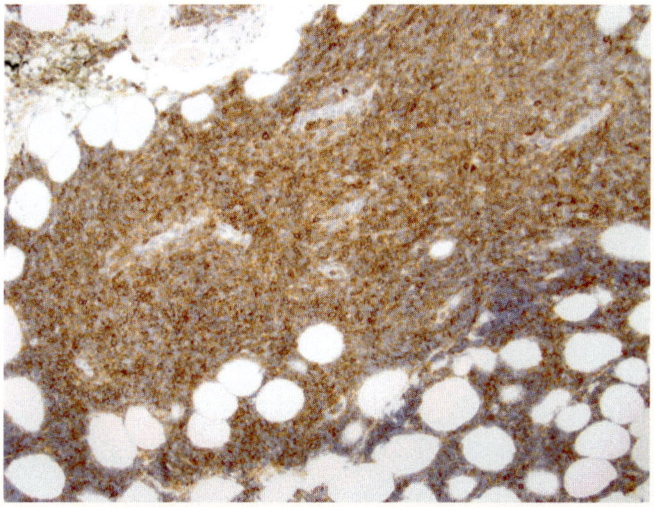

Figure 9.55 They also co-express CD5 (X200).

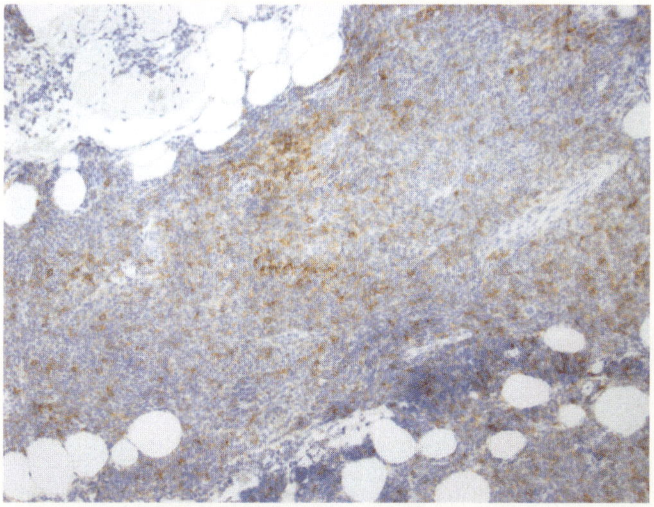

Figure 9.56 Some of the tumor cells express CD23 (X200).

Diagnosis: Cutaneous involvement by chronic lymphocytic leukemia.

Discussion: The co-expression of B-cell markers (CD20, Pax5, and CD79a) and T-cell marker (CD5) is supportive of cutaneous involvement by chronic lymphocytic leukemia/small lymphocytic leukemia. Diffuse and high Ki67 proliferation index is indicative of Richter transformation.[167] Upregulation of LEF1 (lymphocyte-enhancer-binding factor-1), a transcription factor important to the development and proliferation of B- and T-cells, has been reported in CLL by gene expression profiling. Nuclear LEF1 expression has been reported invariably in all B-cells of CLL/SLL (both CD5+ and CD5-) cases and with 92% sensitivity and 70% specificity.[126] Whereas LEF1 expression has not been documented in other small B-cell lymphomas such as mantle cell lymphoma and follicle cell lymphoma.[168]

Case 9.3

Clinical history: A 16-year-old male with a history of acute myelogenous leukemia and recently completed chemotherapy now presented with a new eruption of multiple subcutaneous papules and nodules on trunk and extremities.

Description: A skin biopsy from the patient right forearm showed an infiltrate of atypical hematolymphoid cells in the dermis and subcutaneous tissue (**Figures 9.57 and 9.58**). The tumors were strongly positive for CD56 (**Figure 9.59**) and CD23 (**Figure 9.60**), weakly for CD4, and focally for CD34 (**Figure 9.61**). They were negative for CD3, CD8, CD19, and myeloperoxidase. These findings were similar to those seen in the patient's prior bone marrow biopsy. Flow cytometric analyses performed at the time of initial diagnosis three months ago revealed 73% myeloblasts that are CD33+ CD13+ CD34+ CD14+/- CD11c+ CD64+ CD11b+ CD23+ CD4+ CD56+ myeloperoxidase- CD117- CD10-.

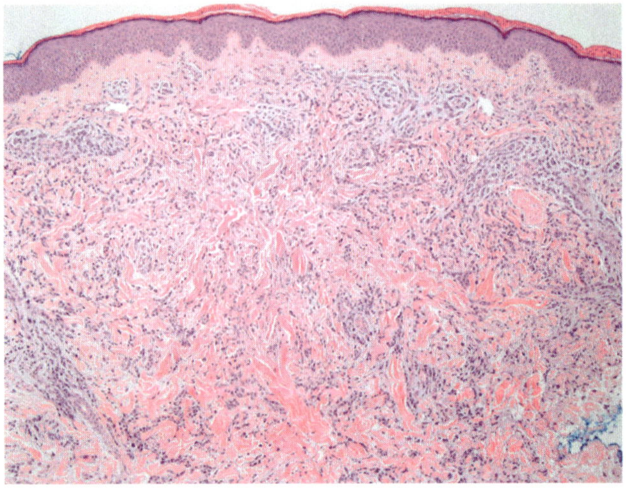

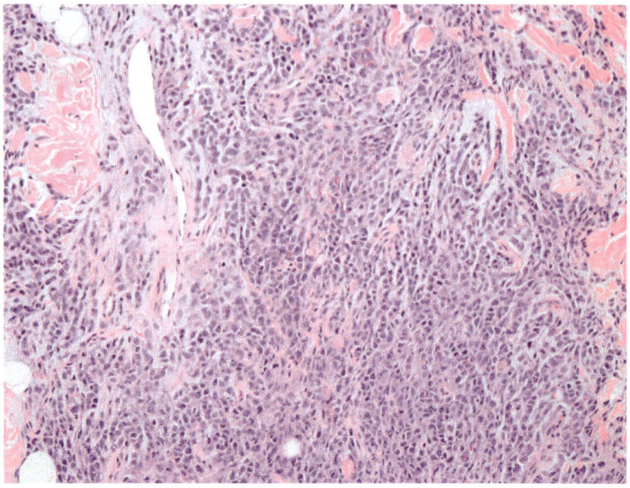

Figures 9.57 and 9.58 Atypical hematolymphoid cells are seen infiltrating the dermis (X100, X200).

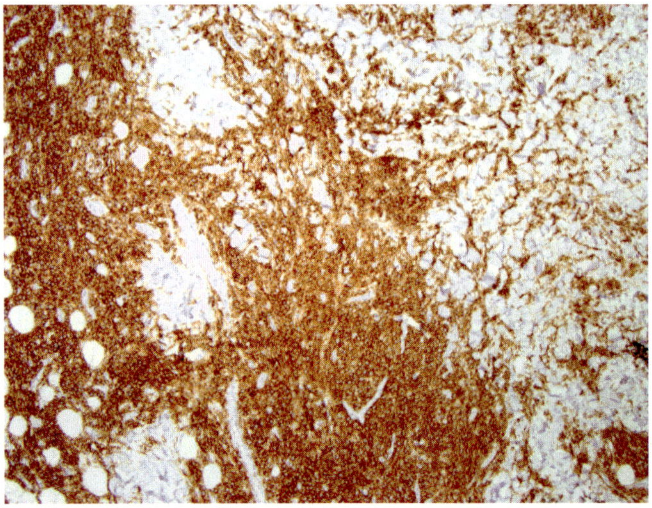

Figure 9.59 The tumor cells strongly express CD56 (X100).

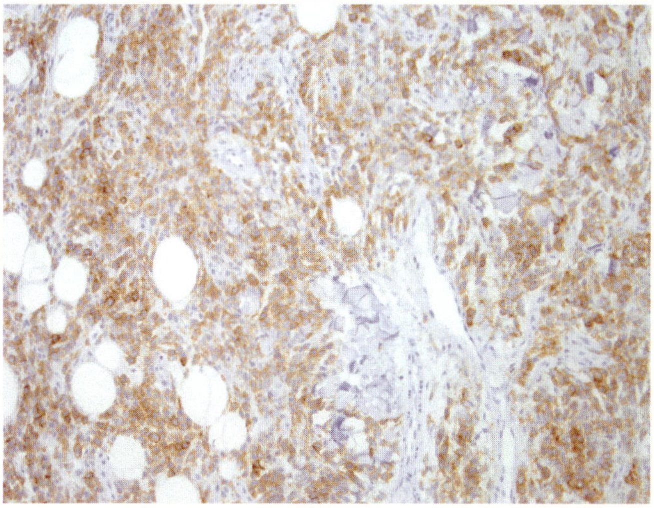

Figure 9.60 They also express CD23 (X400).

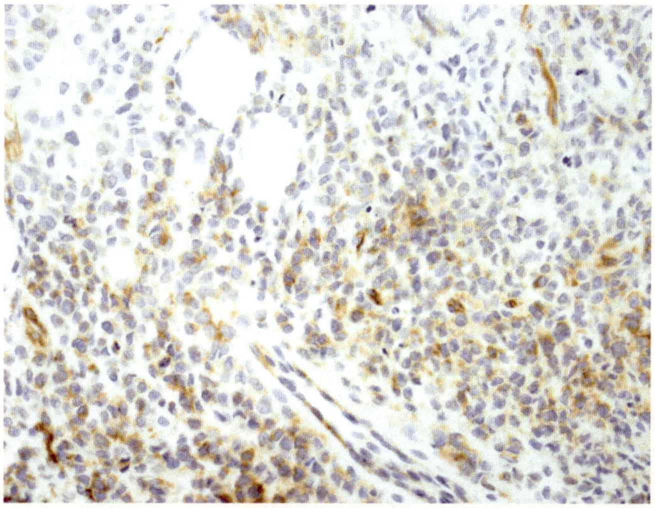

Figure 9.61 The myeloblasts within the infiltrate are CD34 positive (X400).

Diagnosis: Acute myeloid leukemia in dermis with aberrant CD56 expression.

Discussion: CD56 expression can be seen within an atypical hematolymphoid infiltrate and should not be mistaken as a natural-killer cell proliferation.[151] Since variable CD56 and CD4 expression has been reported in myeloid leukemia cases, CD123 would be a helpful stain to distinguish AML from blastic plasmacytoid dendritic cell neoplasm which would express CD4, CD56, and CD123.

Case 9.4

Clinical history: A 56-year-old woman presented with diffuse telangiectatic and erythematous macules on her trunk and extremities.

Description: Beneath an unremarkable epidermis ectatic capillaries are seen within the superficial dermis surrounded by a mild inflammatory infiltrate (**Figure 9.62**). Tryptase immunostain highlights an increased number of spindle mast cells in a perivascular distribution (**Figure 9.63**).

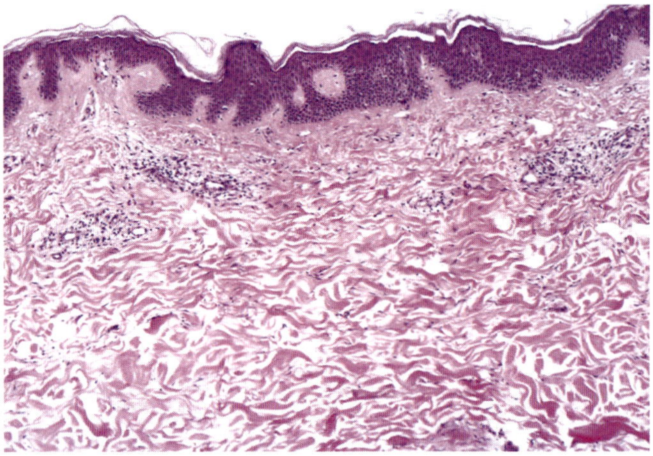

Figure 9.62 Only sparse superficial perivascular inflammatory infiltrate is noted (X100).

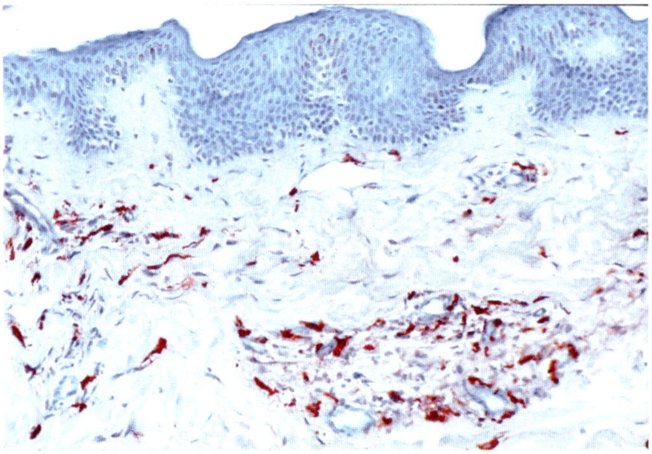

Figure 9.63 Tryptase immunostain highlights an increased number of mast cells around the superficial dermal blood vessels (X200).

Diagnosis: Telangiectasia macularis eruptiva perstans.

Discussion: In the WHO classification cutaneous mastocytosis is subdivided into three variants: urticaria pigmentosa, diffuse cutaneous mastocytosis, and mastocytoma. Urticaria pigmentosa is the most common form and typically presents with widespread red-brown macules and papules. A Darier's sign is characterized by a reddening and whealing reaction caused by mast cells degranulation upon physical stroking of the lesions. Systemic symptoms including diarrhea, wheezing, and syncope can be seen up to 20% of cases.[169]

Diagnostic criteria for cutaneous involvement include a major criterion (typical skin lesion associated with Darier's sign) and two minor criteria (histologically confirmed mast cell infiltrate and an activating *KIT* mutation).[169] Telangiectasia macularis eruptiva perstans accounts for 14% of cutaneous mastocytosis cases and can progress to systemic disease in approximately 50% of cases.[170] Serum tryptase levels are often within normal range. The skin biopsy shows only sparse superficial perivascular infiltrate of dermal mast cells and their presence can be missed without the help of ancillary immunostains such as tryptase and CD117.

Case 9.5

Clinical history: A 73-year-old female with a history of hip replacement 4 years prior presented for full skin examination and an incidental large dusky plaque was discovered on the left buttock. The patient was unaware of its presence.

Description: Sections showed dense superficial and deep neutrophilic and lymphoplasmacytic inflammation and intravascular epithelioid histiocytes (**Figure 9.64**). Vascular markers CD31 and D240 highlighted endothelial cells while CD68 highlighted intraluminal histiocytes (**Figure 9.65**), confirming intralymphatic histiocytic aggregates.

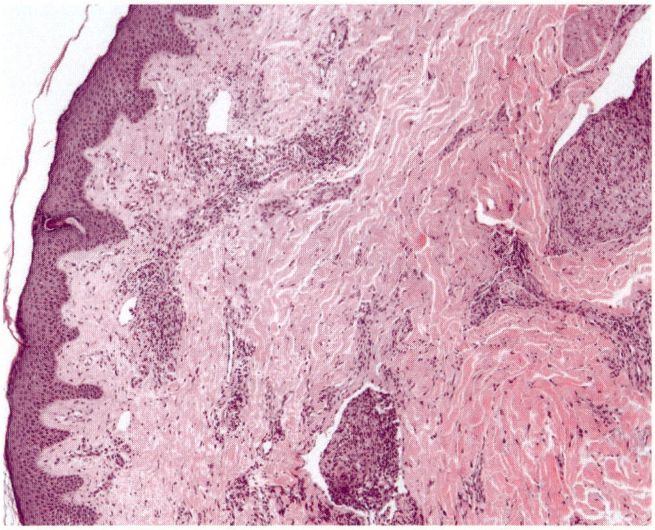

Figure 9.64 Collections of histiocytes are seen within vascular spaces in the dermis (X100).

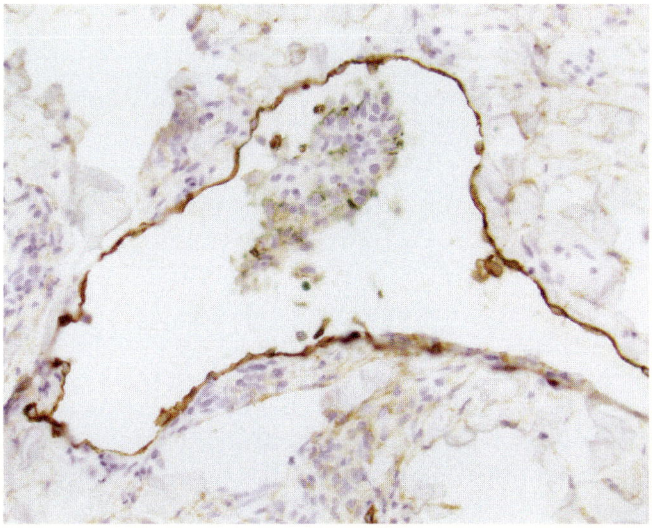

Figure 9.65 D2-40 immunostain demonstrates the vascular space to be lymphatic in nature (X400).

Diagnosis: Intralymphatic histiocytosis.

Discussion: Intralymphatic histiocytosis is a rare disorder manifesting as poorly demarcated erythematous plaques and livedo reticularis-like lesions and typically affecting adult or elderly patients. There is an association with rheumatoid arthritis or prosthetic joint replacement.[130] The histopathologic differential diagnosis includes intravascular lymphoma, leukemia, and inflammatory conditions with accumulation of intralymphatic histiocytes. Intravascular lymphomas can be excluded by lack of immunostaining for B or T cell markers. Benign angioendotheliomatosis may also be considered on the differential diagnosis but the lesional cells would exhibit staining with endothelial markers. While Rosai-Dorfman disease may also show collections of intralymphatic histiocytosis, the absence of emperipolesis and S100 immunostaining would favor intralymphatic histiocytosis.

Case 9.6

Clinical history: A male over the age of 80 presents with a solitary violaceous thin papule on the dorsum of the foot.

Description: A skin biopsy from the dorsal foot showed a dermal-based, bland appearing tumor of spindled to epithelioid cells in a myxoid tumor stroma. The cells show areas of whorled growth and some areas of perineurioma-like growth (**Figure 9.66**). Immunostains for CD34 and S100 were variably positive in the tumor cells. A pan-TRK immunostain highlighted the tumor cells with moderate membranous/cytoplasmic staining (**Figures 9.67 and 9.68**). RNA-based next-generation sequencing demonstrates *PPFIBP1*::*NTRK3* fusion, involving *PPFIBP1* exon 9 and *NTRK3* exon 14 (**Figure 9.69**).

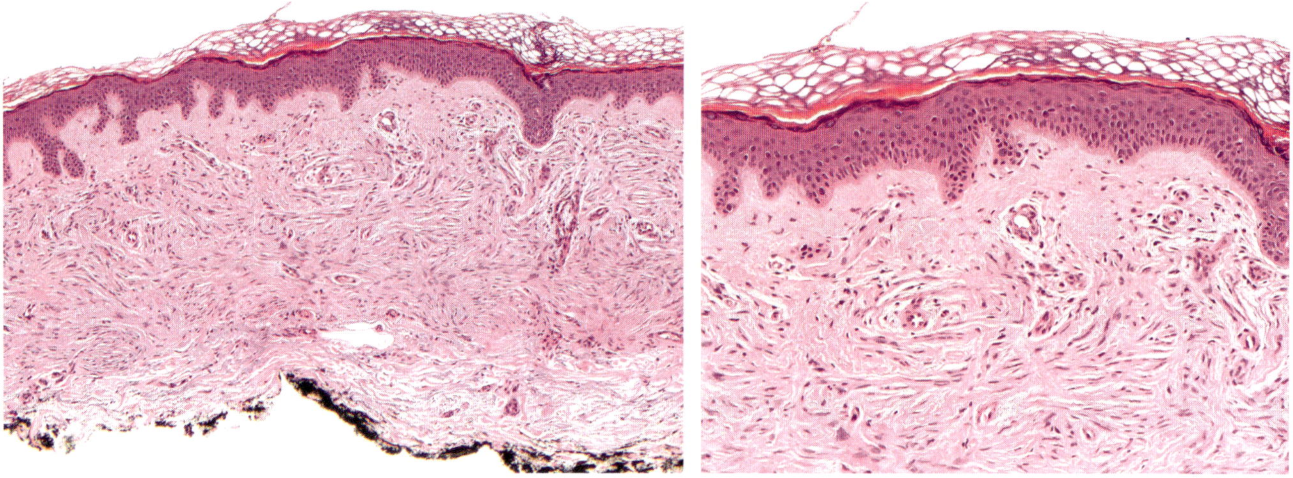

Figures 9.66 and 9.67 A proliferation of slender and spindle cells is seen in the dermis (X100, X200).

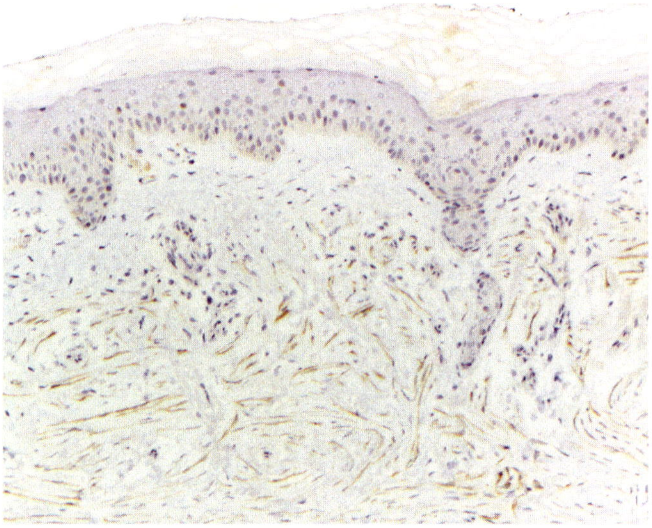

Figure 9.68 pan-TRK immunostain highlights the lesional cells (X200).

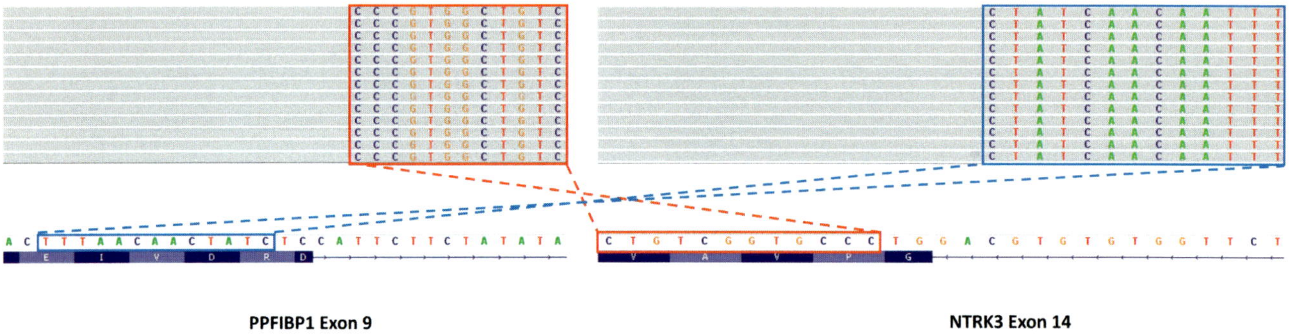

Figure 9.69 *PPFIBP1::NTRK3* fusion (Integrated Genome Viewer).

Diagnosis: *NTRK*-rearranged spindle cell neoplasm.

Discussion: A CD34+ S100+ spindle cell neoplasm with Pan-TRK expression by immunohistochemistry and *NTRK* fusion on molecular testing is most consistent with an *NTRK*-rearranged spindle cell neoplasm. *NTRK*-rearranged spindle cell neoplasms are classified as emerging entity in the 5th edition of the World Health Organization (WHO) Classification of Soft Tissue and Bone Sarcomas. Integration of clinical, histopathologic, and clinical data is needed for establishing the diagnosis. The differential diagnosis includes other tumors potentially harboring *NTRK* rearrangements such as inflammatory myofibroblastic tumor (IMT) and infantile fibrosarcoma.[171] The hypercellular variant of IMT could have spindle cell proliferation but would also show a prominent inflammatory infiltrate of plasma cells, lymphocytes, and eosinophils. Infantile fibrosarcoma typically occurs in patients less than two years of age.

References

1. Feng H, Shuda M, Chang Y, et al. Clonal integration of a polyomavirus in human Merkel cell carcinoma. *Science* 2008; **319**: 1096–100.
2. Ogawa T, Donizy P, Wu CL, et al. Morphologic diversity of Merkel cell carcinoma. *Am J Dermatopathol* 2020; **42**: 629–40.
3. Harms KL, Zhao L, Johnson B, et al. Virus-positive Merkel cell carcinoma is an independent prognostic group with distinct predictive biomarkers. *Clin Cancer Res* 2021; **27**: 2494–504.
4. Kervarrec T, Appenzeller S, Samimi M, et al. Merkel cell polyomavirus-negative Merkel cell carcinoma originating from in situ squamous cell carcinoma: a keratinocytic tumor with neuroendocrine differentiation. *J Invest Dermatol* 2022; **142**: 516–27.
5. Rocamora A, Badia N, Vives R, Carrillo R, Ulloa J, Ledo A. Epidermotropic primary neuroendocrine (Merkel cell) carcinoma of the skin with Pautrier-like microabscesses: report of three cases and review of the literature. *J Am Acad Dermatol* 1987; **16**: 1163–8.
6. Buresh CJ, Oliai BR, Miller RT. Reactivity with TdT in Merkel cell carcinoma: a potential diagnostic pitfall. *Am J Clin Pathol* 2008; **129**: 894–8.
7. Byrd-Gloster AL, Khoor A, Glass LF, et al. Differential expression of thyroid trancription factor 1 in small cell lung carcinoma and Merkel cell tumor. *Hum Pathol* 2000; **31**: 58–62.
8. Dong HY, Liu W, Cohen P, Mahle CE, Zhang W. B-cell specific activation protein encoded by the PAX-5 gene is commonly expressed in merkel cell carcinoma and small cell carcinomas. *Am J Surg Pathol* 2005; **29**: 687–92.
9. Drijkoningen M, de Wolf-Peeters C, van Limbergen E, Desmet V. Merkel cell tumor of the skin: an immunohistochemical study. *Hum Pathol* 1986; **17**: 301–7.
10. Filtenborg-Barnkob BE, Bzorek M. Expression of anaplastic lymphoma kinase in Merkel cell carcinomas. *Hum Pathol* 2013; **44**: 1656–64.
11. He H, Fang W, Liu X, Weiss LM, Chu PG. Frequent expression of glypican-3 in Merkel cell carcinoma: an immunohistochemical study of 55 cases. *Appl Immunohistochem Mol Morphol* 2009; **17**: 40–6.
12. Jensen K, Kohler S, Rouse RV. Cytokeratin staining in Merkel cell carcinoma: an immunohistochemical study of cytokeratins 5/6, 7, 17, and 20. *Appl Immunohistochem Mol Morpphol* 2000; **8**: 310–15.
13. Kolhe R, Reid MD, Lee JR, Cohen C, Ramalingam P. Immunohistochemical expression of PAX5 and TdT by Merkel cell carcinoma and pulmonary small cell carcinoma: a potential diagnostic pitfall but useful discriminatory marker. *Int J Clin Exp Pathol* 2013; **6**: 142–7.
14. Llombart B, Monteagudo C, Lopez-Guerrero JA, et al. Clinicopapthological and immunohistochemical analysis of 20 cases of Merkel cell carcinoma in search of prognostic markers. *Histopathology* 2005; **46**: 622–34.
15. Ly TY, Walsh NM, Pasternak S. The spectrum of Merkel cell polyomavirus expression in Merkel cell carcinoma, in a variety of cutaneous neoplasms, and in neuroendocrine carcinomas from different anatomic sites. *Hum Pathol* 2012; **43**: 557–66.
16. Matsushita M, Nonaka D, Iwasaki T, et al. A new in situ hybridization and immunohistochemistry with a novel antibody to detect small T-antigen expressions of Merkel cell polyomavirus (MCPyV). *Diagn Pathol* 2014; **9**: 65. doi: 10.1186/1746-1596-9-65.
17. McNiff JM, Cowper SE, Lazova R, Subtil A, Glusac EJ. CD56 staining in Merkel cell carcinoma and natural killer-cell lymphoma: magic bullet, diagnostic pitfall, or both? *J Cutan Pathol* 2005; **32**: 541–5.
18. Mhawech-Fauceglia P, Saxena R, Zhang S, et al. Pax-5 immunoexpression in various types of benign and malignant tumours: a high-throughput tissue microarray analysis. *J Clin Pathol* 2007; **60**: 709–14.
19. Paik JY, Hall G, Clarkson A, et al. Immunohistochemistry for Merkel cell polyomavirus is highly specific but not sensitive for the diagnosis of Merkel cell carcinoma in the Australian population. *Hum Pathol* 2011; **42**: 1385–90.
20. Molina-Ruiz AM, Santonja C, Rütten A, Cerroni L, Kutzner H, Requena L. Immunohistochemistry in the diagnosis of cutaneous viral infections- part II: cutaneous viral infections by parvoviruses, poxviruses, paramyxoviridae, picornaviridae, retroviruses and filoviruses. *Am J Dermatopathol* 2015; **37**: 93–106.
21. Rajagopalan A, Browning D, Salama S. CD99 expression in Merkel cell carcinoma: a case series with an unusual paranuclear dot-like staining pattern. *J Cutan Pathol* 2013; **40**: 19–24.
22. Sangoi AR, Cassarino DS. PAX-8 expression in primary and metastatic Merkel cell carcinoma: an immunohistochemical analysis. *Am J Dermatopathol* 2013; **35**: 448–51.
23. Sidiropoulos M, Hanna W, Raphael SJ, Ghorab Z. Expression of TdT in Merkel cell carcinoma and small cell lung carcinoma. *Am J Clin Pathol* 2011; **135**: 831–8.
24. Stetsenko GY, Malekirad J, Paulson KG, et al. p63 expression in Merkel cell carcinoma predicts poorer survival yet may have limited clinical activity. *Am J Clin Pathol* 2013; **140**: 838–44.
25. Su LD, Fullen DR, Lowe L, Uherova P, Schnitzer B, Valdez R. CD117 (kit receptor) expression in Merkel cell carcinoma. *Am J Dermatopathol* 2002; **24**: 289–93.
26. Sur M, AlArdati H, Ross C, Alowami S. TdT expression in Merkel cell carcinoma: potential diagnostic pitfall with blastic hematological malignancies and expanded immunohistochemical analysis. *Mod Pathol* 2007; **20**: 1113–20.
27. McCalmont TH. Paranuclear dots of neurofilament reliably identify Merkel cell carcinoma. *J Cutan Pathol* 2010; **37**: 821–3.
28. Hanly AJ, Elgart GW, Jorda M, Smith J, Nadji M. Analysis of thyroid transcription factor-1 and cytokeratin 20 separates merkel cell carcinoma from small cell carcinoma of lung. *J Cutan Pathol* 2000; **27**: 118–20.
29. Karpinski P, Mendez-Pena JE, Wu C-L, et al. POU4F3 is a sensitive and specific marker of Merkel cell carcinoma. *Modern Pathol* 2025; **38**: 100627. doi: 10.1016/j.modpat.2024.100627.
30. Calder KB, Coplowitz S, Schlauder S, Morgan MB. A case series and immunophenotypic analysis of CK20-/CK7+ primary neuroendocrine carcinoma of the skin. *J Cutan Pathol* 2007; **34**: 918–23.
31. Shalin SC, Cifarelli CP, Suen JY, Gao L. Loss of cytokeratin 20 and acquisition of thyroid transcription factor-1 expression in a merkel cell carcinoma metastasis to the brain. *Am J Dermatopathol* 2014; **36**: 904–6.
32. Zur Hausen A, Rennspiess D, Winnepenninckx V, Speel EJ, Kurz AK. Early B-cell differentiation in Merkel cell carcinomas: clues to cellular ancestry. *Cancer Res* 2013; **15**: 4982–7.
33. Kutzner H, Mentzel T, Kaddu S, Soares LM, Sangueza OP, Requena L. Cutaneous myoepithelioma: an under-recognized cutaneous neoplasm

composed of myoepithelial cells. *Am J Surg Pathol* 2001; **25**: 348–55.

34. Hornick JL, Fletcher CD. Myoepithelial tumors of soft tissue: a clinicopathologic and immunohistochemical study of 101 cases with evaluation of prognostic parameters. *Am J Surg Pathol* 2003; **27**: 1183–96.
35. Jo VY, Fletcher CD. Myoepithelial neoplasms of soft tissue: an updated review of the clinicopathologic, immunophenotypic, and genetic features. *Head Neck Pathol* 2015; **9**: 32–8.
36. Gleason BC, Fletcher CD. Myoepithelial carcinoma of soft tissue in children: an aggressive neoplasm analyzed in a series of 29 cases. *Am J Surg Pathol* 2007; **31**: 1813–24.
37. Folpe AL, Schoolmeester JK, McCluggage WG, et al. SMARCB1-deficient vulvar neoplasms: a clinicopathologic, immunohistochemical, and molecular genetic study of 14 cases. *Am J Surg Pathol.* 2015; **39**: 836–49.
38. Jo VY, Antonescu CR, Dickson BC, et al. Cutaneous syncytial myoepithelioma is characterized by recurrent EWSR1-PBX3 fusions. *Am J Surg Pathol* 2019; **43**: 1349–54.
39. Antonescu CR, Zhang L, Chang NE, et al. EWSR1-POU5F1 fusion in soft tissue myoepithelial tumors: a molecular analysis of sixty-six cases, including soft tissue, bone, and visceral lesions, showing common involvement of the EWSR1 gene. *Genes Chromosomes Cancer* 2010; **49**: 1114–24.
40. Suurmeijer AJH, Dickson BC, Swanson D, et al. A morphologic and molecular reappraisal of myoepithelial tumors of soft tissue, bone, and viscera with EWSR1 and FUS gene rearrangements. *Genes Chromosomes Cancer* 2020; **59**: 348–56.
41. Bahrami A, Dalton JD, Krane JF, Fletcher CDM. A subset of cutaneous and soft tissue mixed tumors are genetically linked to their salivary gland counterpart. *Genes Chromosomes Cancer* 2012; **51**: 140–8.
42. Miettinen M, Farnburg-Smith JV, Virolainen M, Shmookler BM, Fetsch JF. Epithelioid sarcoma: an immunohistochemical analysis of 112 classical and variant cases and a distinction of the differential diagnosis. *Hum Pathol* 1999; **30**: 934–42.
43. Oda Y, Tsuneyoshi M. Extrarenal rhabdoid tumors of the soft tissue: clinicopathological and molecular genetic review and distinction from other soft tissue sarcomas with rhabdoid features. *Pathol Int* 2006; **56**: 287–95.
44. Hornick JL, Dal Cin P, Fletcher CD. Loss of INI1 expression is characteristic of both conventional and proximal-type epithelioid sarcoma. *Am J Surg Pathol* 2009; **33**: 542–50.
45. Kohashi K, Yamada Y, Hotokebuchi Y, et al. ERG and SALL4 expression in SMARCB1/INI1-deficient tumors: a useful tool for distinguishing epithelioid sarcoma from malignant rhabdoid tumor. *Hum Pathol* 2015; **46**: 225–30.
46. Hollmann TJ, Hornick JL. INI1-deficient tumors: diagnostic features and molecular genetics. *Am J Surg Pathol* 2011; **35**: e47–e63.
47. Kohashi K, Oda Y, Yamamoto H, et al. Reduced expression of SMARCB1/INI1 protein in synovial sarcoma. *Mod Pathol* 2010; **23**: 981–90.
48. Gounder MM, Agaram NP, Trabucco SE, et al. Clinical genomic profiling in the management of patients with soft tissue and bone sarcoma. *Nat Commun* 2022; **13**: 3406. doi: 10.1038/s41467-022-30496-0.
49. Sullivan LM, Folpe AL, Pawel BR, Judkins AR, Biegel JA. Epithelioid sarcoma is associated with a high percentage of SMARCB1 deletions. *Mod Pathol* 2013; **26**: 385–92.
50. Jamshidi F, Bashashati A, Shumansky K, et al. The genomic landscape of epithelioid sarcoma cell lines and tumours. *J Pathol* 2016; **238**: 63–73.
51. Rossi S, Orvieto E, Furlanetto A, et al. Utility of the immunohistochemical detection of FLI-1 expression in round cell and vascular neoplasm using a monoclonal antibody. *Mod Pathol* 2004; **17**: 547–52.
52. Folpe AL, Hill CE, Parham DM, O'Shea PA, Weiss SW. Immunohistochemical detection of FLI-1 protein expression: a study of 132 round cell tumors with emphasis on CD99-positive mimics of Ewing's sarcoma/primitive neuroectodermal tumor. *Am J Surg Pathol* 2000; **24**: 1657–62.
53. Tomlins SA, Palanisamy N, Brenner JC, et al. Usefulness of a monoclonal ERG/FLI1 antibody for immunohistochemical discrimination of Ewing family tumors. *Am J Clin Pathol* 2013; **139**: 771–9.
54. Hung YP, Fletcher CDM, Hornick JL. Evaluation of NKX2-2 expression in round cell sarcomas and other tumors with EWSR1 rearrangement: imperfect specificity for Ewing sarcoma. *Mod Pathol* 2016; **29**: 370–80.
55. Llombart-Bosh A, Navarro S. Immunohistochemical detection of EWS and FLI-1 proteinss in Ewing sarcoma and primitive neuroectodermal tumors: comparative analysis with CD99 (MIC-2) expression. *Appl Immunohistochem Mol Morphol* 2001; **9**: 255–60.
56. Wang WL, Patel NR, Caragea M, et al. Expression of ERG, an Ets family transcription factor, identifies ERG-rearranged Ewing sarcoma. *Mod Pathol* 2012; **25**: 1378–83.
57. Mhawech-Fauceglia P, Herrmann F, Penetrante R, et al. Diagnostic utility of FLI-1 monoclonal antibody and dual-colour, break-apart probe fluorescence in situ (FISH) analysis in Ewing's sarcoma/primitive neuroectodermal tumour (EWS/ PNET): a comparative study with CD99 and FLI-1 polyclonal antibodies. *Histopathology* 2006; **49**: 569–75.
58. Miettinen M, Ekfors T. Alveolar soft part sarcoma: immunohistochemical evidence for muscle cell differentiation. *Am J Clin Pathol* 1990; **93**: 32–8.
59. Argani P, Lal P, Hutchinson B, Lui MY, Reuter VE, Ladanyi M. Aberrant nuclear immunoreactivity for TFE3 in neoplasms with TFE3 gene fusions: a sensitive and specific immunohistochemical assay. *Am J Surg Pathol* 2003; **27**: 750–61.
60. Rekhi B, Ingle A, Agarwal M, Puri A, Laskar S, Jambhekar NA. Alveolar soft tissue sarcoma "revisited": clinicopathologic review of 47 cases from a tertiary cancer referral centre, including immunohistochemical expression of TFE3 in 22 cases and 21 other tumours. *Pathology* 2012; **44**: 11–17.
61. Williams A, Bartle G, Sumathi VP, et al. Detection of ASPL/TFE3 fusion transcripts and the TFE3 antigen in formalin-fixed, paraffin-embedded tissue in a series of 18 cases of alveolar soft part sarcoma: useful diagnostic tools in cases with unusual histological features. *Virchows Arch* 2011; **458**: 291–300.
62. Argani P, Antonescu CR, Couturier J, et al. PRCC-TFE3 renal carcinomas: morphologic, immunohistochemical, ultrastructural, and molecular analysis of an entity associated with the t(X;1)(p11.2;q21). *Am J Surg Pathol* 2002; **26**: 1553–66.
63. Pang LJ, Chang B, Zou H, et al. Alveolar soft part sarcoma: a bimarker diagnostic strategy using TFE3 immunoassay and ASPL-TFE3 fusion transcripts in

paraffin-embedded tumor tissues. *Diagn Mol Pathol* 2008; **17**: 245–52.

64. Tsuji K, Ishikawa Y, Imamura T. Technique for differentiating alveolar soft part sarcoma from other tumors in paraffin-embedded tissue: comparison of immunohistochemistry for TFE3 and CD147 and of reverse transcription polymerase chain reaction for ASPSCR1-TFE3 transcript. *Hum Pathol* 2012; **43**: 356–63.
65. Dickson BC, Chung CTS, Hurlbut DJ, et al. Genetic diversity in alveolar soft part sarcoma: a subset contain variant fusion genes, highlighting broader molecular kinship with other MiT family tumors. *Genes Chromosomes Cancer* 2020; **59**: 23–9.
66. Miettinen M, Limon J, Niezabitowski A, Lasota J. Patterns of keratin polypeptides in 110 biphasic, monophasic, and poorly differentiated synovial sarcomas. *Virchows Arch* 2000; **437**: 275–83.
67. O'Sullivan MJ, Kyriakos M, Zhu X, et al. Malignant peripheral nerve sheath tumors with t(X;18): a pathologic and molecular genetic study. *Mod Pathol* 2000; **13**: 1253–63.
68. Baranov E, McBride MJ, Bellizzi AM, et al. A Novel SS18-SSX Fusion-specific antibody for the diagnosis of synovial sarcoma. *Am J Surg Pathol* 2020; **44**: 922–33.
69. Foo WC, Cruise MW, Wick MR, Hornick JL. Immunohistochemistry staining for TLE1 distinguishes synovial sarcoma from histologic mimics. *Am J Clin Pathol* 2011; **135**: 839–44.
70. Valente AL, Tull J, Zhang S. Specificity of TLE1 expression in unclassified high-grade sarcomas for the diagnosis of synovial sarcoma. *Appl Immunohistochem Mol Morphol* 2013; **21**: 408–13.
71. Fletcher CDM, Bridge JA, Hogendoorn P, Mertens F. WHO classification of tumours editorial board: soft tissue and bone tumours. 5th ed. Lyon, France: IARC; 2020.
72. Agaram NP, Zhang L, Sung YS, et al. Recurrent NTRK1 Gene fusions define a novel subset of locally aggressive lipofibromatosis-like neural tumors. *Am J Surg Pathol* 2016; **40**: 1407–16.
73. Suurmeijer AJH, Davis JL. NTRK-rearranged spindle cell neoplasm. In: WHO classification of tumours editorial board: soft tissue and bone tumours. 5th ed. Lyon, France: IARC; 2020.
74. Bautista-Wong C, Mojica-Gonzalez Z, Hop-Garcia K, Quevedo LB. The pan-TRK antibody is a sensitive and specific tool for the detection of NTRK fusion genes. *Appl Immunohistochem Mol Morphol* 2023; **31**: 213–16.
75. Davis JL, Lockwood CM, Stohr B, et al. Expanding the spectrum of pediatric NTRK-rearranged mesenchymal tumors. *Am J Surg Pathol* 2019; **43**: 435–45.
76. Browne TJ, Fletcher CDM. Haemosiderotic fibrolipomatous tumour (so-called haemosiderotic fibrohistiocytic lipomatous tumour): analysis of 13 new cases in support of a distinct entity. *Histopathology* 2006; **48**: 453–61.
77. Antonescu CR, Zhang L, Nielsen GP, et al. Consistent t(1;10) with rearrangements of TGFBR3 and MGEA5 in both myxoinflammatory fibroblastic sarcoma and hemosiderotic fibrolipomatous tumor. *Genes Chromosomes Cancer* 2011; **50**: 757–64.
78. Carter JM, Sukov WR, Montgomery E, et al. TGFBR3 and MGEA5 rearrangements in pleomorphic hyalinizing angiectatic tumors and the spectrum of related neoplasms. *Am J Surg Pathol* 2014; **38**: 1182–92.
79. Folpe AL, Weiss SW. Pleomorphic hyalinizing angiectatic tumor: analysis of 41 cases supporting evolution from a distinctive precursor lesion. *Am J Surg Pathol* 2004; **28**: 1417–25.
80. Emile JF, Abla O, Fraitag S, et al. Revised classification of histiocytoses and neoplasms of the macrophage-dendritic cell lineages. *Blood* 2016; **127**: 2672–81.
81. Khoury JD, Solary E, Abla O, et al. The 5th edition of the World Health Organization classification of haematolymphoid tumours: myeloid and histiocytic/dendritic neoplasms. *Leukemia* 2022; **36**: 1703–19.
82. Friedman JS, Durham BH, Reiner AS, et al. Mixed histiocytic neoplasms: a multicenter series revealing diverse somatic mutations and responses to targeted therapy. *Br J Haematol* 2024; **205**:127–137.
83. Hervier B, Haroche J, Arnaud L, et al. Association of both Langerhans cell histiocytosis and Erdheim-Chester disease linked to the BRAFV600E mutation. *Blood* 2014; **124**: 1119–26.
84. Kapur P, Erickson C, Rakheja D, Carder KR, Hoang MP. Congenital self-healing reticulohistiocytosis (Hashimoto-Pritzker disease): ten-year experience at Dallas Children's Medical Center. *J Am Acad Dermatol* 2007; **56**: 290–4.
85. Go H, Jeon YK, Huh J, et al. Frequent detection of BRAFV600E mutation in histiocytic and dendritic cell neoplasms. *Histopathology* 2014; **65**: 261–72.
86. Wang CJ, Cui L, Li SS, et al. Genetic landscape and its prognostic impact in children with Langerhans cell histiocytosis. *Arch Pathol Lab Med* 2025; **149**: 175-190.
87. Shao H, Xi L, Raffeld M, et al. Clonally related histiocytic/dendritic cell sarcoma and chronic lymphocytic leukemia/small lymphocytic lymphoma: a study of seven cases. *Mod Pathol* 2011; **24**: 1421–32.
88. West DS, Dogan A, Quint PS, et al. Clonally related follicular lymphomas and Langerhans cell neoplasms: expanding the spectrum of transdifferentiation. *Am J Surg Pathol* 2013; **37**: 978–86.
89. McDermott R, Ziylan U, Spehner D, et al. Birbeck granules are subdomains of endosomal recycling compartment in human epidermal Langerhans cells, which form where Langerin accumulates. *Mol Biol Cell* 2002; **13**: 317–35.
90. Massoth LR, Hung YP, Ferry JA, et al. Histiocytic and dendritic cell sarcomas of hematopoietic origin share targetable genomic alterations distinct from follicular dendritic cell sarcoma. *Oncologist* 2021; **26**: e1263–e1272. doi: 10.1002/onco.13801.
91. Hornick JL, Jaffe ES, Fletcher CD. Extranodal histiocytic sarcoma: clinicopathologic analysis of 14 cases of a rare epithelioid malignancy. *Am J Surg Pathol* 2004; **28**: 1133–44.
92. Egan C, Lack J, Skarshaug S, et al. The mutational landscape of histiocytic sarcoma associated with lymphoid malignancy. *Mod Pathol* 2021; **34**: 336–47.
93. Pileri SA, Grogan TM, Harris NL, et al. Tumours of histiocytes and accessory dendritic cells: an immunohistochemical approach to classification from the International Lymphoma Study Group based on 61 cases. *Histopathology* 2002; **41**: 1–29.
94. Emile JF, Abla O, Fraitag S, et al. Revised classification of histiocytoses and neoplasms of the macrophage-dendritic cell lineages. *Blood* 2016; **127**: 2672–81.
95. Kobic A, Shah KK, Schmitt AR, et al. Erdheim-Chester disease: expanding the spectrum of cutaneous manifestations. *Br J Dermatol* 2020; **182**: 405–9.
96. Estrada-Veras JI, O'Brien KJ, Boyd LC, et al. The clinical spectrum of Erdheim-Chester disease: an observational cohort study. *Blood Adv* 2017; **1**: 357–66.

97. Foucar E, Rosai J, Dorfman R. Sinus histiocytosis with massive lymphadenopathy (Rosai-Dorfman disease): review of the entity. *Semin Diagn Pathol* 1990; **7**: 19–73.

98. Dhrif O, Litaiem N, Lahmar W, Fatnassi F, Slouma M, Zeglaoui F. Cutaneous Rosai-Dorfman disease: a systematic review and reappraisal of its treatment and prognosis. *Arch Dermatological Res* 2024; **316**: 393. doi: 10.1007/s00403-024-02982-6.

99. Levine PH, Jahan N, Murari P, Manak M, Jaffe ES. Detection of human herpesvirus 6 in tissues involved by sinus histiocytosis with massive lymphadenopathy (Rosai-Dorfman disease). *J Infect Dis* 1992; **166**: 291–5.

100. Mehraein Y, Wagner M, Remberger K, et al. Parvovirus B19 detected in Rosai-Dorfman disease in nodal and extranodal manifestations. *J Clin Pathol* 2006; **59**: 1320–6.

101. Al-Daraji W, Anandan A, Klassen-Fischer M, Auerbach A, Marwaja JS, Fanburg-Smith JC. Soft tissue Rosai-Dorfman disease: 29 new lesions in 18 patients, with detection of polyomavirus antigen in 3 abdominal cases. *Ann Diagn Pathol* 2010; **14**: 309–16.

102. Delacretaz F, Meuge-Moraw C, Anwar D, Borisch B, Chave JP. Sinus histiocytosis with massive lymphadenopathy (Rosai Dorfman disease) in an HIV-positive patient. *Virchows Arch A Pathol Anat Histopathol* 1991; **419**: 251–4.

103. Perrin C, Michiels JF, Lacour JP, Chagnon A, Fuzibet JG. Sinus histiocytosis (Rosai-Dorfman disease) clinically limited to the skin. An immunohistochemical and ultrastructural study. *J Cutan Pathol* 1993; **20**: 368–74.

104. Slone SP, Fleming DR, Buchino JJ. Sinus histiocytosis with massive lymphadenopathy and Langerhans cell histiocytosis express the cellular adhesion molecule CD31. *Arch Pathol Lab Med* 2003; **127**: 341–4.

105. Ravindran A, Goyal G, Go RS, Rech KL; Mayo Clinic Histiocytosis Working Group. Rosai-Dorfman disease displays a unique monocyte-macrophage phenotype characterized by expression of OCT2. *Am J Surg Pathol* 2021; **45**: 35–44.

106. Koh KN, Yoon SH, Kang SH, Kim H, Im HJ. Advancements in the understanding and management of histiocytic neoplasms. *Blood Res* 2024; **59**: 22. doi: 10.1007/s44313-024-00022-w.

107. Garces S, Medeiros LJ, Patel KP, et al. Mutually exclusive recurrent KRAS and MAP2K1 mutations in Rosai-Dorfman disease. *Mod Pathol* 2017; **30**: 1367–77.

108. Chang KTE, Tay AZE, Kuick CH, et al. ALK-positive histiocytosis: an expanded clinicopathologic spectrum and frequent presence of KIF5B-ALK fusion. *Mod Pathol* 2019; **32**: 598–608.

109. Chan J, Yoshida A, Emile F, et al. ALK-positive histiocytosis. In: WHO Classification of Tumours Series. Haematolymphoid tumours. 5th ed,; vol.11. Lyon (France): International Agency for Research on Cancer; 2024. https://publications.iarc.who.int/

110. Kemps PG, Picarsic J, Durham BH, et al. ALK-positive histiocytosis: a new clinicopathologic spectrum highlighting neurologic involvement and responses to ALK inhibition. *Blood* 2022; **139**: 256–80.

111. Zhang XY, Li J, Chen SL, Li Y, Wang H, He JH. Malakoplakia with aberrant ALK expression by immunohistochemistry: a case report. *Diagn Pathol* 2023; **18**: 97. doi: 10.1186/s13000-023-01383-z.

112. Polat Ekinci A, Buyukbabani N, Baykal C. Novel clinical observations on benign cephalic histiocytosis in a large series. *Pediatr Dermatol* 2017; **34**: 392–7.

113. Gianotti R, Alessi E, Caputo R. Benign cephalic histiocytosis: a distinct entity or a part of a wide spectrum of histiocytic proliferative disorders of children? A histopathological study. *Am J Dermatopathol* 1993; **15**: 315–19.

114. Requena C, Requena L, Traves V, Sanmartin O. Hereditary progressive mucinous histiocytosis: 3 different phenotypes in 3 family members. *J Cutan Pathol* 2017; **44**: 781–5.

115. Schlegel C, Metzler G, Burgdorf W, Schaller M. Hereditary progressive mucinous histiocytosis: first report in a male patient. *Acta Derm Venereol* 2010; **90**: 65–7.

116. Salari B, Dehner LP. Juvenile and adult xanthogranuloma: a 30-year single-center experience and review of the disorder and its relationship to other histiocytoses. *Ann Diagn Pathol* 2022; **58**: 151940.

117. Oza VS, Stringer T, Campbell C, et al. Congenital-type juvenile xanthogranuloma: a case series and literature review. *Pediatr Dermatol* 2018; **35**: 582–7.

118. Dehner LP. Juvenile xanthogranulomas in the first two decades of life: a clinicopathologic study of 174 cases with cutaneous and extracutaneous manifestations. *Am J Surg Pathol* 2003; **27**: 579–93.

119. Janssen D, Harms D. Juvenile xanthogranuloma in childhood and adolescence: a clinicopathologic study of 129 patients from the Kiel pediatric tumor registry. *Am J Surg Pathol* 2005; **29**: 21–8.

120. Zou T, Wei A, Ma H, et al. Systemic juvenile xanthogranuloma: a systemic review. *Pediatr Blood Cancer* 2023; **70**: e30232. doi: 10.1002/pbc.30232.

121. Sangueza OP, Salmon JK, White CR Jr, Beckstead. Juvenile xanthogranuloma: a clinical, histopathologic and immunohistochemical study. *J Cutan Pathol* 1995; **22**: 327–35.

122. Umphress B, Kuhar M, Kowal R, et al. NTRK expression is common in xanthogranuloma and is associated with the solitary variant. *J Cutan Pathol* 2023; **50**: 991–1000.

123. Ungureanu IA, Cohen-Aubart F, Heritier S, Haroche J, Donadieu J, Emile JF. PU.1 is useful nuclear marker to distinguish between histiocytosis and histiocyte-rick tumours. *Histopathology* 2023; **83**: 320–5.

124. Sanchez-Alvarez C, Sandhu AS, Crowson CS, et al. Multicentric reticulohistiocytosis: the Mayo Clinic experience (1980–2017). *Rheumatology* 2020; **59**: 1898–905.

125. Zelger B, Cerio R, Soyer HP, Misch K, Orchard G, Wilson-Jones E. Reticulohistiocytoma and multicentric reticulohistiocytosis. Histopathologic and immunophenotypic distinct entities. *Am J Dermatopathol* 1994; **16**: 577–84.

126. Tashiro A, Takeuchi S, Nakahara T, et al. Aberrant expression of CD10 in ground-glass-like multinucleated giant cells of multicentric reticulohistiocytosis. *J Dermatol* 2010; **37**: 995–7.

127. Kucukardali Y, Solmazgul E, Kunter E, et al. Kikuchi-Fujimoto disease: analysis of 244 cases. *Clin Rheumatol* 2007; **26**: 50–4.

128. Wang W, Huang S, Nong L, Li X, Li D, Zhang B, Li T. Clinicopathologic analysis of Kikuchi-Fujimoto disease and etiologic exploration using metagenomic next-generation sequencing. *Arch Pathol Lab Med* 2023; **147**: 767–73.

129. Marshall EH, Brumbaugh B, Holt A, Chen ST, Hoang MP. Cutaneous intravascular hematolymphoid entities: a review. *Diagnostics* 2024; **14**: 679. doi: 10.3390/diagnostics14070679.

130. Requena L, El-Shabrawi-Caelen L, Walsh SN, et al. Intralymphatic histiocytosis: a clinicopathologic study of 16 cases. *Am J Dermatopathol* 2009; **31**: 140–51.

131. Zanella S, Berti E, Bonometti A ; for Associazione Italiana Ricerca Istiocitosi ONLUS. Indeterminate cell histiocytosis: A systematic review of the literature with a comprehensive revision of clinical, histopathological, and molecular features. *J Eur Acad Dermatol Venereol* 2023; Apr 5. doi: 10.1111/jdv.19095. Online ahead of print. PMID: 37016977

132. Rowden G, Phillips TM, Lewis MG. Ia antigens on indeterminate cells of the epidermis: immunoelectron microscopic studies of surface antigens. *Br J Dermatol* 1979; **100**: 531–42.

133. O'Malley DP, Agrawal R, Grimm KE, et al. Evidence of BRAF V600E in indeterminate cell tumor and interdigitating dendritic cell sarcoma. *Ann Diagn Pathol* 2015; **19**: 113–16.

134. Chan JK, Fletcher CD, Nayler SJ, Cooper K. Follicular dendritic cell sarcoma: clinicopathologic analysis of 17 cases suggesting a malignant potential higher than currently recognized. *Cancer* 1997; **79**: 294–313.

135. Dainese E, Cimetti L, Pozzi B, et al. Primary cutaneous interdigitating dendritic cell sarcoma (IDCS): report of a new case and literature review. *Pathol Res Pract* 2023; **247**: 154559. doi: 10.1016/j.prp.2023.154559.

136. Horny HP, Sillaber C, Menke D, et al. Diagnostic value of immunostaining for tryptase in patients with mastocytosis. *Am J Surg Pathol* 1998; **22**: 1132–40.

137. Hollman TJ, Brenn T, Hornick JL. CD25 expression on cutaneous mast cells from adult patients presenting with urticaria pigmentosa is predictive of systemic mastocytosis. *Am J Surg Pathol* 2008; **32**: 139–45.

138. Soilleux EJ, Bowling J, Hollowood K. CD4 expression by mast cells in mastocytosis: a case report. *J Clin Pathol* 2009; **62**: 564–6.

139. Sotlar K, Cerny-Reiterer S, Petat-Dutter K, et al. Aberrant expression of CD30 in neoplastic mast cells in high-grade mastocytosis. *Mod Pathol* 2011; **24**: 585–95.

140. Parsi M, Go MS, Ahmed A. Leukemia cutis. StatPearls 2023 PMID: 31082180.

141. Stolzel F, Luer T, Lock S, et al. The prevalence of extramedullary acute myeloid leukemia detected by 18FDG-PET/CT: final results from the prospective PETAML trial. *Haematologica* 2020; **105**: 1552–8.

142. Bakst RL, Stallman MS, Douer D, Yahalom J. How I treat extramedullary acute myeloid leukemia. *Blood* 2011; **118**: 3785–93.

143. Hurley MY, Ghahramani GK, Frisch S, et al. Cutaneous myeloid sarcoma: natural history and biology of an uncommon manifestation of acute myeloid leukemia. *Acta Derm Venereol* 2013; **93**: 319–24.

144. Wilson CS, Medeiros LJ. Extramedullary manifestations of myeloid neoplasms. *Am J Clin Pathol* 2015; **144**: 219–39.

145. Pileri SA, Ascani S, Cox MC, et al. Myeloid sarcoma: clinicopathologic, phenotypic and cytogenetic analysis of 92 adult patients. *Leukemia* 2007; **21**: 340–50.

146. Falini B, Lenze D, Hasserjian R, et al. Cytoplasmic mutated nucleophosmin (NPM) defines the molecular status of a significant fraction of myeloid sarcomas. *Leukemia* 2007; **21**: 1566–70.

147. Zhou J, Bell D, Medeiros LJ. Myeloid sarcoma of the head and neck region. *Arch Pathol Lab Med* 2013; **137**: 1560–8.

148. Sangle NA, Schmidt RL, Patel JL, et al. Optimized immunohistochemical panel to differentiate myeloid sarcoma from blastic plasmacytoid dendritic cell neoplasm. *Mod Pathol* 2014; **27**: 1137–43.

149. Kaur V, Swami A, Alapat D, et al. Clinical characteristics, molecular profile and outcomes of myeloid sarcoma: a single institution experience over 13 years. *Hematology* 2018; **23**: 17–24.

150. Sukswai N, Aung PP, Yin CC, et al. Dual expression of TCF4 and CD123 is highly sensitive and specific for blastic plasmacytoid dendritic cell neoplasm. *Am J Surg Pathol* 2019; **43**: 1429–37.

151. Cronin DM, George TI, Sundram UN. An updated approach to the diagnosis of myeloid leukemia cutis. *Am J Clin Pathol* 2009; **132**: 101–10.

152. Lee WJ, Moon HR, Won CH, et al. Precursor B- or T-lymphoblastic lymphoma presenting with cutaneous involvement: a series of 13 cases including 7 cases of cutaneous T-lymphoblastic lymphoma. *J Am Acad Dermatol* 2014; **70**: 318–25.

153. Boccara O, Laloum-Grynberg E, Jeudy G, et al. Cutaneous B-cell lymphoblastic lymphoma in children: a rare diagnosis. *J Am Acad Dermatol* 2012; **66**: 51–7.

154. Schmitt IM, Manente L, Di Matteo A, Felici F, Giangiacomi M, Chimenti S. Lymphoblatic lymphoma of the pre-B phenotype with cutaneous presentation. *Dermatology* 1997; **195**: 289–92.

155. Wright D, McKeever P, Carter R. Childhood non-Hodgkin lymphomas in the United Kingdom: findings from the UK Children's Cancer Study Group. *J Clin Pathol* 1997; **50**: 128–34.

156. Alaggio R, Wood BL, Akkari Y, et al. B-lymphoblastic leukaemis/lymphomas. Introduction. In: WHO Classification of Tumours Editorial Board. Haematolymphoid tumours [Internet; beta version ahead of print]. Lyon (France): International Agency for Research on Cancer; 2022. (WHO classification of tumours series, 5th ed.; vol. 11).

157. Shafer D, Wu H, Al-Saleem T, et al. Cutaneous precursor B-cell lymphoblastic lymphoma in 2 adult patients: clinicopathologic and molecular cytogenetic studies with a review of the literature. *Arch Dermatol* 2008; **144**: 1155–62.

158. Ozdemirli M, Fanburg-Smith JC. Hartmann DP, et al. Precursor B-Lymphoblastic lymphoma presenting as a solitary bone tumor and mimicking Ewing's sarcoma: a report of four cases and review of the literature. *Am J Surg Pathol* 1998; **22**: 795–804.

159. Maitra A, McKenna RW, Weinberg AG, Schneider NR, Kroft SH. Precursor B-cell lymphoblastic lymphoma: a study of nine cases lacking blood and bone marrow involvement and review of the literature. *Am J Clin Pathol* 2001; **115**: 868–75. PMID: 11392884

160. Millot F, Robert A, Bertrand Y, et al. Cutaneous involvement in children with acute lymphoblastic leukemia or lymphoblastic lymphoma. The Children's Leukemia Cooperative Group of the European Organization of Research and Treatment of Cancer (EORTC). *Pediatrics* 1997; **100**: 60–4.

161. Patel JL, Smith LM, Anderson J, et al. The immunophenotype of T-lymphoblastic lymphoma in children and adolescents: a Children's Oncology Group report. *Br J Haematol* 2012; **159**: 454–61. doi: 10.1111/bjh.12042.

162. Muljono A, Graf NS, Arbuckle S. Primary cutaneous lymphoblastic lymphoma in children: a series of eight

cases with review of the literature. *Pathology* 2009; **41**: 223–8.

163. Pilozzi E, Muller-Hermelink HK, Falini B, et al. Gene rearrangements in T-cell lymphoblastic lymphoma. *J Pathol* 1999; **188**: 267–70.

164. T Szczepański 1, M J Pongers-Willemse, A W Langerak, et al. Ig heavy chain gene rearrangements in T-cell acute lymphoblastic leukemia exhibit predominant DH6-19 and DH7-27 gene usage, can result in complete V-D-J rearrangements, and are rare in T-cell receptor alpha beta lineage. *Blood* 1999; **93**: 4079–85.

165. Bonifazi E, Caputo R, Ceci A, Meneghini C. Congenital self-healing histiocytosis. Clinical, histologic, and ulstrastructural study. *Arch Dermatol* 1982; **118**: 267–72.

166. Hashimoto K, Takahashi S, Lee RG, Krull EA. Congenital self-healing reticulohistiocytosis. Report of the seventh case with histochemical and ultrastructural studies. *J Am Acad Dermatol* 1984; **11**: 447–54.

167. Melo J, Catovsky D, Galton DAG. The relationship between chronic lymphocytic leukaemia and prolymphocytic leukaemia. I. Clinical and laboratory features of 300 patients and characterization of an intermediate group. *Br J Haematol* 1986; **63**: 377–87.

168. Menter T, Dirnhofer S, Tzankov A. LEF1: a highly specific marker for the diagnosis of chronic lymphocytic B cell leukaemia/small lymphocytic B cell lymphoma. *J Clin Pathol* 2015; **68**: 473–8.

169. Hartmann K, Escribano L, Grattan C, et al. Cutaneous manifestations in patients with mastocytosis: Consensus report of the European Competence Network on Mastocytosis; the American Academy of Allergy, Asthmas & Immunology; and the European Academy of Allergology and Clinical Immunology. *J Allergy Clin Immunol* 2016; **137**: 35–45.

170. Severino M, Chandesris MO, Barete S, et al. Telangiectasis macularis eruptiva perstans (TMEP): a form of cutaneous mastocytosis with potential systemic involvement. *J Am Acad Dermatol* 2016; **74**: 885–91.

171. Antonescu CR. Emerging soft tissue tumors with kinase fusions: an overview of the recent literature with an emphasis on diagnostic criteria. *Genes Chromosomes Cancer* 2020; **59**: 437–44.

Chapter

10

Detection of Genetic Syndromes

Mai P. Hoang

Introduction

In the setting of multiple cutaneous tumors including adnexal, melanocytic, and mesenchymal ones, these tumors can be associated with a hereditary syndrome that predispose to internal malignancy. Early diagnosis would allow timely genetic counseling and appropriate cancer surveillance. Although a definitive diagnosis would require molecular confirmation, immunohistochemistry is cost effective as a first-line screening test.

10.1 Muir-Torre Syndrome

Lynch syndrome is the most frequent form of hereditary colorectal cancer syndrome, accounting for approximately 5% of all colorectal cancers, and also predispose to the development of endometrial cancers.[1] It is now molecularly characterized as a cancer-predisposing syndrome due to germline mutations in one of the DNA mismatch repair (MMR) genes including *MLH1* (mutL homolog 1) (OMIM 120436) in 40% of the cases, *MSH2* (mutS homolog 2) (OMIM 609309) in 40% of the cases, and less frequently *MSH6* (mutS homolog 6) (OMIM 600678) and *PMS2* (postmeiotic segregation increased 2) (OMIM 185535). The abnormality of the MMR genes leads to accumulation of errors during DNA replication, especially in repetitive sequences known as microsatellites, resulting in microsatellite instability, which is the hallmark of this disorder.[1]

In 1967 Dr. Edgar G. Muir reported the association of internal malignancy with multiple keratoacanthomas.[2] Similar association of internal malignancy and sebaceous neoplasms was noted by Dr. Douglas P. Torre the following year.[3] Germline mutations in DNA mismatch repair genes are also present in the autosomal-dominant Muir-Torre syndrome (MTS) (OMIM 158320), a phenotypic variant of Lynch syndrome. It is defined clinically by the presence of an internal malignancy, most commonly colorectal carcinoma and genitourinary carcinomas, together with at least one sebaceous neoplasm.[4] The cutaneous lesions of Lynch syndrome can include sebaceous adenomas (43%), sebaceous carcinomas (27%), keratoacanthomas (16%), sebaceomas (13%), squamous cell carcinomas (23%), and basal cell carcinomas (10%).[5] Sebaceous neoplasms are cutaneous markers for MTS, and can represent the initial manifestation in 22–41% of cases.[6,7] The sebaceous neoplasms are most often adenomas, but can be sebaceomas, sebaceous carcinoma, and rarely cystic sebaceous tumors.[8,9] Cystic sebaceous tumors have been thought to be a marker of MTS,[4,8,9] although rare sporadic tumor has been reported.[10] The sebaceous carcinomas in Muir-Torre syndrome are not associated with more aggressive biologic behavior.[11] Keratoacanthomas are associated with MTS when they are multiple, associated with two or greater internal malignancies, and with sebaceous differentiation histopathologically.[12] Seborrheic keratosis can have sebaceous differentiation and does not appear to be associated with MTS.[13]

Muir-Torre syndrome is usually the result of germline mutation in one or more of the DNA mis-match repair (MMR) genes including *MSH-2*, *MLH-1*, *MSH-6*, and *PMS2*. The mutational spectrum of MTS appears different from hereditary nonpolyposis colorectal cancer (HNPCC) since *MSH2* mutations are seen in 92% and *MLH1* mutation in 8% of MTS cases; whereas, *MLH1* mutation in 53% and *MSH2* mutation are seen in 37% of HNPCC cases.[14] Mutations of *MSH6* and *PMS2* which can be seen in HNPCC have not been reported in MTS.[14]

Most of the centers now recognize the importance of widespread screening strategies in all patients with colorectal cancer and patients suspected of having MTS, independent of age, histology of the tumor, or other clinical criteria.[15,16] However, in routine practice, screening for mutation is expensive and time-consuming, and often difficult to perform due to the heterogeneity of the mutation spectrum of the MMR genes. Such difficulties make preselection of high-risk patients necessary to narrow the number of patients requiring further genetic testing.[1,17]

In a population-based study of 1077 patients with sebaceous carcinoma, Cook et al.[18] reported low rates of mismatch repair deficiency screening. The Mayo-Clinic risk scoring system includes age at sebaceous neoplasm diagnosis (1 for younger than 60 years), total number of sebaceous neoplasms (2 for 2 tumors or more), personal history of any Lynch-related cancer (1 for yes), and family history of any Lynch-related cancer (1 for yes).[19] A total score of 2 has 100% sensitivity and 81% specificity for predicting a germline mutation.[19] However, patients with score 1 could still have MTR. Recently Sinson et al.[20] reported that immunostaining of patients with score 1 or higher with initial Mayo-Clinic-risk-score might be a better strategy in screening for MTS in patients with sebaceous neoplasms.

Among the most utilized screening tool, the relative usefulness of MSI testing versus immunohistochemistry (MLH1, MSH2, MSH6, and PMS2 immunostains) has been the topic of intensive investigation, with virtually equivalent sensitivity and specificity in predicting germline mutation between the two techniques and a high sensitivity of IHC in predicting germline mutations (around 94% when the four antibodies are tested). Mutation of *MLH1* or *MSH2* will result in concurrent loss of MLH1/PMS2 or MSH2/MSH6 by IHC, respectively (**see** Case Study 1); whereas mutation of *PMS2* or *MSH6* will result in isolated loss of PMS2 or MSH6.[1,17] In sebaceous neoplasms, the loss of MLH1 or MSH2 expression correlated with a known germline mutation in 89% of cases.[21] Therefore, given that IHC is more readily available and less expensive, it is often the first choice in screening patients for genetic testing.[1,17,22] When IHC findings are indicative of a MMR mutation, germline mutation analyses of *MLH-1*, *MSH*-2, and *MSH-6* then are done for confirmation.[21]

Currently there is no data to support testing basal cell carcinoma, keratoacanthoma with sebaceous differentiation, and sebaceous hyperplasia in screening for Muir-Torre syndrome. In 216 consecutive sebaceous neoplasms seen at a community practice, 66% (143/216) showed MMR deficiency – 63% (90/143) with MSH2/MSH6, 19% (27/143) with MLH1/PMS2, 15% (22/143) with MSH6, and 3% (4/143) with PMS2 loss of expression.[23] Everett et al.[24] reported germline mutation in 29% of their patients with abnormal IHC results. Recently a subtype of MTS has been identified which displays microsatellite stability and autosomal recessive mode of inheritance due to biallelic inactivation of *MYH*, a base excision repair gene;[25] however, MYH immunohistochemistry has not been shown to be helpful screening test.[26] Some authors have recommended that MMR IHC performed on sebaceous neoplasms from "below the head and neck" region.[27] Some have recommended that an IHC panel should include at least MLH1, MSH6, and PMS2, with or without MSH2.[16] It is recommended that genetic evaluation is warranted for patients with abnormal IHC results, with personal or family history of Lynch syndrome-associated cancer yet normal IHC results, and/or more than one sebaceous neoplasm.[24]

Immunohistochemical screening panels

Muir-Torre syndrome: MSH–2, MLH–1, MSH–6, PMS2

Lynch syndrome: MSH–2, MLH–1, MSH–6, PMS2, BRAFV600E

10.2 BAP1-Tumor Predisposition Syndrome

Mutations of *BAP1* (BRCA1-Associated Protein 1), a tumor suppressor gene, have been reported recently to increase susceptibility to the development of uveal and cutaneous melanomas, cutaneous atypical and epithelioid melanocytic lesions, lung adenocarcinoma, mesotheliomas, meningioma, clear cell renal cell carcinoma, mesothelioma, and other tumors.[28–36] There is increased risk of developing multiple cancer types which possess more aggressive growth and earlier onset in comparison to sporadic tumors. Tumor formation results from a loss of heterozygosity due to a second mutation or deletion. The BAP1-tumor predisposition syndrome (OMIM #614327) is autosomal dominant with variable penetrance and individuals with heterozygous *BAP1* mutation are at high risk of developing the above-mentioned tumors.

Early recognition of this syndrome has both prognostic and management implications. Screening for individuals who may carry germline *BAP1* mutations can be accomplished through BAP1 IHC on syndrome-associated tumors. All atypical melanocytic lesions and basal cell carcinomas in individuals with germline *BAP1* mutations typically show loss of BAP1 nuclear expression (**Figures 10.1–10.2**) (**Tables 10.1 and 10.2**).[30,31,33–36] Interestingly, a combined BAP1 loss and BRAFV600E positive immunophenotype can be seen in 67% of BAP1 tumor syndrome-associated atypical melanocytic proliferations and appears to be a characteristic feature (**Figures 10.3–10.6**).[33,36] The loss of BAP1 nuclear expression has been shown to correlate with bi-allelic *BAP1* mutation, with positive and negative predictive values of 100% and 98.6%, respectively.[37] Ladanyi et al.[38] have reported absence of BAP1 nuclear expression in 25% of mesotheliomas without *BAP1* mutation. These findings suggest that in a subset of tumors other molecular mechanisms such as inactivation of *BAP1* are responsible for BAP1 loss of

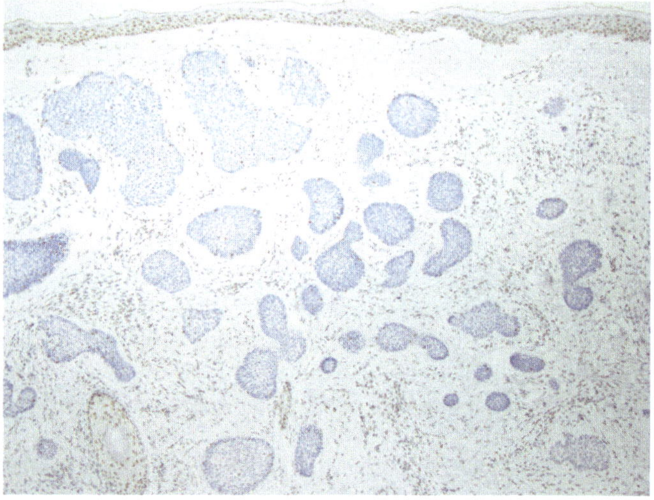

Figure 10.1 While the keratinocytes within the epidermis exhibit nuclear BAP1 expression, the tumor cells of a syndrome-associated basal cell carcinoma exhibit loss of nuclear BAP1 expression (X200).

Table 10.1 Loss of BAP1 expression in benign and malignant melanocytic proliferations[31,33,36]

	Loss of BAP1 expression
BAP1-tumor syndrome-associated lesions	100%
Nevi (dermal, congenital, Spitz, atypical Spitz)	0%
Atypical Spitz tumor	0–28%
Epithelioid Spitz tumor	79%
Proliferative nodules	8%
Primary and non-desmoplastic melanoma	2.5–3%
Desmoplastic melanoma	2.5–22%
Metastatic melanoma	9%

Table 10.2 Loss of BAP1 expression in basal cell carcinoma

References	Number of family	Number of patients	BAP1 nuclear staining of syndrome-associated basal cell carcinoma	Control basal cell carcinomas
de la Fouchardiere 2014 [34]	2	4	0/19	22/22
Wadt 2014 [30]		2	0/2	53/53
Mochel 2015 [35]	1	2	0/7	30/31

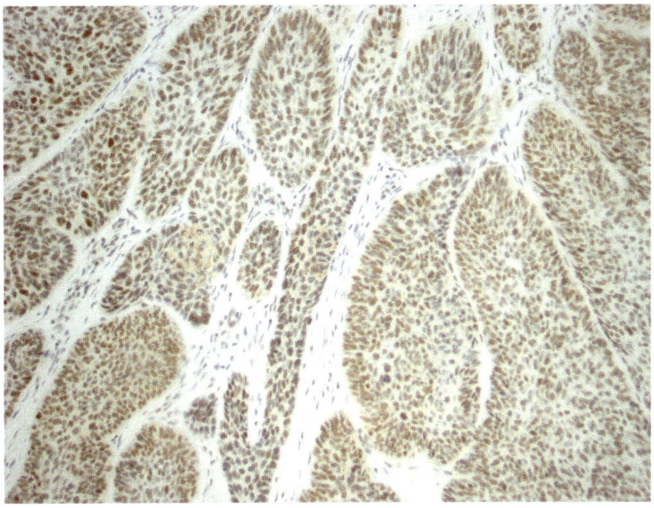

Figure 10.2 A sporadic basal cell carcinoma with diffuse nuclear BAP1 expression (X200).

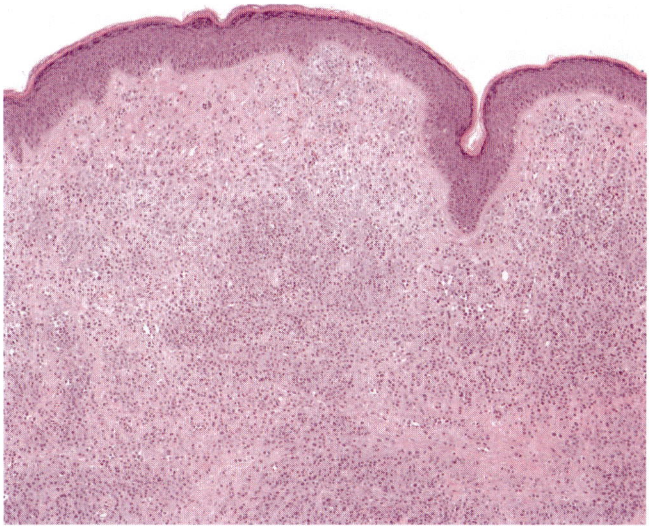

Figure 10.3 A BAP1-tumor syndrome melanocytic lesion is characterized by a proliferation of epithelioid melanocytes in the dermis (X100).

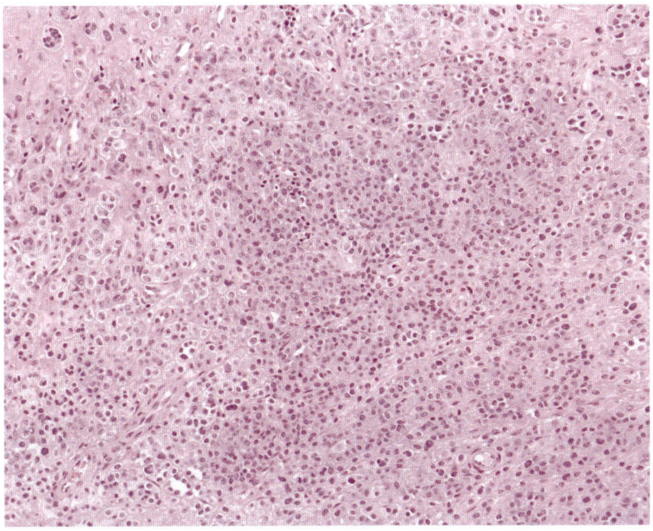

Figure 10.4 These tumor cells have eosinophilic cytoplasm with well-demarcated cytoplasmic borders (X200).

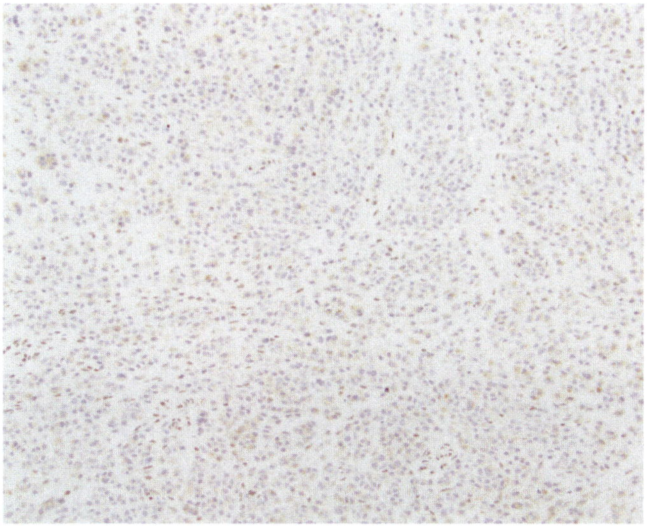

Figure 10.5 Loss of nuclear BAP1 expression is noted (X200).

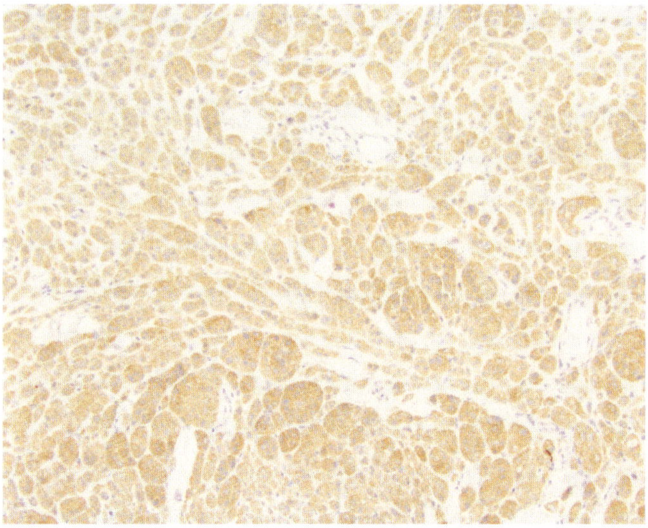

Figure 10.6 The tumor cells diffusely express BRAFV600E (X200).

Table 10.3 Loss of BAP1 expression in melanomas not associated with BAP1-tumor predisposition syndrome

	Primary melanoma	Desmoplastic melanoma	Metastatic melanoma
Murali et al 2013 [40]	4/135 (3%)	5/18 (22%)	
Piris et al 2015 [36]	1/40 (2.5%)	1/40 (2.5%)	2/23 (9%)
Aung et al 2019 [39]	4/4 (100%)		

expression. It is of note that loss of BAP1 expression has been reported in melanomas of patients without BAP1-tumor syndrome (**Table 10.3**).[36,39,40] BAP1 expression loss is also noted in melanoma arising in blue nevi.[41]

10.3 PTEN Hamartoma Tumor Syndrome/ Cowden Syndrome

PTEN (phosphatase and tensin homolog, deleted on chromosome 10) is a tumor suppressor gene that maps to 10q23.3 and encodes a 403 amino acid dual specificity (lipid and protein) phosphatase that localizes to the nucleus and cytoplasm and regulates cell migration, cell growth, apoptosis, and cell cycle arrest.[42,43] Inherited mutations in *PTEN* lead to syndromes of dysfunctional cell growth, so called *PTEN* hamartoma tumor syndromes that include PTEN hamartoma tumor syndrome/ Cowden syndrome, Bannayan-Riley Ruvalcaba syndrome, Proteus syndrome, and Proteus-like syndrome.[44]

Cowden syndrome is autosomal dominant. It has a predilection for Caucasian and females and an incidence of approximately 1:200,000 individuals.[43] The syndrome is diagnosed when the patient exhibits either three or more major criteria (gastrointestinal hamartomas, macrocephaly, and Lhermitte-Duclos disease) or two major and three minor criteria.[45] While the diagnosis of Cowden syndrome is based mainly on clinical criteria, the syndrome is associated with germline *PTEN* mutations. In a cohort of 368 patients with Cowden syndrome by Tan et al.,[46] the risk of developing female breast cancer was 85%, thyroid cancer 35%, kidney cancer 34%, endometrial cancer 28%, colorectal cancer 9%, and malignant melanoma 6%.[46]

Cutaneous tumors are often the first clinical presentation of Cowden syndrome, raising the suspicion and prompting further workup. The characteristic mucocutaneous manifestations include multiple trichilemmomas, sclerotic fibromas, palmo-plantar keratoses, oral mucosal papillomatosis, cutaneous facial papules, benign genital melanosis, lipomas, and hemangiomas.[47] Although it is a rare syndrome early diagnosis is crucial so appropriate cancer screening and genetic counseling can be performed. In fact, the cutaneous presentations manifest up to 30 years prior to internal malignancies, with almost all patients developing at least one skin finding by their 20s to 30s, in contrast to thyroid cancer around age 37, endometrial cancer around age 40, and breast cancer which manifests around age 50.[43]

PTEN expression by IHC has been evaluated in a number of Cowden syndrome-associated lesions and has been shown to be a good screening test for functional PTEN loss.[47–50] It has been described as lost or decreased in dysplastic gangliocytoma of the cerebellum (Lhermitte–Duclos disease) and in synchronous bilateral breast carcinoma.[47,51] Recently, it has been shown that loss of PTEN expression in adenomatous thyroid nodules can aid in the identification of patients with Cowden syndrome.[52] In a series of 21 thyroidectomy specimens, the sensitivity and specificity of PTEN immunostain in detecting Cowden syndrome were 100% and 92%, respectively.[52] In addition, Al-Zaid et al.[53] and Shon et al.[49] demonstrated complete loss of PTEN expression in 83–100% Cowden syndrome-associated trichilemmomas and in only 3–5% sporadic trichilemmomas, further supporting that PTEN immunostain can be a helpful screening test for Cowden syndrome (**Figures 10.7 and 10.8**) (**Table 10.4**).[47,48,49,52] Loss of PTEN expression is frequently noted in

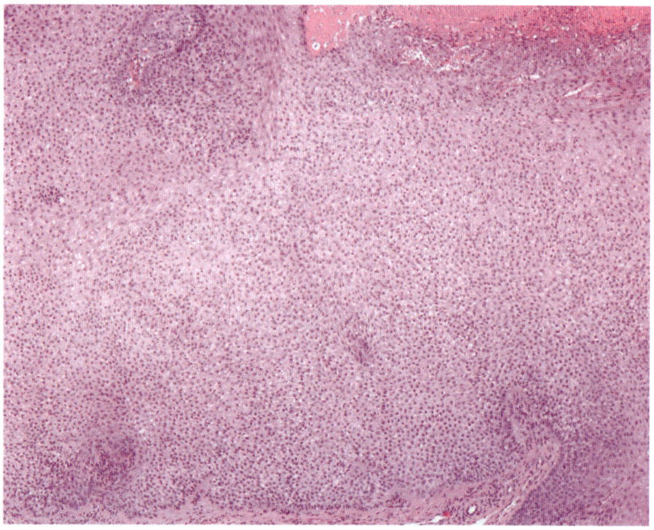

Figure 10.7 Trichilemmoma in a patient with Cowden syndrome is characterized by epithelial proliferation of neoplastic cells with clear cytoplasm (X100).

Table 10.4 Loss of PTEN expression in tumors associated with Cowden syndrome

References	N	Tumor type	Cowden syndrome	Non-Cowden syndrome	Sensitivity	Specificity
Peiro 2010 [51]	1	trichilemmoma	1/1		100%	
Zabetian 2012 [50]	2	trichilemmoma	2/2		100%	
Al-Zaid 2012 [53]	39	trichilemmoma	5/6	1/33	83%	97%
Jin 2013 [47]	89	trichilemmoma	ND	13/89	ND	85%
Shon 2014 [49]	32	trichilemmoma	13/13	1/19	100%	95%
Hartsough 2024 [48]	15	trichilemmoma	6/6	0/9	100%	100%
	12	sclerotic fibroma	5/7	0/5	71%	100%

ND: not done

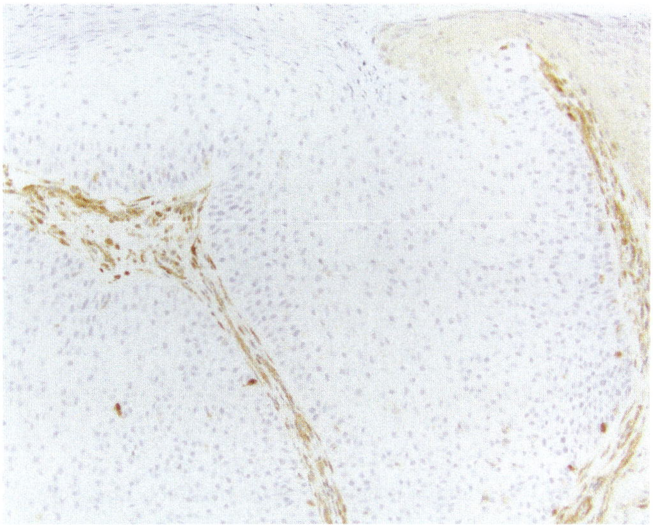

Figure 10.8 Loss of PTEN cytoplasmic expression by the tumor cells in contrast to the positive dermal blood vessels (X200).

Cowden syndrome-associated trichilemmomas as well as sclerotic fibromas. [47,49,52] In our recent study, PTEN expression was lost in 43 of 45 (96%) Cowden syndrome-associated lesions and retained in 30/31 sporadic tumors. The overall sensitivity and specificity of PTEN loss of expression are 96% and 97%, respectively.[48]

10.4 Hereditary Leiomyomatosis and Renal Cell Carcinoma

Reed's syndrome or the multiple cutaneous and uterine leiomyomatosis (MCUL) syndrome is an autosomal dominant disease characterized by cutaneous leiomyomatosis in both gender and multiple leiomyomas in women.[54] Germline heterozygous loss-of-function mutations of fumarate hydratase (*FH*) gene, located on chromosome 1q42.3, have been detected in both MCUL (OMIM 150800) and hereditary leiomyomatosis and renal cell cancer (HLRCC, OMIM 605839) demonstrating that both are allelic manifestation of the same underlying molecular abnormality.[55] Fumarate hydratase catalyzes the conversion of fumarate to malate. Fumarate hydratase mutations appear to promote tumor development via activation of the hypoxia pathway.[56] Papillary renal cell carcinoma can be seen in 14% of patients with MCUL.[57] The renal carcinomas associated with HLRCC often have an early onset, unilateral and biologically aggressive.[58] Up to 77% of women with HLRCC have uterine leiomyomas.[56] The uterine leiomyomas associated with HLRCC often exhibited increased cellularity, multinucleated tumor cells, and cytologic atypia.[59]

Currently there is no consensus regarding diagnostic criteria for HLRCC. Molecular testing for germline *FH* mutation is recommended in patients having multiple cutaneous leiomyomas without a family history of HLRCC, a single cutaneous leiomyoma with a family history of HLRCC, or one or more tubulopapillary, collecting duct, or papillary type 2 renal carcinomas with or without a family history of HLRCC. Since cutaneous and uterine leiomyomas are frequent in MCUL and HLRCC syndromes, initial screening with immunohistochemistry is important for identification and surveillance in patients with a personal or family history of multiple leiomyomas. Clinical awareness is important due to the associated risk of uterine fibroids and renal cell carcinoma.[60]

2-succinocysteine (2SC) and fumarate hydratase (FH) immunostains have shown good concordance with *FH* mutation in uterine leiomyomas.[61] In a recent study by Ahvenainen et al.,[62] 2SC and FH IHC were initially performed 90 uterine leiomyomas from HLRCC patients and 65 sporadic uterine leiomyomas, then confirmed on a second set of 22 leiomyomas with FH alteration and 20 with wildtype FH. 2SC exhibited 100% sensitivity and 100% specificity, while FH had 91% sensitivity and 100% specificity.[62] Another study by Llamas-Velasco et al[63] demonstrated sensitivity of 83.3% and specificity of 75% for FH immunostaining. [63] 2SC positivity and loss of FH staining were seen in 11/11 (100%) and 6/11 (55%) tumors in the multiple cutaneous leiomyomas setting (**Figures 10.9 and 10.10**).[64] Therefore, 2SC and FH immunostains can be helpful screening test with further investigation regarding an underlying genetic syndrome such as HLRCC in cases with loss of FH staining. However, confirmation with genetic testing is needed.

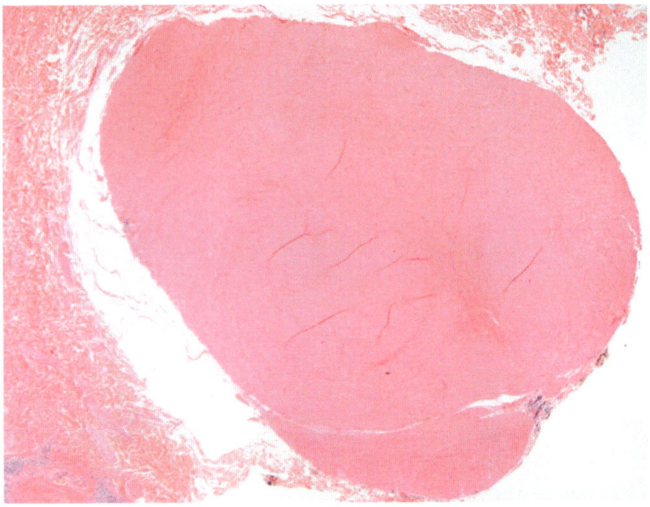

Figure 10.9 A 31-year-old man of Asian or Indian descent presented with multiple painful nodules on his trunk that clinically thought to be neurofibromas. The first lesion appeared when the patient was 17 years of age. These lesions had been progressively painful. The lesion is comprised of a circumscribed proliferation of intersecting smooth muscle bundles.

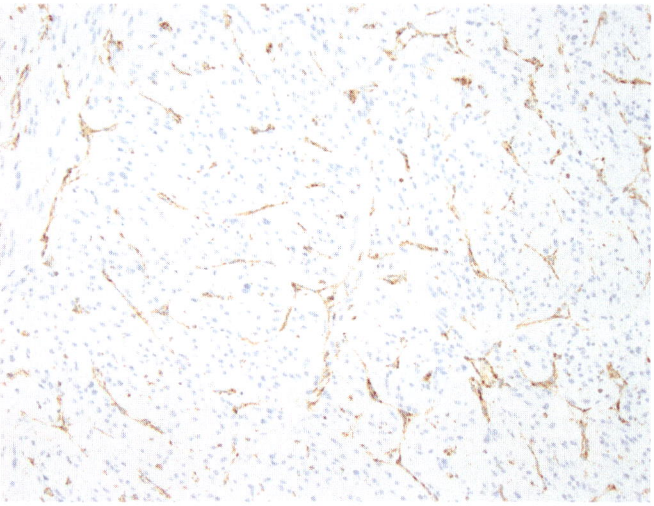

Figure 10.10 FH immunostain highlights the intratumoral vessels while the tumor cells are negative (X200).

10.5 Case Studies

Case 10.1

Case history and description: A 46-year-old man presented with a lesion on his upper chest that clinically thought to be a cyst. The patient has a history of colonic adenocarcinoma. Histologic sections show a cystic lesion that is lined by a basaloid epithelium showing sebaceous differentiation (**Figure 10.11**). At high magnification the basaloid cells do not exhibit atypia and well-differentiated sebocytes are seen (**Figure 10.12**). The tumor cells exhibit loss of MSH2 and MSH6 nuclear expression (**Figure 10.13**). The nuclear expression of MHL1 and PMS2 is preserved (**Figure 10.14**).

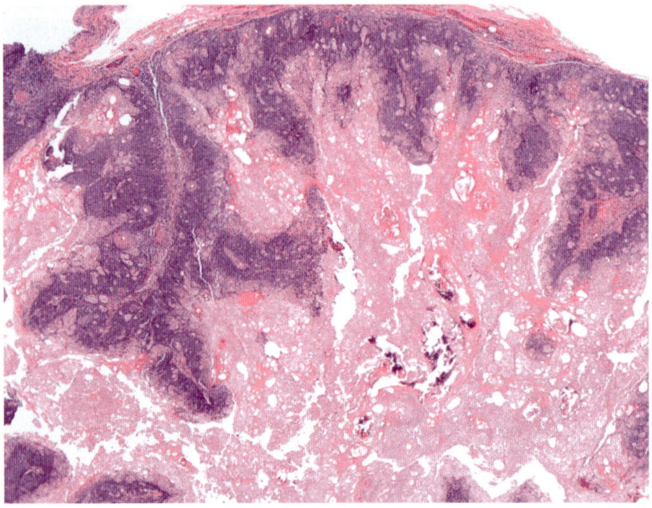

Figure 10.11 A cystic lesion lined by a basaloid epithelium showing sebaceous differentiation consistent with cystic sebaceous tumor (X40).

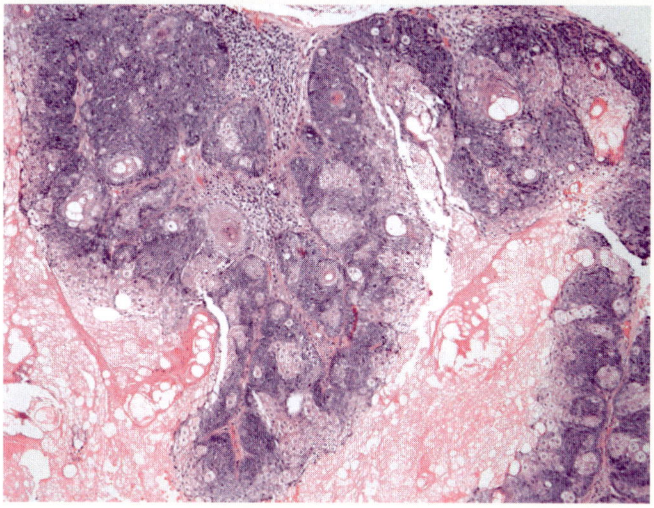

Figure 10.12 The non-atypical basaloid cells and well-differentiated sebocytes are seen (X100).

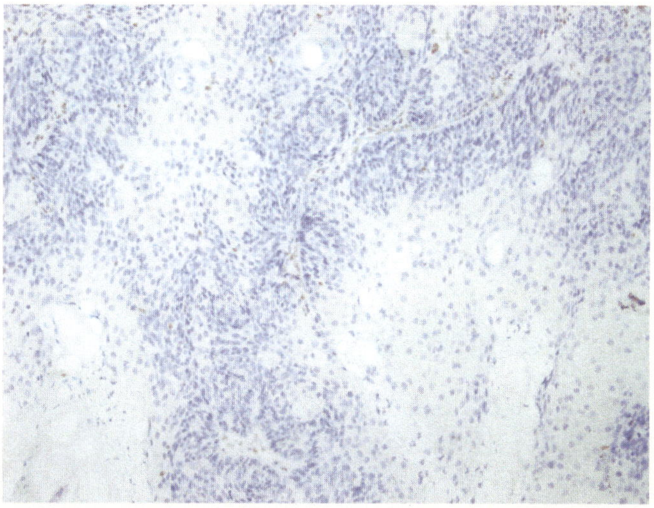

Figure 10.13 The tumor cells exhibit loss of nuclear MSH2 expression (X200).

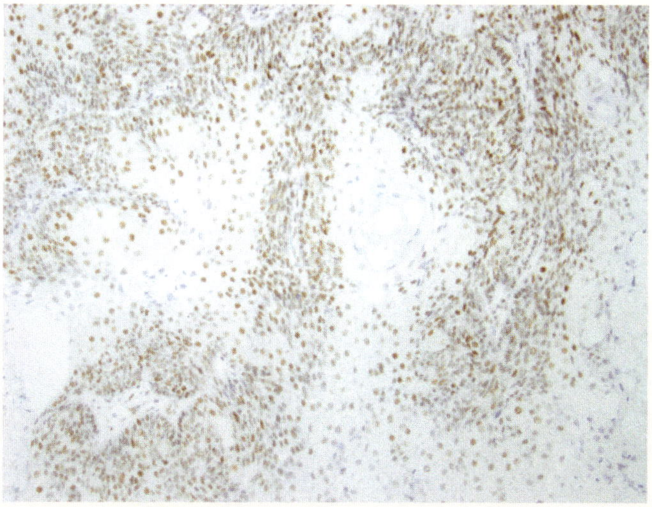

Figure 10.14 MLH1 nuclear expression is intact (X200).

Diagnosis: Cystic sebaceous neoplasm associated with Muir-Torre syndrome.

Discussion: Cystic sebaceous tumors display a spectrum of morphology ranging from benign to proliferative and atypical cystic sebaceous tumors.[4,8,9] These tumors are often deep seated, well circumscribed, and have cytologic atypia.[8,9] Cystic sebaceous adenomas have a thin cyst wall lined with basaloid cells exhibiting sebaceous differentiation. Proliferative cystic sebaceous tumors have a lobulated as well as cystic growth pattern with atypical basaloid cells and prominent mitotic figures. Some consider cystic sebaceous tumors to be well-differentiated sebaceous carcinoma due to their deep location, large size and cytologic atypia; however, neither recurrences nor metastases have been reported in cystic sebaceous neoplasms.[9]

Case 10.2

Case history and description: A 79-year-old woman had a history of an invasive mucinous adenocarcinoma involving her right colon one year ago. The colonic mucinous adenocarcinoma at that time showed loss of MLH1 and PMS2 expression and preserved expression of MSH2 and MSH6 by immunohistochemistry. Although HNPCC was suspected clinically, MLH1 promoter methylation analysis was negative. She now presents with one-month history of zosteriform lesions on her left lower abdomen. A skin biopsy shows a proliferation of mucin producing neoplastic cells with signet-ring cell appearance in the dermis (**Figures 10.15 and 10.16**). These tumor cells are positive for MSH2, MSH6, and BRAFV600E (**Figures 10.17 and 10.18**). They show loss of MLH1 and PMS2 nuclear expression (**Figure 10.19**).

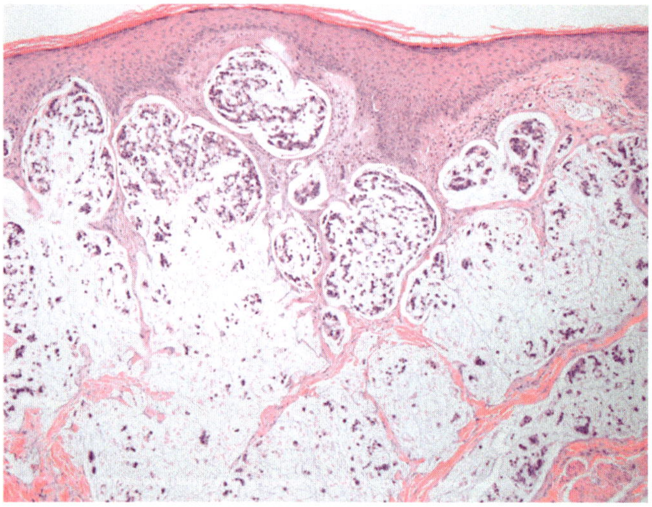

Figure 10.15 A mucin producing carcinoma is present in the dermis consistent with metastatic adenocarcinoma (X100).

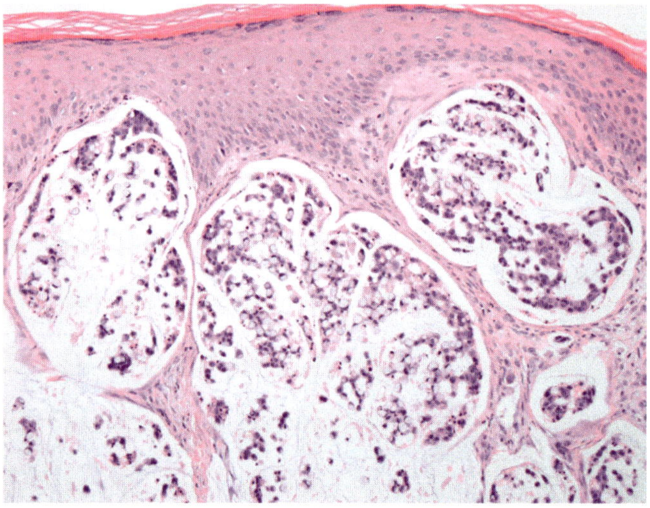

Figure 10.16 Intracytoplasmic mucin imparts a signet ring cell appearance (X200).

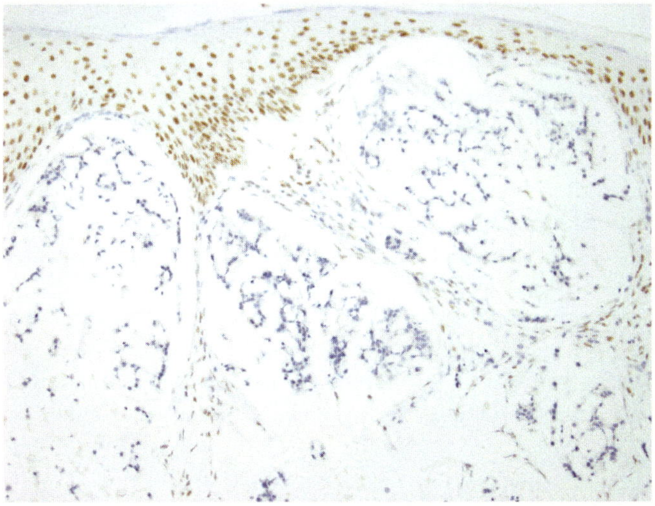

Figure 10.17 The tumor cells exhibit loss of MSH6 nuclear expression (X200).

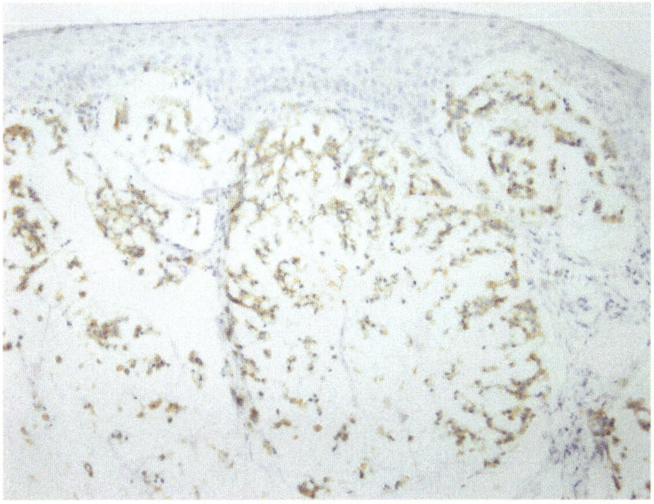

Figure 10.18 The tumor cells express BRAFV600E (X200).

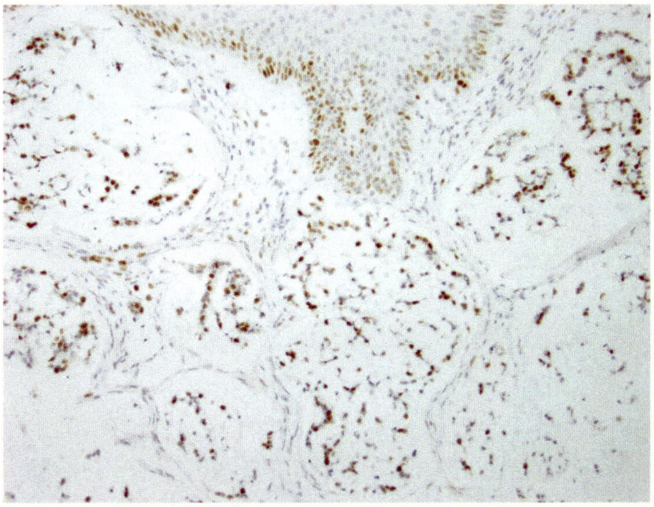

Figure 10.19 PMS2 nuclear expression is intact (X200).

Diagnosis: Metastatic colonic signet ring cell carcinoma, sporadic or not associated with Lynch syndrome.

Discussion: This case illustrates the cost effectiveness of BRAFV600E immunostain in screening for HNPCC or Lynch syndrome. The positive BRAFV600E expression supports this tumor to be sporadic and negates the need for additional mutational analyses. *BRAF* mutations occur at a frequency of 8–10% in sporadic colorectal cancers and in up to 60% of colorectal cancer with *MLH1* silencing due to somatic hypermethylation but virtually absent in hereditary colorectal cancer or Lynch syndrome. The implementation of *BRAF* mutation analysis into Lynch syndrome screening has been suggested for the exclusion of patients from germline MMR gene mutational analysis.[15] Since the presence of *BRAFV600E* mutation in microsatellite-unstable (MSI) colorectal carcinomas invariable excludes Lynch syndrome, an algorithm of IHC analysis with MLH1, MSH2, MSH6, PMS2, with subsequent BRAFV600E in all newly diagnosed cases of colorectal cancer has been proposed (**Figure 10.20**).[15,65] Recently Cornejo et al.[21] examined the role of *BRAF* mutational analysis in identifying sporadic sebaceous neoplasms, analogous to colorectal carcinoma. However, *BRAF* mutational analysis for sebaceous neoplasms with loss of MMR protein expression does not appear to be useful in distinguishing between patients with somatic from germline *MLH1* mutations.

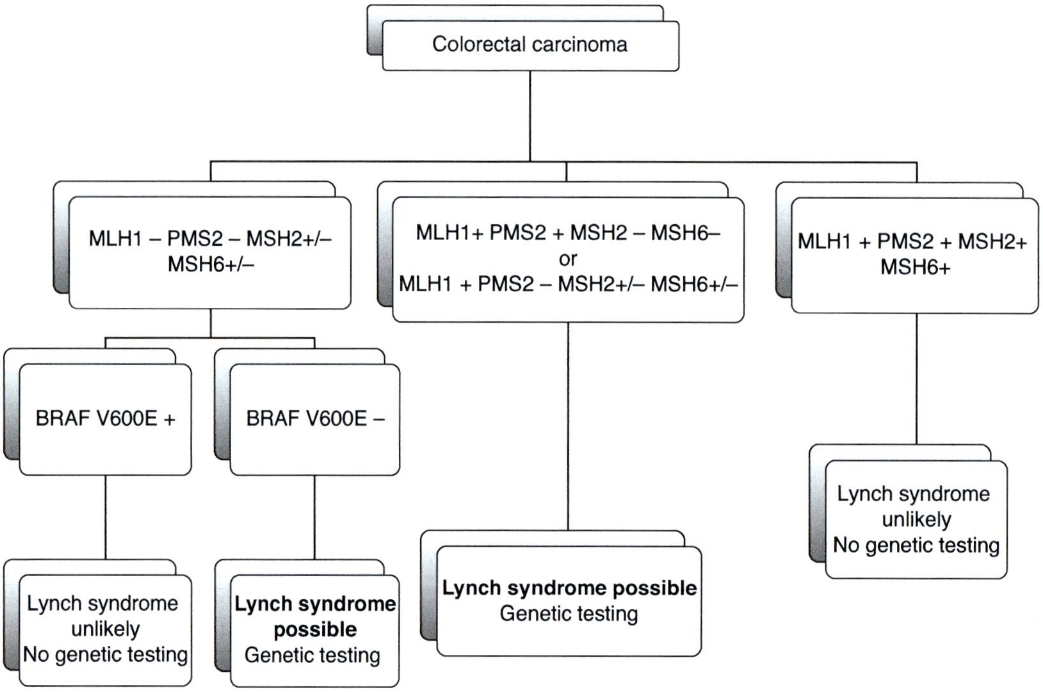

Figure 10.20 A screening algorithm for Lynch syndrome using immunohistochemistry.

Case 10.3

Case history and description: A 52-year-old man presented with a 6 × 6 mm brown-pink papule on his left forearm. The patient has a history of many atypical melanocytic nevi and a family history of uveal melanoma. Histologically the lesion is characterized by an expansile, nodular or sheet-like, dermal aggregate of epithelioid melanocytes with well- demarcated cytoplasmic borders and ample and amphophilic or eosinophilic cytoplasm (**Figures 10.21 and 10.22**). Their nuclei show vesicular chromatin with regular nuclear membrane and prominent nucleoli (**Figure 10.23**). There is an associated background dermal nevus component. The tumor cells are positive for BRAFV600E (**Figure 10.24**) and negative for BAP1 (**Figure 10.25**).

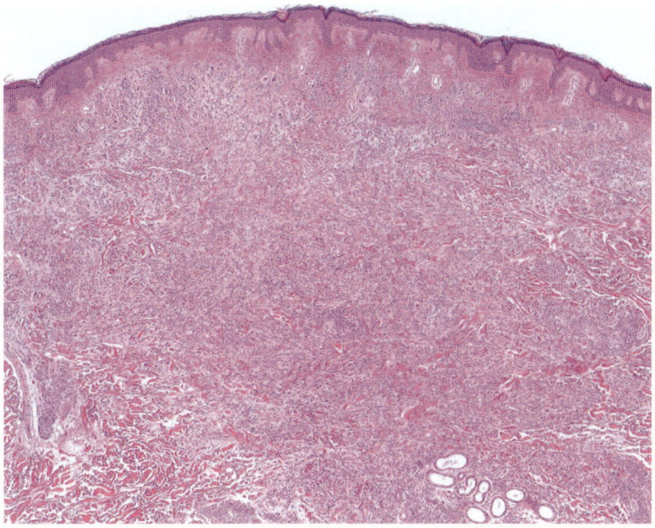

Figure 10.21 A BAP1-tumor syndrome melanocytic lesion is characterized by an expansile and nodular proliferation of melanocytes in the dermis (X40).

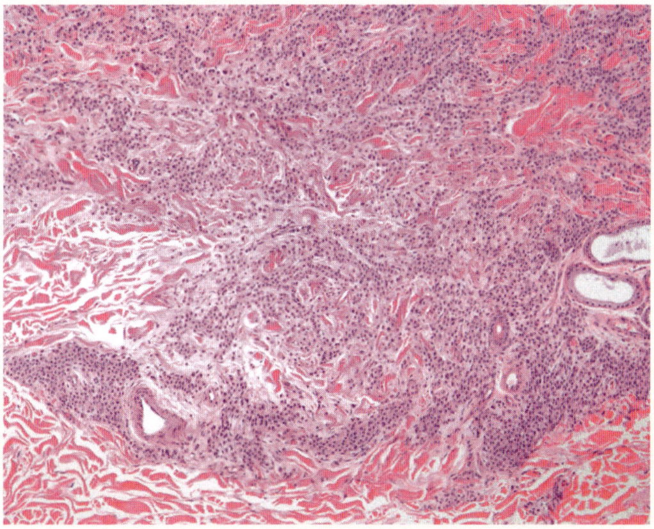

Figure 10.22 These epithelioid melanocytes have eosinophilic cytoplasm with well-demarcated cytoplasmic borders (X100).

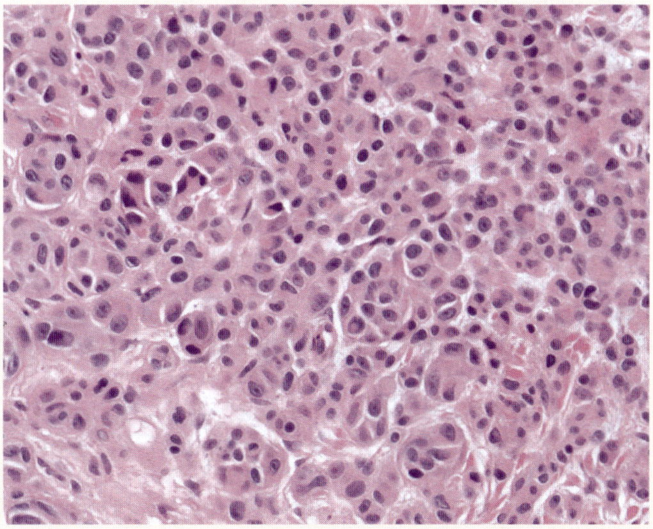

Figure 10.23 The nuclei have vesicular chromatin and prominent nucleoli (X400).

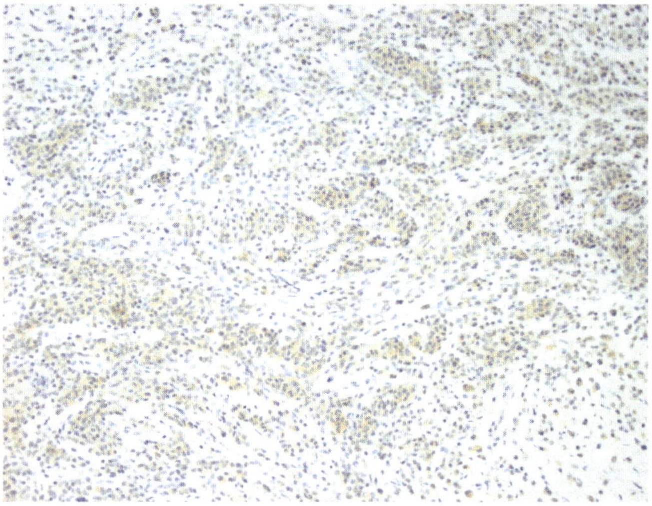

Figure 10.24 BRAFV600E immunostain is positive (X200).

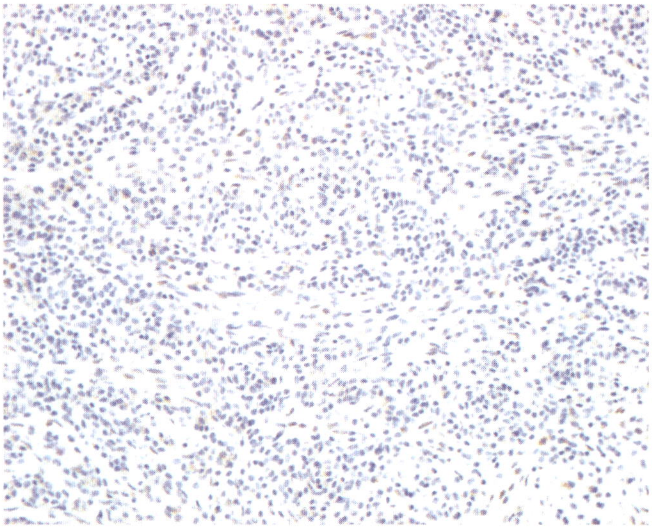

Figure 10.25 Loss of BAP1 nuclear expression is seen (X200).

Diagnosis: BAP1 tumor syndrome-associated melanocytic proliferation.

Discussion: The BAP1 tumor syndrome-associated melanocytic lesions are typically dome-shaped, 5mm in size and located on the head and neck, trunk and extremities; and the number ranged from 5 to over 50.[29–31] Histopathologically, there are two observed growth patterns: (1) a single well-demarcated dermal nodule comprised of epithelioid melanocytes and (2) more than one nest of epithelioid melanocytes in a background of a diffuse dermal melanocytic nevus, often with features of congenital onset. In the second pattern, the number and density of these "atypical" nests was variable. When the nests were prominent, the pattern was a diffuse growth in the dermis. When only a few nests were seen, the pattern was that of a dermal nevus-like proliferation with features of congenital onset.

Case 10.4

Case history: A 34-year-old woman presented with multiple "hamartomas" over her chest, back, and left shoulder. The patient has a known history of multinodular goiter status post left thyroidectomy with thyroid adenomatous nodules, intestinal hamartomatous polyps, and ductal carcinoma *in situ* of both breasts. Previous genetic testing showed a germline pathogenic *PTEN* mutation. Biopsies of several "hamartomas" were performed.

Description: Histologic sections of these lesions show a similar storiform proliferation of dermal collagen bundles (**Figure 10.26**). PTEN immunostain shows lack of staining in the dermal fibroblasts (**Figures 10.27 and 10.28**).

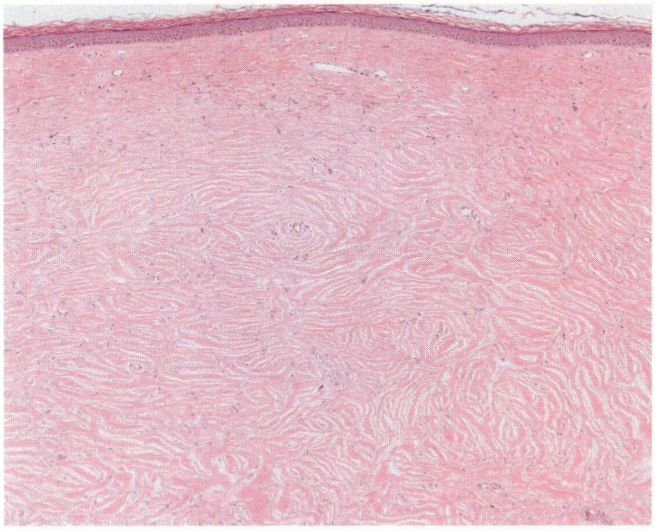

Figure 10.26 A hypocellular and storiform proliferation of collagen in the dermis (X100).

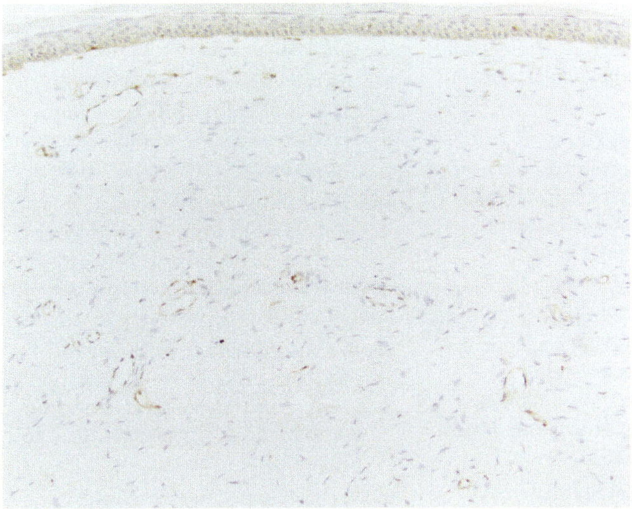

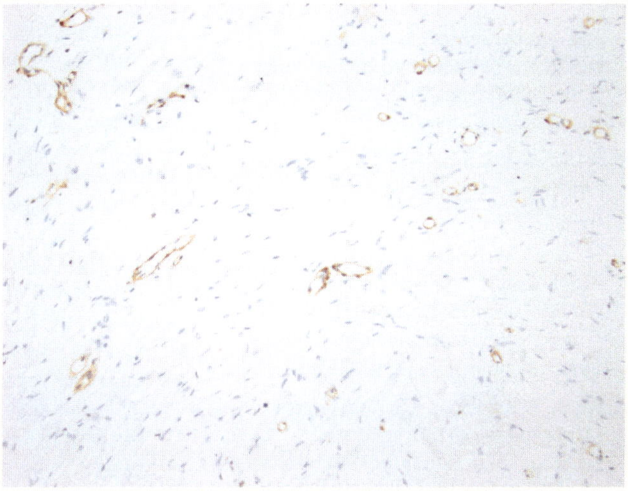

Figures 10.27 and 10.28 PTEN immunostain highlights the dermal blood vessels but not the lesional stellate fibroblasts (X200, X400).

Diagnosis: Multiple sclerotic fibromas in the setting of Cowden syndrome.

Discussion: Although trichilemmomas are the more common cutaneous tumor, this case illustrates that multiple sclerotic fibromas can be the cutaneous presentation of Cowden syndrome. The association of sclerotic fibromas and Cowden syndrome/ PTEN hamartoma syndrome was first reported by Weary and colleagues in 1972.[6] Sclerotic fibromas can present as the only cutaneous tumor type in patients with Cowden syndrome.[48] Similar to trichilemmomas, sclerotic fibromas are often sporadic tumors in healthy individuals, but they are more likely to represent Cowden syndrome in the setting of multiple lesions.[48,67-69]

References

1. Moreira L, Balaguer F, Lindor N, et al. Identification of Lynch syndrome among patients with colorectal cancer. *JAMA* 2012; **308**: 1555–65.
2. Muir EG, Bell AJ, Barlow KA. Multiple primary carcinomata of the colon, duodenum, and larynx associated with keratoacanthomata of the face. *Br J Surg* 1967; **54**: 191–5.
3. Torre D. Multiple sebaceous tumors. *Arch Dermatol* 1968; **98**: 549–51.
4. Lachiewicz AM, Wilkinson TM, Groben P, Ollila DW, Thomas NE. Muir-Torre syndrome. *Am J Clin Dermatol* 2007; **8**: 315–19.
5. Aziz S, O'Sullivan H, Heelan K, Alam A, McVeigh TP. Characterization of sebaceous and non-sebaceous cutaneous manifestations in patients with lynch syndrome: a systematic review. *Fam Cancer* 2023; **22**: 167–75.
6. Ponti G, Losi L, Di Gregorio C, et al. Identification of Muir-Torre syndrome among patients with sebaceous tumors and keratoacanthomas: role of clinical features, microsatellite instability, and immunohistochemistry. *Cancer* 2005; **103**: 1018–25.

7. Cohen PR, Kohn SR, Kurzrock R. Association of sebaceous gland tumors and internal malignancy: the Muir-Torre syndrome. *Am J Med* 1991; **90**: 606–13.
8. Abbott JJ, Hernandez-Rios P, Amirkhan RH, Hoang MP. Cystic sebaceous neoplasms in Muir-Torre syndrome. *Arch Pathol Lab Med* 2013; **127**: 614–17.
9. Rutten A, Burgdorf W, Hugel H, et al. Cystic sebaceous tumors a marker lesions for the Muir-Torre syndrome: a histopathologic and molecular genetic study. *Am J Dermatopathol* 1999; **21**: 405–13.
10. Al-Shobaili HA, AlGhamdi KM, Al-Ghamdi WA. Cystic sebaceous carcinoma: is it a constant pathognomic marker for Muir-Torre syndrome? *J Drugs Dermatol* 2007; **6**: 540–3.
11. Maloney NJ, Zacher NC, Hirotsu KE, Rajan N, Aasi SZ, Kibbi N. Comparison of clinicopathologic features, survival, and demographics in sebaceous carcinoma patients with and without Muir-Torre syndrome. *J Am Acad Dermatol* 2023; **89**: 269–73.
12. Schwartz RA, Torre DP. The Muir-Torre syndrome: a 25-year retrospect. *J Am Acad Dermatol* 1995; **33**: 90–104.
13. Hayani KM, Zelger BG, Kind P, Zelger B. Seborrheic keratosis with sebaceous differentiation, a series of 8 cases and critical review of the literature. *Am J Dermatopathol* 2021; **43**: 801–10.
14. Kruse R, Ruzicka T. DNA mismatch repair and the significance of a sebaceous skin tumor for visceral cancer prevention. *Trends Mol Med* 2004; **10**: 136–41.
15. Toon CW, Walsh MD, Chou A, et al. BRAFV600E immunohistochemistry facilitates universal screening of colorectal cancers for Lynch syndrome. *Am J Surg Pathol* 2013; **37**: 1592–602.
16. Kalloger SE, Allo G, Mulligan AM, et al. Use of mismatch repair immunohistochemistry and microsatellite instability testing: exploring Canadian practices. *Am J Surg Pathol* 2012; **36**: 560–9.
17. Shia J. Immunohistochemistry versus microsatellite instability testing for screening colorectal cancer patients at risk for hereditary nonpolyposis colorectal cancer syndrome. *J Mol Diagn* 2008; **10**: 293–300.
18. Cook S, Pethick J, Kibbi N, et al. Sebaceous carcinoma epidemiology, associated malignancies and Lynch/Muir-Torre syndrome screening in England from 2008 to 2018. *J Am Acad Dermatol* 2023: **89**: 1129–35.
19. Roberts ME, Riegert-Johnson DL, Thomas BC, et al. A clinical scoring system to identify patients with sebaceous neoplasms at risk for the Muir-Torre variant of Lynch syndrome. *Genet Med* 2014: **16**: 711–16.
20. Sinson H, Karayan-Tapon L, Godet J, Rivet P, et al. Immunohistochemistry, molecular biology and clinical scoring for the detection of Muir-Torre syndrome in cutaneous sebaceous tumors: which strategy? *Dermatology* 2023; **239**: 889–97.
21. Cornejo KM, Hutchinson L, Deng A, et al. *BRAF/KRAS* gene sequencing of sebaceous neoplasms after mismatch repair protein analysis. *Hum Pathol* 2014; **45**: 1213–20.
22. Musulén E, Sanz C, Muñoz-Mármol AM, Aurelio Ariza A. Mismatch repair protein immunohistochemistry: a useful population screening strategy for Lynch syndrome. *Hum Pathol* 2014; **45**: 1388–96.
23. Jessup CJ, Redston M, Tilton E, Reimann JD. Importance of universal mismatch repair protein immunohistochemistry in patients with sebaceous neoplasia as an initial screening tool for Muir-Torre syndrome. *Hum Pathol* 2016; **49**: 1–9.
24. Everett JN, Raymond VM, Dandapani M, et al. Screening for germline mismatch repair mutations following diagnosis of sebaceous neoplasm. *JAMA Dermatol* 2014; **150**: 1315–21.
25. Ponti G, Ponz de Leon M, Maffei S, et al. Attenuated familial adenomatous polyposis and Muir-Torre syndrome linked to compound biallelic constitutional MYH gene mutations. *Clin Genet* 2005; **68**: 442–7.
26. O'Shea AM, Cleary SP, Croitoru MA, et al. Pathological features of colorectal carcinomas in MYH-associated polyposis. *Histopathology* 2008; **53**: 184–94.
27. Singh RS, Grayson W, Redston M, et al. Site and tumor type predicts DNA mismatch repair status in cutaneous sebaceous neoplasia. *Am J Surg Pathol* 2008; **32**: 936–42.
28. Abdel-Rahman MH, Pilarski R, Cebulla CM, et al. Germline BAP1 mutation predisposes to uveal melanoma, lung adenocarcinoma, meningioma, and other cancers. *J Med Genet* 2011; **48**: 856–9.
29. Carbone M, Ferris LK, Baumann F, et al. BAP1 cancer syndrome: malignant mesotheliomas, uveal and cutaneous melanoma, and MBAITs. *J Transl Med* 2012; **10**: 179. doi: 10.1186/1479-5876-10-179.
30. Wadt K, Choi J, Chung JY, et al. A cryptic BAP1 splice mutation in a family with uveal and cutaneous melanoma, and paraganglioma. *Pigment Cell Melanoma Res* 2012; **25**: 815–18.
31. Wiesner T, Obenauf AC, Murali R, et al. Germline mutations in BAP1 predispose to melanocytic tumors. *Nat Genet* 2011; **43**: 1018–21.
32. Popova T, Hebert L, Jacquemin V, et al. Germline BAP1 mutations predispose to renal cell carcinomas. *Am J Hum Genet* 2013; **92**: 974–80.
33. Busam KJ, Sung J, Wiesner T, von Deimling A, Jungbluth A. Combined BRAFV600E-positive melanocytic lesions with large epithelioid cells lacking BAP1 expression and conventional nevomelanocytes. *Am J Surg Pathol* 2013; **37**: 193–9.
34. de la Fouchardiere A, Cabaret O, Savin L, et al. Germline BAP1 mutations predispose also to multiple basal cell carcinomas. *Clin Genet* 2015; **88**: 273–7.
35. Mochel MC, Piris A, Nose V, Hoang MP. Loss of BAP1 expression in basal cell carcinomas in patients with germline BAP1 mutations. *Am J Clin Pathol* 2015; **143**: 901–4.
36. Piris A, Mihm MC Jr, Hoang MP. BAP1 and BRAFV600E expression in benign and malignant melanocytic proliferations. *Hum Pathol* 2015; **46**: 239–45.
37. Pena-Llopis S, Vega-Rubin-de-Celis S, Liao A, et al. BAP1 loss defines a new class of renal cell carcinoma. *Nat Genet* 2011; **44**: 1018–21.
38. Ladanyi M, Zauderer MG, Krug LM, et al. New strategies in pleural mesothelioma: BAP1 and NF2 as novel targets for therapeutic development and risk assessment. *Clin Cancer Res* 2012; **18**: 4485–90.
39. Aung P, Nagarajan P, Tetzlaff M, et al. Melanoma with loss of BAP1 expression in patients with no family history of BAP1-associated cancer susceptibility syndrome: a case series. *Am J Dermatopathol* 2019; **41**: 167–79.
40. Murali R, Wilmott JS, Jakrot V, et al. BAP1 expression cutaneous melanoma: a pilot study. *Pathology* 2013; **45**: 606–9.
41. Costa S, Byrne M, Pissaloux D, et al. Melanomas associated with blue nevi or mimicking cellular blue nevi: clinical, pathologic, and molecular study of 11 cases displaying a high frequency of

GNA11 mutations, BAP1 expression loss, and a predilection for the scalp. *Am J Surg Pathol* 2016; **40**: 368–77.

42. Pilarski R. PTEN hamartoma tumor syndrome: a clinical overview. *Cancers* 2019; **11**. doi:10.3390/cancers11060844.
43. Yehia L, Keel E, Eng C. The clinical spectrum of PTEN mutations. *Annu Rev Med* 2020; **71**: 103–16.
44. Nelen MR, Padberg GW, Peeters EA, et al. Localization of the gene for Cowden disease to chromosome 10q22-23. *Nat Genet* 1996; **13**: 114–16.
45. Pilarski R, Burt R, Kohlman W, Pho L, Shannon KM, Swisher E. Cowden syndrome and the PTEN hamartoma tumor syndrome: systematic review and revised diagnostic criteria. *J Natl Cancer Inst* 2013; **105**: 1607–16.
46. Tan MH, Mester JL, Ngeow J, Rybicki LA, Orloff MS, Eng C. Lifetime cancer risks in individuals with germline PTEN mutations. *Clin Cancer Res* 2012; **18**: 400–7.
47. Jin M, Hampel H, Pilarski R, et al. Phosphatase and tensin homolog immunohistochemical staining and clinical criteria for Cowden syndrome in patients with trichilemmoma or associated lesions. *Am J Dermatopathol* 2013; **35**: 637–40.
48. Hartsough E, DeSimone MS, Lorenzo ME, et al. Utilizing PTEN immunohistochemistry as a screening test for Cowden syndrome. *Am J Clin Pathol* 2024; **161**: 490–500.
49. Shon W, Wolz MM, Sukov WR, Wieland CN, Gibson LE, Peters MS. Phosphatase and tensin homologue status in sporadic and Cowden syndrome-associated trichilemmomas: evaluation of immunohistochemistry and fluorescence in situ hybridization. *Br J Dermatol* 2014; **170**: 1201–4.
50. Zabetian S, Mehregan D. Cowden syndrome: report of two cases with immunohistochemical analysis for PTEN expression. *Am J Dermatopathol* 2012; **34**: 632–4.
51. Peiro G, Adrover E, Guijarro J, et al. Synchronous bilateral breast carcinoma in a patient with Cowden syndrome: a case report with morphologic, immunohistochemical and genetic analysis. *Breast J* 2010; **16**: 77–81.
52. Barletta JA, Bellizzi AM, Hornick JL. Immunohistochemical staining of thyroidectomy specimens for PTEN can aid in the identification of patients with Cowden syndrome. *Am J Surg Pathol* 2011; **35**: 1505–11.
53. Al-Zaid T, Ditelberg JS, Prieto VG, et al. Trichilemmomas show loss of PTEN in Cowden syndrome but only rarely in sporadic tumors. *J Cutan Pathol* 2012; **39**: 493–9.
54. Reed WB, Walker R, Horowitz R. Cutaneous leiomyomata with uterine leiomyomata. *Acta Dermatologica Venerologica* 1973; **53**: 406–16.
55. Tomlinson IP, Alam NA, Rowan AJ, et al. Germline mutations in FH predispose to dominantly inherited uterine fibroids, skin leiomyomata and papillary renal cell cancer. *Nat Genet* 2002; **30**: 406–10.
56. Bayley JP, Launonen V, Tomlinson IP. The fumarate hydratase mutation database: an online database of fumarate hydratase mutations involved in the MCUL (HLRCC) tumor syndrome and congenital fumarase deficiency. *BMC Med Genet* 2008; **9**: 20. doi: 10.1186/1471-2350-9-20.
57. Chan I, Wong T, Martinez-Mir A, Christiano AM, McGrath JA. Familial multiple cutaneous and uterine leiomyomas associated with papillary renal cell cancer. *Clin Exp Dermatol* 2005; **30**: 75–8.
58. Merino MJ, Torres-Cabala C, Pinto P, et al. The morphologic spectrum of kidney tumors in hereditary leiomyomatosis and renal cell carcinoma (HLRCC) syndrome. *Am J Surg Pathol* 2007; **31**: 1578–85.
59. Sanz-Ortega J, Vocke C, Stratton P, Linehan WM, Merino MJ. Morphologic and molecular characteristics of uterine leiomyomas in hereditary leiomyomatosis and renal cancer (HLRCC) syndrome. *Am J Surg Pathol* 2013; **37**: 74–80.
60. Alam NA, Barclay E, Rowan AJ, et al. Clinical features of multiple cutaneous and uterine leiomyomatosis: an underdiagnosed tumor syndrome. *Arch Dermatol* 2005; **141**: 199–206.
61. Joseph NM, Solomon DA, Frizzell N, Rabban JT, Zaloudek C, Garg K. Morphology and immunohistochemistry for 2SC and FH aid in detection of fumarate hydratase gene aberrations in uterine leiomyomas from young patients. *Am J Surg Pathol* 2015; **39**: 1529–39.
62. Ahvenainen T, Kaukomaa J, Kämpjärvi K, et al. Comparison of 2SC, AKR1B10, and FH antibodies as potential biomarkers for FH-deficient uterine leiomyomas. *Am J Surg Pathol* 2022; **46**: 537–46.
63. Llamas-Velasco M, Requena L, Kutzner H, et al. Fumarate hydratase immunohistochemical staining may help to identify patients with multiple cutaneous and uterine leiomyomatosis (MCUL) and hereditary leiomyomatosis and renal cell cancer (HLRCC) syndrome. *J Cutan Pathol* 2014; **41**: 859–65.
64. Bueow B, Cohen J, Zoltan N, et al. Immunohistochemistry for 2-succinocysteine (2SC) and fumarate hydratase (FH) in cutaneous leiomyomas may aid in identification of patients with HLRCC (hereditary leiomyomatosis and renal cell carcinoma syndrome). *Am J Surg Pathol* 2016; **40**: 982–988.
65. Jin M, Hampel H, Zhou X, et al. BRAF V600E mutation analysis simplifies the testing algorithm for Lynch syndrome. *Am J Clin Pathol* 2013; **140**: 177–83.
66. Weary PE, Gorlin RJ, Gentry WC, Comer JE, Greer KE. Multiple hamartoma syndrome (Cowden's disease). *Arch Dermatol* 1972; **106**: 682–90.
67. Requena L, Gutiérrez J, Sánchez Yus E. Multiple sclerotic fibromas of the skin: a cutaneous marker of Cowden's disease. *J Cutan Pathol* 1992; **19**: 346–51.
68. Al-Daraji WI, Ramsay HM, Ali RBM. Storiform collagenoma as a clue for Cowden disease or PTEN hamartoma tumour syndrome. *J Clin Pathol* 2007; **60**: 840–2.
69. Kieselova K, Santiago F, Henrique M, Cunha MF. Multiple sclerotic fibromas of the skin: an important clue for the diagnosis of Cowden syndrome. *BMJ Case Rep* 2017; 2017. doi:10.1136/bcr-2017-221695.

Chapter 11

Immunobullous Disorders

Mai P. Hoang

Introduction

The technique of immunofluorescence pioneered by Coon, Kaplan, and Jordon[1–3] is broadly used in clinical and research laboratories. In 1941 Albert Coons and his team demonstrated that antibodies that were labeled with fluorescent tag maintained specificity for their antigen.[1] Beutner and Jordon[4] in 1964 demonstrated by indirect immunofluorescence the presence of autoantibodies in the sera of pemphigus patients. Jordon et al.[3] subsequently demonstrated the patterns of immunoglobulin deposition of pemphigus and pemphigoid by direct immunofluorescence in 1971. Improvement in cryostat sectioning, fluorescent microscopy, fluorochromes, and automated staining systems has advanced the role of immunofluorescence in clinical and research laboratories.[5] Direct immunofluorescence (DIF) is an invaluable aid in classifying immunobullous disorders. When the histologic features are inconclusive or not available, the diagnosis can often be made based solely on the DIF findings. In addition to blistering disorders, immunofluorescence studies can be helpful in the diagnosis of vasculitis and connective tissue disease including lupus erythematosus, dermatomyositis, and mixed connective tissue disease (**Table 11.1**).

Table 11.1 Summary of target antigens, direct and indirect NaCl-split skin immunofluorescence results

	Target antigen	Direct immunofluorescence results	Indirect immunofluorescence or NaCl-split skin results
Subcorneal			
IgA pemphigus	Dsc1	IgA intercellular deposition	Intercellular deposition
Pemphigus foliaceus	Dsg1	IgG, C3 intercellular deposition	IgG intercellular deposition
Intraepidermal			
Pemphigus vulgaris		IgG, C3 intercellular deposition	IgG intercellular deposition
Mucosal dominant type	Dsg3		
Mucocutaneous type	Dsg3, Dsg1		
Cutaneous type	Dsg3, Dsg1		
Pemphigus vegetans		IgG, C3 intercellular deposition	IgG intercellular deposition
Hallopeau type	Dsg3, Dsg1, Dsc1, Dsc3		
Neumann type	Dsg3, Dsg1, Dsc1, Dsc3		
Pemphigus erythematosus	Desmoglein 1	IgG, C3 intercellular and granular basement membrane deposition	IgG intercellular deposition
Paraneoplastic pemphigus	Plectin, epiplakin, desmoplakin I/II, A2ML1, periplakin, envoplakin, Dsg1, Dsg3, Dsc1–3, BP180, BP230, transglutaminase 1	IgG, C3 intercellular and granular basement membrane deposition	IgG intercellular deposition

Table 11.1 (cont.)

	Target antigen	Direct immunofluorescence results	Indirect immunofluorescence or NaCl-split skin results
Pemphigus herpetiformis	Dsg1, Dsg3, Dsc1–3	IgG, C3 intercellular deposition	IgG intercellular deposition
Drug-induced pemphigus	Dsg1	IgG, C3 intercellular deposition	IgG intercellular deposition
Subepidermal			
Bullous pemphigoid	NC16A domain of BPAg2 (180 kDa or collagen XVII) and BPAg1 (230 kDa) LAD1 (ladinin)	IgG and C3 linear basement membrane deposition	Linear IgG on epidermal side or on both side of blister
Mucous membrane pemphigoid	C-terminal domain of BPAg2 (180 kDa or collagen XVII)	IgG, IgA, C3, and infrequently IgM linear basement membrane deposition	Linear IgG on epidermal side of blister
Laminin 5	Linear IgG on dermal side of blister		
Mucous membrane pemphigoid, oral subtype	Alpha–6-integrin		Linear IgG on epidermal side of blister
Mucous membrane pemphigoid, ocular subtype	Beta–4-integrin	IgA > C3 and IgG linear basement membrane deposition	Linear IgG on epidermal side of blister
Pemphigoid gestationis	NC16A domain of BPAg2 and BPAg1	C3 > IgG linear basement membrane deposition	Linear C3 on epidermal side of blister
Anti-p200 pemphigoid	Laminin gamma–1 Laminin beta 4	IgG, C3 linear basement membrane deposition	Linear IgG on dermal side of blister
Linear IgA disease	97-kDa and 1200kDa LAD1 (ladinin)	IgA > IgG ≫ C3 linear basement membrane deposition	Linear IgG on epidermal side of blister
Collagen VII	Linear IgG on dermal side of blister		
Epidermolysis bullosa acquisita	Collagen VII	IgG > C3 linear basement membrane deposition	Linear IgG on dermal side of blister
Bullous lupus erythematosus	Collagen VII	IgG, IgM, C3 > IgA linear or granular basement membrane deposition	Linear IgG on dermal side of blister
Chronic cutaneous lupus erythematosus		IgM, IgG, C3 granular basement membrane deposition of involved skin	
Dermatomyositis		IgM and C3 granular basement membrane deposition	
Connective tissue disease		IgM and C3 granular basement membrane deposition	
Porphyria cutanea tarda		IgG, IgM, IgA and C3 linear basement membrane and dermal vascular deposition	
Dermatitis herpetiformis	Epidermal transglutaminase	IgA > C3 granular papillary dermal deposition	
Lichen planus pemphigoid	NC16A4 domain of BP180 BP230	IgG, C3 linear basement membrane deposition	Linear IgG on epidermal side of blister
Vasculitis			
Vasculitis		IgG and/or IgM, IgA, C3 in early lesions	
IgA vasculitis (Henoch–Schonlein purpura)	none	IgA and C3 vascular deposition	

NC: noncollagenous, Dsg: desmoglein, Dsc: desmocollin

Methodology

Contrary to immunohistochemistry, immunofluorescence techniques utilize fluorescent-labeled antibodies in detecting target antigens. Either a single fluorophore-labeled antibody or a fluorophore-labeled secondary antibody against the Fc domain of an unlabeled primary antibody is used. When irradiated at certain wavelength, the molecules of certain fluorochrome become "excited" and jump to a higher yet less stable energy level. When spontaneously returning to their basic state, the emitted fluorescence has a lower energy thus longer wavelength than the excitation light. This shift in wavelength from short to long during fluorescence was described by Sir George Stokes in 1852.[6] The ideal fluorochrome would possess an absorption peak at an excitation wavelength and emission spectrum that would fall within the range of the detection instrument. Currently used fluorochromes, fluorescein isothiocyanate (FITC) and tetramethyl rhodamine isothiocyanate (TRITC), produce apple-green color and red color, respectively. The fluorochromes are chemically conjugated to antibodies which bind to the antigen of interest. Most frequently used is the following method: the primary and unlabeled antibody binds to the molecule of interest. A secondary antibody or anti-immunoglobulin antibody is tagged with the fluorescent dye and binds to the constant region of the primary antibody. The markers are detected visually by a fluorescence or confocal microscope. A fluorescence microscope has a mercury-vapor or xenon light source, exciter filter to shine light with appropriate wavelength on the tissue slide, and barrier filter to allow only fluorescent light.

Autofluorescence in cells due to flavin coenzymes (FAD and FMN) and reduced pyridine nucleotides (NADH) can interfere with interpretation. Autofluorescence can be over-interpreted as being positive, especially scalp biopsy for connective tissue disease or discoid lupus erythematosus. Other limiting factors of immunofluorescence techniques include the specificity of the antibodies, the specimen preparation, and photobleaching. Since fluorescence excitation generates reactive oxygen species, the fluorochrome is photochemically destroyed.

In DIF, the fluorescent-tagged antibodies bind the target antigens. A fluorophore-labeled secondary antibody would bind to the Fc portion of the autoantibody, allowing visualization with a fluorescent microscope. DIF studies require fresh tissue and specialized equipment. Outdated transported media can have a wide range in pH which can interfere with results. Transported media include Zeus's fixative, Michel's media (both contain ammonium sulfate, citrate buffer, and cysteine protease inhibitor) and saline. Skin samples are washed in saline to remove excess salts from the transport medium. Inadvertent exposure to formalin appears to affect immunofluorescence results for pemphigus more than pemphigoid cases.[7] The skin samples are then frozen in liquid nitrogen prior to sectioning. The tissue sections are incubated with fluorescence tagged antibodies (fluorescein isothiocyanate, FITC) directed against IgG, IgA, IgM, C3, fibrinogen, and albumin. The slides are examined under a microscope with an ultraviolet light source and appropriate filters.

Indirect immunofluorescence (IIF) studies screen blood samples for circulating autoantibodies and monitors treatment such as pemphigus vulgaris. Serum is submitted for IIF in a red top tube. In detecting circulating autoantibodies in immunobullous diseases, sections of normal human skin or monkey esophagus is incubated with the patient's serum. The present autoantibodies would bind to the target antigen. Monkey or guinea pig esophagus or rat bladder is the substrate for indirect assay. In salt-split skin indirect assay, normal skin is the substrate of IIF and is incubated with a 1-M solution of sodium chloride creating a subepidermal blister. The upper aspect of lamina lucida and the hemidesmosomes including bullous pemphigoid antigens are attached to the epidermis, whereas the laminin 5, the lamina densa, and anchoring fibrils are attached to the dermal side.[8]

11.1 Biopsy Procurement

For most cases, perilesional skin or mucosa would be the best site for biopsy. Biopsy from areas of erosions, ulcers, and bullae would best be avoided. For bullous pemphigoid, lesional nonbullous skin biopsy is preferred over perilesional or normal skin. In the setting of lupus erythematosus and connective tissue disease, involved skin or active borders would be the preferred sites. One should indicate on the requisition form whether the site is involved or uninvolved, exposed, or nonexposed skin. For vasculitis, the erythematous or active border of a new lesion, less than 48 hours old, is preferred to minimize false negative DIF results. The older the lesions the greater the chance of the DIF results being falsely negative. Involved skin would be the preferable site for porphyria cutanea tarda and lichen planus.

11.2 Components of the Basement Membrane Zone

Two major cell adhesion structures are desmosomes which connect epidermal keratinocytes and hemidesmosomes which connect epidermal keratinocytes to underlying basement membrane (**Figure 11.1**). Desmosomal cadherins are transmembrane glycoproteins, critical components of desmosomes. They include desmogleins 1–4 (Dsg 1–4), desmocollins 1–3 (Dsc 1–3), and plakin family (epiplakin, desmoplakin I/II, envoplakin and periplakin, plakoglobin and plakophilins.[9] Components of hemidesmosomes include plectin and BP230 at intracellular attachment plaques, BP180 and alpha6 beta4 integrin linking keratinocytes and extracellular matrix proteins (laminin 332, laminin gamma-1, type IV collagen, type VII collagen). BPAg1 (BP230) is intracellular and associated with hemidesmosomes. BPAg2 (BP180) has both intracellular and extracellular components. Laminin 5 (laminin 332) locates in the lamina lucida. Ladinin (LAD-1), a component of anchoring filaments, is located in the lamina lucida beneath the hemidesmosomes. Epidermolysis bullosa acquisita antigen, noncollagenous domain of type VII collagen (145 kDa and 290 kDa), locates within and subjacent to the lamina densa.

11.3 Pemphigus

IgA pemphigus

IgA pemphigus is a rare vesiculopustular disease caused by IgA autoantibodies directed against desmosomal or non-desmosomal antigens present in the epidermis. It has been reported under a number of names: intercellular IgA dermatosis, intercellular IgA vesiculopustular dermatosis, intraepidermal neutrophilic IgA dermatosis, intraepidermal IgA pustulosis, IgA pemphigus foliaceus, and IgA herpetiform pemphigus.[10] IgA pemphigus is currently divided into two subtypes with the first being subcorneal pustular dermatosis-type (SPD-type) with desmocollin 1 as target antigen.[10] The second subtype is intraepidermal neutrophilic IgA dermatosis-type (IEN-type). Although the target antigen of IEN-type has not been fully characterized, studies have reported IgA antibodies directed against desmoglein-1, desmoglein-3, desmocollin 1–3, and non-desmosomal cell surface proteins. It is likely an unknown non-desmosomal protein documented by immunoelectron microscopy.[11]

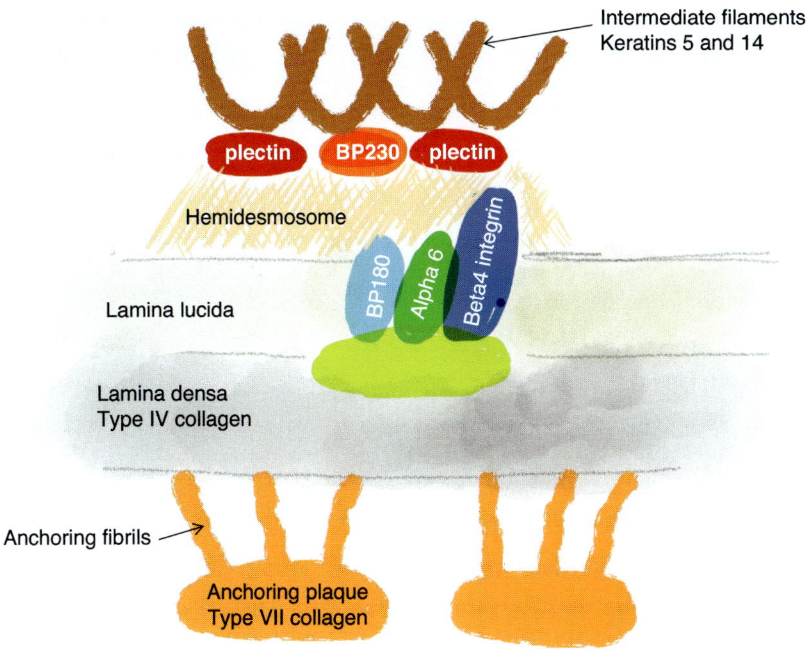

Figure 11.1 Components of the basement membrane zone.

IgA pemphigus affects individuals between 40 and 60 years of age and more women than men.[11] The trunk is the most affected site, followed by the extremities.[10] Initial pustules are seen at the periphery of erythematous annular plaques. These lesions on trunk and proximal extremities often develop into annular or circinate lesions with central crusts. The scalp, postauricular, and intertriginous areas may be affected as well as mucosal sites.[10]

There is an association of IgA pemphigus with various solid tumor, hematologic malignancies including multiple myeloma and diffuse large B-cell lymphoma, and lymphoproliferative disorders.[10,12,13] Association with ulcerative colitis, rheumatoid arthritis, Sjogren syndrome, Crohn's disease, myasthenia gravis, and other systemic diseases has been reported.[10] It can be a cutaneous side effect of immune checkpoint inhibitor.[14]

Histologic Features

Subcorneal pustules containing neutrophils are seen in SPD-type IgA pemphigus while pustules are noted in the entire, mid, or lower epidermis in IEN-type IgA pemphigus. Acantholysis is not a prominent feature as in other types of pemphigus. A mixed infiltrate of neutrophils and eosinophils can be seen.[10]

Direct Immunofluorescence

On DIF intercellular IgA deposition is noted within the epidermis. IgG and C3 can sometimes be present but with weaker intensity. The IgA deposition is seen the upper aspect of the epidermis in the SPD-type in contrast to lower aspect or full-thickness epidermis in the IEN-type.[15] DIF patterns include intercellular IgA alone; combined intercellular IgA and IgG; combined intercellular IgA, IgG, and C3; combined intercellular IgA and C3; and combined intercellular IgA and IgM.[10]

Indirect Immunofluorescence

IIF using the patient's sera and monkey esophagus, or other epithelial substrate would show an intercellular pattern; however, the sensitivity of IIF has been reported to be approximately 50–67%.[10,16] Enzyme linked immunosorbent assay (ELISA) would be the better diagnostic test.[15]

IgG/IgA Pemphigus

Since some patient with clinical features of IgA pemphigus yet with autoantibodies to both epidermal (desmoglein 1, desmoglein 3, and desmocollins 1–3) and basement membrane-associated (BP180) antigens has been reported, Geller et al.[17] have proposed that there exists a spectrum of IgA pemphigus-like diseases. In 2005 Bruckner et al.[18] reported a case of both IgA and IgG anti-desmoglein 3 antibodies in a child raising the possibility of an atypical IgG/IgA pemphigus. Since then, there have been additional reports; however, whether IgG/ IgA pemphigus is a distinct entity remains unclear.[19,20] Mentink et al.[21] performed anti-desmoglein-1 and anti-desmoglein-3 IgA ELISA tests on sera of 100 patients with pemphigus (34 pemphigus foliaceus, 58 pemphigus vulgaris, and 8 paraneoplastic pemphigus). Positive IgA anti-desmoglein results were noted in a high number of these supposedly IgG-mediated pemphigus cases. The authors concluded that perhaps there is a spectrum ranging from IgG to mixed IgG/IgA to mainly IgA pemphigus.[21] On the other hand, in a 20-year retrospective review at the Mayo Clinic, Toosi and colleagues[22] compared the clinical, histologic, and immunopathologic features of 13 patients with IgG/IgA pemphigus, 7 with IgA pemphigus, and 26 with pemphigus vulgaris. The clinical features and treatment response of IgG/IgA pemphigus were more similar to those of pemphigus vulgaris, whereas patients with IgA pemphigus invariably presented with pustular lesions and more frequent intertriginous involvement. The authors concluded that IgG/IgA pemphigus behaves similarly to pemphigus vulgaris and clinicopathologically distinct from IgA pemphigus.

Reported cases have clinical features resembling IgA pemphigus, pemphigus vulgaris, pemphigus foliaceus, or mixed. There are two main presentations: (1) annular erythema with blisters in 30–45% of patients, and (2) discrete erosions or blisters. There can be mucosal involvement in 40–61% of IgG/IgA pemphigus patients, while it is seen in about 13% and 8% of IgA pemphigus and pemphigus herpetiformis, respectively.[23] In a series of 30 cases Hashimoto et al.[24] reported the mean age of 55.6 years, no gender predilection, and common affected sites being trunk and extremities.

IgG and IgA antibodies in patients with IgG/IgA pemphigus could target desmoglein 1, desmoglein 3, and/or desmocollins 1–3 to a different extent, which may account for the mixed clinical presentations of the disease.[25]

Histologic Features

Histopathology of these cases varies from subcorneal to intraepidermal bullous dermatosis to subepidermal bullous dermatosis, parallels with the varied clinical presentation. In a series of 22 patients with IgG/IgA pemphigus by Cho et al.,[23] an intraepidermal vesiculation is the most common histologic appearance. Both neutrophils and eosinophils can be seen within the blister space and in the dermis in IgG/IgA pemphigus, while eosinophils are predominant in pemphigus herpetiformis.

Direct Immunofluorescence

IgG and IgA intercellular deposition is seen within the epidermis on DIF studies.[22] IgA deposition can be seen at the epidermis, lower epidermis, or the entire epidermis.[24] C3 deposition can be seen in 80–100% of cases.[23] In contrast, IgG and C3 deposition is noted in 20% and 14%, respectively, in IgA pemphigus.[23]

Indirect Immunofluorescence

Circulating IgG and IgA autoantibodies to epidermal intracellular spaces can be detected with IIF method against monkey esophageal epithelium. In NaCl-split human skin, IgG and IgA reactivity is seen at the epidermal side of the blister in 12% and 19%, respectively.[24]

Pemphigus Foliaceus

Both nonendemic and endemic pemphigus foliaceus is caused by autoantibodies against extracellular domains 1 and 2 of desmoglein 1.[26] Recently, endemic pemphigus foliaceus (*fogo selvagem*) has been suggested to be triggered by environmental antigen with molecular mimicry with desmoglein 1.[27] Exposure to sand flies (*Lutzomyia longipalpis*), kissing bugs (reduviids), and black flies (simuliids) is likely linked to endemic pemphigus foliaceus.[27] There is a strong association with HLA-DRB1*0102, 0404, and 1402 alleles.[28]

Pemphigus foliaceus typically presents as a generalized eruption. Uncommonly the disease can be localized affecting the face, scalp, and trunk.[29] Rarely pemphigus foliaceus can present as generalized erythroderma.[30]

Histologic Features

The histology of endemic cases is diverse and can be typical, lupus erythematosus-like, chronic dermatosis-like, polymorphous light eruption-like, psoriasis-like, and subcorneal pustular dermatosis-like.[31] In the typical presentation, acantholysis is noted at the granular layer of the epidermis (**Figure 11.2**).

Direct Immunofluorescence

Epidermal intercellular IgG and C3 depositions are seen on DIF studies (**Figure 11.3**).

Indirect Immunofluorescence

Circulating IgG autoantibodies to epidermal intracellular spaces can be detected with IIF method against monkey esophageal epithelium.

Pemphigus Vulgaris

Pemphigus vulgaris, the most frequent type of pemphigus, is characterized by development of blisters above the basal layer of the epidermis because of autoantibodies against desmoglein 3, a 130-kDa glycoprotein, and less commonly desmoglein 1, a 160-kDa, components of desmosomes. Loss of keratinocyte-to-keratinocyte interactions result in epidermal acantholysis and subsequently blisters. While desmoglein 1 is expressed throughout the epidermis, desmoglein 3 is expressed mainly in basal layer of the epidermis. Factors that can induce or exacerbate pemphigus are thiol group drugs (penicillamine, captopril, and rifampicin), vaccines, infections, food, radiation therapy, pregnancy, emotional distress, and physical injury.[32] While there is a genetic predisposition with strong association with some HLA

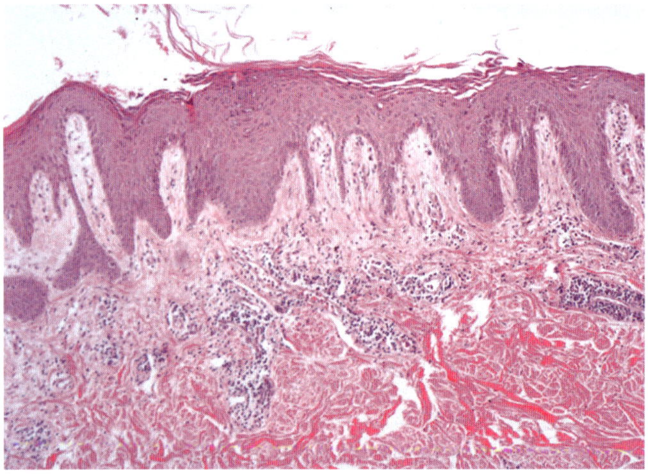

Figure 11.2 Pemphigus foliaceus. Acantholysis is noted at the granular layer of the epidermis (×100).

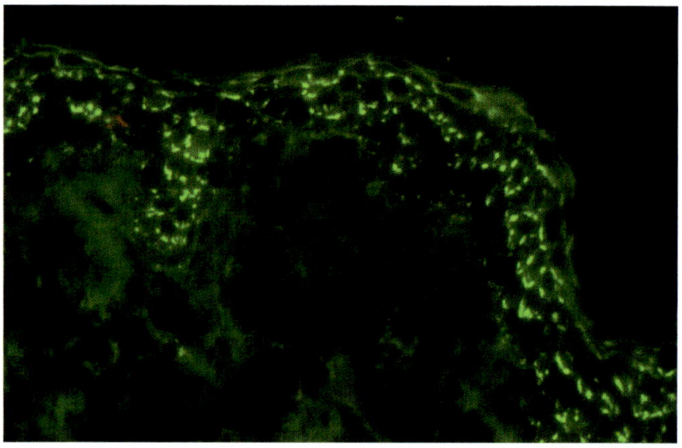

Figure 11.3 Pemphigus foliaceus. Intercellular IgG deposition is seen within the epidermis in direct immunofluorescence studies.

antigens, several drugs such as captopril, penicillamine, aspirin, and rifampin; autoimmune thyroid disease, rheumatoid arthritis, and type I diabetes have also been reported as etiologic factors.[33,34]

Pemphigus vulgaris typically affects women in their fifth or sixth decade. Pemphigus vulgaris patients can have mainly mucosal disease or mucocutaneous disease. Flaccid, thin-walled, and easily ruptured blisters resulting in erosions are seen on scalp, face, and upper trunk. Nikolsky's sign (detachment of the superficial epidermis from the underlying dermis when the examining finger is slid over the skin surface) is present. Genital involvement can be seen in 44% of patients in a series of pemphigus vulgaris patients from Turkey.[35] Pediatric pemphigus vulgaris affects the genital area and eyes more frequently than adults' cases.[36] Atypical presentations of pemphigus vulgaris include pemphigus vegetans, pemphigus herpetiformis, and paraneoplastic pemphigus. In a meta-analysis of 6,679 patients from 16 studies, malignant tumors were seen in 8% of patients with pemphigus (pemphigus vulgaris, 7%; pemphigus foliaceus, 10%; other types of pemphigus, 12%).[37]

In a retrospective review of 170 patients from 134 studies in the literature, Ghaedi et al.[38] reported pemphigus vulgaris to be the most common drug-induced pemphigus, followed by pemphigus foliaceus, and then paraneoplastic pemphigus. The most commonly offending drugs are penicillamine, captopril, and bucillamine.[38]

Histologic Features

In classic cases of pemphigus vulgaris, histologic sections would show intraepidermal acantholysis resulting in a blister right above the basal keratinocytes imparting a "tombstoning" appearance. The acantholysis often extends into hair follicular epithelium (**Figure 11.4**). Striking epidermal papillomatosis or pseudoepitheliomatous hyperplasia, and prominent intraepidermal microabscesses containing eosinophils and neutrophils associated with necrotic keratinocytes are seen in pemphigus vegetans.

Direct Immunofluorescence

Epidermal intercellular IgG and C3 depositions are seen on DIF studies. When the epidermis is not present for evaluation,

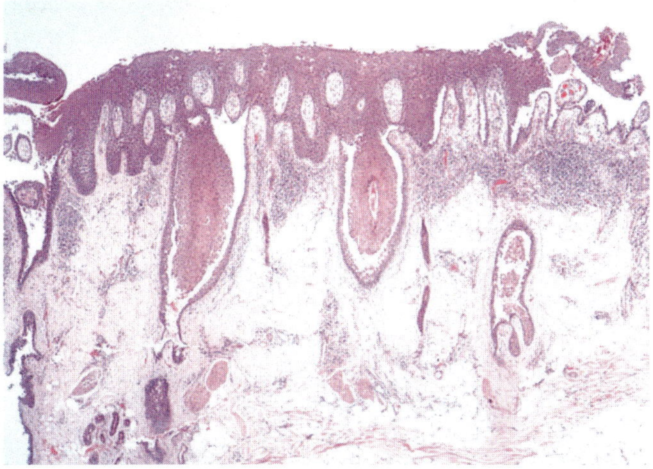

Figure 11.4 Pemphigus vulgaris. Suprabasilar acantholysis is noted within the epidermis and hair follicular epithelium (×100).

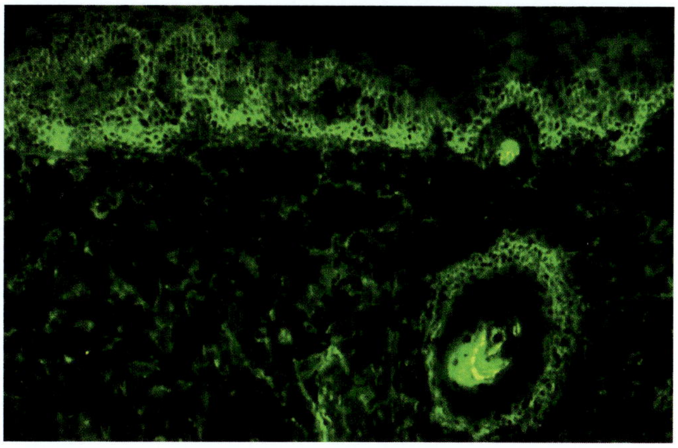

Figure 11.5 Pemphigus vulgaris. Intercellular IgG deposition is seen within the epidermis and within hair follicular epithelium in direct immunofluorescence studies.

the epithelium of hair follicles and/or eccrine glands do exhibit intercellular IgG and C3 deposition (**Figure 11.5**); thus, these findings can be of help in rendering a diagnosis.[39] DIF can be performed on plucked hair follicles as an alternative test since immunofluorescence of outer root sheath of hair follicles can be of diagnostic help.[40,41] In a recent retrospective study by Giurdanella et al.[42] of 233 pemphigus patients with available DIF results and serum for analyses, 9% and 6% of cases would be misdiagnosed if relying mainly on IIF or ELISA, respectively; thus, this study highlights the diagnostic importance of DIF studies.

Indirect Immunofluorescence

Circulating autoantibodies to epidermal intracellular spaces can be detected with IIF method against monkey esophageal epithelium in approximately 80% of cases; and the titer correlates with the clinical activity of the disease. Treatment response and disease activity can be monitored by ELISA for IgG antibodies to desmoglein 1 and desmoglein 3.

Immunohistochemistry

IgG4 immunostain has been shown to be a sensitive and specific test for diagnosing pemphigus in the setting of active lesions when additional frozen tissue is not available for DIF examination.[43] C4d immunostain showed similar sensitivity (77%) and specificity (98%) as IgG4.[44] C3d exhibited low sensitivity (21%); thus, it is not of diagnostic help (**Table 11.2**).[43–47]

Pemphigus Vegetans

Pemphigus vegetans is least common variant of pemphigus vulgaris, comprising of approximately 1–2%.[48] Vegetative plaques are seen in the intertriginous areas (groins, inguinal area, and axilla) and oral mucosa.[48] Less commonly affected sites include scalp, soles of feet, nose, vagina, and even conjunctiva.[49] There are two clinical forms, Hallopeau and Neumann types. While Hallopeau type presents with pustules which heal as vegetative plaques, the Newmann type is characterized as vegetation developed during a blister eruption. Desmoglein 3 and desmoglein 1 are the most common offending autoantibodies, but desmocollins 1–3 have been reported.[50,51]

Table 11.2 Immunostains in the diagnosis of pemphigus[43-47]

	N	Antibody clone	Sensitivity	Specificity
IgG4 (Zhang 2012)[43]	18 (12 PV, 6 PF)		72%	97%
C4d (Villani 2016)[44]	22 (19PV, 3 PNP)		77%	98%
C3d (Pfaltz 2009)[45]	14 PV		21%	
IgG4 (Karabag 2024)[46]	11 pemphigus	MRQ–44, Cell Marque	9.1%	97.4%
IgG (Karabag 2024)[46]	11 pemphigus	Cell Marque	70%	89.6%
C3d (Wu 2024)[47]	63 pemphigus	Abcam, ab136916	71%	96.4%

PV: pemphigus vulgaris, PF: pemphigus foliaceus, PNP: paraneoplastic pemphigus

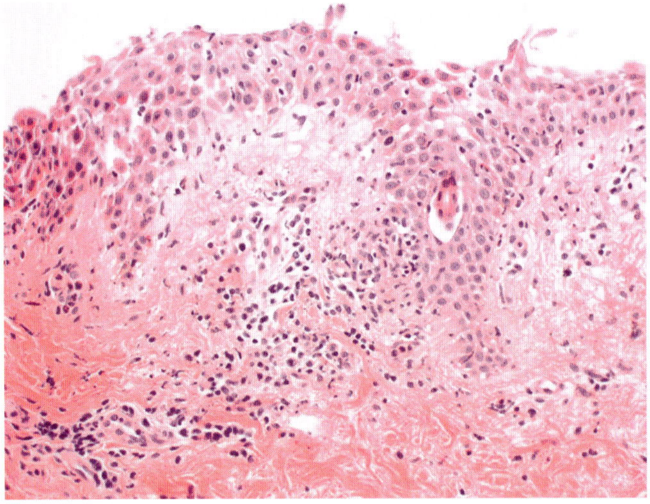

Figure 11.6 Pemphigus erythematosus. Histologic features resembling pemphigus foliaceus with superficial acantholysis noted within the epidermis (×200).

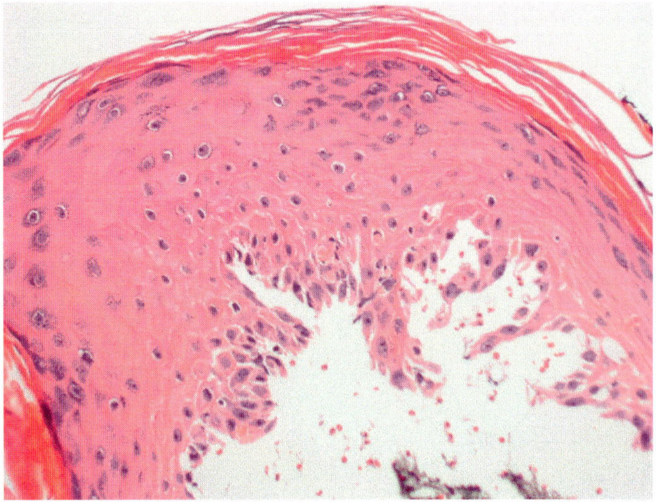

Figure 11.7 Pemphigus erythematosus. Necrotic keratinocyte are noted at the basal aspect of the detached epidermis (×200).

Histologic Features

Hyperkeratosis, epidermal papillomatosis, and hyperplasia with acantholysis are the typical histologic features. Follicular involvement is common. A prominent eosinophilic response characterized by eosinophilic spongiosis, intraepidermal eosinophilic microabscesses, and dermal eosinophils is seen, especially in the Hallopeau type. Neutrophils are more prominent in the Newmann type.[48]

Direct Immunofluorescence

Similar to pemphigus vulgaris, intercellular IgG and C3 deposition within the epidermis is seen in pemphigus vegetans.

Pemphigus Erythematosus

It was first described in 1926 by Senear and Usher as a combination of pemphigus vulgaris and lupus erythematosus.[52] When antibodies to desmosomal cadherin desmoglein 1 versus desmoglein 3 were characterized for pemphigus foliaceus and pemphigus vulgaris, respectively; pemphigus erythematosus was classified as a variant of pemphigus foliaceus with features of both pemphigus and lupus erythematosus.[53] High doses of ultraviolet irradiation have been postulated to induce cleavage of the desmoglein 1 ectodomain.[54] HLA haplotype (A10, A26, and DRW6) associations in some patients have raised the possibility of genetic predisposition. A variety of drugs (penicillamine, propanolol, captropril, and others) and co-existing autoimmune diseases such as myasthenia gravis and thymoma have been reported as etiologic factors.[55]

Pemphigus erythematosus exhibits clinical as well as histologic features of both pemphigus foliaceus (flaccid blisters on erythematous base on photodistributed areas, superficial epidermal acantholysis) and those typical of lupus erythematosus (positive antinuclear antigen, lupus band tests, and interface dermatitis). In a retrospective review of over 100 cases in the literature, Hobbs et al.[56] reported a median age of 57 years (range: 5–84 years) and a slight female predominance. The cutaneous lesions of pemphigus erythematosus are scaly erythematous plaques mimicking those of lupus erythematosus or seborrheic keratosis. The location of skin involvement in descending order includes trunk, face, extremities, and scalp. Oral involvement was noted in approximately 9%.

Histologic Features

Skin lesions can show acantholysis at the granular layer of the epidermis typical of pemphigus foliaceus (**Figure 11.6**). Taken from other areas, the skin biopsies can show an interface dermatitis evidenced by necrotic keratinocytes at the dermal-epidermal junction, follicular plugging and dermal mucin deposition characteristic of lupus erythematosus (**Figures 11.7 and 11.8**).

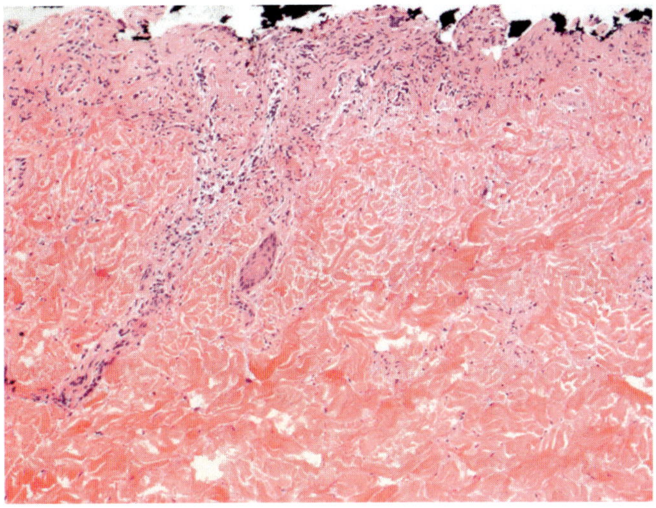

Figure 11.8 Pemphigus erythematosus. Perivascular inflammation and dermal mucin deposition are noted within the dermis (×100).

Direct Immunofluorescence

DIF studies show epidermal and intercellular IgG and C3 deposition. Concurrent granular and linear IgG and C3 (sometimes IgM and IgA) deposition, similar to the "lupus band," are also noted at the basement membrane zone in 83% of uninvolved and sun-exposed skin biopsies and in 23–40% of uninvolved and non-sun-exposed skin biopsies.[55,57] This mixed pattern of DIF findings is similar to that seen in paraneoplastic pemphigus (**Figure 11.9**).

Indirect Immunofluorescence

Intercellular pattern is seen on IIF when sera are examined for autoantibodies. Serum autoantibodies by ELISA assays can be used to monitor disease activity and treatment response.

Paraneoplastic Pemphigus

The term "paraneoplastic pemphigus" was first coined in 1990 by Anhalt et al. when they reported five cases of pemphigus associated with an underlying lymphoproliferative disease. Others have suggested the name paraneoplastic autoimmune multiorgan syndrome since the disease does not only involve the skin but also other organ systems.[59,60] There is invariably an association with malignancy. Non-Hodgkin lymphoma, chronic lymphocytic leukemia, and Castleman disease are the most associated neoplasm with lymphoproliferative disorders noted in 84% of patients.[61,62] There may be a genetic predisposition with increased susceptibility with HLA-DRB1*03 allele in French Caucasian patients and HLA-Cw*14 allele in Chinese patients.[62] The detection of anti-plakin antibodies by immunofluorescence, immunoblotting, immunoprecipitation, or enzyme-linked immunosorbent assay (ELISA) is needed for diagnosis.[60] Svodoba et al.[60] reviewed 265 cases in the literature and proposed modification of the diagnostic criteria established by Camisa and Helm[59] in 1993 which require either three major criteria, or two major and two minor for diagnosis. The major criteria include: (1) mucous membrane involvement with or without cutaneous lesions, (2) associated internal malignancy, and (3) serologic evidence of anti-plakin antibodies. The minor criteria include: (1) histologic features of acantholysis and/or interface lichenoid dermatitis, and (2) intercellular and basement membrane immunoreactant deposition on DIF.[59,60]

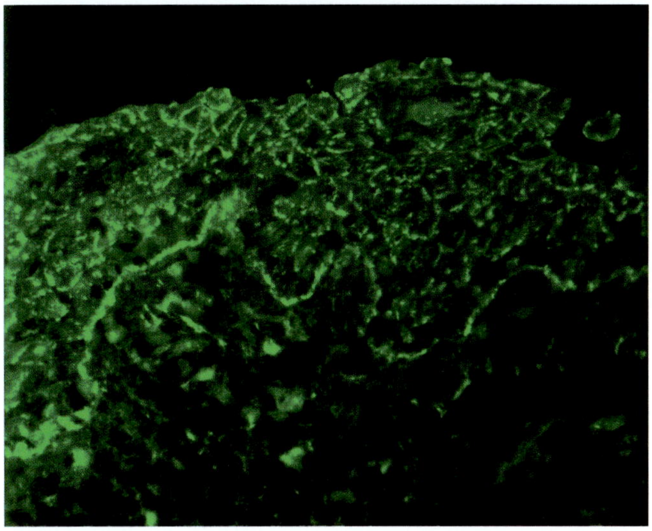

Figure 11.9 Pemphigus erythematosus. Intercellular IgG deposition is noted within the epidermis as well as granular band at the basement membrane zone in direct immunofluorescence studies.

A painful and progressive stomatitis is often the initial presentation. Ocular involvement can be seen in 70% of cases. The cutaneous presentation is polymorphic and can be pemphigus-like, bullous pemphigoid-like, erythema multiforme-like, and graft-versus-host disease-like. In addition to the skin, the disease can affect the gastrointestinal, pulmonary, renal and neurologic system.[63] Nail involvement including onycholysis, onychomadesis, anonychia, and periungual edema can rarely be seen.[62]

Histologic Features

The histologic features would correspond to the varied clinical appearance (**see Case Study 1**). An intraepidermal blister would be seen in the pemphigus-like cases, a subepidermal blister in the bullous pemphigoid-like cases, and an interface dermatitis without epidermal separation in the erythema multiforme-like and graft-versus-host like cases.[64] Fifty-two percent and fifteen percents of patients showed intraepidermal and subepidermal blisters, respectively, in available histologic sections from 61 patients.[61] In a retrospective review of 265 cases by Svodoba et al.,[60] only interface changes, only acantholysis, and both interface and acantholytic changes are seen in 21%, 29%, and 42% of cases, respectively.

Direct Immunofluorescence

Direct immunofluorescence studies show IgG and C3 intercellular deposition within the epidermis as well as at the basement membrane zone (**see Case Study 1**). In a recent study of paraneoplastic pemphigus, 1/11 showed only linear IgG deposition at the basement membrane zone, 6/11 with intercellular IgG within the epidermis and 3/11 with both patterns.[65]

Indirect Immunofluorescence

The majority of cases (15/22) have IgG intercellular staining on IIF on monkey esophagus while both intercellular and basement membrane staining was seen in 12/22 cases on IIF of rat bladder.[65]

Immunoblotting and Immunoprecipitation

Desmoplakin 1 (250 kD), bullous pemphigoid antigen (230 kD), desmoplakin 2 (210 kD), periplakin (190 kD), and alpha-1-macroglobulin-like-1 antigen (170 kD) are detected by immunoblots.[60]

Pemphigus Herpetiformis

Pemphigus herpetiformis is a rare variant of pemphigus with an incidence of 7.3% in a series of 205 pemphigus patients.[66] In a recent literature review of 167 reported cases, Higashida et al.[67] reported a slight female predominance (1.1:1). Pediatric cases have been reported.[68] There is an association with drugs, malignancy, and rheumatoid arthritis.[67] It typically follows a benign clinical course with good response to systemic steroids or dapsone treatment.[69]

The disease presents with herpetiform vesicles and pruritus resembling dermatitis herpetiformis yet with epidermal acantholysis on histology, intercellular immunoglobulin deposition, and circulating autoantibodies to desmoglein 1.[70] Recently autoantibodies against desmoglein 3, both desmogleins 1 and 3, desmocollin 1, desmocollin 3, envoplakin, and periplakin have been reported.[69,71]

Histologic Features

Distinctive histologic feature is the presence of intraepidermal infiltrate of eosinophils, reported in 74–83% of literature review.[67,69] The blisters can be subcorneal, intraepidermal, or suprabasilar. Neutrophils in addition to eosinophils can be seen in some cases.[72] The histologic features can be nonspecific with epidermal acantholysis being minimal or absent in this rare variant of pemphigus.[70]

Direct Immunofluorescence

Intercellular IgG and C3 deposition within superficial epidermis is seen on DIF studies.[73] IgA deposition is typically negative.

Indirect Immunofluorescence

IgG autoantibodies exhibit an intercellular pattern on IIF studies.[72]

11.4 Pemphigoid

Bullous Pemphigoid

Bullous pemphigoid is the most frequent autoimmune blistering disorder in adults as well as the most common one within the pemphigoid group. Its incidence is approximately 10 per one million persons, increasing parallel to age. The cutaneous presentation of bullous pemphigoid is very polymorphic with the initial non-bullous phase with associated generalized pruritus which can mimic a number of inflammatory dermatoses.[74,75] The clinical morphology of this initial non-specific presentation can be targetoid, lichenoid, nodular, eczematous, or urticarial; and can be the only sign of the disease up to 20% of cases.[74,76] The bullous stage presents initially as tense blisters on erythematous base without Nikolsky's sign. Erythema and urticaria can be prodromal changes. Trunk, groin, and flexural areas are commonly affected sites.[77] Mucosal involvement is seen in 10–30% of patients. Drug hypersensitivity reaction, radiation therapy, ultraviolet radiation, thermal or electrical burns, and surgical procedures have been reported as inducers.[74] In recent years exposure to checkpoint inhibitors is another risk factor of developing bullous pemphigoid.[78]

Both idiopathic and drug-induced bullous pemphigoid are caused by autoantibodies against components of hemidesmosomes (230-kDa BPAg1 and 180-kDa BPAg2 or collagen XVII) resulting in damage of the basement membrane and subsequent loss of adhesion between the dermis and epidermis. In rare cases there are overlapping features between linear IgA and the childhood form of bullous pemphigoid, since autoantibodies against 120-kDa have been reported in these cases.[79,80]

Histologic Features

The histology of an established blister is characterized by a subepidermal vesiculation containing serum, fibrin, and a variable number of eosinophils and neutrophils (**Figure 11.10**). The lesion of the urticarial stage shows spongiotic dermatitis, papillary dermal edema, perivascular and interstitial eosinophils admixed with a minor component of neutrophils, lymphocytes, and histiocytes (**Figure 11.11**).

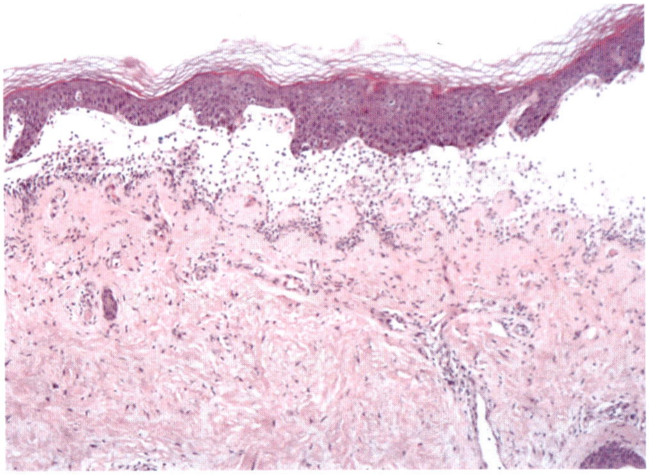

Figure 11.10 Bullous pemphigoid is characterized by a subepidermal blister containing prominent eosinophils (×100).

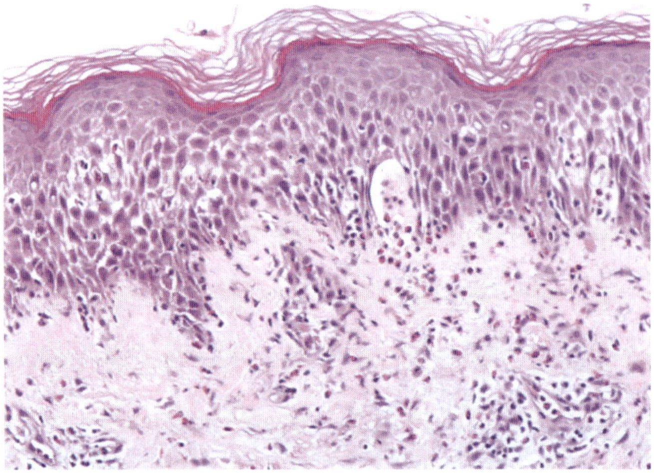

Figure 11.11 A spongiotic dermatitis with prominent eosinophils is seen in urticarial stage of bullous pemphigoid (×200).

Table 11.3 Immunostains in the diagnosis of pemphigoid[44-46,84-88]

	N	Antibody clone	Sensitivity	Specificity
C3d (Magro 2008)[84]	17 BP	Dako-A0063	100%	96%
C3d (Pfaltz 2009)[45]	35 (32 BP, 3 PG)	Abcam, ab15981	97%	100%
C3d (Glauser 2016)[86]	51 BP	Abcam, ab15981	45%	38%
C3d (Karabag 2024)[46]	36 pemphigoid	Cell Marque	69.4%	99%
C3d (Thakur 2023)[88]	74 BP	Cell Marque	59%	100%
	18 MMP	Catalog# 403A–76	41.2%	100%
C4d (Magro 2008)[84]	17BP	Alpco-BI-RC4D	24%	98%
C4d (Kwon 2013)[85]	20 (12 BP, 8 PG)	Cell Marque, catalog# 404A–16	90%	100%
C4d (Villani 2016)[44]	29 BP	Biomedica Gruppe	86%	98%
C4d (Kamyab 2019)[87]	30 BP	Biomedica Gruppe	90%	87%
C4d (Karabag 2024)[46]	36 pemphigoid	SP91, Cell Marque	81%	100%
C4d (Thakur 2023)[88]	74 BP	Cell Marque	26%	100%
	18 MMP	Catalog# 404–14	50%	100%

BP: bullous pemphigoid, PG: pemphigoid gestationis

Direct Immunofluorescence

DIF studies usually demonstrate a linear IgG (70–90%) and C3 (90–100%) deposition at the basement membrane zone. Deposition of IgA and/or IgM is rarely present.[81] DIF findings around hair follicles have been reported to be a helpful clue (**Figure 11.12**).[82] Positive DIF has been shown to be a better predictive value for relapse than ELISA.[83]

Indirect Immunofluorescence

IIF studies performed on salt split skin usually demonstrates the presence of circulating IgG autoantibodies in 60%–80% of patients' serum and they are associated with the roof or epidermal side of the blister.[8] Circulating IgA, IgE, and IgM autoantibodies can be seen.

Immunohistochemistry

When fresh tissue is not available for DIF, C3d and C4d immunostain has been shown to be helpful **(Table 11.3)**.[44–46,84–88] Studies have shown C3d and C4d to exhibit 97% and 86–90% sensitivity, respectively; and 100% and 98–100% specificity, respectively (**Table 11.3**).[44–46,84–88]

Mucous Membrane Pemphigoid

Mucous membrane pemphigoid is also known as cicatricial pemphigoid, anti-laminin 5 cicatricial pemphigoid, anti-epiligrin cicatricial pemphigoid, and ocular pemphigoid. It is a group of autoimmune bullous diseases which has a predilection for mucosal sites including conjunctivae, oral mucosa, nose, larynx, esophagus, rectum, vagina, and penis.[89] The incidence has been estimated to be one to two per one million people affecting most frequently women in the sixth to seventh decade of life.[90] The mouth (gingiva, buccal mucosa, palate, tongue) is the most commonly affected site, followed by conjunctiva, skin, nasal cavity, anogenital area, pharynx, larynx, and esophagus.[91] The disease results in scarring of skin, mucous membrane, or both; therefore, it can potentially cause blindness and esophageal and laryngeal strictures. Oral cavity and conjunctiva are affected in 85% and 65% of patients, respectively. Only conjunctival involvement or ocular pemphigoid is seen in approximately 20% of patients.[89] The rare Brunsting-Perry variant occurs predominantly on the scalp and head with minimal mucosal involvement.[92] Anti-laminin 5 pemphigoid is associated with malignancy. Mucous membrane pemphigoid can develop after immune checkpoint inhibitor therapy.[93]

BPAg2 (BP180) and laminin 5 (laminin 332 or epiligrin) are the major antigens involved in mucous membrane pemphigoid.[94] Other targeted antigens include alpha-6 and beta-4 integrin subunits, laminin 6 (laminin 311), BPAg1 (BP230), the 97/120-kDa linear IgA bullous disease antigen, collagen VII, 168-kDa protein, and 450kDa protein.[94] Patients with autoantibodies to alpha-6 integrin and beta-4 integrin have oral or exclusively ocular disease involvement, respectively.[94] An

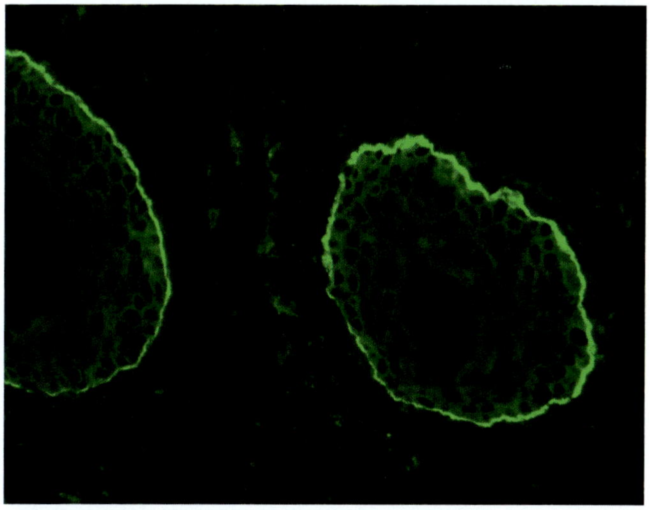

Figure 11.12 Bullous pemphigoid. Strong linear IgG deposition is noted at the basement membrane zone around hair follicles in direct immunofluorescence studies.

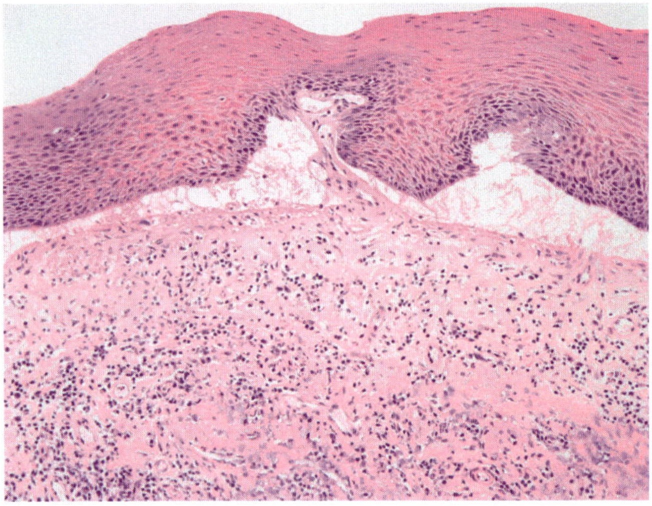

Figure 11.13 Cicatricial pemphigoid. A subepidermal blister containing minimal inflammatory cells and underlying dermal fibrosis and chronic inflammation are noted (×100).

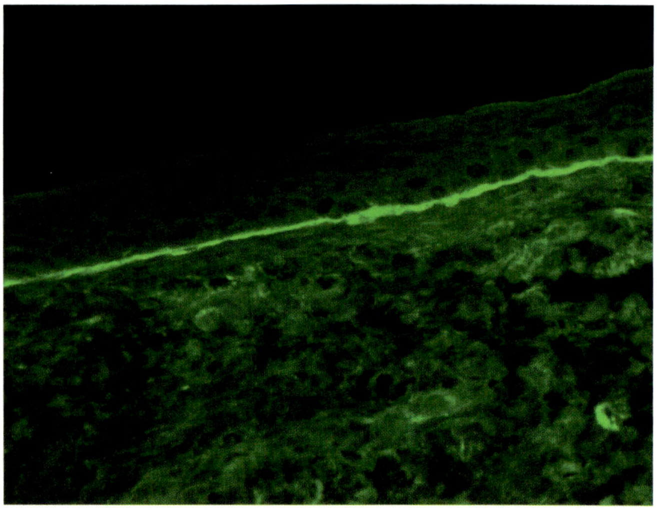

Figure 11.14 Cicatricial pemphigoid. Linear IgG deposition is noted at the basement membrane zone.

increased risk for malignancy is associated with anti-laminin 5 (laminin 332) disease.[95] Dual circulating IgG and IgA antibodies have been reported to be associated with a more severe disease course.[96]

Histologic Features

Histologic sections show a subepithelial separation. Marked chronic inflammation and scarring are seen in the underlying dermis or soft tissue (**Figure 11.13**). In early lesions, dermal neutrophilic microabscesses can be seen. In addition, the subepidermal and perifollicular separation can be focal. All these features can result in a misdiagnosis as a neutrophilic scarring alopecia.[97]

Direct Immunofluorescence

Linear deposition of IgG, IgA, and/or C3 can be seen at the basement membrane zone on DIF (**Figure 11.14**), often with n-serrated pattern of IgG deposition at the basement membrane zone. In contrast, IgA deposition is not seen in BP cases. In cases involving mainly the ocular area, DIF results can be negative up to 40% of cases.[98] In ocular cases, IgA (91%) deposition is seen in a higher frequency than C3 (54%) and IgG (47%) deposition at the basement membrane zone.[98] Rare case of IgM mucous membrane pemphigoid has been reported.[99]

Indirect Immunofluorescence

Although with low sensitivity IIF staining of either the roof or floor of the blister space can help differentiating epidermal/lamina lucida antigens (BP180, alpha-6 beta-4 integrins) from dermal/lamina densa antigens (laminin-5, laminin-6, type VII collagen). IIF can be used to monitor serum IgG and IgA titers as indicator of disease activity and for diagnosis when DIF is negative.

Pemphigoid Gestationis

Pemphigoid gestationis is an autoimmune vesiculobullous dermatosis of pregnancy with an incidence of 1 in 50,000–60,000 pregnancies.[100,101] The etiology of pemphigoid gestationis is still known, but there is a strong association with hydatidiform mole, trophoblastic tumors, choriocarcinoma, and HLA-B8, HLA-DR3, and HLA-DR4.[100] The placenta and amniotic epithelia express BP180. Most patients have circulating autoantibodies against BP180 (BPAg1), type XVII collagen, and not as often BP230 (BPAg2).[100] Collagen XVII is exposed to the maternal immune system and results in antiplacental IgG antibodies which cross react with BP180 and BP230 in the skin.[101]

The initial presentation, usually in the second or third trimester of pregnancy or in the immediate postpartum period, includes severe pruritus and polymorphous papulovesicular eruptions on legs and trunk that leads to blistering and superficial ulcerations. Spontaneous resolution follows soon after delivery, although it may occur during the late third trimester. Known to carry an increased risk for preterm labor and fetal growth restriction, pemphigoid gestationis has been shown to be associated with an increased risk for adverse pregnancy outcomes including gestational hypertension without significant proteinuria, preeclampsia, eclampsia, abnormal liver function, gestational diabetes, among others.[101] There is a tendency for pemphigoid gestationis to recur with subsequent pregnancies, sometimes with an earlier onset and a more severe course.[101] Recognition of pemphigoid gestationis is important due to its association with intrauterine growth retardation.[101] In rare instances, due to passive transplacental transfer of maternal anti-bullous pemphigoid 180 (BP180) or 230 (BP230) immunoglobulin G (IgG), newborns of mothers with pemphigoid gestationis may develop neonatal pemphigoid.[102] An anti-BP180 IgG antibody ELISA value of >150IU in combination with the clinical presence of blisters were found to be associated with higher risk of adverse pregnancy outcomes.[103]

Histologic Features

The diagnostic biopsies would show a subepidermal vesiculation with associated eosinophilic spongiosis, papillary dermal edema, and prominent dermal infiltrate of eosinophils (**see Case Study 2**). However, the histopathology can vary greatly depending on the timing of the biopsy and the nature of the primary lesion; thus nonspecific histologic features are often seen and a diagnosis relies mainly on the DIF results.[104] In a histologic comparison of 21 PG versus 10 polymorphic eruption of pregnancy (PEP), helpful distinguishing histologic features of PG include eosinophilic spongiosis, eosinophilic epitheliotropism, and prominent superficial dermal infiltrate of eosinophils.[105]

Direct Immunofluorescence

DIF studies invariably demonstrate linear C3 (100%) deposition at the basement membrane zone and IgG (25–50%) and infrequently IgA, with C3 having the highest diagnostic sensitivity.[104] Often only linear C3 is seen on DIF in the classic presentation (**see Case Study 2**). Intercellular C3 and/or IgG deposition within the epidermis has been reported.[106]

Indirect Immunofluorescence

IIF and NaCl-slit skin demonstrated circulating IgG autoantibodies in approximately 92% of cases.[106] C3 reactivity is seen on the epidermal side of the blister. ELISA of the NC16a domain of BP180 exhibits greater sensitivity (93%) and specificity (96%) than IIF testing.[107]

Immunohistochemistry

C4d and C3d immunostains have been reported to be helpful in diagnosing pemphigoid on formalin-fixed paraffin-embedded tissue.[45,84] Recently C4d expression was demonstrated in all eight cases of pemphigoid gestationis. C4d immunostain is potentially helpful in the distinction of pemphigoid gestationis versus polymorphic eruption of pregnancy.[85]

Anti-p200 Pemphigoid

Anti-p200 pemphigoid is an uncommon immunobullous disease that is often misclassified as bullous pemphigoid and epidermolysis bullosa acquisita. It has been characterized as anti-laminin gamma-1 pemphigoid in many cases.[108] First described in 1996, the identity of the 200-kDa antigen has been identified as laminin gamma-1, a non-collagenous N-linked glycoprotein that promotes adhesion in the lower lamina lucida of the basement membrane.[109] However, reactivity with laminin gamma-1 is not demonstrated in all patients with anti-p200 pemphigoid. Recently, laminin-beta4 has been described to be an additional target antigen.[110]

The disease presents with tense, pruritic, and urticarial bullae that can resemble bullous pemphigoid or linear IgA dermatosis clinically. In 20% of the patients, predominant mucosal disease can be seen.[108] There is a male predominance. Oral lesions are the most common mucosal lesions, followed by genital then ocular lesions.[111] Epitope spreading, reactivity against another antigen besides p200, is a common occurrence in anti-p200 pemphigoid.[112] Anti-p200 pemphigoid patients with epitope spreading have been reported to have frequent mucosal involvement (even ocular and laryngeal), diverse clinical presentations, treatment resistance, and a more severe disease course.[113] There appears to be a strong association with psoriasis and in some cases malignancy.[108,109,114] The most common used therapy for anti-p200 pemphigoid includes combined systemic corticosteroids and adjuvant immunomodulatory agents.[115]

Histologic Features

Histologic sections would show a subepidermal blister accompanied by an infiltrate comprised predominantly of neutrophils or a mixture of neutrophils and eosinophils in some cases (**see Case Study 3**).[116] These histologic features, more commonly seen in linear IgA disease, together with the clinical presentation would prompt further workup.

Direct Immunofluorescence

Linear IgG and/or C3 are typically seen at the basement membrane zone on DIF (**see Case Study 3**). However, this DIF profile is also seen in bullous pemphigoid and epidermolysis bullosa acquisita. An inverted "u" serration pattern was reported to be present in some anti-p200 pemphigoid cases.[117]

Indirect Immunofluorescence

Using NaCl-split normal human skin as substrate, circulating autoantibodies would bind of the dermal side of the blister whereas an epidermal pattern would be seen in bullous pemphigoid and linear IgA dermatosis.[118] To further differentiate epidermolysis bullosa acquisita from anti-laminin gamma-1 pemphigoid, immunoblotting analysis would be necessary. Since immunoblotting analysis is only available in specialized laboratory, a sensitive and specific ELISA for anti-laminin gamma-1 pemphigoid has been reported and might facilitate timely diagnosis.[119] Immunofluorescence overlay antigen mapping in the identification of autoantigen has recently been reported.[120]

Lichen Planus Pemphigoid

Lichen planus pemphigoid is a rare immunobullous disease with clinical features resembling lichen planus yet immunohistological features of bullous pemphigoid. It has an incidence of 1 per 1,000,000 patients per year.[121] Lichen planus pemphigoid can be triggered by immune checkpoint inhibitors.[122]

The majority of patients with lichen planus pemphigoid present initially with lichenified lesions of lichen planus on upper and lower extremities then subsequently develop tense blisters not associated with the lichenoid lesions, unlike bullous lichen planus. The average time interval between onset of lichenoid dermatitis and the development of blisters is reported to be 8.3 months.[123] Oral lesions can develop with or without cutaneous lesions and tend to affect the gingiva and buccal mucosa most frequently.[124] Uncommon clinical presentation includes palmoplantar keratoderma.[125]

Although the pathogenesis is still not understood, the epitope of lichen planus pemphigoid is within the C-terminal NC16A domain of BP180 antigen.[126] The report of a 200-kD antigen on the epidermal side of NaCl-split skin supports that lichen planus pemphigoides is a distinct entity and not a co-existence of lichen planus and bullous pemphigoides.[127] Although most cases are idiopathic, there are reports of association with malignancy, phototherapy, drugs, and infections including varicella and Hepatitis B and C.[128]

Histologic Features

On histologic sections, a lichenoid dermatitis with vacuolar degeneration of the basal layer or a subepidermal blister containing eosinophils indistinguishable from bullous pemphigoid can be seen.[124]

Direct Immunofluorescence

IgG and C3 linear deposition at the basement membrane zone is seen on DIF. IgA and IgM deposition can be seen infrequently.

Indirect Immunofluorescence

On IIF by NaCl-split skin, IgG is seen binding to the epidermal side of the blister.

11.5 Linear IgA Disease

Characterized as an entity in 1979 by Chorzelski,[129] linear IgA disease or linear IgA bullous dermatosis affects all ages, and specifically in children it is known as chronic bullous dermatosis of childhood or linear IgA disease of childhood. While the adult linear IgA disease affects females between the ages of 60 and 65 years old, the childhood form most often occurs in children of preschool age with a peak incidence at 4.5 years.[130] Of the idiopathic cases, the median age is 54 years and 60% have mucosal involvement.[130] Patients older than 70 years and without mucosal involvement were more likely to have complete remission.[130] While the majority of cases are idiopathic, a subset of cases can be associated with a number of drugs, mainly vancomycin, and malignancy.[131] In a recent French series of 69 patients with drug-induced linear IgA, antibiotics are the main offenders with Vancomycin being the most frequent.[131]

Historically linear IgA disease can be divided into major lamina lucida-type and minor sublamina densa-type. Most lamina lucida-type sera react against 97 kDa (LABD-97) and 120 kDa (LAD1) antigens, both are proteolytic cleavage products of BP180 (BPAg2) ectodomain.[132] On the other hand, the sera of sublamina densa-type, which is now called IgA epidermolysis bullosa acquisita, react against collagen VII.[133] These patients are currently classified as epidermolysis bullosa acquisita due to autoantibodies against collagen VII.[134]

Histologic Features

A subepidermal blister containing predominantly neutrophils, sometimes with admixed eosinophils, is seen (**Figure 11.15**). While neutrophils are the predominant inflammatory type, eosinophils or pauci-inflammatory can be seen.[135] There are no significant differences in the histopathologic features of the idiopathic versus drug-induced groups. The predominance of neutrophils helps to distinguish this entity from bullous pemphigoid, though eosinophils have been reported to be more prominent in drug-induced linear IgA disease. The histologic features can be indistinguishable from anti-p200 pemphigoid. The differential diagnosis would include dermatitis herpetiformis, anti-p200 pemphigoid, bullous pemphigoid, mucosal membrane pemphigoid, epidermolysis bullosa acquisita, and bullous systemic lupus erythematosus.

Direct Immunofluorescence

DIF examination of lesional and perilesional skin demonstrates a linear IgA deposition at the basement membrane zone. Both linear IgA and IgG/C3 can be seen. IgM linear deposition

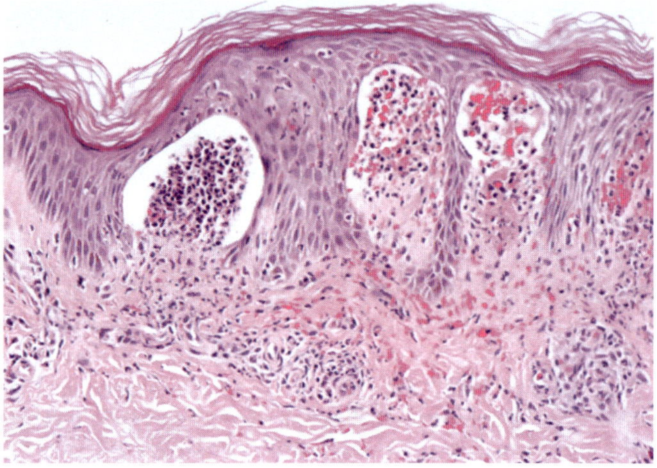

Figure 11.15 Linear IgA disease is characterized by a subepidermal blister containing neutrophils (×200).

is rarely seen. Of note, linear IgA and IgG/C3 can be seen in other autoimmune bullous disorders. Granular IgA deposition at the basement membrane zone can be seen in about 20% of cases.[136] The n-serrated pattern is seen in the lamina lucida-type, whereas u-serrated pattern is seen in the sublamina densa-type (now classified as IgA epidermolysis bullosa acquisita.[137]

Indirect Immunofluorescence

Circulating autoantibodies can be detected in up to 70% of cases by IIF using salt-split normal human skin (preferred method) or monkey esophagus.[138] In about 50% of cases with negative DIF findings, IgG antibodies can be detected by ELISA or immunoblotting.[138] IgA deposition can be detected on the epidermal (BPAg2), dermal (LAD1), or both sides of the salt-induced blister.[139]

Immunohistochemistry

Laminin 5 and collagen IV immunostains highlighted the floor of the blister space in 65% and 90% of 20 adult linear IgA disease cases.[140]

11.6 Epidermolysis Bullosa Acquisita

Epidermolysis bullosa acquisita is a rare autoimmune bullous disorder in which autoantibodies to collagen VII (290-kDa), a component of anchoring fibrils of the dermal epidermal junction resulting in blisters on skin and mucous membrane.[141] Its incidence is 0.2–0.5 new cases per million per year, affecting men and women equally. The disease is very uncommon in adults and exceedingly rare in pediatric patients.[142] Epidermolysis bullosa acquisita is associated with major histocompatibility complex (MHC), especially HLA-DRB1*15 and HLA-DRB1*16.[141] There is an association with malignancy and various systemic diseases most commonly inflammatory bowel disease, and also systemic lupus erythematosus, rheumatoid arthritis, chronic lymphocytic leukemia, and others.[143]

Clinically, epidermolysis bullosa acquisita can resemble hereditary dystrophic epidermolysis bullosa and classified clinically as noninflammatory (classical or mechanobullous) and inflammatory (non-mechanobullous) subtypes. The majority of cases are non-mechanobullous type (55%). The mechanobullous and combined subtypes are comprised of 38% and 7%, respectively.[141] In the mechanobullous subtype, blisters with subsequent scarring develop on trauma-prone skin sites. Scarring alopecia and nail dystrophy can be seen.[141] In the non-mechanobullous subtype, generalized urticarial plaques with blisters form and subsequent scarring and milia formation are not seen. Mucosal involvement can be seen in 23% of patients. The clinical presentations are diverse including classic porphyria cutanea tarda-like, bullous pemphigoid-like, cicatricial pemphigoid-like, Brunsting-Perry like, and IgA bullous dermatosis-like. Co-morbidities with other systemic diseases such as Crohn's disease, ulcerative colitis, rheumatoid arthritis, multiple endocrinopathy syndrome, pulmonary fibrosis, and others have been reported. [141]

Collagen VII, a 290 kDa protein, is the main component of hemidesmosome anchoring fibrils. [141] IgG autoantibodies to collagen VII are the most commonly detected in the serum, but IgA, IgM, and IgE autoantibodies have also been identified.[141]

Histologic Features

Although a subepidermal blister is seen in diagnostic biopsies, the degree of dermal inflammatory infiltrate varies with more inflammation (a mixture of lymphocytes, histiocytes, neutrophils, and eosinophils) seen in the inflammatory or nonclassical variant. Dermal fibrosis and milia are seen in biopsies of late lesions.

Direct Immunofluorescence

DIF shows linear IgG and C3 deposition at the basement membrane zone. There is variable IgA and IgM deposition. C3 deposition is most commonly seen, followed by IgG, IgA, then IgM.[144] Only IgA deposits are seen in 2% of cases, corresponding to IgA-EBA. Vascular deposition is not seen as in porphyria cutanea tarda which can have similar histologic features as epidermolysis bullosa acquisita. A u-serrated pattern, finger-like structures or spikes, seen on DIF is characteristic for either epidermolysis bullosa acquisita or bullous systemic lupus erythematosus. This pattern distinguishes EBA from BP, MMP, LABD, p200 pemphigoid, and anti-laminin 332 pemphigoid with up to 100% specificity.[145]

Indirect Immunofluorescence

IIF detects circulating IgG antoantibodies targeting the basement membrane zone. EBA can be distinguished from bullous pemphigoid by IF using salt-split skin in which staining is seen on the floor of the blister. However, IIF and salt-split skin IF cannot help distinguishing EBA from anti-laminin 5 mucous membrane pemphigoid and anti-p200, pemphigoid. Recently developed full-length-collagen VII ELISA has been shown to be significantly more sensitive than collagen VII-non-collagenous domains 1 and 2 ELISA and IIF.[146]

11.7 Connective Tissue Disease

The "lupus band test," deposition of IgG, IgA, and IgM at the basement membrane zone of lesional skin, was coined in 1970 by Burnham et al.[147] It is thought that these deposits represent circulating immune complexes of deoxyribonucleic acid (DNA) and antinuclear antibodies trapped within the basement membrane zone.

Direct Immunofluorescence

Lupus erythematosus. Positive DIF finding or "lupus band" is positive in 70–80% of sun-exposed non-lesional and 55% of sun-protected non-lesional skin biopsies of systemic lupus erythematosus (SLE) patients (**Figure 11.16**). Positive DIF result in non-lesional and sun-protected skin in patients with SLE correlates with antibodies to double-stranded DNA and extracutaneous disease.[148] However, immune deposits at the dermal epidermal junction can be seen in both sun-exposed and normal skin in a number of conditions.[149]

The immune deposition, often three or more immunoreactants, is granular but occasionally homogeneous linear band at the basement membrane zone and in half of the cases around hair follicles.[150] Nuclear staining can sometimes be seen. The various reported patterns of immune deposition include homogeneous, linear, granular, stippled, fibrillar, and lumpy. 98% of bullous SLE cases have positive DIF. [150] Linear or granular IgG (91%), IgA (72%), IgM (68%), and C3 (67%) deposition was seen in bullous SLE cases.[150] A u-serrated pattern is typically noted for bullous LE (Barker 2024).[151] IgM is most commonly identified, followed by C3, IgG, and IgA, in discoid lupus erythematosus (DLE) lesions.[152] While in sun-protected skin weak IgM or IgG is indicative of positivity, IgM deposit has to be at least moderate in intensity and encompasses at least half of the width of the biopsy in sun-exposed skin.[153] IgG is less frequently seen than IgM and IgA is the least frequently identified. The more immunoreactants detected at the basement membrane zone, the greater predictive value and better specificity would be.[153]

In *mixed connective tissue disease*, various staining patterns can be seen. IgG staining of keratinocytes can be seen on DIF including speckled nuclear pattern, peripheral nuclear rim pattern, and granular cytoplasmic pattern.[154] Vascular IgM, C3 and fibrinogen deposition is seen in lesions with vasculitis. [154] Granular cytoplasmic and nuclear staining of keratinocytes for C5b-9 is seen in all cases. [154]

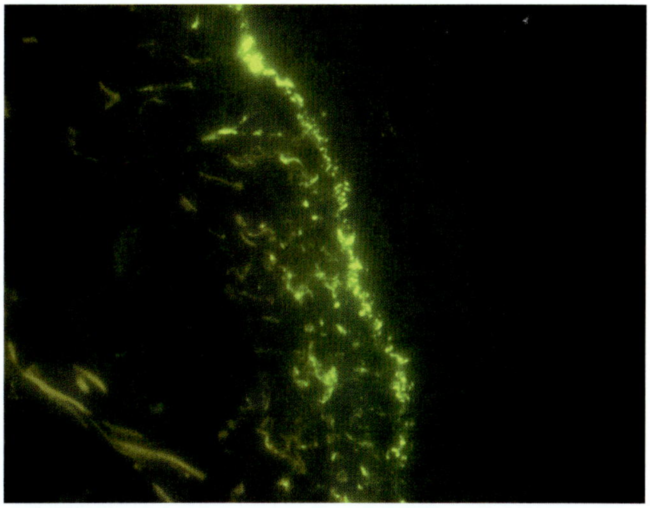

Figure 11.16 Lupus band is characterized by granular IgG deposition at the basement membrane zone.

In *dermatomyositis*, granular IgG and C5b-9 staining is seen at the basement membrane zone. A lupus band at the basement membrane zone (IgG, IgM, or C3) with colloid bodies in some cases was seen in 19/35 cases reported by Jones et al.[155] The presence of C5b-9 deposition at the basement membrane zone and within vessels together with a negative lupus band test has been shown to be predictive of dermatomyositis.[153] Granular nuclear staining of keratinocytes for Cb5-9 is seen in patients with positive nuclear antinuclear antibody (ANA).[156]

Immunohistochemistry

C3d and C4d immunostains have recently been reported to be helpful in diagnosing lupus erythematosus.[84] Both C3d and C4d are stable component of complement cascade. Granular C3d staining at the dermal epidermal junction was seen in all DLE cases, whereas C4d staining was noted in only 15% of DLE cases.[84] Staining was negative for all subacute cutaneous lupus erythematosus (SCLE) cases. Staining for both C3d and C4d was seen in all SLE cases.[84]

11.8 Porphyria Cutanea Tarda

Porphyria cutanea tarda (PCT) is a bullous disease that can be associated with a hereditary disorder of porphyrin metabolism (partial deficiency of uroporphyrinogen decarboxylase), hepatitis C, and human immunodeficiency virus infection.[157] Although possessing similar clinical and histologic features, porphyrin metabolism is normal in pseudo-PCT, a condition induced by drug, chronic renal failure, and hemodialysis.[158] The clinical features of PCT and pseudo-PCT are similar – blisters, skin fragility, milia, and scarring are seen on sun-exposed skin.

Histologic Features

A subepidermal blister is seen with minimal associated inflammatory infiltrate (**Figure 11.17**).[159] The walls of the superficial blood vessels are thickened and hyalinized which highlighted by periodic acid-Schiff (PAS) stain with diastase digestion (**Figure 11.18**). The projection of dermal papillae with thickened vessel walls into the blister space imparts a "festooning" appearance. Caterpillar bodies, PAS-positive globules, are seen within the blister roof and represent degenerated keratinocytes and basement membrane. Dermal sclerosis similar to scheroderma histopathologically can be seen.

Direct Immunofluorescence

C3 (69%), IgM (56%), IgG (44%), IgA (25%), and fibrinogen (44%) vascular deposition was noted in the majority of cases.[159] In addition, granular C3 (56%), IgG (25%), IgM (12%), and fibrinogen (38%) deposition was seen at the basement membrane zone.[159] By performing DIF with antibodies against laminin and collagen IV, the level of separation appears to be at the level of lamina lucida.[160]

11.9 Dermatitis Herpetiformis

Dermatitis herpetiformis (DH), a chronic severely pruritic dermatosis, affects mainly Caucasians with disease onset most common in the third decade. DH is rarely seen in Asian patients and exceedingly rarely in African Americans.[161] It is a disease seen mainly in adulthood (30–40 years, mean 43 years), although cases in childhood and adolescence have been reported. It is considered to be an extraintestinal manifestation of celiac disease. The incidence of dermatitis herpetiformis ranges from 11 to 66 per 100,000 in Europe.[162] The disease has a strong association with HLA-DQ2 (80–90%) and HLA-DQ8 (10–20%). A complex interaction of genetic, immunologic, and environmental factors is thought to be the disease pathogenesis. [161]

Tissue transglutaminase (TG2/tTG) present in the gut is the autoantigen responsible for celiac disease. TG2 modifies glutamine to glutamic acid within gliadin, an alcohol-soluble portion of gluten. This modification step results in stronger affinity of gliadin to HLA DQ2 and DQ8 on antigen presenting cells. Via epitope spreading, circulating IgA autoantibodies are also formed against epidermal transglutaminase (TG3/eTG) in dermatitis herpetiformis. Anti-TG3 antibodies deposited in the papillary dermal papillae triggered a neutrophilic response. [161]

The disease has a polymorphous presentation characterized clinically as episodes of intensely pruritic erythematous papules and /or urticarial plaques grouped on extensor surfaces of extremities (elbows and knees), shoulders, midline of back,

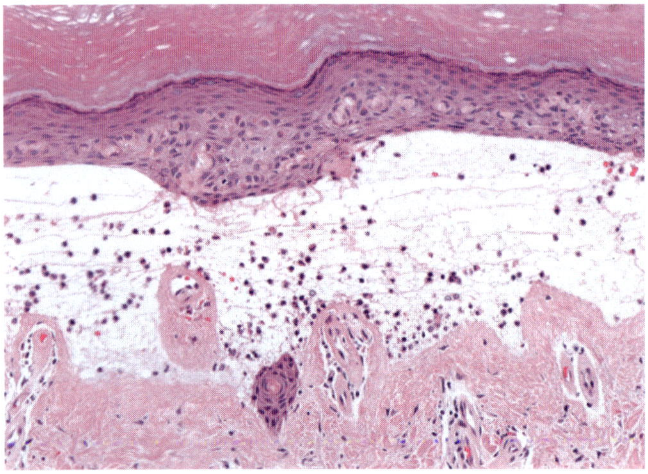

Figure 11.17 Porphyria cutanea tarda. Papillary dermal papillae project into the blister space as the result of thickened dermal blood vessel walls (×200).

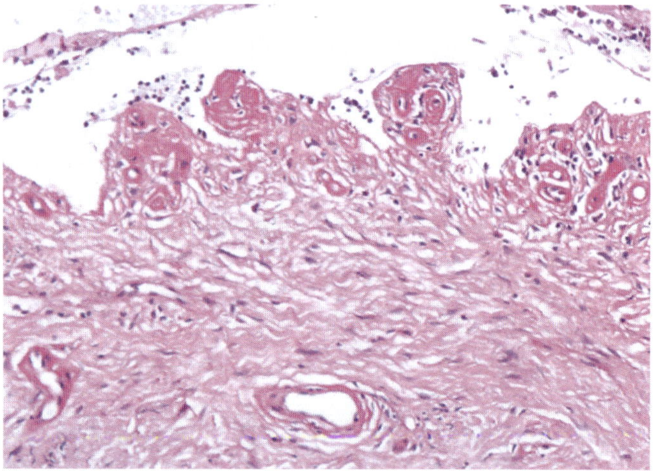

Figure 11.18 Porphyria cutanea tarda. A periodic acid-Schiff test would highlight the perivascular deposit (×200).

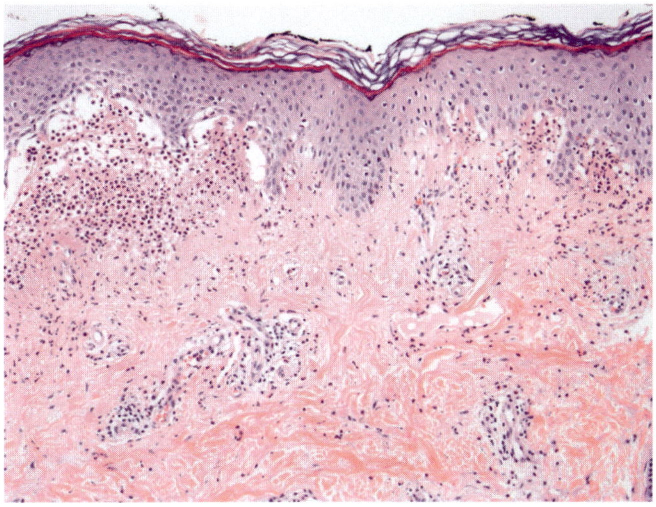

Figure 11.19 Dermatitis herpetiformis. A subepidermal blister containing neutrophils is noted.

buttocks, sacral area, and scalp.[161] Blisters are more frequently detected in patients older than 65.[163] Although all DH patients have gluten sensitivity, only 3–10% of patients with celiac disease will develop DH.[161] IgA autoantibodies are directed against epidermal transglutaminase in DH.[164]

Histologic Features

Due to the intense pruritus, erosions remain clinically. The histologic features of DH can be non-specific such as a perivascular lymphocytic infiltrate up to 40% of cases. The typical histologic features are neutrophilic infiltrate at the dermal epidermal junction resulting in a subepidermal blister containing neutrophils (**Figure 11.19**). This histologic pattern can be seen in linear IgA disease and bullous systemic lupus erythematosus. Intraepidermal eosinophils may be occasionally seen.

Direct Immunofluorescence

DIF is the gold standard in diagnosing dermatitis herpetiformis. Uninvolved perilesional skin is recommended for DIF since lesion biopsy has a high false negative rate. On DIF studies granular IgA deposition can be seen within the dermal papillae, continuous at the basement membrane zone, or both (**Figure 11.20**).[165] A fibrillary pattern (linear streaks) of IgA deposition at the basement membrane zone can be seen which can result in misdiagnosis.[165,166] C3 and/or IgM deposition can be seen in lower frequency.[116] Granular IgA deposition in the skin of celiac patients with inflammatory dermatoses without dermatitis herpetiformis can be seen in 64% yet none in skin of control patients, which can be considered a marker of celiac disease.[167] In some patients with a cutaneous eruption resembling dermatitis herpetiformis, a deposition of only C3 at the dermal epidermal junction is seen. The term "granular C3 dermatosis" has been proposed.[168]

11.10 Epidermolysis Bullosa

Epidermolysis bullosa (EB), a group of hereditary bullous disorders, is classified based on the level of the blister. It is considered to be a mechanobullous disorder. Mutations affecting 18 genes encoding the elements responsible for the attachment of the epidermis to the dermis result in damage of the basement membrane zone.[169] There are four major categories classified based on the ultrastructural location of the skin cleavage and underpinning molecular alteration: EB simplex, junctional EB, dystrophic EB, and Kindler EB. EB simplex, the most common (70%), has an autosomal dominant inheritance pattern. Junctional EB has an autosomal recessive inheritance and the blister locates within the lamina lucida of the basement membrane. Dystrophic EB has an autosomal dominant or autosomal recessive pattern and the separation occurs below the lamina densa of the basement membrane zone. Kindler EB is autosomal recessive and has variable ultrastructural separation within the basement membrane zone.[170]

Keratin 5 (*KRT5*) and keratin 14 (*KRT14*) gene mutations affect 75% of EB simplex patients.[170] Other genes encoding hemidesmosomal proteins such as plectin (*PLEC*), dystonin (*DST*), and exophilin 5 (*EXPH5*) have also been implicated. In junctional EB, genes encoding type XVII collagen (*COL17A1*), laminin 332 (*LAMA3*, *LAMB3*, and *LAMC2*), integrin alpha6beta4 (*ITGA6* and *ITGB4*), and the integrin alpha3 subunit (*IGTA3*) are affected.[170] COL7A1 mutations are seen in dystrophic EB. Kindlin 1 protein, encoded by *FERMT1*, is affected in Kindler EB.

Histologic Features

These lesions invariably show a subepidermal blister on histologic sections (**Figure 11.21**). Immunofluorescent mapping of laminin 332, collagen VII, and collagen XVII has been replaced by ultrastructural examination for definitive classification.

Ultrastructural Findings

Three areas of the basement membrane zone important for EB pathogenesis include: (1) hemidesmosomes, (2) lamina lucida (electron lucent), and (3) lamina densa (electron dense). The separation is within the basal keratinocytes in EB simplex

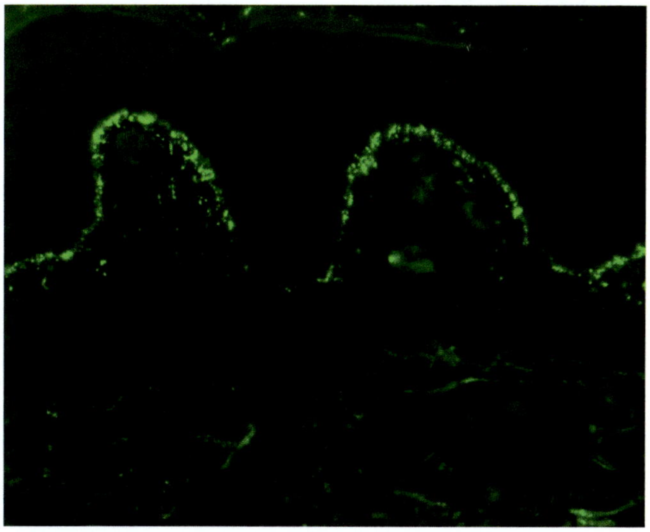

Figure 11.20 Dermatitis herpetiformis. Granular IgA deposition is seen within the dermal papillae.

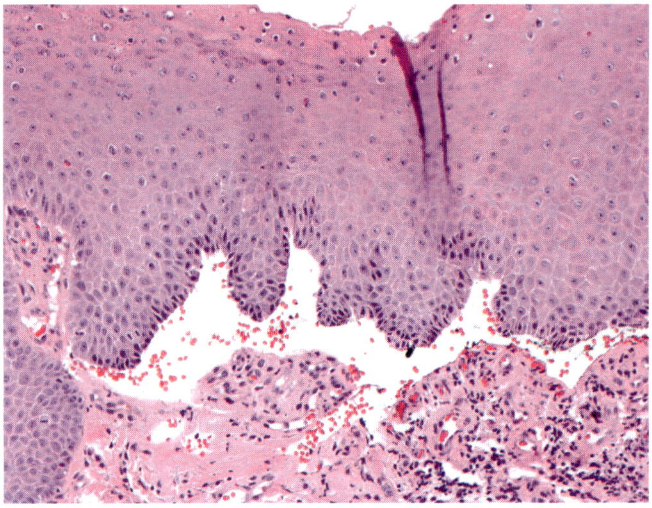

Figure 11.21 Epidermolysis bullosa. A subepidermal blister containing minimal inflammatory cells is noted (×200).

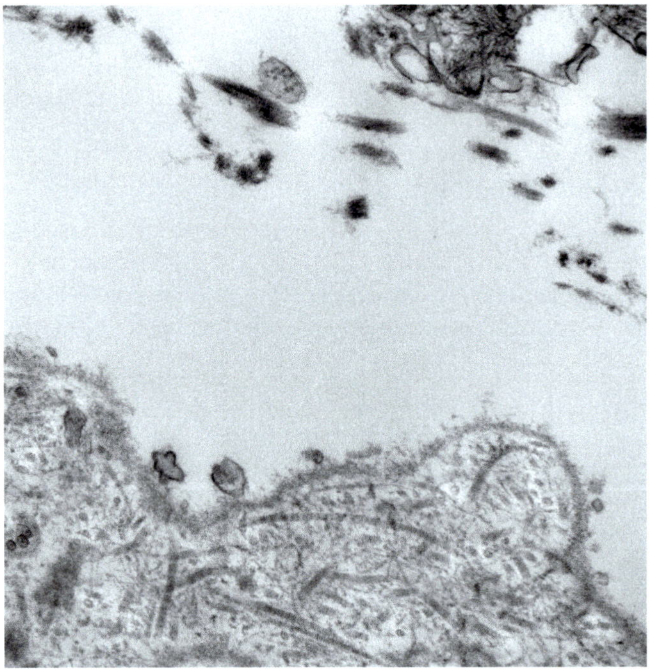

Figure 11.23 Junctional epidermolysis bullosa. The separation is at the lamina lucida with lamina densa seen at the floor of the blister (×36,000).

(EBS) (**Figure 11.22**), lamina lucida in junctional EB (JEB) (**Figure 11.23**), and below the lamina densa in the dystrophic EB (DEB) (**Figure 11.24**).

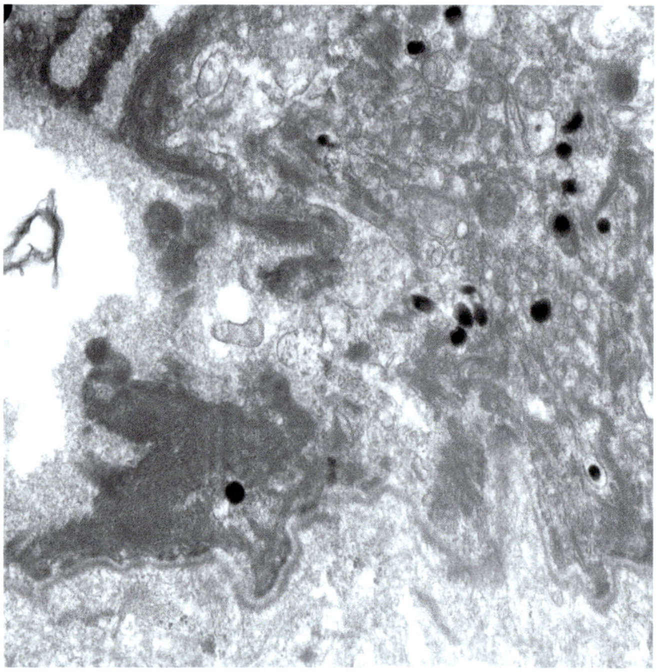

Figure 11.22 Epidermolysis bullosa simplex. The separation is within the basal keratinocytes with basement membrane and hemidesmosomes seen at the floor of the blister (×25,000).

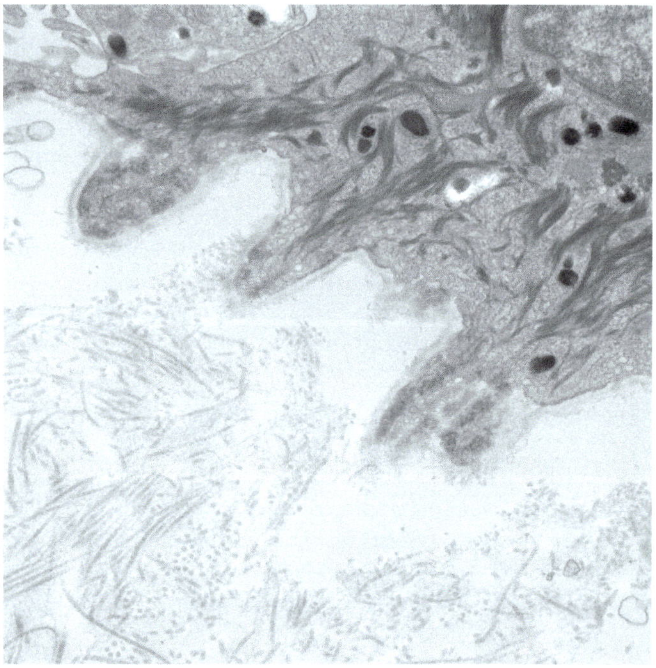

Figure 11.24 Dystrophic epidermolysis bullosa. The separation is at the lamina densa with basement membrane seen attached to the roof of the blister (×14,000).

11.11 IgA Vasculitis

IgA vasculitis, formerly known as Henoch–Schonlein purpura (HSP), the most common IgA vasculitis, typically occurs in the pediatric population, is triggered by infection and associated with IgA deposition in the skin, kidney, and intestine.[171–173] The main morbidity associated with HSP results from glomerulonephritis and the risk of chronic renal failure; therefore, distinguishing HSP from hypersensitivity vasculitis is important. Systemic symptoms, proteinuria, and hematuria are more common in patients with IgA small vessel vasculitis in comparison to non-IgA cases.[174,175] The antecedent infection can be caused by group A or C streptococcal infection, *Mycoplasma pneumoniae*, *Yersinia*, *Salmonella hirshfeldii*, Hepatitis A or C, and Parvovirus B19.[173] IgA vasculitis can develop following COVID-19 vaccination.[176] The purpuric cutaneous eruption often involves the upper and lower extremities, buttocks, and abdomen.

Histologic Features

The skin biopsy typically shows fibrinoid necrosis of the vessel walls, perivascular infiltrate of neutrophils, and extravasated erythrocytes (**Figure 11.25**).[173]

Direct Immunofluorescence

Granular vascular IgA deposition has been reported in lesional skin of 83–100% HSP patients (**Figure 11.26**).[177–179] Concurrent vascular IgM, C3, and fibrinogen, and uncommonly IgG deposition, can be seen in 37%, 87%, 92%, and 3%, respectively.[179] Some reports have suggested that cutaneous IgA predicts renal and gastrointestinal involvement.[177] However, vascular IgA deposition is not diagnostic of HSP since it can be seen in cryoglobulinemia, drug hypersensitivity reaction, inflammatory bowel disease, rheumatoid arthritis, and others.[173] Granular and vascular IgA deposition can be seen in uninvolved skin of IgA nephropathy patients and alcohol liver disease patients.[180,181]

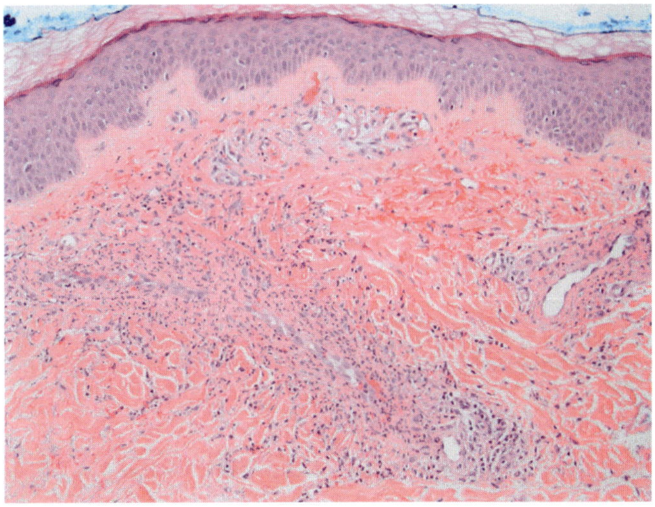

Figure 11.25 Fibrinoid necrosis of vessel walls and perivascular infiltrate of neutrophils are noted in this example of leukocytoclastic vasculitis (×200).

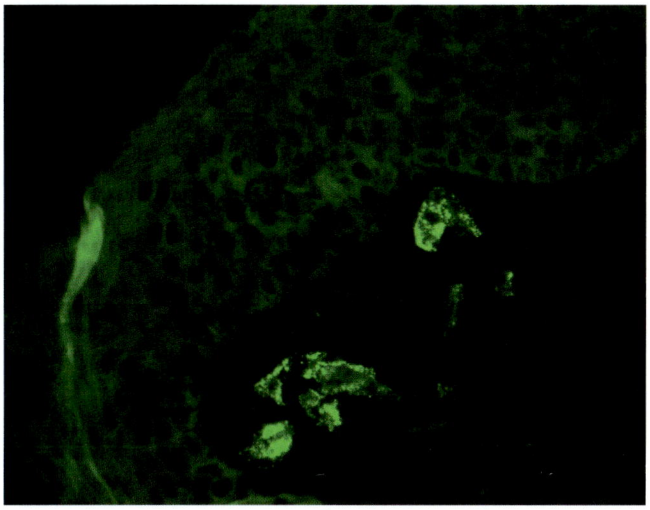

Figure 11.26 Henoch–Schonlein purpura is characterized by vascular IgA deposition on direct immunofluorescence examination.

11.12 Case Studies

Case 11.1

Case history: A 69-year old man with B-cell chronic lymphocytic leukemia presented with a progressively worsened skin eruption that has resulted in extensive skin sloughing over his trunk (**Figure 11.27**). There was oral as well ocular involvement.

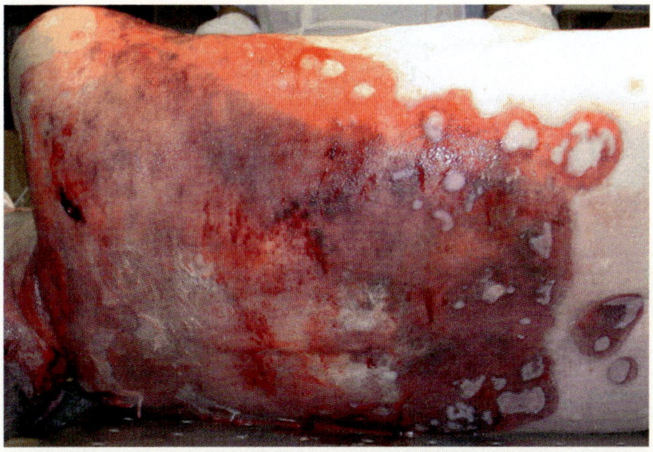

Figure 11.27 Extensive skin sloughing is noted on trunk of a patient with B-cell chronic lymphocytic leukemia.

Description: Skin biopsies from left posterior thigh showed two histology appearances. While one biopsy showed an interface dermatitis with associated full-thickness epidermal necrosis, suprabasilar acantholysis was noted on the other biopsy punch (**Figures 11.28 and 11.29**). DIF studies demonstrated intercellular IgG deposition within the epidermis as well as granular IgG and C3 deposition at the basement membrane zone (**Figure 11.30**). Immunoblotting studies of the patient's serum showed bands corresponding to 210-kDa envoplakin and the 190-kDa periplakin, supportive of paraneoplastic pemphigus.

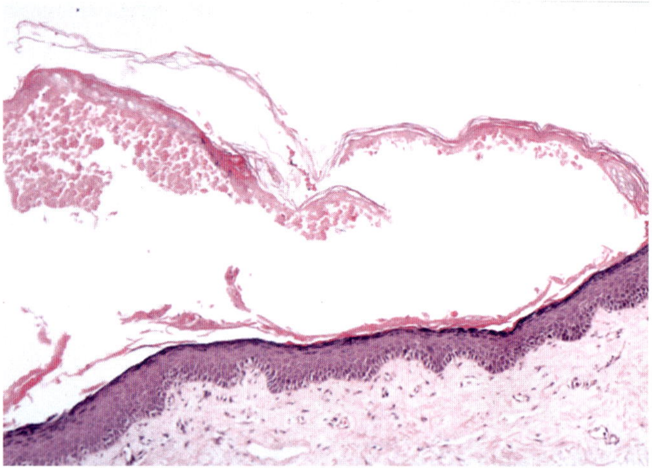

Figure 11.28 Full-thickness epidermal necrosis is noted in one skin biopsy (×100).

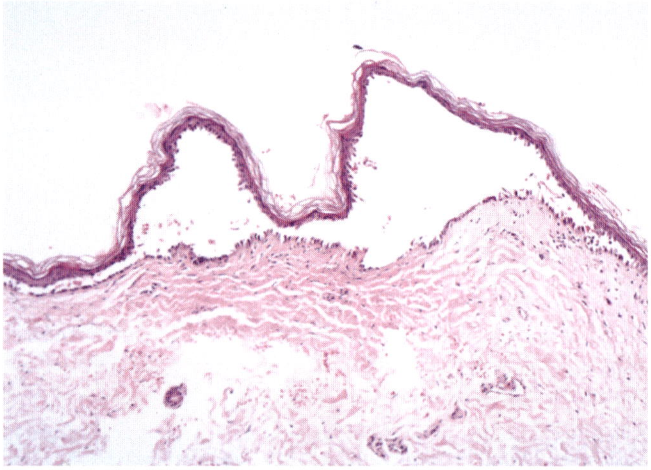

Figure 11.29 Suprabasilar acantholysis is noted in another skin biopsy (×100).

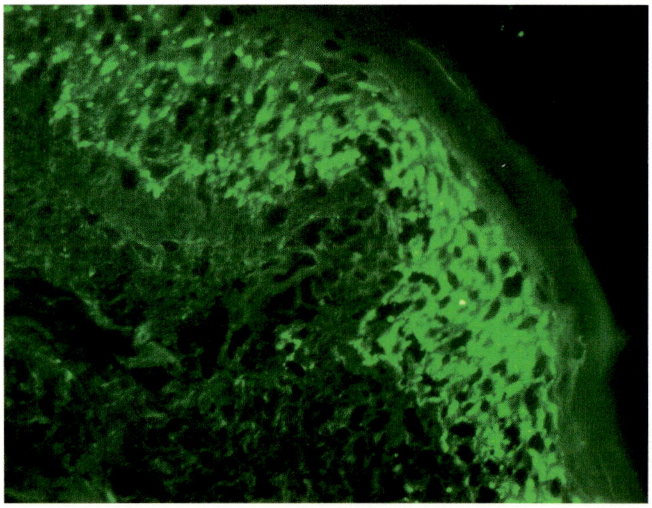

Figure 11.30 Direct immunofluorescence studies demonstrate intercellular IgG deposition within the epidermis as well as granular IgG and C3 deposition at the basement membrane zone.

Diagnosis: Paraneoplastic pemphigus.

Discussion: The clinical presentation and histopathologic features of paraneoplastic pemphigus are polymorphic and varied from case to case. Due to the phenotypic heterogeneity of this disease the diagnosis relies on the demonstration of serum autoantibodies against desmosomal plakin proteins: desmoplakin I (250 kDa), desmoplakin II (210 kDa), envoplakin (210 kDa), periplakin (190 kDa), alpha-2-macroglobulin-like protein 1 (170 kDa), and plectin by immunoprecipitation or immunoblotting. Autoantibodies against desmoglein 1, desmoglein 3, and BPAg1 (230 kDa) can be detected.[182] In a recent series Ohzono and colleagues [133] demonstrated antibodies to desmocollin 1, desmocollin 2, and desmocollin 3 in 18.6%, 41.2%, and 60.8% of 102 patients, respectively, by ELISA. Sixty percent of 53 patients had antibodies to alpha-2-macroglobulin-like protein 1. These authors concluded that antibodies to desmocollins and A2ML1 are helpful.[61]

Case 11.2

Case history: A 30-year-old gravida 1 para 0 presented at 29 weeks' gestation complaining of pruritus and a rash that started on her thighs, then spreading to back, upper extremities and periumbilical area.

Description: A skin biopsy showed a subepidermal blister. Many dermal eosinophils were noted within the epidermis and the dermis (**Figure 11.31**). DIF examination demonstrated linear C3 deposition at the basement membrane zone (**Figure 11.32**). Examination for IgG, IgA, IgM, and fibrinogen deposition was negative.

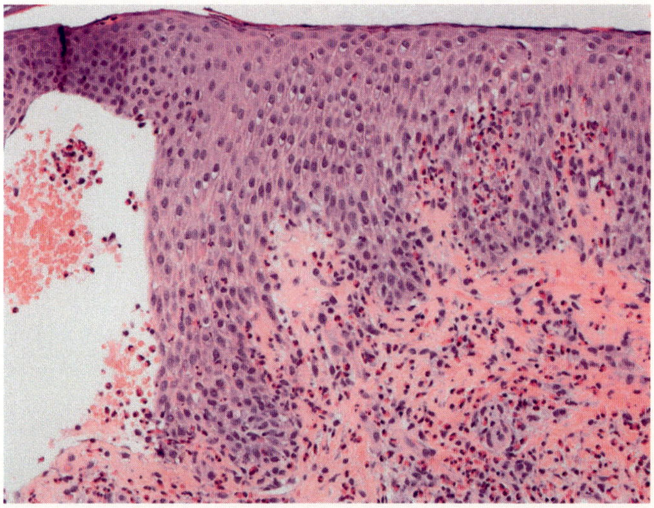

Figure 11.31 A subepidermal blister containing prominent eosinophils is noted (×200).

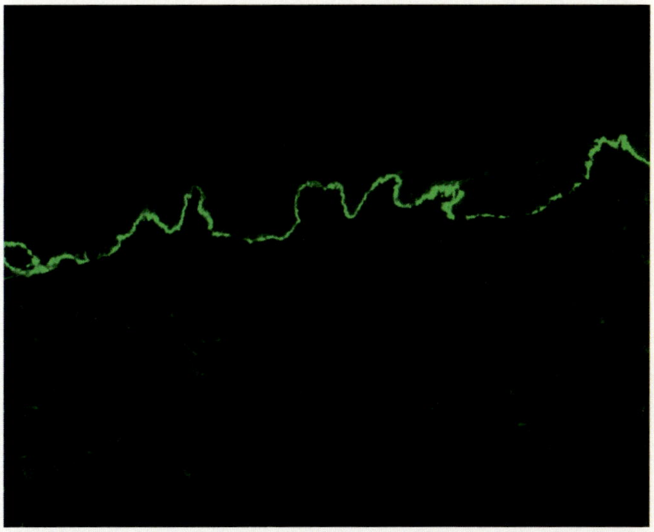

Figure 11.32 Linear C3 deposition is noted the basement membrane zone on direct immunofluorescence studies.

Diagnosis: Pemphigoid gestationis.

Discussion: Pemphigoid gestationis is the only condition associated with pregnancy and positive DIF findings. Pemphigoid gestationis presents in the second or third trimester as pruritic periumbilical plaques that evolve into bullae, often sparing the palms, soles, mucous membrane, and face. The main differential diagnosis is pruritic urticarial plaques and papules of pregnancy/ polymorphic eruption of pregnancy. Most cases begin in the last three months, especially the last five weeks, when the stretching is greatest. It is rare for pruritic urticarial plaques and papules of pregnancy to begin after delivery. DIF examination would be negative.

Case 11.3

Case history: A 75-year-old man was started on finasteride and developed an itchy rash on his chest 5 days later. A morbilliform drug eruption was favored clinically at that time. He then developed a bullous and urticarial eruption. Over the next couple of days he continued to develop new oral lesions and bullae on his neck, trunk and extremities. On physical examination, raised erythematous plaques and bullae were seen on his back, abdomen, upper and lower extremities involving approximately 30% of his total body surface area. Some of the blisters were tense (**Figure 11.33**). Two to three-millimeter vesicles were seen on his lips.

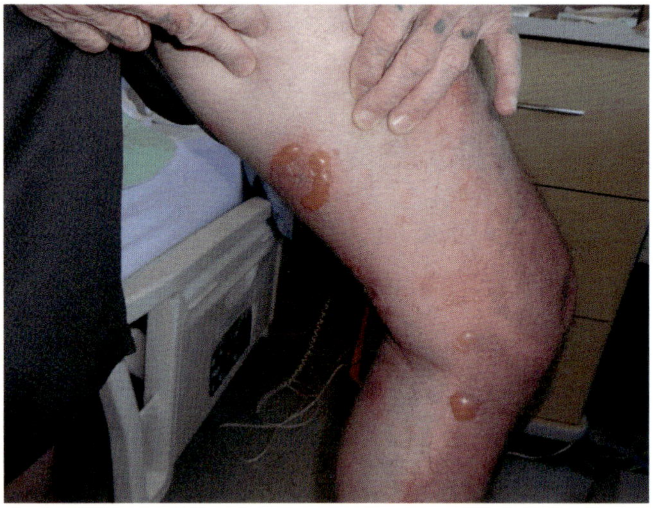

Figure 11.33 Tense blisters are noted on erythematous plaques on the patient's lower extremity (courtesy of Keith W. Morley, M.D., Department of Dermatology, Massachusetts General Hospital, Boston, Massachusetts, USA).

Description: A skin biopsy from right anterior thigh showed a subepidermal blister containing many neutrophils (**Figure 11.34**). DIF studies showed linear IgG and C3 deposition at the basement membrane zone (**Figure 11.35**). Examination for IgA, IgM, and fibrinogen deposition was negative. On NaCl-split skin indirect immunofluorescence examination, IgG positivity was noted on the dermal side or floor of the blister (**Figure 11.36**). Immunoblotting studies of the patient's serum showed a 200-kDa band corresponding to laminin gamma-1. There was no reaction observed for epidermolysis bullosa acquisita (EBA) antigen (290 kDa type VII collagen), bullous pemphigoid antigens (BP230 and BP180), paraneoplastic pemphigus antigens (210 kDa envoplakin and 190 kDa periplakin), pemphigus vulgaris antigen (130 kDa desmoglein 3), and pemphigus foliaceus antigen (160 kDa desmoglein 1).

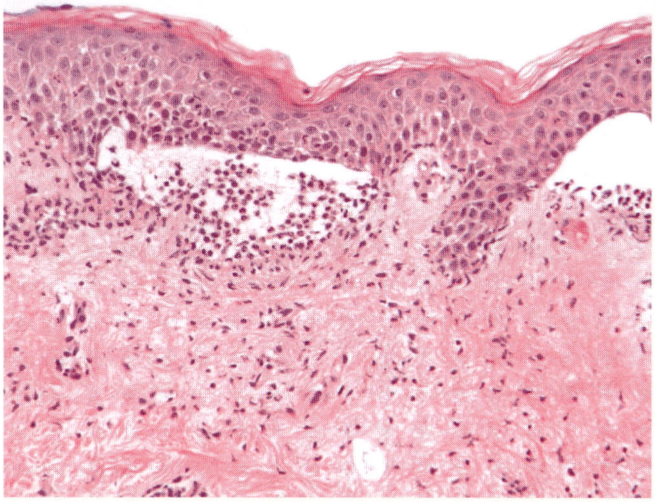

Figure 11.34 Histologic section demonstrates a subepidermal blister containing numerous neutrophils (original magnification ×200).

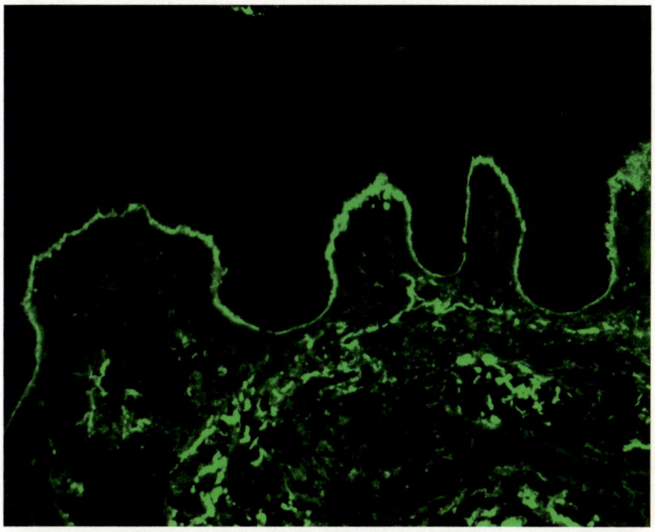

Figure 11.35 On direct immunofluorescence examination, there is IgG deposition at the basement membrane zone.

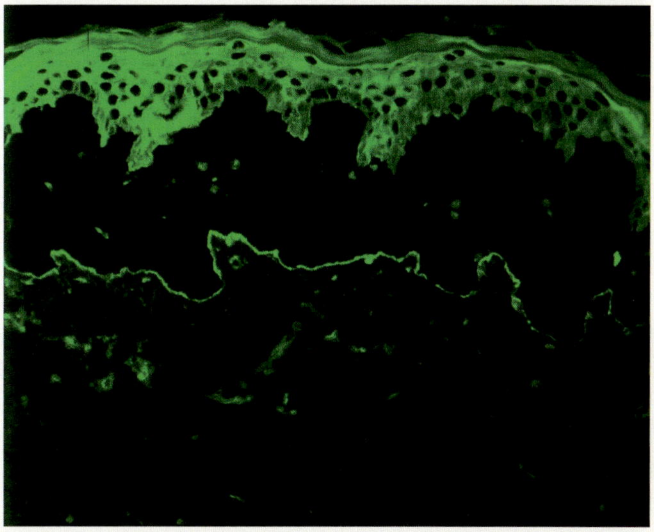

Figure 11.36 On NaCl-split skin indirect immunofluorescence examination, the patient's IgG reacts on dermal side of the blister.

Diagnosis: Anti-p200 pemphigoid.

Discussion: Although the histologic features are those commonly seen in linear IgA disease, the DIF results, linear IgG and C3 deposition at the basement membrane zone, together with the clinical presentation would prompt further workup (**Figure 11.37**). NaCl-split skin indirect immunofluorescence would help distinguish bullous pemphigoid from epidermolysis bullosa acquisita and anti-p200 pemphigoid. Circulating autoantibodies would bind to epidermal aspect or roof of the blister in the setting of bullous pemphigoid, whereas IgG deposition would be seen on the dermal side or floor of the blister in the setting of EBA and anti-p200 pemphigoid. For the entities with dermal staining on IIF, immunoblotting analysis would be needed for definitive diagnosis.

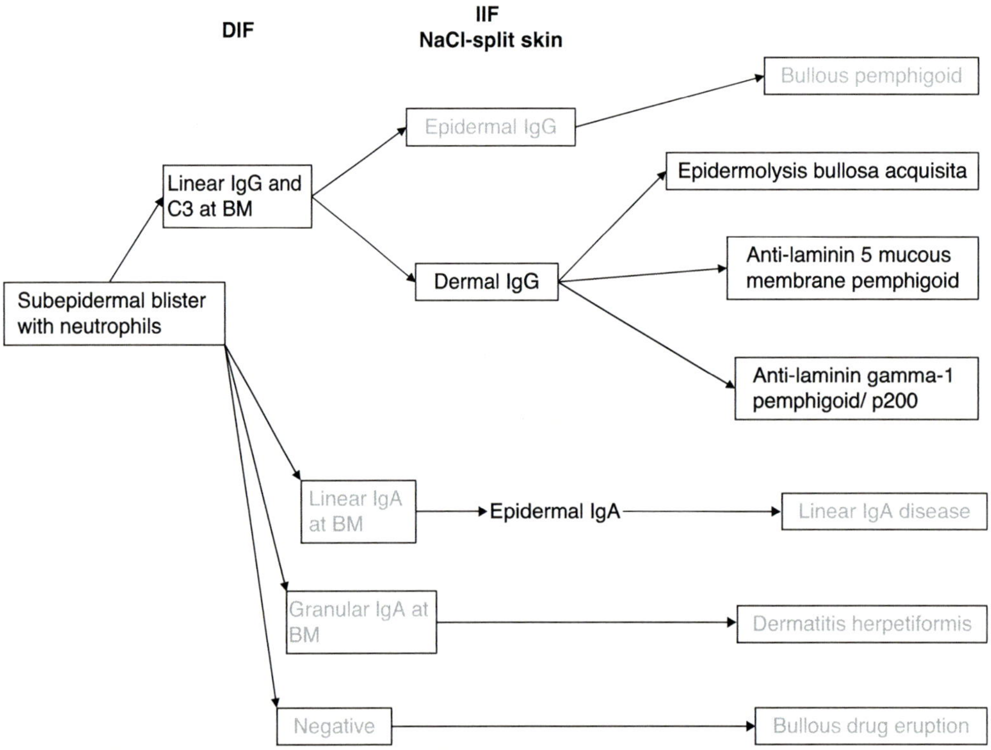

Figure 11.37 An algorithm of how to approach a skin biopsy showing subepidermal blister containing neutrophils.

Case 11.4

Case history: A 56-year-old man presented with a one-year history of pruritus which started on his abdomen. Excoriated and scaly clusters of papules are seen on bilateral elbows, posterior waistline, and gluteal cleft.

Description: Two skin biopsies of his right arm were performed. One submitted for histologic section shows a subepidermal blister containing neutrophils (**Figure 11.38**). Neutrophils are seen lining up at the dermal epidermal junction adjacent to the blister (**Figure 11.39**). Another biopsy submitted for direct immunofluorescence examination shows granular IgA deposition within the papillary dermis (**Figure 11.40**).

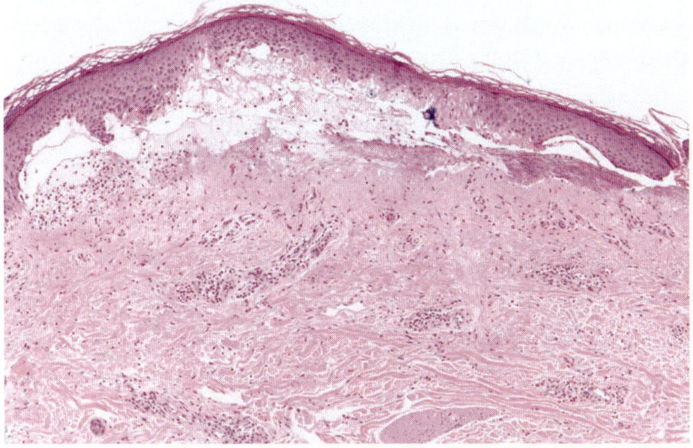

Figure 11.38 A subepidermal blister is seen at low magnification.

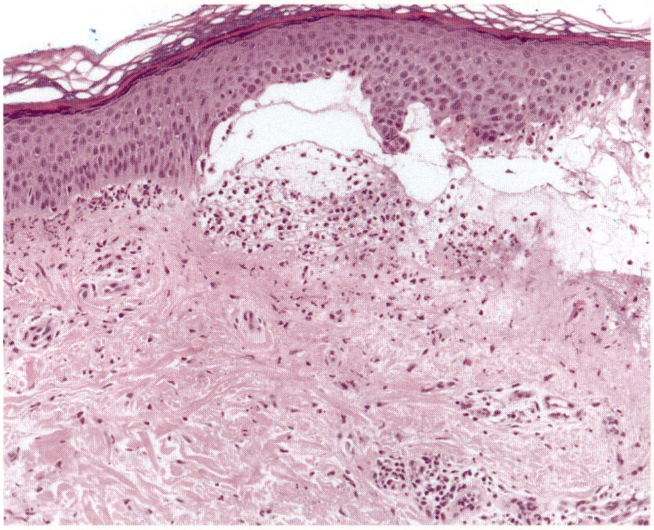

Figure 11.39 Neutrophils are seen within the blister space and at the adjacent dermal epidermal junction.

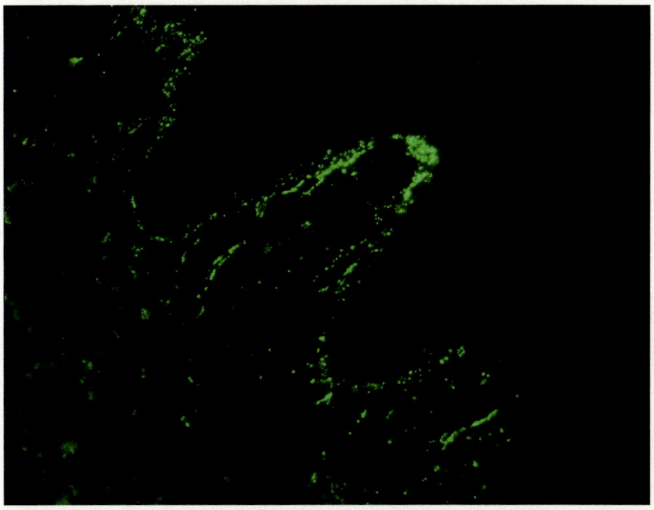

Figure 11.40 Granular IgA deposition is seen within the dermal papillae and at the dermal epidermal junction.

Diagnosis: Dermatitis herpetiformis.

Discussion: Due to intense pruritus, epidermal erosion is often seen on histologic sections. Biopsy of a new blister would be helpful to demonstrate the characteristic subepidermal bullous dermatosis containing neutrophils. The histologic features can often be nonspecific; therefore, the diagnosis is often rested on the DIF findings. DIF is considered to be the gold standard in diagnosing dermatitis herpetiformis. Uninvolved perilesional skin is recommended for DIF since lesional biopsy exhibits a high false negative rate.

Case 11.5

Case history: A 63-year-old man presented with a 2-week history of erythematous vesicles with crust on his right thigh (**Figures 11.41 and 11.42**).

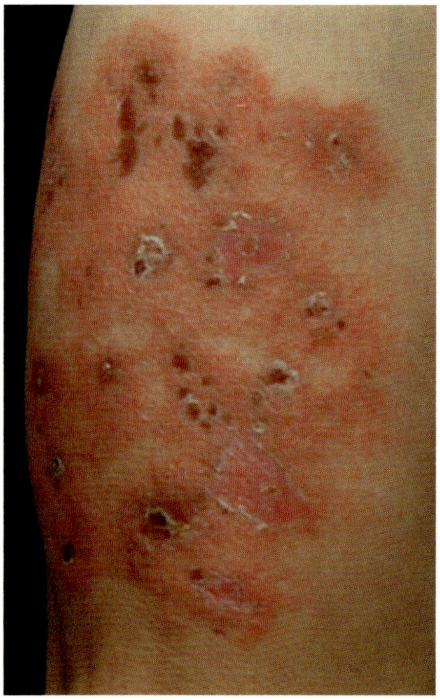

Figure 11.41 Clinical presentation of vesicles on erythematous base (courtesy of Dr. Joonsoo Park, Department of Dermatology, School of Medicine and the Catholic University of Daegu, Daegu, South Korea).

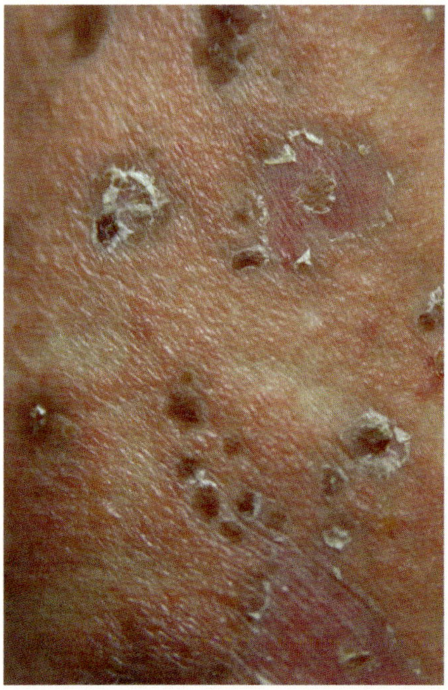

Figure 11.42 Vesicles with associated crust are seen (courtesy of Dr. Joonsoo Park, Department of Dermatology, School of Medicine and the Catholic University of Daegu, Daegu, South Korea).

Description: A skin biopsy shows a subepidermal separation with mild inflammation in a fibrotic superficial dermis (**Figure 11.43**). Direct immunofluorescence examination demonstrates strong and linear band of IgG (**Figure 11.44**) and C3 at the basement membrane zone. On salt-split skin indirect immunofluorescence examination, immunoreactact is seen at the floor of the blister.

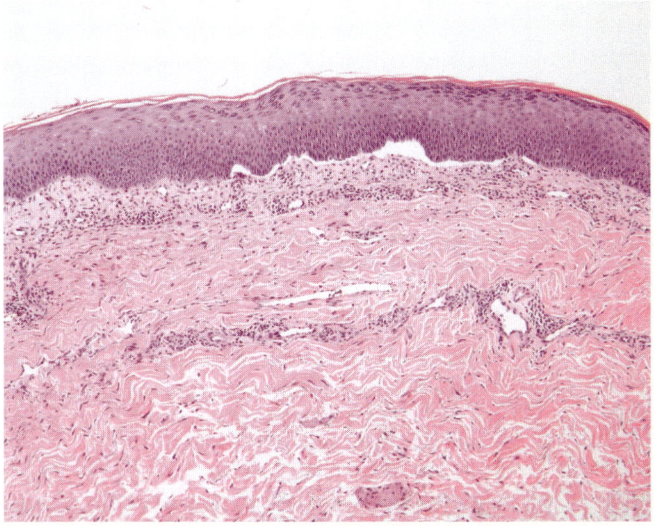

Figure 11.43 Histologic section of the skin biopsy shows a subepidermal blister (×100).

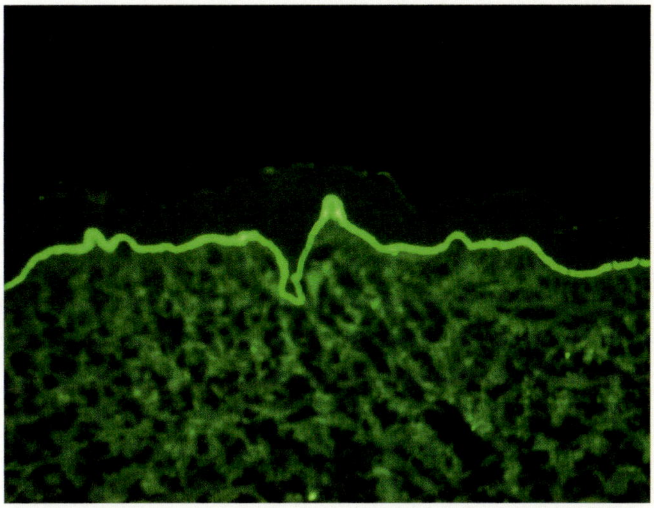

Figure 11.44 Direct immunofluorescence examination shows strong linear IgG deposition at the basement membrane zone.

Diagnosis: Epidermolysis bullosa acquisita.

Discussion: With a subepidermal blister seen on histologic section and linear IgG and C3 deposition at the basement membrane zone, epidermolysis bullosa acquista is often mistaken for bullous pemphigoid. Indirect immunofluorescence examination by salt split skin is helpful since the patient's circulating IgG autoantibodies would bind to the floor of the blister instead of the roof as in bullous pemphigoid. However, immunoblot would be needed to separate epidermolysis bullosa acquisita from anti-p200 pemphigoid.

References

1. Coons AH, Creech HJ, Jones RN. Immunological properties of an antibody containing fluorescent group. *Pro Soc Exp Biol Med* 1941; **47**: 200–2.
2. Coons AH, Kaplan MH. Localization of antigen in tissue cells. II. Improvements in a method for the detection of antigen by means of fluorescent antibody. *J Exp Med* 1950; **91**: 1–13.
3. Jordon RE, Triftshauser CT, Schroeter AL. Direct immunofluorescent studies of pemphigus and bullous pemphigoid. *Arch Dermatol* 1971; **103**: 486–91.
4. Beutner EH, Jordon RE. Demonstration of skin antibodies in sera of pemphigus vulgaris patients by indirect immunofluorescent staining. *Proc Soc Exp Biol Med* 1964; **117**: 505–10.
5. Lemcke S, Sokolowski S, Rieckhoff N, et al. Automated direct immunofluorescence analyses of skin biopsies. *J Cutan Pathol* 2016; **43**: 227–35.
6. Stokes GG. On the change of refrangibility of light. *Trans Cambridge Philos Soc* 1852; **9**: 399.
7. Arbesman J, Grover R, Helm TN, Beutner EH. Can direct immunofluorescence testing still be accurate if performed on biopsy specimens after brief inadvertent immersion in formalin? *J Am Acad Dermatol* 2011; **65**: 106–11.
8. Gammon WR, Briggarman RA, Imman AO 3rd, Quenn LL, Wheeler CE. Differentiating anti-lamina lucida and anti-sublamina dense anti-BMZ antibodies by indirect immunofluorescence on 1.0 M sodium chloride-separated skin. *J Invest Dermatol* 1984; **82**: 139–44.
9. Desai BV, Harmon RM, Green KJ. Desmosomes at a glance. *J Cell Sci* 2009; **122**: 4401–7.
10. Kridin K, Patel PM, Jones VA, Cordova A, Amber KT. IgA pemphigus: a systematic review. *J Am Acad Dermatol* 2020; **82**: 1386–92.
11. Manjaly P, Sanchez K, Gregoire S, Ly S, Kamal K, Mostaghimi A. Superficial and bullous neutrophilic dermatoses: Sneddon-Wilkinson, IgA pemphigus, and bullous lupus. *Dermatol Clin* 2024; **42**: 307–15.
12. Espana A, Gimenez-Azcarate A, Ishii N, et al. Antidesmocollin 1 autoantibody negative subcorneal pustular dermatosis-type IgA pemphigus associated with multiple myeloma. *Br J Dermatol* 2015; **172**: 296–8.
13. Asashina A, Koga H, Suzuki Y, Hashimoto T. IgA pemphigus associated with diffuse large B-cell lymphoma showing unique reactivity with desmocollins: unusual clinical and histopathologic features. *Br J Dermatol* 2013; **168**: 224–6.
14. Bruijn TVM, Geraedts A, Vlahu CA, Jaspars LH, Elshot YS. IgA pemphigus as an immune checkpoint inhibitor-associated skin manifestation. *JAAD Case Rep* 2024; **47**: 41–3.
15. Hashimoto T, Ebihara T, Nishikawa T. Studies of autoantigens recognized by IgA anti-keratinocyte cell surface antibodies. *J Dermatol Sci* 1996; **12**: 10–17.
16. Hashimoto T, Komai A, Futei Y, Nishikawa T, Amagai M. Detection of IgA autoantibodies to desmogleins by an enzyme-linked immunosorbent assay: the presence of new minor subtypes of IgA pemphigus. *Arch Dermatol* 2001; **137**: 735–8.
17. Geller S, Gat A, Zeeli T, et al. The expanding spectrum of IgA pemphigus: a case report and review of the literature. *Br J Dermatol* 2014; **171**: 650–6.
18. Bruckner AL, Fitzpatrick JE, Hashimoto T, Weston WL, Morelli JG. Atypical IgA/IgG pemphigus involving the skin, oral mucosa, and colon in a child: a novel variant of IgA pemphigus? *Pediatr Dermatol* 2005; **22**: 321–7.
19. Zaraa I, Kerkeni N, Sellami M, et al. IgG/IgA pemphigus with IgG and IgA antidesmoglein 3 antibodies and IgA antidesmoglein 1 antibodies detected by enzyme-linked immunosorbent assay: a case report and review of the literature. *Int J Dermatol* 2010; **49**: 293–302.
20. Kowalewski C, Hashimoto T, Amagai M, Jablonska S, Mackiewicz W, Wozniak K. IgA/IgG pemphigus: a new atypical subset of pemphigus? *Acta Derm Venereol* 2006; **86**: 357–8.
21. Mentink LF, de Jong MC, Kloosterhuis GJ, Zuiderveen J, Jonkman MF, Pas HH. Coexistence of IgA antibodies to desmogleins 1 and 3 in pemphigus vulgaris, pemphigus foliaceus and paraneoplastic pemphigus. *Br J Dermatol* 2007; **156**: 635–41.
22. Toosi S, Collins JW, Lohse CM, et al. Clinicopathologic features of IgG/IgA pemphigus in comparison with classic (IgG) and IgA pemphigus. *Int J Dermatol* 2016; **55**: e184–90.
23. Cho YT, Fu KT, Chen KL, Chang YL, Chu CY. Clinical, histopathologic, and immunohistochemical features of patients with IgG/IgA pemphigus. *Biomedicines* 2022; **10**: 1197. doi: 10.3390/biomedicines10051197.
24. Hashimoto T, Teye K, Hashimoto K, et al. Clinical and immunological study of 30 cases with both IgG and IgA anti-keratinocyte cell surface autoantibodies toward the definition of intercellular IgG/IgA dermatosis. *Front Immunol* 2018; **9**: 994. doi: 10.3389/fimmu.2018.00994.
25. Criscito MC, Cohen JM, Toosi S, et al. A retrospective study on the clinicopathologic features of IgG/IgA pemphigus. *J Am Acad Dermatol* 2021; **85**: 237–40.
26. Barcelos VM, Vale ECSD, Araujo MG, Bittencourt FV. Epidemiological and clinical study of cases of endemic pemphigus foliaceus and pemphigus vulgaris in a reference center in the state of Minas Gerais, Brazil. *An Bras Dermatol* 2024; **99**: 43–52.
27. Qian Y, Jeong JS, Maldonado M, et al. Cutting edge: Brazilian pemphigus foliaceus anti-desmoglein 1 autoantibodies cross-react with sand fly salivary LJM11 antigen. *J Immunol* 2012; **189**: 1535–9.
28. Moraes ME, Fernandez-Vina M, Lazaro A, et al. An epitope in the third hypervariable region of the DRB1 gene is involved in the susceptibility to endemic pemphigus foliaceus (fogo selvagem) in three different Brazilian populations. *Tissue Antigens* 1997; **49**: 35–40.
29. Kunadia A, Moschella S, McLemore J, Sami N. Localized pemphigus foliaceus: diverse presentations, treatment, and review of the literature. *Indian J Dermatol* 2023; **68**: 123. doi: 10.4103/ijd.ijd_324_22.
30. Norikawa N, Igari S, Ishikawa M, et al. Six cases of erythrodermic pemphigus foliaceus: a case report. *Case Rep Dermatol* 2022; **14**: 258–63.
31. Howard MS, Yepes MM, Maldonado-Estrada JG, et al. Broad histopathologic patterns of non-glabrous skin and glabrous skin from patients with a new variant of endemic pemphigus foliaceus – part 1. *J Cutan Pathol* 2010; **37**: 222–30.
32. Moro F, Sinagra JLM, Salemme A, et al. Pemphigus: trigger and predisposing factors. *Front Med* 2023; **10**: 1326359. doi: 10.3389/fmed.2023.1326359.
33. Brenner S, Goldberg I. Drug-induced pemphigus. *Clin Dermatol* 2011; **29**: 455–7.
34. Parameswaran A, Attwood K, Sato R, Seiffert-Sinha K, Sinha AA.

Identification of a new disease cluster of pemphigus vulgaris with autoimmune thyroid disease, rheumatoid arthritis and type I diabetes. *Br J Dermatol* 2015; **172**: 7129–38.

35. Kavala M, Topaloqlu Demir F, Zindanci I, et al. Genital involvement in pemphigus vulgaris (PV): correlation with clinical and cervicovaginal Pap smear findings. *J Am Acad Dermatol* 2015; **73**: 655–9.

36. Sriram S, Hasan S, Mansoori S, Saeed S, Banerjee A, Ramalingam K. Juvenile pemphigus vulgaris: Literature review and a rare case report. *Clin Case Rep* 2024; **12**: e8954. doi: 10.1002/ccr3.8954.

37. Luo Y, Fei X, Wang M, et al. Epidemiology of malignant tumors in patients with pemphigus: an analysis of trends from 1955 to 2021. *Clin Exp Med* 2024; **24**: 100. doi: 10.1007/s10238-024-01354-8.

38. Ghaedi F, Etesami I, Aryanian Z, et al. Drug-induced pemphigus: a systematic review of 170 patients. *Int Immunopharmacol* 2021; **92**: 107299. doi: 10.1016/j.intimp.2020.107299.

39. Zhou C, Yu Y, Elston DM. Diagnostic value of eccrine glands and hair follicles in direct immunofluorescent analysis of pemphigus vulgaris and bullous pemphigoid. *J Cutan Pathol* 2016; **43**: 334–8.

40. Alexandru A, Zurac S, Salavastru CM, et al. Direct immunofluorescence on hair follicles: present and future perspectives. *Am J Dermatopathol* 2013; **35**: 472–6.

41. Kamaresan M, Rai R, Sandhya V. Immunofluorescence of the outer root sheath: an aid to diagnosis in pemphigus. *Clin Exp Dermatol* 2011; **36**: 298–301.

42. Giurdanella F, Diercks GF, Jonkman MF, Pas HH. Laboratory diagnosis of pemphigus: direct immunofluorescence remains the gold standard. *Br J Dermatol* 2016; **175**: 185–6.

43. Zhang X, Hyjek E, Soltani K, Petronic-Rosic V, Shea CR. Immunohistochemistry for immunoglobulin G4 on paraffin sections for the diagnosis of pemphigus. *Arch Pathol Lab Med* 2012; **136**: 1402–7.

44. Villani AP, Chouvet B, Kanitakis J. Application of C4d immunohistochemistry on routinely processed tissue sections for the diagnosis of autoimmune bullous dermatoses. *Am J Dermatopathol* 2016; **38**: 186–8.

45. Pfaltz K, Mertz K, Rose C, Scheidegger P, Pfaltz M, Kempf W. C3d immunohistochemistry on formalin-fixed tissue is a valuable tool in the diagnosis of bullous pemphigoid of the skin. *J Cutan Pathol* 2010; **37**: 654–8.

46. Karabağ S, Zorlu Ö. Diagnosis of autoimmune bullous dermatoses: comparative analysis of immunohistochemical staining using C4d, C3d, IgG, and IgG4 in lesional tissues and perilesional frozen skin samples. *Ann Diagn Pathol* 2024; **73**: 152367. doi: 10.1016/j.anndiagpath.2024.152367.

47. Wu N, Cai Y, Wu F, Liang Y, Liu S, Zhang P, Liu Y. C3d Immunohistochemical staining on paraffin-embedded tissue for diagnosis of pemphigus. *Arch Pathol Lab Med* 2024; **148**: 1022–7.

48. Mergler R, Kerstan A, Schmidt E, Goebeler M, Benoit S. Atypical clinical and serological manifestation of pemphigus vegetans: a case report and review of the literature. *Case Rep Dermatol* 2017; **9**: 121–30.

49. Jain VK, Dixit VB, Mohan H. Pemphigus vegetans in an unusual site. *Int J Dermatol* 1989; **28**: 352–3.

50. Cozzani E, Christana K, Mastrogiacomo A, et al. Pemphigus vegetans Neumann type with anti-desmoglein and anti-periplakin autoantibodies. *Eur J Dermatol* 2007; **17**: 530–3.

51. Kimura A, Makino T, Kitayama S, et al. Immunohistopathological analyses of a case of pemphigus vegetans with antibodies against desmoglein 1 and desmocollins 1–3. *J Dermatol* 2024; Jul 29. doi: 10.1111/1346-8138.17410.

52. Senear FE, Usher B. An unusual type of pemphigus combining features of lupus erythematosus. *Arch Derm Syphilol* 1926; **13**: 761–81.

53. Hacker-Foegen MK, Janson M, Amagai M, Fairley JA, Lin MS. Pathogenicity and epitope characteristics of anti-desmoglein-1 from pemphigus foliaceus patients expressing only IgG1 autoantibodies. *J Invest Dermatol* 2003; **121**: 1373–8.

54. Oktarina DA, Poot AM, Kramer D, Diercks GF, Jonkman MF, Pas HH. The IgG "lupus-band" deposition pattern of pemphigus erythematosus. *Arch Dermatol* 2012; **148**: 1173–8.

55. Amerian ML, Ahmed AR. Pemphigus erythematosus. *J Am Acad Dermatol* 1984; **10**: 215–22.

56. Hobbs LK, Noland MB, Raghavan SS, Gru AA. Pemphigus erythematosus: a case series from a tertiary academic center and literature review. *J Cutan Pathol* 2021; **48**: 1038–50.

57. Chorzelski T, Jablonska S, Blaszczyk M. Immunopathological investigations in the Senear-Usher syndrome (coexistence of pemphigus and lupus erythematosus). *Br J Dermatol* 1968; **80**: 211–17.

58. Anhalt GJ, Kim SC, Stanley JR, et al. Paraneoplastic pemphigus: an autoimmune mucocutaneous disease associated with neoplasia. *N Engl J Med* 1990; **323**: 1729–35.

59. Camisa C, Helm TN. Paraneoplastic pemphigus is a distinct neoplasia induced autoimmune disease. *Arch Dermatol* 1993; **129**: 883–6.

60. Svoboda SA, Huang S, Liu X, Hsu S, Motaparthi K. Paraneoplastic pemphigus: revised diagnostic criteria based on literature analysis. *J Cutan Pathol* 2021; **48**: 1133–8.

61. Ohzono A, Sogame R, Li X, et al. Clinical and immunological findings in 104 cases of paraneoplastic pemphigus. *Br J Dermatol* 2015; **173**: 1447–52.

62. Anderson HJ, Huang S, Lee JB. Paraneoplastic pemphigus/paraneoplastic autoimmune multiorgan syndrome: part I. Clinical overview and pathophysiology. *J Am Acad Dermatol* 2024; **91**: 1–10.

63. Czernik A, Camilleri M, Pittelkow MR, Grando SA. Paraneoplastic autoimmune multiorgan syndrome: 20 years after. *Int J Dermatol* 2011; **50**: 905–14.

64. Horn TD, Anhalt GJ. Histologic features of paraneoplastic pemphigus. *Arch Dermatol* 1992; **128**: 1091–5.

65. Poot AM, Siland J, Jonkman MF, Pas HH, Diercks GF. Direct and indirect immunofluorescence staining patterns in the diagnosis of paraneoplastic pemphigus. *Br J Dermatol* 2016; **174**: 912–15.

66. Maciejowska E, Jablonska S, Chorzelski T. Is pemphigus herpetiformis an entity? *Int J Dermatol* 1987; **26**: 571–7.

67. Higashida S, Nishimura K, Muneishi Y, et al. A case of refractory pemphigus herpetiformis with positive anti-desmoglein 1 antibody: case report and literature review to revisit the disease characteristics of 167 cases. *Indian J Dermatol* 2024; **69**: 283. doi: 10.4103/ijd.ijd_1015_23.

68. Hayder F, Bahloul E, Sellami K, et al. Pemphigus herpetiformis in a 4-year-old child: case report and review of the literature. *Clin Case Rep* 2022; **10**: e05567. doi: 10.1002/ccr3.5567.

69. Costa LMC, Cappel MA, Keeling JH. Clinical, pathologic, and immunologic features of pemphigus herpetiformis: a

literature review and proposed diagnostic criteria. *Int J Dermatol* 2019; **58**: 997–1007.

70. Robinson ND, Hashimoto T, Amagai M, Chan LS. The new pemphigus variants. *J Am Acad Dermatol* 1999; **40**: 649–71.
71. Ohata C, Koga H, Teye K, et al. Concurrence of bullous pemphigoid and herpetiform pemphigus with IgG antibodies to desmogleins 1/3 and desmocollins 1–3. *Br J Dermatol* 2013; **168**: 879–81.
72. Duarte IB, Bastazini I Jr, Barreto JA, Carvalho CV, Nunes AJ. Pemphigus herpetiformis in childhood. *Pediatr Dermatol* 2010; **27**: 488–91.
73. Ishii K, Amagai M, Komai A, et al. Desmoglein 1 and desmoglein 3 are the target autoantigens in herpetiform pemphigus. *Arch Dermatol* 1999; **135**: 943–7.
74. Schiavo AL, Ruocco E, Brancaccio G, Caccavale S, Ruocco V, Wolf R. Bullous pemphigoid: etiology, pathogenesis, and inducing factors: facts and controversies. *Clin Dermatol* 2013; **31**: 391–9.
75. Hertl M, Schmidt T. Underrecognition of the heterogeneous clinical spectrum of bullous pemphigoid. *JAMA Dermatol* 2013: **149**: 954–5.
76. Cozzani E, Gasparini G, Buriando M, Drago F, Parodi A. Atypical presentations of bullous pemphigoid: clinical and immunopathological aspects. *Autoimmun Rev* 2015; **14**: 438–45.
77. Marren P, Wojnarowska F, Venning V, Wilson C, Nayar M. Vulvar involvement in auto-immune bullous diseases. *J Reprod Med* 1993; **38**: 101–7.
78. Kawsar A, Edwards C, Patel P, et al. Checkpoint inhibitor-associated bullous cutaneous immune-related adverse events: a multicentre observational study. *Br J Dermatol* 2022; **187**: 981–7.
79. Arechalde A, Braun RP, Calza AM, et al. Childhood bullous pemphigoid associated with IgA antibodies against BP180 or BP230 antigens. *Br J Dermatol* 1999; **140**: 112–18.
80. Collier P, Wojnarowska F, Allen J, Kirtschiq G. Molecular overlap of the IgA target antigens in the subepidermal blistering diseases. *Dermatology* 1994; **189**: 105–7.
81. Korman NJ. Bullous pemphigoid. The latest in diagnosis, prognosis, and therapy. *Arch Dermatol* 1998; **134**: 1137–41.
82. Lehman JS, Carnilleri MJ. Diagnostic utility of direct immunofluorescence findings around hair follicles and sweat glands in immunobullous disease. *J Cutan Pathol* 2013; **40**: 230–5.
83. Ingen-Housz-Oro S, Plee J, Belmondo T, et al. Positive direct immunofluorescence is of better value than ELISA-BP180 and ELISA-BP230 values for the prediction of relapse after treatment cessation in bullous pemphigoid: a retrospective study of 97 patients. *Dermatology* 2015; **231**: 50–5.
84. Magro CM, Dyrsen ME. The use of C3d and C4d immunohistochemistry on formalin-fixed tissue as a diagnostic adjunct in the assessment of inflammatory skin disease. *J Am Acad Dermatol* 2008; **59**: 822–33.
85. Kwon EJ, Ntiamoah P, Shulman KJ. The utility of C4d immunohistochemistry on formalin-fixed paraffin-embedded tissue in the distinction of polymorphic eruption of pregnancy from pemphigoid gestationis. *Am J Dermatopathol* 2013; **35**: 787–91.
86. Glauser S, Rutz M, Cazzaniga S, Hegyi I, Borradori L, Beltraminelli H. Diagnostic value of immunohistochemistry on formalin-fixed paraffin-embedded skin biopsy specimens for bullous pemphigoid. *Br J Dermatol* 2016; **175**: 988–93.
87. Kamyab K, Abdolreza M, Ghanadan A, et al. C4d immunohistochemical stain of formalin-fixed paraffin-embedded tissue as a sensitive method in the diagnosis of bullous pemphigoid. *J Cutan Pathol* 2019; **46**: 723–8.
88. Thakur N, Chatterjee D, Dev A, et al. Utility of C3d and C4d immunohistochemical staining in formalin-fixed skin or mucosal biopsy specimens in diagnosis of bullous pemphigoid and mucous membrane pemphigoid. *Sci Rep* 2023; **13**: 11283. doi: 10.1038/s41598-023-38193-8.
89. Carey B, Setterfield J. Mucous membrane pemphigoid and oral blistering diseases. *Clin Exp Dermatol* 2019; **44**: 732–9.
90. Schmidt E, Zillikens D. Pemphigoid diseases. *Lancet* 2013; **381**: 320–32.
91. Boch K, Ludwig RJ, Zillikens D, Schmidt E. Penile mucous membrane pemphigoid. *J Dtsch Dermatol Ges* 2020; **18**: 727–9.
92. Daito J, Katoh N, Asai J, et al. Brunsting-Perry cicatricial pemphigoid associated with autoantibodies to the C-terminal domain of BP180. *Br J Dermatol* 2008; **159**: 984–6.
93. Fässler M, Rammlmair A, Feldmeyer L, et al. Mucous membrane pemphigoid and lichenoid reactions after immune checkpoint inhibitors: common pathomechanisms. *J Eur Acad Dermatol Venereol* 2020; **34**: e112–e115. doi: 10.1111/jdv.16036.
94. Rahid H, Lamberts A, Borradori L, et al. European guidelines (S3) on diagnosis and management of mucous membrane pemphigoid, initiated by the European Academy of Dermatology and Venereology – Part I. *J Eur Acad Dermatol Venereol* 2021; **35**: 1750–64.
95. Egan CA, Lazarova Z, Darling TN, et al. Anti-epiligrin cicatricial pemphigoid and relative risk for cancer. *Lancet* 2001; **357**: 1850–1.
96. Setterfield J, Shirlaw PJ, Kerr-Muir M, et al. Mucous membrane pemphigoid: a dual circulating antibody response with IgG and IgA signified a more severe and persistent disease. *Br J Dermatol* 1998; **138**: 602–10.
97. Rahbar Z, Cohen JN, McCalmont TH, et al. Cicatricial pemphigoid Brunsting-Perry variant masquerading as neutrophil-mediated cicatricial alopecia. *J Cutan Pathol* 2022; **49**: 408–11.
98. Mehra T, Guenova E, Dechent F, et al. Diagnostic relevance of direct immunofluorescence in ocular mucous membrane pemphigoid. *J Dtsch Dermatol Ges* 2015; **13**: 1268–74.
99. Yilmaz K, Hammers CM, Boch K, Zillikens D, Shimanovich I, Schmidt E. Immunoglobulin M mucous membrane pemphigoid. *J Dtsch Dermatol Ges* 2023; **21**: 285–7.
100. Lipozencic J, Ljubojevic S, Bukvic-Mokos Z. Pemphigoid gestationis. *Clin Dermatol* 2012; **30**: 51–5.
101. Preuß SL, Vorobyev A, Moderegger EL, et al. Pemphigoid gestationis is associated with an increased risk for adverse pregnancy outcomes: a large-scale propensity-matched retrospective cohort study. *J Am Acad Dermatol* 2024; **91**:748–750.
102. Jimenez A, Blain K, Khalighi M, Clarke JT, Snook J, Cipriano SD. Neonatal pemphigoid gestationis: an atypical presentation of a rare disease. *Pediatr Dermatol* 2021; **38**: 1575–6.
103. Cordel N, Flament J, Jouen F, et al; French study Group on autoimmune bullous skin diseases. Anti-BP180 IgG antibody ELISA values correlate with adverse pregnancy outcomes in pemphigoid gestationis. *J Eur Acad Dermatol Venereol* 2023; **37**: 1207–14.

104. Castro LA, Lundell RB, Krause PK, Gibson LE. Clinical experience in pemphigoid gestationis: report of 10 cases. *J Am Acad Dermatol* 2006; **55**: 823–8.

105. Baban F, Xie F, Lehman JS, Theiler R, Todd A, Davis DM, Johnson EF. Histopathological features of pemphigoid gestationis and polymorphic eruption of pregnancy: A blinded retrospective comparative study of 31 cases. *J Cutan Pathol* 2023; **50**: 358–63.

106. Tani N, Kimura Y, Koga H, et al. Clinical and immunological profiles of 25 patients with pemphigoid gestationis. *Br J Dermatol* 2015; **172**: 120–9.

107. Barnadas MA, Rubiales V, Gonzalez MJ, et al. Enzyme-linked immunosorbent assay (ELISA) and indirect immunofluorescence testing in a bullous pemphigoid and pemphigoid gestationis. *Int J Dermatol* 2008; **47**: 1245–9.

108. Dilling A, Rose C, Hashimoto T, Zillikens D, Shimanovich I. Anti-p200 pemphigoid: a novel autoimmune subepidermal blistering disease. *J Dermatol* 2007; **34**: 1–8.

109. Dainichi T, Kurono S, Ohyama B, et al. Anti-laminin gamma-1 pemphigoid. *Proc Natl Acad Sci USA* 2009; **106**: 2800–5.

110. Goletz S, Pigors M, Lari TR, et al. Laminin beta4 is a constituent of the cutaneous basement membrane zone and additional autoantigen of anti-p200 pemphigoid. *J Am Acad Dermatol* 2024; **90**: 790–7.

111. Gao Y, Qian H, Hashimoto T, Li X. Potential contribution of anti-p200 autoantibodies to mucosal lesions in anti-p200 pemphigoid. *Front Immunol* 2023; **14**: 1118846. doi: 10.3389/fimmu.2023.1118846.

112. Holtsche MM, Goletz S, von Georg A, et al. Serologic characterization of anti-p200 pemphigoid: epitope spreading as a common phenomenon. *J Am Acad Dermatol* 2021; **84**: 1155–7.

113. Wang Y, Li S, Li Z, et al. Clinical and immunoserological characteristics of anti-p200 pemphigoid: Comparisons of patients with epitope spreading and non-epitope spreading. *Int J Dermatol* 2025; **64**:359–366.

114. Goetze S, Dumke AK, Zillikens D, Hipler UC, Elsner P. Anti-p200/laminin gamma1 pemphigoid associated with metastatic oesophageal cancer. *J Eur Acad Dermatol Venereol* 2017; **31**: e219–e221.

115. Laufer Britva R, Amber KT, Cohen AD, Kridin K. Treatment and clinical outcomes in anti-p200 pemphigoid: a systematic review. *J Eur Acad Dermatol Venereol* 2020; **34**: 465–72.

116. Rose C, Weyers W, Denisjuk N, et al. Histopathology of anti-p200 pemphigoid. *Am J Dermatopathol* 2007; **29**: 119–24.

117. Senatore S, Maglie R, Montefusco F, et al. Inverted-U serration pattern: a novel clue for the diagnosis of anti-laminin-gamma1 pemphigoid. *Int J Dermatol* 2021; **60**: 1547–9.

118. Lau I, Goletz S, Holtsche MM, Zillikens D, Fechner K, Schmidt E. Anti-p200 pemphigoid is the most common pemphigoid disease with serum antibodies against the dermal side by indirect immunofluorescence microscopy on human salt-split skin. *J Am Acad Dermatol* 2019; **81**: 1195–7.

119. Groth S, Recke A, Vafia K, et al. Development of a simple enzyme-linked immunosorbent assay for the detection of autoantibodies in anti-p200 pemphigoid. *Br J Dermatol* 2011; **164**: 76–82.

120. Kitayama S, Makino T, Hayashi M, et al. Usefulness of immunofluorescence overlay antigen mapping in the identification of autoantigen in anti-p200 pemphigoid. *J Dermatol* 2023; **50**: 1194–8.

121. Hubner F, Langan EA, Recke A. Lichen planus pemphigoides: from lichenoid inflammation to autoantibody-mediated blistering. *Front Immunol* 2019; **10**: 1389. https://doi.org/10.3389/fimmu.2019.01389

122. Wang S, Sun J, Deng S, et al. Lichen planus pemphigoides induced by anti-PD-1 antibody: a case only involved in oral mucosa with excellent topical treatment efficiency. *J Cutan Pathol* 2024; **51**: 114–18.

123. Zaraa I, Mahfoudh A, Sellami MK, et al. Lichen planus pemphigoides: four new cases and a review of the literature. *Int J Dermatol* 2013; **52**: 406–12.

124. Solomon LW, Helm TN, Stevens C, et al. Clinical and immunopathologic findings in oral lichen planus pemphigoides. *Oral Surg Oral Med Oral Pathol Oral Radiol Endod* 2007; **103**: 808–13.

125. Mansfield PK, Moody R, Li Y, Heinecke G. A rare case of lichen planus pemphigoides with palmoplantar hyperkeratotic plaques. *JAAD Case Rep* 2024; **49**: 14–16. doi: 10.1016/j.jdcr.2024.04.001.

126. Zillikens D, Caux F, Mascaro JM, et al. Autoantibodies in lichen planus pemphigoides react with a novel epitope within the C-terminal NC16A domain of BP180. *J Invest Dermatol* 1999; **113**: 117–21.

127. Okochi H, Nashiro K, Tsuchida T, Seki Y, Tamaki K. Lichen planus pemphigoides: case report and results of immunofluorescence and immunoelectron microscopic study. *J Am Acad Dermatol* 1990; **22**: 626–31.

128. Jang SH, Yun SJ, Lee SC, Lee JB. Lichen planus pemphigoides associated with chronic hepatitis B virus infection. *Clin Exp Dermatol* 2015; **40**: 868–71.

129. Chorzelski TP, Jablonska S. IgA linear dermatosis of childhood (chronic bullous disease of childhood). *Br J Dermatol* 1979; **101**: 535–42.

130. Gottlieb J, Ingen-Housz-Oro S, Alexandre M, et al. Idiopathic linear IgA bullous dermatosis: prognostic factors based on a case series of 72 adults. *Br J Dermatol* 2017; **177**: 212–22.

131. Garel B, Ingen-Housz-Oro S, et al. Drug-induced linear immunoglobulin A bullous dermatosis: a French retrospective pharmacovigilance study of 69 cases. *Br J Clin Pharmacol* 2019; **85**: 570–9.

132. Ishiko A, Shimizu H, Masunaga T, et al. 97-kDa linear IgA bullous dermatosis angigen localizes in the lamina lucida between the NC16A and carboxyl terminal domain of the 180 kDa bullous permphigoid antigen. *J Invest Dermatol* 1998; **111**: 93–6.

133. Caux F, Patsatsi A, Karakioulaki M, et al. S2 k guidelines on diagnosis and treatment of linear IgA dermatosis initiated by the European Academy of Dermatology and Venereology. *J Eur Acad Dermatol Venereol* 2024; **38**: 1006–23.

134. Becker M, Schumacher N, Schmidt E, Zillikens D, Sadik CD. Evaluation and comparison of clinical and laboratory characteristics of patients with IgA epidermolysis Bullosa Acquisita, Linear IgA Bullous Dermatosis, and IgG Epidermolysis Bullosa Acquisita. *JAMA Dermatol.* 2021; **157**: 917–23.

135. Wang KL, Todd A, Davis DMR, Lehman JS. Histopathologic features in drug-induced, malignancy-associated, or idiopathic linear IgA bullous dermatosis: a retrospective comparative cohort study of 65 patients. *J Cutan Pathol* 2025; **52**:254–258.

136. Egan CA, Taylor TB, Meyer LJ, Petersen MJ, Zone JJ. The immunoglobulin A antibody response in clinical subsets

of mucous membrane pemphigoid. *Dermatology* 1999; **198**: 330–5.

137. Vodegel RM, Jonkman MF, Pas HH, de Jong MC. U-serrated immunodeposition pattern differentiates type VII collagen targeting bullous diseases from other subepidermal bullous autoimmune diseases. *Br J Dermatol* 2004; **151**: 112–18.
138. Ohata C, Ishii N, Koga H, Nakama T. A clinical and serological study of linear IgA bullous dermatosis without linear immunoglobulin deposition other than IgA at the basement membrane zone using direct immunofluorescence. *Br J Dermatol* 2017; **177**: 152–7.
139. Willsteed E, Bhogal BS, Black MM, McKee P, Wojnarowska F. Use of 1 M NaCl split skin in the direct immunofluorescence of the linear IgA bullous dermatoses. *J Cutan Pathol* 1990; **17**: 144–8.
140. El-Domyati M, Abdel-Wahab H, Ahmad H. Immunohistochemical localization of basement membrane laminin 5 and collagen IV in adult linear IgA disease. *Int J Dermatol* 2015; **54**: 922–8.
141. Kridin K, Kneiber D, Kowalski EH, Valdebran M, Amber KT. Epidermolysis bullosa acquisita: a comprehensive review. *Autoimmun Rev* 2019; **18**: 786–95.
142. Hignett E, Sami N. Pediatric epidermolysis bullosa acquisita: a review. *Pediatr Dermatol* 2021; **38**: 1047–50.
143. Hundorfean G, Neurath MF, Sitaru C. Autoimmunity against type VII collagen in inflammatory bowel disease. *J Cell Mol Med* 2010; **14**: 2393–403.
144. Miyamoto D, Gordilho JO, Santi CG, Porro AM. Epidermolysis bullosa acquisita. *An Bras Dermatol* 2022; **97**: 409–23.
145. Meijer JM, Atefi I, Diercks GFH, et al. Serration pattern analysis for differentiating epidermolysis bullosa acquisita from other pemphigoid diseases. *J Am Acad Dermatol* 2018; **78**: 754–59.e6. doi: 10.1016/j.jaad.2017.11.029.
146. Seta V, Aucouturier F, Bonnefoy J, et al. Comparison of 3 type VII collagen (C7) assays for serologic diagnosis of epidermolysis bullosa acquisita (EBA). *J Am Acad Dermatol* 2016; **74**: 1166–72.
147. Burnham TK, Neblett TR, Fine G. Immunofluorescent "band" test for lupus erythematosus. II. Employing skin lesions. *Arch Dermatol* 1970; **102**: 42–50.
148. Cardinali C, Caproni M, Fabbri P. The utility of the lupus band test on sun-protected non-lesional skin for the diagnosis of systemic lupus erythematosus. *Clin Exp Rheumatol* 1999; **17**: 427–32.
149. Leibold AM, Bennion S, David-Bajar K, Schleve MJ. Occurrence of positive immunofluorescence in the dermo-epidermal junction of sun-exposed skin of normal adults. *J Cutan Pathol* 1994; **21**: 200–6.
150. de Risi-Pugliese T, Cohen Aubart F, Haroche J, et al. Clinical, histological, immunological presentations and outcomes of bullous systemic lupus erythematosus: 10 new cases and a literature review of 118 cases. *Semin Arthritis Rheum* 2018; **48**: 83–9.
151. Barker CS, Bruner E, Self S, Elston DM. U-serrated and n-serrated patterns in bullous pemphigoid, epidermolysis bullosa acquisita, and bullous lupus: a retrospective observational study. *J Am Acad Dermatol* 2024; **90**: 1282–4.
152. Kontos AP, Jirsari M, Jacobsen G, et al. Immunoglobulin M predominance in cutaneous lupus erythematosus. *J Cutan Pathol* 2005; **32**: 352–5.
153. Magro CM, Crowson AN. The immunofluorescent profile of dermatomyositis: a comparative study with lupus erythematosus. *J Cutan Pathol* 1997; **24**: 543–52.
154. Magro CM, Crowson AN, Regauer S. Mixed connective tissue disease: a clinical, histologic, and immunofluorescence study of eight cases. *Am J Dermatopathol* 1997; **19**: 206–13.
155. Jones SA, Black MM. The value of direct immunofluorescence as a diagnostic aid in dermatomyositis: a study of 35 cases. *Clin Exp Dermatol* 1997; 22: 77–81.
156. Magro CM, Crowson AN, Harrist TJ. The use of antibody to C5b-9 in the subclassification of lupus erythematosus. *Br J Dermatol* 1996; **134**: 855–62.
157. Kakoullis L, Louppides S, Papachristodoulou E, Panos G. Porphyrias and photosensitivity: pathophysiology for the clinician. *Postgrad Med* 2018; **130**: 673–86.
158. 110. Green JJ, Manders SM. Pseudoporphyria. *J Am Acad Dermatol* 2001; **44**: 100–8.
159. Maynard B, Peters MS. Histologic and immunofluorescence study of cutaneous porphyrias: histologic and immunofluorescence study of cutaneous porphyrias. *J Cutan Pathol* 1992; **19**: 40–7.
160. Dabski C, Beutner EH. Studies of laminin and type IV collagen in blisters of porphyria cutanea tarda and drug-induced pseudoporphyria. *J Am Acad Dermatol* 1991; **25**: 28–32.
161. Nguyen CN, Kim SJ. Dermatitis herpetiformis: an update on diagnosis, disease monitoring, and management. *Medicina* 2021; **57**: 843. doi: 10.3390/medicina57080843.
162. Mobacken H, Kastrup W, Nilsson LA. Incidence and prevalence of dermatitis herpetiformis in western Sweden. *Acta Derm Venereol* 1984; **64**: 400–4.
163. Verdelli A, Corrà A, Mariotti EB, et al. Skin gluten-related disorders: new and old cutaneous manifestations to be considered. *Front Med* 2023; May 17; **10**: 1155288. doi: 10.3389/fmed.2023.1155288.
164. Sardy M, Karpati S, Merkl B, Paulsson M, Smyth N. Epidermal transglutaminase (Tgase 3) is the autoantigen of dermatitis herpetiformis. *J Exp Med* 2002; **195**: 747–57.
165. Barnadas MA. Dermatitis herpetiformis: a review of direct immunofluorescence findings. *Am J Dermatopathol* 2016; **38**: 283–8.
166. Drozdowski R, Stewart C, Murphy M. Fibrillary "fern-like" immunoglobulin A deposition in dermatitis herpetiformis. *Am J Dermatopathol* 2022; **44**: 389–90.
167. Antiga E, Maglie R, Lami G, et al. Granular deposits of IgA in the skin of coeliac patients without dermatitis herpetiformis: a prospective multicentric analysis. *Acta Derm Venereol.* 2021; **101**: adv00382. doi: 10.2340/00015555-3742.
168. Hashimoto T, Tsuruta D, Yasukochi A, et al. Granular C3 dermatosis. *Acta Derm Venereol* 2016; **96**: 748–53.
169. Fine JD, Bruckner-Tuderman L, Eady RAJ, et al. Inherited epidermolysis bullosa: updated recommendations on diagnosis and classification. *J Am Acad Dermatol* 2014; **70**: 1103–26.
170. Bardhan A, Bruckner-Tuderman L, et al. Epidermolysis bullosa. *Nat Rev Dis Primers* 2020; **6**: 78. doi: 10.1038/s41572-020-0210-0.
171. Carmona-Cruz SA, Durán-McKinster LC, García-Romero MT. Atypical purpura and other features associated with unfavorable outcomes of IgA vasculitis (Henoch–Schonlein purpura) in children: a retrospective study. *Pediatr Dermatol* 2022; **39**: 369–71.

172. Hammad H, Krausz J, Barcan M, Fisher S, Edison N, Ziv M. Adult Henoch–Schönlein purpura: comprehensive assessment of demographic, clinical, and histopathological features as predictors for systemic involvement. *Dermatology* 2023; **239**: 609–15.

173. Magro CM, Crowson AN. A clinical and histologic study of 37 cases of immunoglobulin A associated vasculitis. *Am J Dermatopathol* 1999; **21**: 234–40.

174. Hirt PA, Nanda S, Ogunbufunmi F, Dorizas A, Maderal A. Increased systemic symptoms in patients with positive direct immunofluorescence of skin biopsies with Henoch–Schonlein purpura/IgA vasculitis: a retrospective chart review. *Am J Dermatopathol* 2023; **45**: 861–2.

175. Gambichler T, Bui D, Domin B, et al. Comparison of clinical and laboratory data of adult patients with cutaneous IgA vasculitis and non-IgA vasculitis. *Clin Exp Dermatol* 2024; **49**: 859–65.

176. Ramdani Y, Bettuzzi T, Bouznad A, et al. IgA vasculitis following COVID-19 vaccination: a French multicenter case series including 12 patients. *J Rheumatol* 2023; **50**: 252–7.

177. Barnadas MA, Perez E, Gich I, et al. Diagnostic, prognostic and pathogenic value of the direct immunofluorescence test in cutaneous leukocytoclastic vasculitis. *Int J Dermatol* 2004; **43**: 19–26.

178. Linskey KR, Kroshinsky D, Mihm MC Jr, Hoang MP. Immunoglobulin A-associated small-vessel vasculitis: a 10-year experience at the Massachusetts General Hospital. *J Am Acad Dermatol* 2012; **66**: 813–22.

179. Poterrucha TJ, Wetter DA, Gibson LE, Camilleri MJ, Lohse CM. Correlates of systemic disease in adult Henoch–Schonlein purpura: a retrospective study of direct immunofluorescence and skin lesion distribution in 87 patients at Mayo Clinic. *J Am Acad Dermatol* 2012; **67**: 612–16.

180. Thompson AJ, Chan YL, Woodroffe AJ, et al. Vascular IgA deposits in clinically normal skin of patients with renal disease. *Pathology* 1980; **12**: 407–13.

181. Saklayen MG, Schroeter AL, Nafz MA, Jalik K. IgA deposition in the skin of patients with alcoholic liver disease. *J Cutan Pathol* 1996; **23**: 12–18.

182. Schepens I, Jaunin F, Begre N, et al. The protease inhibitor alpha-2-macroglobulin-like-1 is the p170 antigen recognized by paraneoplastic pemphigus autoantibodies in human. *PLoS One* 2010; **5**: e12250.

Chapter 12

Cutaneous Infections

Wun Ju Shieh and Mai P. Hoang

Introduction

Healthy and intact skin provides an effective barrier against invasion by microorganisms. Clinical skin infection usually results from breakdown of this natural barrier due to injury, loss of local immunity, or disturbances within the normal flora on skin surface. Skin infections can be caused by a wide variety of microorganisms, including bacteria, viruses, parasites, and fungi. Clinical manifestations of skin infection can vary greatly in presentations, such as size, shape, number, localization, and severity. In some cases, infections can spread beyond the skin into the bloodstream and involve other organ systems. Some of the infections can be self-limited without treatment, whereas others can be fatal if no appropriate diagnosis and management are made. A crucial step toward making the etiologic diagnosis of infection is sample collection with pertinent laboratory testing. Direct examination of material obtained from skin lesions, such as vesicular fluid or scraps from smear or touch preparation can be a useful noninvasive method for a quick diagnosis. However, most of the time, a definitive diagnosis relies on other ancillary tests, such as culture, special stains, serology, molecular techniques, and others. Skin biopsy is an important tool for diagnosis of skin infections. It allows the examination of the histologic changes due to infectious process and host responses, as well as localization of the causative microorganisms in tissue. In conjunction with special stains, immunohistochemistry, electron microscopy, and molecular assays, a skin biopsy can provide useful diagnostic information with clinicopathologic correlation.

Immunohistochemistry (IHC) has been widely used in all aspects of pathology diagnosis in the past three decades. There are IHC assays readily available for the diagnosis of skin infections (**Table 12.1**). By using a variety of antibodies, IHC can detect the presence of microbial antigens in skin biopsies, whether they represent the intact or degraded pathogens, and whether they are intracellular or extracellular. Many of the antibodies used in IHC are commercially available and are widely used in diagnostic pathology laboratories. Others, especially those antibodies for detecting emerging or unusual pathogens, are available only at highly specialized laboratories such as the Centers for Disease Control and Prevention. Similar to all other laboratory assays, the sensitivity and specificity of any immunostain always require a careful evaluation before establishing its status as a diagnostic assay.

There are many advantages of using formalin-fixed tissues and IHC to detect etiologic pathogens. It is particularly useful in detecting those fastidious or slow-growing organisms, such as mycobacteria or *Tropheryma whipplei*, and can improve the speed, sensitivity, and specificity of microbial diagnosis. It is also valuable for characterizing emerging infections or pathogens with high biosafety concern, such as those caused by *Bacillus anthracis* or Ebola virus. IHC performed on fixed tissues can minimize laboratory worker's potential risk of exposure to infectious agents because of the deactivation of pathogens by formalin fixation. Additionally, immunolocalization of antigens with IHC provides histomorphologic correlation between the infectious pathogen and host tissue responses, which is not only crucial for diagnosis but also important to study the pathogenesis of those emerging infections.

12.1 Bacteria

A wide range of bacteria, including mycobacteria, rickettsiae, and spirochetes, can affect the skin and subcutaneous tissue. They represent the largest proportion of pathogens causing emerging and travel-associated skin infections. Clinically, they can present as folliculitis, furuncles, carbuncles, abscess, erysipelas, cellulitis, ecthyma, or impetigo. A limited number of histopathologic patterns are seen with bacterial infections in the skin, and none of these reaction patterns are specific for any pathogens. Definitive diagnosis of most bacterial diseases depends on identification of the pathogens with appropriate cultures or molecular techniques. Cultures from actual biopsies have a higher yield than cultures from aspirates or superficial swabs. An ideal method to maximize the yield of etiologic diagnosis for deeper skin infections is to send half of the biopsy for culture and molecular testing, while the other half for histopathologic evaluation, special stains, and IHC. The location of the bacteria in the skin biopsy is important to note. Gram-positive cocci and coccobacilli, such as staphylococci and corynebacteria,

Table 12.1 Summary of available immunostains for detecting infectious agents

Immunostain	Clone	Source
Bacteria		
Bacillus anthracis	polyclonal	Xceltis
Bacillus anthracis (capsule)	FDF1B9	CDC
Bacillus anthracis (cell wall)	EAII6G6	CDC
Bartonella henselae	H2A10	Acris Antibodies
Clostridium species	polyclonal	Meridian Life Science
Franciscella tularensis	FT–03-A-G3	CDC
Mycobacterium bovis	polyclonal	Dako
Mycobacterium tuberculosis	polyclonal	Zytomed Systems
Neisseria gonorrhea	polyclonal	Xceltis
Neisseria meningitidis	polyclonal	Thermo Fisher Scientific
Neisseria meningitides group C	7H9–4	CDC
Orientia tsutsugamushi	polyclonal	CDC
Rickettsia rickettsii	polyclonal	CDC
Staphylococcus aureus	KPL 29740	BacTrace QED Bioscience
Streptococcus pyogenes	polyclonal	Biorbyt
Treponema pallidum	polyclonal	Biocare Medical
Yersinia pestis	F1–04-A-G1	Naval Research Institute
Virus		
Herpes simplex virus I	polyclonal	Dako, Cell Marque
Herpes simplex virus II	polyclonal	Dako, Cell Marque
Varicella zoster virus	SG1–1, SG1-SG4, NCP–1 and IE–62	Cell Marque
Cytomegalovirus	CCH2 + DDG9 8B1.2, iG5.2 and 2D4.2	Dako Cell Marque
Epstein Barr virus	ish probe	Novocastra
Human herpes virus 8	13B10	Novocastra
Human papillomavirus 6 and 11 (low risk)	DNA and RNA ish probes	Leica Biosystems, Roche, Biocare Medical, Advanced Cell Diagnostics
Human papillomavirus 16, 18, and 33 (high risk)	DNA and RNA ish probes	Leica Biosystems, Roche, BioCare Medical, Advanced Cell Diagnostics
Human papillomavirus 42	RNA ish probes	Advanced Cell Diagnostics
Parvovirus B19	R92F6	Sigma Aldrich
Merkel cell polyomavirus	CM2B4, 4B3	Santa Cruz Biotechnology
Human T-cell lymphotropic virus 1 Tax antibody	1A3	Santa Cruz Biotechnology
Enterovirus (Coxsackievirus)	2E11	Chemicon
Orthopoxvirus (smallpox, monkeypox)	polyclonal	CDC
Parapoxvirus (Orf)	polyclonal	CDC
Ebola virus	polyclonal	CDC
Dengue virus	polyclonal	CDC
Lassa fever virus	B1001–52–2085–0006-BG12	CDC
Parasite		
Acanthamoeba species	polyclonal	CDC
Balamuthia mandrillaris	polyclonal	CDC
Leishmania species	polyclonal	CDC
Fungus		
Aspergillus species	MAB-WF-AF–1	Dako
Cryptococcus	polyclonal	Dako
Mucormycetes	MAB-WSSA-RA–1	Dako

CDC: Centers for Disease Control and Prevention

are usually normal flora within the follicles or on the skin surface. They are often seen in crusted, eroded, or ulcerated skin lesions. On the contrary, gram-positive cocci in the dermis or subcutaneous tissue indicate a true significant infectious process such as panniculitis, cellulitis or fasciitis. Special stains, including Gram, acid-fast bacilli (AFB), Warthin-Starry silver, Steiner silver, and Grocott's methenamine (GMS) stains may help highlight certain bacteria, but none of them is specific. IHC are available for the detection of some pathogens, while molecular technique offers a more sensitive and specific method for a definitive identification of etiologic agent. However, many of these specialized tests are available only in research laboratories or special facilities.

Bacillus Anthracis

Anthrax is an infection caused by *Bacillus anthracis*, a gram-positive rod that is enzootic in many countries and human infections are usually associated with exposure to animals or animal products, such as wool or hides.[1] The organism was used as a biological weapon in 2001 through mails intentionally contaminated with spores of *Bacillus anthracis*.[2] There are three clinical forms of anthrax: inhalational, gastrointestinal, and cutaneous. Only a small proportion (~5%) of human cases are inhalation anthrax or gastrointestinal disease from eating infected meat. The majority of natural human infections occur one to seven days after primary inoculation of the skin with the bacteria from animals or animal products. During the 2001 incidence, 11 confirmed inhalational anthrax with 5 deaths and 11 cutaneous anthrax with no fatalities were identified from October to November.

The skin lesion usually starts as a red macule, sometimes pruritic, and evolves from papular and vesicular stages into hemorrhagic pustule. The pustule eventually ulcerates, and the lesion will be covered by a thick, black eschar (the name anthrax comes from the Greek word for "coal"). The eschar is usually surrounded by marked edema and erythema, which is more extensive on the head or neck than on the trunk or extremities. Pain is mild or absent in cutaneous anthrax, and patients are usually afebrile; however, tender regional lymphadenopathy, fatigue, fever, or chills may develop in some cases. Clinical lesions of anthrax may resemble impetigo, sporotrichosis, orf, arthropod bites, plague, rickettsialpox, scrub typhus, or tularemia.

The skin lesions usually heal spontaneously in one to two weeks, leaving very little scarring. Fatality from untreated cutaneous anthrax used to be as high as 25% but is now very rare with appropriate early treatment. Confirmatory laboratory diagnosis includes cultures, serologic assays, and polymerase chain reaction (PCR) testing, which are available through the public health network.[3,4]

The organism is best demonstrated when the lesion is in the acute vesicular stage, so swab exudates for Gram stain and biopsy should be taken for suspected cases. Cultures and full-thickness punch biopsies should be taken from the edges of both vesicle and eschar if present. Histopathologic features can vary according to the stages of infection and sites of biopsy. At the site of the eschar, the epidermis is destroyed, and the ulcerated surface is covered with necrotic tissue. The dermis is markedly edematous with necrosis and variable lymphocytes and neutrophils (**Figure 12.1**). Vasculitis, vascular necrosis, and hemorrhage can be observed. In acute stage of untreated cases, abundant gram-positive bacilli with characteristic capsule are usually present in upper dermis (**Figure 12.2**). However, typical bacilli are rarely seen in skin biopsies obtained from a later stage of infection with antibiotic treatment. In general, the longer the duration of illness and treatment course, the less chance of detecting *B. anthracis* organism by culture and special stains. Steiner's silver-impregnation stain appears to be more sensitive than Gram stain for highlighting these bacilli in cutaneous lesion obtained at a later stage (**Figure 12.3**).[3]

IHC assay provides a more sensitive and specific way to establish the diagnosis of cutaneous anthrax because of its capability to detect bacterial antigens in tissues regardless of the treatment (**Figure 12.4**). IHC was used as a crucial diagnostic tool during the investigation of the 2001 intentional release of Bacillus anthracis spores.[3,5]

Bartonella Henselae

Bartonella henselae is a gram-negative bacillus, which causes Cat-scratch disease. It is closely related to *Bartonella quintana*, the etiologic agent of louse-borne trench fever. The cat was

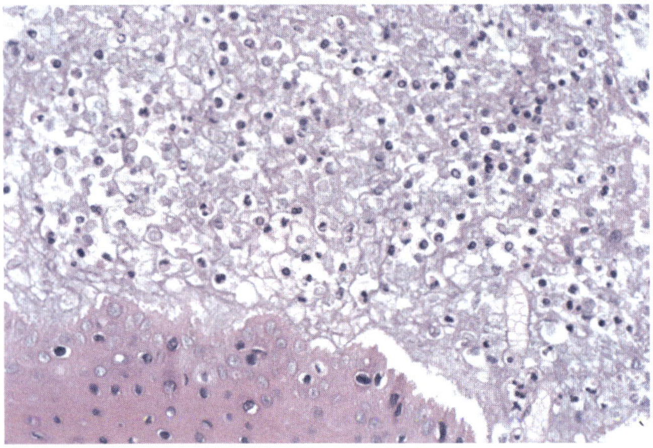

Figure 12.1 Cutaneous anthrax. The dermis is markedly edematous with necrosis and variable lymphocytes and neutrophils.

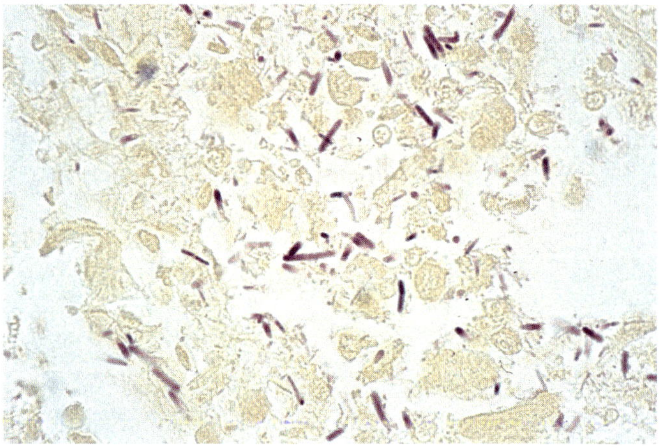

Figure 12.2 Cutaneous anthrax. Abundant gram-positive bacilli with characteristic capsule are usually present in upper dermis.

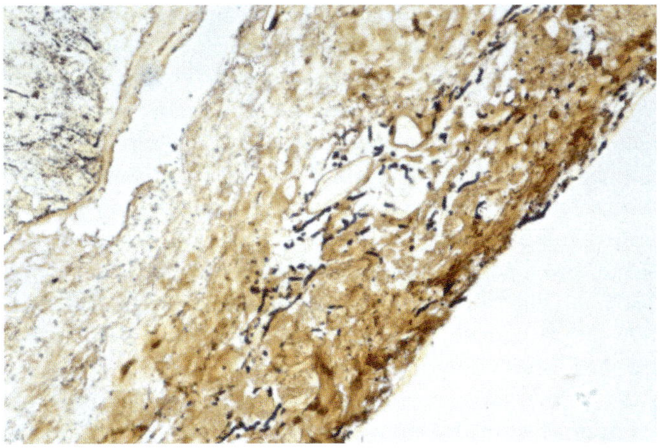

Figure 12.3 Steiner's silver-impregnation stain appears to be more sensitive than Gram stain for highlighting Bacillus anthracis in skin biopsies obtained at a later stage.

recognized as the natural reservoir of the disease in 1950. The organism is usually carried in the blood or oral cavities of cats. Kittens are more likely to carry the bacteria in their blood and may therefore be more likely to transmit the disease than adult cats. Many studies showed the transmission of *B. henselae* from cats to humans is very likely through a contaminated cat scratch wound or across a mucosal surface with flea feces containing bacteria.[6]

The skin lesion develops two to four days after a scratch or bite from a cat; it may appear as macular, papular, or nodular lesions, and more often on the forearm or hand. A single or a group of large, tender swelling lymph nodes may develop in the drainage area of the skin lesion two to three weeks later. The skin lesion usually heals in a normal fashion and resolves spontaneously, but the affected lymph nodes may become fluctuant as a result of suppuration and may persist for several months after other symptoms disappear.[7] About one-third of patients develop fever or constitutional symptoms. In immunocompromised patients more severe complications sometimes occur. There are other clinical forms of *B. henselae* infections, such as bacillary angiomatosis, bacillary peliosis, optic neuritis, and acute encephalopathy. Bacillary angiomatosis is primarily a vascular skin lesion more commonly associated with human immunodeficiency virus (HIV) or severe immunocompromised patients. The infection may extend to bone or other areas of the body. The diagnosis can be established by the cat-scratch skin test (Hanger-Rose test). The skin test is reliable when performed one week after infection; however, it is not readily available in most of the laboratories. *B. henselae* is extremely difficult to culture. Serologic and PCR assays have been used to confirm the diagnosis.[8,9]

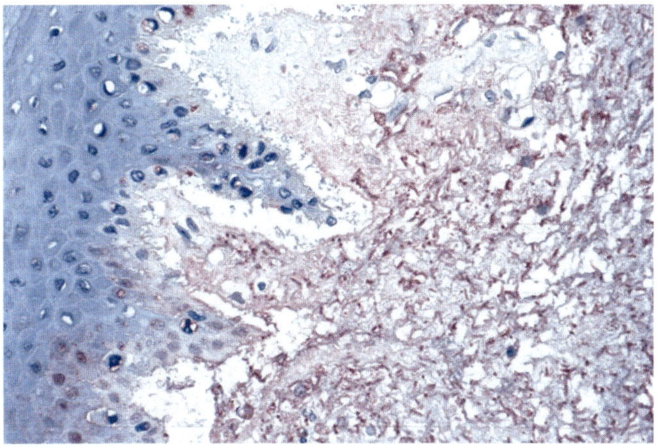

Figure 12.4 Immunostaining of *Bacillus anthracis* in dermis.

Biopsies of the primary papular lesion at the site of the scratch show one or several areas of necrosis with variable shapes in the dermis. There are usually several layers of lymphohistiocytic and epithelioid cells surrounding the necrosis, with the innermost layer exhibiting a palisading arrangement (**Figure 12.5**). Scattered multinucleated giant cells may be present. Other microscopic features, such as perivascular lymphoplasmacytic or neutrophilic infiltrates can also be present.[10] The histopathologic findings in the lymph node is similar to those observed in the skin, except microabscess formation in the central necrotic areas of the epithelioid granulomas is more commonly seen due to the accumulation of numerous neutrophils. The palisading granulomas in the skin biopsies of patients with cat-scratch disease need to be differentiated from granulomatous inflammation caused by other infectious agents, such as mycobacteria, fungi, *Leishmania spp.*, *F. tularenis*, and so on. Warthin-Starry stain may occasionally demonstrate small, pleomorphic, gram-negative bacilli at the periphery of central necrosis in involved skin and lymph node. IHC is an excellent method to demonstrate the coccobacilli and bacterial antigens in tissues (**Figure 12.6**). PCR can be performed on paraffin-embedded skin biopsies to confirm the diagnosis.[8,9]

Clostridium Species

Clostridium is a genus of gram-positive bacteria, which includes several significant human pathogens, such as C. *botulinum*, C. *difficile*, C. *perfringens*, C. *tetani*, C. *sordellii*, and C. *novyi*.

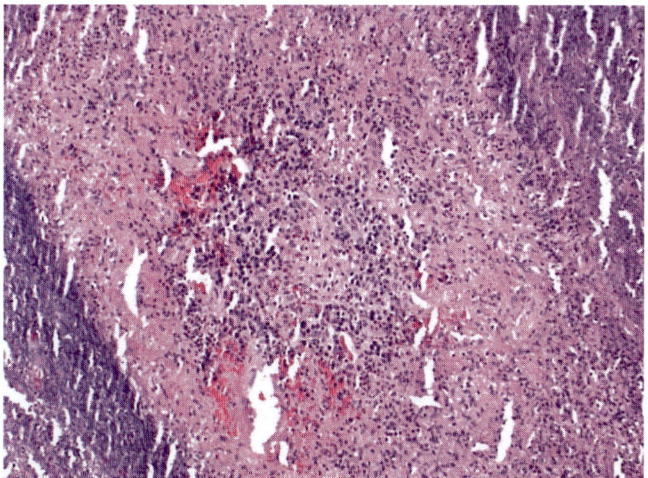

Figure 12.5 Cat-scratch disease. There are usually several layers of lymphohistiocytic and epithelioid cells surrounding the necrosis, with the innermost layer exhibiting a palisading arrangement.

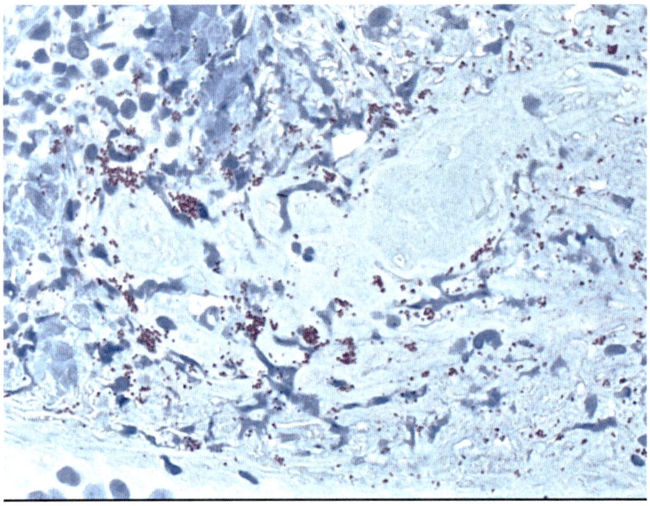

Figure 12.6 Immunostaining of *Bartonella henselae* adjacent to necrosis in dermis.

They are obligate anaerobes capable of producing endospores. *Clostridium* species inhabit soils and the intestinal tract of animals and humans. Clostridial infections of skin and soft tissues, including cellulitis, myositis, or myonecrosis usually occur after trauma. These infections are also common among injection drug users. Subcutaneous and intramuscular injection ("skin-popping") and the injection of "speedballs" (a mixture of heroin and cocaine) are important risk factors for clostridial infections of skin and soft tissues in this patient population. Pathogenic Clostridium species may contaminate the materials used in the injection of drugs and cause subsequent serious or life-threatening diseases. C. *novyi* type A was implicated in an outbreak of severe infection with high mortality in injection drug users who injected heroin extravascularly.[11]

Laboratory diagnosis of clostridial infection can be made by isolation of organisms from wound, pus, or blood, along with toxin and serological assays. PCR assay has been developed to detect Clostridium species in tissue samples; it is a sensitive and rapid diagnostic method and also allows further speciation.[12]

Histopathologic findings in most cases show marked subepithelial fibrosis and edema with a variable lymphocytic and plasma cell infiltrate. Full-thickness epidermal necrosis with ulceration can be present. Necrosis may extend to involve the underlying dermis and is associated with fibrosis, granulation tissue, and a polymorphonuclear neutrophil infiltrate (**Figure 12.7**). Acellular debris, fibrinous exudates, and abscess formation are prominent in some cases. Necrotizing fasciitis and myonecrosis can be seen in more severe and deeper infections. In addition, dermal vessels may show focal vasculitis, and there was fat necrosis of the subcutaneous tissue. Clostridial bacilli may not be readily demonstrated by special stains because the lesions are mainly caused by exotoxin and most of the bacteria may have degenerated at the time of biopsy or autopsy.[13] However, IHC assay can highlight the remaining bacterial antigens in tissue samples and help establishing the etiologic diagnosis (**Figure 12.8**).[14] The limitation is the specificity of the antibodies used in IHC assay because most of the anti-clostridia antibodies are cross-reactive and cannot provide further speciation.

Francisella Tularensis

Francisella tularensis is a small, gram-negative, pleomorphic coccobacillus that causes tularemia. Human infection is usually acquired through direct contact with animal reservoirs harboring the bacteria. The disease can also be transmitted by insects, such as mosquitoes, ticks, or deer flies, and so on. The disease is endemic in North America, and parts of Europe and Asia. The bacterium has several subspecies with varying degrees of virulence. *F. tularensis tularensis* (Type A) is the most important one, which is highly pathogenic in humans and domestic rabbits. *F. tularensis palaearctica* (Type B) occurs mainly in aquatic rodents, and is less virulent for humans and rabbits.[15]

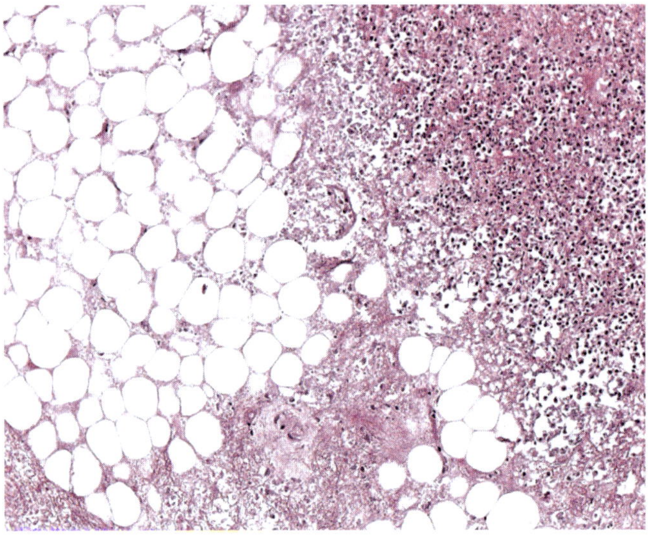

Figure 12.7 Cutaneous clostridial infection. Necrosis may extend to involve the underlying dermis and subcutaneous tissue with abundant polymorphonuclear neutrophil infiltrate.

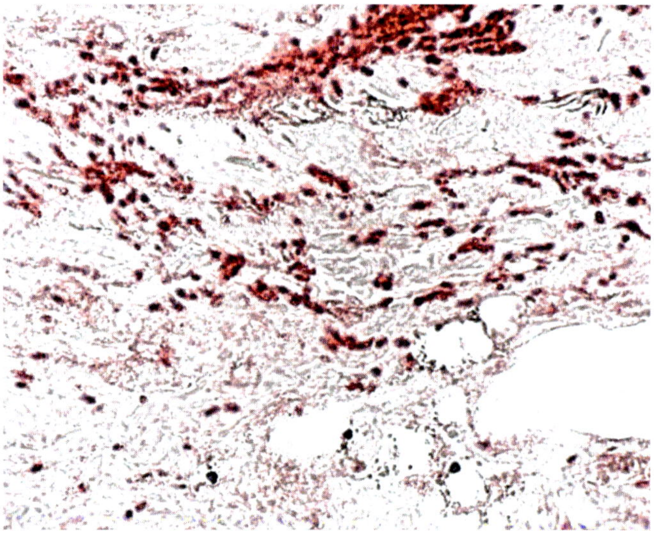

Figure 12.8 Immunostaining of clostridial bacterial antigens in tissue (X1,000).

Tularemia is a rare infectious disease that typically attacks the skin, eyes, lymph nodes and lungs. The disease can occur as sporadic cases or small epidemics. The usual incubation period is three to five days. There are several forms of clinical disease, and the most common one is ulceroglandular tularemia, which represents about 80% of cases.[16] Usually, the finger or hand is the primary site of the inoculation, where a rapidly growing papulonodular lesion develops followed by painful ulceration and necrosis. Tender subcutaneous nodes may form along the lymph vessels that drain the primary lesion. Swelling of the regional lymph nodes with marked constitutional symptoms can become very prominent. A black eschar appears within three to five days after contact. Complete healing of the lesion may occur in two to five weeks. Other important forms of tularemia include oropharyngeal, oculoglandular, pulmonary, gastrointestinal, and typhoidal. Mortality of pneumonic tularemia ranges from 30% to 60% if untreated. Laboratory diagnosis can be challenging because *F. tularensis* is a category A bioterroristic agent; even culture of the organism can confirm the diagnosis, laboratory biosafety is a concern. Serologic diagnosis is safer and more effective. PCR testing also provides a sensitive and rapid method for confirmatory diagnosis.[17]

Skin biopsies typically show ulceration, extravasated erythrocytes, and necrosis surrounded by palisading neutrophils. Suppurative granuloma formation eventually develops with central necrosis and nuclear debris (**Figure 12.9**). Some of the lesions may appear with caseous necrosis similar to mycobacterial infections. There are also rare reports describing the cutaneous manifestations of tularemia may appear vesicular similar to those lesions seen in herpesvirus infections.[18] The lymph nodes along the lymphatic distribution show multiple necrotizing granulomas deep in the dermis and extending into the subcutaneous tissue. Gram stain are rarely useful to demonstrate the organisms. Steiner or Warthin-Starry silver-impregnation stain may be more sensitive in highlighting the bacteria. IHC with a specific anti-*F. tularensis* antibody provides a sensitive method for confirmatory diagnosis because of its capability to detect bacterial antigens in skin and lymph node biopsies (**Figure 12.10**).[19]

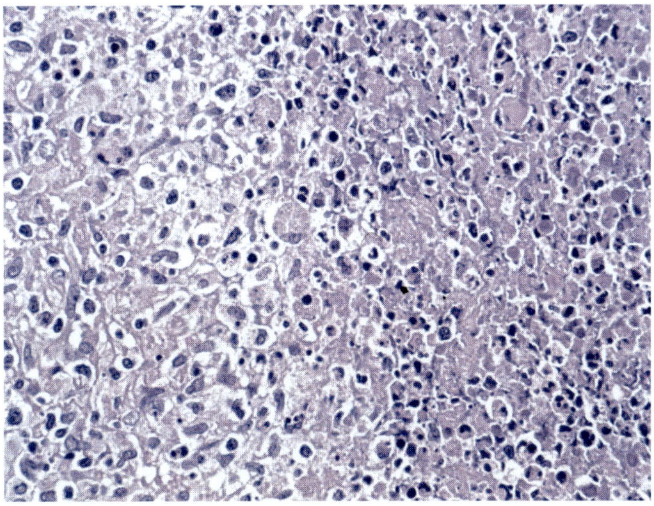

Figure 12.9 Ulceroglandular tularemia. Suppurative granuloma formation with lymphohistiocytic infiltrate, necrosis, and nuclear debris in dermis (X400).

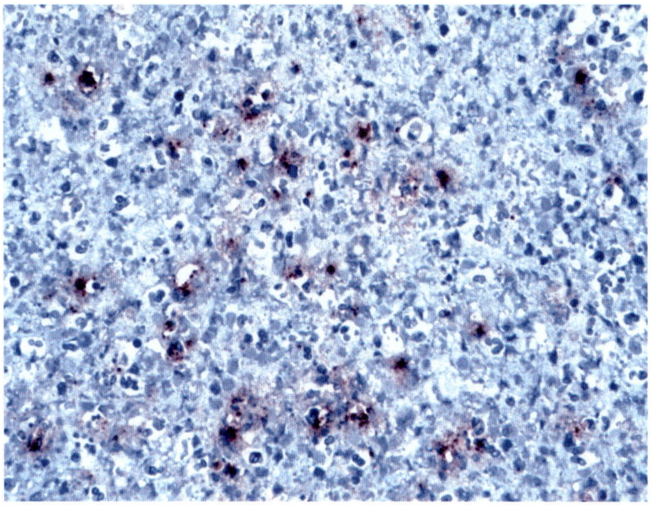

Figure 12.10 Immunostaining of *Francisella tularensis* antigens in dermis with inflammation and necrosis (X400).

Mycobacterium Tuberculosis

Mycobacterium tuberculosis primarily affects the lungs, but skin and many other organs can be involved as well. The incidence of tuberculosis (TB) was decreasing in North America and Europe until the advent of acquired immunodeficiency syndrome (AIDS). The strains with antibiotics resistance have been a growing concern. Skin testing with tuberculin purified-protein derivative is commonly used as a reliable means of confirming previous mycobacterial infection in patients who have not been vaccinated with bacille Calmette-Guérin (BCG). Cultures and acid-fast stains of biopsies, sputum, or other fluids are required to make a diagnosis of active disease. When these results are negative, PCR assays may be helpful.[20]

Cutaneous TB almost always means a long-standing active disease in other organs, with the rare exception of primary inoculation. There are many different clinical forms of cutaneous tuberculosis, including primary-inoculation, military, TB cutis orificialis, scrofuloderma, tuberculosis verrucosa cutis, lupus vulgaris, and tuberculids.[21,22]

Histopathologically, *M. tuberculosis* infection typically causes caseating granulomas and suppuration or purulence may be more prominent, depending on the stage of lesion and patient's immune status (**Figure 12.11**).[22–24] IHC can highlight acid-fast bacilli or bacterial antigens in skin biopsy (**Figure 12.12**), and is usually more sensitive than acid-fast stain. Differential diagnosis should include atypical mycobacteriosis, leprosy, deep fungal infections, cat-scratch disease, granuloma inguinale, lymphogranuloma venereum, tularemia, brucellosis, leishmaniasis, and other noninfectious granulomas.[23]

Nontuberculosis Mycobacteria

Nontuberculosis mycobacteria (NTM) are abundant in soil and water, and human exposure is frequent in most parts of the world. There are many different NTMs that may cause skin

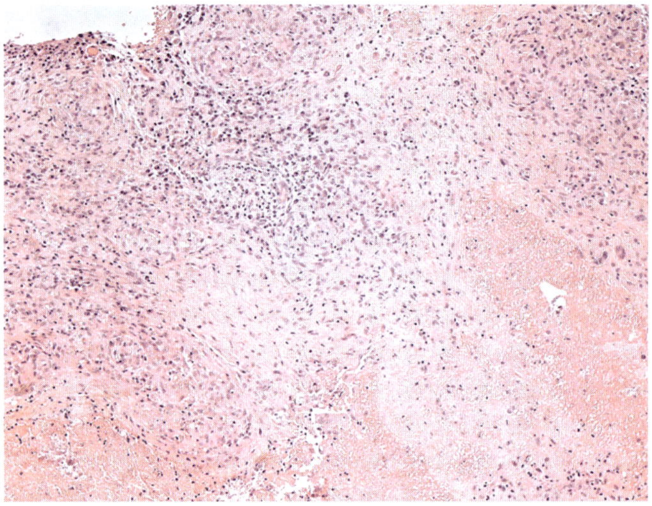

Figure 12.11 Cutaneous tuberculosis. Lymphohistiocytic granulomatous inflammation with scattered multinucleated cells and necrosis (X100).

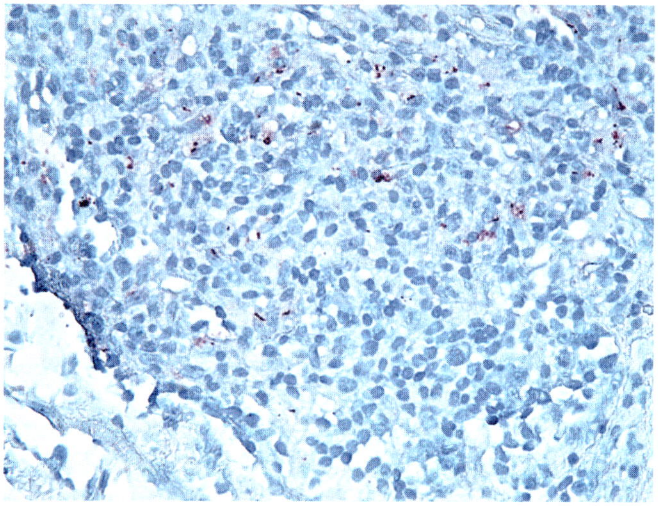

Figure 12.12 Immunostaining of *M. tuberculosis* (X400).

infections. Common organisms include *M. marinum* ("swimming pool granuloma"), *M. ulcerans* (Buruli ulcer), *M. avium-intracellulare* (MAI, especially with AIDS), and *M. fortuitum* and *M. chelonei* (rapid growers). These skin infections may be acquired by direct inoculation into the skin or by hematogenous spread from other visceral foci.[25,26] Increased use of immunosuppression in medicine, such as those for organ transplant and cancer chemotherapy and the pandemic of HIV have resulted in many more NTM skin infections.[27,28]

Clinical lesions of NTM infections are variable, including solitary or multiple erythematous nodules, abscesses, ulcers, verrucous plaques, cysts, or sinus tracts. Sometimes lesions can spread in a sporotrichoid pattern. NTMs can be identified by culture and biochemical methods. The slow growers include *M. avium complex*, *M. marinum*, *M. kansasii*, and *M. ulcerans*. The rapid growers include *M. fortuitum* and *M. chelonei*. In addition to culture, multiple PCR assays have been established for detection of these NTM organisms.[26,29]

The histopathologic features in cutaneous lesions caused by NTM are widely variable and may show nonspecific acute and chronic inflammation, suppuration and abscess formation, or granulomas with or without caseation.[25,26,28] The presence or absence of AFB depends on the tissue reaction and treatment modalities. Various modifications of the Ziehl-Neelson acid-fast stain or Fite stain may reveal AFB. The bacilli are most frequently found in microabscesses or within vacuoles in the sections rather than within multinucleated giant cells (**Figure 12.13**).[30] These AFB can be highlighted by IHC (**Figure 12.14**).

Mycobacterium Leprae

M. leprae is the etiologic pathogen of leprosy (Hansen disease), which affects millions of people worldwide. The disease is endemic in many tropical and subtropical countries but is declining in prevalence as a result of multidrug therapy.[31,32] In the United States, it occurs mainly in immigrants from endemic areas, but some cases have been reported in Texas and Louisiana,

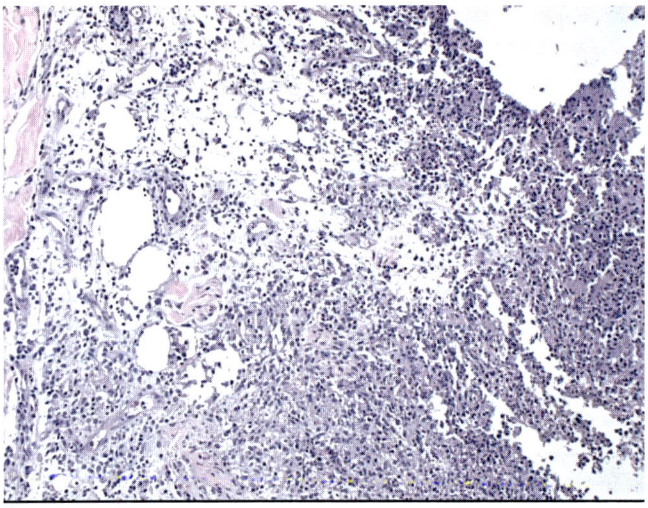

Figure 12.13 Mycobacterium marinum. Suppurative lymphohistiocytic inflammation in dermis (X100).

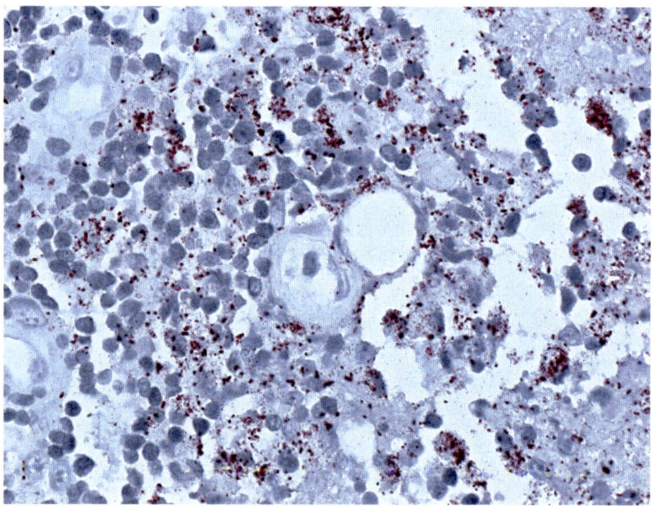

Figure 12.14 Immunostaining of numerous *M. marinum* antigens.

perhaps from armadillo exposure. The mode of transmission of leprosy is largely unknown; however, the bacilli may be inhaled from the nasal excretion of a multibacillary patient, or possibly implanted from organisms in the soil. Direct person-to-person infection through skin contact occurs rarely. Leprosy can affect various organs, but clinical manifestations are most commonly present in the skin, eyes, and peripheral nerves.

Leprosy is divided into several types in the Ridley-Jopling classification system based on the immune status of the patient.[33,34] Patients with lepromatous leprosy are anergic, and they tend to develop widespread cutaneous lesions. Lepromatous leprosy initially has cutaneous and mucosal lesions, with neural changes occurring later. The lesions usually are numerous and are symmetrically arranged. Lepromatous lesions include hypopigmented or erythematous macules, infiltrated erythematous nodules or plaques, leonine (lion-like) facies with a loss of eyebrows and eyelashes, and diffuse macular involvement of the skin resulting in a smooth surface. The skin lesions of tuberculoid leprosy are scanty, dry, erythematous, hypopigmented

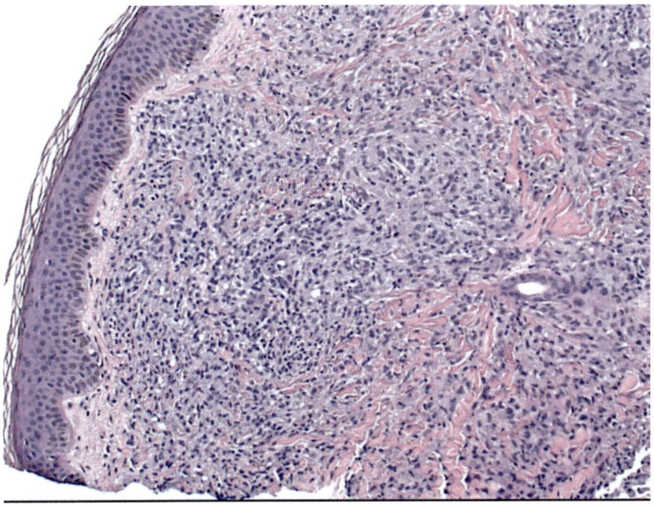

Figure 12.15 Lepromatous leprosy. Dermal infiltrate with abundant lymphocytes and macrophages underneath the narrow grenz zone (X400).

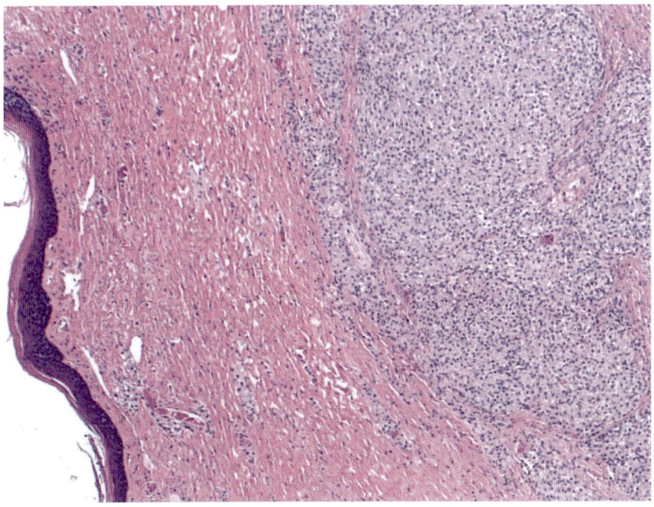

Figure 12.16 Tuberculoid leprosy. No prominent grenz zone is present. Granulomas are often linear and follow distribution of nerves in dermis (X100).

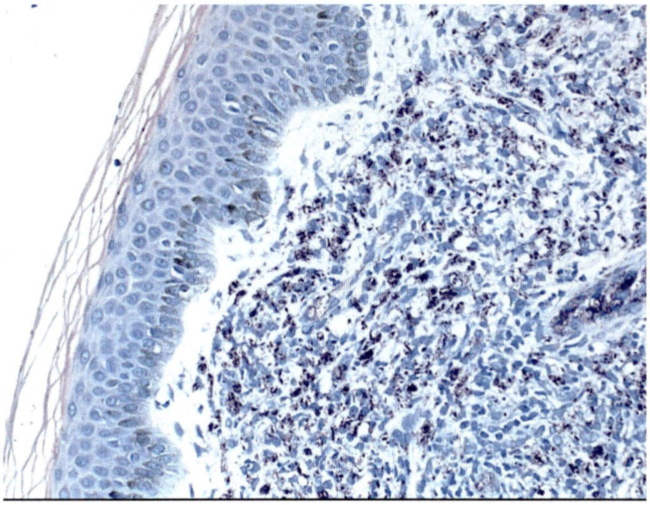

Figure 12.17 Immunostaining of numerous *M. leprae* antigens (X400).

papules, or plaques with sharply defined edges. The tuberculoid form occurs in those with intact immunity, and patients tend to develop one or a few lesions with prominent hypoesthesia and palpable thickened peripheral nerves. In borderline leprosy, combined features of tuberculoid and lepromatous disease are seen.

The histopathologic findings of leprosy vary in different forms.[35,36] The typical lepromatous form shows diffuse dermal infiltrate of foamy macrophages with grenz zone separating the macrophages from the epidermis (**Figure 12.15**). Numerous acid-fast bacilli are often present in clumps or in endothelial cells. Tuberculoid form shows granulomas without grenz zone. These granulomas are often linear and follow distribution of nerves (**Figure 12.16**). Acid-fast bacilli are usually rare or absent. The Fite stain is recommended because the conventional AFB stain methods, such as Ziehl-Neelson stain do not work as well. Immunostaining for AFBs can enhance the ability to diagnose lesions containing bacilli (**Figure 12.17**). *In situ* hybridization and PCR analysis of specimens are more sensitive and are available at a few specialized laboratories.[37–39]

Neisseria Meningitides

Acute infections with the Gram negative bacteria *Neisseria meningitides* are still the worldwide leading cause of meningitis and rapidly fatal sepsis.[40] Depending on the clinical setting and patients' background (congenital deficiencies of immunoglobulin, complement deficiencies, and young age) the mortality of meningococcal sepsis ranges from 20% to 80%.[40]

The clinical presentation of meningococcal meningitis includes fever, rash, meningeal signs, and altered mental status. The diagnosis is confirmed by cerebrospinal fluid (CSF) pleocytosis, Gram stain with or without culture of CSF, blood or skin lesions.[41] However, the sensitivity of cultures is decreased due to antimicrobial treatment. Alterative diagnostic tests including antigen detection with latex agglutination assays and PCR assays on CSF, blood, and serum samples have been developed.[42]

Histologic findings in the skin were documented in only few studies. In two surviving patients with *Neisseria meningitides*

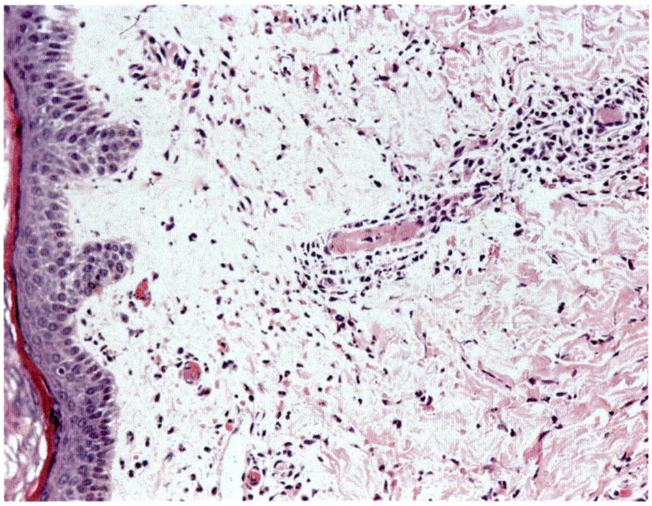

Figure 12.18 Skin with *Neisseria meningitides* infection showing dermal edema and leukocytoclastic vasculitis (X200).

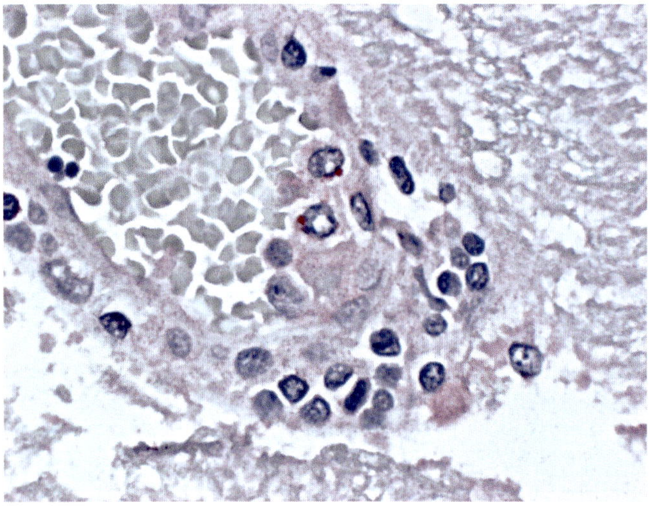

Figure 12.19 Immunostains highlighted meningococci and granular meningococcal antigens within circulating monocytes attached to the vascular wall (X1000).

cutaneous findings were leukocytoclastic vasculitis and cellulitis (**Figure 12.18**).[42] The diagnostic sensitivity of Gram stain performed on skin biopsies was reported to be 36%; therefore, the detection of the organisms in formalin-fixed paraffin-embedded tissues by immunostains can be helpful.[43] In a series of 14 cases, 2 of which had skin biopsies, intracellular and extracellular cocci were identified in various tissues in pairs in in clumps in all cases.[42] Immunostains highlighted meningococci and granular meningococcal antigens within monocytes, neutrophils, and endothelial cells (**Figure 12.19**).[42]

Neisseria Gonorrhoeae

Gonorrhea is a sexually or perinatally transmitted bacterial infection affecting the mucous membrane of the urethra, cervix, rectum, oropharynx, and conjunctivae. Sepsis, neonatal conjunctivitis, meningitis, and arthritis are the most severe complications of neonatal gonococcal infection. The highest prevalence occurs in adolescents and young adults living in densely populated areas.[44] In several days to two weeks after primary genital infections bacteremic dissemination of *N. gonorrhoeae* occurs. Disseminated gonococcal infection can present in the skin as vasculitis.[45] Visualization of the organisms by either Gram stain or immunostain using commercially available antibody is difficult since O'Brien and colleagues were unable to culture the organisms in all 10 skin lesions.[44]

Spotted Fever Group Rickettsiae

Rickettsiae are obligate intracellular parasites that are transmitted from infected arthropods to humans. Rickettsia species usually infect and damage endothelial cells, leading to cutaneous and systemic lymphohistiocytic vasculitis, the hallmark and major pathogenesis of vasculotropic rickettsioses. There are a variety of rickettsial and rickettsial-like organisms. Skin lesions are more commonly seen in infections caused by spotted fever group rickettsiae and *Orientia tsutsugamushi*.

Depending on the vectors and geographic areas, spotted fever group rickettsiae are associated with many diseases, such as Rocky Mountain spotted fever (RMSF) caused by *Rickettsia rickettsia*, Mediterranean spotted fever or Boutonneuse fever caused by *R. conorii*, African tick bite fever caused by *R. africae*, Maculatum disease caused by *R. Parkeri*, and rickettsialpox caused by *R. akari*. The rickettsial disease of greatest importance in the United States is RMSF, which is acquired after the bite of infected Dermacentor subspecies ticks.[46,47] Maculatum disease and rickettsialpox are other spotted fever group rickettsioses that occur in local areas of the United States.[48] Rickettsialpox is unique because the bacteria is transmitted to humans from a bite by infected mite, not tick. The detection of rickettsialpox has been increased due to increasing awareness of the disease and development of diagnostics.[49]

There are many similar clinical features shared among vasculotropic rickettsioses. In RMSF, a short period of malaise and headache followed by high fever and chills usually occurs after an incubation period of one to two weeks after the tick bite.[50] The skin rash starts as maculopapular eruptions on the wrists and ankles after three or four days and soon spreads centrally to limbs, trunk, and face. The palms and soles are usually involved. The lesions at first are macular to papular but become purpuric within two to three days. The degree of cutaneous involvement is highly variable and sometimes transient; approximately 10% to 15% of infected patients do not develop a prominent rash.[51] Localized petechiae can be present, but widespread ecchymoses are usually more common in fatal cases. Acral gangrene may result from small vessel occlusion. Mortality of RMSF exceeds 10% because initial recognition and diagnosis may not be made and the course may progress rapidly, despite the effectiveness of antibiotics. Eschar is usually more prominent in Mediterranean spotted fever, African tick bite fever, and rickettsialpox. Although serologic assay has been used for clinical diagnosis, the titer may not rise in the acute phase up to 10 days. PCR testing is a more sensitive and rapid method to confirm the diagnosis.[52]

The histopathologic features are similar among various vasculotropic rickettsioses. Significant findings are usually confined within the dermis. The early changes include a mild to moderate lymphohistiocytic infiltrate that surrounds and penetrates the walls of the dermal vessels (**Figure 12.20**). Erythrocyte extravasation, endothelial swelling, and edema are commonly seen. Vascular damage with leukocytoclastic vasculitis frequently occurs at a later stage, and the inflammation is predominantly lymphohistiocytic admixed with occasional neutrophilic infiltrate and karyorrhectic nuclear debris. Microthrombi and vessel wall necrosis can be present. These later changes are often associated clinically with petechiae or hemorrhagic, purpuric rashes.[53,54] The rickettsial organism is too small to be visible by light microscopy using regular stains. IHC can readily demonstrate rickettsial antigens in endothelial cells in association with perivascular lymphocytic infiltration (**Figure 12.21**).[55,56]

Orientia Tsutsugamushi

Orientia tsutsugamushi is a rickettsial-like organism that causes scrub typhus. It is transmitted from natural rodent reservoir by the bites of the mites, *Trombicula akamushi* and *T. deliensis*. It is a common disease in endemic areas of Southeast Asia and western Pacific islands. During the Vietnam war, it was a common cause of fever in American soldiers.[57]

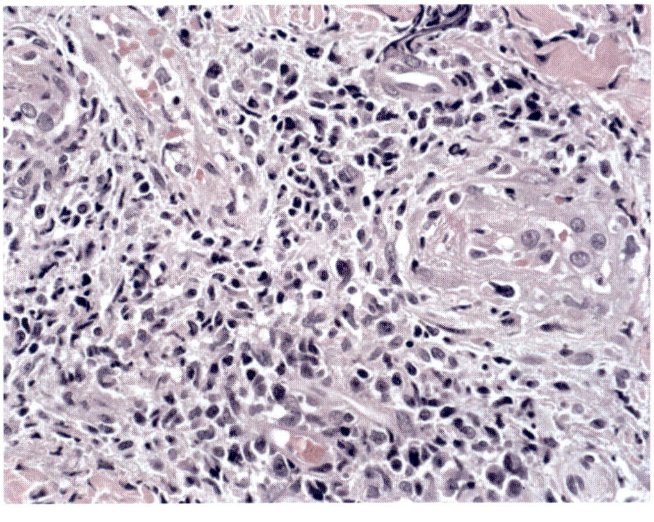

Figure 12.20 Spotted fever group rickettsioses. Vasculitis, microthrombi and vessel wall necrosis (X400).

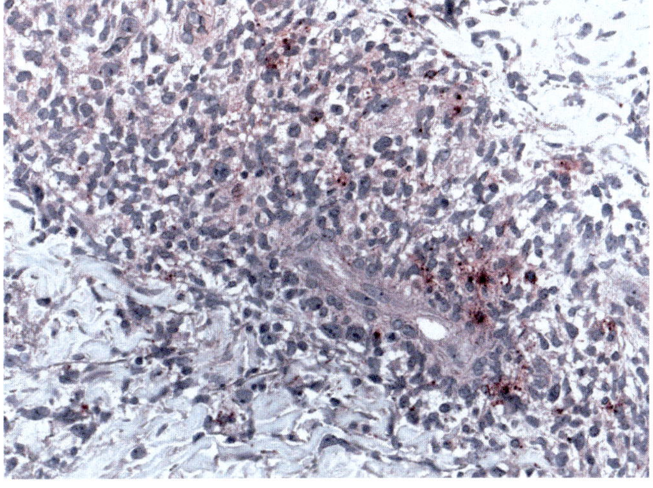

Figure 12.21 Immunostaining of rickettsial antigens in endothelial cells in association with perivascular lymphocytic infiltration (X400).

Scrub typhus usually presents as an acute febrile illness after an incubation period of about 10 days (6–21 days). Primary skin lesion usually develops in conjunction with fever, headache, and conjunctivitis. The primary lesion is a firm papule surmounted by a vesicle, which eventually dries to form a black eschar crust. Eschar lesions of scrub typhus may resemble impetigo, anthrax, orf, arthropod bite, plague, rickettsialpox, or tularemia.[58] Travel history to endemic areas should raise the index of suspicion. The regional lymph nodes are enlarged and tender. A generalized macular or maculopapular eruption may develop after about a week, and may fade rapidly or persist for one to two weeks. More severe clinical complications, such as pneumonitis and myocarditis can occur and the mortality in cases without treatment can be as high as 60%.[59] In mild or treated cases, the fever subsides and recovery occurs during the second or third week. Serologic and PCR assays have been used for confirmatory diagnosis.[60,61]

Histopathologic findings of eschar lesion show ulceration with prominent epidermal and dermal necrosis. A lymphohistiocytic vasculitis of small vessels with microthrombi and vascular necrosis is typically present in the dermis (**Figure 12.22**). Various degrees of perivascular infiltrate with lymphocytes and occasional neutrophils are seen.[62] IHC assay can demonstrate the organisms in endothelial cells and macrophages (**Figure 12.23**).[63]

Streptococcus Pyogenes

Streptococcus pyogenes is a beta-hemolytic bacterium that belongs to Lancefield serogroup A, also known as the group A streptococci (GAS). GAS has a wide tissue tropism in humans, causing different diseases depending on the bacterial strains' virulence factor repertoire and the tissue involved.[64] These diseases range from a mild skin infection or a sore throat to severe, life-threatening conditions. GAS is the most common bacterial cause of acute pharyngitis, accounting for 15–30% of cases in children and 5–10% of cases in adults.[65] Other severe or systemic diseases include pneumonia, bacteremia, necrotizing fasciitis, osteomyelitis, meningitis, acute rheumatic fever, and acute

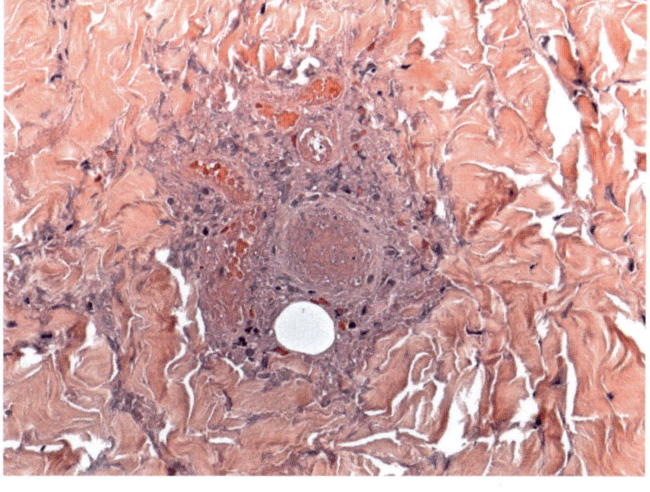

Figure 12.22 Scrub typhus caused by *Orientia tsutsugamushi*. Lymphohistiocytic vasculitis of small vessels with microthrombi and vascular necrosis in the dermis.

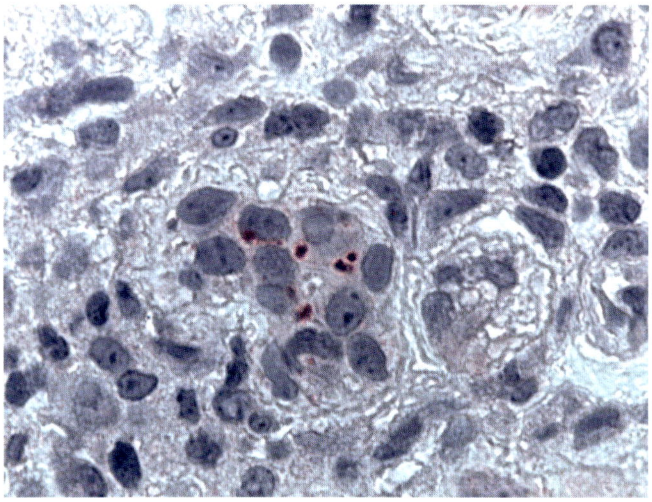

Figure 12.23 Immunostaining of *O. tsutsugamushi* in endothelial cells and macrophages (X1000).

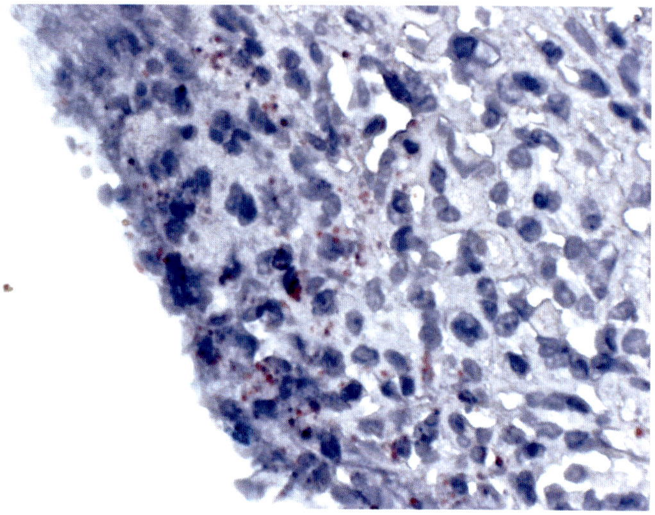

Figure 12.25 Immunostaining of *S. pyogenes* (X630).

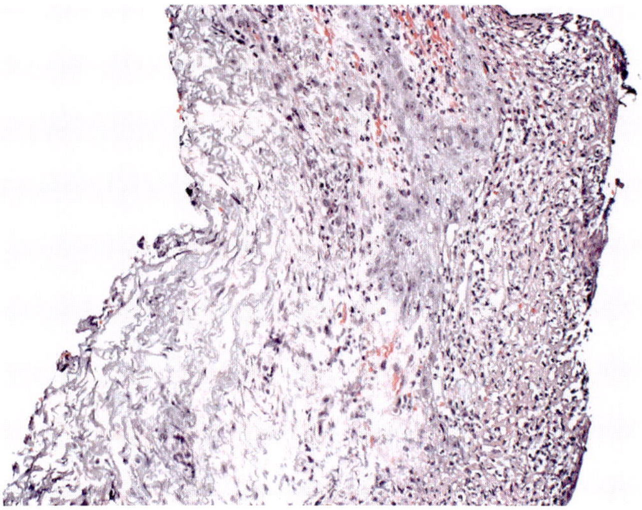

Figure 12.24 Impetigo caused by *Streptococcus pyogenes*. Ulceration and subcorneal pustules containing neutrophils with occasional acantholytic keratinocytes (X100).

glomerulonephritis.[66,67] Skin infections with *S. pyogenes* also span a wide range, such as impetigo, ecthyma, cellulitis, erysipelas, blistering distal dactylitis, and others.[67,68]

To identify GAS in clinical samples, blood agar plates are screened for the presence of β-hemolytic colonies. Subsequent serologic grouping by the Lancefield method is the standard for differentiation of pathogenic streptococcal species. GAS can also be identified more cost effectively by other methods, such as latex agglutination, coagglutination, or enzyme immunoassay procedures.[69,70]

Histopathologic features of GAS skin infections vary depending on their clinical presentations. Impetigo is one of the common superficial bacterial infections that occurs more frequently in children, especially around the mouth, nose, and groin.[71] The etiologic agents are *GAS* and *Staphylococcus aureus*. There are two types of impetigo: impetigo contagiosa, or nonbullous impetigo, usually caused by *Staphylococcus aureus or* GAS; and bullous impetigo, caused by *S. aureus*, which may also cause the staphylococcal scalded-skin syndrome. Impetigo is often diagnosed on clinical grounds, with or without culture, and biopsies are frequently not performed. In skin biopsy of impetigo, subcorneal pustules containing neutrophils are present with occasional acantholytic keratinocytes (**Figure 12.24**). Gram-positive cocci may be identified in the pustule or on the surface of ulcers, if the lesion is acute and the biopsy is performed before antibiotics treatment. Older lesions have a crust with neutrophils and parakeratosis instead of pustules. The dermal infiltrate is usually composed of lymphocytes and neutrophils in a perivascular distribution. IHC can readily demonstrate the presence of cocci or remaining bacterial antigens (**Figure 12.25**), thus providing an excellent tissue diagnosis if no culture or other laboratory methods are performed.[72]

Staphylococcus Aureus

Staphylococci are normal inhabitants of the skin surface and mucous membranes of humans. Despite being harmless in most individuals, *S. aureus* can cause various infections of the skin and other organ systems. S. aureus skin infections are common in people with skin injury, and more frequently in pre-pubertal children and adolescent.[73] As GAS, Staphylococcus aureus is a common etiologic pathogen of impetigo. However, it can cause staphylococcal scalded-skin syndrome (SSSS), also known as *Ritter disease*.[74] SSSS is a generalized systemic illness caused by certain strains of *S. aureus* (phage group II, especially type 71) that produce an exfoliative exotoxin A or B.[75] The exfoliative toxins are superantigens that stimulate T-cell proliferation.[76] SSSS most commonly affects children younger than five years of age. It is rare in adults, and most adults with SSSS are either immunosuppressed or have renal insufficiency. SSSS can be self-limited, resolving in a few weeks without scarring. Mortality in children beyond the neonatal period is low, and long-term complications are rare.

Histopathologic findings in biopsies of Staphylococcal impetigo cases are similar to those caused by GAS (**Figure 12.26**). Gram-positive cocci may be identified in the pustules, on skin surface, or in dermis. IHC can help identify the presence

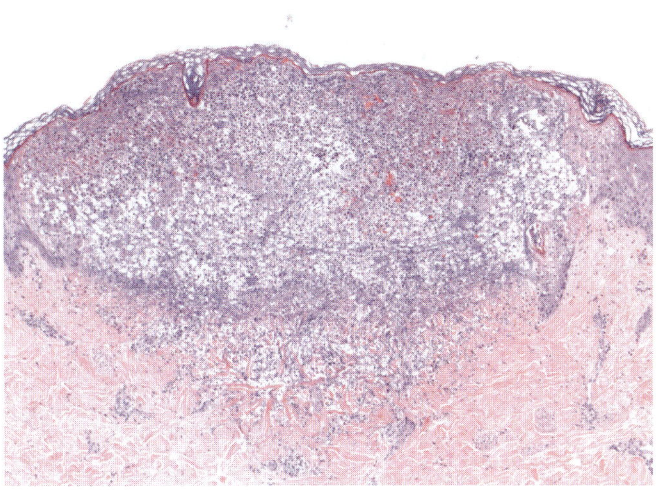

Figure 12.26 Impetigo caused by *Staphylococcus aureus*. Ulceration and subcorneal pustules containing neutrophils (X50).

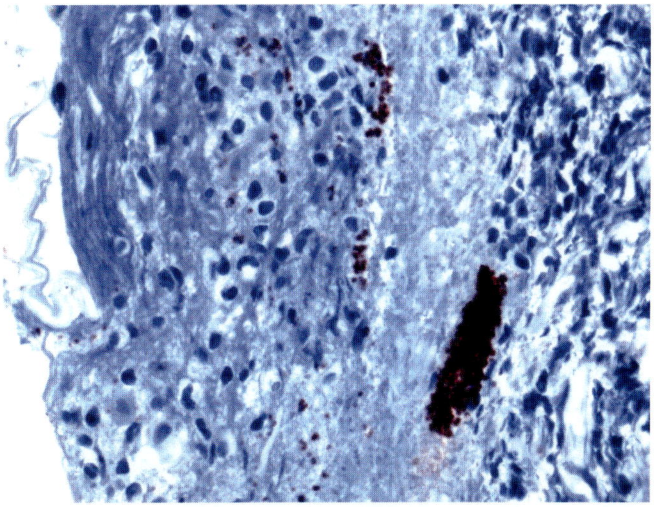

Figure 12.27 Immunostaining of *S. aureus* (X630).

of bacterial antigens (**Figure 12.27**). In biopsies of SSSS, the level of blistering is in the subcorneal zone through the granular layer. Inflammatory response is usually minimal, and epidermal necrosis generally is absent. Acantholytic keratinocytes and dermal edema may be seen.[77] Since bacteria are not present in skin lesion, diagnostic tests on skin biopsies, including culture, special stains, IHC, or PCR testing are usually negative.

Treponema Pallidum

Syphilis, the great mimicker both clinically and histopathologically, is caused by the spirochete *Treponema pallidum* which cannot be cultured. The disease can present in four stages: primary, secondary, latent, and tertiary.[78] Painless, indurated, and shallow ulcers on genital sites within three weeks of initial contact are the presenting signs of chancres or primary lesions.[78] The chancre will resolve within two to six weeks without treatment. Correct diagnosis is important since approximately one third of untreated individuals will develop secondary syphilis via hematogenous dissemination. The lesions of secondary syphilis present as a generalized cutaneous eruption on the trunk, genital area, extremities, and palms and soles. They can assume diverse clinical morphology ranging from urticarial to macular, papular, nodular, and pustular. Atypical clinical presentations such as annular lesions and pruritic erythematous scaly plaques can be seen in up to a quarter of secondary syphilis cases.[79] It can mimic pemphigus even with positive direct immunofluorescence.[80] Both primary and secondary lesions enter a latent stage even without treatment. Only a small number of patients with latent syphilis will progress to tertiary syphilis whose manifestations due to exuberant systemic immune response include neurosyphilis, cardiovascular disease, and gummata (lesions of skin, bones, or viscera).[78]

Diagnosis can be made by dark-field and bright-field microscopic examination, serologic studies, or polymerase chain reaction (PCR). Serologic studies are comprised of nontreponemal (rapid plasma reagin or Venereal Disease Research Laboratory) and treponemal tests (*T. pallidum* hemagglutination assay or *T. pallidum* particle agglutination).

The histologic appearance of syphilis under the microscope can be as diverse as its clinical presentation. There are epidermal as well as dermal changes. On histologic sections proliferation of endothelial cells and perivascular lymphocytic infiltrate would be seen in early lesions. The epidermis becomes acanthotic and can ulcerate centrally with associated dermal infiltrate of plasma cells, lymphocytes and histiocytes in later stage. Although plasma cells can be absent or present sparsely in 25% of cases, they are helpful histologic clue to distinguish syphilis from histologic differential diagnoses.[81]

Although serologic testing is the gold standard, false negative results in early primary syphilis, some cases of secondary syphilis, coinfection with HIV, and immunosuppressed conditions. The organisms can be visualized on skin biopsy by direct immunofluorescence, special stain, or immunohistochemistry. In comparison to special stain techniques such as Warthin-Starry and Steiner silver stains immunostains have been shown to exhibit better sensitivity (71%–80%) and specificity in the detection of *T. pallidum*.[81,82] Using immunohistochemistry with a polyclonal antibody, the organisms were visualized in the epidermis and dermis with a sensitivity of 91% in comparison to 75% by PCR.[83] While higher density and vascular and perivascular distribution of spirochetes were noted in primary syphilis, basal aspect of the epidermis and superficial dermis are the localization of the organisms in secondary syphilis (**Figure 12.28**).[81,82] In some cases the organisms can be prominent within follicular and adnexal epithelium. In the study by Buffet et al.,[83] skin biopsies from three patients presented with erythema chronicum migrans of Lyme disease were negative when tested with T. pallidum immunostain. However, cross reactivity of the antibody with other spirochetal infections and borreliosis have been reported. In the latent and tertiary stages where PCR tests are expected to be better methods, IHC has been shown to have better sensitivity (**Figure 12.29**). It was thought that while the antigens are preserved, the *T. pallidum*-specific DNA is degraded.[83]

Yersinia Pestis

Yersinia pestis is a small, gram-negative, non-sporing, and nonmotile bacillus that causes plague. It is a zoonotic infection that

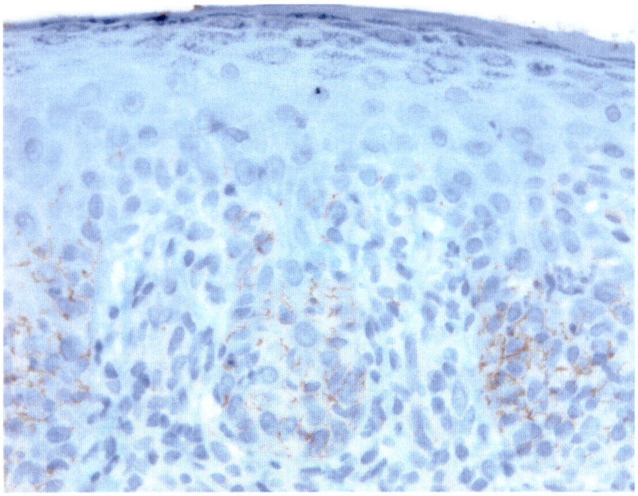

Figure 12.28 *T. pallidum* immunostain demonstrates many spirochetes at the basal aspect of the epidermis (X600).

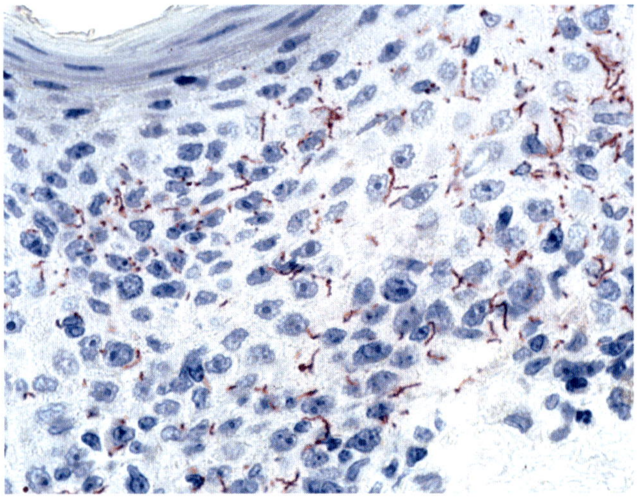

Figure 12.29 Immunostaining of *T. pallidum* (X630).

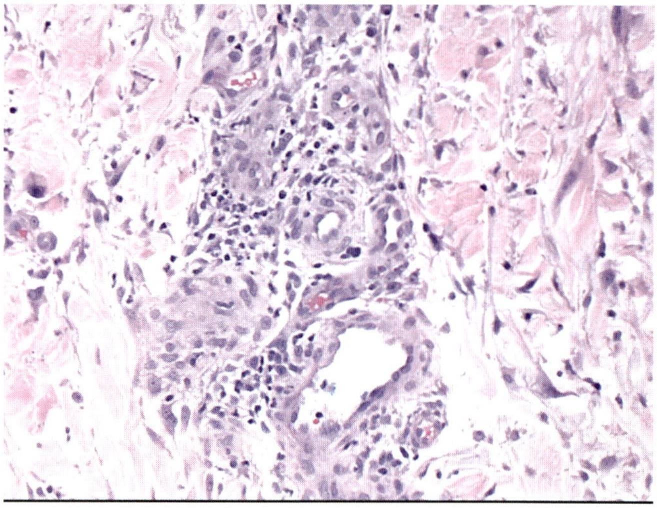

Figure 12.30 Cutaneous plague. Vasculitis and vascular necrosis with mixed inflammatory infiltrate (X400).

affects a wide variety of rodents, particularly the urban and domestic rats. The bacteria are usually transmitted from infected rodents to humans by the bites of fleas. Human-to-human transmission rarely occurs in pneumonic plague through inhalation of infectious droplets or other contaminated material. Plague is still endemic in many regions of the world, including India and the Far East, and in Southern and Central Africa. Sporadic outbreaks occur in North Africa, including small endemic areas in the USA. Occasional cases have been reported elsewhere in travelers from the endemic areas.[84]

There are various clinical forms of plague, including bubonic, septicemic, pneumonic, pharyngeal, and meningeal plague. The incubation period is usually three or four days, but it may occasionally be longer than seven days. Following inoculation of the organism by a flea bite, the regional lymph node becomes swollen, and systemic dissemination with a severe febrile illness can quickly develop, leading to death within days if untreated. Primary pulmonary infection occurs if *Y. pestis* is inhaled, which is almost always fatal within three or four days.[85]

Clinical cutaneous manifestations of plague are usually nonspecific. Typically, there is no distinct lesion at the site of the initial flea bite; however, an erythematous plaque may appear, becomes bullous, and subsequently forms crust like an eschar. Such primary cutaneous lesions may occur in 10% of patients. The involved regional lymph nodes become painfully swollen several days later. A macular, erythematous, or petechial rash may develop during the bacteremic phase. Aspiration of a bubo and direct examination of smears and culture can confirm the diagnosis. The culture of blood and sputum should also be undertaken if septicemic or pneumonic plague is suspected. Serologic and PCR assays can establish the diagnosis as well.[86,87]

The histopathologic features of the skin lesions are generally nonspecific and vary according to the type of lesion associated with their clinical presentations. The purpuric and petechial lesions, especially in those associated with shock, may show vasculitis, vascular necrosis with microthrombi, hemorrhage, and other signs of disseminated intravascular coagulation (**Figure 12.30**). Septal panniculitis and perivascular lymphocytic infiltrate can be seen in biopsies taken from erythematous lesion or morbilliform rash. Giemsa and Gram stains may highlight bacilli with characteristic bipolar staining. Bacilli are usually more abundant in vessels and perivascular areas in biopsy samples obtained at septicemic stage. IHC with a specific anti-*Y. pestis* antibody provides a sensitive method for confirmatory diagnosis because of its capability to detect bacilliform and granular antigens in areas of inflammation and necrotic debris (**Figure 12.31**).[88]

12.2 Virus

Many viral infections produce prominent skin manifestations. Some appear with characteristic lesions suggesting a specific viral illness, such as chickenpox or measles. Viral cytopathic effects, including alterations of cellular functions and host responses to the presence of viruses are factors that lead to the manifestations of viral disease. Before viruses can enter a cell, they must attach to specific receptors on the cell surface. Thus, viral infection

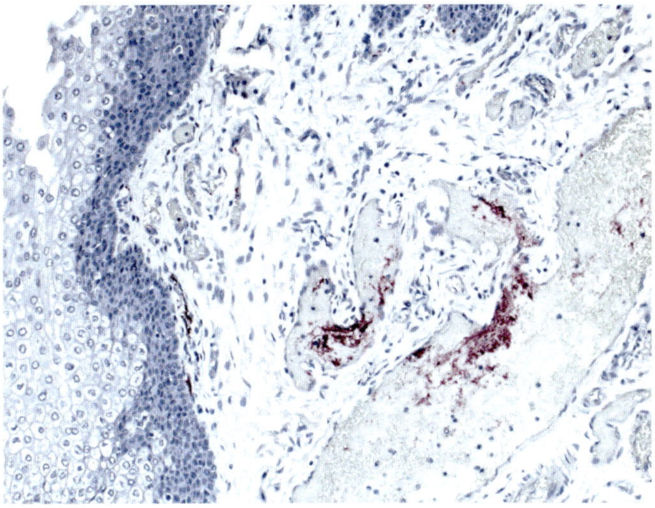

Figure 12.31 Immunostaining of *Y. pestis* in vessels (X100).

is a receptor-mediated, species- and cell type-specific process. The virus families that commonly affect the skin include *Herpesviridae*, *Poxviridae*, *Papovaviridae*, *Picornaviridae*, and *Retroviridae*. In addition to these common ones, exanthems can occur following infection with many other virus families, such as *Adenoviridae, Togaviridae, Reoviridae, Parvoviridae, Paramyxoviridae, Flaviviridae, and Hepadnaviridae,* and *Filoviridae*. Lesions from the *Herpesviridae*, *Poxviridae*, and *Papovaviridae*, usually contain viral inclusions and cytopathic effects helpful for diagnosis. Infections from the other virus families often produce rather nonspecific histologically changes with superficial perivascular dermatitis and occasional apoptotic cells in the epidermis.

Clinical diagnosis can be established by isolation of virus in cell culture, detection of viral particle by immunoassays or electron microscopy, and detection of viral nucleic acid by molecular assays. IHC assays are available for the detection of some common viral pathogens, such as those in *Herpesviridae* and *Papovaviridae*.

Enteroviruses

The human enterovirus genus is a member of the Picornaviridae family of small, icosahedral, single-stranded, positive-sense RNA viruses. More than 100 serotypes are currently recognized. Enteroviruses can cause a wide spectrum of illness, including respiratory tract infections, conjunctivitis, myocarditis, meningitis, encephalitis, and skin infections. Seasonal distribution is a characteristic feature of enteroviral infections. In temperate climates, they are more commonly seen in the summer and autumn, whereas in tropical areas, they tend to occur year-round.[89,90]

Enteroviral skin infections are usually caused by coxsackieviruses, echoviruses, or enterovirus 71 (EV71). Infection of these enteroviruses can manifest as exanthems, which is a symptom of a more general disease or enanthems, which involve the mucous membranes. Coxsackieviruses are separated into two groups, A and B. Coxsackie A viruses are the primary etiologic agents of herpangina and hand-foot-and-mouth disease (HFMD). Coxsackie B viruses are less dermatotropic and are associated with epidemic pleurodynia, myocarditis, and pericarditis. Echoviruses include 34 distinct serotypes, and at least half of them can cause skin rash. The two skin diseases specifically associated with echoviruses are Boston exanthem disease (BED), caused by echovirus type 16, and eruptive pseudoangiomatosis (EP) caused by echovirus types 25 and 32. EV71 71 has caused several large outbreaks of HFMD associated with severe complications, such as brainstem encephalitis, acute flaccid paralysis, and fatal cardiopulmonary failure.[91]

HFMD is most associated with coxsackie A viruses, echoviruses, and EV71. The incubation time is one to seven days. A brief prodromal period is characterized by low-grade fever, malaise, nonspecific respiratory or gastrointestinal symptoms, and occasional lymphadenopathy. After 24–48 hours, vesicles appear on buccal mucosa, tongue, and pharyngeal wall, associated with oral pain and odynophagia. Painless papules and vesicles can be seen on the hands, feet, and some other parts of the body. A morbilliform eruption on the buttocks can also occur. The oral enanthem is an important clinical manifestation to help distinguish HFMD from other viral causes. Uncomplicated HFMD usually resolves in five to seven days.[92]

Skin lesions from HFMD or other enteroviral infections are rarely biopsied; however, atypical presentation of HFMD which is often associated with coxsackievirus A6, can prompt a skin biopsy.[93] Histopathologic features usually show a mixture of neutrophilic and lymphocytic infiltrate in epidermis with keratinocyte necrosis, dyskeratosis, and intraepidermal vesiculation because of epidermal edema (**Figure 12.32**). Various degrees of perivascular infiltrate and edema are usually present in the dermis. Confirmatory diagnosis can be made by using IHC (**Figure 12.33**) or PCR essays.[94,95]

Hemorrhagic Fever Viruses

A disparate group of viruses can cause fever with prominent hemorrhagic manifestations, or viral hemorrhagic fevers (VHF). These viruses are collectively called hemorrhagic fever

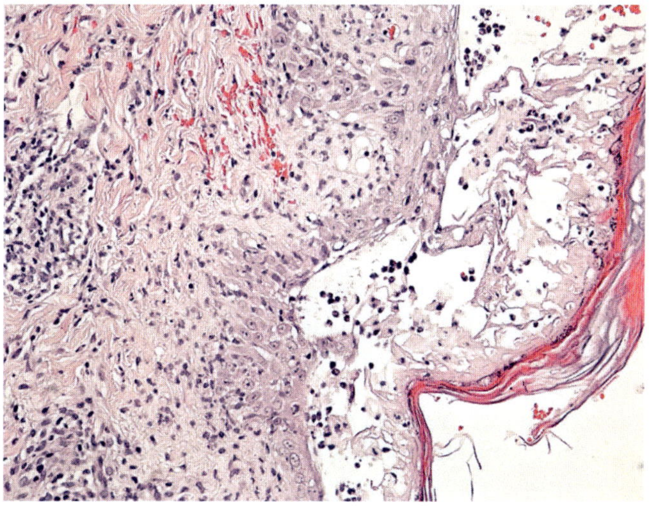

Figure 12.32 Hand, foot, and mouth disease caused by enteroviruses. Mixed inflammatory infiltrate in epidermis with keratinocyte necrosis, dyskeratosis, and intraepidermal vesiculation (X200).

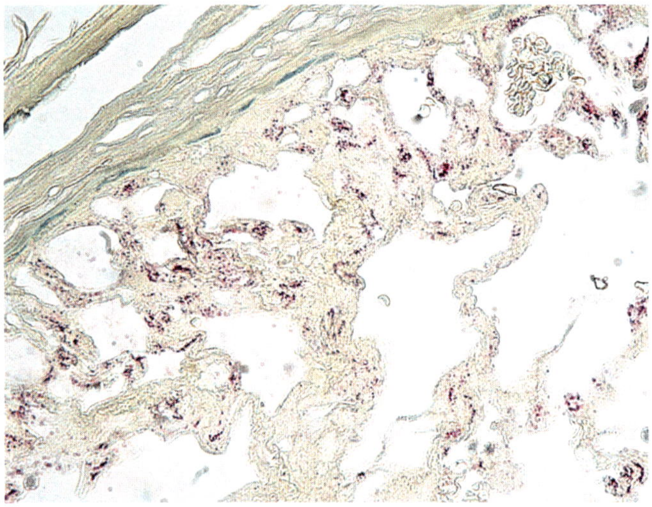

Figure 12.33 Immunostaining of enteroviruses in infected keratinocytes (X400).

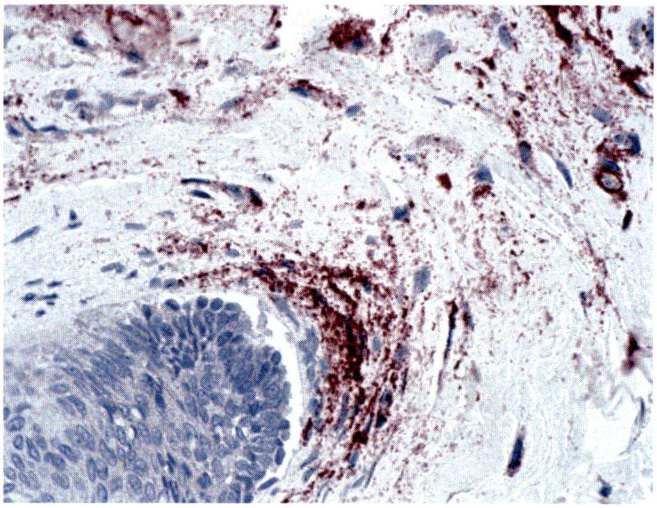

Figure 12.34 Ebola hemorrhagic fever. Immunostaining of Zaire strain of Ebola virus in dermis (X400).

viruses and mainly from four virus families: 1) Filoviridae, such as Ebola virus and Marburg virus; 2) Arenaviridae. such as Lassa virus (Lassa HF), Junin virus (Argentinian HF), Machpo virus (Bolivian HF), and Guanarito virus (Venezuelan HF); 3) Flaviviridae, such as yellow fever virus and dengue virus; 4) Bunyaviridae, such as Rift Valley fever virus (RVF), Crimean-Congo hemorrhagic fever virus (CCHF), and hantavirus (hemorrhagic fever with renal syndrome and hantavirus pulmonary syndrome). These viruses produce a substantial global public health impact with very limited effective vaccines or antiviral agents available. Although VHFs are generally regarded as emerging diseases, most of them have existed for many years in different parts of the world. The human exposure to these viruses has been increasing to an alarming level, especially with the recent large Ebola virus outbreak in West Africa. The hemorrhagic fever viruses are maintained in different species of reservoir in nature, such as insect, arthropod, or animal populations. They are transmitted from these reservoir populations to humans by direct or indirect exposure. Typical vectors include rodents, ticks, or mosquitoes, but person-to-person transmission in health care settings or through sexual contact can also occur. The incidence and prevalence of VHFs vary widely due to many factors, such as the population density of reservoir and human, mode of transmission, geoclimatic alterations, environmental changes, and virulence of viruses. The hemorrhagic fever viruses most commonly exist in tropical locations; however, some of them can exist in cooler climates.[96,97]

The incubation period of these VHFs varies from three days to three weeks. The clinical symptoms and signs are usually nonspecific and often start as flu-like illness with fever, headache, backache, generalized myalgia, and arthralgia. These symptoms may be accompanied by nausea, vomiting, diarrhea, and abdominal pain. Hemorrhagic manifestations can appear early as petechiae, purpura, subconjunctival hemorrhage, or mucosal bleeding from oral cavity and gastrointestinal tract. Case fatality varies widely according to the different family of viruses, ranging from 15% to > 90%.

The skin lesions of VHFs usually reflect the systemic involvement and hemorrhagic manifestations of the viral infection. There is no specific histopathologic finding in skin biopsies of VHFs. Occasionally, mild perivascular lymphocytic infiltrate and subtle endothelial hyperplasia may be seen, but they do not provide any diagnostic value. IHC assay is a sensitive method for diagnosis of Zaire strain of Ebola virus infection in skin biopsies (**Figure 11.34**).[98] However, the sensitivity of using skin biopsies and IHC assay is generally too low to diagnose dengue virus, Lassa virus, or Marburg virus.[99,100]

Herpesviruses

Herpes simplex virus, varicella-zoster virus, cytomegalovirus, Epstein-Barr virus, human herpes virus 6, human herpes virus 7, and human herpes virus 8 belong to the herpes family Herpesviridae. All are comprised of double-stranded linear deoxyribonucleic acid (DNA) within an icosahedral capsid. They all rely on the host cell nucleus for DNA replication and RNA transcription thus giving rise to characteristic nuclear inclusions. All cause irreversible destruction of infected cells and have the ability to remain latent and reactivate in appropriate settings.

Herpes Simplex Virus Types 1 and 2 (Human Herpes Virus 1 and 2)

Herpes simplex virus (HSV) types 1 and 2 can induce primary infection, latency, and recurrent oral and genital diseases. HSV type 1 is very common with a seroprevalence of greater than 90% in many countries. HSV type 2 has been estimated to infect approximately 500 millions worldwide. HSV type 1 is acquired during childhood whereas HSV type 2 is invariably transmitted sexually. Being the most frequently sexually transmitted disease worldwide, genital herpes infection can be caused by HSV type 2 as well as HSV type 1 in younger women.[101] Neonatal HSV infection, a rare infection with high morbidity and mortality in infants less than 6 weeks of age, is caused by HSV1 in 84% of cases.[102]

A prodrome of fever, myalgias, and malaise develops three to five days after exposure in a primary infection. Clusters of painful vesicles on erythematous base then develop which progress to pustules and erosions. These lesions typically resolve without scarring unless there is secondary infection. The virus replicates at the site of infection, travels retrograde to axonal neurons in the dorsal root ganglia, establishes a latent phase, and can reactivate. Recurrences occur in approximately 57% and 89% of individuals with primary HSV type 1 and HSV type 2, respectively.[103] Lymphadenopathy and systemic symptoms are features of recurrent disease rather than primary infection. The infection can present as a severe disseminated infection on sites of skin damage induced by atopic dermatitis and burns known as eczema herpeticum.

Histologic sections of a vesicle typically show ballooning degeneration of keratinocytes resulting in acantholysis. Commonly the affected keratinocytes show multinucleation, nuclear molding, blue-gray nuclei, and margination of nuclear chromatin or "ground glass" appearance (**Figure 12.35**). Eosinophilic intranuclear Cowdry A inclusions which are 3–8 micrometer and eosinophilic intranuclear inclusions and surrounded by a halo can occasionally be identified. The inclusions can be identified within hair follicles (77%), sebaceous glands (67%), and rarely eccrine epithelium.[104] Herpes infections can cause a pseudolymphomatous response with prominent CD30-positive cells as well as CD56-positive infiltrate mimicking CD56-positive NK/T-cell lymphoma.[105] In patients with HIV/AIDS prominent lymphoplasmacytic infiltrate can be seen.[105] Immunohistochemistry using HSV-specific antibodies can be of help in confirming the diagnosis and to distinguish HSV from VZV infection (**Figure 12.36**).

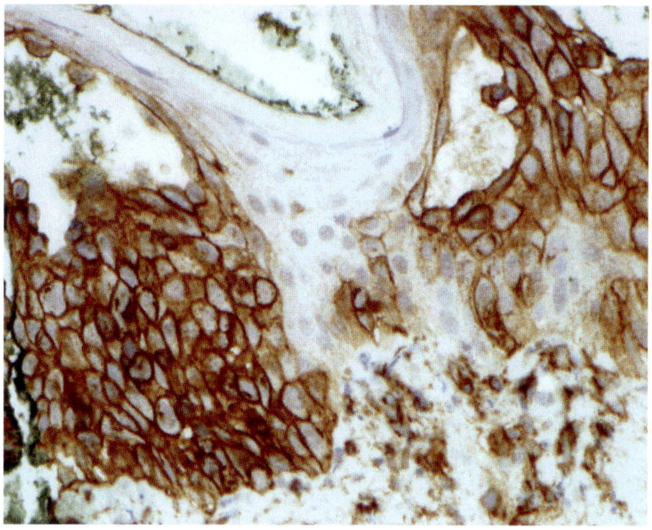

Figure 12.36 A combined HSVI and II immunostain demonstrates staining of infected epidermal keratinocytes (X400).

Varicella Zoster Virus (Human Herpes Virus 3)

Varicella zoster virus (VZV) is an alpha herpesvirus with a linear, double-stranded DNA genome. Following a primary infection, varicella or chickenpox clinically, a latent infection is established within cranial or sensory dorsal root ganglia. Herpes zoster or shingles occur when the virus is reactivated. Reactivation occurs at higher frequency in immunocompetent individuals older than 50 years and in immunocompromised individuals.[106] The zoster vaccine has been shown to reduce infection and severity.[107]

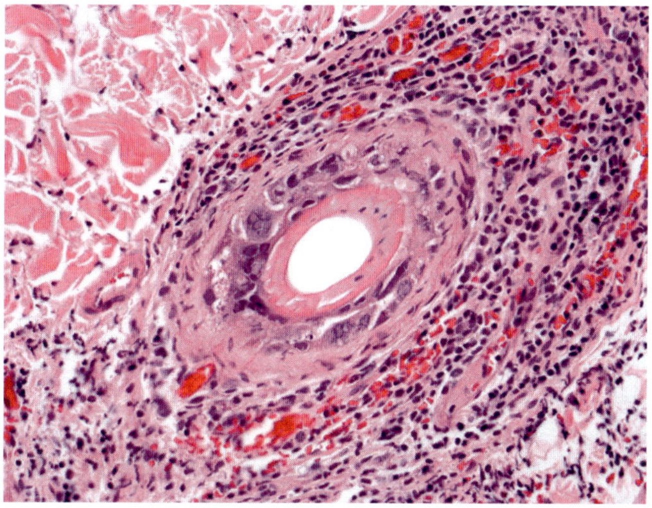

Figure 12.37 Varicella-zoster infection. Keratinocytes with characteristic nuclear inclusions are seen within follicular epithelium (X400).

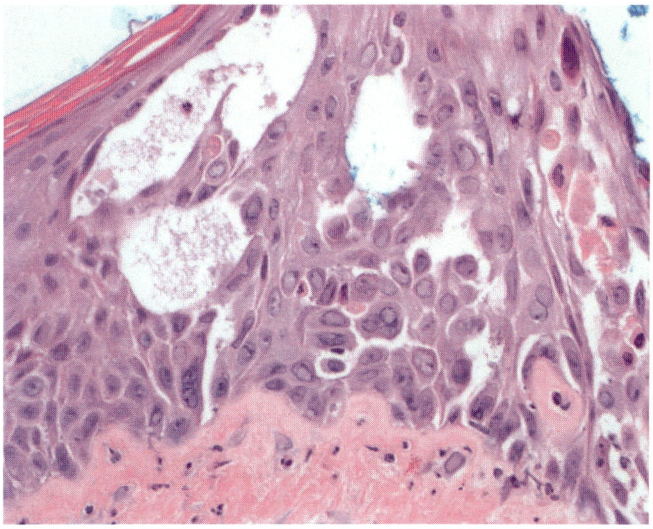

Figure 12.35 Herpes simplex virus infection. Intraepidermal blister associated with multinucleated keratinocytes possessing nuclear molding and chromatin margination (X400).

Symptoms of reactivation begin with a prodrome of pain, pruritus, or tingling in a unilateral distribution limited to one to three dermatomes. Clusters of papules soon appear and progress into vesicles on an erythematous base within 12 to 24 hours then pustular or hemorrhagic lesions in three to four days. Crusting of lesions occurs in seven to ten days but resolution might not occur till four to six weeks. Postherpetic neuralgia, the most frequent complication of herpes zoster, can cause long-term debilitating pain.[106] Satellite cutaneous lesions have been reported to be indicative of disseminated zoster often requiring hospitalization and development of systemic signs.[108]

Viral cultures are definitive for diagnosis; however, it would take one to two weeks for results.[109] A skin biopsy would show intraepidermal acantholysis, necrotic keratinocytes, and keratinocytes with viral cytopathic effects including intranuclear inclusions, steel gray nuclei, multinucleation, and nuclear molding (**Figure 12.37**). The viral inclusions can be seen in endothelial cells of capillaries, fibroblasts, and epithelial cells of hair follicles and eccrine coils. In addition, a denser inflammatory response, often vasculitis, and involvement of hair follicles are seen in zoster infection than HSV infection. Zoster folliculitis, more commonly seen with VZV than HSV, might not be associated with epidermal changes typically seen in herpes infection and the diagnosis can be missed.[110]

VZV immunostain is a cost and time effective test to distinguish VZV from HSV infection (**Figure 12.38**). Using monoclonal antibodies against VZV, viral antigens can be detected in keratinocytes, dermal fibroblasts, histiocytes, endothelial and perineurial cells. Positive VZV staining of epidermal keratinocytes is seen mainly during vesicular stage.[111] Whether VZV glycoprotein E is detected in keratinocytes, hair follicle epithelium, or eccrine glands by immunostain would be dependent upon the stages of the herpes zoster lesions. VZV glycoprotein E staining of epidermal keratinocytes is seen in vesicular stage whereas staining of eccrine epithelium is identified in late stage.[112] Cross reactivity with different types of myocytes (smooth, skeletal, and cardiac) and arteries (temporal, coronary, and vertebral) has been reported with Millipore MAB8612 antibody.[113]

Epstein Barr Virus (Human Herpes Virus 4)

Epstein-Barr virus (EBV) causes infectious mononucleosis and associated with hydroa vacciniforme, Gianotti-Crosti syndrome, Kikuchi histiocytic necrotizing lymphadenitis, oral hairy leukoplakia, and others. It is associated a number of neoplastic processes including nasopharyngeal lymphoepithelial carcinoma, smooth muscle tumors in immunosuppressed individuals, and lymphoproliferative processes. The lymphoid lesions include post-transplant lymphoproliferative disorders, angioimmunoblastic T-cell lymphoma, extranodal NK/T-cell lymphoma, and diffuse large B-cell lymphoma in elderly patients (**see Chapter 6**).[114]

Cutaneous lesions are uncommon and often in immunocompromised individuals.[115] A maculopapular or morbilliform eruption will show nonspecific histologic findings. An eruption of pruritic pink to red papules on extensor surfaces of extremities, cheeks, and buttocks. A spongiotic, lichenoid, or lymphocytic vasculitis reaction pattern can be seen on histologic sections. Ballooning and pale keratinocytes may contain atypical nuclear changes are seen within the squamous epithelium in oral hairy leukoplakia.[116]

EBV possesses a latent phase in memory B lymphocytes; therefore, the presence of EBV DNA does not correlate with disease. Immunohistochemical stains against latent membrane protein (LMP) 1 and EBV-encoded nuclear antigen 1 (EBNA1) have not been shown to have good sensitivity and specificity.[117] Detection of Epstein-Barr-encoded RNAs (EBERs) by *in situ* hybridization has high sensitivity and specificity in demonstrating the presence of viral RNA in tumor nuclei and currently the diagnostic gold standard (**Figure 12.39**).[118] EBV latency membrane protein 1 (LMP1) immunostain can identify EBV infection in normal, inflammatory, and neoplastic tissues, especially EBV-associated Hodgkin lymphoma.[119]

Cytomegalovirus (Human Herpes Virus 5)

Cytomegalovirus (CMV) is a member of the Herpesviridae family. The clinical presentation can be characterized by primary infection, latent phase, and reactivation/ reinfection. The viral sources in the primary infection can be prenatal, postnatal, blood transfusion, and organ transplant. After primary infection, CMV persists as latent infection and can be reactivated due to alteration of host immunological defenses. Reactivation is not distinguishable from reinfection with a different antigenic virus type.[120]

In immunocompromised individuals CMV infection is a common systemic infection involving the lung, central nervous system, eye, gastrointestinal tract and often fatal. Cutaneous involvement can rarely be seen in immunocompromised individuals, especially those with acquired immune deficiency syndrome (AIDS), most commonly as anogenital ulcers. It has been thought that likely colonization of endothelial cells during CMV viremia. Concurrent infection with other viruses such as HSV and VZV is not uncommon. The cutaneous lesions can be nonspecific or specific. The nonspecific lesions are often comprised

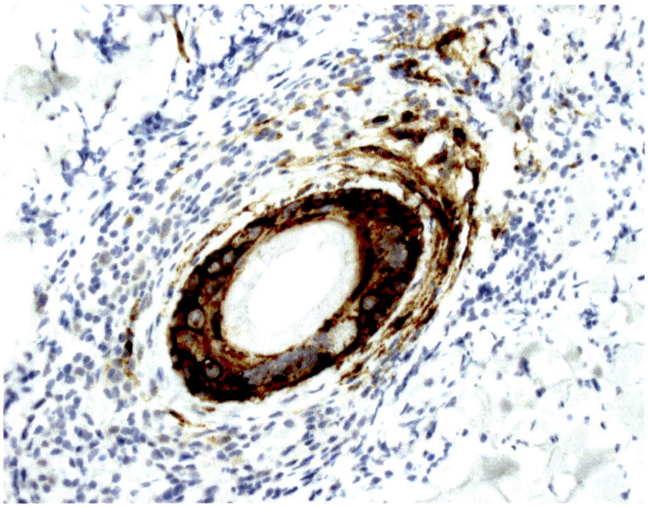

Figure 12.38 VZV immunostain is strongly positive (X400).

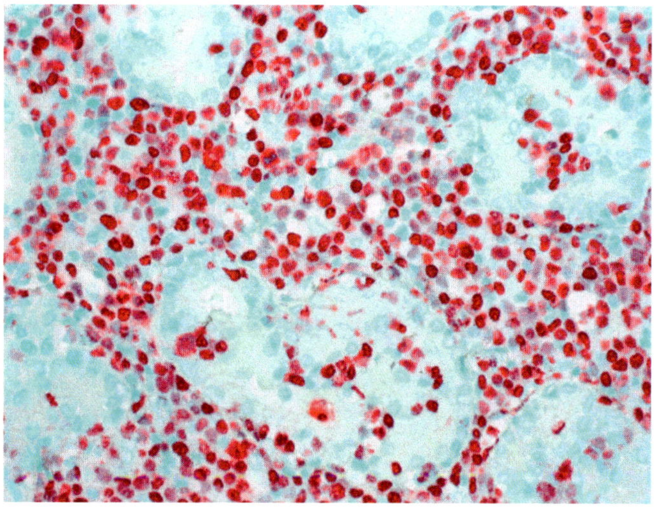

Figure 12.39 EBER *in situ* hybridization demonstrates strong nuclear staining (X200).

of maculopapular and urticarial eruption.[120] Congenital or CMV inclusion disease occurs as a result of transplacental transmission of the virus and present with petechiae, purpura, jaundice and blueberry muffin lesions.[121] In immunosuppressed individuals, the skin may be the initial involvement and a clue to systemic infection. The cutaneous infection can be localized as oral or cutaneous ulcerations or widespread as morbilliform or papulopustular eruptions.[122]

CMV infection in immunocompetent host most often presents with mononucleosis-like symptoms and rarely with cutaneous lesions. Specific lesions have been reported only in case reports as purpuric rash with bullae in an adult and purpuric papules and plaques in a background of livedo in a child.[120]

IgG and IgM antibody titers can be determined by using either enzyme-linked immunosorbent assay or complement fixation. Elevated IgM and IgG antibody titers are indicative of recent infection and latent infection, respectively. Rising levels of both IgM and IgG antibodies are indicative of reactivation. Although with easy serologic tests can give both false positive and false negative results since immunocompromised and transplant patients may not mount an IgM response to active or recurrent infection. In these settings histopathology and IHC play an important role.

The histopathology of cutaneous CMV infection can be variable and non-specific. Cytomegaly, irregular shape, nuclear hyperchromatism, and smudging appearance can be seen.[123] The pathognomonic histologic features are characteristic enlarged, 10 micrometer, irregular shaped endothelial cells containing eosinophilic intranuclear inclusions with clear halo also known as Cowdry type A intranuclear inclusions or owl's eye inclusions (**Figure 12.40**).[122] These inclusions can be seen within dermal fibroblasts, histiocytes, keratinocytes, and eccrine epithelium.[123,124] Intracytoplasmic inclusion and vacuolated cytoplasm can be seen as well. The appearance of the viral inclusions varies from nuclear enlargement in the initial stage, then cytoplasmic enlargement and cytoplasmic/nuclear inclusion, and lastly with nuclear inclusion fragmentation.[123]

These viral inclusions can be labeled by IHC using monoclonal antibody directed against the virus in paraffin-embedded

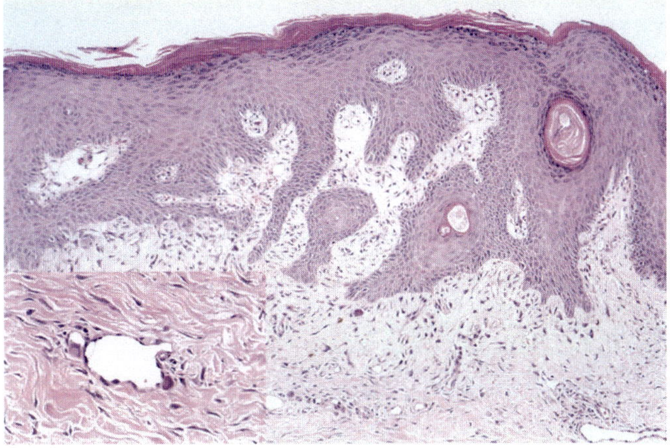

Figure 12.40 Cytomegalovirus infection. Beneath a hyperplastic epidermis intranuclear inclusions are identified within endothelial cells of ectatic vascular channels within a fibrotic dermis (X100).

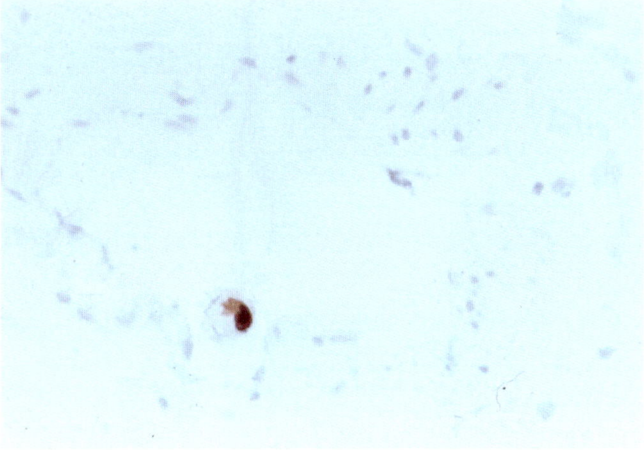

Figure 12.41 CMV immunostain highlights the rare nuclear inclusion (X400).

tissue (**Figure 12.41**). Though specific, histopathologic findings and immunostains are not as sensitive as indirect immunofluorescence studies or viral cultures.

Human Herpes Virus 6 and Human Herpes Virus 7

Human herpesvirus (HHV) 6 and HHV-7 cause exanthem subitum or roseola infantum. A prodrome of three to five days of high fever would typically follow by diffuse erythematous macules and papules. Resolution then develops one to two days after. HHV6 has been reported in association with infectious mononucleosis, pityriasis rosea, Rosai-Dorfman disease, and malignancy. HHV7 has been reported in association with pityriasis rosea. The cutaneous histopathologic findings of HHV-6 and HHV-7 are nonspecific.[125] HHV6 staining of infected lymphocytes by IHC in the skin of two patients with mononucleosis-like syndrome has been reported.[126] HHV6 and HHV7 antigen were demonstrated in dermal fibroblasts and follicular keratinocytes in skin of 15% and 67% of 15 patients with pityriasis rosea, respectively.[127] However, these monoclonal antibodies have not been validated for clinically use. By *in situ* hybridization HHV6 was detected in seven of nine cases of extracutaneous Rosai-Dorfman disease; however, this finding has not been confirmed in cutaneous Rosai-Dorfman disease.[128,129] Currently, PCR assays are used to detect the presence of HHV6 and HHV7 in the clinical setting.

Human Herpes Virus 8

Human herpes virus 8 (HHV8) is the causative organism of Kaposi sarcoma. Since HHV-8 exhibits tropism for endothelial cells, some authors have proposed that the endothelial cells are site of latency of the virus. Kaposi sarcoma is characterized by a proliferation of ectatic vascular channels dissecting the dermis and adnexal structures associated with hemosiderin deposition and infiltrate of plasma cells in the early patch stage. The lesion progresses to a plaque and then nodular/tumor stage which is a cellular spindled-cell proliferation with erythrocytes extravasation (**Figure 12.42**).[130]

A commercially available monoclonal antibody directed against the C-terminus of the latent nuclear antigen-1 (LNA-1) encoded by the ORF-73 gene has facilitated clinical diagnosis.[131] The sensitivity of the antibody in detecting Kaposi sarcoma

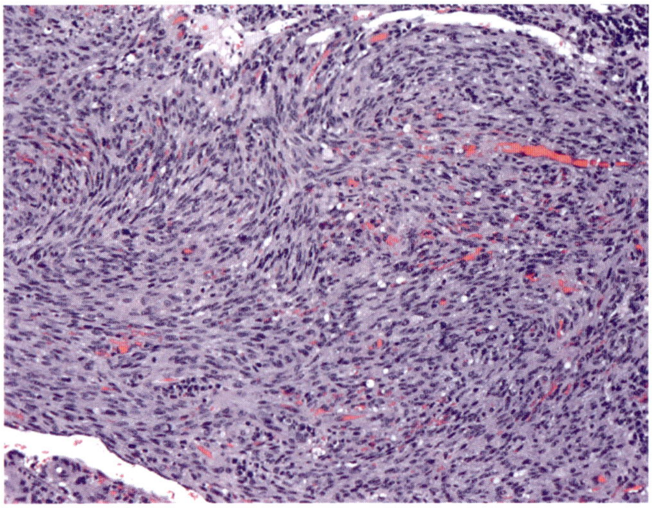

Figure 12.42 Kaposi sarcoma. Intersecting fascicles of spindle tumor cells are seen characteristic of tumor stage (X200).

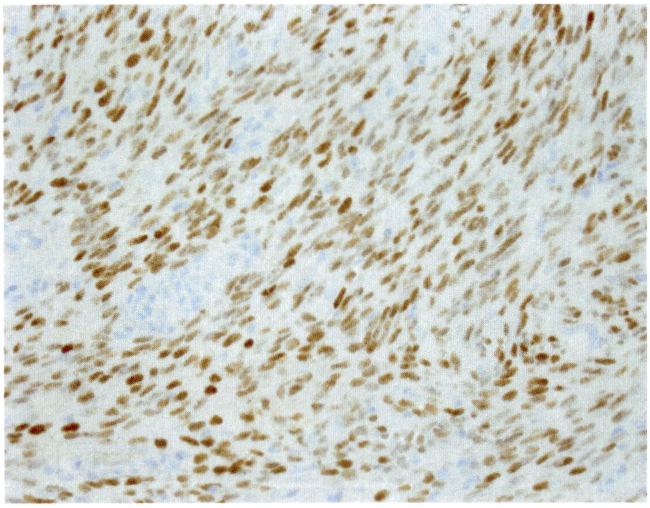

Figure 12.43 Kaposi sarcoma. HHV8 immunostain demonstrates strong nuclear staining within tumor cells (X400).

has been reported to be approximately 78%.[131] The presence of HHV8 can be demonstrated in the nuclei of neoplastic cells in early patch as well as tumor stages of KS and is a very helpful marker in distinguishing KS from histologic mimickers including angiosarcoma, radiation induced angiosarcoma, kaposiform hemangioendothelioma, benign lymphangioendothelioma, and others (**Figure 12.43**).[132] However, HHV8 expression can be seen in a subset of angiosarcoma.[133]

Human Papilloma Virus

Human papilloma virus (HPV) is a family of non-enveloped, circular, double-stranded DNA viruses. HPV is the causal agent for verruca vulgaris, condyloma acuminata, and subsequent SCC. Genital warts or condyloma acuminata can affect the genital sites and perianal skin. There are approximately 40 types of HPV that can cause genital lesions. HPV type 6 and HPV type 11, also known as "low risk," are the common types present in condyloma acuminate.[134] HPV types 16 and 18 are "high risk" since they are identified in vulva/penile/anal intraepithelial lesions and associated SCC. A quadrivalent (HPV types 6, 11, 16, and 18) or bivalent (HPV types 6 and 11) vaccines are available in recent years.

Condyloma acuminata present clinically as multiple verrucous, filiform, or flat lesion on the skin or mucosa of genital sites. They are typically asymptomatic unless superinfection occurs. In immunocompromised individuals, they present as large masses with frequent recurrences.[135] On histologic sections, condylomata present as polypoid lesions whose epidermis exhibit acanthosis, papillomatosis, and prominent granular layer (**Figure 12.44**). Koilocytes with irregular, enlarged, and hyperchromatic nuclei with surrounding cytoplasmic halos are seen. Binucleated and multinucleated keratinocytes can be seen (**Figure 12.45**).

p16 immunostain is commonly used as a surrogate marker for high-risk HPV infection in the anogenital tract. In HPV-driven tumors production of E6 and E7 viral oncoprotein is activated by integration of the virus into host cell genome. E7

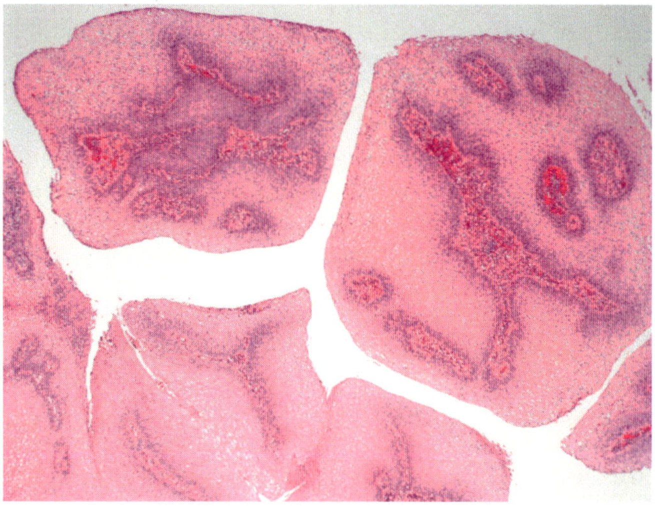

Figure 12.44 Condyloma acuminatum. A polypoid growth is seen (X40).

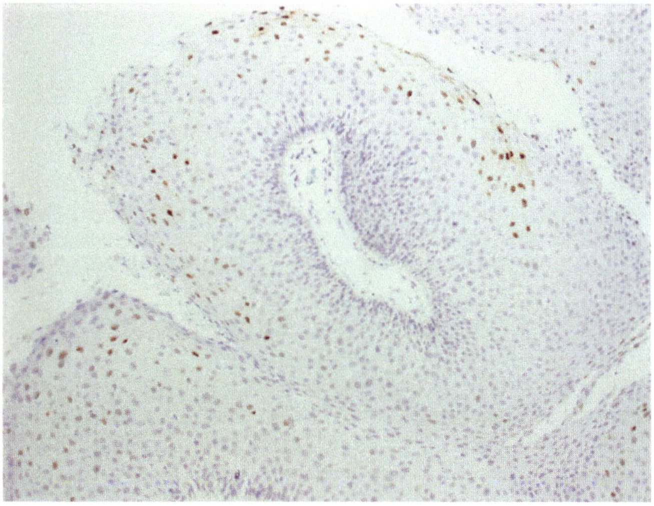

Figure 12.45 Condyloma acuminatum. HPV6 and 11 *in situ* hybridization demonstrate nuclear staining within keratinocytes (X100).

oncoprotein inactivates the function of phospho-Rb which results in degradation of p53 and an increased expression of p16. Studies have shown that transcriptionally active HPV results in very high levels of p16 expression. Diffuse strong nuclear staining or nuclear and cytoplasmic staining involving the majority of the area of interest ("block" staining) is considered as positive staining (**see Chapter 3**).[136] However, there is a subset of high-grade intraepithelial lesion that has been reported to be negative for p16 immunostain; therefore, immunostain finding must be interpreted in conjunction with histopathologic findings.[137] In the vulva, p16 immunostain is helpful in detecting high-grade dysplasia at cauterized surgical margin. Positive p16 staining is helpful to exclude the possibility of differentiated vulvar intraepithelial neoplasia which occurs in the setting of lichen sclerosus.[138]

Although HPV PCR assays are sensitive methods approved by the FDA and considered as gold standards for the detection and typing of HPV, visualization of viral transcripts within the tissues cannot be determined, unlike immunohistochemical stain such as p16 or *in situ* hybridization (ISH) assay using either DNA or RNA probes.[139] Studies have shown similar sensitivity and specificity between RNA ISH and DNA ISH using commercially available probes detecting HPV (**Figure 12.46**). RNA ISH assay (RNAscope) targeting high-risk HPV E6/E7 mRNA transcript has been reported to be a sensitive assay. Recently HPV mRNA ish probes targeting E6 and E7 mRNA transcript of HPV6, HPV11, HPV16, HPV18, HPV33, and HPV42 have shown to be helpful tests in detecting papillomavirus in formalin-fixed paraffin-embedded tissue.[140]

Human T-Cell Lymphotropic Virus Type 1

Human T-cell lymphotropic virus type 1 (HTLV-1), also known as adult T-cell lymphoma virus type 1, is endemic in the Caribbean islands and southern Japan. The virus can cause an eczematous dermatitis involving the scalp, axillae, and groin.[141] HTLV-1 is more known for its association with adult T-cell leukemia/lymphoma (ATLL) (**see Chapter 6**). Four variants of ATLL are recognized by WHO classification including acute leukemic, chronic leukemic, lymphomatous, and smoldering types. Cutaneous manifestations are commonly seen in the smoldering form and the histologic findings are similar to those of mycosis fungoides; therefore, the demonstration of HTLV-1 is important for diagnostic distinction. Although there is report of using IHC to detect HTLV-1 proviral DNA pX region p40Tax protein and pX p27Rex protein; these immunostains have not been validated for clinical use and serologic testings remain the gold standard.[142] Recently, multiplexed fluorescence imaging of DNA, RNA, and protein has been reported in detecting HTLV-1; however, this technique is currently mainly for research.[143]

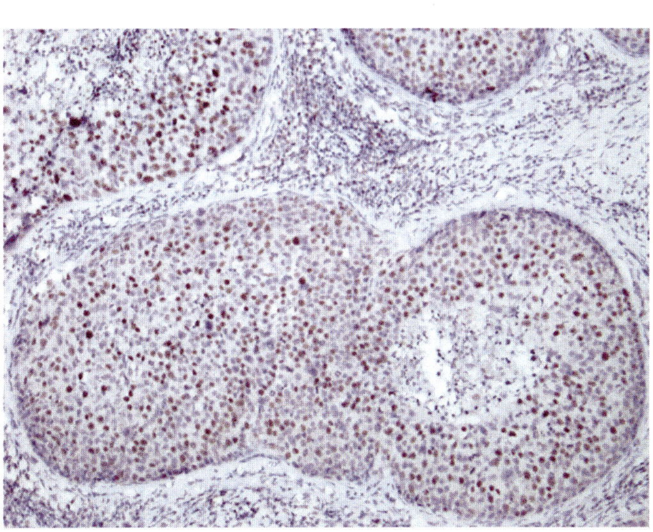

Figure 12.46 Diffuse and strong nuclear staining on HPV 16 and 18 *in situ* hybridization (X200).

Parvovirus B19

Parvoviruses are single-stranded DNA viruses and etiologic agent of two dermatologic diseases: the more common erythema infectiosum (fifth disease) and the rare purpuric "gloves-and-socks" syndrome. Papular-purpuric "gloves and socks" syndrome is a transient febrile dermatosis characterized by acral pruritus, edema, and petechiae. Persistent Parvovirus B19 infection occurs in patients with hereditary of acquired immunodeficiency syndromes. The cutaneous histologic findings of both entities are nonspecific and often comprised of epidermal spongiosis and superficial perivascular infiltrate of lymphocytes in the dermis.[144]

Parvovirus B19 DNA has been identified by PCR in 25% in skin with unrelated diseases and from healthy individuals; thus, it has been questioned whether the virus is a true pathogen.[145] Some authors have reported the presence of virus in epidermal keratinocytes by indirect immunofluorescence and *in situ* hybridization tests.[146] By immunohistochemistry Parvovirus B19 can be demonstrated in the cytoplasm of endothelial cells of dermal capillaries by other authors.[144,147] At the CDC, immunohistochemical staining has been documented in cases of hydrops fetalis, bone marrow, and placenta, but not in skin to date (personal observation by W-J Shieh).

Merkel Cell Polyomavirus

Polyomaviruses are double-stranded DNA viruses that are typically non-oncogenic but can be oncogenic in certain settings. The Merkel cell polyomavirus (MCPyV) genome integrates clonally into the host chromosomes resulting in expression of small T antigen and truncated large T antigen. The association between Merkel cell carcinoma and Merkel cell polyomavirus have been well established.[148] The presence of Merkel cell polyomavirus has also been documented in seborrheic keratosis and rare cases of squamous cell carcinomas in immunosuppressed patients by PCR.[149,150]

A monoclonal antibody CM2B4 directed against the MCPyV T antigen exon 2 was developed by Shuda and colleagues[151] to detect Merkel cell polyomavirus expression in tumor cells. The nuclear expression of CM2B4 immunostain was reported in 77% of Merkel cell carcinoma harboring the virus demonstrated by PCR. Using a combination of CM2B4 and CM5E1 immunostains the sensitivity increased to 92%.[152] A recent mouse monoclonal antibody Ab3 has been reported to have better sensitivity (97%, 56/58) than CM2B4 antibody in detection Merkel

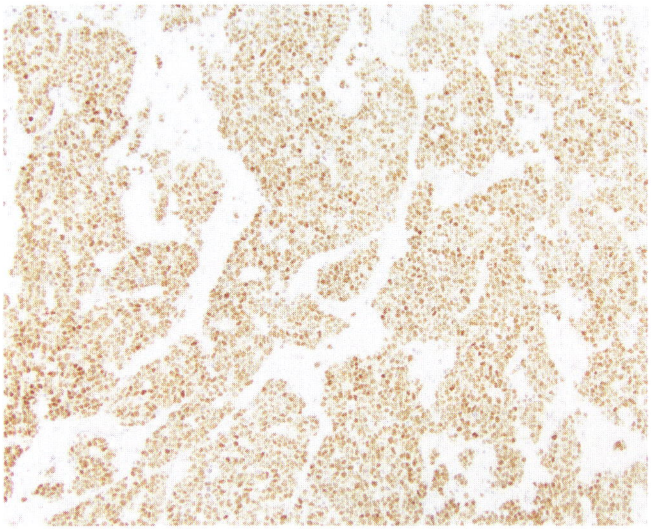

Figure 12.47 Nuclear expression of Merkel cell polyomavirus immunostain in a Merkel cell carcinoma (X400).

cell polyomavirus large T antigen (**Figure 12.47**).[153] These monoclonal antibodies can be a helpful diagnostic adjunct in distinguishing Merkel cell carcinoma from histologic mimics such as pulmonary neuroendocrine carcinomas.[154]

Poxviruses

The Poxviridae are double-stranded DNA viruses with two subfamilies that can infect both vertebrate and invertebrate animals. Four genera of poxviruses may infect humans: 1) orthopoxviruses such as those causing variola (smallpox), mpox, and vaccinia; 2) parapoxviruses such as those causing orf (ecthyma contagiosum) and milker's nodule; 3) Molluscipoxvirus, mainly molluscum contagiosum virus; and 4) Yatapoxviruses, such as tanapox. These are complex DNA viruses that replicate in the cytoplasm and are highly adapted to proliferation in keratinocytes. Spread of poxviruses is primarily by direct contact with infectious material from an infected human or animal. Transmission can also occur via fomites or aerosolized droplets, such as smallpox virus. After the eradication of smallpox, the most common poxvirus infections in humans are vaccinia in Indian subcontinent, orf, and molluscum contagiosum; however, mpox in west and central African countries and some unusual parapoxvirus infections worldwide have become emerging diseases with various degrees of public health impact.

Mpox (Monkeypox) Virus

Mpox virus belongs to the genus Orthopoxvirus. There are two known clades of mpox virus – one that originated in Central Africa (Clade I) and one that originated in West Africa (Clade II). It is a zoonotic pathogen that causes a febrile rash disease in humans. It was first identified as a pathogen of laboratory macaque monkeys in 1958, and the first human cases were reported in 1970, in Democratic Republic of the Congo.[155] A variety of African mammals may serve as a natural reservoir for mpox virus, while humans and primates are possibly incidental hosts and do not readily transmit infection to others.[156] The first reported outbreak in the United States occurred in 2003 in several midwestern states. Most of the patients became sick after having contact with pet prairie dogs infected with mpox virus, through contact with imported rodents from Ghana.[157] No evidence of human-to-human transmission was identified during the outbreak, and most of the confirmed human cases presented with scattered skin lesions. However, the global outbreak of mpox in 2022 redefined its epidemiology. The transmission route of this global outbreak was mainly through intimate human-to-human contact, and many cases showed abundant skin lesions with mucosal involvement. The outbreak has brought alarming challenges to the healthcare professionals and public health agencies in many non-endemic areas because of its unusual mode of transmission and atypical presentation on top of the general unfamiliarity of the disease.[158]

Mpox virus has an average incubation period of approximately 12 days, with a range of 7 to 17 days. The signs and symptoms of mpox in humans are very similar to those of smallpox, but usually milder. Clinical manifestations often start with several days of high fever, general malaise, myalgia, and headache followed by the development of a maculopapular rash. The rash appears first on the oropharyngeal mucosa, face, forearms, and spreads to the trunk and legs, similar to smallpox. The rash becomes vesicular and then pustular within one to two days of appearance, and usually evolves through several stages before eventual crusting and detaching. The main distinguishing characteristic between mpox and smallpox is the prominent involvement of lymph nodes in mpox. Generalized or regional lymphadenopathy with tenderness can appear and usually develops concurrently with or shortly after the onset of the fever. Most of the mpox cases resolve spontaneously within two to four weeks. However, a small number of patients, especially in pediatric population, may present with a more severe course with respiratory distress or neurologic disorders. Complications reported from African outbreaks include deforming scars, bronchopneumonia, secondary bacterial infection with septicemia, respiratory failure, ulcerative keratitis, blindness, and encephalitis.[159] The diagnosis of human mpox requires a high index of suspicion in correlation with pertinent clinical and epidemiologic information.[159] The most common laboratory diagnosis for mpox is usually established based on molecular testing or viral isolation from non-tissue material obtained with noninvasive methods. PCR assays have been developed to provide a rapid confirmatory diagnosis.[160] Electron microscopy, if available, can be a very useful tool for morphologic diagnosis on clinical samples, such as skin scraps or vesicular fluid.[161]

Skin biopsy is an important tool for diagnosis of mpox infection. Microscopic examination of the skin lesion shows a spectrum of histopathologic changes corresponding to the progression of disease. At early stage, epidermis with mild acantholysis, spongiosis, and ballooning degeneration of basal keratinocytes is observed.[162] The epidermal changes progress to marked acantholysis and full thickness necrosis later, especially in vesiculopustular lesions. A mixed inflammatory cell infiltrate is usually present in the epidermis and around the perivascular areas, eccrine glands, and follicles in the dermis. Viral cytopathic effect can be seen with multinucleated syncytial keratinocytes and eosinophilic intracytoplasmic inclusions (**Figure 12.48**).

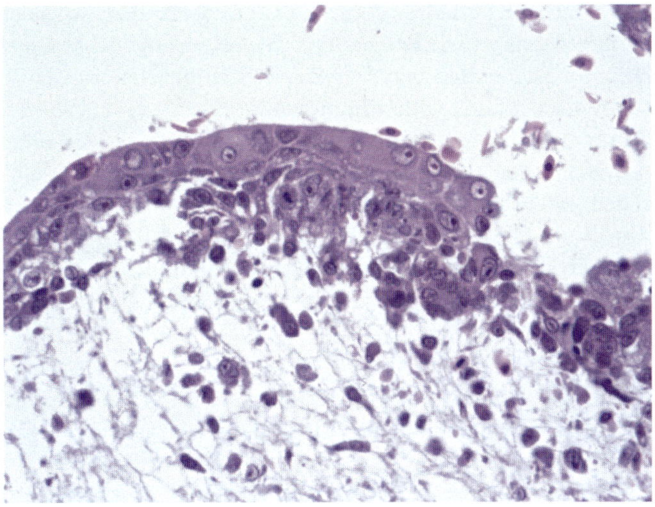

Figure 12.48 Monkeypox. Viral cytopathic effect with multinucleated syncytial keratinocytes and intracytoplasmic inclusions (X400).

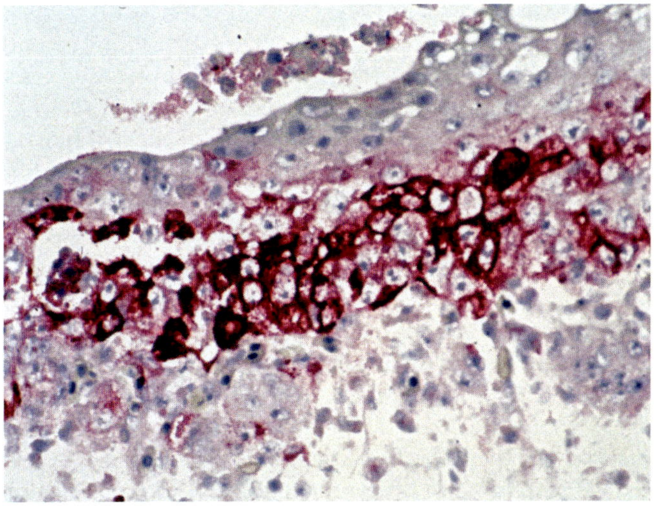

Figure 12.49 Immunostaining of monkeypox virus antigens within the infected keratinocytes (X400).

Eosinophilic inclusions, the so-called "Guarnieri bodies," can be observed in the cytoplasm. IHC is a useful method for tissue diagnosis that can demonstrate viral antigens within the infected keratinocytes and dermal adnexae (**Figure 12.49**). The viral inclusions, although distinctive, are not specific to mpox because other orthopoxviruses, such as variola virus or vaccinia virus can cause similar cytopathic effects.

Parapoxviruses

Parapoxviruses infect many vertebrates, such as cows, sheep, goats, and red squirrels worldwide.[163] They cause skin lesions with a wide spectrum of clinical presentations that vary in size, shape, location, and distribution. Orf and Milker's nodule are the two most common human infections caused by parapoxvirus. There are many emerging parapoxviruses identified in the past decade because of increasing awareness of the disease and availability of diagnostic techniques, especially molecular assays.[164]

Orf virus is widespread in sheep and goats. Human infections are caused by direct inoculation of infected material from animals and are more common among shepherds, veterinarians, and other individuals with animal exposure. Butchers, meat porters, and cooks are sometimes infected from infected carcasses. Incubation period is usually five to six days; a small, firm, red or reddish-blue papule enlarges to form an umbilicated hemorrhagic pustule or bulla. In the fully developed lesion, the central crust is surrounded by a grayish to violaceous ring encircled by a zone of erythema. The lesions are usually solitary and are located most commonly on the fingers, hands, or forearms. Mild fever with lymphangitis or regional tender lymphadenopathy may be present. Spontaneous recovery usually occurs within three to six weeks.[165,166]

Milker's nodule is caused by a parapoxvirus that most commonly leads to infection of the teats and mouths of cattle. Milkers, farmers, and veterinarians with a direct exposure to these lesions are accidental hosts. After an incubation period of about five days to two weeks, flat, red papules are formed. Within a week they appear as reddish-blue, firm, slightly tender nodules. The epidermis becomes opaque and grayish, and soon after, a crust develops centrally. Similar to orf, central umbilication is usually present. Many cases develop lymphangitis but there are rarely any constitutional symptoms. Lesions resolve over four to six weeks without scarring. In contrast to orf, lesions are usually multiple. The most common sites of involvement are the hands and fingers. Rarely, a more widespread papulovesicular eruption of the extremities and neck may develop.[167,168] Other acute inflammatory infections that may resemble parapoxvirus infections include primary tuberculosis, sporotrichosis, pyogenic granulomas, anthrax, impetigo, arthropod bites, plague, rickettsialpox, scrub typhus, and tularemia. These lesions can usually be differentiated by histopathologic examination.

Parapoxvirus infections share some common histopathologic features. The epidermis usually shows prominent parakeratosis, marked inter- and intracellular edema, vacuolization, ballooning degeneration, epidermolysis, and focal necrosis. Keratinocytes with eosinophilic cytoplasmic and intranuclear inclusions can be observed (**Figure 12.50**). A dense infiltrate is

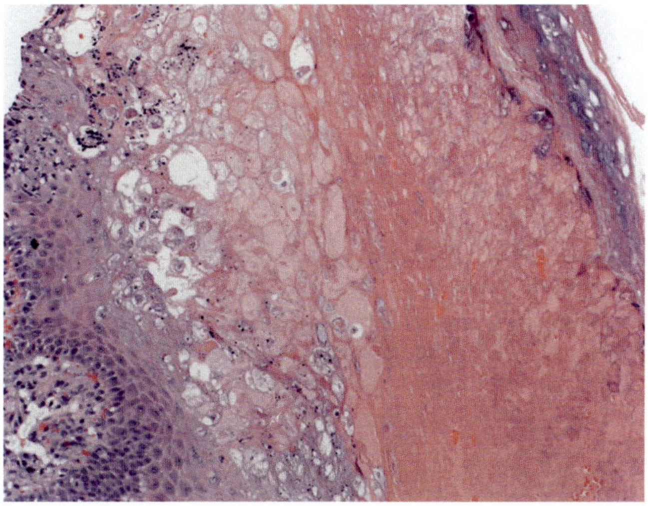

Figure 12.50 Orf. Prominent parakeratosis, marked epidermal edema, vacuolization, ballooning degeneration, epidermolysis, focal necrosis, and keratinocytes with eosinophilic inclusions (X200).

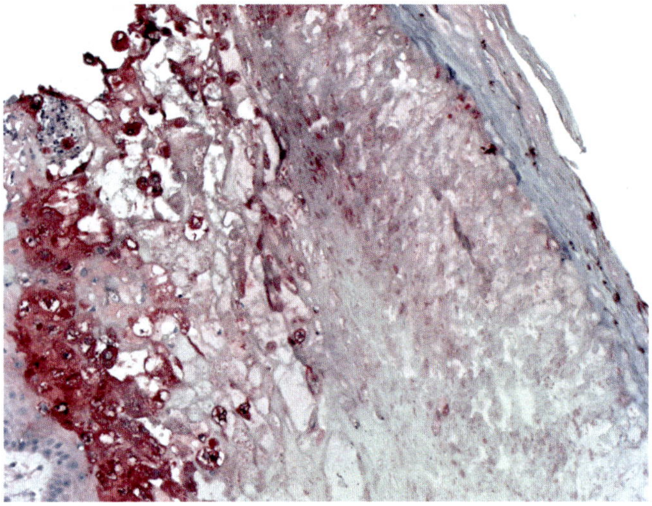

Figure 12.51 Immunostaining of parapoxvirus antigens (X200).

present in the dermis that consists mainly of macrophages at the center with lymphocytes and plasma cells at the periphery. There are usually very few neutrophils. The dermis may contain many newly formed, dilated capillaries with perivascular mononuclear infiltrate.[169] IHC is a useful ancillary assay that can demonstrate the parapoxviruses antigens in skin biopsies to establish the diagnosis (**Figure 12.51**).[170]

12.3 Parasite

Parasitic infections of skin are more commonly seen in tropical and subtropical countries. However, the increase in international travel from endemic regions has brought these infectious diseases to North America and Europe. Immigrants from Asia, Africa, and South America represent another contingent of patients afflicted by diseases that are normally not prevalent in the United States and Western Europe. In addition, HIV infection and other causes of immunosuppression have become important cofactors in the emergence of these rare infections in the developed world. The key to the recognition of these parasitic infections is knowledge of epidemiological risk factors such as the parasite's geographic distribution and the major modes of clinical presentation. Parasitic organisms are usually readily recognizable by their morphology; however, the diagnosis can be challenging due to the unfamiliarity of the organisms to the dermatologists and pathologists. Laboratory diagnosis is usually established by direct visualization, including gross examination, light microscopy, and electron microscopy. Molecular assays have been developed for the diagnosis of a variety of parasitic organisms; however, they're not readily available in most of the conventional laboratories. IHC assays are also limited to specialized laboratories. The best examples by using IHC assay as ancillary diagnostics are cutaneous protozoal infections caused by free-living amoebae and Leishmania species.

Free-Living Amoebae

Free-living amoebae (FLA) are important pathogens of human and animal diseases. These organisms are commonly found in soil and water throughout the world. Species that are able to tolerate temperatures above 37°C are most likely to cause human disease, such as *Naegleria fowleri*, *Acanthamoeba species*, and *Balamuthia mandrillaris*. These organisms can cause severe encephalitis with a high fatality rate. *Naegleria fowleri* causes primary amoebic meningoencephalitis (PAM); while *Acanthamoeba spp.* and *Balamuthia mandrillaris* are associated with granulomatous amoebic encephalitis (GAE). *Acanthamoeba species* and *Balamuthia mandrillaris* can also produce skin infections, especially in immunocompromised patients.

Acanthamoeba Species

Acanthamoeba spp. is the most common FLA organism capable of producing cutaneous lesions, especially in HIV, organ transplant, and other immunocompromised patients.[171,172] Acanthamoeba spp. can be isolated from soil, dust, air, natural and treated water, and so on. These organisms can also be found in nasal and pharyngeal mucosa of healthy individuals. They have a worldwide distribution with many genotypes that can cause skin infections. T4 is the most common genotype in the environment and causes most cases of corneal and cutaneous infections. *Acanthamoeba spp.* exists in two forms: 1) cysts, measuring 12 to 20 μm in diameter, are resistant to desiccation and transform to trophozoites only in a favorable environment; 2) trophozoites, measuring 15 to 45 μm in size, representing the infectious and invasive form of the organism. Both cyst and trophozoite stages exist in nature and can be identified in tissue sections. Transmission occurs via the respiratory mucosa or contamination of skin lesions. The organisms can infect other organs through hematogenous spread.[173]

The skin lesions in acanthamoebiasis are nonspecific and may present as macules, papules, nodules, or chronic ulcers. The ulcers are poorly demarcated with elevated borders that may form eschar. The lesions are usually multiple and may appear in crops involving trunk, face, and extremities. Disseminated form have been reported in transplant patients.[174,175] Clinical laboratory diagnosis can be made by culture, direct fluorescent antibody (DFA), or PCR assays.

The skin biopsies usually demonstrate multifocal or diffuse perivascular inflammatory infiltrate, composed mostly of neutrophils and histiocytes admixed with extensive tissue necrosis, sometimes evolving into abscess formation. A predominant neutrophilic infiltrate may be present in the pustules, acute ulcers, or abscesses. Leukocytoclastic vasculitis with fibrin deposits in the vessel wall and vascular necrosis can also been observed. Lobular panniculitis with necrotizing vasculitis has been reported in cases with deep dermal and subcutaneous lesions.[175,176] Variable numbers of amoebic organisms can be seen throughout the skin lesion and are often more abundant in perivascular areas (**Figure 12.52**). The cyst forms display a double wall, with the outer wall wavy and wrinkled in appearance and the inner wall shallow and scalloped surrounding the cytoplasm. The cyst walls can be highlighted with PAS and GMS. The round trophozoites usually present with projecting acanthopodia, vacuolated cytoplasm, and a central large nucleus with a single prominent karyosome mixed within the inflammatory infiltrate (**Figure 12.53**). The trophozoite forms are relatively inconspicuous and can be missed easily, because their morphology closely resembles macrophages. The genus and species cannot be determined by morphologic features. IHC is a useful ancillary assay to help demonstrate the amoebic organisms in tissue samples, especially when the organisms are mixed with abundant macrophages with similar morphology (**Figure 12.54**).[177]

Balamuthia Mandrillaris

B. mandrillaris is the only known species of this genus and was originally isolated from the brain of a mandrill baboon. *B. mandrillaris* is found in the environment and can infect human beings through skin wounds or by inhaling the dust containing the organisms. The life cycle consists of the trophozoite and cyst stages, both of which are infectious. *B. mandrillaris* trophozoites have a diameter ranging from 12 – 60 μm; cysts have a diameter ranging from 12–30 μm with a wavy and irregular outer wall that is composed of three layers. On H&E–stained slides, the

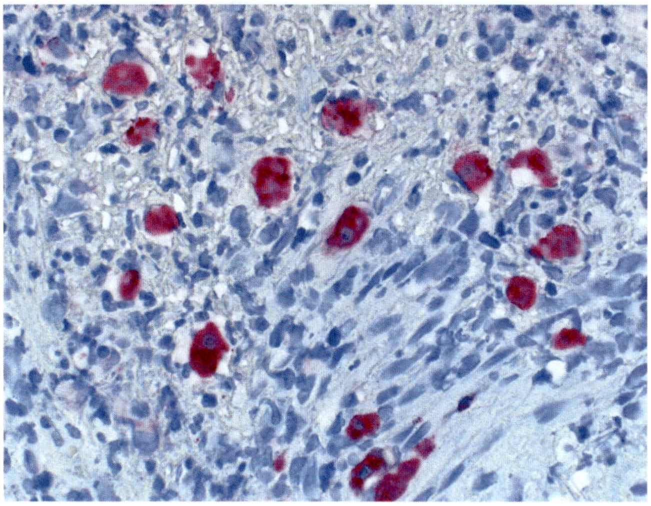

Figure 12.54 Immunostaining of antigens of Acanthamebic organisms (X630).

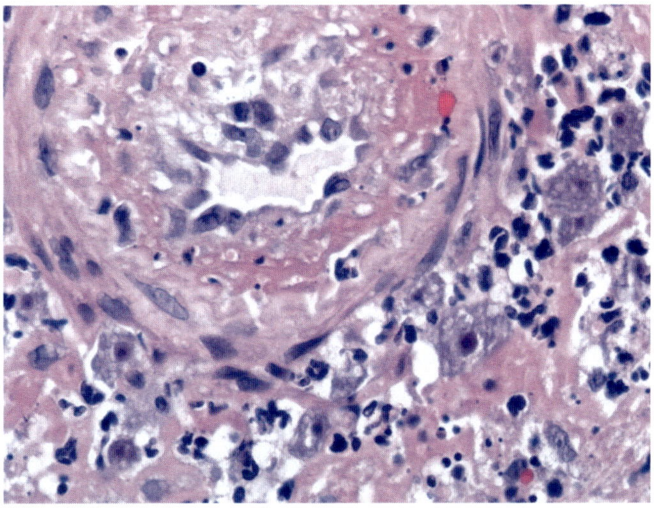

Figure 12.52 Cutaneous Acanthamebiasis. Variable numbers of amebic organisms in the dermis, often more abundant in perivascular areas (X630).

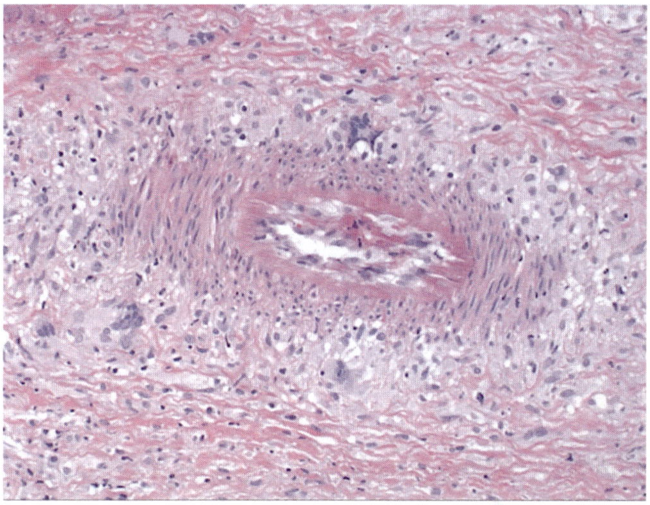

Figure 12.55 Balamuthia mandrillaris infection. Perivascular granulomatous inflammatory infiltrate, vasculitis, and vascular necrosis in dermis (X400).

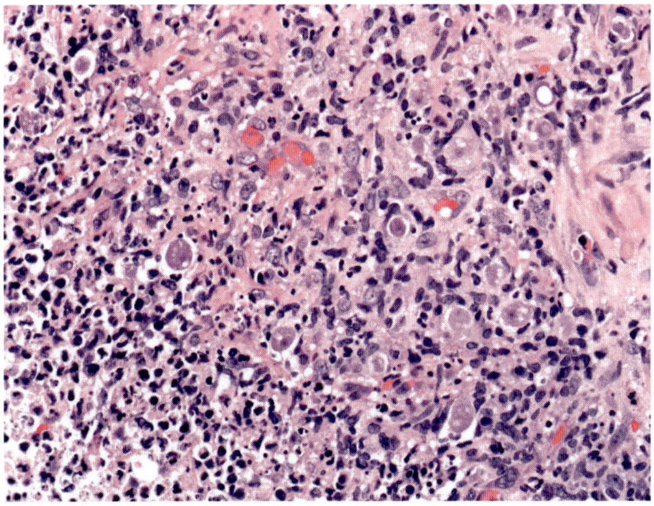

Figure 12.53 Cutaneous Acanthamebiasis. The round trophozoites usually present with projecting acanthopodia, vacuolated cytoplasm, and a central large nucleus with a single prominent karyosome mixed within the inflammatory infiltrate (X200).

organism cannot be reliably differentiated from *Acanthamoeba species*.[178]

Balamuthia can cause disease in both immunocompetent and immunocompromised hosts. Cutaneous Balamuthia infection has been particularly common in Peruvian patients.[179] These skin lesions are usually solitary, nodular, and often appear on the central portion of face, although lower face, abdomen, and extremities have also been reported. Balamuthia skin lesions frequently precede central nervous system involvement. Clinical laboratory diagnosis can be made by DFA or PCR assays.[180]

The skin lesions caused by *B. mandrillaris* are similar to those caused by Acanthamoeba species with a broader spectrum. The inflammatory responses can range from an acute or neutrophilic infiltrate to a lymphocytic or granulomatous response. Perivascular inflammatory infiltrate, vasculitis, and vascular necrosis are usually present (**Figure 12.55**). Unlike in cases of GAE, cysts and trophozoites of *B. mandrillaris* are not readily appreciable in skin biopsies.[181] IHC is a useful ancillary assay

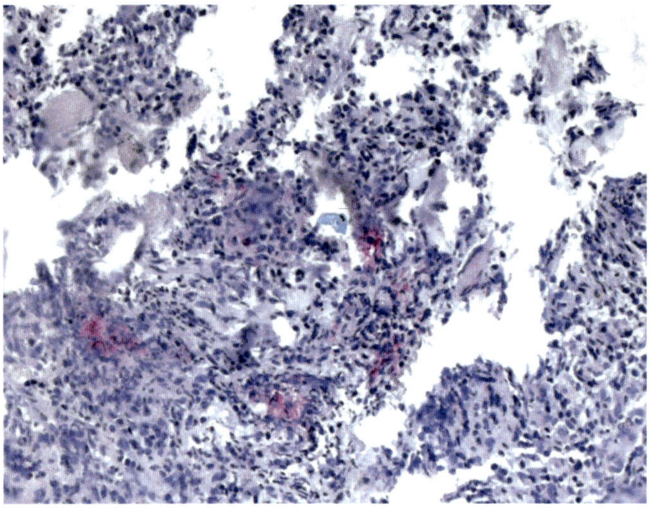

Figure 12.56 Immunostaining of antigens of *B. mandrillaris*. Unlike in cases of granulomatous amoebic encephalitis, cysts and trophozoites of *B. mandrillaris* are not readily appreciable in skin lesions (X100).

to help highlight the antigens of *B. Mandrillaris* in skin biopsy samples for etiologic diagnosis (**Figure 12.56**).[182]

Leishmania Species

Leishmaniasis is caused by the protozoon *Leishmania* with a wide spectrum of clinical illness, including cutaneous, mucosal, or visceral diseases. Leishmaniasis is a prevalent infectious disease worldwide, with a higher incidence in countries with warmer climate. There are many species of *Leishmania* but most cases seen in travelers returning from tropical areas are due to *L. tropica*, *L. major*, and *L. aethiopica*. The infection is usually zoonotic; one species of Leishmania may be associated with one, or many, natural vertebrate hosts, which provide the reservoir of infection. Humans are usually accidental hosts.[183,184]

Leishmania spp. have both flagellar (promastigote) and aflagellar (amastigote) stages during their life cycle. In sandfly or in artificial culture media, the organisms are present at the elongated motile promastigote stage with an anterior flagellum. Human infection is transmitted by the bite of the infected sandfly, usually outdoors at night. After the promastigotes have entered the skin of the human host, they transform into amastigotes, which primarily affect cells of mononuclear phagocytic system in its vertebrate host. Skin lesions develop if the host response to Leishmania spp. is confined to the skin. However, internal organs can become involved if dissemination of the protozoa occurs. The amastigote is round or oval, 2–3 μm in diameter, with a prominent kinetoplast.[185]

Leishmaniasis used to be classified into a cutaneous, mucocutaneous, and visceral form; however, this simplistic classification has been abandoned in favor of a classification that recognizes the overlap in the clinical spectrum and complexity of host-vector-parasite relationship in different forms of leishmaniasis.[186] These different forms include localized acute cutaneous leishmaniasis, diffuse acute cutaneous leishmaniasis, chronic cutaneous leishmaniasis, mucocutaneous leishmaniasis, post-kala-azar dermal leishmaniasis, and visceral leishmaniasis. The most common form of skin involvement is the localized acute cutaneous leishmaniasis. This form usually affects the exposed parts of the body, such as face, scalp, and arms. It initially appears as a painless, erythematous papule that enlarges to a nodule or a plaque over a period of 4 to 12 weeks. Ulceration is common. The lesion usually spontaneously regresses after several months, starting from the center and progressing outwards. Eventually, the lesion is replaced by a scar with hypo- or hyper- pigmentation.[187,188] The diagnosis of leishmaniasis depends on isolation or identification of the organism from tissue.[189] Species-specific PCR assays have been developed to provide a rapid confirmatory diagnosis, especially in lesions that organisms cannot be identified in histologic sections.[190]

The characteristic histopathologic change is a dense and diffuse lymphohistiocytic infiltrate throughout the dermis with varying numbers of organisms, depending on the stage of the infection and the immunologic status of the host. Eosinophils and neutrophils are rare; and more commonly seen in ulcerated lesion. In routine H&E sections, amastigotes with dull blue-grey, round to oval bodies measuring 2 to 4 μm in diameter are seen in the cytoplasm of the histiocytes (**Figure 12.57**). Typical organisms also show a round basophilic nucleus and a rod-shaped paranuclear kinetoplast, a specialized mitochondrial structure containing extracellular DNA. These intracellular bodies stain red or dark blue with Giemsa stain but not with PAS or GMS stains. They are more abundant in early lesions and in immunocompromised hosts. Extracellular distribution can be present when there are numerous organisms. The number of both organisms and histiocytes tend to gradually decrease as the lesions progress. A granulomatous reaction containing epithelioid cells and multinucleated giant cells often develops with no caseous necrosis (**Figure 12.58**). The epidermal changes are nonspecific and consist of hyperkeratosis, parakeratosis, and epidermal atrophy or hyperplasia.[191–193]

The morphology of intracytoplasmic amastigotes can appear similar to other organisms, such as *Histoplasma capsulatum*,

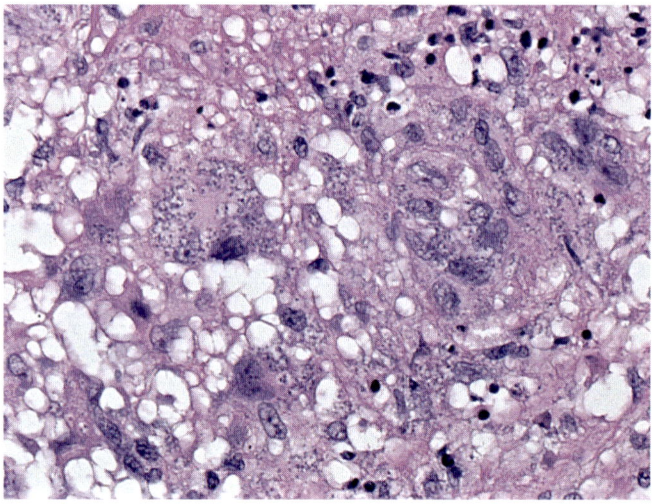

Figure 12.57 Cutaneous Leishmaniasis. Amastigotes with a round basophilic nucleus and a rod-shaped paranuclear kinetoplast (X630).

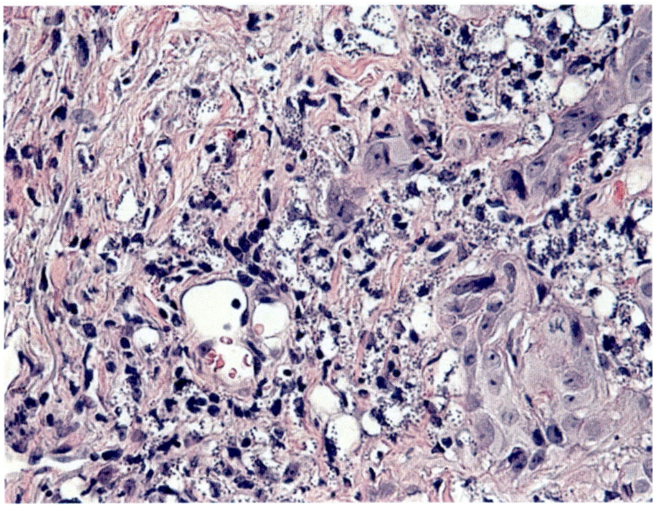

Figure 12.58 Cutaneous Leishmaniasis. A granulomatous reaction containing epithelioid cells and multinucleated giant cells with no caseous necrosis (X200).

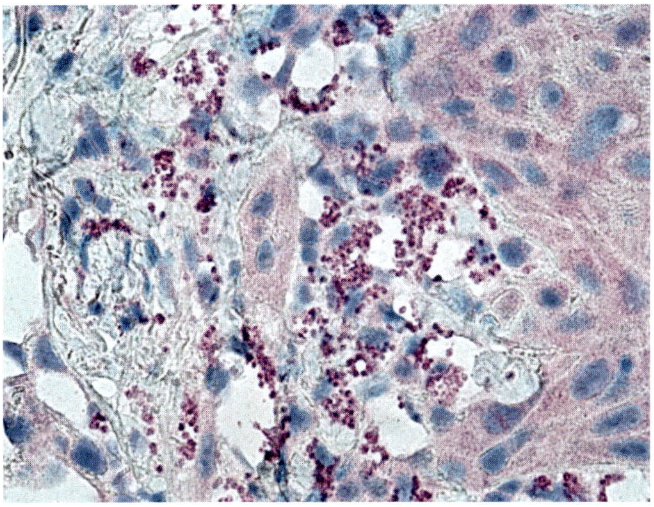

Figure 12.59 Immunostaining of intracellular and extracellular leishmanial antigens (X630).

Toxoplasma gondii, *Trypanosoma cruzi*, *Sarcocystis species*, and *microsporidia*. IHC with specific anti-Leishmania antibodies is a useful assay to highlight Leishmania organisms and antigens in skin biopsies to establish the diagnosis (**Figure 12.59**).[194] Extracellular parasites can be noted in the connective tissue or in capillary lumens.

12.4 Fungus

Fungal diseases affect a considerable number of people worldwide and can cause significant morbidity and mortality. Similar to parasitic infections, the incidence of fungal infections has multiplied with the increase in global travel and immunosuppression. The primary cutaneous fungal infections can be divided into superficial and deep infections according to their nature of the fungus and locations of the lesions they produced. The basic histopathologic pattern of cutaneous fungal infection is relatively uniform because of similar host responses. The degree of inflammatory response varies according to the host immune status. Deep cutaneous fungal infections are clinically more significant because of their detrimental local or systemic consequence. These infections typically demonstrate a mixed dermal inflammatory infiltrate associated with pseudoepitheliomatous hyperplasia and occasionally with dermal fibrosis. Deep cutaneous fungal infections have also been associated with traumatic wound or iatrogenic injection. These rare instances are caused by environmental fungi that penetrate into host tissue due to breakdown of cutaneous barrier. The laboratory diagnosis of fungal infections relies on culture, histopathologic evaluation, and other ancillary tests. Multiple special stains have been used to highlight various fungal organisms. These histochemical stains can be helpful, especially when the overall histologic pattern is suspicious for a fungal infection but fungi are not readily recognizable on routine H&E-stained sections. These special stains include PAS, GMS, Gram, Fontana-Masson, mucicarmine, Alcian blue, India ink, and acid-fast stains. IHC assays, albeit their usefulness in demonstrating fungal antigens in tissues, are unfortunately very limited in clinical practice due to the broad cross-reactivity of those antibodies raised against fungal organisms.[195,196] Currently, only three IHC assays developed at CDC are rather specific for diagnosis of fungal organisms: Aspergillus species, Cryptococcus species, and Mucormycetes. IHC for Aspergillus species is helpful to differentiate them from other fungi with similar morphologic features, such as hyalohyphomycetes. A number of *in situ* hybridization and PCR assays have been developed to provide more specific diagnosis for fungal infections.[197–199]

Aspergillus Species

Aspergillus species are ubiquitous saprophytes found in soil, air, and decaying organic matter. They are the leading cause of opportunistic infection among immunocompromised patients, especially those with leukemia and solid organ or bone marrow transplant recipients. *A. fumigatus* is the most common human pathogen of the genus. They usually present as 2–4 μm septate hyphae with dichotomous branching at 45-degree angle in skin biopsies. Primary infection usually shows granulomatous inflammation, while secondary infection from a systemic source shows angioinvasion, ischemic necrosis, neutrophilic infiltrate, and hemorrhage (**Figures 12.60 and 12.61**).

Cryptococcus Species

Cryptococcus neoformans and C. gattii are present in soil contaminated with bird and bat excreta. Skin manifestation is variable with papules, pustules, nodules, plaques, and cellulitis. *C. neoformans* is one of the most common systemic fungal infections in AIDS patients. *C. gattii* is more commonly seen in immunocompetent patients. The fungi usually present as 5–15 μm spore with wide capsule in gelatinous reaction, or 2–4 μm spore in granulomatous reaction. Gelatinous reaction is commonly seen with many spores, while granulomatous reaction shows fewer spores (**Figures 12.62 and 12.63**).

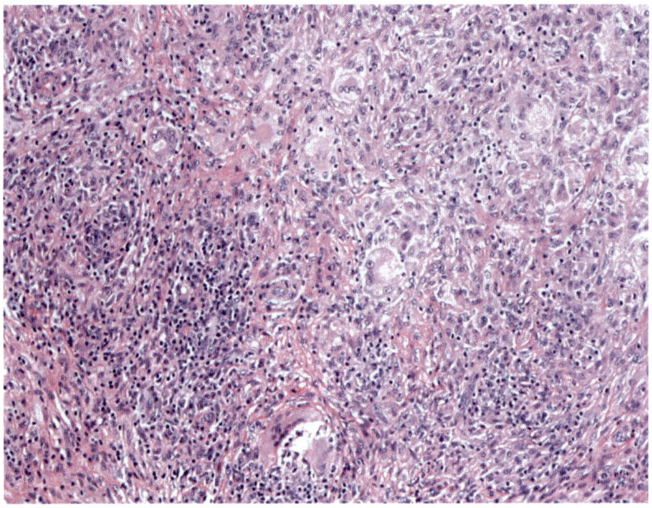

Figure 12.60 Cutaneous aspergillosis. Primary infection with granulomatous inflammation. Fungal hyphae may not be readily visible on routine histologic section (X200).

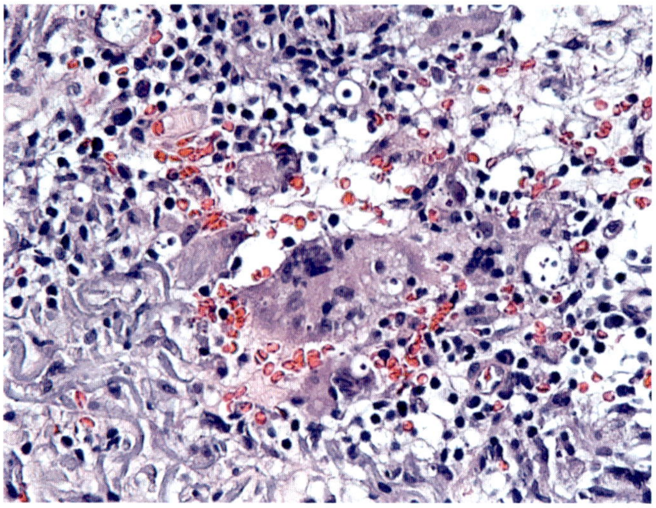

Figure 12.62 Cutaneous cryptococcosis. Granulomatous inflammation in the dermis with scattered yeast-form organisms (X200).

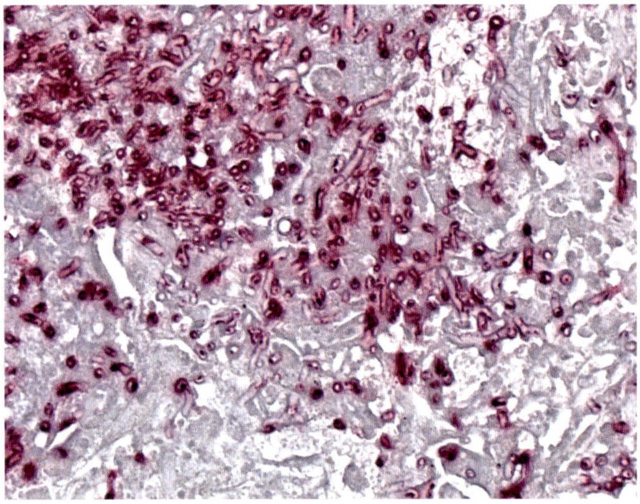

Figure 12.61 Immunostaining of Aspergillus hyphae (X400).

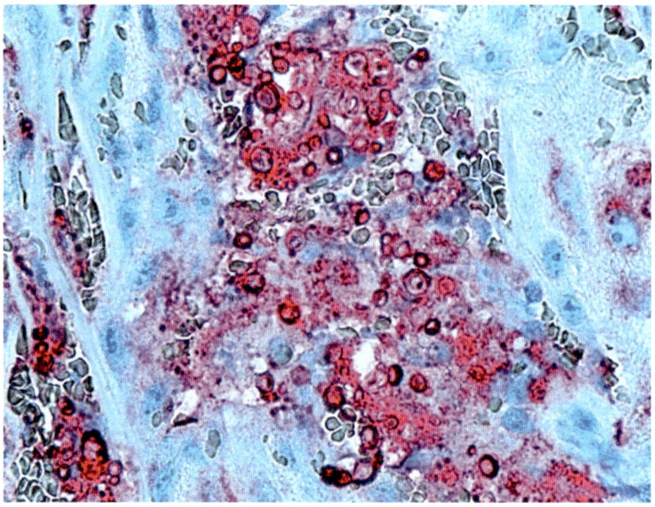

Figure 12.63 Immunostaining of Cryptococcus yeasts and antigens (X630).

Mucormycetes

Similar to Aspergillus species, mucormycetes are also ubiquitous saprophytic organisms found in soil and decomposing organic material. The two major orders of Mucormycetes causing human diseases are:1) Order Mucorales, including *Rhizopus*, *Mucor*, *Absidia*, *Rhizomucor*, *Apophysomyces*, and *Cunninghamella bertholletiae;* 2) Order Entomophthorales, including *Conidiobolus* and *Basidiobolus*. There is a wide spectrum of clinical forms associated with Mucormycetes infection, such as rhinocerebral, pulmonary, GI, cutaneous, and disseminated. The fungi usually present as 8–30 μm hyphae with pauciseptation and branching at haphazardly arranged angles. The wall is variably thin and often collapsed or twisted. Primary infection usually shows granulomatous inflammation, while secondary infection from a systemic source shows angioinvasion with thrombosis, infarction, necrosis, and mild neutrophilic infiltrate (**Figures 12.64 and 12.65**).

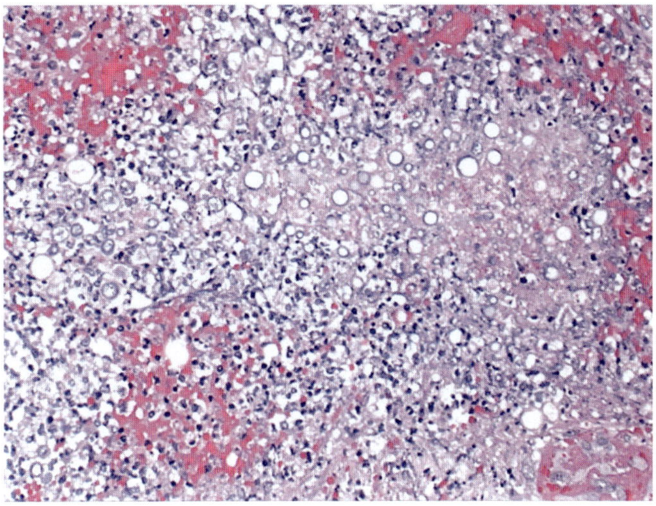

Figure 12.64 Cutaneous mucormycosis. Primary infection with granulomatous inflammation. Fungal hyphae may not be readily visible on routine histologic section (X400).

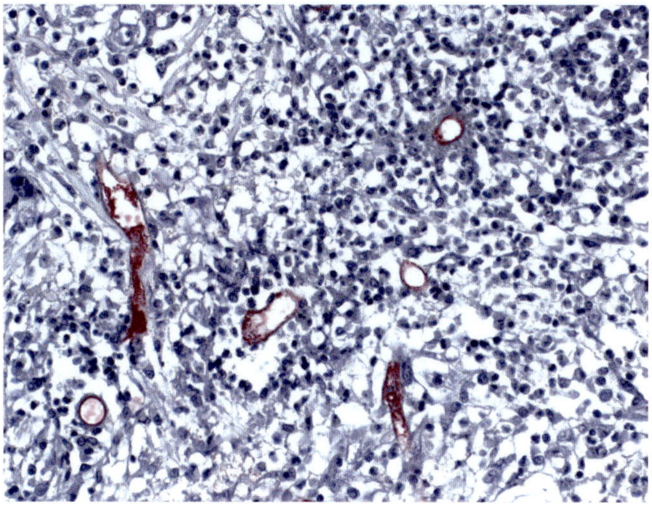

Figure 12.65 Immunostaining of Mucormycetes mixed within inflammation (X400).

12.5 Case Studies

Case 12.1

Case history: A 54-year-old man presented with a 10-day history of an eruption of pink papules some with micaceous scale on his back, chest, abdomen, extremities, and face; fever and myalgia (**Figure 12.66**). The clinical impression was pityriasis lichenoides et varioliformis acuta or Mucha-Habermann disease. A skin biopsy from right forearm was obtained.

Description: Histologic sections of the skin biopsy show a band-like and perivascular infiltrate in the superficial and deep dermis (**Figure 12.67**). The inflammation obscures the dermal epidermal junction and is comprised of lymphocytes, histiocytes and prominent plasma cells (**Figure 12.68**). Many spirochetes were highlighted within the epidermis and superficial dermis by a *T. pallidum* immunostain (**Figure 12.69**).

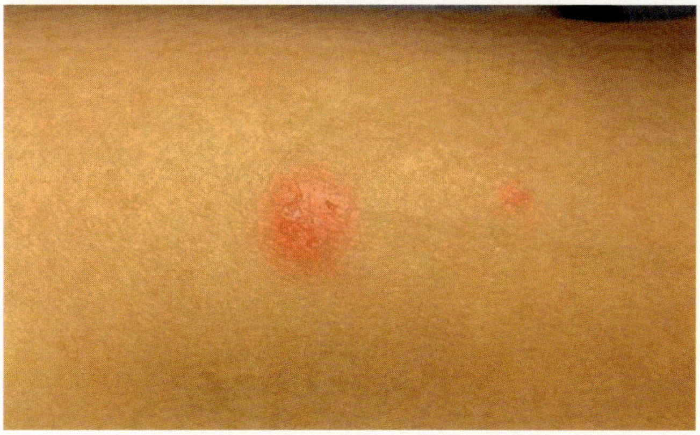

Figure 12.66 Pink papules are noted on the patient's arm (courtesy of Drs. Avery Lachance and Molly Plovanich, Dermatology, Massachusetts General Hospital, Boston, MA).

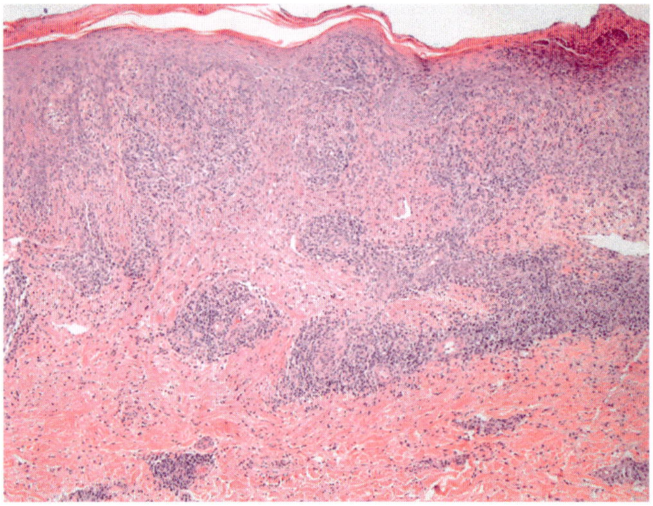

Figure 12.67 A lichenoid and perivascular dermatitis is noted on histologic section (X200).

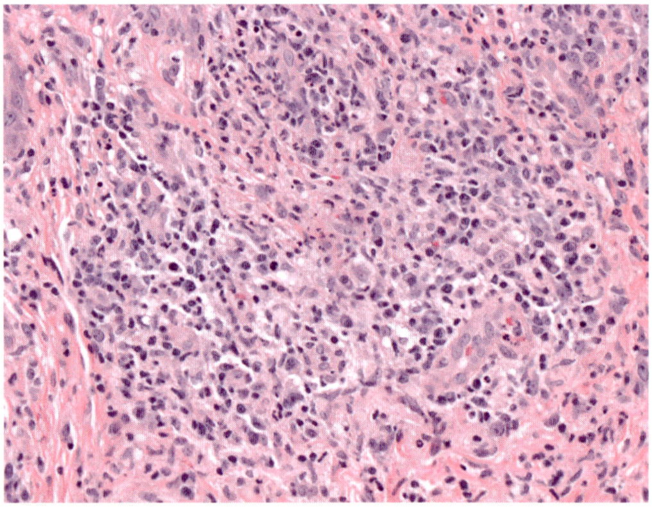

Figure 12.68 Prominent number of plasma cells is seen within the dermal infiltrate (X400).

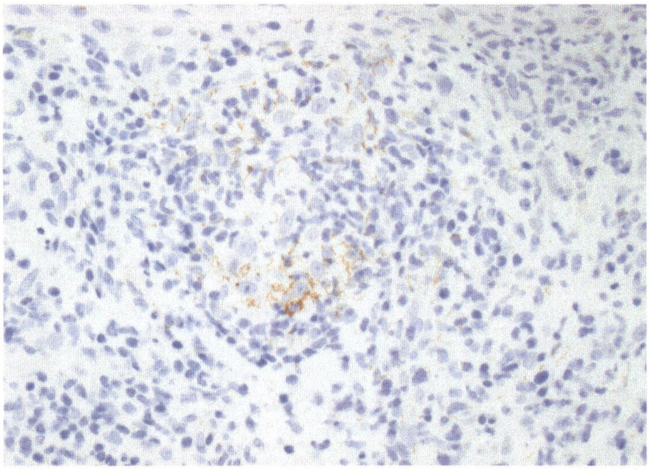

Figure 12.69 *Treponema pallidum* immunostain highlights many spirochetes within the basal aspect of the epidermis and superficial dermis (X400).

Diagnosis: Secondary syphilis.

Discussion: This case illustrates that secondary syphilis can mimic other entities both clinically and histopathologically. The presence of dermal plasma cells at a site that is not genital nor mucosal should raise the suspicion for secondary syphilis. *T. pallidum* immunostain is superior to special stains such Warthin-Starry and Steiner silver stains since the organisms can be readily visualized due to minimal background staining.[79,80]

Case 12.2

Case history: A 60-year-old man presented with a history of fever for three weeks while in Africa and developed skin lesions on his right flank about 1 cm in size with central eschar and surrounding erythema (**Figure 12.70**). A skin biopsy from the skin lesion was obtained.

Description: Histologic sections of the skin biopsy shows focal epidermal and superficial dermal necrosis with neutrophilic infiltration and overlying inflammatory crust. Dense perivascular mononuclear infiltrates are seen throughout the deeper and adjacent dermis (**Figure 12.71**). Variable endothelial hyperplasia, vasculitis, and occasional thrombosis of affected vessels are present (**Figure 12.72**). IHC shows positive immunostaining of spotted fever group rickettsiae (**Figure 12.73**) and PCR was positive for *Rickettsia africae*.

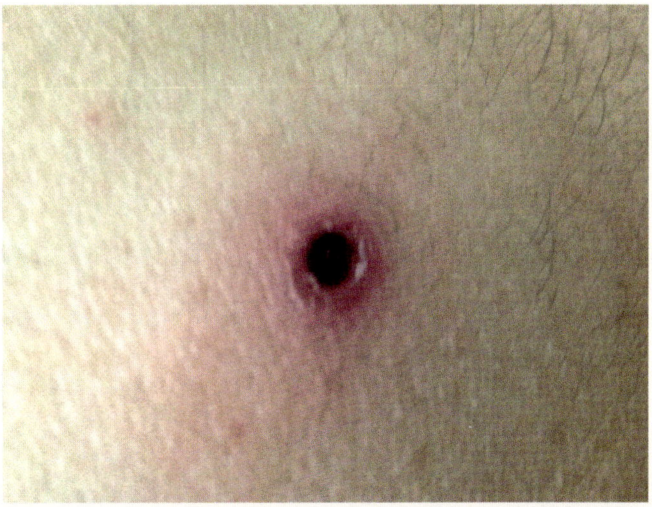

Figure 12.70 Skin lesion with central eschar and surrounding erythema.

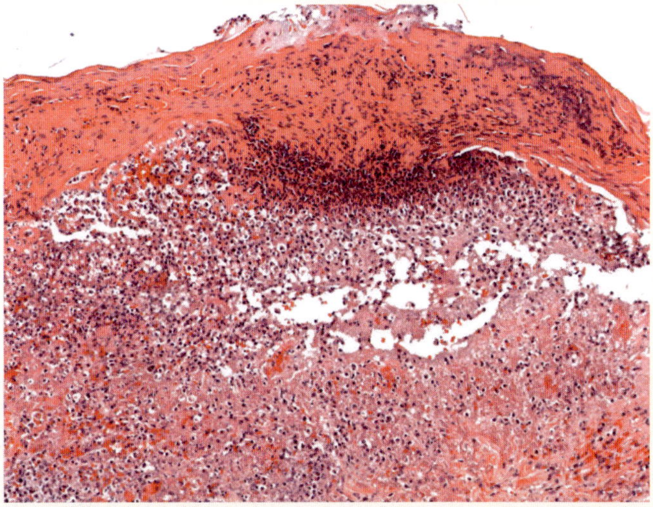

Figure 12.71 Focal epidermal and superficial dermal necrosis with neutrophilic inflammation and overlying serum crust. Dense perivascular mononuclear infiltrates throughout the deeper dermis (X50).

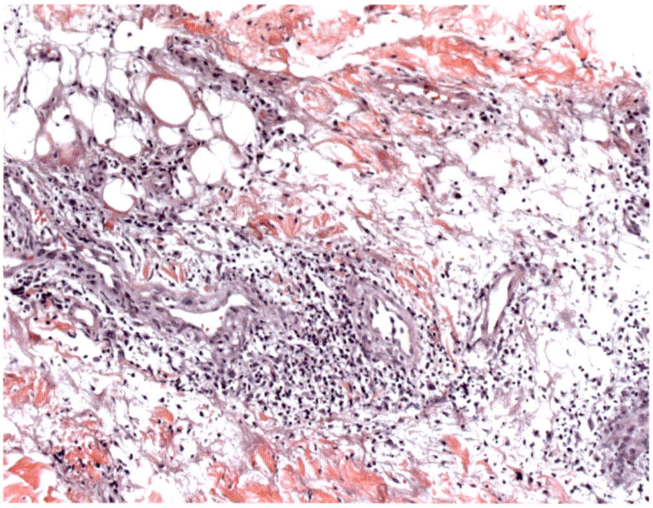

Figure 12.72 Endothelial hyperplasia, vasculitis, and occasional thrombosis of affected vessels (X100).

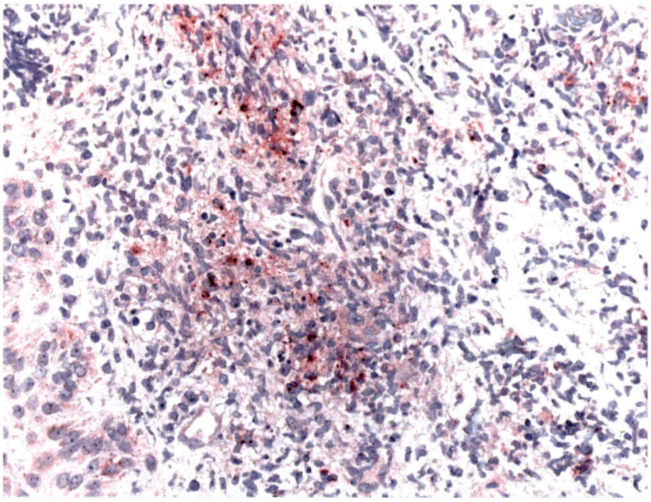

Figure 12.73 Immunostaining of spotted fever group rickettsiae (X200).

Diagnosis: African tick-bite fever.

Discussion: Skin lesions are one of the top medical concerns in travelers returning from tropical regions. Infection is the most common cause of these lesions and usually develops before the travelers return home. Many of these infections are rare in developed countries and a definite diagnosis often needs special testing. This case illustrates such scenario and underscores the importance to keep alert on those travel-associated skin infections. Other skin lesions that can present with eschar include anthrax, impetigo, sporotrichosis, orf, arthropod bites, plague, rickettsialpox, scrub typhus, and tularemia.

Case 12.3

Case history: A 77-year-old woman who had contact with fresh meat from the butcher and developed a solitary nodular lesion with pustular formation on the left third finger (**Figure 12.74**). No other systemic symptoms were reported.

Description: Histologic sections of the skin biopsy show focal necrotic epithelium and extensive amounts of overlying serum crust. Prominent neutrophilic inflammatory infiltrates, hemorrhage, and collections of fibrin are associated with damaged epithelial surface (**Figure 12.75**). Keratinocytes with ballooning degenerative and apoptotic changes are seen (**Figure 12.76**). There are abundant lymphohistiocytic inflammatory infiltrates in the underlying dermis. IHC shows positive immunostaining for parapoxvirus (**Figure 12.77**) and PCR was positive for Orf virus.

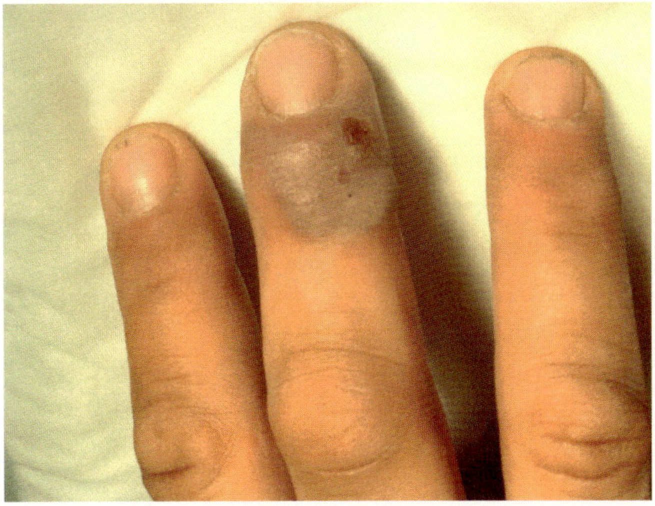

Figure 12.74 A solitary nodular lesion with pustular formation on the left third finger

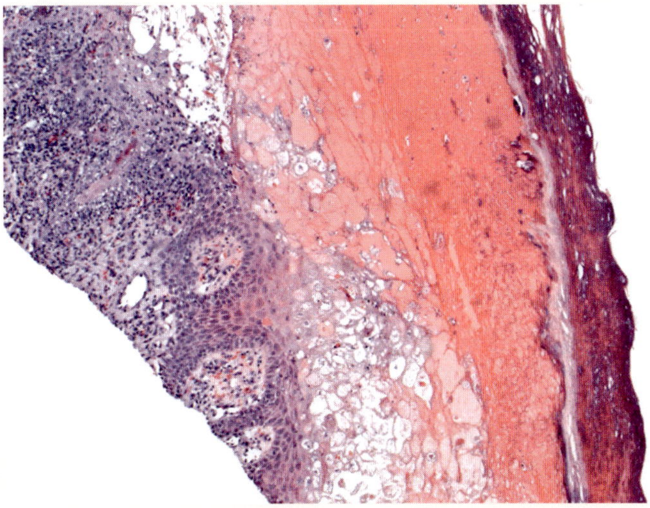

Figure 12.75 Prominent neutrophilic inflammatory infiltrates, hemorrhage, and collections of fibrin with damaged epithelial surface (X100).

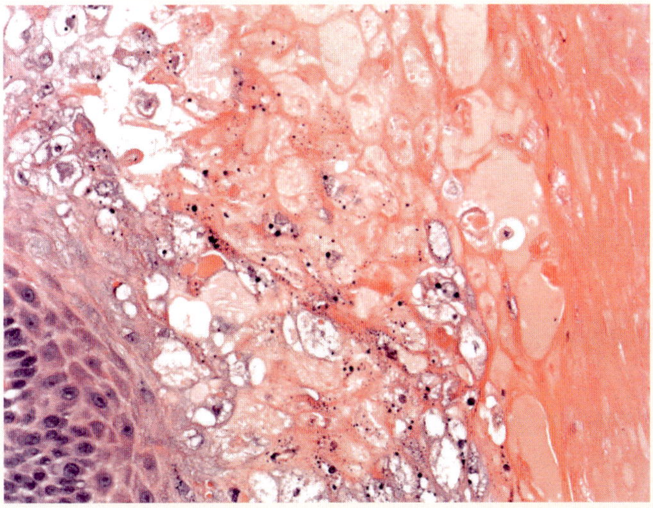

Figure 12.76 Keratinocytes with ballooning degenerative and apoptotic changes (X400).

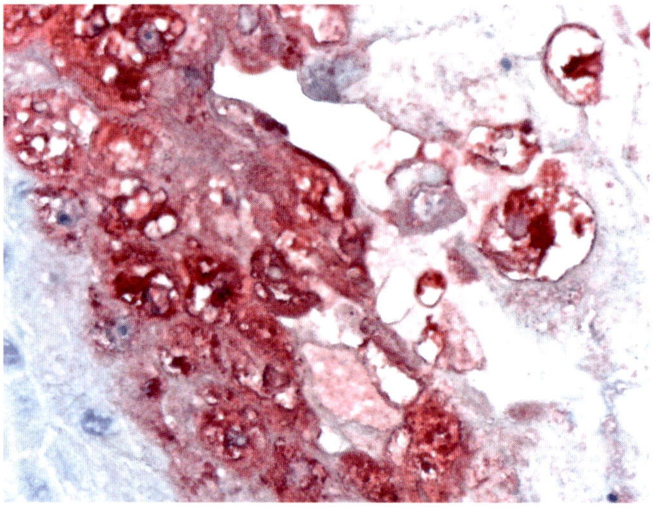

Figure 12.77 Immunostaining of parapoxvirus (X400).

Diagnosis: Orf.

Discussion: Emerging zoonotic infectious diseases are common causes for public health alert and concern. With the magnitude of complexity, the challenge of zoonoses has become a formidable task for healthcare professionals working in different subspecialties, including dermatologists and dermatopathologists. This case illustrates the importance of increasing awareness and utilization of modern diagnostic capability to deal with the challenge of these emerging infections.

Case 12.4

Case history: A 55-year-old woman with a history of acute myelogenous leukemia presented with acute onset violaceous plaques on her right upper thigh. A skin biopsy was performed.

Description: Histologic sections show acute inflammation with abscess formation and necrosis in the deep dermis and subcutaneous tissue, respectively (**Figures 12.78 and 12.79**). GMS stain (**Figure 12.80**) and Aspergillus immunostain (**Figure 12.81**) highlight the fungal forms within the subcutaneous necrotic area.

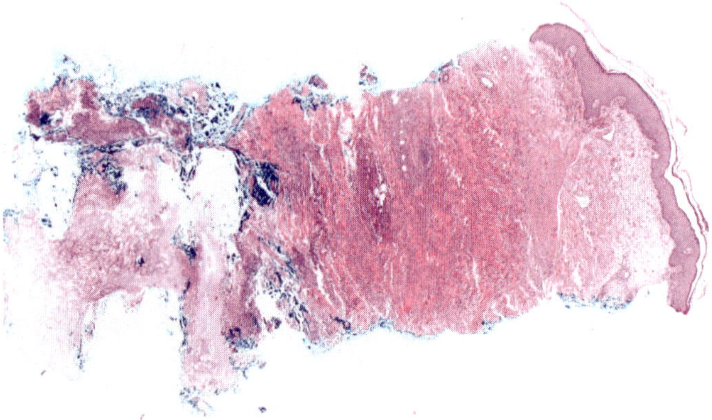

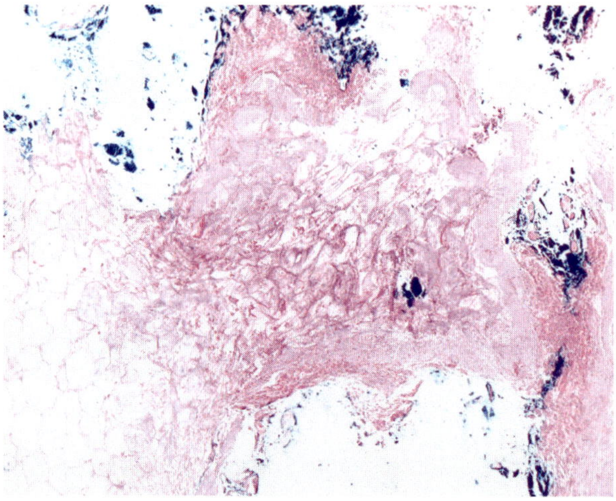

Figures 12.78 and 12.79 Acute inflammation with abscess formation and necrosis in the deep dermis and subcutaneous tissue, respectively (X20, X100).

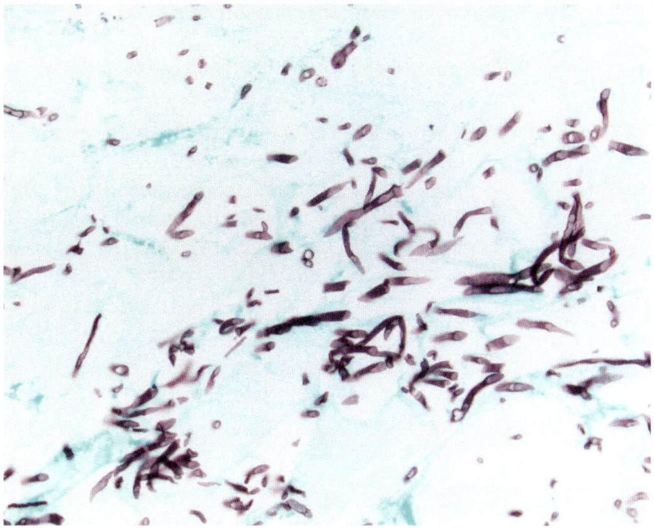

Figure 12.80 Septate fungal hyphae are seen on GMS stain (X600).

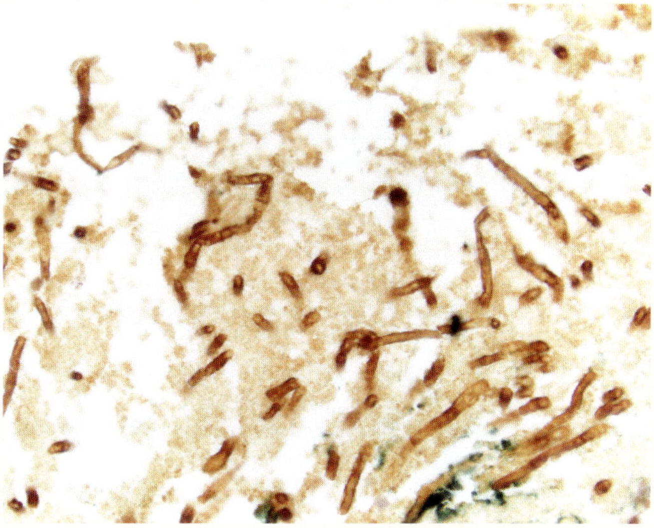

Figure 12.81 Aspergillus immunostain is positive (X600).

Diagnosis: Aspergillosis.

Discussion: Primary cutaneous Aspergillosis usually occurs in immunocompromised patients, although it can be seen in immunocompetent individuals. Angioinvasive fungal infections pose high risk for severe morbidity and high mortality, therefore prompt therapy is of clinical importance. On histologic sections, it is difficult to identify the fungal forms and the fungal cultures require some time for growth. This case illustrates that Aspergillus immunostain can facilitate a timely diagnosis.

References

1. Godyn JJ, Siderits R, Dzaman J. Cutaneous anthrax. *Arch Pathol Lab Med* 2004; **128**: 709–10.
2. Shieh W-J, Guarner J, Paddock C, et al. The critical role of pathology in the investigation of bioterrorism-related cutaneous anthrax. *Am J Pathol* 2003; **163**: 1901–10.
3. Quinn C, Dull P, Semenova V, et al. Immune responses to *Bacillus anthracis* protective antigen in patients with bioterrorism-related cutaneous or inhalation anthrax. *J Infect Dis* 2004; **190**: 1228–36.
4. Dauphin LA, Marston CK, Bhullar V, et al. Swab protocol for rapid laboratory diagnosis of cutaneous anthrax. *J Clin Microbiol* 2012; **50**: 3960–7.
5. Tatti KM, Greer P, White E, et al. Morphologic, immunologic, and molecular methods to detect bacillus anthracis in formalin-fixed tissues. *Appl Immunohistochem Mol Morphol* 2006; **14**: 234–43.
6. Murakawa GJ. American Academy of Dermatology 1997 awards for young investigators in Dermatology: pathogenesis of Bartonella henselae in

cutaneous and systemic disease. *J Am Acad Dermatol* 1997; **37**: 775–6.

7. Pierard-Franchimont C, Quatresooz P, Pierard GE. Skin diseases associated with Bartonella infection: facts and controversies. *Clin Dermatol* 2010; **28**: 483–8.
8. Maass M, Schreiber M, Knobloch J. Detection of Bartonella bacilliformis in cultures, blood, and formalin preserved skin biopsies by use of the polymerase chain reaction. *Trop Med Parasitol* 1992; **43**: 191–4.
9. Hansmann Y, DeMartino S, Piemont Y, et al. Diagnosis of cat scratch disease with detection of Bartonella henselae by PCR: a study of patients with lymph node enlargement. *J Clin Microbiol* 2005; **43**: 3800–6.
10. Czarnetzki BM, Pomeranz JR, Khandekar PK, Wolinsky E, Belcher RW. Cat-scratch disease skin test: studies of specificity and histopathologic features. *Arch Dermatol* 1975; **111**: 736–9.
11. Brazier JS, Duerden BI, Hall V, et al. Isolation and identification of Clostridium spp. from infections associated with the injection of drugs: experiences of a microbiological investigation team. *J Med Microbiol* 2002; **51**: 985–9.
12. Bhatnagar J, Deleon-Carnes M, Kellar KL, et al. Rapid, simultaneous detection of Clostridium sordellii and Clostridium perfringens in archived tissues by a novel PCR-based microsphere assay: diagnostic implications for pregnancy-associated toxic shock syndrome cases. Infect Dis Obstet Gynecol 2012; **2012**: 972845. doi: 10.1155/2012/972845.
13. Tsokos M, Schalinski S, Paulsen F, Sperhake JP, Püschel K, Sobottka I. Pathology of fatal traumatic and nontraumatic clostridial gas gangrene: a histopathological, immunohistochemical, and ultrastructural study of six autopsy cases. *Int J Legal Med* 2008; **122**: 35–41.
14. Guarner J, Bartlett J, Reagan S, et al. Immunohistochemical evidence of Clostridium sp, Staphylococcus aureus, and group A Streptococcus in severe soft tissue infections related to injection drug use. *Hum Pathol* 2006; **37**: 1482–8.
15. Eliasson H, Broman T, Forsman M, Bäck E. Tularemia: current epidemiology and disease management. *Infect Dis Clin North Am* 2006; **20**: 289–311.
16. Syrjala H, Karvonen J, Salminen A. Skin manifestations of tularemia: a study of 88 cases in northern Finland during 16 years (1967–1983). *Acta Derm Venereol* 1984; **64**: 513–16.
17. Splettstoesser WD, Tomaso H, Dahouk Al S, Neubauer H, Schuff-Werner P. Diagnostic procedures in tularaemia with special focus on molecular and immunological techniques. *J Vet Med B Infect Dis Vet Public Health* 2005; **52**: 249–61.
18. Byington CL, Bender JM, Ampofo K, et al. Tularemia with vesicular skin lesions may be mistaken for infection with herpes viruses. *Clin Infect Dis* 2008; **47**: e4–6. doi: 10.1086/588843.
19. Asano S, Mori K, Yamazaki K, et al. Temporal differences of onset between primary skin lesions and regional lymph node lesions for tularemia in Japan: a clinicopathologic and immunohistochemical study of 19 skin cases and 54 lymph node cases. *Virchows Arch* 2012; **460**: 651–8.
20. Degitz K. Detection of mycobacterial DNA in the skin: etiologic insights and diagnostic perspectives. *Arch Dermatol* 1996; **132**: 71–5.
21. Beyt BEJ, Ortbals DW, Santa Cruz DJ, Kobayashi GS, Eisen AZ, Medoff G. Cutaneous mycobacteriosis: analysis of 34 cases with a new classification of the disease. *Medicine* 1981; **60**: 95–109.
22. Farina MC, Gegundez MI, Pique E, et al. Cutaneous tuberculosis: a clinical, histopathologic, and bacteriologic study. *J Am Acad Dermatol* 1995; **33**: 433–40.
23. Jordaan HF, Van Niekerk DJ, Louw M. Papulonecrotic tuberculid: a clinical, histopathological, and immunohistochemical study of 15 patients. *Am J Dermatopathol* 1994; **16**: 474–85.
24. Min K-W, Ko JY, Park CK. Histopathological spectrum of cutaneous tuberculosis and non-tuberculous mycobacterial infections. *J Cutan Pathol* 2012; **39**: 582–95.
25. Dodiuk-Gad R, Dyachenko P, Ziv M, et al. Nontuberculous mycobacterial infections of the skin: a retrospective study of 25 cases. *J Am Acad Dermatol* 2007; **57**: 413–20.
26. Sia TY, Taimur S, Blau DM, et al. Clinical and pathological evaluation of mycobacterium marinum group skin infections associated with fish markets in New York City. *Clin Infect Dis* 2016; **62**: 590–5.
27. Mahaisavariya P, Chaiprasert A, Khemngern S, et al. Nontuberculous mycobacterial skin infections: clinical and bacteriological studies. *J Med Assoc Thai* 2003; **86**: 52–60.
28. Lee WJ, Kang SM, Sung H, et al. Non-tuberculous mycobacterial infections of the skin: a retrospective study of 29 cases. *J Dermatol* 2010; **37**: 965–72.
29. Cook SM, Bartos RE, Pierson CL, Frank TS. Detection and characterization of atypical mycobacteria by the polymerase chain reaction. *Diagn Mol Pathol* 1994; **3**: 53–8.
30. Mahaisavariya P, Manonukul J, Khemngern S, Chaiprasert A. Mycobacterial skin infections: comparison between histopathologic features and detection of acid fast bacilli in pathologic section. *J Med Assoc Thai* 2004; **87**: 709–12.
31. Noordeen SK. Eliminating leprosy as a public health problem; why the optimism is justified. *Int J Lepr Other Mycobact Dis* 1995; **63**: 559–66.
32. Declercq E. Guide to eliminating leprosy as a public health problem. Lepr Rev 2001; **72**: 106–7.
33. Ridley DS, Jopling WH. Classification of leprosy according to immunity: a five-group system. *Int J Lepr Other Mycobact Dis* 1966; **34**: 255–73.
34. Skinsnes OK. Immuno-pathology of leprosy: the century in review. Pathology, pathogenesis, and the development of classification. *Int J Lepr Other Mycobact Dis* 1973; **41**: 329–60.
35. Ridley DS. Histological classification and the immunological spectrum of leprosy. *Bull World Health Organ* 1974; **51**: 451–65.
36. Fine PE, Job CK, Lucas SB, et al. Extent, origin, and implications of observer variation in the histopathological diagnosis of suspected leprosy. *Int J Lepr Other Mycobact Dis* 1993; **61**: 270–82.
37. Fleury RN, Bacchi CE. S-100 protein and immunoperoxidase technique as an aid in the histopathologic diagnosis of leprosy. *Int J Lepr Other Mycobact Dis* 1987; **55**: 338–44.
38. de Wit MY, Faber WR, Krieg SR, et al. Application of a polymerase chain reaction for the detection of Mycobacterium leprae in skin tissues. *J Clin Microbiol* 1991; **29**: 906–10.

39. Nishimura M, Kwon KS, Shibuta K, et al. Methods in pathology: an improved method for DNA diagnosis of leprosy using formaldehyde-fixed, paraffin-embedded skin biopsies. *Mod Pathol* 1994; **7**: 253–6.

40. van Deuren M, Brandtzaeg P, van der Meer JW. Update on meningococcal disease with emphasis on pathogenesis and clinical management. *Clin Microbiol Rev* 2000; **13**: 144–66.

41. Stephens DS, Greenwood B, Brandtzaeg P. Epidemic meningitis, meningococcaemia, and Neisseria meningitides. *Lancet* 2007; **369**: 2196–210.

42. Guarner J, Greer PW, Whitney A, et al. Pathogenesis and diagnosis of human meningococcal disease using immunohistochemical and PCR assays. *Am J Clin Pathol* 2004; **122**: 754–64.

43. Arend SM, Lavrijsen AP, Kuijken I, van der Plas RN, Kuijper EJ. Prospective controlled study of the diagnostic value of skin biopsy in patients with presumed meningococcal disease. *Eur J Clin Microbiol Infect Dis* 2006; **25**: 643–9.

44. O'Brien JP, Goldenberg DL, Rice PA. Disseminated gonococcal infection: a prospective analysis of 49 patients and a review of pathophysiology and immune mechanisms. *Medicine* 1983; **62**: 395–406.

45. Jain S, Win HN, Chalam V, Yee L. Disseminated gonococcal infection presenting as vasculitis: a case report. *J Clin Pathol* 2007; **60**: 90–1.

46. Walker DH. Rocky Mountain spotted fever: a seasonal alert. *Clin Infect Dis* 1995; **20**: 1111–17.

47. Chapman AS, Murphy SM, Demma LJ, et al. Rocky Mountain spotted fever in the United States, 1997–2002. *Vector Borne Zoonotic Dis* 2006; **6**: 170–8.

48. Paddock CD, Finley RW, Wright CS, et al. Rickettsia parkeri rickettsiosis and its clinical distinction from Rocky Mountain spotted fever. *Clin Infect Dis* 2008; **47**: 1188–96.

49. Koss T, Carter EL, Grossman ME, et al. Increased detection of rickettsialpox in a New York City hospital following the anthrax outbreak of 2001: use of immunohistochemistry for the rapid confirmation of cases in an era of bioterrorism. *Arch Dermatol* 2003; **139**: 1545–52.

50. Sexton DJ, Kaye KS. Rocky mountain spotted fever. *Med Clin North Am* 2002; **86**: 351–60.

51. Sexton DJ, Corey GR. Rocky Mountain "spotless" and "almost spotless" fever: a wolf in sheep's clothing. *Clin Infect Dis* 1992; **15**: 439–48.

52. Dumler JS, Walker DH. Diagnostic tests for Rocky Mountain spotted fever and other rickettsial diseases. *Dermatol Clin* 1994; **12**: 25–36.

53. Walker DH, Herrero-Herrero JI, Ruiz-Beltran R, Bullon-Sopelana A, Ramos-Hidalgo A. The pathology of fatal Mediterranean spotted fever. *Am J Clin Pathol* 1987; **87**: 669–72.

54. Kao GF, Evancho CD, Ioffe O, Lowitt MH, Dumler JS. Cutaneous histopathology of Rocky Mountain spotted fever. *J Cutan Pathol* 1997; **24**: 604–10.

55. Vyas NS, Shieh WJ, Phelps RG. Investigating the histopathological findings and immunolocalization of rickettsialpox infection in skin biopsies: a case series and review of the literature. *J Cutan Pathol* 2020; **47**: 451–8.

56. Paddock CD, Greer PW, Ferebee TL, et al. Hidden mortality attributable to Rocky Mountain spotted fever: immunohistochemical detection of fatal, serologically unconfirmed disease. *J Infect Dis* 1999; **179**: 1469–76.

57. Seong SY, Choi MS, Kim IS. Orientia tsutsugamushi infection: overview and immune responses. *Microbes Infect* 2001; **3**: 11–21.

58. Kim D-M, Won KJ, Park CY, et al. Distribution of eschars on the body of scrub typhus patients: a prospective study. *Am J Trop Med Hyg* 2007; **76**: 806–9.

59. Lee J-H, Lee J-H, Chung KM, et al. Dynamics of clinical symptoms in patients with scrub typhus. *Jpn J Infect Dis* 2013; **66**: 155–7.

60. Koraluru M, Bairy I, Varma M, Vidyasagar S. Diagnostic validation of selected serological tests for detecting scrub typhus. *Microbiol Immunol* 2015; **59**: 371–4.

61. Kim CM, Cho MK, Kim DM, et al. Accuracy of conventional PCR targeting the 16S rRNA gene with the Ot-16sRF1 and Ot-16sRR1 primers for diagnosis of scrub typhus: a case-control study. *J Clin Microbiol* 2016; **54**: 178–9.

62. Park JH, Hart MS. The pathology of scrub typhus. *Am J Clin Pathol* 1946; **16**: 139–49.

63. Kim D-M, Lim S-C, Won KJ, Choi Y-J, Park K-H, Jang W-J. Severe scrub typhus confirmed early via immunohistochemical staining. *Am J Trop Med Hyg* 2007; **77**: 719–22.

64. Brouwer S, Rivera-Hernandez T, Curren BF, et al. Pathogenesis, epidemiology and control of Group A Streptococcus infection. Nat Rev Microbiol 2023; **21**: 431–47.

65. Nelson GE, Pondo T, Toews K-A, et al. Epidemiology of invasive group A streptococcal infections in the United States, 2005–2012. *Clin Infect Dis* 2016; **63**: 478–86.

66. Hoge CW, Schwartz B, Talkington DF, Breiman RF, MacNeill EM, Englender SJ. The changing epidemiology of invasive group A streptococcal infections and the emergence of streptococcal toxic shock-like syndrome: a retrospective population-based study. *JAMA* 1993; **269**: 384–9.

67. Low DE, McGeer A. Skin and soft tissue infection: necrotizing fasciitis. *Curr Opin Infect Dis* 1998; **11**: 119–23.

68. Parks T, Smeesters PR, Steer AC. Streptococcal skin infection and rheumatic heart disease. *Curr Opin Infect Dis* 2012; **25**: 145–53.

69. Shulman ST, Bisno AL, Clegg HW, et al. Clinical practice guideline for the diagnosis and management of group a streptococcal pharyngitis: 2012 update by the Infectious Diseases Society of America. *Clin Infect Dis* 2012; **55**: e86–e102.

70. Cohen JF, Chalumeau M, Levy C, et al. Effect of clinical spectrum, inoculum size and physician characteristics on sensitivity of a rapid antigen detection test for group A streptococcal pharyngitis. *Eur J Clin Microbiol Infect Dis* 2013; **32**: 787–93.

71. Hartman-Adams H, Banvard C, Juckett G. Impetigo: diagnosis and treatment. *Am Fam Physician* 2014; **90**: 229–35.

72. Guarner J, Sumner J, Paddock CD, et al. Diagnosis of invasive group a streptococcal infections by using immunohistochemical and molecular assays. *Am J Clin Pathol* 2006; **126**: 148–55.

73. Cohen PR. Community-acquired methicillin-resistant Staphylococcus aureus skin infections: implications for patients and practitioners. *Am J Clin Dermatol* 2007; **8**: 259–70.

74. Lyell A. The staphylococcal scalded skin syndrome in historical perspective: emergence of dermopathic strains of Staphylococcus aureus and discovery of the epidermolytic toxin. A review of events up to 1970. *J Am Acad Dermatol* 1983; **9**: 285–94.

75. Rieger-Fackeldey E, Plano LRW, Kramer A, Schulze A. Staphylococcal scalded skin syndrome related to an exfoliative toxin A- and B-producing strain in preterm infants. *Eur J Pediatr* 2002; **161**: 649–52.
76. Ladhani S. Understanding the mechanism of action of the exfoliative toxin of *Staphylococcus aureus*. *FEMS Immunol Med Microbiol* 2003; **39**: 181–9.
77. Singh G. Pathogenesis of staphylococcal infections of the skin. *Int J Dermatol* 1975; **14**(10): 755–60.
78. Peeling RW, Hook EW. The pathogenesis of syphilis: the Great Mimicker, revisited. *J Pathol* 2006; **208**: 224–32.
79. Ciccarese G, Facciorusso A, Mastrolonardo M, Herzum A, Parodi A, Drago F. Atypical manifestations of syphilis: a 10-year retrospective study. *J Clin Med* 2024; **13**: 1603. doi10.3390/jcm13061603.
80. Stone CJ, Nicholson L, Florell SR, Khalighi MA, Lewis BKH. A case of secondary syphilis presenting like pemphigus with positive direct immunofluorescence. *JAAD Case Rep* 2023; **42**: 38–41.
81. Hoang MP, High WA, Molberg KH. Secondary syphilis: a histologic and immunohistochemical evaluation. *J Cutan Pathol* 2004; **31**: 595–9.
82. Martin-Ezquerra G, Fernandez-Casado A, Barco D, et al. Treponema pallidum distribution patterns in mucocutaneous lesions of primary and secondary syphilis: an immunohistochemical and ultrastructural study. *Hum Pathol* 2009; **40**: 624–30.
83. Buffet M, Grange PA, Gerhardt P, et al. Diagnosing Treponema pallidum in secondary syphilis by PCR and immunohistochemistry. *J Invest Dermatol* 2007; **127**: 2345–50.
84. Stenseth NC, Atshabar BB, Begon M, et al. Plague: past, present, and future. *PLoS Med* 2008; **5**: e3. doi: 10.1371/journal.pmed.0050003.
85. Perry RD, Fetherston JD. *Yersinia pestis*: etiologic agent of plague. *Clin Microbiol Rev* 1997; **10**: 35–66.
86. Butler T, Hudson BW. The serological response to *Yersinia pestis* infection. *Bull World Health Organ* 1977; **55**: 39–42.
87. Radnedge L, Gamez-Chin S, McCready PM, et al. Identification of nucleotide sequences for the specific and rapid detection of *Yersinia pestis*. *Appl Environ Microbiol* 2001; **67**: 3759–62.
88. Guarner J, Shieh W-J, Greer PW, et al. Immunohistochemical detection of Yersinia pestis in formalin-fixed, paraffin-embedded tissue. *Am J Clin Pathol* 2002; **117**: 205–9.
89. st NR, Bell EJ, Assad F. Enteroviruses in human disease. *Prog Med Virol* 1978; **24**: 114–57.
90. Strikas RA, Anderson LJ, Parker RA. Temporal and geographic patterns of isolates of nonpolio enteroviruses in the United States. *J Infect Dis* 1986; **153**: 346–51.
91 Ooi MH, Wong SC, Lewthwaite P, Cardosa MJ, Solomon T. Clinical features, diagnosis, and management of enterovirus 71. *Lancet Neurol* 2010; **9**: 1097–105.
92. Aswathyraj S, Arunkumar G, Alidjinou EK, Hober D. Hand, foot and mouth disease (HFMD): emerging epidemiology and the need for a vaccine strategy. *Med Microbiol Immunol* 2016; **205**: 397–407.
93. Starkey SY, Mar K, Khaslavsky S, et al. Atypical cutaneous findings of hand-foot-mouth disease in children: a systematic review. *Pediatr Dermatol* 2024; **41**: 23–7.
94. Bubba L, Pellegrinelli L, Pariani E, Primache V, Amendola A, Binda S. A novel multiplex one-step real-time RT-PCR assay for the simultaneous identification of enterovirus and parechovirus in clinical fecal samples. *J Prev Med Hyg* 2015; **56**: E57–60.
95. Shieh WJ, Jung SM, Hsueh C, et al. Pathologic studies of fatal cases in outbreak of hand, foot, and mouth disease, Taiwan. *Emerg Infect Dis* 2001; 7: 146–8.
96. Guerrant RL, Walker DH, Weller PF. *Tropical Infectious Diseases: Principles, Pathogens and Practice*. Elsevier Health Sciences, Oxford, 2011.
97. Singh SK, Ruzek D. *Viral Hemorrhagic Fevers*. CRC Press, Boca Raton, 2013.
98. Zaki SR, Shieh WJ, Greer PW, et al. A novel immunohistochemical assay for the detection of Ebola virus in skin: implications for diagnosis, spread, and surveillance of Ebola hemorrhagic fever. Commission de Lutte contre les Epidémies à Kikwit. *J Infect Dis* 1999; **179**: S36–47.
99. Shieh WJ, Demby A, Jones T, et al. Pathology and pathogenesis of Lassa fever: novel immunohistochemical findings in fatal cases and clinico-pathologic correlation. *Clin Infect Dis* 2022; **74**: 1821–30.
100. Saadiah S, Sharifah BI, Robson A, Greaves MW. Skin histopathology and immunopathology are not of prognostic value in dengue haemorrhagic fever. *Br J Dermatol* 2008; **158**: 836–7.
101. Bernstein DI, Bellamy AR, Hook EW, et al. Epidemiology, clinical presentation, and antibody response to primary infection with herpes simplex virus type 1 and type 2 in young women. *Clin Infect Dis* 2013; **56**: 344–51.
102. Bouthry E, Portet-Sulla V, Bouokazi MM, et al. Neonatal herpes: case series in two obstetric centres over a 10-year period (2013–2023), France. *Eur J Pediatr* 2024; **183**: 3183–3191.
103. Benedetti J, Corey L, Ashley R. Recurrence rates in genital herpes after symptomatic first-episode infection. *Ann Intern Med* 1994; **121**: 847–54.
104. Leinweber B, Kerl H, Cerroni L. Histopathologic features of cutaneous herpes virus infections (herpes simplex, herpes varicella/zoster): a broad spectrum of presentations with common pseudolymphomatous aspects. *Am J Surg Pathol* 2006; **30**: 50–8.
105. Hoyt B, Bhawan J. Histological spectrum of cutaneous herpes infections. *Am J Dermatopathol* 2014; **36**: 609–19.
106. Weinberg JM. Herpes zoster: epidemiology, natural history, and common complications. *J Am Acad Dermatol* 2007; **57**: S130–5.
107. Oxman MN, Levin MJ, Johnson GR, et al, Shingles Prevention Study Group. A vaccine to prevent herpes zoster and postherpetic neuralgia in older adults. *N Engl J Med* 2005; **352**: 2271–84.
108. el Hayderi L, Bontems S, Nikkels-Tassoudji N, et al. Satellite lesions accompanying herpes zoster: a new prognostic sign for high-risk zoster. *Br J Dermatol* 2015; **172**: 1530–4.
109. Wilson DA, Yen-Lieberman B, Schindler S, Asamoto K, Schold JD, Procop GW. Should varicella-zoster virus culture be eliminated? A comparison of direct immunofluorescence antigen detection, culture, and PCR, with a historical review. *J Clin Microbiol* 2012; **50**: 4120–2.
110. Boer A, Herder N, Winter K, Falk T. Herpes folliculitis: clinical,

histopathological, and molecular pathologic observations. *Br J Dermatol* 2006; **154**: 743–6.

111. Muraki R, Baba T, Iwasaki T, Sata T, Kurata T. Immunohistochemical study of skin lesions in herpes zoster. *Virchows Arch A Pathol Anat Histopathol* 1992; **420**: 71–6.

112. Horie C, Mizukawa Y, Yamazaki Y, Shiohara T. Varicella-zoster virus antigen expression of eccrine gland and duct epithelium in herpes zoster lesions. *Br J Dermatol* 2011; **165**: 802–7.

113. Pisapia DJ, Lavi E. VZV, temporal arteritis, and clinical practice: false positive immunohistochemical detection due to antibody cross-reactivity. *Exp Mol Pathol* 2016; **100**: 114–15.

114. Fernandez Flores A. Epstein-Barr virus in cutaneous pathology. *Am J Dermatopathol* 2013; **35**: 763–86.

115. Tan HH, Goh CL. Viral infections affecting the skin in organ transplant recipients: epidemiology and current management strategies. *Am J Clin Dermatol* 2006; **7**: 13–29.

116. Chisholm C, Lopez L. Cutaneous infections caused by Herpesviridae: a review. *Arch Pathol Lab Med* 2011; **135**: 1357–62.

117. Hennard C, Pfuhl T, Buettner M, et al. The antibody 2B4 directed against the Epstein-Barr virus (EBV)-encoded nuclear antigen 1 (EBNA1) detects MAGE-4: applications for studies on the EBV association of human cancers. *J Pathol* 2006; **209**: 430–5.

118. Kempf W, Flaig MJ, Kutzner H. Molecular diagnostics in infectious skin diseases. *J Dtsch Dermatol Ges* 2013; **11**: 50–8.

119. Aravinth SP, Rajendran S, Li Y, et al. Epstein-Barr virus-encoded LMP1 induces ectopic CD137 expression on Hodgkin and Reed-Sternberg cells via the PI3 K-AKT-mTOR pathway. *Leuk Lymphoma* 2019; **60**: 2697–704.

120. Drago F, Aragone MG, Lugani C, Rebora A. Cytomegalovirus infection in normal and immunocompromised humans. A review. *Dermatology* 2000; **200**: 189–95.

121. Fine JD, Arndt KA. The TORCH syndrome: a clinical review. *J Am Acad Dermatol* 1985; **12**: 697–706.

122. Pariser RJ. Histologically specific skin lesions in disseminated cytomegalovirus infection. *J Am Acad Dermatol* 1983; **9**: 937–46.

123. Resnik KS, DiLeonardo M, Maillet M. Histopathologic findings in cutaneous cytomegalovirus infection. *Am J Dermatopathol* 2000; **22**: 397–407.

124. Choi YL, Kim JA, Jang KT, et al. Characteristics of cutaneous cytomegalovirus infection in non-acquired immune deficiency syndrome, immunocompromised patients. *Br J Dermatol* 2006; **155**: 977–82.

125. Boutolleau D, Fernandez C, Andre E, et al. Human herpesvirus (HHV)-6 and HHV-7: two closely related virus with different infection profiles in stem cell transplantation recipients. *J Infect Dis* 2003; **187**: 179–86.

126. Sumiyoshi Y, Akashi K, Kikuchi M. Detection of human herpes virus 6 (HHV6) in the skin of a patient with primary HHV 6 infection and erythroderma. *J Clin Pathol* 1994; **47**: 762–3.

127. Broccolo F, Drago F, Careddu AM, et al. Additional evidence that pityriasis rosea is associated with reactivation of human herpesvirus-6 and -7. *J Invest Dermatol* 2005; **124**: 1234–40.

128. Levine PH, Jahan N, Murari P, Manak M, Jaffe ES. Detection of human herpesvirus 6 in tissues involved by sinus histiocytosis with massive lymphadenopathy (Rosai-Dorfman disease). *J Infect Dis* 1992; **166**: 291–5.

129. Ortonne N, Fillet AM, Kosuge H, Bagot M, Frances C, Wechsier J. Cutaneous Destombes-Rosai-Dorfman disease: absence of detection of HHV-6 and HHV-8 in skin. *J Cutan Pathol* 2002; **29**: 113–18.

130. Hiatt KM, Nelson AM, Lichy JH, Fandburg-Smith JC. Classic Kaposi sarcoma in the United States over the last two decades: a clinicopathologic and molecular study of 438 non-HIV-related Kaposi sarcoma patients with comparison to HIV-related Kaposi sarcoma. *Mod Pathol* 2008; **21**: 572–82.

131. Hong A, Davies S, Lee CS. Immunohistochemical detection of the human herpes virus 8 (HHV8) latent nuclear antigen-1 in Kaposi's sarcoma. *Pathology* 2003; **35**: 448–50.

132. Cheuk W, Wong KO, Wong CS, et al. Immunostaining for human herpesvirus 8 latent nuclear antigen-1 helps distinguish Kaposi sarcoma from its mimickers. *Am J Clin Pathol* 2004; **121**: 335–42.

133. McDonagh DP, Liu J, Gaffey MJ, et al. Detection of Kaposi's sarcoma-associated herpesvirus-like DNA sequence in angiosarcoma. *Am J Pathol* 1996; **149**: 1363–8.

134. Nuovo GJ, Friedman D, Richart DM. In situ hybridization analysis of human papillomavirus DNA segregation patterns in lesions of the female genital tract. *Gynecol Oncol* 1990; **36**: 256–62.

135. Marshburn PB, Trofatter KF. Recurrent condyloma acuminatum in women over age 40: association with immunosuppression and malignant disease. *Am J Obstet Gynecol* 1988; **159**: 429–33.

136. Mahajan A. Practical issues in the application of p16 immunohistochemistry in diagnostic pathology. *Hum Pathol* 2016; **51**: 64–74.

137. Kostopoulou E, Samara M, Kollia P, et al. Different patterns of p16 immunoreactivity in cervical biopsies: correlation to lesion grade and HPV detection, with a review of the literature. Eur J Gynaecol Oncol 2011; **32**: 54–61.

138. O'Neill CJ, McCluggage WG. p16 expression in the female genital tract and its value in diagnosis. *Adv Anat Pathol* 2006; **13**: 8–15.

139. Lenhoff A. Five FDA-approved HPV assays. *MLO Med Lab Obs* 2012; **44**: 14, 16, 18.

140. Luk PP, Selinger CI, Cooper WA, et al. Clinical utility of in situ hybridization assays in head and neck neoplasms. *Head Neck Pathol* 2019; **13**: 397–414.

141. La Grenade L, Manns A, Fletcher V, et al. Clinical, pathologic, and immunologic features of human T-lymphotropic virus type I-associated infective dermatitis in children. *Arch Dermatol* 1998; **134**: 439–44.

142. Hasui K, Wang J, Tanaka Y, et al. Development of ultra-super sensitive immunohistochemistry and its application to the etiological study of adult T-cell leukemia/lymphoma. *Acta Histochem Cytochem* 2012; **45**: 83–106.

143. Shah R, Lan S, Puray-Chavez MN, et al. Single-cell multiplexed fluorescence imaging to visualize viral nucleic acids and proteins and monitor HIV, HTLV, HBV, HCV, Zika virus, and influenza infection. *J Vis Exp* 2020; **164**: 10.3791/61843. doi: 10.3791/61843.

144. Santonja C, Nieto-Gonzalez G, Santos-Briz A, et al. Immunohistochemical detection of parvovirus B19 in

"gloves and socks" papular purpuric syndrome: direct evidence for viral endothelial involvement. Report of three cases and review of the literature. *Am J Dermatopathol* 2011; **33**: 790–5.

145. Bonvicini F, La Placa M, Manaresi E, et al. Parvovirus B19 DNA is commonly harboured in human skin. *Dermatology* 2010; **220**: 138–42.
146. Schwarz TF, Wiersbitzky S, Pambor M. Case report: detection of parvovirus B19 in a skin biopsy of a patient with erythema infectiosum. *J Med Virol* 1994; **43**: 171–4.
147. Takahashi M, Ito M, Sakamoto F, et al. Human parvovirus B19 infection: immunohistochemical and electron microscopic studies of skin lesions. *J Cutan Pathol* 1995; **22**: 168–72.
148. Feng H, Shuda M, Chang Y, et al. Clonal integration of a polyomavirus in human Merkel cell carcinoma. *Science* 2008; **319**: 1096–100.
149. Andres C, Belloni B, Puchta U, Sander CA, Flaig MJ. Prevalence of MCPyV in Merkel cell carcinoma and non-MCC tumors. *J Cutan Pathol* 2010; **37**: 28–34.
150. Mertz KD, Pfaltz M, Junt T, et al. Merkel cell polyomavirus is present in common warts and carcinoma in situ of the skin. *Hum Pathol* 2010; **41**: 1369–79.
151. Shuda M, Arora R, Kwun HJ, et al. Human Merkel cell polyomavirus infection I. MCV T antigen expression in Merkel cell carcinoma, lymphoid tissues and lymphoid tumors. *Int J Cancer* 2009; **125**: 1243–9.
152. Shuda M, Kwun HJ, Feng H, et al. Human Merkel cell polyomavirus small T antigen is an oncoprotein targeting the 4E-BP1 translation regulator. *J Clin Invest* 2011; **121**: 3623–34.
153. Rodig SJ, Cheng J, Wardzala J, et al. Improved detection suggests all Merkel cell carcinomas harbor Merkel polyomavirus. *J Clin Invest* 2012; **122**: 4645–53.
154. Busam JK, Jungbluth AA, Rekthman N, et al. Merkel cell polyomavirus expression in Merkel cell carcinomas and its absence in combined tumors and pulmonary neuroendocrine carcinomas. *Am J Surg Pathol* 2009; **33**: 1378–85.
155. Levine RS, Peterson AT, Yorita KL, Carroll D, Damon IK, Reynolds MG. Ecological niche and geographic distribution of human monkeypox in Africa. *PLoS One* 2007; **2**: e176. doi: 10.1371/journal.pone.0000176.
156. Fleischauer AT, Kile JC, Davidson M, et al. Evaluation of human-to-human transmission of monkeypox from infected patients to health care workers. *Clin Infect Dis* 2005; **40**: 689–94.
157. Reed KD, Melski JW, Graham MB, et al. The detection of monkeypox in humans in the Western Hemisphere. *N Engl J Med* 2004; **350**: 342–50.
158. Rahi M, Joy S, Sharma A. Public health challenges in the context of the global spread of mpox infections. *Am J Trop Med Hyg* 2023; **108**: 641–5.
159. Gupta AK, Talukder M, Rosen T, Piguet V. Differential diagnosis, prevention, and treatment of mpox (monkeypox): a review for dermatologists. *Am J Clin Dermatol* 2023; **24**: 541–56.
160. Li Y, Olson VA, Laue T, Laker MT, Damon IK. Detection of monkeypox virus with real-time PCR assays. *J Clin Virol* 2006; **36**: 194–203.
161. Goldsmith CS, Ksiazek TG, Rollin PE, et al. Cell culture and electron microscopy for identifying viruses in diseases of unknown cause. *Emerg Infect Dis* 2013; **19**: 864–9.
162. Labrandero Hoyos C, Grau Echevarría A, Peñuelas Leal R, Casanova Esquembre A, Lorca Spröhnle J, Hernández Bel P, et al. Monkeypox biopsy: early cutaneous changes. *Am J Dermatopathol* 2023; **45**: 509–10.
163. Hessami M, Keney DA, Pearson LD, Storz J. Isolation of parapox viruses from man and animals: cultivation and cellular changes in bovine fetal spleen cells. *Comp Immunol Microbiol Infect Dis* 1979; **2**: 1–7.
164. Tondury B, Kuhne A, Kutzner H, et al. Molecular diagnostics of parapox virus infections. *J Dtsch Dermatol Ges* 2010; **8**: 681–4.
165. Leavell UWJ, McNamara MJ, Muelling R, et al. Orf. Report of 19 human cases with clinical and pathological observations. *JAMA* 1968; **204**: 657–64.
166. Johannessen JV, Krogh HK, Solberg I, et al. Human orf. *J Cutan Pathol* 1975; **2**: 265–83.
167. Kuokkanen K, Launis J, Mörttinen A. Erythema nodosum and erythema multiforme associated with milker's nodules. *Acta Derm Venereol* 1976; **56**: 69–72.
168. Groves RW, Wilson-Jones E, MacDonald DM. Human orf and milkers' nodule: a clinicopathologic study. *J Am Acad Dermatol* 1991; **25**: 706–11.
169. Evins S, Leavell UWJ, Phillips IA. Intranuclear inclusions in milker's nodules. *Arch Dermatol* 1971; **103**: 91–3.
170. Sanchez RL, Hebert A, Lucia H, Swedo J. Orf. A case report with histologic, electron microscopic, and immunoperoxidase studies. *Arch Pathol Lab Med* 1985; **109**: 166–70.
171. Helton J, Loveless M, White CRJ. Cutaneous acanthamoeba infection associated with leukocytoclastic vasculitis in an AIDS patient. *Am J Dermatopathol* 1993; **15**: 146–9.
172. Tan B, Weldon-Linne CM, Rhone DP, Penning CL, Visvesvara GS. Acanthamoeba infection presenting as skin lesions in patients with the acquired immunodeficiency syndrome. *Arch Pathol Lab Med* 1993; **117**: 1043–6.
173. Gullett J, Mills J, Hadley K, Podemski B, Pitts L, Gelber R. Disseminated granulomatous acanthamoeba infection presenting as an unusual skin lesion. *Am J Med* 1979; **67**: 891–6.
174. Wortman PD. Acanthamoeba infection. *Int J Dermatol* 1996; **35**: 48–51.
175. Galarza C, Ramos W, Gutierrez EL, et al. Cutaneous acanthamebiasis infection in immunocompetent and immunocompromised patients. *Int J Dermatol* 2009; **48**: 1324–9.
176. Rosenberg AS, Morgan MB. Disseminated acanthamoebiasis presenting as lobular panniculitis with necrotizing vasculitis in a patient with AIDS. *J Cutan Pathol* 2001; **28**: 307–13.
177. Guarner J, Bartlett J, Shieh W-J, Paddock CD, Visvesvara GS, Zaki SR. Histopathologic spectrum and immunohistochemical diagnosis of amebic meningoencephalitis. *Mod Pathol* 2007; **20**: 1230–7.
178. Lobo SA, Patil K, Jain S, et al. Diagnostic challenges in Balamuthia mandrillaris infections. *Parasitol Res* 2013; **112**: 4015–19.
179. Martinez DY, Seas C, Bravo F, et al. Successful treatment of Balamuthia mandrillaris amoebic infection with extensive neurological and cutaneous involvement. *Clin Infect Dis* 2010; **51**: e7–11.

180. Qvarnstrom Y, Visvesvara GS, Sriram R, da Silva AJ. Multiplex real-time PCR assay for simultaneous detection of Acanthamoeba spp., Balamuthia mandrillaris, and Naegleria fowleri. *J Clin Microbiol* 2006; **44**: 3589–95.

181. Pritzker AS, Kim BK, Agrawal D, Southern PMJ, Pandya AG. Fatal granulomatous amebic encephalitis caused by Balamuthia mandrillaris presenting as a skin lesion. *J Am Acad Dermatol* 2004; **50**: S38–41.

182. Farnon EC, Kokko KE, Budge PJ, et al. Balamuthia Transplant Investigation Teams: Transmission of Balamuthia mandrillaris by organ transplantation. *Clin Infect Dis* 2016; **63**: 878–88.

183. Grevelink SA, Lerner EA. Leishmaniasis. *J Am Acad Dermatol* 1996; **34**: 257–72.

184. Pavli A, Maltezou HC. Leishmaniasis, an emerging infection in travelers. *Int J Infect Dis* 2010; **14**: e1032–9.

185. Ryan ET, Maguire JH, Strickland GT, Solomon T, Hill DR. *Hunter's Tropical Medicine and Emerging Infectious Disease*. W B Saunders Company, Philadelphia, 2012.

186. Sangueza OP, Sangueza JM, Stiller MJ, Sangueza P. Mucocutaneous leishmaniasis: a clinicopathologic classification. *J Am Acad Dermatol* 1993; **28**: 927–32.

187. Goihman-Yahr M. American mucocutaneous leishmaniasis. *Dermatol Clin* 1994; **12**: 703–12.

188. Salman SM, Rubeiz NG, Kibbi AG. Cutaneous leishmaniasis: clinical features and diagnosis. *Clin Dermatol* 1999; **17**: 291–6.

189. Gazozai S, Iqbal J, Bukhari I, Bashir S. Comparison of diagnostic methods in cutaneous Leishmaniasis (histopathology compared to skin smears). *Pak J Pharm Sci* 2010; **23**: 363–6.

190. de Almeida ME, Steurer FJ, Koru O, et al. Identification of Leishmania spp. by molecular amplification and DNA sequencing analysis of a fragment of rRNA internal transcribed spacer 2. *J Clin Microbiol* 2011; **49**: 3143–9.

191. Kurban AK, Malak JA, Farah FS, Chaglassian HT. Histopathology of cutaneous leishmaniasis. *Arch Dermatol* 1966; **93**: 396–401.

192. Gutierrez Y, Salinas GH, Palma G, Valderrama LB, Santrich CV, Saravia NG. Correlation between histopathology, immune response, clinical presentation, and evolution in Leishmania braziliensis infection. *Am J Trop Med Hyg* 1991; **45**: 281–9.

193. Mehregan DR, Mehregan AH, Mehregan DA. Histologic diagnosis of cutaneous leishmaniasis. Clin Dermatol 1999; **17**: 297–304.

194. Kenner JR, Aronson NE, Bratthauer GL, et al. Immunohistochemistry to identify Leishmania parasites in fixed tissues. *J Cutan Pathol* 1999; **26**: 130–6.

195. Neblett Fanfair R, Benedict K, Bos J, et al. Necrotizing cutaneous mucormycosis after a tornado in Joplin, Missouri, in 2011. *N Engl J Med* 2012; **367**: 2214–25.

196. Ritter JM, Muehlenbachs A, Blau DM, et al; Exserohilum Infections Working Group. Exserohilum infections associated with contaminated steroid injections: a clinicopathologic review of 40 cases. *Am J Pathol* 2013; **183**: 881–92.

197. Bialek R, Konrad F, Kern J, et al. PCR based identification and discrimination of agents of mucormycosis and aspergillosis in paraffin wax embedded tissue. *J Clin Pathol* 2005; **58**: 1180–4.

198. Lau A, Chen S, Sorrell T, et al. Development and clinical application of a panfungal PCR assay to detect and identify fungal DNA in tissue specimens. *J Clin Microbiol* 2007; **45**: 380–5.

199. Muñoz-Cadavid C, Rudd S, Zaki SR, et al. Improving molecular detection of fungal DNA in formalin-fixed paraffin-embedded tissues: comparison of five tissue DNA extraction methods using panfungal PCR. *J Clin Microbiol* 2010; **48**: 2147–53.

Index